ROSEN'S DIAGNOSIS OF

Breast
Pathology

By Needle Core Biopsy

ROSEN'S DIAGNOSIS OF
Breast Pathology

By Needle Core Biopsy

▲ **Edi Brogi, MD**
Professor of Pathology
Weill Medical College of Cornell University
Attending Pathologist
Memorial Sloan-Kettering Cancer Center
New York, New York

▲ **Syed A. Hoda, MD**
Professor of Clinical Pathology
Weill Medical College of Cornell University
Attending Pathologist
New York Presbyterian Hospital–Weill Cornell
Center
New York, New York

▲ **Frederick C. Koerner, MD**
Associate Professor of Pathology
Harvard Medical School
Attending Pathologist
Massachusetts General Hospital
Boston, Massachusetts

▲ **Paul P. Rosen, MD**
Emeritus Professor of Pathology
Weill Medical College of Cornell University
Formerly, Chief of Breast Pathology
New York Presbyterian Hospital–Weill Cornell
Center
New York, New York

FOURTH EDITION

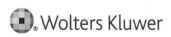
. Wolters Kluwer

Philadelphia • Baltimore • New York • London
Buenos Aires • Hong Kong • Sydney • Tokyo

Acquisitions Editor: Ryan Shaw
Development Editor: Kate Heaney
Production Project Manager: David Saltzberg
Design Coordinator: Joan Wendt
Manufacturing Coordinator: Beth Welsh
Marketing Manager: Dan Dressler
Prepress Vendor: S4Carlisle Publishing Services

4th edition

9 8 7 6 5 4 3 2 1

Printed in China

Library of Congress Cataloging-in-Publication Data

Names: Brogi, Edi, author. | Hoda, Syed A., author. | Koerner, Frederick C., author. | Rosen, Paul Peter, author. | Preceded by (expression): Rosen, Paul Peter. Breast pathology. 3rd ed. | Complemented by (expression): Rosen, Paul Peter. Rosen's breast pathology. 4th ed.
Title: Rosen's diagnosis of breast pathology by needle core biopsy / Edi Brogi, Syed A. Hoda, Frederick C. Koerner, Paul Peter Rosen.
Other titles: Diagnosis of breast pathology by needle core biopsy
Description: 4th edition. | Philadelphia, PA : Wolters Kluwer Health, [2017] | Preceded by: Breast pathology : diagnosis by needle core biopsy / Paul Peter Rosen, Syed A. Hoda. 3rd ed. c2010. | Includes bibliographical references and index.
Identifiers: LCCN 2016047762 | ISBN 9781496307255 (hardback)
Subjects: | MESH: Breast Neoplasms—pathology | Breast—pathology | Biopsy, Needle
Classification: LCC RG493.5.B56 | NLM WP 870 | DDC 616.99/44907—dc23 LC record available at https://lccn.loc.gov/2016047762

LWW.com

Contributors

Edi Brogi, MD
Professor of Pathology
Weill Medical College of Cornell University
Attending Pathologist
Memorial Sloan-Kettering Cancer Center
New York, New York

Judith A. Ferry, MD
Professor of Pathology
Harvard Medical School
Director of Hematopathology
Attending Pathologist
Massachusetts General Hospital
Boston, Massachusetts

Syed A. Hoda, MD
Professor of Clinical Pathology
Weill Medical College of Cornell University
Attending Pathologist
New York Presbyterian Hospital–Weill Cornell Center
New York, New York

Frederick C. Koerner, MD
Associate Professor of Pathology
Harvard Medical School
Attending Pathologist
Massachusetts General Hospital
Boston, Massachusetts

Paul P. Rosen, MD
Emeritus Professor of Pathology
Weill Medical College of Cornell UniversityFormerly,
Chief of Breast Pathology
New York Presbyterian Hospital–Weill Cornell Center
New York, New York

Preface to First Edition (Updated)

Prior to the widespread implementation of breast conservation therapy, the role of the pathologist in breast cancer care was limited to making the diagnosis from tissue obtained by surgical biopsy and documenting the extent of the tumor after a mastectomy was performed. These two events typically centered around a single operative procedure in which the diagnosis made with a frozen section was followed by a mastectomy and axillary lymph node dissection. Presently, considerably more information is required to recommend breast cancer treatment that may employ more than one of the major existing therapeutic modalities: surgery, radiation, and chemotherapy. An important part of the data used for therapeutic decisions is generated by the pathologist using routine histopathologic procedures and immunohistochemistry.

The complex multifactorial description of breast pathology now considered to be standard practice has expanded the diagnostic report from a brief one- or two-line statement, such as "Infiltrating duct carcinoma, grade II; negative lymph nodes," to a catalog of data one or more pages in length, often including many statements indicating the absence as well as the presence of features regarded as relevant to therapeutic decisions and to prognosis. A partial list of this information includes classification of the carcinoma, histologic grade, nuclear grade, tumor size, and statements about vascular invasion, the proportion of the in situ component in invasive lesions, subtype of in situ carcinoma, multifocality, and proximity of carcinoma to margins of excision. Immunohistochemistry is used to characterize the distribution of estrogen and progesterone receptors, as well as other biomarkers and oncogene expression which are part of pathology reports. Proliferative activity may be estimated by the pathologist using immunohistochemistry.

Other advances have added to the complexity of the pathologist's role in breast cancer treatment. Primary among these is the widespread use of needle core biopsy procedures, especially for the diagnosis of nonpalpable mammographically detected lesions. Stereotactic needle core biopsy is an extremely valuable tool in planning breast conservation therapy because it can establish the diagnosis of nonpalpable lesions before operative surgical intervention. Needle core biopsy procedures often yield diagnostic samples, but in a significant number of cases, the material obtained offers ambiguous findings that do not provide a specific diagnosis on which to base therapy. This is a limitation of the procedure and not a failure on the part of the pathologist or radiologist. When this situation arises, it is necessary for physicians caring for the patient to consider the entire clinical situation. This process of reflection is often referred to as "clinical correlation."

Many mammographically detected nonpalpable lesions present the pathologist with challenging diagnostic problems when excised intact and viewed in context with surrounding tissues. The appearance of such lesions in the incomplete and often disrupted form of needle core biopsy samples can substantially increase the degree of difficulty. The major differential diagnostic problems encountered in these specimens include:

- reactive changes versus recurrent carcinoma after lumpectomy
- benign sclerosing lesions (radial scar) versus infiltrating carcinoma
- papilloma versus papillary carcinoma
- fibroadenoma versus cystosarcoma
- atypical duct hyperplasia versus intraductal carcinoma (DCIS)
- DCIS versus DCIS with (micro)invasion
- spindle cell tumors (metaplastic carcinoma vs. sarcoma)
- vascular lesions (angioma vs. angiosarcoma)

Although self-evident, it is important to understand that the diagnosis made with a needle core biopsy specimen can be based only on the samples available to the pathologist and that these samples are not always representative of all of the pathologic findings in a given case. Consequently, carcinoma may be found in up to 50% of surgical biopsies after a needle core biopsy diagnosis of atypical hyperplasia, and microinvasion may be present in about 20% of surgical excisions after a needle core diagnosis of intraductal carcinoma. Three principles offer guidance in the use of the needle core biopsy procedure for the diagnosis and treatment of breast lesions:

- Anything can turn up.
- What you see is what you have, and it may not be all there is.
- What you have may be all there is.

The emergence of the needle core biopsy procedure as a major diagnostic tool epitomizes the growing complexity of the interaction of radiologists, surgeons, and pathologists in the diagnosis and management of mammary diseases, especially in the era of breast conservation therapy. Specialization in medicine has created circumstances in which the specialist physician is increasingly dependent on the assistance of colleagues who have acquired complementary expertise. This evolving situation has contributed to the team approach to disease management reflected in this volume. The intentional limited scope of this presentation, which focuses on diagnosis, does not permit the inclusion of contributions from other important members of the team, including surgeons, radiotherapists, and medical oncologists who depend on these diagnoses to implement therapy.

Paul P. Rosen, MD

Introduction to the Third Edition (Updated)
Breast Imaging and the Origin of Needle Core Biopsy

Noninvasive techniques have been employed to study breast lesions since the beginning of the 20th century. The usefulness of this approach in the clinical setting has been dependent on technical advances that permitted the radiologist to detect lesions that were inapparent to the patient and physician, including clinically occult carcinomas. A consequence of this advance has been the need for a close working relationship between the practitioners of several medical specialties. The result is certainly one of the important examples of "team" management that requires the cooperative efforts of medical specialists to provide effective patient care.

The Beginning of Breast Imaging

Two methods of nonsurgical investigation of the breast were studied in the 1920s and early 1930s, namely, transillumination and radiography. As Cutler (1) reported, the idea for transillumination as a means of diagnosis "was first developed among the members of the laboratory staff of Memorial Hospital during the routine examination of breast specimens." Cutler also stated that "at the suggestion of Dr. Ewing, . . . Adair attempted to transilluminate breasts but encountered technical difficulties, chiefly due to the excessive heat developed by the transilluminating lamp." Although Cutler improved upon the light source, it is clear that transillumination offered little as a method of diagnosis except possibly as a way to distinguish between cystic and solid lesions. With widespread acceptance of needle aspiration of cysts, transillumination was abandoned and has now been replaced by ultrasonography.

The earliest radiologic studies of the breast reported in the United States in the 1930s by Fray and Warren, by Seabold, and by Lockwood were contemporaneous with similar investigations in Europe (2–7). When first employed clinically, it was apparent that roentgenography might prove helpful in the diagnosis of so-called early breast carcinoma. The definition of "early" has changed appreciably since this concept was introduced. This change is exemplified in a 1932 report by Fray and Warren (2) that described a 54-year-old woman who, on clinical examination, was thought to have chronic cystic mastitis. Roentgenologic examination revealed "a small area of dense tissue with irregular margins . . . in the left breast." The lesion proved on biopsy to be a carcinoma "the size of a walnut." It was concluded by the authors that the early status (of the tumor) was reflected not only by its small size but also by the absence of macroscopic involvement of pectoral muscles. Today, the case described by Fray and Warren would be considered operable and potentially curable, but not "early."

Within a relatively short period, the term "early" has come to be used for lesions of microscopic dimensions, often detectable only by imaging techniques that include mammography, ultrasonography, and magnetic resonance imaging (MRI).

The initial mammography studies were met with skepticism. In 1931, Seabold (5) described the mammographic findings in a series of cases presented to the Philadelphia Academy of Surgery. The summary of the discussion that followed his report included the following comment:

> Dr. J. Stewart Rodman said that any attempt to make the diagnosis more exact is certainly praiseworthy. Being a surgeon, however, he is not sure but that sometimes x-ray men have somewhat vivid imaginations. . . . The clinical diagnosis of carcinoma of the breast and chronic cystic mastitis is not ordinarily difficult, and therefore until we have x-ray evidence of a more positive value we had best go a little slow in accepting evidence which is contrary to clinical findings.

Gunsett and Sichel (7) stated in 1934 that their x-ray images might be useful in some cases, but that radiologic distinctions between benign and malignant lesions were not precise enough to form a basis for surgical treatment. They concluded that mammography would not replace biopsy as a diagnostic procedure. The warning offered in these comments is applicable today. The clinician faced with a palpable abnormality in the breast should not depend only on mammography to decide whether biopsy is required. On the other hand, advances in clinical mammography and the development of stereotactic biopsy instruments have made it possible to detect and perform biopsies on nonpalpable lesions found by "x-ray men" who "have vivid imaginations" (5).

The Beginning of Pathology–Radiology Correlation

The need to relate radiologic findings to the histopathologic examination of breast tissue has been appreciated since the earliest x-ray images of the breast were obtained. In 1913, Albert Salomon (8), a surgeon at the University of Berlin, described a method for obtaining roentgenograms of serial sections of surgical breast specimens in order to correlate histologic observations with the specimen x-rays. The histologic appearance of calcification within a mammary carcinoma was described in his paper. Salomon may be credited with the first reported example of breast specimen radiography, and he deserves recognition for investigations that anticipated later developments in mammography and specimen radiography.

Detailed pathologic–radiologic correlations were carried out in the late 1920s by Dominguez (9–11) in Montevideo, Uruguay. Dominguez was especially interested in studying the properties of calcifications in breast lesions. In addition to specimen radiography, he undertook biochemical analyses of the calcium content of breast tissue. Conway (12) described the clinical radiologic appearance of calcification in breast cysts and sarcomatous tumors, but failed to appreciate the potential usefulness of calcification as an x-ray marker for carcinoma. Lockwood (3) stressed the importance of correlating pathologic and radiologic findings, but did not obtain x-rays of specimens, nor was there any mention of mammary calcification as an indicator of carcinoma in his report. Warren (6) described two cases thought roentgenologically to be carcinoma but reported to be benign on pathologic examination that "could not be studied because the specimens were thrown out before films could be made to locate the supposed small area of malignancy seen at the original examination."

The observations of Salomon, and later Dominguez, that calcium deposits in mammary carcinoma could be visualized radiologically remained largely unappreciated for nearly two decades. They were again brought to attention by Leborgne (13,14) in Montevideo, who developed a technique for soft tissue roentgenography that made it possibly to identify small tumors and calcifications in clinical mammograms. He noted that "the roentgenographic study of the operative specimen also permitted the localization of the tiny calcifications for histopathologic study, and thus aided in finding a small cancer that would otherwise have been overlooked." As had Gershon-Cohen and Colcher (15) some years earlier, Leborgne anticipated the role of mammography for detecting preclinical cancer when he stated:

> We firmly believe that the recognition and demonstration of this roentgenographic sign constitutes one of the easily observed aspects in which mammary cancer is presented, especially in its ductal form . . . and (is) therefore susceptible of detection in prophylactic examinations of women who do not yet present clinical tumor symptomology. With a systematic prophylactic roentgenographic examination of all women with antecedents of cancer in their family, we enter a new stage in the fight against mammary cancer.

The Origins of Needle Core Biopsy

The origin of modern needle core biopsy sampling of the breast to obtain a tissue specimen for histologic diagnosis is entwined with the history of needle aspiration biopsy and parallels the development of clinical mammography. Needles have been used to obtain samples for diagnosis from various anatomic sites since the middle of the 19th century (16). Needle aspiration sampling of the lung (17,18) and lymph nodes (19–21) was described by 1914. Many of the early biopsy attempts involved aspirating cells with a needle attached to a syringe. The aspirated blood and cellular material were expressed onto a slide and spread thinly to create a cytologic preparation.

The application of the needle aspiration biopsy technique to the diagnosis of neoplastic conditions attracted attention early in the 20th century. In 1921, Guthrie (22) reported that needle aspiration could be employed to evaluate the causes of lymph node enlargement. A method for aspirating cells from lymph nodes and the preparation of stained slides from this material was described in detail by Forkner (23,24), who also reported his experience using these samples for the diagnosis of cancer, including three women with adenocarcinoma in axillary lymph nodes.

The first concerted effort to employ the needle aspiration technique to the diagnosis of cancer was undertaken at Memorial Hospital in New York. In 1922, Ellis (25), a technician working under Dr. James Ewing, described cancer cells in cell block specimens of pleural fluid. Ellis concluded that "the diagnosis of cancer from direct smears is hazardous, but when one has made thin paraffin sections of suspected material and their evidence is fortified by some confirmatory clinical data, positive diagnosis may often be obtained." Four years later, Hayes Martin, a surgeon at Memorial Hospital; Fred Stewart, then the junior associate of Dr. Ewing; and Ellis began to use the aspiration biopsy technique in patients with head and neck cancer (26). In succeeding publications, they documented the applicability of the aspiration biopsy technique to a variety of tumors and defined the role of this procedure in the clinical management of cancer patients (27,28).

The Memorial Hospital technique proved to be the forerunner of what are now two largely separate methods of diagnosis: fine-needle aspiration (FNA) and needle core biopsy. The specimens obtained by Martin and his clinical colleagues included disaggregated cells for cytologic examination, equivalent to FNA today, and fragments of tissue that they described as the clot, a counterpart of the modern needle core biopsy specimen. Ewing, Stewart, and their colleagues were not prepared to rely entirely on cytologic smears, as evidenced by the importance they attached to the "clot," described in the following commentary by Godwin (29):

> After the material is obtained in the syringe, the negative pressure is released to obviate splattering of the aspirate in the syringe. With the rake, the material is placed on several slides and gently smeared by approximating two slides and pulling them apart. The remaining material is placed on a small piece of blotting paper or fibrin foam and put in formalin for later paraffin section. This is designated as the clot.

The clot was "helpful in many instances where the smear is not diagnostic and in making a more definitive diagnosis as to the type of tumor" (29).

The system of aspirating tumors for diagnosis implemented at Memorial Hospital in the 1920s and 1930s evolved as a result of experience gained by the participants in this effort. In a later review, Godwin (30) observed:

> The interpretation of aspirates, as with other pathological material, is certainly not without pitfalls. It requires experience. It is necessary that a sufficient number of cases be available for both clinician and pathologist to maintain their efficiency. The

pathologist must know the clinical setting, the normal cells of the region, and the nature of lesions to be anticipated in the area.

Breast Specimen Radiography

Technologic developments in imaging have played a major role in advancing the use of needles to obtain tissue samples from lesions in superficial and visceral locations. The impetus for improving needle biopsy techniques for breast lesions began with the increasing utilization of mammography in the 1960s and 1970s. The mammographic detection of nonpalpable lesions presented a diagnostic challenge to the radiologist, surgeon, and pathologist, and led to the development of methods to localize nonpalpable lesions so that they could be found and excised by surgeons and sampled in the pathology laboratory. Various localizing procedures were introduced, employing needles, wires, dyes, and other markers placed in or near the lesion under mammographic or ultrasound guidance. After localization by the radiologist, the surgeon was guided by the marker. Radiographic examination of the specimen (specimen radiography) has been employed to confirm excision of a nonpalpable abnormality and to help the pathologist pinpoint the lesion for histologic examination (31–33). Specimen radiography has been particularly useful for lesions containing calcifications.

Under optimal conditions where a surgical biopsy was recommended for mammographic abnormalities with calcifications that were considered to be suspicious for carcinoma, 25% to 30% of the excised lesions proved to be carcinoma (32,33). Thus, for each patient with a biopsy sample that revealed carcinoma, three underwent surgical excision of a benign lesion. The surgical management of nonpalpable breast lesions without calcifications was more difficult because specimen radiography was not very reliable for confirming the adequacy of excision. The availability of the modern needle core biopsy procedure to sample nonpalpable mammographically detected lesions made it possible to avoid surgical biopsy in a substantial number of women. Friese et al. (34) analyzed Surveillance, Epidemiology, and End Results (SEER)-Medicare data for 45,542 patients with intraductal and invasive stage I to II breast carcinoma diagnosed between 1991 and 1999. The frequency of needle core biopsy as the first procedure increased from approximately 20% in 1991 to 30.9% in 1999 ($p < 0.0001$), and there was a concomitant decrease in initial surgical biopsy procedures. Women who had a needle core biopsy procedure initially tended to have fewer surgical procedures overall than those whose first biopsy specimen was obtained surgically.

Modern Needle Core Biopsy Techniques

The introduction of stereotaxic devices in the 1970s resulted in improved needle localization and made it possible to obtain needle biopsy samples from nonpalpable lesions more efficiently (35,36). One of the first papers described a "stereotaxic instrument" that facilitated "percutaneous needle biopsy of the breast for microscopic diagnosis" (37). The authors reported that "the sampling site can be located at a precision of ±1 mm."

The instrument can also be used for positioning of metal and dye indicators for guiding surgery and for postoperative identification of excised tumors." Linkage of this computer-guided localization system with the automated biopsy gun introduced in the 1980s (38) led to the development of modern stereotaxic core biopsy instruments (39). Ultrasound-guided core biopsy has proven to be particularly effective for nonpalpable lesions without calcifications. Stereotaxic MRI and ultrasound-guided core biopsy procedures are now widely used for the diagnosis of breast diseases. These technologies provide efficient methods for sampling small areas rapidly, with less morbidity and expense than surgical excision (40–42). Multifocal lesions are also accessible with this approach (43).

The use of needle biopsies for the diagnosis of breast lesions has expanded greatly in the past 25 years. A study based on Medicare patient data from 1990s found that only 24% of patients had undergone a needle biopsy (34). A population-based study from Florida published in 2011 reported that 70% of breast biopsies were needle biopsies (44). Analysis of Medicare data for the period 2003 to 2007 revealed that needle biopsy had been used in 68.7% of the 89,712 patients surveyed (45). In the latter study of Medicare patients, the likelihood of multiple carcinoma-related procedures was significantly ($p < 0.001$) lower among patients diagnosed by a needle biopsy (33.7%) than for those who did not have a diagnostic needle biopsy (69.6%) with an adjusted relative risk in the non-needle biopsy group of 2.08.

The Pathologic Examination of Needle Core Biopsy Specimens

Needle core biopsy procedures provide the pathologist with tissue specimens that are processed to produce histologic sections. While satisfying the preference of surgical pathologists for a tissue sample rather than a cytology specimen, needle core biopsy samples create new diagnostic problems and challenges. To some extent, these difficulties arise from the partial view of a lesion in the core biopsy specimen. This problem can be compounded by the heterogeneous nature of some tumors such as papillary and fibroepithelial lesions as well as carcinomas (46). The context of surrounding tissue afforded by sections of surgical biopsy specimens, important in some instances, is largely lacking in needle core biopsy samples. Nonpalpable lesions are frequently small abnormalities that can be difficult to interpret even in a complete excisional biopsy specimen, and they should not be submitted for frozen section examination except in extraordinary circumstances (47).

False-negative results for needle core biopsy samples are lower when specimens are obtained by using techniques that produce larger samples such as 11-gauge and vacuum-assisted instruments (48,49). Failure to sample a carcinoma that is present is more likely to occur in cases where the target is solely microcalcifications than a mass lesion (50). Consequently, intraductal carcinoma, especially the noncomedo type, is more likely to be missed than is invasive carcinoma. False-negative needle core biopsy samples can usually be appreciated prospectively because of discordance between the imaging studies for which the procedure was performed and the pathology diagnosis (51).

Relatively common diagnostic problems encountered in needle core biopsy specimens include the following: columnar cell lesions and atypical hyperplasia, radial sclerosing lesions and papillary tumors, lobular atypia, and lobular carcinoma in situ (LCIS). Unusual tumors previously encountered only in surgical biopsy specimens such as pseudoangiomatous stromal hyperplasia, mucocele-like lesions, myofibroblastoma, metaplastic carcinoma, and hemangiomas are now the targets of stereotaxic needle core biopsy procedures (47,52). Today, virtually any lesion that occurs in the breast may appear on the pathologist's microscope in a needle core biopsy sample. The purpose of this book is to provide guidance in the interpretation of diagnosis of needle core specimens and the pathologic changes that occur in the breast as a result of these procedures.

Lesion Localization

The accuracy of needle core biopsy sampling is so precise that imaging evidence of the target may be lost after the procedure, and in some cases the lesion itself may be entirely extirpated (53,54). When all imaging evidence of carcinoma has been removed, up to nearly 80% of patients have residual carcinoma in a subsequent excisional biopsy. Lee et al. (55) reported that the MRI-targeted lesion was completely extirpated in 30% of carcinomas diagnosed by MRI-guided vacuum-assisted needle core biopsy. Nonetheless, 64% of patients whose MRI-detected lesion had been removed had residual carcinoma. Liberman et al. (56) found that the mammographic target was entirely removed in 100 of 214 (47%) carcinomas and that carcinomas remained in 79% of cases after complete removal of the imaging abnormality.

To assist the surgeon and pathologist in finding the site of a prior needle core biopsy where part, or all, of the lesion may have been removed, a clip may be placed in the biopsy cavity at the conclusion of the procedure. Sometimes, multiple clips are used to bracket a lesion or to mark more than one biopsy site. Clips of differing shapes are available, and various types may be employed with mammographic, sonographic, or MRI-guided biopsy procedures (55,57,58). Migration of clips (59), extraction of the clip during a vacuum-assisted biopsy procedure (60), and loss of the clip during surgical excision have been reported.

Paul P. Rosen, MD

REFERENCES

1. Cutler M. Transillumination as an aid in the diagnosis of breast lesions, with special reference to its value in cases of bleeding nipple. *Surg Gynecol Obstet.* 1929;48:721–729.
2. Fray WW, Warren SL. Stereoscopic roentgenography of breasts: an aid in establishing the diagnosis of mastitis and carcinoma. *Ann Surg.* 1932;95:425–432.
3. Lockwood IH. Roentgen ray evaluation of breast symptoms. *Am J Roentgenol.* 1933;29:145–155.
4. Seabold PS. Roentgenographic diagnosis of diseases of the breast. *Surg Gynecol Obstet.* 1931;53:461–468.
5. Seabold PS. Diagnosis of breast disease by x-ray. *Ann Surg.* 1931;94:443.
6. Warren SL. Roentgenologic study of the breast. *Am J Roentgenol.* 1930;24:113–124.
7. Gunsett A, Sichel G. Sur la valeur pratique de la radiographie du sein. *J de radiol et d´electrol.* 1934;18:611–614.
8. Salomon A. Beiträge zur Pathologie und Klinik der Mammacarcinome. *Archiv für Klin Chirurgie.* 1913;101:573–668.
9. Dominguez CM. Estudio sistematizado del cancer del seno. *Boll Liga Uruguay contra el cancer genit gemen.* 1929;1:23.
10. Dominguez CM. Estudio radiologico de los descalcificadores. *Boll Soc Anatomia Patologica.* 1930;1:175.
11. Dominiguez CM, Lucas A. Investigacion radiografica y quimica sobre el calcio precipitado en tumores del aparato genital feminino. *Boll Soc Anatomia Patologica.* 1930;1:217.
12. Conway JH. Calcified breast tumors. *Am J Surg.* 1936;31:72–76.
13. Leborgne R. Diagnostico de los tumores de la mamma por la radiografia simple. *Boll Cir Uruguay.* 1949;20:407.
14. Leborgne R. Diagnosis of tumors of the breast by simple roentgenography: calcifications in carcinomas. *Am J Roentgenol.* 1951;65:1–11.
15. Gershon-Cohen J, Colcher AE. An evaluation of the roentgen diagnosis of early carcinoma of the breast. *JAMA.* 1937;108:867–871.
16. Webb AJ. Through a glass darkly: the development of needle aspiration biopsy. *Bristol Med Chir J.* 1974;89:59–68.
17. Horder TJ. Lung puncture: a new application of clinical pathology. *Lancet.* 1909;2:1345–1346; 1539–1540.
18. Leyden OO. Ueber infectiöse Pneumonie. *Dtsch Med Wochenschr.* 1883;9:52–54.
19. White WC, Pröscher F. Spirochaetes in acute lymphatic leukemia and in chronic benign lymphomatosis (Hodgkin's disease). *JAMA.* 1907;69:1115.
20. Grieg EDW, Gray ACH. Note on the lymphatic glands in sleeping sickness. *Lancet.* 1914;1:1570.
21. Chatard JA, Guthrie CG. Human trypanosomiasis: report of a case observed in Baltimore. *Am J Trop Dis Prev Med.* 1914;1:493–505.
22. Guthrie CG. Gland puncture as a diagnostic measure. *Bull Johns Hopkins Hosp.* 1921;32:266–269.
23. Forkner CE. Material from lymph nodes in man: I: method to obtain material by puncture of lymph nodes for study with supravital and fixed stains. *Arch Intern Med.* 1927;40:532–537.
24. Forkner CE. Material from lymph nodes of man. Studies on living and fixed cells withdrawn from lymph nodes of man. *Arch Intern Med.* 1927;40:647–660.
25. Ellis EB. Cancer cells in pleural fluid. *Bull Int Assoc Med Museums J Tech Methods.* 1922;8:126–127.
26. Martin HE, Ellis EB. Biopsy by needle puncture and aspiration. *Ann Surg.* 1930;92:169–181.
27. Martin HE, Ellis EB. Aspiration biopsy. *Surg Gynecol Obstet.* 1934;59:578–589.
28. Stewart FW. The diagnosis of tumors by aspiration. *Am J Pathol.* 1933;9:801–812.
29. Godwin JT. Aspiration biopsy: technique and application. *Ann NY Acad Sci.* 1956;63:1348–1373.
30. Godwin JT. Cytologic diagnosis of aspiration biopsies of solid and cystic tumors. *Acta Cytol.* 1964;8:206–215.
31. Rosen PP, Snyder PE, Foote FW, et al. Detection of occult carcinoma in the apparently benign breast biopsy through specimen radiography. *Cancer.* 1970;26:944–953.
32. Rosen PP, Snyder RE, Urban J, et al. Correlation of suspicious mammograms and x-rays of breast biopsies during surgery: results of 60 cases. *Cancer.* 1973;31:656–660.
33. Snyder R, Rosen PP. Radiography of breast specimens. *Cancer.* 1971;28:1608–1611.
34. Friese CR, Neville BA, Edge SB, et al. Breast biopsy patterns and outcomes in Surveillance, Epidemiology, and End Results-Medicare data. *Cancer.* 2009;115:716–724.
35. Fox CH. Innovation in medical diagnosis: the Scandinavian curiosity. *Lancet.* 1979;1:1387–1388.

36. Nordenström B. New instruments for biopsy. *Radiology.* 1975;117:474–475.
37. Bolmgren J, Jacobson B, Nordenström B. Stereotaxic instrument for needle biopsy of the mamma. *Am J Roentgenol.* 1977;129:121–125.
38. Lindgren PG. Percutaneous needle biopsy: a new technique. *Acta Radiol Diagn.* 1982;23:653–656.
39. Burbank F. Stereotactic breast biopsy: its history, its present, and its future. *Am Surg.* 1996;2:128–150.
40. Nields MW. Cost-effectiveness of image-guided core needle biopsy versus surgery in diagnosing breast cancer. *Acad Radiol.* 1996;3:S138–S140.
41. Liberman L, Fahs MC, Dershaw DD, et al. Impact of stereotactic core biopsy on cost of diagnosis. *Radiology.* 1995;195:633–637.
42. Groenewoud JH, Pijnappel RM, vandenAkker-van Marle ME, et al. Cost-effectiveness of stereotactic large-core needle biopsy for nonpalpable breast lesions compared to open-breast biopsy. *Br J Cancer.* 2004;90:383–392.
43. Rosenblatt R, Fineberg SA, Sparano JA, et al. Stereotactic core needle biopsy of multiple sites in the breast: efficacy and effect on patient care. *Radiology.* 1996;201:67–70.
44. Gitwein LG, Ang DN, Liu H, et al. Utilization of minimally invasive biopsy for evaluation of suspicious breast lesions. *Am J Surg.* 2011;202:127–132.
45. Eberth JM, Xu Y, Smith GL, et al. Surgeon influence on use of needle biopsy in patients with breast cancer.: a national Medicare study. *J Clin Oncol.* 2014;32:2206–2216.
46. Morris EA, Lieberman L, Trevisan SG, et al. Histological heterogeneity of masses at percutaneous breast biopsy. *Breast J.* 2002;8:187–191.
47. Association of Directors of Anatomic and Surgical Pathology. Immediate management of mammographically detected breast lesions. *Am J Surg Pathol.* 1993;12:850–851.
48. Hoorntje LE, Peeter PH, Mali WP, et al. Vacuum-assisted breast biopsy: a critical review. *Eur J Cancer.* 2003;39:1676–6183.
49. Kettritz V, Rotter K, Schreer I, et al. Stereotactic vacuum-assisted breast biopsy in 2874 patients: a multicenter study. *Cancer.* 2004;100:245–251.
50. Liberman L, Dershaw DD, Glassman JR, et al. Analysis of cancers not diagnosed at stereotactic core breast biopsy. *Radiology.* 1997;203:151–157.
51. Schueller G, Jaromi S, Ponhold L, et al. US-guided 14-gauge core-needle breast biopsy: results of a validation study in 1352 cases. *Radiology.* 2008;248:406–413.
52. Hoda SA, Rosen PP. Observations on the pathologic diagnosis of selected unusual lesions in needle core biopsies of breast. *Breast J.* 2004;6:522–527.
53. Brenner RJ. Lesions entirely removed during stereotactic biopsy: pre-operative localization on the basis of mammographic landmarks and feasibility of freehand technique-initial experience. *Radiology.* 2000;214:585–590.
54. March DE, Coughlin BF, Barham RB, et al. Breast masses: removal of all US evidence during biopsy using a hand held vacuum-assisted device-initial experience. *Radiology.* 2003;227:549–555.
55. Lee J-M, Kaplan JB, Murray MP, et al. Complete excision of the MRI target lesion at MRI-guided vacuum-assisted biopsy of breast cancer. *AJR.* 2008;191:1198–1202.
56. Liberman L, Kaplan JB, Morris EA, et al. To excise or to sample the mammographic target: what is the goal of stereotactic 11-gauge vacuum-assisted breast biopsy? *AJR.* 2002;179:679–683.
57. Calhoun K. Giuliano A, Brenner RJ. Intraoperative loss of core biopsy clips: clinical implications. *AJR.* 2008;190:W196–W200.
58. Mercado CL, Guth AA, Toth HK, et al. Sonographically guided marker placement for confirmation of removal of mammographically occult lesions after localization. *AJR.* 2008;191:1216–1219.
59. Philpotts LE, Lee CH. Clip migration after 11-gauge vacuum assisted stereotactic biopsy: case report. *Radiology.* 2002;222:794–796.
60. Brenner RJ. Percutaneous removal of post biopsy marking clip in the breast using stereotactic technique. *AJR.* 2001;176:417–419.

DCIS Is DCIS Is DCIS
A Controversial Introduction to the Fourth Edition

As is apparent to most readers, the title to this discussion is a paraphrase of the oft-repeated and celebrated first line of Gertrude Stein's 1913 poem "Sacred Emily," which reads as, "Rose is a rose is a rose is a rose." Some say that Stein drew inspiration for this line from Juliet in Shakespeare's "Romeo and Juliet," who argued that Romeo would be the man she loved regardless of his Montague family ties when she said, "A rose by any other name would smell as sweet." However one puts it and whatever name is applied, a rose is a rose, although some varieties are red and others pink or white, and some roses smell sweeter than others. Apples are apples, although some are sweet and others are tart. Which brings us to ductal carcinoma in situ or DCIS. DCIS is DCIS regardless of the variety.

This discussion offers a rational, fact-based summary of current knowledge about DCIS as it effects treatment. In this space it is not possible, nor probably useful, to attempt a review of all of the voluminous published literature on this subject. The material presented has been selected to emphasize the highlights of the evolution of our understanding of DCIS and how this process led to the current treatment dilemma, and to consider some prospects for the future. Other writers might, in some instances, have selected different material or have chosen to emphasize their own contributions. The absence of any reference here should not be interpreted as an unfavorable opinion of that report.

As will become apparent in what follows, considerable progress made in the treatment of DCIS during the past half century has brought us to a crossroad as expressed by Esserman and Yau (1) in the title of their editorial titled "Rethinking the Standard for Ductal Carcinoma In Situ Treatment". The following essay is devoted to that issue.

The History of the Concept of In Situ Carcinoma

In the mid-19th century, it was widely believed that all neoplasms, including those with epithelial features, were derived from connective tissue cells or primitive mesenchyme (2). The recognition, approximately 160 years ago, that invasive carcinomas were preceded by a phase of growth that originated in epithelium, a stage later referred to as in situ, was a major advance in understanding neoplastic disease. When Robert Remak (3) proposed, in 1854, that epithelial neoplasms were derived from the epithelial germ layer, his suggestion was referred to as an "extravagant hypothesis". In 1865, Thiersch's (4) research led him to conclude that squamous carcinomas of the skin and oral cavity arose from the epithelium at these

sites, thereby anticipating Broder's use of the term *in situ carcinoma* in the oral cavity by 67 years. Coincidentally, the epithelial origin of carcinoma was recognized in France in 1865 by Cornil (5), who used the mammary gland as a model for his research. Cornil's (6) work included illustrations showing the close similarity between cells confined to the epithelium of origin (in situ) in lobules and the characteristic linear growth pattern of the invasive component now referred to as invasive lobular carcinoma. In 1867, Waldeyer (7), a German anatomist, illustrated the origin of mammary carcinoma from hyperplasia to invasion of the lobular and extralobular connective tissue. Writing about "primary acinar carcinoma" of the breast in 1928, Ewing (8) quoted Cornil.

One of the most complete descriptions of the origin of invasive mammary carcinoma from intraepithelial (in situ) carcinoma was published in 1931 by Cheatle and Cutler (9), who stated that:

> There are appearances of malignancy which prove conclusively that the carcinoma process in the breast begins in an epithelial neoplasia in ducts and acini which continues to grow there before and after there has been a transgression of normal boundaries by epithelial cells whose parents are still within the normal but distended structure. In these instances there is no doubt that these epithelial cells inside the normal boundaries are as histologic malignant as those that have transgressed them . . . the new property possessed by the epithelial cells of being able to invade, grow, and metastasize in outside tissues has been acquired and transmitted by their parent cells within normal boundaries.

This quote from Cheatle and Cutler is also notable for its reference to "epithelial neoplasia," which has been in wide use since the 1970s, and the intimation that invasive carcinoma arises when in situ carcinoma cells acquire and are distinguished by the capacity to invade, which is evidenced by their location but not by their appearance. Although the cells of in situ and invasive breast carcinoma may not be distinguishable histologically out of their microanatomic context, it is clear that invasive carcinoma cells have acquired properties that distinguish them from their in situ ancestors and/or that the surrounding host tissue has been altered to permit invasion to occur. Unraveling this puzzle will be a major step toward developing treatment strategies that are targeted at the characteristics of in situ lobular or duct carcinoma and/or the host environment in an individual patient.

Introducing the term in situ carcinoma in 1932 with reference to squamous carcinoma, Albert C. Broders (10) emphasized the clinical importance of treating the in situ stage of carcinoma when he wrote,

> . . . if carcinoma in situ appears alone, its recognition is necessary, for failure to recognize it may constitute an error of omission fraught with grave danger to the patient; if it goes unrecognized carcinoma is allowed to masquerade as a benign or not more than a precancerous process with the possibility of its becoming too far advanced to be amenable to treatment.

The idea that leaving in situ carcinoma *untreated* posed a "grave danger" to the patient was to dominate the treatment of breast carcinoma, leading to the widespread use of mastectomy for LCIS and DCIS for decades thereafter.

Anecdotal Reports of Untreated DCIS Prior to 1978

Untreated in this and other comparable reports means that no intervention other than the original diagnostic biopsy was performed to excise a palpable abnormality. Margins were not cleared, and no further surgery was performed after the initial excision. In most cases, the patients were not under surveillance in this era predating the regular use of mammography. This would not qualify as adequate breast conserving surgery by today's standards, and under these circumstances, it is not surprising that the first evidence of subsequent carcinoma was almost always a mass representing invasive carcinoma.

Prior to 1978, there were no prospective published studies of untreated DCIS and no retrospective studies of a large cohort of consecutive patients. Anecdotal reports before 1978 (11–14) described a total of 48 selected patients, including some with papillary and comedo DCIS, who had not been treated for a variety of reasons. During an interval of 1 to 12 years, 21 of the 48 patients (43.8%) were found to have subsequent carcinoma. The largest series in this group consisted of 25 women with untreated DCIS in a consecutive cohort of 200 DCIS patients treated at a single institution (12). There were various reasons for the absence of treatment other than the diagnostic biopsy. Carcinoma other than the original DCIS was found during follow-up of 1 to 8 years in 5 of the 25 (20%) women. The subsequent carcinomas were described as being "within or nearby the previous excisional site."

A Systematic Study of Untreated LCIS and DCIS

As the basis for a systematic study of the "natural history" of untreated LCIS, Rosen personally reviewed all available histologic slides from breast biopsies interpreted as not showing carcinoma at Memorial Hospital in New York City between 1940 and 1950 (15). The material reviewed consisted of 12,052 slides from 8,609 cases. This exercise uncovered 124 instances of previously undiagnosed and/or untreated in situ carcinoma (99 LCIS and 25 DCIS), representing 1.4% of the entire cohort. Because in this time period it was customary to sample a very limited portion of a grossly benign-appearing biopsy specimen, the average number of slides available per case was 1.4. Consequently, the 1.4% frequency of undiagnosed in situ carcinoma in these patients is probably a low estimate. Follow-up was sought for all of the 124 patients. The results were reported separately for LCIS (15) and DCIS (16).

The Example of LCIS

For nearly 30 years after its recognition, the standard treatment for LCIS was a mastectomy. Beginning in the 1970s, controversy began to swirl around the treatment of LCIS. The Memorial Hospital report (15) and other similar follow-up studies of patients with LCIS in one breast that was not treated after the initial diagnostic biopsy showed that:

a. the risk of subsequent invasive carcinoma was nearly equal in both breasts;
b. the majority of subsequent carcinomas were of the duct rather than lobular type; and
c. the interval to the appearance of subsequent carcinoma was a decade or more in a substantial number of patients.

These observations led some clinicians and researchers:

a. to consider LCIS exclusively to be a "marker" for increased breast carcinoma risk;
b. to urge that the lesion be referred to by such terms as "lobular neoplasia," or as "lobular intraepithelial neoplasia" (LIN), rather than carcinoma; and
c. to recommend that management after diagnosis consists of expectant follow-up limited to clinical and imaging examinations.

Eschewing further surgery and lacking an effective method for preventing invasive carcinoma in untreated women with LCIS, this strategy focused on the "early" diagnosis of DCIS or invasive carcinoma to offer the greatest chance to cure in women with LCIS who were not treated by mastectomy.

Controversy has now largely subsided in regard to LCIS as chemoprevention using selective estrogen receptor modulators and aromatase inhibitors has become available for treatment. The pendulum has now swung to a more rational position, with the understanding that LCIS is both a "marker" for duct-type breast carcinoma risk and a nonobligate precursor to invasive lobular carcinoma, although we have not yet discovered attributes of the lesion that characterize these potentials. As a consequence, prior concerns about LCIS have largely been laid to rest, and there is again relatively widespread acceptance of the term lobular carcinoma in situ. An updated discussion of LCIS can be found in Chapter 18.

"It's Like Déjà Vu All Over Again": Is DCIS a Marker or a Precursor?

Attention has now turned to DCIS, with questions being raised about the use of the word carcinoma for all these lesions and the need for any treatment after a diagnostic biopsy. This state of affairs is represented by the conclusion expressed by

Esserman and Yau (1) that "much of DCIS should be considered a 'risk factor' for invasive breast cancer and an opportunity for targeted prevention," as well as by newspaper articles about DCIS with subtitles such as "Doubt Is Raised Over Value of Surgery for Breast Lesions at Earliest Stage" (17).

It will become apparent in the discussion that follows that the most pressing issue now in the forefront about DCIS is not what to call it or how it "should be considered," but rather to determine the most beneficial therapeutic program for each patient, "Rethinking the treatment of DCIS" is nothing new. The issues were clearly stated almost four decades ago by Hutter (18) in an essay titled "Is Cured Early Cancer Truly Cancer?"

> The real issue here is not whether the pathologic diagnosis of microscopic cancer is valid . . . the real issue is how to manage patients with these lesions today; acknowledging that we do not yet have the diagnostic capability to separate those patients with lesions which will progress from those which will not.

Follow-up of Untreated DCIS Reported in 1978

The Memorial Hospital Study

The 25 DCIS patients identified retrospectively by Rosen represented 0.3% of the cohort of 8,609 patients with a breast biopsy that was diagnosed as benign (15). Two of the 25 also had LCIS. Clinical records were found for 15 patients. The average age of the patients when the biopsy containing DCIS was performed was 48.2 years (range, 34–59 years). The majority presented with a mass that proved to be due to fibrocystic changes. All of the DCIS was low-grade, typically micropapillary type, with focal solid and cribriform areas. Follow-up was available for 10 patients averaging 21.6 years (range, 7–30 years) among whom 7 (70%) were subsequently found to have carcinoma (5 invasive duct, 1 medullary, and 1 DCIS). All subsequent carcinomas developed in the ipsilateral breast, usually in the same quadrant as the original DCIS. Included among the seven were the two women who originally had DCIS and LCIS, one of whom developed invasive duct carcinoma 6 years later whereas the other had non–low-grade DCIS 11 years later. Overall, the interval to subsequent ipsilateral carcinoma averaged 9.7 years (range, 10 months to 24 years).

Subsequently, four of the seven patients developed metastatic carcinoma, including two who died of breast carcinoma and two who were alive with metastases at last follow-up.

Reports of Untreated DCIS After 1978

Other follow-up studies of untreated DCIS appeared between 1978 and 2000 (19,20). The data from these and prior studies were reviewed by Leonard and Swain (21) in 2004 and by Erbas et al. (22) in 2006. The varieties of DCIS included in these reports were papillary, comedo, and noncomedo types. After follow-up ranging from 1 to 28 years, the frequency of progression to invasive carcinoma varied from 14% to 75%, with 50% or greater progression in half of the studies and an average progression rate of 43%.

The Vanderbilt University Study

The most important study after 1978 is that of Page et al. (19), first reported in 1982, with published updates in 1995 (23), 2005 (24), and 2015 (25). In these reports, the authors document more than 40 years of follow-up in a single series of women with untreated DCIS identified at Vanderbilt University and associated hospitals. This series has many features in common with Rosen's study reported in 1978 (12) and will be reviewed in some detail here.

Page's study began with 28 patients found to have untreated DCIS in a retrospective review of slides from nearly 12,000 biopsies previously reported to be benign (19). The 28 DCIS cases represented 0.24% of the reviewed biopsies. The average number of slides reviewed from a reviewed biopsy was 2. The types of DCIS were described as ". . . typical cribriform patterns, micropapillary carcinomas and intermediate forms. . ." Two patients also had LCIS. Age at the time of biopsy ranged from 33 to 80 years (average age, 52 years). Among the 25 women with follow-up of more than 3 years at the time of the initial report, 7, or 28%, had developed invasive breast carcinoma within 10 years of the original biopsy. The average interval to invasive carcinoma was 6.1 years. All subsequent invasive carcinomas were in the breast that harbored DCIS, and five were clearly in the same quadrant.

The second publication from this series, which appeared 13 years later (23), reported that invasive carcinoma had been detected in two additional women in the ipsilateral breast 15 and 31 years, respectively, after the biopsy that harbored DCIS. Consequently, at the time of this second report, 9 of the original 28 patients (32%) had developed invasive carcinoma, which resulted in the deaths of 5 women. In addition, 25 years after the original biopsy with DCIS, one woman required a mastectomy for treatment of extensive noncomedo DCIS in the same quadrant as the original DCIS. Thus, the complete tally of patients who required treatment at the time of the report was 10/28, or 35.7%.

A third publication updating the status of the original 28 patients reported that 11, or 39.3%, had developed invasive carcinoma in the breast that initially harbored DCIS, including three after intervals of 23 to 42 years (24). At this time, the median follow-up of women who did not develop invasive carcinoma was 31 years. If one includes the woman who was treated by mastectomy for extensive DCIS, the 12 subsequent carcinomas represent 42.9% of the study cohort. At the time of this report, 5 of the 11 women who developed an invasive recurrence had died of metastatic carcinoma.

A 2015 report (25) combines the follow-up of the original 28 women with 17 ". . . other more recently identified patients" for a total of 45 patients. The source of the latter group is difficult to discern in this publication, and the updated follow-up status of the initial 28 patients is not presented separately. Overall, it is reported that 16 of the 45 patients (35.6%) developed invasive carcinoma in the same breast as the DCIS over a period of 3 to 42 years with an average interval to invasive carcinoma of 13 years.

At the time of last follow-up in this report, 30 of the 45 women were deceased, including 7 (15.6%) who developed distant metastases and died of breast carcinoma 1 to 7 years after an invasive breast recurrence.

Interim Comment-1

The foregoing unique retrospective studies with long-term follow-up of untreated low and intermediate-grade DCIS demonstrated a substantial risk for progression to invasive carcinoma extending over decades in the absence of clinical and mammographic follow-up. The study by Rosen et al. (15) was significantly hampered by the lack of follow-up for 15 (60%) of the 25 patients with untreated DCIS. Although the 6 women with subsequent invasive carcinoma represented 60% of the 10 patients with follow-up, they were only 24% of the entire study cohort. The actual frequency of subsequent ipsilateral invasive carcinoma most likely lies somewhere in the vicinity of 39.3% reported by Page et al. (23) and 43.8% in collected anecdotal reports prior to 1978 cited earlier.

Some of these patients experienced invasive breast recurrences and eventually died of metastatic breast carcinoma, but the results of these studies do not permit an estimate of the effect of postlumpectomy invasive breast recurrence on survival in the context of current medical practice.

Perhaps influenced by these data and largely anecdotal information about the even greater, accelerated postlumpectomy risk for progression to invasive breast recurrence associated with high-grade DCIS, complete mastectomy remained the standard surgical treatment for DCIS until the advent of breast conserving surgery in the 1980s. Thereafter, data began to accumulate about the results of treatment by lumpectomy alone with close clinical and mammographic surveillance, largely in a prospective, investigational setting. These latter studies differ from those of Rosen, Page, and others described earlier in that the diagnosis of DCIS was known, surgery was usually performed to achieve negative margins to the extent possible, and the patients were carefully followed prospectively with mammography.

Nonrandomized Prospective Studies of DCIS Treated by Breast Conserving Surgery Alone and Mammographic Surveillance

California Study by Lagios et al.

Over a 15-year period, Lagios and his associates assembled 79 patients with DCIS lesions who had no treatment after mammographic and pathologic complete excision of unifocal DCIS no larger than 25 mm (average 6.8 mm). Ninety-two percent of the foci of DCIS had been detected by mammography, and all were followed clinically with mammography. A report published in 1990 (26) described 10 recurrences (12.7%) after a median follow-up of 68 months. Half of the recurrences were invasive and half were DCIS. The rate of recurrence was higher in patients with comedo DCIS or cribriform DCIS with necrosis (9/36, 25%) than in those with low-grade forms of DCIS lacking necrosis (1/43, 2%). These results highlighted the more rapid recurrence rate of high-grade DCIS, even after apparently complete excision of small lesions, and the benefit

of careful clinical surveillance with mammography, which makes it possible to detect some instances of recurrent DCIS before they progress to invasion. Nevertheless, in this series of carefully selected patients, approximately 6% progressed to invasive carcinoma while under surveillance in little more than 5 years.

With follow-up ranging from 1 month to 136 months after a breast recurrence was detected, all of the patients were alive with no evidence of breast carcinoma.

Jefferson University Study by Schwartz et al.

This study of carefully selected patients was conducted by Schwartz et al. (27), who collected 70 patients (72 involved breasts) with 83.3% detected by mammography and 16.7% found incidentally between 1978 and 1990. At the time of the report, follow-up ranged from 18 to 168 months (median 47 months), during which time 11 of the 70 patients (15.3%) had had a recurrence. The mean time to recurrence was 34 months (range, 8–85 months). Eight of the recurrences were in the form of DCIS and three were invasive carcinomas (one with nodal metastases). All recurrences were detected by mammography as new calcifications. The initial DCIS in 10 patients with recurrent DCIS was at least partly of the comedo type, and 8 recurrent DCIS foci at an original biopsy site had comedo features. No patient with incidentally detected DCIS had had a recurrence at the time of the report.

In subsequent years, additional patients with DCIS diagnosed by mammography or found incidentally were enrolled by Schwartz and his colleagues in their study of treatment by lumpectomy alone. A 2004 publication about 151 patients with a median follow-up of 65 months reported 42 (29.8%) recurrences that were detected 11 to 97 months after lumpectomy (28). The median time to recurrence was 28.5 months. Follow-up of patients without recurrence ranged from 15 to 201 months (median 86 months). Among the many prognostic factors analyzed as potential markers of increased risk for recurrence, only lesion size larger than 15 mm and the presence of comedo necrosis were statistically significant.

At the time of the report, all patients who had had a breast recurrence were clinically free of systemic disease, including a woman whose invasive breast recurrence was accompanied by nodal metastases.

Interim Comment-2

The studies by Lagios et al. (26) and Schwartz et al. (27,28) confirm the proclivity of comedo DCIS to rapid invasive recurrence even for foci that measured 1 cm or less in excisions that had negative margins. Although it was possible in both studies to detect the majority of recurrences as DCIS before invasive carcinoma arose, despite careful surveillance with mammography about 5% of patients in both studies had invasive recurrences within about 5 years of the original biopsy (Lagios et al., 5/79 or 6.3%; Schwartz et al., 3/70 or 4.2%).

The studies thus far reviewed do not demonstrate in a systematic way that having a breast recurrence, whether DCIS or invasive, is associated with an increased risk for developing metastatic breast carcinoma or death due to breast carcinoma when compared with women who do not experience a breast recurrence after lumpectomy for DCIS.

Randomized Clinical Trial of DCIS Treated by Conservative Surgery and Surveillance

National Surgical Adjuvant Breast Project (NSABP) Protocol 6

NSABP Protocol 6 was a randomized trial intended to study patients with clinical stage I and stage II invasive breast carcinoma randomized to lumpectomy alone, lumpectomy with breast irradiation, and total mastectomy. All patients had an axillary dissection. During the course of pathology review after randomization had occurred and treatment was begun, it was discovered that 78 of the 2,072 (3.8%) randomized patients only had DCIS, including 2 who also had LCIS (29). Excluding those treated by mastectomy, 29 had been randomized to lumpectomy with radiation and 21 to lumpectomy only. Comedo necrosis was present in 72% of the DCIS specimens; combinations of papillary, cribriform, and solid foci were seen in 58%; and only 6% were classified as having a pure or predominant papillary pattern. The size of DCIS was 2.2 ± 1.3 cm, with only one clinically occult lesion found by mammography.

During follow-up ranging from 32 to 88 months, overall seven patients with DCIS (9%) treated by lumpectomy had breast recurrences all of which developed in or near the quadrant where DCIS had been present previously. Five of these recurrences were found in women treated by lumpectomy alone (5/21, 23.8%) (DCIS-2; invasive-3), and two in women treated by lumpectomy and radiation (2/29, 6.9%) (DCIS-1; invasive-1). The authors reported that "no clinical or pathologic features were recognized to allow for the prediction of local breast recurrence." These results suggested that radiation was helpful for suppressing occult residual DCIS that was responsible for breast recurrences after lumpectomy for DCIS with negative margins.

At the time of last follow-up, six of the patients with a breast recurrence were alive without evidence of breast carcinoma, and one had metastatic breast carcinoma.

Randomized Clinical Trial of DCIS Treated by Conservative Surgery, with or without Radiotherapy, and Surveillance

NSABP B-17 Trial

Following up on the inadvertent randomization of DCIS patients in NSABP Project 6, the NSABP B-17 trial was specifically designed to compare the outcome of DCIS patients treated by lumpectomy alone ($n = 403$) with those who had lumpectomy with breast irradiation ($n = 410$) (30). A requirement for entry into the trial was that lumpectomy margins be microscopically clear. In this trial, about 80% of the DCIS in both arms was detected by mammography only, about 19% by mammography and clinical exam, and only about 3% by clinical exam alone. Slightly more than 75% of the measured DCIS lesions in both arms were 1.0 cm or less.

There were 141 breast recurrences (79 invasive and 62 DCIS) in the lumpectomy only arm (35%; annual failure rate = 3.36), and 81 failures (44 invasive; 37 DCIS) in the lumpectomy plus radiation arm (19.8%; annual failure rate = 1.65). These data reveal a 52% reduction in breast recurrences associated with breast irradiation after lumpectomy for DCIS with negative margins. The cumulative incidence of recurrence at 15 years was reduced from 19.4% in the lumpectomy only arm to 8.9% when radiation was added to lumpectomy.

In the B-17 trial, the addition of radiotherapy to lumpectomy did not result in a significant reduction in deaths during the period of follow-up when compared with lumpectomy alone (hazard ratio = 1.08, 95% CI: 0.79–1.48). Overall, there were 358 deaths in the B-17 trial cohort at the time of the 2011 report. Only 72 (18.7%) of these deaths were breast carcinoma–related, with a 15-year cumulative incidence that was slightly lower in the lumpectomy alone group (3.1%) than in patients who had a lumpectomy plus radiation (4.7%), a difference that was not statistically significant with a hazard ratio of 1.44 (95% CI: 0.71–2.92). Also important was the finding that the cumulative probability of death due to breast carcinoma was 10.4% 10 years after an invasive recurrence, and only 2.7% after recurrence as DCIS.

Nonrandomized Clinical Trial of DCIS Treated by Conservative Surgery Alone and Surveillance Supplemented with Tamoxifen

Eastern Cooperative Oncology Trial

This one-arm prospective study involved two groups of patients who received lumpectomy that was supplemented in some cases by tamoxifen (31). One group consisted of 565 women with low- and/or intermediate-grade DCIS measuring 2.5 cm or less, and the other was composed of 105 women with high-grade DCIS measuring 1 cm or less. Clear margins of at least 3 mm and excision of all mammographic calcifications were required for inclusion in the trial. Mean tumor sizes in the two groups were 6 and 5 mm, respectively. Patients were accrued between 1997 and 2002. Following the release of results of the NSABP B-24 Trial showing that recurrences were reduced by the addition of tamoxifen (30), patients were offered this option, which was chosen by 31.3% in the low/intermediate-grade group and 28.6% in the high-grade group.

The median follow-up for all patients was 6.3 years when the data were analyzed for a report that appeared in 2009 (30). At that time, there were 49 breast recurrences in the low/intermediate-grade group (8.6%) with 53% invasive and 47% DCIS only. The high-grade group had 17 breast recurrences (16.2%), among which 35% were invasive and 65% DCIS only. The 7-year breast recurrence rates were 10.5% and 18% in the low/intermediate-grade and high-grade groups, respectively. Even within the relatively short-term follow-up in this report, breast recurrences continued to occur between the 5th and 7th years after lumpectomy, leading the authors to comment that "the increase in IBE (ipsilateral breast events or recurrences) beyond 5 years warrants caution regarding the clinical implications of our results . . . thus, substantially longer observation is warranted to determine whether omission of radiation is appropriate for some patients with DCIS." The report did not indicate whether tamoxifen had an effect on the rate of breast recurrences in either group.

The 5-year survival rates were 95.7% (95% CI: 94–97.4) and 97% (95% CI: 93.6–100) for the low/intermediate- and high-grade groups, respectively. At the time of the report, there had been no deaths caused by breast carcinoma.

There were 23 (3.8%) new contralateral breast carcinomas in the low/intermediate-grade group (65.2% invasive) with a 7-year rate of 4.8% (95% CI: 2.7–6.9). In the high-grade group, the six (5.8%) new contralateral breast carcinomas were all invasive with a 7-year rate of 7.4% (95% CI: 1.4–13.3).

Randomized Clinical Trial of DCIS Treated by Conservative Surgery and Breast Irradiation, with or without Adjuvant Tamoxifen

NSABP B-24 Trial

In this trial, follow-up was available for 1,799 patients who were randomly assigned to tamoxifen or placebo after treatment by conservative surgery supplemented with breast irradiation (30). The median follow-up was 163 months. About 85% of the measured DCIS lesions in both arms were 1 cm or less, and at least 80% were detected by mammography alone. Margins were reported to be involved or unknown in about 25% of cases in both study groups. When compared with outcome after radiation + placebo, radiation + tamoxifen resulted in a 32% reduction in invasive breast recurrences. The 15-year breast recurrence rate was 10% in the radiation + placebo arm and 8.5% after radiation + tamoxifen. Twenty-two of 39 (54%) deaths after an invasive breast recurrence were due to breast carcinoma. The occurrence of invasive breast recurrence was associated with a significantly increased risk of death (hazard rate of death = 1.75, 95% CI: 1.45–2.96, $p < 0.001$), whereas recurrence of DCIS did not significantly affect mortality in this study. The 15-year cumulative death rates were 2.7% and 2.3% after radiation + placebo and radiation + tamoxifen, respectively.

Interim Comment-3

The following conclusions can be drawn from the results of the preceding clinical trials:

a. Breast recurrences in women previously treated by lumpectomy for DCIS almost always occur in the same quadrant as the initial DCIS, frequently in the same location, regardless of margin status of the original lumpectomy;

b. The addition of breast irradiation to lumpectomy results in an overall reduction of about 50% in the incidence of breast recurrences;

c. Approximately 55% of breast recurrences after lumpectomy are invasive, regardless of whether irradiation was added or not added;

d. Breast irradiation alone probably does not reduce the cumulative incidence of breast carcinoma deaths after DCIS is treated by lumpectomy;

e. The addition of tamoxifen to lumpectomy and breast irradiation resulted in a reduction of invasive breast carcinoma recurrences of about 30% when compared with lumpectomy and irradiation alone;

f. The average time to recurrence after lumpectomy is shorter for high-grade than for low/intermediate-grade DCIS. As a consequence, follow-up of at least 10 years is necessary to reliably gauge the effect of a treatment program on the rate of recurrence;

g. When recurrences are detected after lumpectomy, they are more likely to be invasive if the initial DCIS was low/intermediate grade than if it was high grade. This circumstance probably reflects the frequent presence of more abundant, readily detected calcifications in high-grade DCIS leading to earlier detection of recurrences before invasion has developed;

h. Combined data from the B-17 and B-24 trials revealed that the 15-year cumulative incidence of contralateral breast carcinoma ranged from 10.2% to 10.8% for various treatment groups except those who received breast irradiation and tamoxifen, among whom the incidence was 7.3%. Overall, the majority (67.4%) of contralateral carcinomas were invasive; and

i. Invasive breast recurrences can be a source of fatal metastatic carcinoma, even after low/intermediate-grade DCIS, although most invasive breast recurrences are adequately controlled when detected in the course of clinical surveillance.

Epidemiologic Study of Breast Carcinoma Mortality Following Lumpectomy and Breast Irradiation for DCIS

Narod et al. (32) studied breast carcinoma mortality rates in 108,196 women younger than 70 years with a diagnosis of DCIS recorded from 1988 to 2011 in the Surveillance, Epidemiology, and End Results (SEER) database. No pathology review was conducted. In the entire cohort, consisting of patients treated by mastectomy, lumpectomy alone, and lumpectomy with breast irradiation, breast carcinoma-specific mortality was 3.3% (95 CI: 3.0–3.6) at 20 years. The risk of death due to breast carcinoma in all women with DCIS was 1.8 (95 CI: 1.7–1.9) times greater than expected when compared with the United States population, and the risk decreased with increasing age at diagnosis (17.0 for women diagnosed before age 35 years, and 1.4 for women older than 65 years at diagnosis). Other factors reported to be associated with higher breast carcinoma mortality after DCIS were larger DCIS size, higher grade, and ER-negative DCIS.

After 10 years of follow-up, the risk of ipsilateral invasive recurrence after lumpectomy for DCIS was significantly lower after breast irradiation (2.5%) than in the absence of breast irradiation (4.9%), but this did not translate into a significant reduction in breast carcinoma mortality (0.8% with irradiation vs. 0.9% without irradiation). Among the 956 women with DCIS who reportedly died of breast carcinoma, 210 (22%) had an invasive ipsilateral recurrence, 165 (17.3%) were reported to have had an invasive contralateral carcinoma, 20 (2.1%) had invasive carcinoma of undetermined laterality, and 517

(54.1%) had no documented invasive ipsilateral recurrence or contralateral carcinoma. The latter 517 women represent about 0.05% of the entire study cohort of 108,196 women.

On the basis of their epidemiologic data suggesting that about 0.5% of women who died of breast carcinoma after treatment of DCIS did not have a reported ipsilateral invasive recurrence or invasive contralateral carcinoma, Narod et al. (32) drew the following highly speculative conclusion:

> Cases of DCIS have more in common with small invasive cancers than previously thought. . . . Some cases of DCIS have an inherent potential for distant metastatic spread. It is therefore appropriate to consider these as de facto breast cancers and not as preinvasive markers predictive of subsequent invasive cancer.

Interim Comment-4

The epidemiologic study by Narod et al. (32) included patients treated by mastectomy, lumpectomy followed by breast irradiation, and lumpectomy without breast irradiation. The data confirm the results of previously cited clinical trials indicating that breast irradiation reduces the frequency of invasive breast recurrences after lumpectomy. In this report, invasive breast recurrences were reduced from 4.9% to 2.5% by the addition of breast irradiation after lumpectomy.

The authors concluded that breast carcinoma mortality after treatment of DCIS was inversely related to the patient's age at diagnosis, with the highest mortality among those less than 35 years old. Scrutiny of the data presented reveals that most of this effect was related to 5,253 women less than 39 years of age who constituted only 4.9% of the entire study cohort of 108,196 women. At age 40 and above, age at diagnosis did not appear to have an important effect on mortality after treatment.

The authors' interpretation of data on the effect of DCIS size, grade, and ER-status on breast carcinoma recurrence and mortality is questionable because of the significant numbers of cases recorded as "Unknown" in each category: (estrogen receptor status, 49.2%; grade, 26%; size, 30.6%). In fact, the p-value for the "Unknown" category in each of these parameters was statistically significant ($p < 0.001$). This is a consequence of the fact that a pathology review was not conducted.

The observation that breast irradiation after lumpectomy reduces the risk of invasive recurrences without a commensurate reduction in breast carcinoma mortality was previously recorded in the NSABP B-17 and B-24 trials (30). Although it might be expected that the rate of invasive breast recurrences would be directly related to breast carcinoma mortality, there are reasons why this effect might not be evident in the foregoing studies. One of these factors is the relatively small absolute number of patients with invasive recurrences and the small proportion of deaths attributable to breast carcinoma in each study. For example, in the NSABP B-17 trial, the lumpectomy arm had 79 invasive recurrences (19.6%) compared with 44 in the lumpectomy plus breast irradiation arm (10.7%).

A noteworthy aspect of this epidemiologic study was the data on contralateral invasive carcinoma. The mean annual rate at which invasive contralateral carcinomas occurred was 0.31%. Contralateral invasive breast carcinoma was associated with a significantly increased risk of breast carcinoma mortality (HR, 13.8 [95 CI: 11.5–16.6]; $p < 0.001$). Thus, subsequent fatal metastatic carcinoma could, in a significant number of cases, have arisen from a new contralateral carcinoma rather than from an ipsilateral invasive recurrence. Since this study did not include a pathologic review, it would not be possible to distinguish between an ipsilateral invasive recurrence and a new invasive contralateral carcinoma as the source of fatal metastatic carcinoma in any one case.

Does DCIS Have an Inherent Potential to Metastasize?

Despite the histologic similarity of the cells in DCIS and those of associated invasive duct carcinomas, it is clear that new properties are manifested by the invasive cells, including the ability to metastasize. Although it is possible that there are examples of DCIS that are inherently capable of metastatic spread, the actual occurrence of metastases seeming to arise from DCIS is so exceedingly rare in clinical practice in the absence of an accompanying detectable invasive carcinoma as to make this possibility an insufficient basis for treating the more than 99% of DCIS patients for whom this is not a concern.

The rarity of metastases apparently arising from DCIS alone was documented by Roses et al. (33) in a series of patients with DCIS treated at a single institution over a 13-year period. The cohort of 2,123 patients included 3 with DCIS (0.14%) who had metastatic breast carcinoma in the absence of demonstrated invasive carcinoma in either breast.

The possibility of metastases arising from DCIS in the absence of a documented invasive lesion can also be found among the less than 1% of breast carcinoma patients who present with axillary lymph nodes metastases as the first clinical manifestation of their disease. In one series of such cases, 12% of the primary lesions were DCIS and 3% were DCIS with LCIS (34). Additional rare examples of DCIS presenting with axillary nodal metastases have been described in other reports (35–37).

Documented Phenomena Can Easily Explain Reported Metastases from DCIS

1. Most obvious is the possibility that a small invasive focus or a microinvasive focus was overlooked during pathologic examination or a lesion was inadvertently misclassified as DCIS when invasion was clearly present but not recognized. It is beyond the scope of this discussion to review the extensive literature on discrepant diagnoses uncovered by a second review of breast pathology. Four recently published illustrative examples are cited here (38–41). Attention is also drawn to the previously discussed NSABP Protocol 6 in which pathology review determined that 78 of 2,072 patients (3.8%) enrolled in the trial with a diagnosis of invasive carcinoma had only DCIS (29). This underscores the essential role of pathology review as an integral part of randomized clinical trials and epidemiologic studies.

As an aside, it must be emphasized that observer variability and discrepant diagnoses are not unique to pathologists. In 1990, the National Library of Medicine added the category of "observer variation" to its catalog of search headings. In 1992, Elmore and Feinstein (42) published an article titled "A Bibliography of Publications on Observer Variability (Final Installment)" that listed 29 categories of medically related topics, including "epidemiologic risk factors." Relevant to the current discussion is the listed article titled "A Study of the Accuracy of Cancer Risk Factor Information Reported to a Central Registry Compared with that Obtained by Interview" (43). The absence of a pathology review in the study of Narod et al. (32) based on a central registry casts a dark shadow over their conclusion that DCIS is comparable to small invasive carcinoma.

2. There is also a precedent for an invasive focus to disappear before it can be detected histologically, a phenomenon that can be associated with "healed" DCIS in which the lesion is partially or completely obliterated, probably by some immunologic phenomenon (44). When this occurs, the DCIS is replaced with a scar consisting of circumferential layers of collagen and elastic tissue accompanied by a predominantly lymphocytic inflammatory reaction. Because the end-stage scars produced by this process are not distinguishable from scars formed in advanced periductal mastitis and other obliterative inflammatory conditions, "healing" DCIS can be recognized only when at least some residual DCIS is still present. The phenomenon of a "healed" malignant neoplasm being reduced to a scar is not unique to the breast. It also occurs rarely in malignant melanoma, renal carcinoma, and other neoplasms, where it can be associated with the presence of metastatic disease in the absence of a detectable primary lesion.

3. Invasion might also occur at a submicroscopic level without being apparent in conventional histologic sections examined with the light microscope. Evidence for this is the presence of foci of discontinuity in basement membranes that encircle DCIS that can be detected by electron microscopy (45) and by immunohistochemistry (46). Carcinoma cells have been observed protruding through gaps in the basement membrane by electron microscopy when no invasion was apparent with the light microscope (45,47).

What Does This Tell Us About the "Inherent Potential" of DCIS "for Distant Metastatic Spread"

1. At present, there is incomplete understanding of the following aspects of DCIS:
   a. the factors that control the potential to become invasive;
   b. the acquisition of the ability to give rise to metastatic foci; and
   c. the timing of the acquisition of these properties.

   Based on many decades of experience, it is widely agreed that invasive growth beyond the confines of DCIS, leading to access to the lymphovascular system, is necessary to initiate the process of metastatic spread. This understanding generally assumes that this is a stepwise process in which the acquisition of invasiveness precedes the ability to initiate metastatic spread and to establish metastases. The hypothesis that DCIS might have an inherent potential for metastatic spread before becoming invasive suggests that these attributes need not necessarily be acquired or expressed sequentially. Thus, a particular DCIS lesion could be capable of initiating metastases but not have acquired the ability to become invasive. Such an inherent potential for metastatic spread would necessarily remain latent and clinically undetectable until invasion had occurred or a biologic method were developed to detect this attribute while the carcinoma was in still its in situ state.

2. A latent, inherent potential for metastases might account by itself for exceedingly rare instances of DCIS with metastases without pathologically documented invasive carcinoma in the setting of "healed" DCIS or the theoretical spread of DCIS cells that slipped through the basement membrane at a submicroscopic level. Nonetheless, virtually all patients treated for DCIS do not develop metastases until after invasive growth has appeared, and in the majority, even an adequately treated invasive recurrence does not lead to metastases. It would be irresponsible to predicate the treatment of DCIS on the largely unsubstantiated theory that all or even a portion of DCIS has an "inherent potential . . . for distant metastatic spread" until this potential has been proven to exist and a reliable method for detecting this "potential" becomes available.

Rethinking the Treatment of DCIS

The Historical DCIS Treatment Paradigm

Although it has been stated that ". . . the natural history of ductal carcinoma in situ has never been elucidated" (48), it is apparent from the foregoing discussion of published information that considerable knowledge has accumulated on this subject. These studies have shown that if left untreated by contemporary standards after a diagnostic biopsy, some but not all low/intermediate- and high-grade DCIS lesions are capable of progressing to invasion, and that the time span for this process is on average shorter for high-grade lesions. Even if there is a subset of DCIS lesions, regardless of grade, with an inherent potential for metastatic spread, this property will virtually never be manifested until the DCIS has given rise to invasive carcinoma.

It is this paradigm that has guided the treatment of DCIS, driven by the goal of detecting and eradicating the disease before it becomes invasive. In my nearly 50 years of experience as a physician in the field of breast diseases, I have seen the treatment of DCIS evolve from radical mastectomy to modified mastectomy and then to lumpectomy augmented variously by breast irradiation and/or tamoxifen or other hormone modulators. All of these procedures were designed to prevent the recurrence of DCIS and its evolution into invasive carcinoma with the capacity to metastasize.

As has been demonstrated by the clinical trials summarized above, the panoply of breast conserving therapy has been successful in reducing the frequency of ipsilateral recurrences as DCIS or invasive carcinoma to a level that approximates the occurrence of new carcinomas in the contralateral breasts of treated patients. And, within the time frame of the available follow-up, invasive ipsilateral recurrences do not appear to significantly increase breast carcinoma mortality when they occur in the setting of contemporary posttreatment surveillance and appropriate treatment for the recurrence.

Regardless of the assurances given to a patient who experiences an invasive breast recurrence, the experience can be very unsettling, and it is likely to result in additional treatments that can have significant side effects and may ultimately lead to a mastectomy. Consequently, the primary treatment of DCIS should be designed to minimize the likelihood of a breast recurrence and subject the patient to the least damaging therapy consistent with achieving this goal. A cavalier attitude toward DCIS that is suggested by attempts to eliminate the word carcinoma from the name of the disease denies its inherent malignant potential and is not in the best interests of patients with DCIS.

DCIS Is a Heterogeneous Disease

DCIS is not a single disease. The fact that DCIS is heterogeneous is fully appreciated by pathologists who document the diverse characteristics of these lesions in their reports. Histologic characteristics have been used to develop classification schemes of DCIS that are designed to predict the risk for recurrence and progression to invasion. Most classifications divide DCIS into low, intermediate, and high grades signifying increasing risk. Clinically related factors such as age at diagnosis, race, and the completeness of excision after breast conserving surgery are also important. This aspect of DCIS is thoroughly discussed in Chapter 8.

Predicting the Risk for Progression from the Molecular Constitution of DCIS

In the past decade, attention has turned to the study of the molecular characteristics of DCIS for clues to assessing the risk for progression and to find new treatment options after breast conserving surgery. This approach has led to the development of multiparameter nomograms incorporating pathologic, clinical, and molecular information as well as assays based solely on the molecular constitution of individual DCIS lesions. The goal of this approach is to develop more precise measures of the risk of progression to invasion and to find new therapies that can be applied in a more targeted manner. These topics are covered in detail in Chapter 8 and will not be reviewed here.

Concluding Comment: "Overdiagnosis" and "Overtreatment" of DCIS?

An evolving concept today is that some DCIS lesions may have such a low likelihood for recurrence, progression to invasion, and metastatic spread that they pose little risk to the patient and require no treatment after a diagnostic biopsy. It is suggested that DCIS in this category is most likely to be detected

by screening and that it is currently "overdiagnosed" when referred to as carcinoma and consequently "overtreated." To avoid "overtreatment," the advocates of this view recommend that DCIS be subsumed in a group of "indolent lesions of epithelial origin," or IDLE, to include "precursors that are unlikely to cause harm if left untreated" (48). The goal of this approach is to eliminate the "frightening" words cancer or carcinoma from such low-grade lesions and thus make it more acceptable to leave them untreated.

With this proposal, history repeats itself. IDLE is essentially a repackaging of the now largely dismissed scheme introduced in the 1990s to substitute the term *ductal intraepithelial neoplasia* or "DIN" for DCIS, with the inclusion of atypical duct hyperplasia and subdivisions that parallel conventional grades of DCIS (49). As noted at the outset of this discussion, a similar proposal was put forth nearly 50 years ago to convert LCIS to LIN or LN with the same goal of altering therapy by changing terminology. Now, with the availability of effective chemoprevention therapy, LCIS can be properly viewed as a marker of duct carcinoma risk and as a direct precursor to invasive lobular carcinoma without a name change.

It is very regrettable that proposals to alter the terminology and treatment of DCIS have been disseminated to the public without rigorous investigation. This has led to articles with alarming headlines such as "A surgeon's less-is-more approach challenges conventional wisdom on treating some kinds of breast lesions" (50) highlighting Dr. Laura Esserman, one of the creators of IDLE, and "Doubt is raised on quick surgery on breast lesion; report questions value of aggressive moves at earliest stages," (17) referring to the seriously flawed epidemiologic study by Narod et al. (32) discussed earlier. A reasonably balanced presentation of the current situation appeared in *Time* under the title "Why Doctors Are Rethinking Breast-Cancer Treatment" (51).

Although the time has come to improve the treatment of DCIS using new methodologies now available that offer the potential to tailor therapy more specifically to an individual patient's disease, there are no data-based, clearly established guidelines for modifying the current treatment paradigm to accomplish this goal and avoid "overtreatment." It is possible that there are situations where treatment can be minimized to consist of lumpectomy alone with surveillance, a "watch and wait" scenario, with a high degree of certainty that the patient will not be jeopardized. Without changing terminology, it would be appropriate to clearly determine with reproducible specificity which, if any, forms of DCIS could qualify as sufficiently "indolent" as not to require any treatment after a diagnostic biopsy. In addition to clinical parameters and descriptive histopathology, this will involve thorough molecular analysis of DCIS lesions and follow-up in randomized clinical trials. Despite all the hype that has been created in the press, IDLE should remain idle. It is clear that not all DCIS is the same and that further research is urgently needed to identify the parameters that make a difference for treatment in the 21st century.

Paul P. Rosen, MD

REFERENCES

1. Esserman L, Yau C. Rethinking the standard for ductal carcinoma in situ. *JAMA Oncol.* 2015;1:881–883.

2. Virchow R. Cellular-Pathologie. *Virchows Arch [A].* 1855;8:3–39.

3. Remak R. Beitrag zur Entwickelungsgeschichte der krebshaften Geschuwulste. *Deutshe Klin.* 1854;6:170–174.

4. Thiersch C. *Der Epithelial krebs, namentlich der Haut. Eine anatomischer-klinishe Untersuchung.* Leipzig, Germany: Engelmann; 1865.

5. Cornil A-V. Contributions a l'histoire du development histologique des tumeurs epitheliales (sqirrhe, encephaloide, etc). *J Anat Physiol.* 1865;2:266–276.

6. Cornil A-V. *Les tumeuers du sein.* Paris, France: Libraire Germer Ballaire; 1908.

7. Waldeyer W. Die Entwikelung der Carcinome. *Arch Pathol Anat Phys Klin Chir.* 1913;101:573–668.

8. Ewing J. *Neoplastic Diseases.* 2nd ed. Philadelphia, PA: WB Saunders; 1928.

9. Cheatle GL, Cutler M. *Tumours of the Breast.* Philadelphia, PA: JB Lippincott; 1931.

10. Broders AC. Carcinoma in situ contrasted with benign penetrating epithelium. *JAMA* 1932;99:1670–1674.

11. Dean L, Geschickter CF. Comedo carcinoma of the breast. *Arch Surg.* 1938;36:225–234.

12. Krauss FT, Neubecker RD. The differential diagnosis of papillary tumors of the breast. *Cancer.* 1962;15:444–455.

13. Farrow JH. Current concepts in the detection and treatment of the earliest of the early breast cancers (The James Ewing Lecture). *Cancer.* 1970;25:458–477.

14. Haagensen CD. *Diseases of the Breast.* 2nd ed. New York, NY: WB Saunders; 1971:528–544, 586–590.

15. Rosen PP, Lieberman PH, Braun DW, Jr., et al. Lobular carcinoma *in situ* of the breast. Detailed analysis of 99 patients with average follow-up of 24 years. *Am J Surg Pathol.* 1978;2:225–251.

16. Betsill WL, Rosen PP, Lieberman PH, et al. Intraductal carcinoma: long-term follow-up after treatment by biopsy alone. *JAMA.* 1978;239:1863–1867.

17. Kolata G. Doubt is raised over value of surgery for breast lesions at earliest stage. *New York Times.* August 25, 2015:A1–A13.

18. Hutter RVP. Is cured early cancer truly cancer? *Cancer* 1981;47:1215–1220.

19. Page DL, Dupont WD, Rogers LW, et al. Intraductal carcinoma of the breast: follow up after biopsy only. *Cancer.* 1982;49:751–758.

20. Eusebi V, Fendale E, Foschini MP, et al. Long-term follow-up of in situ carcinoma of the breast. *Semin Diagn Pathol.* 1994;11:223–235.

21. Leonard GD, Swain SM. Ductal carcinoma *in situ*, complexities and challenges. *JNCI.* 2004;96:906–920.

22. Erbas B, Provenzano E, Armes J, et al. The natural history of ductal carcinoma *in situ* of the breast: a review. *Breast Cancer Res Treat.* 2006;97:135–144.

23. Page DL, Dupont WD, Rogers LW, et al. Continued local recurrence of carcinoma 15–25 years after a diagnosis of low grade ductal carcinoma in situ of the breast treated only by biopsy. *Cancer.* 1995;76:1197–1200.

24. Sanders ME, Schuyler PA, Dupont WD, et al. The natural history of low-grade ductal carcinoma in situ of the breast in women treated by biopsy only revealed over 30 years of long-term follow-up. *Cancer.* 2005;103:2481–2484.

25. Sanders ME, Schuyler PA, Simpson JF, et al. Continued observation of the natural history of low-grade ductal carcinoma *in situ* reaffirms the proclivity for local recurrence even after more than 30 years of follow-up. *Mod Pathol.* 2015;28:662–669.

26. Lagios MD, Margolin FR, Westdahl PR, et al. Mammographically detected duct carcinoma in situ. Frequency of local recurrence following tylectomy and prognostic effect of nuclear grade on local recurrence. *Cancer.* 1989;63:618–624.

27. Schwartz GF, Finkel GC, Garcia JC, et al. Subclinical ductal carcinoma in situ: treatment by local excision and surveillance alone. *Cancer.* 1992;70:2468–2474.

28. Cornfield DB, Palazzo JP, Schwartz GF, et al. The prognostic significance of multiple morphologic features and biologic markers in ductal carcinoma in situ of the breast. A study of a large cohort of patients treated by surgery alone. *Cancer.* 2004;100:2317–2327.

29. Fisher ER, Sass R, Fisher B, et al. Pathologic findings from the National Surgical Adjuvant Breast Project (Protocol 6). Intraductal carcinoma (DCIS). *Cancer.* 1986;57:197–208.

30. Wapnir IL, Dignam JJ, Fisher B, et al. Long-term outcomes of invasive ipsilateral breast tumor recurrences after lumpectomy in NSABP B-17 and B-24 randomized clinical trials for DCIS. *J Natl Cancer Inst.* 2011;103:1–11.

31. Hughes LL, Wang M, Page DL, et al. Local excision alone without irradiation for ductall carcinoma in situ of the breast: a trial of the Eastern Cooperative Oncology Group. *J Clin Oncol.* 2009;32:5319–5324.

32. Narod SA, Iqbal S, Giannakeas V, et al. Breast cancer mortality after a diagnosis of ductal carcinoma in situ. *JAMA Oncol.* 2015;1:888–896.

33. Roses RE, Arun BK, Mittendorf EA, et al. Ductal carcinoma-in situ of the breast with subsequent distant metastasis and death. *Ann Surg Oncol.* 2011;10:2873–2878.

34. Rosen PP, Kimmel M. Occult breast carcinoma presenting with axillary lymph node metastases: follow-up study of 48 patients. *Hum Pathol.* 1990;21:518–523.

35. Westbrook KC, Gallager HS. Breast carcinoma presenting as an axillary mass. *Am J Surg.* 1971;122:607–611.

36. Rosen PP. Axillary lymph node metastases in patients with occult noninvasive breast carcinoma. *Cancer.* 1980;46:1298–1306.

37. Bhatia SK, Saclarides TJ, Witt TR, et al. Hormone receptor studies in axillary metastases from occult breast cancers. *Cancer.* 1987;59:1170–1172.

38. Allison KH, Reisch LM, Carney PA, et al. Understanding diagnostic variability in breast pathology: lessons learned from an expert consensus review panel. *Histopathology.* 2014;65:240–251.

39. Khazal L, Middleton LP, Goktepe N, et al. Breast pathology second review identifies clinically significant discrepancies in over 10% of patients. *J Surg Oncol.* 2015;111:192–197.

40. Marco V, Muntal T, Garcia-Hernandez F, et al. Changes in breast cancer reports after pathology second opinion. *Breast J.* 2014;20:295–301.

41. Elmore JG, Longton GM, Carney PA, et al. Diagnostic concordance among pathologists interpreting breast biopsy specimens. *JAMA.* 2015;313:1122–1132.

42. Elmore JG, Feinstein AR. A bibliography of publications on observer variability (final installment). *J Clin Epidemiol.* 1992;45:567–580.

43. Bronson RC, Davis JR, Chang JC, et al. A study of the accuracy of cancer risk factor information reported to a central registry compared with that obtained by interview. *Am J Epidemiol.* 1989;129:616–624.

44. Muir R, Aitkenhead AC. The healing of intraductal carcinoma of the mamma. *J Pathol Bacteriol.* 1943;38:117–127.

45. Ozzello L. Ultrastructure of intraepithelial carcinoma of the breast. *Cancer.* 1971;28:1508–1515.

46. Rajan PB, Perry RH. A quantitative study of patterns of basement membrane in ductal carcinoma in situ (DCIS) of the breast. *Breast J.* 1995;1:315–321.

47. Tamimi SO, Ahmed A. Stromal changes in early invasive and noninvasive breast carcinoma: an ultrastructural study. *J Pathol.* 1986;150:43–49.

48. Esserman LJ, Thompson IM, Reid B, et al. Addressing overdiagnosis and overtreatment in cancer: a prescription for change. *Lancet Oncol.* 2014;15:e234–e242.

49. Tavassoli FA. *Pathology of the Breast.* 2nd ed. Stamford, CT: Appleton & Lange; 1999:205–260.

50. Hafner K. A strong second opinion. A surgeon's less-is-more approach challenges conventional wisdom on treating some kinds of breast lesions. *New York Times.* September 29, 2015:D1–D5.

51. O'Connor S. Why doctors are rethinking breast-cancer treatment. *Time.* October 12, 2015:31–36.

Pathology and the Origin of Specialization in Medicine

The development of modern medical specialism during the latter part of the 19th century and the early part of the present century . . . would hardly have taken place had not physicians accustomed themselves to the idea of distinct disease entities consisting of localized organic lesions connected with certain clinical pictures. . . . The development and application of a concept of localized pathology laid the groundwork for modern specialism by providing a number of foci of interest in the field of medicine. Each such focus of interest, that is, a disease or the diseases of an organ or region of the body, provided a nucleus around which could gather the results of clinical and pathologic investigation.

On the technologic side, the influences represented in specialization manifest themselves in the multiplicity of technical skills, devices, and theories applied to the achievement of human aims in the field of medicine.

From *The Specialization of Medicine*
by George Rosen, MD, 1944.

Acknowledgments

The potential for the team approach to cancer treatment is epitomized in the management of patients with mammographically detected breast lesions, who are the most likely candidates for the needle core biopsy procedure. This effort draws upon the skills of mammographers, pathologists, and surgeons, as well as radiation therapists and medical oncologists. We are grateful to the hundreds of pathologists, surgeons, medical oncologists, and radiologists throughout the United States and abroad who contributed cases for pathology consultation that may be illustrated in this book, and to their patients.

The new illustrations in this book were taken from cases seen in consultation submitted from several institutions or diagnosed and treated at various medical centers with which the authors are affiliated. Each specimen is vitally important to the individual from whom it was obtained, and we endeavor to provide a specific diagnosis that will contribute to the clinical care of that patient. This material is also a priceless resource for research and teaching. Thousands of adult women as well as many hundreds of men and children afflicted with breast diseases who cannot be recognized individually are acknowledged for their anonymous contributions to this and prior editions of *Rosen's Diagnosis of Breast Pathology by Needle Core Biopsy*.

Knowledge gained in the course of providing this clinical service contributes to providing better care to patients with breast diseases. In this sense, each patient who has had a diagnosis made in the nearly 45 years of these consultation practices has participated in the academic undertaking and contributed to improving the diagnostic skill in breast pathology of hundreds of pathologists in training, to the benefit of still more individuals.

We also wish to recognize the superb support of the publisher for this project, most notably Ms. Kate Heaney, Development Editor, and Mr. Ryan Shaw, Acquisitions Editor, from the earliest discussions of the concept for this fourth edition to the final publication.

All photographic images in this edition were digitally processed or reprocessed by Ms. Patricia Kuharic in the Medical Arts Department of the Weill Cornell Medical College. We express our deepest appreciation for her high professional standards that have made an essential contribution to this volume. Drs. Timothy D'Alphonso, Maria Arafah and Esther Cheng are thanked for their help with the preparation of some figures.

Contents

Preface to First Edition (Updated) *vii*
Paul P. Rosen, MD

Introduction to the Third Edition (Updated):
Breast Imaging and the Origin of Needle Core Biopsy *ix*
Paul P. Rosen, MD

DCIS is DCIS is DCIS: A Controversial
Introduction to Fourth Edition *xv*
Paul P. Rosen, MD

Acknowledgments *xxvii*

1 Embryology, Development, Histology, and
   Physiologic Morphology 1
   Syed A. Hoda

2 Inflammatory and Reactive Lesions 13
   Syed A. Hoda

3 Specific Infections 32
   Syed A. Hoda

4 Benign Papillary Tumors 39
   Frederick C. Koerner

5 Myoepithelial Lesions 71
   Edi Brogi

6 Adenosis and Microglandular Adenosis 83
   Edi Brogi

7 Fibroepithelial Neoplasms 104
   Edi Brogi

8 Ductal Hyperplasia, Atypical Ductal
   Hyperplasia, and Ductal Carcinoma
   In Situ 125
   Syed A. Hoda

9 Invasive Ductal Carcinoma 179
   Syed A. Hoda

10 Tubular Carcinoma 199
    Edi Brogi

11 Papillary Carcinoma 215
    Frederick C. Koerner

12 Medullary Carcinoma 232
    Frederick C. Koerner

13 Metaplastic Carcinoma Including
    Low-grade Adenosquamous Carcinoma 238
    Edi Brogi

14 Mucinous Carcinoma 259
    Edi Brogi

15 Apocrine Carcinoma 275
    Edi Brogi

16 Adenoid Cystic Carcinoma 288
    Edi Brogi

17 Other Special Types of Invasive Ductal
    Carcinoma 298
    Frederick C. Koerner

18 Lobular Carcinoma In Situ and Atypical
    Lobular Hyperplasia 320
    Syed A. Hoda

19 Invasive Lobular Carcinoma 349
    Syed A. Hoda

20 Mesenchymal Lesions 364
    Frederick C. Koerner

21 Lymphoid and Hematopoietic Tumors 413
    Judith A. Ferry

22 Metastases in the Breast from
    Nonmammary Malignant Neoplasms 428
    Syed A. Hoda

23 Pathologic Effects of Therapy 440
    Frederick C. Koerner

24 Men and Children 452
    Edi Brogi

25 Pathologic Changes and Clinical
    Complications Associated with
    Needling Procedures 466
    Syed A. Hoda

26 Processing, Pathological Examination,
    and Reporting of Needle Core Biopsy
    Specimens 477
    Syed A. Hoda

List of Abbreviations 499

Index 500

Embryology, Development, Histology, and Physiologic Morphology

SYED A. HODA

EMBRYOLOGY AND DEVELOPMENT

The mammary glands develop from mammary ridges (so-called milk lines). The latter are thickenings of the epidermis that appear on the ventral surface of the 5-week fetus. The bilateral mammary ridges extend from the axilla to the vulva. In humans of either gender, the ridges largely disappear during normal fetal development, except for a pair of thickenings, one on either side of the pectoral region. Persistence of other segments of the milk line results in the development of ectopic mammary glandular tissue, which occurs most often at the extreme ends of the mammary ridge, that is, in the axilla and vulva.

The aforementioned thickening is caused by an epithelial bud that forms around condensed mesenchymal tissue. Columns of epithelial cords grow downward, branch, canalize, and transform into ducts and, ultimately, lobules. Each column eventually forms a lobe of the breast. Obviously, stem cells and molecular mechanisms have roles in mammary development; however, these roles are presently unclear (1–3).

In most girls, functional breast development does not begin until puberty. Premature thelarche is the unilateral or bilateral appearance of a discoid subareolar thickening before puberty (4). The incidence in white female infants and children up to 7 years of age in the United States in 1980 was 20.8 per 100,000 (5). Its prevalence, as reported in 2010, among 318 female children aged between 1 and 4 years in a midwestern American hospital, was calculated to be 4.7% (6). The nodular breast tissue formed in premature thelarche can measure up to 6.5 cm, and tends to slowly regress over a period of 6 months to 6 years. Premature thelarche has been associated with precocious puberty (7), but not with a predisposition to develop breast carcinoma (8). Histologically, the breast glandular tissue in premature thelarche resembles gynecomastia. Both lesions are characterized by ductal epithelial hyperplasia with solid and micropapillary configurations. Branching of proliferating ducts results in an increased number of ducts. The latter are surrounded by moderately cellular stroma. Excisional biopsy, or overzealous sampling via needle core biopsy, of prematurely developed breast tissue is inappropriate, because it could result in impairment of subsequent physical development of the breast or complete failure of the breast to develop.

With the onset of the cyclical production of estrogen and progesterone at puberty, adolescent female breast development begins (**Fig. 1.1**). Growth of ducts and periductal stroma is estrogen dependent (9). As stated above, mammary lobules are derived from solid masses of cells that form at the ends of terminal ducts. Breast glandular differentiation occurs mostly during puberty, but this process can continue into the third decade of life and is enhanced by pregnancy (3). The bulk of lobules in the mature breast are embedded in fibrous tissue; however, normal lobules may also be located amid mammary adipose tissue—usually in postmenopausal women (**Fig. 1.2**).

HISTOLOGY

The functional lobular and ductal elements of the breast are embedded in fibroadipose tissue that forms the bulk of the mammary gland. The relative proportions of fibrous and fatty stroma vary greatly among individuals and with age. The combination of stromal and epithelial components is responsible for the radiologic appearance of breast structure in normal and pathologic states. Magnetic resonance imaging (MRI) provides a relatively precise method for discriminating between fatty and fibroglandular tissue in the breast. By comparing images obtained with mammography and MRI, Lee et al. (10) found a mean fat content of 42.5% (SD ± 30.3%) in mammograms and 66.5% (SD ± 18%) in MRI images. The ranges of fat content obtained by mammography and MRI imaging were 7.5% to 90% and 17% to 89%, respectively. The correlation coefficient for estimates of fat content obtained by both methods was 0.63, with the strongest correlation ($r = 0.81$) in postmenopausal women.

Breast "density" refers to the proportion of more dense (fibroconnective and glandular) to less dense (adipose) tissues as evidenced on mammography. There has been considerable interest in the genetic and hormonal basis of such density and its relationship to the detection, incidence (and even prognosis) of breast carcinoma (11,12). Greater breast density has been associated with advanced tumor stage at diagnosis and increased risk of both local recurrence and second primary

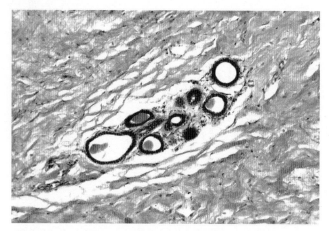

FIGURE 1.1 Immature Breast. Breast tissue at the onset of puberty in an 11-year-old girl showing early lobular differentiation with glandular secretion and developing intralobular stroma.

cancers. The biologic and genetic pathways that modulate mammographic density and its variability during various phases of the menstrual cycle phase remain unresolved (13).

Approximately 20 lactiferous (collecting) ducts terminate in, and exit from, the breast at the nipple. Each lactiferous duct drains a mammary lobe **(Fig. 1.3)**. These lobes vary in extent, and are arranged in a spoke-like manner radiating from the nipple. The individual lobes do not constitute grossly discrete structures, and may overlap with adjacent ones around the edges. The structure of each lobe is simple: the lactiferous duct extends distally from the nipple through a series of branches that diminish in caliber from the nipple to the terminal ductal–lobular units.

The squamocolumnar junction in the lactiferous ducts, where the squamous epithelium joins the glandular duct epithelium, is normally distal to a dilated segment of the lactiferous duct, the lactiferous sinus, located just beneath the nipple surface. Extension of squamous epithelium into or below the lactiferous sinus represents metaplasia of the lining ductal epithelia. This process, when exuberant, may result in obstruction of the affected duct. Lactiferous ducts in the nipple are surrounded by circular and longitudinal arrays of smooth muscle fibers rooted in dense fibrous stroma.

The branching mammary ductal system is embedded in specialized, hormonally responsive stroma. The extralobular ducts are lined mainly by a single layer of epithelium, with underlying myoepithelial cells and basement membrane. In the nonlactating breast, the major ducts cut in cross section have contours marked by numerous folds or indentations that create a stellate structure, with a serrated contour. The epithelium in the bay-like pouches of the duct lumen can give rise to ductular branches. Fully formed lobules originate directly from these pouches in the more distal segments of the mammary duct system—and more rarely in its more proximal segments, that is, the lactiferous ducts of the nipple (14).

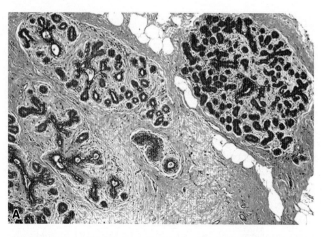

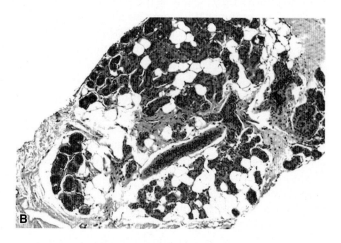

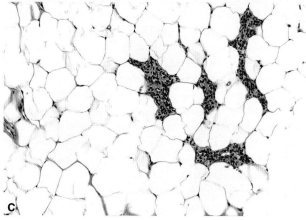

FIGURE 1.2 Normal Lobules. A: A lobule in fibrocollagenous stroma. **B:** A lobule in mammary adipose tissue. **C:** An atrophic lobule amid mammary adipose tissue in a 75-year-old woman.

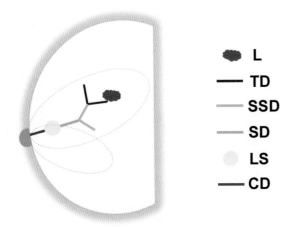

The great majority of epithelial cells that form the lining of the mammary glandular system (ducts and lobules) are cuboidal or columnar cells. Their cytoplasm is endowed with abundant organelles involved in secretory functions. Myoepithelial cells lie between the epithelial layer and the basal lamina (**Fig. 1.4**). The cytoplasm of myoepithelial cells, distributed in a network of slender processes that invest the overlying epithelial cells, is rich in myofibrils. The histologic appearance and immunoreactivity of myoepithelial cells is variable, especially in pathologic conditions, and depends on the degree to which the myoid or epithelial phenotype is accentuated in a particular situation. Myoepithelial cells are typically spindle shaped ("bipolar"), but they may become cuboidal, or undergo "myoid" or clear cell change in certain proliferative or pathologic conditions (**Fig. 1.5**). Myoepithelial cells display nuclear reactivity for p63 and p40 (15). Epithelioid (cuboidal) myoepithelial cells can have absent or reduced p63 reactivity. Glands lined by apocrine epithelia (inactive, hyperplastic, or noninvasive malignant) occasionally show complete lack of myoepithelial cells as evidenced by immunohistochemistry (16–18).

FIGURE 1.3 Diagrammatic Representation of the Glandular Structure of the Adult Female Breast. The lobules *(violet)* open into terminal ducts *(blue)*. The lobules and terminal ducts together constitute the terminal duct–lobular unit (TDLU). Terminal ducts connect in sequence to subsegmental ducts *(green)*, segmental ducts *(orange)*, lactiferous sinus *(yellow)*, collecting duct *(red)*, and nipple. Two (of the 20 or so) lobes are depicted in stippled outline. Note the variable size of lobes. CD, collecting duct; L, lobules; LS, lactiferous sinus; SD, segmental ducts; SSD, subsegmental ducts; TD, terminal ducts.

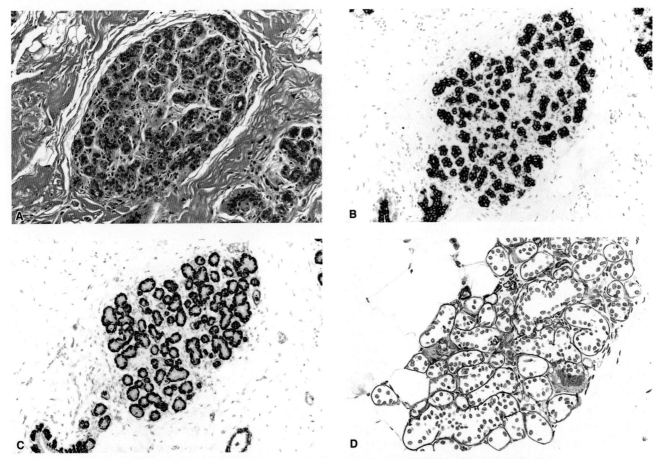

FIGURE 1.4 Myoepithelial Cell Layer and Basement Membrane in a Lobule. A: A typical inactive lobule in a patient of childbearing age. Note the relatively inconspicuous myoepithelial cell layer on H&E-stain. **B:** A cytokeratin AE1/3 immunostain highlights the mammary epithelium in the luminal aspect of the glands. **C:** A smooth muscle myosin immunostain shows the myoepithelial cell layer in the abluminal aspect of the gland. **D:** A laminin immunostain highlights the basement membranes surrounding all glands.

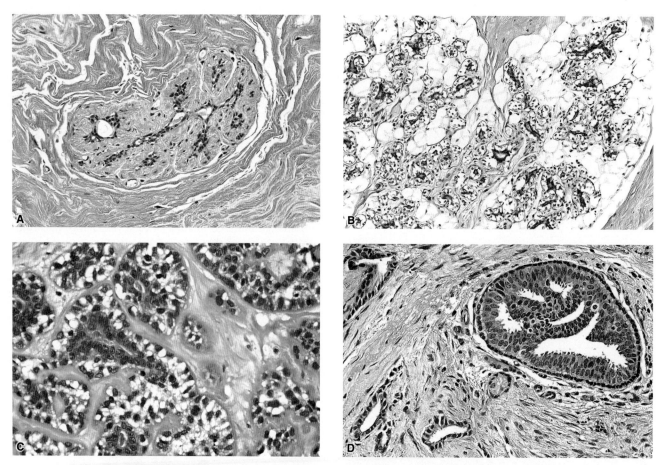

FIGURE 1.5 Variations in Myoepithelial Cells. A: Myoepithelial cells appear "myoid," that is, plump, in atrophic ducts. **B:** Clear cell change in myoepithelial cells in adenosis. **C:** Typical adenomyoepithelioma with clear cell change in the myoepithelial cell component. **D:** Myoepithelial cells appear prominent in the intraductal carcinoma associated with tubular carcinoma.

The normal periductal stroma contains fibroblasts and elastic fibers, as well as scattered sparse lymphocytes, plasma cells, mast cells, and histiocytes. *Ochrocytes* are histiocytes with a cytoplasmic accumulation of lipofuscin pigment **(Fig. 1.6).** These pigmented cells become more numerous in the postmenopausal breast and in association with inflammatory or proliferative conditions (19). In addition to being present in the duct lumen, ochrocytes are found in the ductal epithelium, where they have a "pagetoid-like" distribution, and in periductal stroma. They are easily distinguished from pagetoid and periductal carcinoma cells by immunostains that typically yield the following results: CK7 (−), CK20 (−), and CD68 (+). When restricted to an intraepithelial position, ochrocytes may be confused with epithelioid myoepithelial cells, but they are not reactive with myoepithelial markers such as p63, myosin, and calponin.

Secretion of milk originates in lobules—the distal-most portion of the mammary glandular system. Lobules are composed of alveolar glands encased in specialized vascularized stroma. They are drained by terminal lobular ducts, which in turn open into the extralobular duct system. The resting lobular gland is lined by a single layer of cuboidal epithelial cells supported by loosely connected myoepithelial cells and a basement membrane.

PHYSIOLOGIC MORPHOLOGY

The "normal" microscopic anatomy of the lobules is inconstant because the histologic appearance of the lobule in the mature breast is subject to changes associated with the menstrual cycle, pregnancy, lactation, exogenous hormone administration, aging, and menopause. Furthermore, there is variation in the functional state of individual lobules regardless of physiologic circumstances, an observation that suggests that individual lobules or regions of the breast have intrinsic differences in response to hormonal and other stimuli. This is reflected in the substantial variability in labeling indices, indicating different proliferative rates among lobules in a given individual (20). Immunoreactivity for estrogen and progesterone receptors is also variably expressed in the epithelial cells of the lobules and ducts.

Histologic alterations occur in the normal breast during the menstrual cycle (21). According to some authors, the proliferative phase, days 3 through 7, features the highest rate of epithelial mitoses and of apoptosis (22,23). Other investigators who defined this phase as days 0 to 5 reported that "apoptosis and mitosis were by and large absent in this phase" (22). Lobular glands at this time are lined by crowded, poorly oriented epithelial cells with little or no lumen formation and secretion. Myoepithelial cells are inconspicuous and

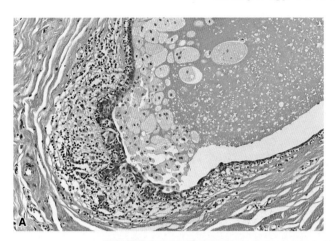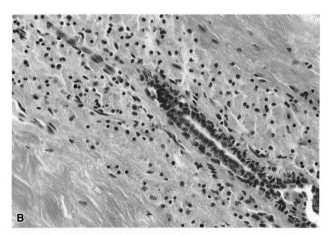

FIGURE 1.6 Histiocytes and Ochrocytes in Ductal Epithelium and Periductal Stroma.
A: Histiocytes with granular, lipofuscin-contaning cytoplasm are present in the periductal stroma and in the ductal epithelium in an example of periductal mastitis associated with duct ectasia. The histiocytes have a "pagetoid-like" distribution and extend into periductal stroma. **B:** Ochrocytes are seen in the stroma after a complete pathologic response to neoadjuvant chemotherapy for breast carcinoma.

difficult to distinguish from epithelial cells. The lobular stroma is relatively dense and hypovascular, with plump fibroblasts ringing the glands.

Mitoses and apoptotic bodies are inconspicuous in the follicular phase (days 8–14). At this stage, the myoepithelial cells have a polygonal shape, clear cytoplasm, and become more apparent. Epithelial cells become columnar, with increasingly basophilic cytoplasm and basally oriented, darkly stained nuclei. An acinar lumen without secretion is evident.

During the luteal phase, comprising days 15 through 20, myoepithelial cells become more prominent with increased glycogen accumulation that results in cytoplasmic clearing. The glandular lumen is clearly defined by epithelial cells with basophilic cytoplasm. Luminal secretion is present in a few glands. Edema and a mixed inflammatory cell infiltrate appear in the intralobular stroma. Mitoses and apoptotic bodies are infrequent.

The secretory phase corresponding to days 21 through 27 features increased secretory activity with distention of glandular lumina. The epithelium consists of columnar epithelial and myoepithelial cells with progressively clear cytoplasm. It is at this stage that mitoses and apoptotic bodies are most conspicuous with maximal intralobular edema and inflammation.

In the menstrual phase, comprising days 28 through 2, the mammary stroma becomes compact with loss of intralobular edema. At this stage, lymphocytes, macrophages, and plasma cells are most conspicuous in the lobular stroma (22). Some glandular lumina remain, and others appear collapsed. Mitotic activity is absent.

The ability to recognize menstrual cycle–related morphologic changes in the breast may be useful in premenopausal women. Evidence suggesting that surgery performed during the luteal phase is advantageous, in prognostic terms, remains controversial (24–28). Nevertheless, it has been proposed that premenopausal women could benefit from higher sensitivity of mammography if they schedule screening mammography during the first week of their menstrual cycle (29).

Estrogen and progesterone receptors (ER and PR) are variably expressed in the nuclei of epithelial cells in the normal breast.

Immunohistochemical staining reveals a higher proportion of positive nuclei in lobular than in ductal cells (30). Considerable heterogeneity exists in nuclear hormone–receptor activity among lobules. Maximal expression of ER and PR is typically observed in the follicular phase (31); however, no consistent menstrual cycle–related pattern has been found in the expression of ER and PR in breast carcinomas in premenopausal women (32,33).

Secretory changes associated with pregnancy occur unevenly throughout the breast **(Fig. 1.7)**. There is progressive recruitment of lobules with advancing stages of pregnancy. Earlier in pregnancy, terminal ducts and lobules grow rapidly, resulting in lobular enlargement with some coincidental depletion of the fibrofatty stroma (34,35). Stromal vascularity increases, accompanied by infiltration by mononuclear inflammatory cells. During the second and third trimesters, lobular growth progresses through epithelial hypertrophy (enlargement of cells) as well as epithelial hyperplasia (proliferation of cells).

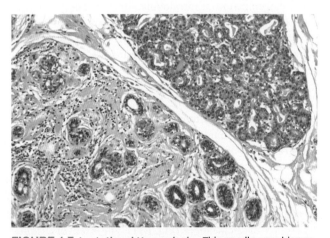

FIGURE 1.7 Lactational Hyperplasia. This needle core biopsy specimen from a 31-year-old woman 34 weeks pregnant shows lactational hyperplasia in one lobule **(upper right)** and another unaltered lobule with fibroadenomatoid change.

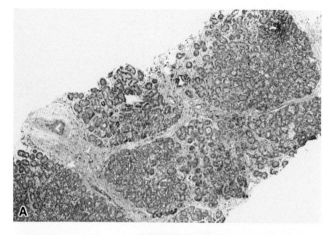

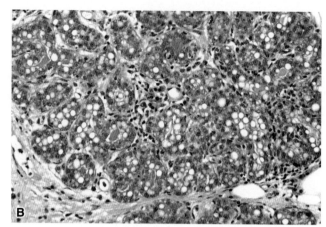

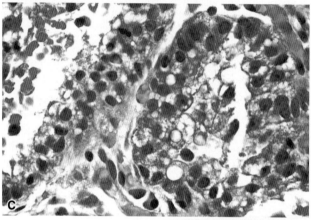

FIGURE 1.8 Lactational Hyperplasia. A: The patient was 8 months pregnant when this needle core biopsy was performed for a mass that proved to be nodular lactational hyperplasia. **B:** The markedly enlarged lobules are composed of a greatly increased number of glands that should not be mistaken for carcinoma. **C:** Basophilic, vacuolated cytoplasm, luminal secretion, and inconspicuous myoepithelial cells are characteristic features.

The cytoplasm of lobular epithelial cells becomes vacuolated, and secretion accumulates in lobular glands **(Fig. 1.8)**. Lactation features markedly distended irregularly shaped lobular glands formed by cells with hyperchromatic nuclei **(Fig. 1.9)**.

Hormonal alterations that occur during and after the menopause are manifested by a decrease in the cellularity and number of lobules, mainly as a result of epithelial atrophy. Coincidental with the loss of glandular epithelium, there is a tendency toward thickening of lobular basement membranes and collagenization of intralobular stroma. The process of menopausal atrophy occurs in a heterogeneous fashion, often leaving some lobules relatively unaffected. Most lobular glands appear to collapse and shrink, but cystic distention may also occur, and calcifications are sometimes formed in atrophic lobular glands **(Fig. 1.10)**. In many elderly women, lobular integrity is progressively lost, leaving ducts and glands that may contain calcifications embedded in fibrocollagenous stroma. Atrophy tends to spare lobular myoepithelial cells that frequently persist, or become even more prominent, in a late stage of the process. The relative proportions of fat and stroma vary in the atrophic breast. In advanced atrophy, calcifications may be found in the stroma unaccompanied by epithelium, and pronounced elastotic change in the stroma can be a source of calcifications **(Fig. 1.11)**. The extent of terminal duct lobular unit (TDLU) involution has been linked to lower breast cancer risk; however, this factor has, thus far, not been fully studied (36).

Mammographic changes suggestive of physiologic proliferative alterations have been observed in women receiving *postmenopausal hormone replacement therapy* (37,38). The effect of hormone replacement therapy on the mammographic appearance of the breast is substantially less in women who have undergone prior breast irradiation (39). In the nonirradiated breast, the effect of hormone replacement is manifested mainly by increased parenchymal density. This has been observed after treatment with estrogen alone and with an estrogen–progesterone combination therapy. Histologic examination does not reveal a consistent pattern. Some patients have lobular differentiation comparable to the premenopausal state, whereas others have prominent cystic or proliferative alterations of ducts and lobules. The findings suggest that the existing epithelial status of the breast is accentuated by exogenous hormone administration.

Pregnancy-like change (pseudolactational metaplasia) is usually a focal microscopic alteration characterized by lobules that resembles the physiologic process of lactation. It occurs in breast tissue from women who are neither pregnant nor lactating. Many such patients are parous, pre- or postmenopausal women, but similar changes have been observed in nulliparous women (40). The reported frequency of pregnancy-like change is 1.7% to 3% in surgical pathology and autopsy series (40,41). The etiology of pregnancy-like change remains unknown. Glands and terminal ducts with pregnancy-like change usually contain little or no secretion, although they may be dilated **(Fig. 1.12)**. The glandular cells are swollen with abundant

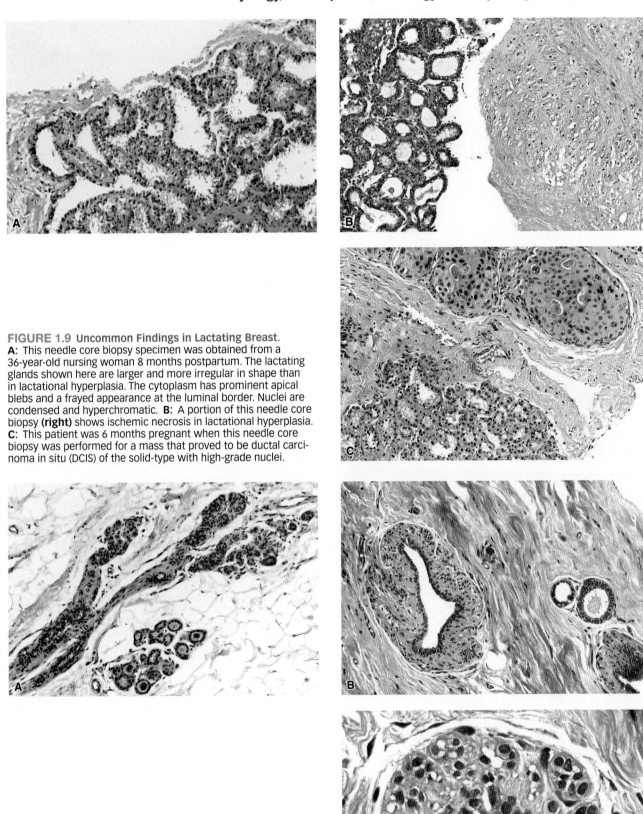

FIGURE 1.9 Uncommon Findings in Lactating Breast.
A: This needle core biopsy specimen was obtained from a 36-year-old nursing woman 8 months postpartum. The lactating glands shown here are larger and more irregular in shape than in lactational hyperplasia. The cytoplasm has prominent apical blebs and a frayed appearance at the luminal border. Nuclei are condensed and hyperchromatic. **B:** A portion of this needle core biopsy **(right)** shows ischemic necrosis in lactational hyperplasia. **C:** This patient was 6 months pregnant when this needle core biopsy was performed for a mass that proved to be ductal carcinoma in situ (DCIS) of the solid-type with high-grade nuclei.

FIGURE 1.10 Atrophy. **A:** An atrophic lobule with a calcification in inactive glands **(lower center)**. The needle core biopsy was performed on a 73-year-old woman with mammographically detected calcifications. **B, C:** Myoid metaplasia of myoepithelial cells is evident around the atrophic duct in this biopsy specimen.

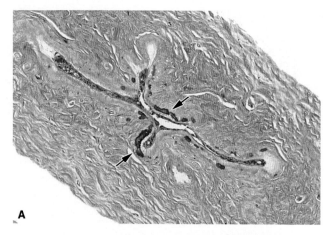

A

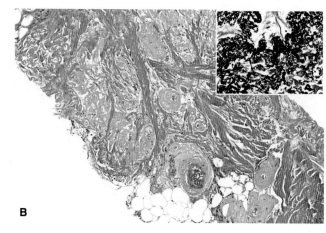

B

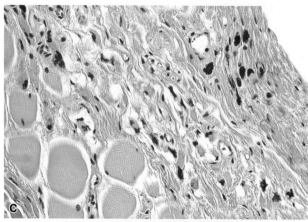

C

FIGURE 1.11 Atrophy. A: Calcifications *(arrows)* are shown in the periductal stroma in a needle core biopsy specimen from a postmenopausal woman. **B:** Diffuse stromal elastosis in a needle core biopsy from an elderly woman with a breast mass. Inset highlights elastic fibers on Verhoeff-van Gieson stain. **C:** Needle core biopsy performed to evaluate a "seroma" (s/p mastectomy) showing atrophy of chest wall skeletal muscle. The altered skeletal muscle fibers appear largely clumped with aggregates of pyknotic nuclei **(right)**. Relatively less affected muscle fibers are seen on left.

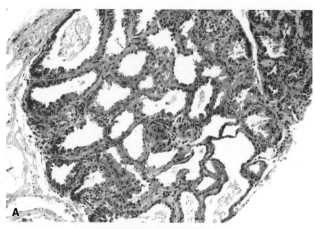

A

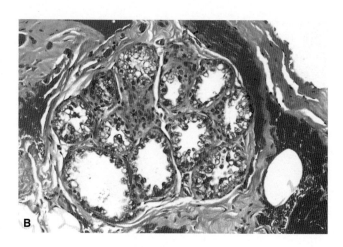

B

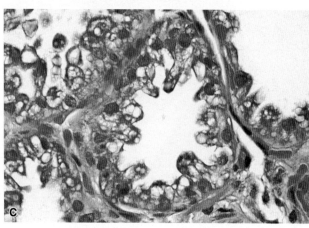

C

FIGURE 1.12 Pregnancy-Like Change. A: This lobule was present in a needle core biopsy specimen from a 49-year-old woman with invasive carcinoma. The enlarged lobule is composed of irregularly shaped glandular acini that contain small amounts of secretion. **B, C:** Pregnancy-like change in the atrophic lobule of a 74-year-old woman who had a needle core biopsy performed for calcifications that were localized to columnar cell duct hyperplasia.

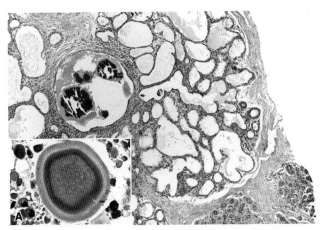
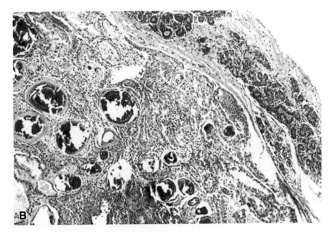

FIGURE 1.13 Pregnancy-Like Change, with Calcification. A: Characteristically large, laminated calcifications are present in pregnancy-like change shown in this needle core biopsy specimen from a 37-year-old nonpregnant, nonlactating woman with mammographically detected calcifications. Inset shows details of calcifications and a dominant Liesegang-like structure. **B:** Lymphocytes are scattered in the stroma of the enlarged lobule with pregnancy-like hyperplasia and calcifications in this needle core biopsy sample from a 34-year-old woman.

pale-to-clear, finely granular, or vacuolated cytoplasm. The nuclei are usually small, uniform, round, and dark. The luminal cytoplasmic borders of glandular cells are frayed, and small cytoplasmic blebs are formed. The nucleus may contain blebs of cytoplasm extruded into the glandular lumen. Calcifications, occasionally of the psammomatous type, can be formed in pregnancy-like change **(Fig. 1.13)**. Diastase-resistant granules that stain positively with periodic acid–Schiff (PAS) are present in the cytoplasm. The affected cells are immunoreactive for α-lactalbumin and S-100 protein (41).

In most instances, the epithelium in lobules altered by pregnancy-like change remains one or two cell layers thick. Pregnancy-like hyperplasia represents the occurrence of pregnancy-like change in hyperplastic epithelium. The hyperplastic epithelial tissue usually assumes papillary or micropapillary configurations **(Fig. 1.14)**. The epithelium is arranged in irregular fronds composed entirely of glandular cells. Although the cytologic appearance may duplicate the findings of pregnancy-like change, some of these lesions feature nuclear atypia, manifested in most instances by nuclear pleomorphism. Rarely, these atypical cytologic changes may warrant a diagnosis of atypical pregnancy-like hyperplasia **(Fig. 1.15)**. Atypical changes are more likely to be present when pregnancy-like hyperplasia coexists with cystic hypersecretory hyperplasia (42) **(Fig. 1.16)**. Rarely, carcinoma has been found to arise from pregnancy-like hyperplasia, usually in combination with cystic hypersecretory hyperplasia (43).

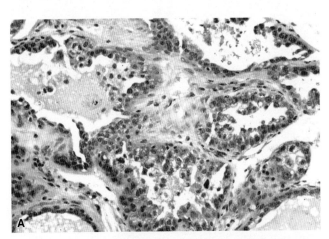
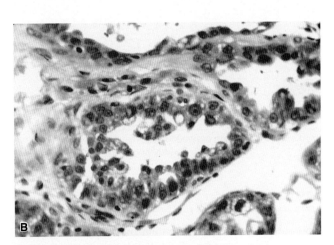

FIGURE 1.14 Pregnancy-Like Hyperplasia. A, B: Micropapillary fronds composed of hyperplastic epithelium protrude into some gland lumina. Note the slightly uneven, crowded distribution of nuclei. Some nuclei have prominent nucleoli. Pale eosinophilic secretion is present. This appearance resembles cystic hypersecretory carcinoma in a lobule, but the epithelium does not have the appearance of micropapillary carcinoma, and the secretion lacks the intense eosinophilia and linear parallel cracks that characterize a cystic hypersecretory lesion.

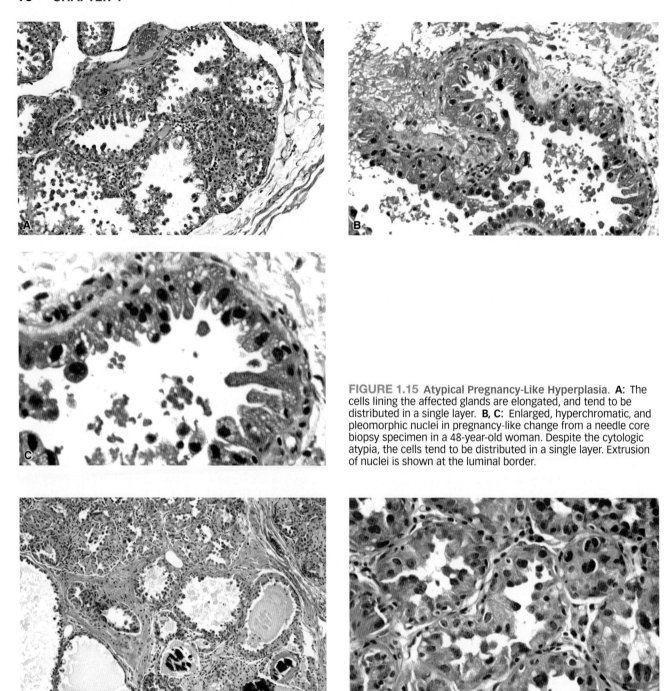

FIGURE 1.15 **Atypical Pregnancy-Like Hyperplasia. A:** The cells lining the affected glands are elongated, and tend to be distributed in a single layer. **B, C:** Enlarged, hyperchromatic, and pleomorphic nuclei in pregnancy-like change from a needle core biopsy specimen in a 48-year-old woman. Despite the cytologic atypia, the cells tend to be distributed in a single layer. Extrusion of nuclei is shown at the luminal border.

FIGURE 1.16 **Atypical Pregnancy-Like Hyperplasia and Cystic Hypersecretory Hyperplasia.** **A:** This needle core biopsy specimen was obtained for calcifications that proved to be at the junction between cystic hypersecretory hyperplasia **(below)** and atypical pregnancy-like hyperplasia **(above)**. **B:** Magnified view of lobular glands in atypical pregnancy-like hyperplasia.

METAPLASIA

Apocrine metaplasia is a common "normal" finding in the glandular epithelia of the adult female breast. The metaplastic apocrine cells of the breast are histologically similar to the apocrine cells that are normally present in cutaneous glands, especially in the axillary, periareolar, and perineal regions. On H&E staining, apocrine cells may appear to be either uniformly pink with extremely fine vacuoles or coarsely granular. The granules are birefringent, and tend to accumulate in the luminal aspect of the cells. Apical snouts can be a prominent feature of apocrine cells. In general, the nuclei of apocrine cells are round and centrally placed with distinct nucleoli. Nucleoli may not be evident in flattened or cuboidal apocrine epithelium. Apocrine cells typically show some nuclear variability, even in putatively inactive cells; however, overt nuclear atypia, mitotic activity, and necrosis are harbingers of apocrine carcinoma. It is notable that radiation-related nuclear changes are relatively more evident in apocrine metaplastic cells.

Apocrine metaplastic cells are immunoreactive for epithelial membrane antigen (EMA), cytokeratins 8 and 18, and androgen receptors (AR). They usually do not express estrogen receptor (ER) or progesterone receptors (PR). Apocrine cells are also immunoreactive with three proteins found in mammary cyst fluids, namely, gross cystic disease fluid protein (GCDFP) 15, 24, and 44 (44).

Clear cell (change) metaplasia is a cytologic alteration in lobular and terminal duct epithelium that has also been referred to as "hellenzellen" (German: clear or bright cells) (45). The affected lobules tend to be larger than adjacent uninvolved lobules. Some glands have dilated lumina in which there is PAS-positive, diastase-resistant secretion, but more often, the lobular gland lumina are obliterated by the swollen cells (46). The lobular gland epithelium is composed of swollen cells with abundant clear or pale cytoplasm **(Fig. 1.17)**. The cells have well-defined borders. The small, round, and dark nuclei are often displaced toward the center of the gland. Calcifications are uncommon in clear cell change. The clear cells are immunoreactive for cytokeratin but not for actin.

The etiology of clear cell change remains unknown. It is encountered in pre- and postmenopausal women. There is no association with pregnancy or exogenous hormone use (46,47). Foci of clear cell change have been identified retrospectively in breast tissue obtained before exogenous hormones were available. Clear cell change is usually multifocal, but can involve both breasts. Viña and Wells (41) reported finding clear cell change in 15 of 934 (1.6%) biopsies. Specimens that contain clear cell change may harbor carcinoma or a variety of benign or atypical changes, there being no association with any particular breast lesions (41). Rarely, clear cell change and pregnancy-like change may coexist in the same breast (47).

The differential diagnosis of clear cell change includes pregnancy-like change as well as cytoplasmic clearing in apocrine metaplastic cells and in myoepithelial cells, and clear cell forms of carcinoma—such as glycogen-rich carcinoma and metastatic renal clear cell carcinoma. Pregnancy-like change is readily distinguished from clear cell change by the presence of "decapitation" secretion at the luminal borders of the cells in the former. Cytoplasmic clearing in apocrine metaplasia is usually a focal change in epithelium that otherwise has the typical features of apocrine metaplasia. Myoepithelial cells with clear cell change retain their position between the epithelium and basement membrane.

Squamous metaplasia of the mammary epithelium occurs in association with inflammatory and reactive conditions, and in current practice is most commonly encountered as a reparative change in epithelium that was damaged by a prior procedure.

REFERENCES

1. Rios AC, Fu NY, Lindeman GJ, et al. In situ identification of bipotent stem cells in the mammary gland. *Nature.* 2014;506:322–327.
2. Cowin P, Wysolmerski J. Molecular mechanisms guiding embryonic mammary gland development. *Cold Spring Harb Perspect Biol.* 2010;2:a003251.
3. Van Keymeulen A, Rocha AS, Ousset M, et al. Distinct stem cells contribute to mammary gland development and maintenance. *Nature.* 2011;479:189–193.
4. Codner E, Román R. Premature thelarche from phenotype to genotype. *Pediatr Endocrinol Rev.* 2008;5:760–765.
5. van Winter JT, Noller KL, Zimmerman D, et al. Natural history of premature thelarche in Olmsted County, Minnesota, 1940 to 1984. *J Pediatr.* 1990;116:278–280.
6. Curfman AL, Reljanovic SM, McNelis KM, et al. Premature thelarche in infants and toddlers: prevalence, natural history and environmental determinants. *J Pediatr Adolesc Gynecol.* 2011;24:338–341.
7. Pasquino AM, Pucarelli I, Passeri F, et al. Progression of premature thelarche to central precocious puberty. *J Pediatr.* 1995;126:11–14.
8. Adriance MC, Inman JL, Peterson OW, et al. Myoepithelial cells: good fences make good neighbors. *Breast Cancer Res.* 2005;7:190–197.
9. Topper YJ, Freeman CS. Multiple hormone interactions in the developmental biology of the mammary gland. *Physiol Rev.* 1980;60:1049–1106.
10. Lee NA, Rusinek H, Weinreb J, et al. Fatty and fibroglandular tissue volumes in the breasts of women 20–83 years old: comparison of x-ray mammography and computer-assisted MR imaging. *AJR: Am J Roentgenol.* 1997;168:501–506.
11. Huo CW, Chew GL, Britt KL, et al. Mammographic density—a review on the current understanding of its association with breast cancer. *Breast Cancer Res Treat.* 2014;144:479–502.
12. Maskarinec G, Pagano IS, Little MA, et al. Mammographic density as a predictor of breast cancer survival: the Multiethnic Cohort. *Breast Cancer Res.* 2013;15:R7.
13. Morrow M, Chatterton RT Jr, Rademaker AW, et al. A prospective study of variability in mammographic density during the menstrual cycle. *Breast Cancer Res Treat.* 2010;121:565–574.
14. Rosen PP, Tench W. Lobules in the nipple: frequency and significance for breast cancer treatment. *Pathol Annu.* 1985;20(pt 1):317–322.
15. Sarda R, Taylor J. p40 (ΔNp63), a lung squamous cell marker, can also be used to label breast myoepithelial cells. *Arch Pathol Lab Med.* 2014;138:584.
16. Cserni G. Lack of myoepithelium in apocrine glands of the breast does not necessarily imply malignancy. *Histopathology.* 2008;52:253–255.
17. Tramm T, Kim JY, Tavassoli FA. Diminished number or complete loss of myoepithelial cells associated with metaplastic and neoplastic apocrine lesions of the breast. *Am J Surg Pathol.* 2011;35:202–211.
18. Cserni G. Benign apocrine papillary lesions of the breast lacking or virtually lacking myoepithelial cells-potential pitfalls in diagnosing malignancy. *APMIS.* 2012;120:249–252.
19. Davies JD. Pigmented periductal cells (ochrocytes) in mammary dysplasias: their nature and significance. *J Pathol.* 1974;114:205–216.

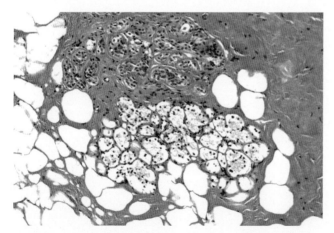

FIGURE 1.17 Clear Cell Change. The lower lobule is composed of cells with clear cytoplasm and small dark nuclei in this needle core biopsy specimen from a 54-year-old woman with mammographically detected calcifications that were associated with intraductal carcinoma.

20. Christov K, Chew KL, Ljung B-M, et al. Proliferation of normal breast epithelial cells as shown by *in vivo* labeling with bromodeoxyuridine. *Am J Pathol.* 1991;138:1371–1377.

21. Ramakrishnan R, Khan S, Badve S. Morphological changes in breast tissue with menstrual cycle. *Mod Pathol.* 2002;15:1348–1356.

22. Longacre TA, Bartow SA. A correlative morphologic study of human breast and endometrium in the menstrual cycle. *Am J Surg Pathol.* 1986;10:382–393.

23. Ferguson DJP, Anderson TJ. Morphological evaluation of cell turnover in relation to the menstrual cycle in the "resting" human breast. *Br J Cancer.* 1981;4:177–181.

24. Donegan W, Shah D. Prognosis of patients with breast cancer related to the timing of operation. *Arch Surg.* 1993;128:309–313.

25. Badwe R, Mittra I, Havaldor R. Timing of surgery during the menstrual cycle and prognosis of breast cancer. *J Biosci.* 2000;25:113–120.

26. Milella M, Nistico C, Ferraresi V, et al. Breast cancer and timing of surgery during menstrual cycle: a 5-year analysis of 248 premenopausal women. *Breast Cancer Res Treat.* 1999;55:259–266.

27. Nomura Y, Kataoka A, Tsuitsui S, et al. Lack of correlation between timing of surgery in relation to the menstrual cycle and prognosis of premenopausal patients with early breast cancer. *Eur J Cancer.* 1999;35:1326–1330.

28. Grant CS, Ingle JN, Suman VJ, et al. Menstrual cycle and surgical treatment of breast cancer: findings from the NCCTG N9431 study. *J Clin Oncol.* 2009;27:3620–3626.

29. Miglioretti DL, Walker R, Weaver DL, et al. Accuracy of screening mammography varies by week of menstrual cycle. *Radiology.* 2011;258:372–379.

30. Petersen OW, Hoyer PE, van Deurs B. Frequency and distribution of estrogen receptor-positive cells in normal, nonlactating human breast tissue. *Cancer Res.* 1987;47:5748–5751.

31. Fabris G, Marchetti E, Marzola A, et al. Pathophysiology of estrogen receptors in mammary tissue by monoclonal antibodies. *J Steroid Biochem Mol Biol.* 1987;27:171–176.

32. Markopoulos C, Berger U, Wilson P, et al. Estrogen receptor content of normal breast cells and breast carcinoma throughout the menstrual cycle. *Br Med J.* 1988;296:1349–1351.

33. Smyth CM, Benn DE, Reeve TS. Influence of the menstrual cycle on the concentrations of estrogen and progesterone receptors in primary breast cancer biopsies. *Breast Cancer Res Treat.* 1988;11:45–50.

34. McCarty KS Jr, Tucker JA. Breast. In: Sternberg SS, ed. *Histology for Pathologists.* New York, NY: Raven Press; 1992:893–902.

35. Salazar H, Tobon H, Josimovich JB. Developmental gestational and postgestational modifications of the human breast. *Clin Obstet Gynecol.* 1975;18:113–137.

36. Figueroa JD, Pfeiffer RM, Patel DA, et al. Terminal duct lobular unit involution of the normal breast: implications for breast cancer etiology. *J Natl Cancer Inst.* 2014;106(10):1–11. pii:dju286.

37. Rand T, Heytmanek G, Seifert M, et al. Mammography in women undergoing hormone replacement therapy: possible effects revealed at routine examination. *Acta Radiol.* 1997;38:228–231.

38. Laya MB, Gallagher JC, Schreiman JS, et al. Effect of postmenopausal hormonal replacement therapy on mammographic density and parenchymal pattern. *Radiology.* 1995;196:433–437.

39. Margolin FR, Denny SR, Gelfand CA, et al. Mammographic changes after hormone replacement therapy in patients who have undergone breast irradiation. *AJR: Am J Roentgenol.* 1999;172:147–150.

40. Kiaer HW, Andersen JA. Focal pregnancy-like changes in the breast. *Acta Pathol Microbiol Scand A.* 1977;85:931–941.

41. Viña M, Wells CA. Clear cell metaplasia of the breast: a lesion showing eccrine differentiation. *Histopathology.* 1989;15:85–92.

42. Shin SJ, Rosen PP. Pregnancy-like (pseudolactational) hyperplasia: a primary diagnosis in mammographically detected lesions of the breast and its relationship to cystic hypersecretory hyperplasia. *Am J Surg Pathol.* 2000;24:1670–1674.

43. Shin S, Rosen PP. Carcinoma arising from preexisting pregnancy-like and cystic hypersecretory hyperplasia lesions of the breast: a clinicopathologic study of 9 patients. *Am J Surg Pathol.* 2004;28:789–793.

44. Wells CA, El-Ayat GA. Nonoperative breast pathology: apocrine lesions. *J Clin Pathol.* 2007;60:1313–1320.

45. Skorpil F. Uber das Vorkommen von sog. hellen Zellen (Lamprocyten) in der Milchdruse [in German]. *Beitrage zur pathol Anat.* 1943;108:378–393.

46. Barwick KW, Kashigarian M, Rosen PP. 'Clear-cell' change within duct and lobular epithelium of the human breast. *Pathol Annu.* 1982;17(pt 1):319–328.

47. Tavassoli FA, Yeh IT. Lactational and clear cell changes of the breast in nonlactating, nonpregnant women. *Am J Clin Pathol.* 1987;87:23–29.

Inflammatory and Reactive Lesions

SYED A. HODA

FAT NECROSIS

Mammary fat necrosis may occasionally result from incidental trauma; however, presently, the most common causes are previous needling procedures (such as fine needle aspiration or needle core biopsy), surgery, and radiation therapy (1,2). Patients with fat necrosis typically present with a painless superficial mass, occasionally associated with retraction or dimpling of the overlying skin. Any part of the breast may be affected. At presentation, the typically solitary mass spans approximately 2 cm. Fat necrosis in the male breast is usually traumatic in origin and has been diagnosed on needle core biopsy (3). Hemorrhagic and fat necrosis of subcutaneous and breast tissue, occasionally progressing to gangrenous necrosis, has been associated with warfarin (Coumadin) anticoagulant treatment (4); however, with better therapeutic monitoring, this iatrogenic complication is now less common (5).

The clinical and radiologic problem of distinguishing fat necrosis from recurrent carcinoma is especially difficult in patients who have undergone breast-conserving surgery and various modalities of radiation therapy (6–8). Mammography of fat necrosis usually reveals a spiculated mass that may contain irregular, punctate, or coarse calcifications (9,10). Less frequently, the lesion appears as an "oil cyst", that is, a circumscribed, oil-filled, partly calcified cyst (11). Both patterns may coexist in a single lesion. Ultrasonography and magnetic resonance imaging (MRI) features of fat necrosis are also variable and may be indistinguishable from carcinoma (10).

The initial histologic change in fat necrosis is adipocyte injury (diminished size, fine vacuolization, and dropout) associated with a neutrophilic infiltrate **(Fig. 2.1)**. Further evolution of the lesion is marked by the progressive appearance of histiocytes, eosinophils, lymphocytes, and plasma cells with deposition of hemosiderin **(Fig. 2.2)**. Some histiocytes that accompany fat necrosis can simulate lipoblasts. Unlike lipoblasts, histiocytes are of relatively uniform size with fine intracytoplasmic vacuoles that do not indent the generally round nucleus. A giant cell granulomatous reaction may develop over time **(Fig. 2.3)**. Fibrosis develops peripherally, demarcating the region of necrotic fat, cellular debris, and calcifications **(Fig. 2.4)**. In late lesions, the reactive inflammatory components are replaced by fibroplasia, which evolves into a dense scar. An exaggerated histiocytic response to fat necrosis may take the form of

a "cellular spindled histiocytic pseudotumor" (12) (arguably, an innovative term for inflammatory pseudotumor), wherein the mitotically active histiocytic spindle cell proliferation has the potential to be mistaken for spindle cell neoplasm, such as metaplastic carcinoma. Reactive squamous metaplasia may develop in the epithelium of ducts and lobules in the vicinity of fat necrosis. Loculated necrotic fat, with dystrophic calcification, may persist for many years **(Fig. 2.5)**. Among patients who develop fat necrosis after radiotherapy, the characteristic histopathologic effects of radiation on epithelial, stromal, and vascular tissues can be identified in the native mammary tissue.

Needle core biopsy is required in all instances wherein clinical and radiologic diagnosis of fat necrosis is uncertain. Careful microscopic examination is warranted in every needle core biopsy of fat necrosis as the process may mask a histologically subtle invasive carcinoma. The use of epithelial (cytokeratin) and histiocytic (CD11c, CD68, and CD163) immunostains can be helpful in this regard.

Erdheim–Chester disease, an extremely infrequent xanthomatous form of non-Langerhans cell histiocytosis of uncertain etiology, rarely involves the breast (13–15). Histologically, the disease can be mistaken for fat necrosis, especially if the initial clinical manifestation is a breast mass (13). Typically, there are synchronous cutaneous, osseous, and orbital lesions that are characterized by infiltrates of histiocytes, Touton-type giant cells (with wreath-like arrangement of nuclei at the perimeter of the giant cell), plasma cells, and infrequent epithelioid granulomata. The lesional histiocytes are immunoreactive for CD68, but are negative for S-100 protein, CD1a, and cytokeratins (13). The disease may simply be interpreted as a benign histiocytic proliferation on needle core biopsy—unless the clinical setting is known and Touton-type giant cells are recognized (14).

BREAST INFARCT

The most frequent form of breast infarct occurs during pregnancy or in the postpartum period. The lesion usually presents as a solitary, discrete, firm mass that can clinically suggest carcinoma. Pain and tenderness are sometimes reported. Hemorrhage and ischemic degeneration with little or no inflammatory cell infiltrate characterize the histologic appearance of

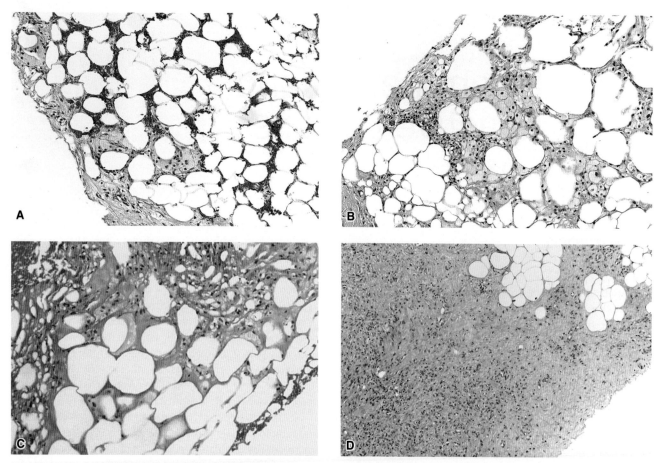

FIGURE 2.1 Fat Necrosis, Phases. A: Early fat necrosis manifested by a histiocytic and eosinophilic infiltrate, associated with hemorrhage. **B:** Early organization in fat necrosis. Note focal presence of lymphocytes amid the histiocytic infiltrate. **C:** Healing fat necrosis. This needle core biopsy specimen obtained from a 1 cm stellate lesion consists of infarcted fat cells, hemorrhage, and a histiocytic reaction. **D:** Late (organized) fat necrosis: fibrosis and hemosiderin deposition are associated with necrotic fat. This needle core biopsy of a breast mass followed a softball injury 6 weeks earlier.

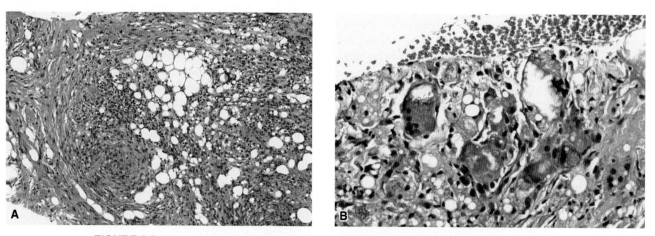

FIGURE 2.2 Fat Necrosis. A: Needle core biopsy specimen from a mammographically detected mass at the site of a prior lumpectomy for intraductal carcinoma. Fibrosis and granulomatous reaction are evident in the fat necrosis. No foreign body material was found. **B:** Multinucleated histiocytes with foreign body material are shown in a needle core biopsy specimen from fat necrosis at a prior surgical site.

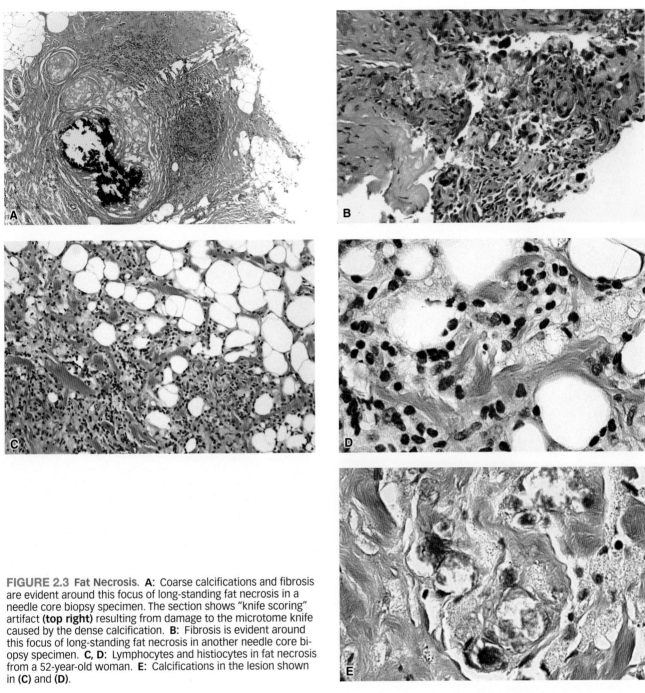

FIGURE 2.3 Fat Necrosis. A: Coarse calcifications and fibrosis are evident around this focus of long-standing fat necrosis in a needle core biopsy specimen. The section shows "knife scoring" artifact **(top right)** resulting from damage to the microtome knife caused by the dense calcification. **B:** Fibrosis is evident around this focus of long-standing fat necrosis in another needle core biopsy specimen. **C, D:** Lymphocytes and histiocytes in fat necrosis from a 52-year-old woman. **E:** Calcifications in the lesion shown in **(C)** and **(D)**.

FIGURE 2.4 Fat Necrosis. Infarcted fat with calcification in a needle core biopsy specimen. Nuclear detail is absent from the fat cells. The lesion was biopsied after calcifications were found on a routine mammogram.

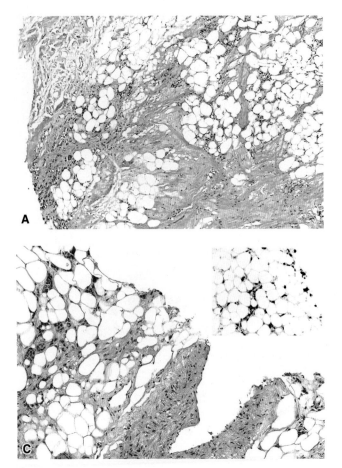

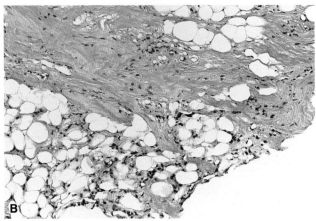

FIGURE 2.5 Invasive Carcinoma in Needle Core Biopsies Simulating Fat Necrosis. A–C: Three examples of invasive lobular carcinoma, all without a history of antecedent trauma or prior needling procedure, are shown. Cursory low-power microscopic examination can misleadingly suggest fat necrosis in each case. Inset in **(C)** shows estrogen receptor positivity in the malignant cells.

early lesions. Later stages feature fully developed coagulative necrosis (i.e., infarct). Bilateral multifocal mammary infarcts involving lactational breast tissue have been reported (16).

Infarction can occur spontaneously in fibroadenomas (17–19) and in benign proliferative lesions. Foci of necrosis may be found in florid sclerosing adenosis, usually during pregnancy, when the epithelium in sclerosing adenosis may also exhibit pronounced hyperplasia, mitotic activity, and cytologic atypia. The latter feature can be striking in fine needle aspirates of breast infarcts (20,21).

Papillomas are susceptible to partial or complete infarction, especially those that occur in major lactiferous ducts. Infarction can occur in papillomas at any age, but tends to be more frequent in postmenopausal women, and there is no known association with pregnancy. Bloody nipple discharge is the most frequent sign of an infarcted papilloma. Acute infarcts in a papilloma exhibit ischemic degeneration progressing to coagulative necrosis. Despite progressive loss of cytologic detail, the architectural integrity of the papilloma is usually maintained **(Fig. 2.6)**. At a late stage, fragmentation of infarcted portions of the papilloma occurs. Occasionally, an infarcted papilloma is reduced to an inflammatory polyp consisting mainly of granulation tissue with little or no epithelium. Chronic ischemia and healing of infarcts are marked by fibrosis that may cause sclerosing entrapment of residual epithelium, producing a pattern that could be mistaken for carcinoma (22). Squamous metaplasia sometimes develops in the proliferating reparative

epithelium within an infarcted papilloma (23,24). Calcifications eventually appear in the infarcted papilloma.

Infarcted carcinoma can be distinguished from infarction of a benign lesion if there is residual viable in situ or invasive carcinoma (25). In such cases, one can display the "ghost" architecture of the lesion upon reticulin staining. In some instances, immunoreactivity for cytokeratin and myoepithelial markers, especially p63, is surprisingly well preserved. When this occurs, it may be possible to "resurrect" the structure of the original lesion to a considerable degree. If a papillary structure can be demonstrated in this circumstance, the lesion was probably a papilloma rather than a papillary carcinoma because infarcts occur considerably more often in benign papillary tumors than in papillary carcinomas.

Excisional biopsy is usually necessary for the diagnosis of a mammary infarct, although the findings in a needle core biopsy specimen may be suggestive of the lesion. In most cases, recognition of the underlying condition hinges on finding a residual histologically viable (i.e., uninfarcted) component. As noted earlier, a reticulin stain and a p63 immunostain may be useful. Rarely, the diagnosis of a totally infarcted lesion remains enigmatic **(Fig. 2.7)**.

Before diagnosing a breast infarct, particularly on the basis of a needle core biopsy sampling, it is prudent to exclude the presence of a centrally necrotizing carcinoma of the breast. These carcinomas typically harbor a large central acellular zone (26). Clinical and radiologic correlation is helpful in this regard.

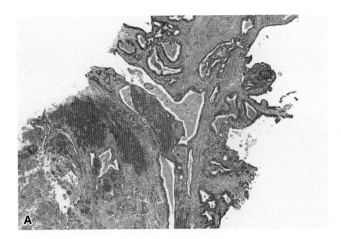

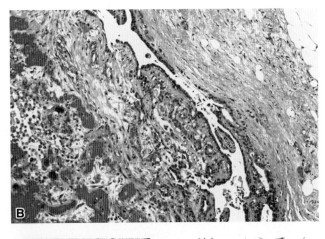

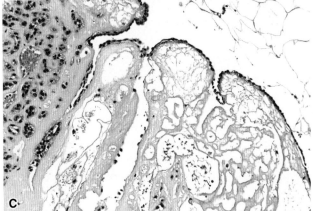

FIGURE 2.6 **Infarcted Papilloma. A:** A needle core biopsy specimen showing an area of hemorrhage and infarction in a papilloma. **B:** A sample from the periphery of the lesion with degenerated papillary tissue fragments. **C:** An area in an excised partially necrotic papilloma showing intact papillary structures. Relatively viable cells are focally evident (**top left**).

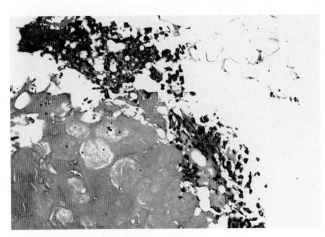

FIGURE 2.7 **Infarct with Atypical Cells.** This needle core biopsy specimen shows a totally infarcted lesion, possible fat necrosis, and an attached fragment of tissue composed of atypical cells. The latter were cytokeratin-positive (not shown here).

GALACTOCELE

A galactocele is a cystically dilated major duct, typically filled with degenerated milky contents. The lesion is most commonly encountered in younger women who are either pregnant or lactating. At presentation, the lesion typically spans about 2 cm; however, much larger lesions (>5 cm)

have been described (27). Mammography reveals a circumscribed density that, in many instances, has a characteristic appearance with two zones demarcated by a "fluid level" (28). The two zones consist of the upper, lighter lipid-containing components over the lower, heavier water-based constituents of the fluid. Comparable differences in echogenicity are observed on ultrasound examination.

Clinically, the firm and usually painless lesion may suggest carcinoma. Necrotic cells and debris, accompanied by inflammatory cells, are present in a fine needle aspiration–derived cytology preparation (29,30). Viable cells with reactive hyperchromatic nuclei may be present and could be mistaken for carcinoma. Excisional biopsy is diagnostic and provides adequate therapy if the lesion does not resolve after the aspiration of cyst contents.

Histologically, a galactocele is composed of a cyst, or an aggregate of cysts, which are lined by simple cuboidal epithelium. The cysts contain milky inspissated secretions in the form of soft caseous material. Intact cysts are encompassed by a variably thick fibrous wall with little or no inflammatory reaction. Leakage from a cyst elicits a chronic inflammatory cell reaction that may be accompanied by fat necrosis and a xanthogranulomatous reaction (31). Peri-implant galactocele formation has been described after breast augmentation procedures (32). In this setting, a galactocele has been reported to develop after a needle core biopsy procedure (33).

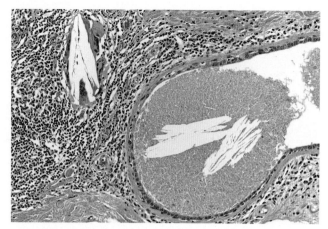

FIGURE 2.8 Galactocele. A cystically dilated gland lined by flattened apocrine-type cells. Cholesterol crystals are present within and outside this galactocele.

DUCT ECTASIA

Duct ectasia (i.e., dilatation) is usually encountered in the breasts of premenopausal women as a localized reaction to inspissated secretions in larger ducts (34). The earliest symptom of the disease is spontaneous, intermittent, mainly watery nipple discharge. Upon disease progression, subareolar induration may lead to the formation of a mass. Nipple retraction

and inversion is generally associated with periductal fibrosis and contracture. In some cases, squamous metaplasia of the terminal lactiferous duct epithelium results in obstruction that contributes to ductal dilatation, and could eventually lead to the formation of lactiferous duct fistulas (35,36). The mammographic abnormalities include microcalcifications, spiculated masses, and lobulated partially smooth masses, and can rarely simulate carcinoma (37).

The composition of the intraluminal contents in duct ectasia is variable, ranging from eosinophilic (granular or amorphous) proteinaceous material to an admixture of lipid-containing histiocytic cells and desquamated duct epithelial cells. Cholesterol crystals and calcifications may be found amid such debris (**Fig. 2.8**). Histiocytes that contain ceroid pigment have been termed *ochrocytes* by Davies (38). Foam cells (histiocytes with finely vacuolated cytoplasm) may be found within ductal lumina, in the epithelial–myoepithelial layer of ducts, and in periductal tissues (**Fig. 2.9**). The presence of neutrophils, lymphocytes, and plasma cells within the ducts indicates a more intense inflammatory reaction (**Fig. 2.10**). Disruption of ectatic ducts is accompanied by discharge of stasis material (including cholesterol crystals) in periductal tissue, causing periductal inflammation. Deposition of cholesterol crystals is the predominant finding in needle core biopsies of mass-forming lesions ("cholesteroloma") (39,40). Plasma cells and granulomata are inconspicuous features of duct ectasia.

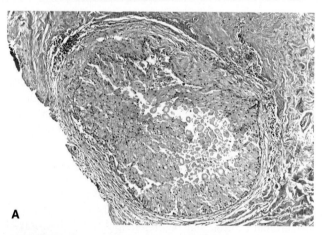

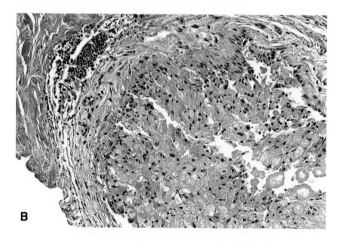

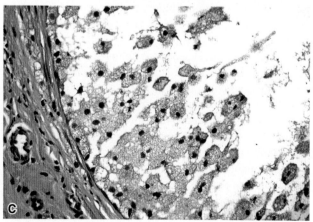

FIGURE 2.9 Duct Ectasia. A, B: Mammographic density led to a needle core biopsy that demonstrated this dilated duct with a dense, mainly intraluminal, histiocytic reaction. **C:** Histiocytes with vacuolated, granular cytoplasm have a micropapillary arrangement in this dilated duct in another case. **D, E:** Ectasia with a solid accumulation of histiocytes and periductal inflammation that mimics clear cell intraductal carcinoma. Residual ductal epithelial cells are highlighted by the cytokeratin immunostain in **(D)**. The histiocytes are cytokeratin-negative. **F:** Histiocytes with finely granular ceroid pigment *(arrow)*, so-called ochrocytes, are present in the duct lumen, the epithelium, and the surrounding tissue.

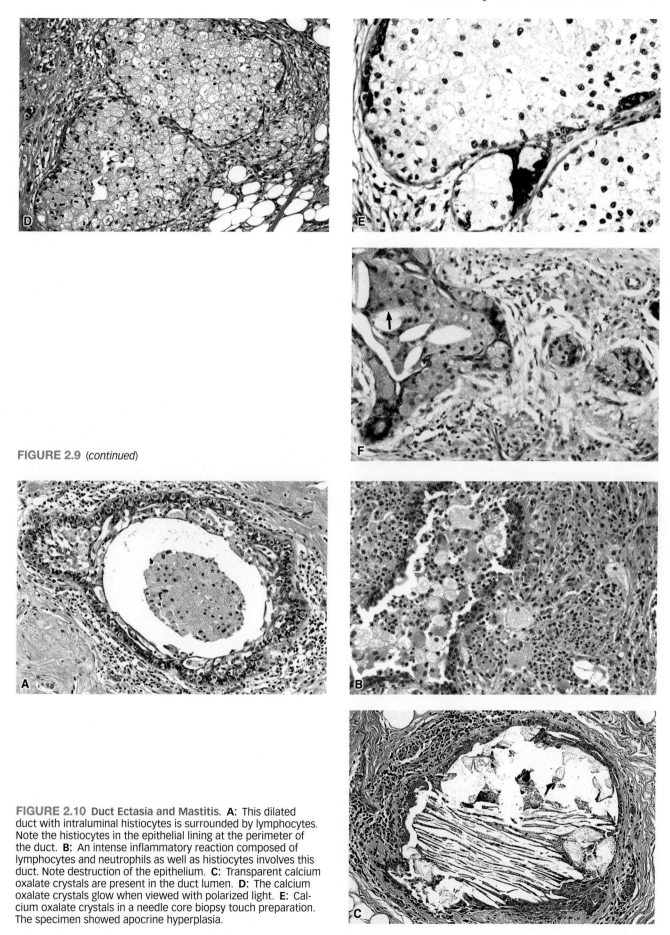

FIGURE 2.9 (*continued*)

FIGURE 2.10 Duct Ectasia and Mastitis. A: This dilated duct with intraluminal histiocytes is surrounded by lymphocytes. Note the histiocytes in the epithelial lining at the perimeter of the duct. **B:** An intense inflammatory reaction composed of lymphocytes and neutrophils as well as histiocytes involves this duct. Note destruction of the epithelium. **C:** Transparent calcium oxalate crystals are present in the duct lumen. **D:** The calcium oxalate crystals glow when viewed with polarized light. **E:** Calcium oxalate crystals in a needle core biopsy touch preparation. The specimen showed apocrine hyperplasia.

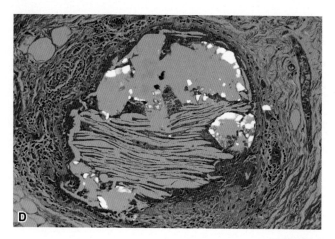

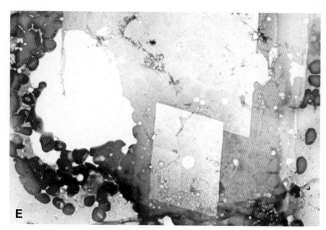

FIGURE 2.10 (*continued*)

Calcium oxalate crystals may be found when stasis occurs in a duct with apocrine epithelium (**Fig. 2.10**).

Histiocytes with clear or "foamy" cytoplasm positioned in ductal epithelia can be confused with pagetoid carcinoma cells. In most instances, the distinction is made with ease on the basis of bland nuclear cytology of these cells, and the associated inflammatory and reactive features, of duct ectasia. The histiocytic phenotype of foam cells can be confirmed by CD68 (KP1) immunoreactivity. These cells are negative for cytoplasmic cytokeratin and actin, but may display misleading

surface cytokeratin staining from the cell membranes of contiguous epithelial cells or weak reactivity for adsorbed antigens such as gross cystic disease fluid protein-15 (GCDFP-15) (41).

In advanced cases of duct ectasia, the development of periductal fibrosis and hyperelastosis, often with a lamellar distribution, leads to mural thickening (**Fig. 2.11**). The inflammatory reaction is less conspicuous, and the ducts are encased in thickened laminated layers of fibrous and elastic tissue (42). The duct lumen can become widely dilated, or even partially obliterated—so-called "mastitis obliterans"

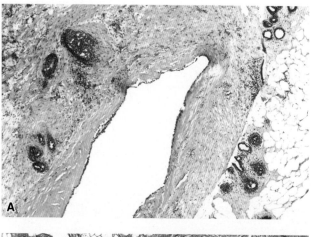

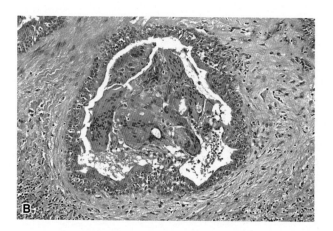

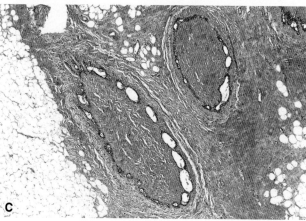

FIGURE 2.11 **Duct Ectasia, Late Phases. A:** A late-stage lesion sampled by needle core biopsy. There is marked periductal fibrosis with a minimal chronic inflammatory cell infiltrate. **B:** Duct ectasia with intraluminal multinucleated histiocytes. **C:** Duct ectasia with mastitis obliterans. A fibrous "polyp" has "obliterated" most of the ductal lumen in this excisional biopsy.

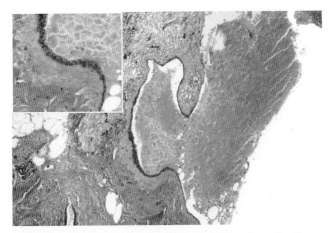

FIGURE 2.12 **Duct Ectasia, without Inflammation.** The dilated duct is lined by flat epithelium. There is no inflammation. Acellular proteinaceous material fills the duct lumen. Inset shows detail of the epithelial cells lining the dilated duct.

(**Fig. 2.12**). In some instances, the periductal reactive process includes proliferating granulation tissue and hyperelastosis that can narrow, and even occlude, ducts (43,44). The affected ducts may eventually be reduced to a fibrous scar. Remnants of persisting epithelium may proliferate to form secondary glands within such sclerotic ducts.

The diagnosis of primary "histiocytoid" breast carcinoma should be considered in cases wherein minimally atypical histiocyte-like cells proliferate with neither admixed inflammatory cell infiltrate nor ductal disruption. Use of epithelial (cytokeratin) and histiocytic (CD68) immunostains can be helpful in confirming the diagnosis (45).

SO-CALLED PLASMA CELL MASTITIS

The disease process known as plasma cell mastitis (PCM) is an extreme form of periductal mastitis that features a prominent plasma cell reaction to retained secretions in ducts. In the early phases of PCM, patients experience the acute onset of redness,

pain, and thick nipple discharge. After the inflammatory symptoms subside, the skin may remain edematous over the lesional mass. The latter may span several centimeters. Nipple discharge is usually persistent, and nipple retraction is observed in most patients. The ipsilateral axillary lymph nodes are often enlarged. In all its phases, PCM can be clinically (and radiologically) difficult to distinguish from mammary carcinoma.

PCM is characterized by a marked, diffuse plasma cell infiltrate surrounding ducts as well as lobules. The lesion is associated with variably hyperplastic ductal epithelium (**Fig. 2.13**). Foci of PCM, which grossly appear to be xanthomatous and necrotic, histologically correspond to histiocytic and granulomatous reaction to the desquamated epithelium and lipid material. Lymphocytes and neutrophils are variably present. Neither periductal fibrosis nor obliterative intraductal proliferation of granulation tissue are features of PCM. Hyperplastic epithelial cells, which may appear to be highly atypical, can be mistaken for carcinoma in a needle core biopsy sample. Plasmacytoma and myeloma should be considered in the differential diagnosis in cases of overwhelming plasma cell infiltration. It is possible for some cases of exuberant duct ectasia to be mistaken for PCM, and vice versa.

DIABETIC MASTOPATHY

The occurrence of tumor-forming stromal proliferations in patients with diabetes mellitus is referred to as diabetic mastopathy (DM) (46). The initial clinical symptom is a palpable, firm-to-hard mass that may suggest carcinoma. The histopathologic alterations are not entirely specific for insulin-dependent diabetes mellitus (47–49), and similar lesions have been reported in patients with autoimmune diseases who did not have diabetes (50,51).

With rare exceptions (52), DM has been limited to females. In six series, the mean age of patients at the time of biopsy varied from 36 to 57 years, with a range of 20 to 77 years (48). Most DM patients with type I insulin-dependent diabetes

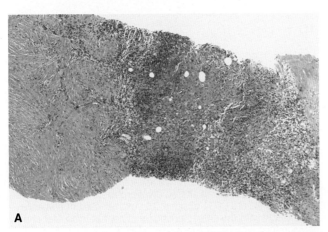

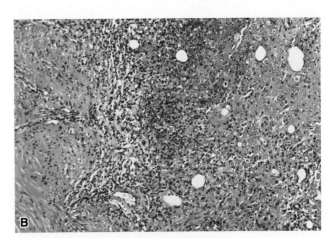

FIGURE 2.13 **So-called Plasma Cell Mastitis. A, B:** A needle core biopsy specimen from a patient with a breast mass suspected to be carcinoma. Plasma cells are a prominent element in the reactive cellular infiltrate around the area of necrosis (**right**).

mellitus are younger than 30 years, and the interval between the onset of diabetes and detection of the breast lesion is about 20 years. Bilateral lesions have been present in nearly 50% of the cases. Most of the DM patients have had complications of juvenile-onset diabetes, with diabetic retinopathy being reported in many instances.

The mammogram in DM often reveals localized, increased density or a heterogeneous parenchymal pattern, but no specific features have been associated with this condition (53,54). The mammographic appearance of the mass can resemble a fibroadenoma or carcinoma (50,55). An irregular hypoechoic mass with variable acoustic shadowing is found on sonographic examination. Ultrasound guidance is the preferred modality

for performing a needle core biopsy procedure (53). Breast density associated with DM could obscure a coexistent lesion such as carcinoma, a setting in which MRI may be useful (56,57). Spontaneous regression and clinical disappearance of DM has been described (58).

The lesional tissue of DM consists of collagenous stroma with keloidal features and a variably increased number of stromal cells when compared with the surrounding breast tissue. Polygonal epithelioid cells are found dispersed in the collagen among the spindly stromal cells in most, but not all, cases. The stromal cells are myofibroblasts with variable fibroblastic and myoid differentiation (**Fig. 2.14**). Multinucleated stromal giant cells and mitotic activity are not part of this proliferative

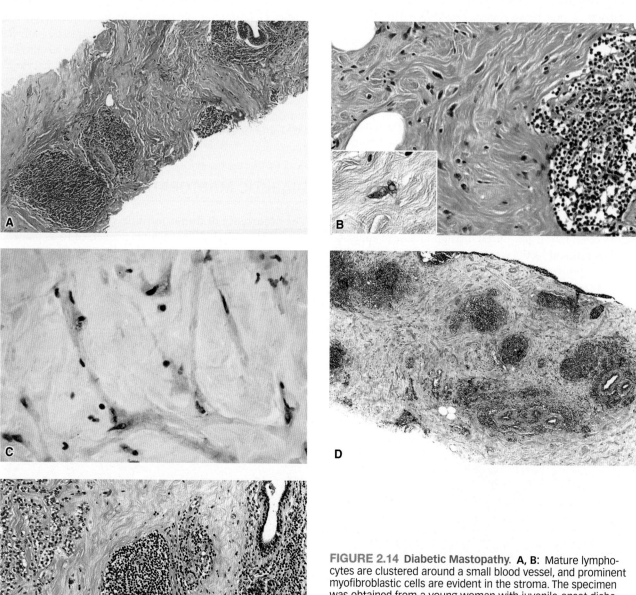

FIGURE 2.14 Diabetic Mastopathy. A, B: Mature lymphocytes are clustered around a small blood vessel, and prominent myofibroblastic cells are evident in the stroma. The specimen was obtained from a young woman with juvenile-onset diabetes mellitus who presented with a unilateral breast mass. Inset in **(B)** shows detail of an altered myofibroblast. **C:** The spindly myofibroblasts are CD34-positive. **D:** Another case of diabetic mastopathy with the characteristic prominent perivascular and periglandular lymphocytic response amid fibrotic stroma.
E: A needle core biopsy showing invasive carcinoma **(left)** and changes characteristic of diabetic mastopathy in a 38-year-old patient with childhood-onset diabetes mellitus.

process. Rarely, CD10-positive atypical myofibroblastic cells may be present (59). Mature perivascular, periductal, and perilobular lymphocytes are clustered throughout the lesion. Few, if any, plasma cells or neutrophils are present in the infiltrates. Lymphoid follicles with germinal centers are rare. When studied by immunohistochemistry, the lymphocytes have a B-cell phenotype. The polymerase chain reaction detected no Ig heavy-chain gene rearrangements in tissue samples from six patients with DM (60).

In one series of 20 patients with DM, 13 (65%) showed all four of its histopathologic characteristics (i.e., keloid-like fibrosis, epithelioid fibroblasts, widespread periductal/lobular lymphocytic infiltration, and widespread perivascular lymphocytic infiltration), but one or more of these typical findings was absent in the remainder of the cases (61). Infarcts, fat necrosis, granulomas, duct stasis, arteritis, and other inflammatory lesions are not features of DM. Stromal collagen fibers are sometimes prominent. Proliferative epithelial changes may be present coincidentally, but are not an integral component of DM. The differential diagnosis of DM includes nonspecific lymphocytic lobulitis (**Fig. 2.15**) and fibromatosis.

DM is generally regarded as a self-limited stromal abnormality. Recurrent tumors have occurred in the ipsilateral breast in a minority of cases, and these patients are prone to asynchronous, as well as synchronous, bilateral involvement. Excisional biopsy is adequate treatment. There is no evidence to suggest that DM predisposes to the development of mammary carcinoma or stromal neoplastic diseases such as fibromatosis. Nonetheless, patients with DM can coincidentally harbor mammary carcinoma (62).

Lymphocytic mastitis and sclerosing lymphocytic mastitis are terms used for immune-mediated, nonspecific lymphocytic infiltrates in the breast. The term lymphocytic mastitis is sometimes used as a synonym for DM. However, the latter term ought to be used only when the disease process forms a palpable mass and is associated with diabetes mellitus.

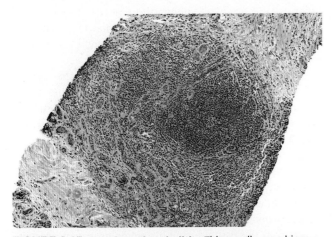

FIGURE 2.15 Lymphocytic Lobulitis. This needle core biopsy was performed to assess a nonpalpable lesion without mammographic evidence of calcifications. The patient had no known systemic illness. A lobule heavily infiltrated by nonneoplastic lymphocytes is shown here. The infiltrate was polyclonal by immunohistochemistry (not shown here).

Lymphocytic mastitis can be diagnosed when there is a dense intralobular, perilobular, and perivascular lymphocytic infiltrate associated with lobular atrophy and sclerosis. When the sclerotic process is intense, the term "sclerosing lymphocytic mastitis" can be used.

GRANULOMATOUS MASTITIS

Numerous pathogenetic processes responsible for granulomatous inflammation are included under the generic heading of *granulomatous mastitis* (GM) (63). The differential diagnosis of GM includes specific entities such as tuberculosis, leprosy, brucellosis and other bacterial infections, and fungal and parasitic infestations (63–66). It is necessary to exclude the presence of acid-fast bacilli (AFB) or other bacteria and fungi with cultures, histochemical stains, polymerase chain reaction (67), and other appropriate clinical tests. Reactive nonnecrotizing epithelioid sarcoid-like granulomatous inflammation that develops in association with breast carcinomas is restricted to intratumoral and peritumoral tissue as well as the ipsilateral axillary lymph nodes (68). Rheumatoid nodules, characterized by noncaseating and nonvasculitic granulomata with fibrinoid necrosis, have been diagnosed on needle core biopsy sampling in a case of mammary involvement with rheumatoid arthritis (69).

Granulomatous lobular mastitis is a clinicopathologic condition characterized by perilobular granulomatous inflammation (70,71). This pattern of distribution of the granulomata suggests a cell-mediated reaction to one or more substances in mammary secretions or in lobular epithelial cells; however, no specific antigen has been identified. The lesion usually appears approximately 2 years after a pregnancy. The age at diagnosis ranges from 17 to 42 years, with a mean of about 33 years (71). Virtually all patients are parous. The distinct, firm-to-hard mass may involve any portion of the breast, but it tends to spare the subareolar region. Granulomatous lobular mastitis can form a mass that can span as much as 8 cm, although it averages approximately 6 cm. The clinical findings often suggest carcinoma, and mammography has been described as "suspicious" (63). In one report, sonograms were characterized by "multiple clustered, often contiguous tubular hypoechoic lesions" (72). The primary histopathologic finding is granulomatous lobulitis (**Fig. 2.16**). The granulomas are composed of epithelioid histiocytes and Langhans giant cells (giant cells with multiple nuclei, typically arranged at the perimeter of the cell) accompanied by lymphocytes, plasma cells, and occasional eosinophils. Fat necrosis and abscesses containing polymorphonuclear leukocytes are occasionally present, and these processes contribute to the effacement of the lobulocentric distribution in confluent lesions. Asteroid bodies are unusual, and Schaumann bodies have not been reported in the giant cells. Spaces that develop in the centers of the abscesses contain no foreign material, demonstrable secretion, or bacteria. Squamous metaplasia of duct and lobular epithelium is unusual. Vasculitis is not present. Stains and cultures for bacteria, AFB, and fungi are negative. The

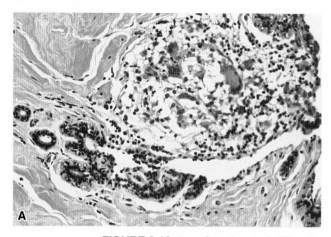 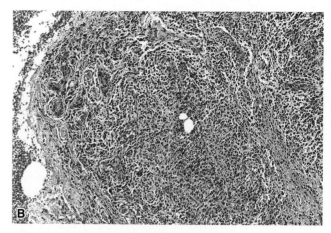

FIGURE 2.16 Granulomatous Lobulitis. A: A granuloma with epithelioid giant cells in a lobule at the edge of a needle core biopsy specimen. No specific etiology was demonstrated in this patient. **B:** This granuloma of undetermined etiology and central necrosis has destroyed much of the lobule in which it resides.

management of nonspecific GM is generally difficult, unless a specific etiology for the process is determined. Needle core biopsies, as the initial diagnostic procedure, can be useful in planning management of GM (73,74). Steroids may be of use in appropriately selected cases, and surgical excision can alleviate chronic pain in cases that are refractory to medical management (75).

Cystic neutrophilic granulomatous mastitis is a particular form of GM characterized by minute cystic spaces in the center of granulomata. A narrow zone of neutrophils usually outlines these spaces. The latter contain rare Gram-positive bacilli (76,77). Microbiologic culture studies have identified *Corynebacterium spp.* that are sensitive to the tetracycline group of antibiotics.

SARCOIDOSIS

Sarcoidosis usually involves the breasts of women in their 20s and 30s, reflecting the overall age distribution of the disease (78–81). Mammary involvement is often detected after the diagnosis of sarcoidosis has been established on biopsy performed on the basis of clinical manifestations of the disease at other sites such as a lymph node or lung. Mammary involvement presenting as the primary manifestation of the disease is extremely rare. In some patients, mammary sarcoidosis produces a firm-to-hard mass that may be clinically mistaken for carcinoma. Occasionally, mammary sarcoidosis is clinically inapparent, and the disease is incidentally discovered in a biopsy performed for an unrelated condition.

The mammographic, ultrasound, MRI, and positron emission tomography (PET) characteristics of mammary sarcoidosis are not specific and can be interpreted as "suggestive" of carcinoma (82,83), especially if a spiculated lesion is seen on mammography (84). Rarely, sarcoidosis produces multiple, bilateral small mammographically detected lesions (80).

Microscopic examination of mammary sarcoidoisis reveals nonnecrotizing epithelioid granulomata in a periductal and perilobular distribution (**Fig. 2.17**). Multinucleated Langhans giant cells within the granulomata may contain cytoplasmic asteroid bodies (eosinophilic stellate forms) or intracellular Schaumann structures (proteinaceous calcified crystals). The lesions usually show no necrosis. A variable lymphoplasmacytic and fibrotic reaction is present. Apart from the dominant mass-forming lesion, minute isolated sarcoid granulomata may be dispersed throughout the breast.

MASTITIS RELATED TO AUGMENTATION PROCEDURES

In the postimplant setting, the ability to detect carcinoma by mammography and ultrasound is usually impaired by GM caused by leakage of implant contents (e.g., silicone) and/or an inflammatory reaction to the coating of the implant (85–87). Calcifications that deposit in the leaked contents of a mammary implant are generally irregular and coarse. Finer calcifications, resembling those of carcinoma, should be biopsied (88). Enhanced MRI is an important procedure for detecting carcinoma in a breast distorted by leakage of implant contents (89).

Mammary implants are usually filled with either foreign chemicals (silicone and other substances) or saline. Upon leakage, silicone and other fillers typically elicit a foreign body giant cell granulomatous reaction associated with fat necrosis (**Fig. 2.18**). Occasionally, this process can mimic liposarcoma because of the presence of numerous enlarged multivacuolated histiocytes that are "disarming replicas of lipoblasts" (90). The accompanying chronic inflammatory reaction and fibrosis varies in intensity. Silicone and other fillers may also enter the lumina of ducts and lobules (91). Some of the foreign material is lost from the tissue during histologic processing, leaving clear spaces of varying size on H&E stained sections. The presence of silicone and other substances can be confirmed by electron microscopy, infrared spectroscopy, atomic absorption spectrophotometry, and other procedures (92).

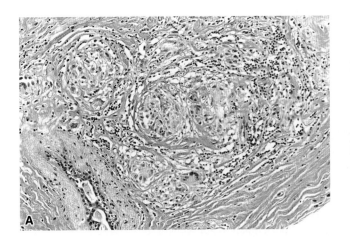

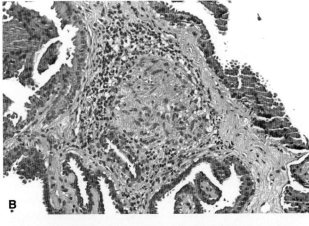

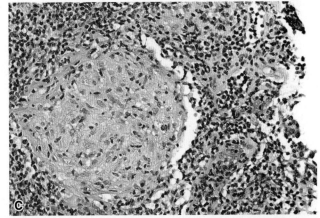

FIGURE 2.17 Sarcoidosis. A: This epithelioid nonnecrotizing granuloma, typical of sarcoidosis, lies adjacent to a mammary duct. **B:** A granuloma amid apocrine cysts in a needle core biopsy sample from a 53-year-old woman known to have sarcoidosis. **C:** Detail of a granuloma in an intramammary lymph node in a 45-year-old woman with sarcoidosis.

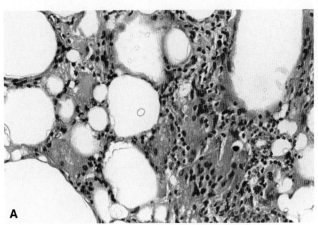

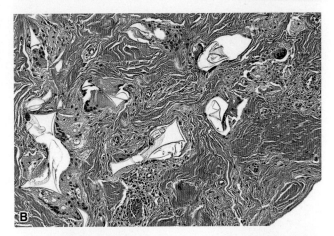

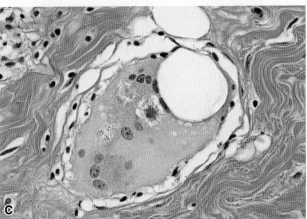

FIGURE 2.18 Implant-Associated Mastitis. A: This chronic inflammatory cell infiltrate surrounds vacuolar spaces that contain silicone material. **B:** Refractile fragments of polyurethane from the outer surface of a silicone cosmetic breast implant were present in this needle core biopsy sample from a 44-year-old woman who presented with a breast mass. **C:** An "asteroid" body **(central)** and cholesterol crystals are present within a multinucleated giant cell in this granulomatous reaction to leaked implant material.

The most common etiology for a mass that forms in the postaugmentation setting is implant leak–related GM; however, it should be noted that mammary implants have been associated with a variety of neoplasms, including *anaplastic large cell lymphoma* (93,94), *fibromatosis*, and other fibroblastic neoplasms (95).

Lastly, cosmetic augmentation of the breasts can also be achieved by direct injection of silicone, other chemicals, and autologous adipose tissue. Such direct injections invariably lead to intramammary granulomatous reaction of the foreign body type. It is notable that free silicone and other such agents migrate under the effect of gravity and can, therefore, be found at sites distant from the site of introduction. The ipsilateral axillary lymph nodes can show a similar reaction owing to drainage or transport of the foreign material. Injection of autologous fat tissue can result in formation of intramammary *liponecrotic pseudocysts* (96).

INFLAMMATORY PSEUDOTUMOR

No well-characterized lesion of the breast qualifies for the specific diagnosis of inflammatory pseudotumor (IPT). This diagnostic term has been erroneously used for a variety of benign and malignant breast lesions including (but not limited to) GM, IgG4 mastitis, and inflammatory myofibroblastic tumors. In most cases, lesions diagnosed as IPT are the result of fat necrosis or duct ectasia associated with mastitis (**Fig. 2.19**). Localized nodular lesions of the breast composed of interlacing bundles of bland myofibroblastic cells with a prominent inflammatory cell infiltrate composed mainly of lymphocytes, plasma cells, and histiocytes are diagnosed as IPT (12,97–101). Typically, needle core biopsy samplings of IPT show nonspecific "inflammatory" features (98). Mammography in one case of IPT revealed a 2-cm round mass with ill-defined borders and no calcifications. The tumor was hypoechoic, homogeneous, and lacked acoustic shadowing on ultrasound (99).

The differential diagnosis of IPT includes the aforementioned lesions as well as PCM, Erdheim–Chester disease, and adult type "juvenile" xanthogranuloma. The latter lesion consists of a prominent spindle cell proliferation associated with lymphocytes, plasma cells, xanthomatous histiocytes, and multinucleated giant cells, including those of the Touton type (102).

IPT is a benign lesion but may recur. One patient with IPT had a unilateral lesion that did not recur after excision (98).

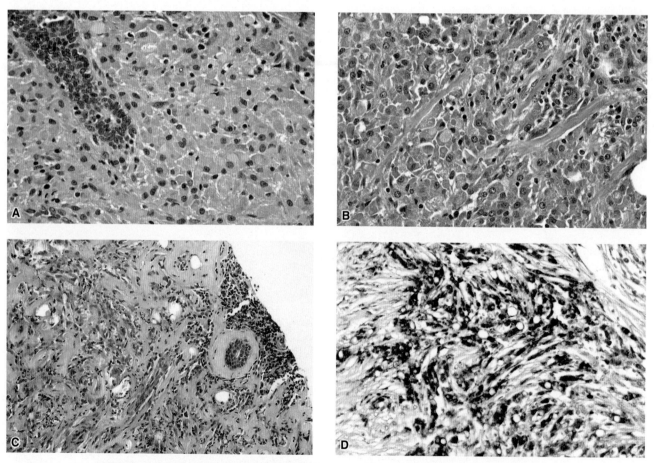

FIGURE 2.19 Inflammatory Pseudotumor. A, B: This specimen is from a 2-cm tumor that probably represents resolving fat necrosis. The lesion is composed of numerous epithelioid histiocytes and sparse fibroblasts and lymphocytes. **C:** A needle core biopsy specimen from another, more fibrotic inflammatory pseudotumor. Note the duct at the border of the specimen. **D:** Histiocytes in the lesion shown in **(C)** are highlighted by Mac 387 immunostain (a macrophage marker).

Another patient with bilateral tumors developed recurrences in both breasts (97).

IgG4-related disease is a relatively recently defined entity characterized by mass-forming IgG4-dominant plasma cells associated with fibrosclerosis and obliterative phlebitis. The prototype of this disease is sclerosing pancreatitis (autoimmune pancreatitis). Mammary involvement with this disease has been described. Most patients with IgG4 mastitis are premenopausal women who present with unilateral, palpable, painless mass. The histopathologic features of the disease are variable; however, a combination of prominent lymphocytic and plasma (pseudolymphomatous) cell infiltrate, phlebitis, sclerosis, and glandular atrophy is usually present (103). Giant cells and granulomata are usually, but not always, absent (104). Core biopsy sampling may show severe lymphoplasmacytic infiltration (105). Predictably, IgG4-immunoreactive plasma cells are prominent within the mass, and the proportion of IgG4+ plasma cells to IgG+ plasma cells is of diagnostic significance (>40% in most organs). Serum IgG4 levels are elevated. It is possible that some cases diagnosed as IPT or PCM may be examples of IgG4-related sclerosing mastitis. Excision of the mass and steroid therapy is usually curative.

Inflammatory myofibroblastic tumor (IMT) is best regarded as a low-grade neoplasm with recurrent potential, rather than a reactive inflammatory condition. IMTs are usually encountered in the abdominopelvic region in younger patients (106), although several cases have been reported in the breast—including one that was encountered on needle core biopsy sampling (107). The tumors are composed of myofibroblasts accompanied by plasma cells, lymphocytes, and eosinophils. Approximately one-half of IMTs harbor clonal rearrangements of the *ALK* gene at 2p23 and approximately as many are immunoreactive for anaplastic lymphoma kinase (ALK). ALK immunoreactivity is regarded as being relatively specific for IMT within the range of myofibroblastic tumors. There is no histologic difference between IMTs harboring *ALK* gene abnormalities and those that do not. The histogenesis of

IMT is uncertain, although a clonal origin is favored. Most mammary IMTs are usually treated successfully by excision (although *ALK*-targeted therapy has potential). Recurrences are rare, and metastases are even rarer.

AMYLOID TUMOR (AMYLOIDOMA)

Amyloid tumor (AT), also referred to as amyloidoma, is a mass-forming amyloid deposition. AT in the breast has been described in patients with systemic diseases that predispose to amyloid deposition. These diseases include immunocytic dyscrasias (such as multiple myeloma and plasmacytoid lymphoma), rheumatoid arthritis, and primary amyloidosis. More than one-half of patients with mammary amyloidosis have a concurrent hematologic disorder—most commonly mucosa-associated lymphoid tissue (MALT) lymphoma, followed by plasma cell neoplasm (108).

AT limited to the breast are uncommon (109–111). AT in the breast typically presents as a unilateral solitary mass in middle-aged or older women. Bilateral involvement has been described (112,113). ATs have been reported at the site of insulin injections (114). This is notable because the underside of the breast is a favored site for insulin injection in some diabetic women. Clinical examination reveals a discrete, hard mass that mimics carcinoma. Mammography of AT typically shows calcifications (115–118). MRI features of mammary amyloidosis have not been fully characterized; however, one reported case of bilateral mammary amyloidosis demonstrated a high signal on T2 imaging (generally, a low signal is indicative of a benign lesion) (119). Concurrent mammary carcinoma and amyloidosis have been described (120–122).

Histologically, AT is characterized by amorphous, faintly eosinophilic, homogeneous deposits of amyloid in intramammary adipose tissue, fibrous stroma, and in walls of blood vessels (**Fig. 2.20**). Deposits of amyloid around ducts and in lobules are associated with atrophy and obliteration of the affected structures. In adipose tissue, thin ribbons of amyloid

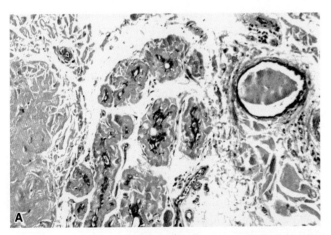
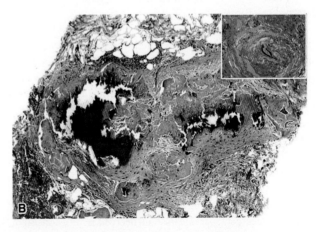

FIGURE 2.20 Amyloidosis. A: A thick layer of amyloid has been deposited in the basement membranes of the glands in a lobule next to a nodule of amyloid in the stroma on the left. **B:** This amyloid tumor is composed of masses of amyloid, fibrosis, and calcification with ossification. Inset shows apple-green birefringence of amyloid with Congo red stain (under polarized light) in periductal tissue.

("rings") may be formed around individual adipocytes. These amyloid rings are accentuated when Congo red–stained sections are examined with polarized light (123). Varying numbers of lymphocytes, plasma cells, and multinucleated giant cells are usually present in association with the amyloid deposits. The latter can show punctate or irregular calcifications. Rarely, osseous metaplasia of AT is evident (116,124). Amyloid is periodic acid Schiff-positive, appears to be metachromatic with the crystal violet stain, and exhibits apple-green birefringence when the Congo red–stained section is examined under polarized light. As determined by immunohistochemistry and mass spectrometry–based proteomics, the majority of breast amyloid depositions are of the AL (usually kappa) type (108), although the deposits can be of AA, AL, and β2-microglobulin types. Mammary amyloidosis can be readily diagnosed on needle core biopsy material (110,117,118).

The lesion can be treated by excisional biopsy. When limited to the breast, AT has proven to be an innocuous condition (in the limited follow-up reported so far). Notably, one woman who presented with bilateral mammary AT developed systemic amyloidosis 1 year later (125). The prognosis of patients with mammary lesions and systemic amyloidosis depends on the clinical course of the underlying disease.

VASCULITIS

Inflammatory lesions of blood vessels (i.e., vasculitis) are encountered in a variety of systemic disorders that are broadly grouped under the heading of collagen-vascular disease. Vasculitis in the breast may present as an isolated process or with multiorgan involvement. The clinical manifestations of mammary vasculitis sometimes resemble those of carcinoma.

Although there are subtle differences in the pathologic features of the vasculitides associated with various collagen–vascular diseases, the diagnosis of a specific condition is more often rendered on the composite basis of the clinical and histopathologic findings. Some of these conditions may be manifested by a tumor formation or mammographically detected calcifications (126).

Giant cell arteritis clinically limited to the breast has been reported in postmenopausal women who presented with one or more palpable breast tumors (127–130). The lesions can be bilateral. The firm tumors range from less than 1 to 4 cm, and carcinoma is clinically suspected in most patients (131). Axillary nodal enlargement has been noted in some cases (128). Systemic symptoms reported by patients with giant cell arteritis of the breast include headache, muscle and joint pain, fever, and night sweats. Mild anemia and an elevated erythrocyte sedimentation rate are found in most cases. Microscopically, transmural inflammation involves small- and medium-sized arteries throughout the affected tissue **(Fig. 2.21)**. Veins and arterioles are largely spared. Fibrinoid necrosis is not a consistent feature, but fragmentation of the intramural elastic fibers is demonstrable with an elastic stain. Multinucleated giant cells tend to be oriented around the disrupted elastic fibers. The vascular lumen may be narrowed or occluded. Perilesional

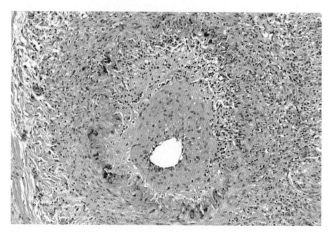

FIGURE 2.21 Giant Cell Arteritis. The patient presented with a mass, and biopsy revealed fat necrosis due to diffuse arteritis. This artery is almost totally occluded by the inflammatory process. The elastic layer is fragmented. No giant cells are evident in this particular area.

breast tissue exhibits edema, fibrosis, fat necrosis, and atrophy of glandular elements. The differential diagnosis includes other types of arteritis, phlebitis, traumatic fat necrosis, and infarction related to pregnancy or lactation.

Breast involvement has also been reported in patients with Wegener granulomatosis (132,133), polyarteritis (134,135), scleroderma (136), dermatomyositis (137), lupus erythematosis (138–140), and Churg–Strauss syndrome (i.e., allergic granulomatous angiitis) (141). Core biopsy can reveal vasculitis involving various types and sizes of vessels, and different kinds of inflammatory cell infiltrates, with or without granulomas or necrosis (142). The lesions in several of these vasculitides may be manifested by a mass with vascular calcifications or with irregular dystrophic calcifications (126). Fat necrosis is often present. Patients with one of these forms of systemic vasculitis may develop coincidental breast carcinoma in the absence of mammary vasculitis, but there is no evidence that the vasculitis *per se* predisposes to breast carcinoma (143–145).

Lupus mastitis is a rare complication of lupus erythematosus (138,146). In some cases, this disease is manifested by lymphocytic mastopathy distributed mainly in and around lobules, but a perivascular component may also be detected. Lupus mastitis is a form of lupus panniculitis characterized clinically by nodular lesions and histologically by fat necrosis in various stages of evolution (147). Concentric perivascular fibrosis and hyalinized stromal fibrosis extending around ducts and lobules were described in a woman who had recurrent lupus mastitis over an 8-year period starting at 40 years of age (139). The patient had clinically documented systemic lupus with elevated serum antinuclear antibody (ANA) titers. Core biopsy of lupus mastitis may show a "dense lymphoplasmacytic infiltrate with no normal breast ducts or lobules" (129). Advanced lesions may show considerable calcification. Immunoglobulin deposits can be demonstrated around blood vessels in lesional tissue, and serum ANAs are present. Clinical findings in the skin may mimic inflammatory carcinoma (148).

OTHER INFLAMMATORY AND REACTIVE LESIONS

Needle core biopsies of the breast are generally performed to evaluate palpable masses or lesions detected on various radiologic modalities including mammograms, sonograms, CTs, MRIs, and PET scans (149). The consequent biopsies yield a variety of neoplastic and inflammatory/reactive conditions. Many of the latter have been described in this chapter. Several additional lesions (including some that have been recently described, such as eosinophilic mastitis (150) and nephrogenic systemic fibrosis (151)) can be encountered in needle core biopsies. This possibility highlights the need to be constantly on the alert for unanticipated and novel findings even in these limited samplings.

Lastly, a type of reactive process that follows the performance of needle core biopsies of breast (152) deserves mention. This type of lesion follows the deployment of various types of marking devices ("clips") at the biopsied site. Placement of the clip at the time of needle core biopsies facilitates surgical and radiologic localization of the site at a later date. The titanium clips are placed admixed with some form of "plug" (either a resorbable chemical or bovine collagen). The "plug" minimizes the risk of "clip migration," but invariably elicits a prominent nonspecific mixed inflammatory cell and granulation tissue response. Over time, there is fibrous scarring of the site. These findings are, of course, evident in excisional biopsies and mastectomies performed *after* needle core biopsies, but can be encountered in needle core biopsy samples in cases wherein the biopsy is repeated at the same site for any reason.

REFERENCES

1. Layfield LJ, Frazier S, Schanzmeyer E. Histomorphologic features of biopsy sites following excisional and core needle biopsies of the breast. *Breast J.* 2015;21:370–376.
2. Tan PH, Lai LM, Carrington EV, et al. Fat necrosis of the breast—a review. *Breast.* 2006;15:313–318.
3. Akyol M, Kayali A, Yildirim N. Traumatic fat necrosis of male breast. *Clin Imaging.* 2013;37:954–956.
4. Hogge JP, Robinson RE, Magnant CM, et al. The mammographic spectrum of fat necrosis of the breast. *Radiographics.* 1995;15:1347–1356.
5. Martin BF, Phillips JD. Gangrene of the female breast with anticoagulant therapy: report of two cases. *Am J Clin Pathol.* 1970;53:622–626.
6. Clarke D, Curtis JL, Martinez A, et al. Fat necrosis of the breast simulating recurrent carcinoma after primary radiotherapy in the management of early breast cancer. *Cancer.* 1983;52:442–445.
7. Rostom AY, el-Sayed ME. Fat necrosis of the breast: an unusual complication of lumpectomy and radiotherapy in breast cancer. *Clin Radiol.* 1987;38:31.
8. Girling AC, Hanby AM, Millis RR. Radiation and other pathological changes in breast tissue after conservation treatment for carcinoma. *J Clin Pathol.* 1990;43:152–156.
9. Isenberg JS, Tu Q, Rainey W. Mammary gangrene associated with warfarin ingestion. *Ann Plast Surg.* 1996;37:553–555.
10. Taboada JL, Stephens TW, Krishnamurthy S, et al. The many faces of fat necrosis in the breast. *AJR Am J Roentgenol.* 2009;192:815–825.
11. Bargum K, Moller Nielsen S. Case report: fat necrosis of the breast appearing as oil cysts with fat-fluid levels. *Br J Radiol.* 1993;66:718–720.
12. Sciallis AP, Chen B, Folpe AL. Cellular spindled histiocytic pseudotumor complicating mammary fat necrosis: a potential diagnostic pitfall. *Am J Surg Pathol.* 2012;36:1571–1578.
13. Barnes PJ, Foyle A, Hache KA, et al. Erdheim–Chester disease of the breast: a case report and review of the literature. *Breast J.* 2005;11:462–467.
14. Provenzano E, Barter SJ, Wright PA, et al. Erdheim–Chester disease presenting as bilateral clinically malignant breast masses. *Am J Surg Pathol.* 2010;34:584–588.
15. Guo S, Yan Q, Rohr J, et al. Erdheim–Chester disease involving the breast—a rare but important differential diagnosis. *Hum Pathol.* 2015;46:159–164.
16. Aggon AA, Eakin LO, Desimone N, et al. Extensive multifocal mammary infarction—a case report. *Breast Care (Basel).* 2013;8:143–145.
17. Oh YJ, Choi SH, Chung SY, et al. Spontaneously infarcted fibroadenoma mimicking breast cancer. *J Ultrasound Med.* 2009;28:1421–1423.
18. Toy H, Esen HH, Sonmez FC, et al. Spontaneous infarction in a fibroadenoma of the breast. *Breast Care (Basel).* 2011;6:54–55.
19. Skenderi F, Krakonja F, Vranic S. Infarcted fibroadenoma of the breast: report of two new cases with review of the literature. *Diagn Pathol.* 2013;8:38. 23445683.
20. Kavdia R, Kini U. WCAFTI: worrisome cytologic alterations following tissue infarction: a mimicker of malignancy in breast cytology. *Diagn Cytopathol.* 2008;36:586–588.
21. Agnihotri M, Naik L, Kothari K, et al. Fine-needle aspiration cytology of breast lesions with spontaneous infarction: a five-year study. *Acta Cytol.* 2013;57:413–417.
22. Flint A, Oberman HA. Infarction and squamous metaplasia of intraductal papilloma: a benign breast lesion that may simulate carcinoma. *Hum Pathol.* 1984;15:764–767.
23. Ginter PS, Hoda SA, Ozerdem U. Exuberant squamous metaplasia in an intraductal papilloma of breast. *Int J Surg Pathol.* 2015;23:125–126.
24. Murad TM, Contesso G, Mouriesse H. Papillary tumors of large lactiferous ducts. *Cancer.* 1981;48:122–133.
25. Jones EL, Codling BW, Oates GD. Necrotic intraduct breast carcinomas simulating inflammatory lesions. *J Pathol.* 1973;110:101–103.
26. Yu L, Yang W, Cai X, et al. Centrally necrotizing carcinoma of the breast: clinicopathological analysis of 33 cases indicating its basal-like phenotype and poor prognosis. *Histopathology.* 2010;57:193–201.
27. Golden GT, Wangensteen SL. Galactocele of the breast. *Am J Surg.* 1972;123:271–273.
28. Salvador R, Salvador M, Jimenez JA, et al. Galactocele of the breast: radiologic and ultrasonographic findings. *Br J Radiol.* 1990;63:140–142.
29. Novotny DB, Maygarden SJ, Shermer RW, et al. Fine needle aspiration of benign and malignant breast masses associated with pregnancy. *Acta Cytol.* 1991;35:676–686.
30. Heymann JJ, Halligan AM, Hoda SA, et al. Fine needle aspiration of breast masses in pregnant and lactating women: experience with 28 cases emphasizing Thinprep findings. *Diagn Cytopathol.* 2015;43:188–194.
31. Adams EG, Kemp JD, Holcomb KZ, et al. Xanthogranulomatous reaction to a ruptured galactocele. *J Cutan Pathol.* 2010;37:973–976.
32. Tung A, Carr N. Postaugmentation galactocele: a case report and review of literature. *Ann Plast Surg.* 2011;67:668–670.
33. Taylor D, Kulawansa ST, McCallum DD, et al. Peri-implant galactocele following vacuum-assisted core biopsy of the breast: a cautionary tale. *BMJ Case Rep.* 2013;2013. pii:bcr2012007127. doi:10.1136/bcr-2012-007127.
34. Rahal RM, de Freitas-Júnior R, Carlos da Cunha L, et al. Mammary duct ectasia: an overview. *Breast J.* 2011;17:694–695.
35. Habif DV, Perzin KH, Lipton R, et al. Subareolar abscess associated with squamous metaplasia of lactiferous ducts. *Am J Surg.* 1970;119:523–526.
36. Passaro ME, Broughan TA, Sebek BA, et al. Lactiferous fistula. *J Am Coll Surg.* 1994;178:29–32.
37. Sweeney DJ, Wylie EJ. Mammographic appearances of mammary duct ectasia that mimic carcinoma in a screening programme. *Australas Radiol.* 1995;39:18–23.
38. Davies JD. Pigmented periductal cells (ochrocytes) in mammary dysplasias: their nature and significance. *J Pathol.* 1974;114(4):205–216.
39. Seidman MA, Scognamiglio T, Hoda SA. "Cholesteroloma": a rare cause of "indeterminate" microcalcifications on mammography. *Breast J.* 2009;15:303–304.
40. Bezić J, Piljić-Burazer M. Breast cholesterol granuloma: a report of two cases with discussion on potential pathogenesis. *Pathologica.* 2013;105:349–352.
41. Tashiro T, Hirokawa M, Sano T. Are mammary pagetoid foam cells histiocytic or epithelial? *Virchows Arch.* 2001;439:102–103.

42. Davies JD. Inflammatory damage to ducts in mammary dysplasia: a cause of duct dilatation. *J Pathol.* 1975;117:47–54.

43. Davies JD. Hyperelastosis, obliteration and fibrous plaques in major ducts of the human breast. *J Pathol.* 1973;110:13–26.

44. Wang Z, Leonard MH Jr, Khamapirad T, et al. Bilateral extensive ductitis obliterans manifested by bloody nipple discharge in a patient with long-term diabetes mellitus. *Breast J.* 2007;13:599–602.

45. Tan PH, Harada O, Thike AA, et al. Histiocytoid breast carcinoma: an enigmatic lobular entity. *J Clin Pathol.* 2011;64:654–659.

46. Tomaszewski JE, Brooks JSJ, Hicks D, et al. Diabetic mastopathy: a distinctive clinicopathologic entity. *Hum Pathol.* 1992;23:780–786.

47. Chan CL, Ho RS, Shek TW, et al. Diabetic mastopathy. *Breast J.* 2013;19:533–538.

48. Dorokhova O, Fineberg S, Koenigsberg T, et al. Diabetic mastopathy, a clinicopathological correlation of 34 cases. *Pathol Int.* 2012;62:660–664.

49. Seidman JD, Schnaper LA, Phillips LE. Mastopathy in insulin-requiring diabetes mellitus. *Hum Pathol.* 1994;25:819–824.

50. Ashton MA, Lefkowitz M, Tavassoli FA. Epithelioid stromal cells in lymphocytic mastitis—a source of confusion with invasive carcinoma. *Mod Pathol.* 1994;7:49–54.

51. Love JE, Lawton TJ. Diabetic mastopathy in patients with non-diabetic autoimmune disease. *Mod Pathol.* 2005;18(suppl 1):41A.

52. Weinstein SP, Conant EF, Orel SG, et al. Diabetic mastopathy in men: imaging findings in two patients. *Radiology.* 2001;219:797–799.

53. Tang DA, Diamond AB, Rogers L, et al. Diabetic mastopathy: adjunctive use of ultrasound and utility of core biopsy in diagnosis. *Breast J.* 2000;6:183–188.

54. Camuto PM, Zetrenne E, Ponn T. Diabetic mastopathy: a report of 5 cases and a review of the literature. *Arch Surg.* 2000;135:1190–1193.

55. Byrd BF Jr, Hartmann WH, Graham LS, et al. Mastopathy in insulindependent diabetics. *Ann Surg.* 1987;205:529–532.

56. Gabriel HA, Feng C, Mendelson EB, et al. Breast MRI for cancer detection in a patient with diabetic mastopathy. *AJR Am J Roentgenol.* 2004;182:1081–1083.

57. Tuncbilek N, Karakas HM, Okten O. Diabetic fibrous mastopathy: dynamic contrast-enhanced magnetic resonance imaging findings. *Breast J.* 2004;10:359–362.

58. Bayer U, Horn LC, Schulz HG. Bilateral, tumor-like diabetic mastopathy: progression and regression of the disease during a 5-year follow-up: case report. *Eur J Radiol.* 1998;26:248–253.

59. Shousha S. Diabetic mastopathy: strong CD10⁺ immunoreactivity of the atypical stromal cells. *Histopathology.* 2008;52:648–650.

60. Valdez R, Thorson J, Finn WG, et al. Lymphocytic mastitis and diabetic mastopathy: a molecular, immunophenotypic, and clinicopathologic evaluation of 11 cases. *Mod Pathol.* 2003;16:223–228.

61. Morgan MC, Weaver MG, Crowe JP, et al. Diabetic mastopathy: a clinicopathologic study of palpable and nonpalpable breast lesions. *Mod Pathol.* 1995;8:349–354.

62. Coyne JD, Baildam AD, Asbury D. Lymphocytic mastopathy associated with ductal carcinoma in situ of the breast. *Histopathology.* 1995;26:579–580.

63. Fitzgibbons PL. Granulomatous mastitis. *N Y State J Med.* 1990;90:287.

64. Cooper NE. Rheumatoid nodule of the breast. *Histopathology.* 1991;19:193–194.

65. Lacambra M, Thai TA, Lam CC, et al. Granulomatous mastitis: the histological differentials. *J Clin Pathol.* 2011;64:405–411.

66. Pandhi D, Verma P, Sharma S, et al. Borderline-lepromatous leprosy manifesting as granulomatous mastitis. *Lepr Rev.* 2012;83:202–204.

67. Nalini G, Kusum S, Barwad A, et al. Role of polymerase chain reaction in breast tuberculosis. *Breast Dis.* 2015;35(2):129–132.

68. Bässler R, Birke F. Histopathology of tumour associated sarcoid-like stromal reaction in breast cancer: an analysis of 5 cases with immunohistochemical investigations. *Virchows Arch [A].* 1988;412:231–239.

69. Iqbal FM, Ali H, Vidya R. Breast lumps: a rare site for rheumatoid nodules. *BMJ Case Rep.* 2015;2015. pii:bcr2014208586. doi:10.1136/bcr-2014-208586.

70. Fletcher A, Magrath IM, Riddell RH, et al. Granulomatous mastitis: a report of seven cases. *J Clin Pathol.* 1982;35:941–945.

71. Going JJ, Anderson TJ, Wilkinson S, et al. Granulomatous lobular mastitis. *J Clin Pathol.* 1987;40:535–540.

72. Han B-K, Choe YH, Park JM, et al. Granulomatous mastitis: mammographic and sonographic appearances. *AJR Am J Roentgenol.* 1999;173:317–320.

73. Oran EŞ, Gürdal SÖ, Yankol Y, et al. Management of idiopathic granulomatous mastitis diagnosed by core biopsy: a retrospective multicenter study. *Breast J.* 2013;19:411–418.

74. Joseph KA, Luu X, Mor A. Granulomatous mastitis: a New York public hospital experience. *Ann Surg Oncol.* 2014;21:4159–4163.

75. Hovanessian Larsen LJ, Peyvandi B, Klipfel N, et al. Granulomatous lobular mastitis: imaging, diagnosis, and treatment. *AJR Am J Roentgenol.* 2009;193:574–581.

76. Renshaw AA, Derhagopian RP, Gould EW. Cystic neutrophilic granulomatous mastitis: an underappreciated pattern strongly associated with gram-positive bacilli. *Am J Clin Pathol.* 2011;136:424–427.

77. D'Alfonso TM, Cheng E, Moo T, et al. Cystic neutrophilic granulomatous mastitis: further characterization of a distinctive histopathologic entity not always demonstrably attributable to *Corynebacterium* infection. *Am J Surg Pathol.* 2015;39:1440–1447.

78. Fitzgibbons PL, Smiley DF, Kern WH. Sarcoidosis presenting initially as breast mass: report of two cases. *Hum Pathol.* 1985;16:851–852.

79. Banik S, Bishop PW, Ormerod LP, et al. Sarcoidosis of the breast. *J Clin Pathol.* 1986;39:446–448.

80. Nicholson BT, Mills SE. Sarcoidosis of the breast: an unusual presentation of a systemic disease. *Breast J.* 2007;13:99–100.

81. Zujić PV, Grebić D, Valenčić L. Chronic granulomatous inflammation of the breast as a first clinical manifestation of primary sarcoidosis. *Breast Care (Basel).* 2015;10:51–53.

82. Kenzel PP, Hadijuana J, Hosten N, et al. Boeck sarcoidosis of the breast: mammographic, ultrasound, and MR findings. *J Comput Assisted Tomogr.* 1997;21:439–441.

83. Ito T, Okada T, Murayama K, et al. Two cases of sarcoidosis discovered accidentally by positron emission tomography in patients with breast cancer. *Breast J.* 2010;16:561–563.

84. Kirshy D, Gluck B, Brancaccio W. Sarcoidosis of the breast presenting as a spiculated lesion. *AJR Am J Roentgenol.* 1999;172:554–555.

85. Venkataraman S, Hines N, Slanetz PJ. Challenges in mammography: part 2, multimodality review of breast augmentation—imaging findings and complications. *AJR Am J Roentgenol.* 2011;197:W1031–W1045.

86. Destouet JM, Monsees BS, Oser RF, et al. Screening mammography in 350 women with breast implants: prevalence and findings of implant complications. *AJR Am J Roentgenol.* 1992;159:973–978.

87. Cheung YC, Su MY, Ng SH. Lumpy silicone-injected breasts: enhanced MRI and microscopic correlation. *Clin Imaging.* 2002;26:397–404.

88. Morgenstern L, Gleischman SH, Michel SL, et al. Relation of free silicone to human breast carcinoma. *Arch Surg.* 1986;120:573–577.

89. Maijers MC, Niessen FB, Veldhuizen JF, et al. MRI screening for silicone breast implant rupture: accuracy, inter- and intraobserver variability using explantation results as reference standard. *Eur Radiol.* 2014;24:1167–1175.

90. Goldblum JR, Weiss SW, Folpe AL. In: *Enzinger and Weiss's Soft Tissue Tumors.* 6th ed. Philadelphia, PA: Saunders; 2013:496.

91. Leibman AJ, Kossoff MB, Kruse BD. Intraductal extension of silicone from a ruptured breast implant. *Plast Reconstr Surg.* 1992;89:546–547.

92. Travis WE, Balogh K, Abraham JL. Silicone granulomas: report of three cases and review of the literature. *Hum Pathol.* 1985;16:19–27.

93. Taylor CR, Siddiqi IN, Brody GS. Anaplastic large cell lymphoma occurring in association with breast implants: review of pathologic and immunohistochemical features in 103 cases. *Appl Immunohistochem Mol Morphol.* 2013;21:13–20.

94. Hoda RS, Rao R, Hoda SA. Breast implant-associated anaplastic large cell lymphoma. *Int J Surg Pathol.* 2015;23:209–210.

95. Balzer BL, Weiss SW. Do biomaterials cause implant-associated mesenchymal tumors of the breast? Analysis of 8 new cases and review of the literature. *Hum Pathol.* 2009;40:1564–1570.

96. Kim H, Yang EJ, Bang SI. Bilateral liponecrotic pseudocysts after breast augmentation by fat injection: a case report. *Aesthetic Plast Surg.* 2012;36:359–362.

97. Yip CH, Wong KT, Samuel D. Bilateral plasma cell granuloma (inflammatory pseudotumour) of the breast. *ANZ J Surg.* 1997;67:300–303.

98. Pettinato G, Manivel JC, Insabato L, et al. Plasma cell granuloma (inflammatory pseudotumour) of the breast. *Am J Clin Pathol*. 1988;90:627–632.

99. Haj M, Weiss M, Loberant N, et al. Inflammatory pseudotumor of the breast: case report and literature review. *Breast J*. 2003;9:423–425.

100. Hill PA. Inflammatory pseudotumor of the breast: a mimic of breast carcinoma. *Breast J*. 2010;16:549–550.

101. Sari A, Yigit S, Peker Y, et al. Inflammatory pseudotumor of the breast. *Breast J*. 2011;17:312–314.

102. Shin SJ, Scamman W, Gopalan A, et al. Mammary presentation of adult-type 'juvenile' xanthogranuloma. *Am J Surg Pathol*. 2005;29:827–831.

103. Cheuk W, Chan AC, Lam WL, et al. IgG4-related sclerosing mastitis: description of a new member of the IgG4-related sclerosing diseases. *Am J Surg Pathol*. 2009;33:1058–1064.

104. Ogura K, Matsumoto T, Aoki Y, et al. IgG4-related tumour-forming mastitis with histological appearances of granulomatous lobular mastitis: comparison with other types of tumour-forming mastitis. *Histopathology*. 2010;57:39–45.

105. Ogiya A, Tanaka K, Tadokoro Y, et al. IgG4-related sclerosing disease of the breast successfully treated by steroid therapy. *Breast Cancer*. 2014;21:231–235.

106. Coffin CM, Hornick JL, Fletcher CD. Inflammatory myofibroblastic tumor: comparison of clinicopathologic, histologic, and immunohistochemical features including ALK expression in atypical and aggressive cases. *Am J Surg Pathol*. 2007;31:509–520.

107. Kovács A, Máthé G, Mattsson J, et al. ALK-positive inflammatory myofibroblastic tumor of the nipple during pregnancy—an unusual presentation of a rare disease. *Breast J*. 2015;21:297–302.

108. Said SM, Reynolds C, Jimenez RE, et al. Amyloidosis of the breast: predominantly AL type and over half have concurrent hematologic disorders. *Mod Pathol*. 2013;26:232–238.

109. Charlot M, Seldin DC, O'hara C, et al. Localized amyloidosis of the breast: a case series. *Amyloid*. 2011;18:72–75.

110. Huerter ME, Hammadeh R, Zhou Q, et al. Primary amyloidosis of the breast presenting as a solitary nodule: case report and review of the literature. *Ochsner J*. 2014;14:282–286.

111. Luo J-H, Rotterdam H. Primary amyloid tumor of the breast: a case report and review of the literature. *Mod Pathol*. 1997;10:735–738.

112. Silverman JF, Dabbs DJ, Norris HT, et al. Localized primary (AL) amyloid tumor of the breast: cytologic, histologic, immunocytochemical and ultrastructural observations. *Am J Surg Pathol*. 1986;10:539–545.

113. Fleury AM, Buetens OW, Campasi C, et al. Pathologic Quiz Case: a 77-year old woman with bilateral breast masses. *Arch Pathol Lab Med*. 2004;128:e67.

114. Yumlu S, Barany R, Eriksson M, et al. Localized insulin-derived amyloidosis in patients with diabetes mellitus: a case report. *Hum Pathol*. 2009;40:1655–1660.

115. Liaw Y-S, Kuo S-H, Yang P-C, et al. Nodular amyloidosis of the lung and the breast mimicking breast carcinoma with pulmonary metastasis. *Eur Respir J*. 1995;5:871–873.

116. Lynch LA, Moriarty AT. Localized primary amyloid tumor associated with osseous metaplasia presenting as bilateral breast masses: cytologic and radiologic features. *Diagn Cytopathol*. 1993;9:570–575.

117. Eghtedari M, Dogan BE, Gilcrease M, et al. Imaging and pathologic characteristics of breast amyloidosis. *Breast J*. 2015;21:197–199.

118. Ngendahayo P, Faverly D, Hérin M. Primary breast amyloidosis presenting solely as nonpalpable microcalcifications: a case report with review of the literature. *Int J Surg Pathol*. 2013;21:177–180.

119. O'Brien J, Aherne S, McCormack O, et al. MRI features of bilateral amyloidosis of breast. *Breast J*. 2013;19:338–339.

120. Sabate JM, Clotet M, Torrubia S, et al. Localized amyloidosis of the breast associated with invasive lobular carcinoma. *Br J Radiol*. 2008;81:e252–e254.

121. Rocken C, Kronsbein H, Sletten K, et al. Amyloidosis of the breast. *Virchows Arch*. 2002;440:527–535.

122. Munson-Bernardi BD, DePersia LA. Amyloidosis of the breast coexisting with ductal carcinoma in situ. *AJR Am J Roentgenol*. 2006;186:54–55.

123. Libbey CA, Skinner M, Cohen AS. The abdominal fat aspirate for the diagnosis of systemic amyloid. *Arch Intern Med*. 1983;143:1549–1552.

124. Yokoo H. Nakazato Y. Primary localized amyloid tumor of the breast with osseous metaplasia. *Pathol Int*. 1998;48:545–548.

125. Hecht AH, Tan A, Shen JF. Case report: primary systemic amyloidosis presenting as breast masses, mammographically simulating carcinoma. *Clin Radiol*. 1991;44:123–124.

126. Kim SM, Park JM, Moon WK. Dystrophic breast calcifications in patients with collagen diseases. *Clin Imaging*. 2004;28:6–9.

127. Clement PB, Senges H, How AR. Giant cell arteritis of the breast: case report and literature review. *Hum Pathol*. 1987;18:1186–1189.

128. Lau Y, Mak YF, Hui PK, et al. Giant cell arteritis of the breast. *ANZ J Surg*. 1996;66:259–261.

129. Kadotani Y, Enoki Y, Itoi N, et al. Giant cell arteritis of the breast: a case report with a review of literatures. *Breast Cancer*. 2010;17:225–232.

130. Marie I, Audeguy P, François A, et al. Giant cell arteritis presenting as a breast lesion: report of a case and review of the literature. *Am J Med Sci*. 2008;335:489–491.

131. Pappo I, Beglaibter N, Amir G. Mammary arteritis mimicking cancer. *Eur J Surg*. 1992;158:191–193.

132. Jordan JM, Rowe TW, Allen NB. Wegener's granulomatosis involving the breast: report of three cases and review of the literature. *Am J Med*. 1987;83:159–164.

133. Allende DS, Booth CN. Wegener's granulomatosis of the breast: a rare entity with daily clinical relevance. *Ann Diagn Pathol*. 2009;13:351–357.

134. Yamashina M, Wilson TK. A mammographic finding in focal polyarteritis nodosa. *Br J Radiol*. 1985;58:91–92.

135. Dhaon P, Bansal N, Das SK, et al. Cutaneous polyarteritis nodosa presenting with digital gangrene and breast ulcer. *Int J Rheum Dis*. 2013;16:774–776.

136. Harrison GO, Elliott RL. Scleroderma of the breast: light and electron microscopy study. *Am Surg*. 1987;53:526–531.

137. Gyves-Ray KM, Adler DD. Dermatomyositis: an unusual cause of breast calcifications. *Breast Dis*. 1989;2:195–201.

138. Cernea SS, Kihara SM, Sotto MN, et al. Lupus mastitis. *J Am Acad Dermatol*. 1993;29:343–346.

139. Nigar E, Contractor K, Singhal H, et al. Lupus mastitis—a cause of recurrent breast lumps. *Histopathology*. 2007;51:847–849.

140. Kinonen C, Gattuso P, Reddy VB. Lupus mastitis: an uncommon complication of systemic or discoid lupus. *Am J Surg Pathol*. 2010;34:901–906.

141. Visentin MS, Salmaso R, Modesti V, et al. Parotid, breast, and fascial involvement in a patient who fulfilled the ACR criteria for Churg–Strauss syndrome. *Scand J Rheumatol*. 2012;41:319–321.

142. Hernández-Rodríguez J, Tan CD, Molloy ES, et al. Vasculitis involving the breast: a clinical and histopathologic analysis of 34 patients. *Medicine*. 2008;87:61–69.

143. Bonnetblanc JM, Bernard P, Fayol J. Dermatomyositis and malignancy: a multicenter cooperative study. *Dermatologica*. 1990;180:212–216.

144. Sigurgeirsson B, Lindelöf B, Edhag O, et al. Risk of cancer in patients with dermatomyositis or polymyositis: a population-based study. *N Engl J Med*. 1992;326:363–367.

145. Kontos M. Fentiman I. Systemic lupus erythematosus and breast cancer. *Breast J*. 2008;14:81–86.

146. Chen X, Hoda SA, Delellis RA, et al. Lupus mastitis. *Breast J*. 2005;11:283–284.

147. Holland NW, McKnight K, Challa VR, et al. Lupus panniculitis (profundus) involving the breast: report of 2 cases and review of the literature. *J Rheumatol*. 1995;22:344–346.

148. Fernandez-Flores A, Crespo LG, Alonso S, et al. Lupus mastitis in the male breast mimicking inflammatory carcinoma. *Breast J*. 2006;12:272–273.

149. Adejolu M, Huo L, Rohren E, et al. False-positive lesions mimicking breast cancer on FDG PET and PET/CT. *AJR Am J Roentgenol*. 2012;198:W304–W314.

150. Singh A, Kaur P, Sood N, et al. Bilateral eosinophilic mastitis: an uncommon unheard entity. *Breast Dis*. 2015;35:33–36.

151. Solomon GJ, Wu E, Rosen PP. Nephrogenic systemic fibrosis mimicking inflammatory breast carcinoma. *Arch Pathol Lab Med*. 2007;131:145–148.

152. Guarda LA, Tran TA. The pathology of breast biopsy site marking devices. *Am J Surg Pathol*. 2005;29:814–819.

3

Specific Infections

SYED A. HODA

A wide variety of microbial infections caused by bacteria, fungi, parasites, and viruses can afflict the breast. Most forms of infectious mastitis are a manifestation of a systemic infection. It is rare for the breast to be the only organ involved in an infectious disease process outside of the settings of pregnancy and lactation or an underlying compromised immune status.

The presence of most specific infectious processes in needle core biopsy specimens is unexpected. More often than not, the only clinical information available in such cases is either a mass or radiographic abnormality, and the pathologist is usually unaware of any concurrent systemic, or suspicion of any current local, infection. Thus, pathologists ought to be alert to the possibility of encountering infectious disease processes in needle core biopsies.

BACTERIAL INFECTION

Abscess

Bacterial infections are the commonest cause of mastitis and are most frequent during lactation and pregnancy. *Staphylococcus aureus* is the usual cause of bacterial abscesses, including those that occur during lactation (**Fig. 3.1**). A minor (approximately 10%) proportion of *S. aureus* that cause mammary abscess are due to the methicillin-resistant variety (1), and antibiotic use ought to be guided by results of bacterial cultures.

Rare instances of mammary abscesses due to *Nocardia* (2), *Salmonella* (3–5), *Pseudomonas* (6), and brucellosis (7) have been reported. Mammary lesions owing to cat-scratch disease caused by *Bartonella* present as a mass with inflammatory signs, often accompanied by axillary nodal enlargement that may mimic inflammatory carcinoma (8). The mammary lesion of bartonellosis is in an intramammary lymph node rather than in mammary glandular or stromal parenchyma.

The existence of an immunodeficiency or immunocompromised state (including HIV/AIDS) can predispose to infections including those caused by *Salmonella* and *Pseudomonas aeruginosa* (9). Mammary gangrene has been reported in HIV-positive patients in the absence of prior trauma or other injury to the breast (10). Among other predisposing factors for mammary bacterial infections are the performance of needle core biopsy (11) and insertion of nipple rings purportedly for adornment purposes (12).

Actinomycotic infection of the breast typically presents as an abscess near the nipple and areola. Predisposing factors include lactation, diabetes, nipple piercing, and immunosuppressive therapy (13–15). Sinus tracts can develop following incision and drainage of an actinomycotic abscess, or with progression of the untreated lesion. A chronic abscess may form, creating a hard mass that can simulate carcinoma (13). Axillary lymph node enlargement generally reflects reaction to the mammary inflammatory process rather than spread of actinomycosis to the lymph nodes; however, primary actinomycotic axillary lymphadenitis has been reported (14,15). In advanced cases, the infection can spread to the chest wall. Extension of pulmonary actinomycosis to the breast has also been described (16). The diagnosis of actinomycosis is rendered by the demonstration of the Gram-positive organism in filaments or colonies ("sulfur" granules). Isolates from mammary actinomycosis include *Actinomyces meyeri* (17), *A. viscosus* (18), *A. radingae, A. turicensis* (15), and *A. israelli* (19). Treatment with penicillin has reportedly been effective (14), but recurrent or advanced infections may require multiple antibiotics (15) and rarely wide local excision or mastectomy.

Mycobacterial Infections

Mycobacterium tuberculosis infection of the breast, in immunosuppressed as well as immunocompetent men and women, is not an uncommon condition in many regions of the world (20–23). Tuberculous mastitis has been reported as a manifestation of AIDS, and this presentation is encountered with increasing frequency in HIV-positive individuals (9,24).

Mammary tuberculosis unassociated with HIV infection is primarily a disease of premenopausal women with a predilection for the lactating breast, but it can affect the adult female breast at any age. Infection of the breast may be the primary manifestation of tuberculosis, but the breasts are probably infected secondarily in most patients even when the primary nonmammary focus remains clinically inapparent.

It is difficult to make a clinical diagnosis of tuberculous mastitis because the disease has multiple patterns of clinical presentation. The most common form is nodular mastitis in which the patient develops a slowly growing solitary mass. The mammographic presentation of these lesions resembles carcinoma (25,26). Microcalcifications are typically absent. Advanced nodular lesions become fixed to the skin and may develop draining sinuses. An acute and diffuse type of tuberculous mastitis is characterized by development of multiple painful nodules throughout the breast producing a pattern

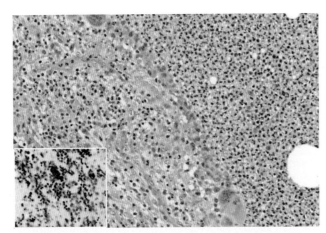

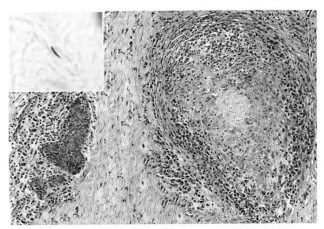

FIGURE 3.1 Staphylococcal Abscess. Purulent mastitis in a 35-year-old woman who had been nursing until a few weeks prior to the biopsy. The abscess contained Gram-positive cocci (inset). *S. aureus* was cultured.

FIGURE 3.3 Tuberculous Mastitis. A granuloma with central "caseous" necrosis is present in the vicinity of inactive mammary glands. Inset shows an acid-fast bacillus on a Ziehl–Neelsen preparation.

that can clinically and mammographically mimic inflammatory carcinoma (26). A third, sclerosing variety of infection occurs predominantly in elderly women, resulting in diffuse induration of the breast and diffusely increased density on mammography. The clinical distinction between tuberculous mastitis and mammary carcinoma can be complicated by the occasional coexistence of both conditions (27). Rarely, tuberculosis of the chest wall can present as a breast lump (20).

Microscopically, granulomatous lesions in tuberculous mastitis do not always feature "caseous" necrosis, and fibrosis may be prominent in chronic cases. The granulomas are associated with ducts and lobules (**Fig. 3.2**). Acid-fast bacteria are histologically detected in fewer cases (**Fig. 3.3**). Neutrophils can obscure the granulomatous character of the process in specimens from patients with necrotizing abscesses or sinus tracts. Calcifications are uncommon. The finding of necrotizing granulomas in a needle core biopsy specimen may be considered presumptive evidence of mammary tuberculosis in the appropriate clinical setting. If mammary infection is suspected clinically, an aspirate or tissue sample should be submitted for microbiological culture or polymerase chain reaction (PCR) study.

A wide variety of *atypical (nontuberculous) mycobacteria* can infect breast tissue in acute, recurrent, and chronic forms (28) and can simulate a neoplasm (29). Breast abscess formation attributable to atypical mycobacterial infection such as *Mycobacterium fortuitum* (12,30) and *M. abscessus* (31) has been observed following nipple piercing. *M. fortuitum* infections have also complicated prosthetic breast implants (32).

The diagnosis of mammary mycobacterial and atypical (nontuberculous) mycobacterial infection and other granulomatous conditions is facilitated by PCR technique (21,28,33).

Cystic Neutrophilic Granulomatous Mastitis

A particular type of granulomatous mastitis associated with cystic degeneration and marked neutrophilic infiltrate has been associated with *Corynebacterium*, a Gram-positive bacterium (33–36) (**Fig. 3.4**). Cystic neutrophilic granulomatous mastitis can present as a mass. In general, tuberculous granulomata

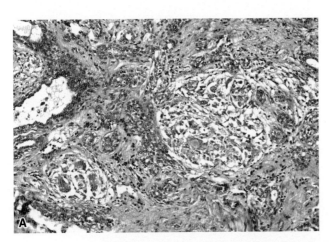

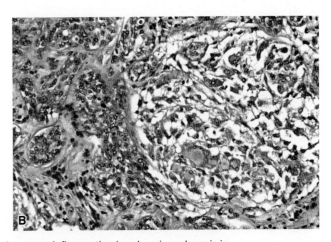

FIGURE 3.2 Tuberculous Mastitis. A, B: Granulomatous inflammation in sclerosing adenosis in a patient with active pulmonary tuberculosis. The needle core biopsy was performed to evaluate a breast mass. No acid-fast bacteria were found with the acid-fast (Ziehl–Neelsen) stain.

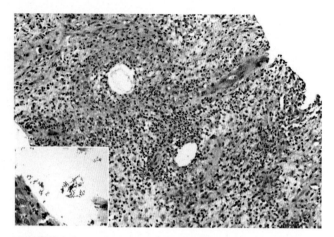

FIGURE 3.4 Cystic Neutrophilic Granulomatous Mastitis. Mammary glandular and stromal tissue has been destroyed by abscess formation with the characteristic central cystic structure. Neutrophils are predominant amid the inflammatory cell infiltrate. Inset shows Gram-positive rods. *Corynebacterium sp.* was cultured.

show more necrosis and less cystic change. Other forms of granulomatous mastitis are discussed in detail in Chapter 2.

FUNGAL INFECTIONS

Infection with *Histoplasma capsulatum* is endemic in the Ohio and Mississippi river valleys of the United States and in many geographic zones in all continents. Calcified granulomata have not been described in the breast, but there have been rare instances of localized mammary *Histoplasma* infection. The latter can present as a solitary unilateral mass that may clinically simulate a neoplasm (37,38). Histologically, the lesions consist of confluent necrotizing granulomas in which *H. capsulatum* is demonstrated by a methenamine silver reaction. The granulomatous reaction is essentially similar to that of nonspecific granulomatous lobular mastitis (38,39).

Rare instances of other fungal infections of the breast have also been reported. These include *Cryptococcus* (40,41),

Aspergillus (42), *Coccidioides* (43), and *Blastomyces* (44). *Aspergillus* infection has been reported at the site of breast augmentation implants (45). Notably, and inexplicably, coccidioidomycosis can "flare up" during pregnancy—occasionally with breast involvement (46,47).

PARASITIC INFESTATION

A variety of parasites can infest female and male breast tissue. In almost all instances, the mammary involvement is part of a systemic disease process.

Mammary filariasis is caused most frequently by *Wuchereria bancrofti* and has been reported from tropical and semitropical regions in South America, China, and South Asia, where infection with this organism is endemic. Involvement of the breast occurs in the chronic phase of the disease, sometimes more than a decade after last exposure to infection.

The patient with mammary filariasis usually presents with a solitary, nontender, painless unilateral breast mass. Multiple lesions occur in a minority of cases. Many lesions involve subcutaneous tissue, and they may be fixed to the skin. The resultant hard mass with cutaneous attachment, sometimes accompanied by inflammatory changes including edema, appears to be clinically indistinguishable from carcinoma (48). In this setting, axillary lymph nodal enlargement caused by filarial lymphadenitis further complicates the differential diagnosis. Viable microfilariae can be detected in the breast by ultrasound examination if they produce a distinctive pattern of movement referred to as the "filaria dance" sign (49). Mammographically detected calcifications attributed to *W. bancrofti* and *Loa loa* infection have been described as having a spiral or serpiginous configuration (50). Microscopic examination of fine needle aspiration or tissue biopsy samples reveals adult filarial worms that may be well preserved or in different stages of degeneration (51) (**Fig. 3.5**). Granulomatous reaction with eosinophilia is present in tissues around the parasites. Fully degenerated worms are likely to become calcified. Microfilariae are not always detected in the peripheral blood (52).

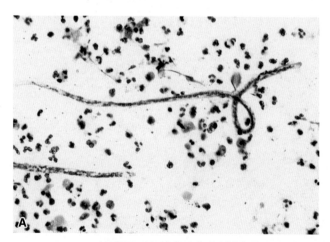

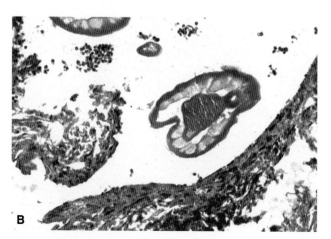

FIGURE 3.5 Mammary Filariasis. A: Microfilariae in a fine needle aspiration specimen with *W. bancrofti* infection. **B:** Biopsy specimen from a mammary filarial abscess showing a microfilaria in cross section and fragments of the surrounding tissue. (Courtesy of Dr. Kusum Kapila, Kuwait.)

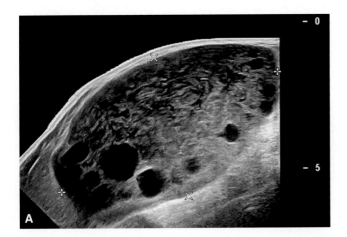

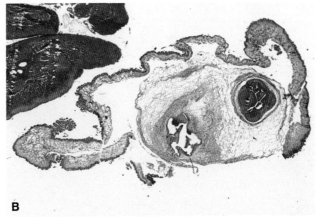

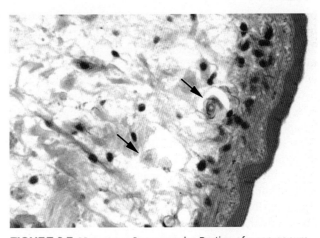

FIGURE 3.6 Echinococcal (Hydatid) Diseases. A: Ultrasound image of a breast showing a mass with multiple internal anechoic cysts. (Courtesy of Dr. Abdulmohsen Alkushi, Saudi Arabia.) **B:** Part of an echinococcal cyst wall and a cross section of the larval tapeworm in another breast specimen. (Courtesy of Dr. Kusum Kapila, Kuwait.) **C:** A portion of yet another mammary hydatid (echinococcal) cyst wall with numerous echinococcal scolices. Inset shows detail of a scolex.

Adult worms and microfilariae may also be found in axillary lymph nodes (53).

Several cases of mammary *cysticercosis*, an infection caused by larvae of tapeworms, that have been described have mimicked a neoplasm (54–56). Most instances of mammary cysticercosis are caused by *Taenia solium*, and such a case diagnosed by needle core biopsy in a *male* breast has been reported (57). *T. solium* is typically acquired by ingesting undercooked pork; however, mammary infection has been reported in a vegetarian presumably by ingestion of *T. solium* eggs in contaminated food (56).

The breast can also be the site of hydatid cyst formation caused by *Echinococcus granulosus*. The lesion typically presents as a firm, discrete mobile mass. Mammography reveals a dense, well-circumscribed tumor within which internal ring structures representing air fluid levels may be seen. Ultrasound evaluation displays air fluid levels and multiple cysts to better advantage (58,59) **(Fig. 3.6A)**. Rarely, mammographically detected calcifications in clinically inapparent cysts have been the first evidence of mammary cysticercosis (60,61). Mammary hydatid disease can be recognized by finding fragments of the adult worm, the hydatid membranes, and hooklets in aspirated cyst contents or a tissue biopsy specimen (62) **(Fig. 3.6B and C)**.

The diagnosis of mammary *sparganosis* by needle core biopsy caused by the tapeworm *Spirometra* has been described (63) **(Fig. 3.7)**. Complete excision is the treatment of choice (64,65).

FIGURE 3.7 Mammary Sparganosis. Portion of a sparganum larva obtained by needle core biopsy of the breast. Note the presence of whorled calcifications in the larva *(arrows)*. (Courtesy of Dr. Amy Bik-Wan Chan, Hong Kong.)

Calcified ova of *schistosomiasis* can simulate a carcinoma on mammograms (66) **(Fig. 3.8),** or the inflammatory nodule may be mistaken for a fibroadenoma (67).

Microcalcifications attributed to *trichinellosis*, that is, *Trichinella* infection, have been found in the pectoral muscles by mammography (68).

Cutaneous *myiasis* caused by larvae of the botfly *Dermatobia hominis* results in a mass lesion accompanied by local

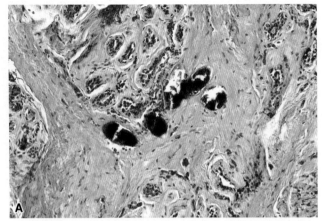

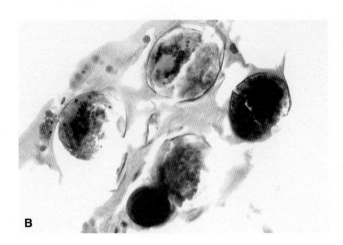

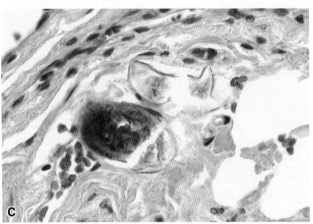

FIGURE 3.8 Mammary Schistosomiasis. This young woman with gastrointestinal symptoms was found to have numerous calcifications in the breast by mammography. **A:** The needle core biopsy sample shown here has five calcified ova of *Schistosoma mansoni* in the stroma next to a lobule. **B:** Five calcified ova in fat from the same specimen. **C:** Magnified view showing the characteristic spine. (Courtesy of Dr. Rhonda Yantiss, New York.)

inflammation. The mammographic and ultrasound findings in five patients with mammary lesions were reported by de Barros et al. (69). The mammographically ill-defined tumors measured 0.7 to 2.0 cm. Paired linear microcalcifications were visualized in three lesions. Oval larvae outlined by a hypoechoic zone were demonstrated by ultrasound examination. Although the diagnosis of myiasis could be suggested by a history of origin from or a visit to an endemic area, the clinical signs, the ultrasound findings, the presence of an ill-defined mass with calcification, and inflammation may mimic inflammatory carcinoma clinically (70). Another form of cutaneous myiasis that manifests as abscesses with draining sinuses is caused by infestation by larvae of the Tumbu fly (*Cordylobia anthropophaga*), which is found in sub-Saharan West Africa (71).

VIRAL INFECTION

Although a variety of secondary infections can involve the breast in patients with *human immunodeficiency virus (HIV)* infection (*vide supra*), the disease can manifest itself in an intramammary lymph node (72). The characteristic findings in this setting are florid follicular hyperplasia with "follicle-lysis."

Infection of the mammary skin, and rarely of the nipple, with a variety of viruses including *Human papillomavirus*

(causing verruca vulgaris), *Herpes simplex*, and *H. zoster* has been reported (73); however, these infectious processes are unlikely to be encountered in needle core biopsy specimens.

REFERENCES

1. Dabbas N, Chand M, Pallett A, et al. Have the organisms that cause breast abscess changed with time? Implications for appropriate antibiotic usage in primary and secondary care. *Breast J.* 2010;16:412–415.
2. Simpson AJH, Jumaa PA, Das SS. Breast abscess caused by *Nocardia asteroides. J Infect.* 1995;30:266–267.
3. Banu A, Hassan MM, Anand M. Breast abscess: sole manifestation of *Salmonella typhi* infection. *Indian J Med Microbiol.* 2013;31:94–95.
4. Vattipally V, Thatigotla B, Nagpal K, et al. *Salmonella typhi* breast abscess: an uncommon manifestation of an uncommon disease in the United States. *Am Surg.* 2011;77:E133–E135.
5. Singh S, Pandya Y, Rathod J, et al. Bilateral breast abscess: a rare complication of enteric fever. *Indian J Med Microbiol.* 2009;27:69–70.
6. Harji DP, Rastall S, Catchpole C, et al. Pseudomonal breast infection. *Ann R Coll Surg Engl.* 2010;92:W20–W22.
7. Gurleyik E. Breast abscess as a complication of human brucellosis. *Breast J.* 2006;12:375–376.
8. Povoski SP, Spigos DG, March WL. An unusual case of cat-scratch disease from *Bartonella quintana* mimicking inflammatory breast cancer in a 50-year old woman. *Breast J.* 2003;9:497–500.
9. Pantanowitz L, Connolly JL. Pathology of the breast associated with HIV/AIDS. *Breast J.* 2002;8:234–243.
10. Venkatramani V, Pillai S, Marathe S, et al. Breast gangrene in an HIV-positive patient. *Ann R Coll Surg Engl.* 2009;91:W13–W14.
11. Roque DR, MacLaughlan S, Tejada-Berges T. Necrotizing infection of the breast after core needle biopsy. *Breast J.* 2013;19:201–202.

12. Bengualid V, Singh V, Singh H, et al. *Mycobacterium fortuitum* and anaerobic breast abscess following nipple piercing: case presentation and review of the literature. *J Adolesc Health.* 2008;42:530–532.

13. Thambi R, Devi L, Sheeja S, et al. Primary breast actinomyces simulating malignancy: a case diagnosed by fine-needle aspiration cytology. *J Cytol.* 2012;29(3):197–199.

14. Jain BK, Sehgal VN, Jagdish S, et al. Primary actinomycosis of the breast: a clinical review and a case report. *J Dermatol.* 1994;21:497–500.

15. Attar KH, Waghorn D, Lyons M, et al. Rare species of *Actinomyces* as causative pathogens in breast abscess. *Breast J.* 2007;13:501–505.

16. Pinto MM, Longstreth GB, Khoury GM. Fine needle aspiration of *Actimomyces* infection of the breast: a novel presentation of thoracopleural actinomycosis. *Acta Cytol.* 1991;35:409–411.

17. Allen JN. *Actinomyces meyeri* breast abscess. *Am J Med.* 1987;83:186–187.

18. Capobianco G, Dessole S, Becchere MP, et al. A rare case of primary actinomycosis of the breast caused by *Actinomyces viscosus*: diagnosis by fine needle aspiration cytology under ultrasound guidance. *Breast J.* 2005;11:57–59.

19. Akhlaghi M, Ghazvini RD. Clinical presentation of primary actinomycosis of the breast. *Breast J.* 2009;15:102–103.

20. Teo TH, Ho GH, Chaturverdi A, et al. Tuberculosis of the chest wall: unusual presentation as a breast lump. *Singapore Med J.* 2009;50: e97–e99.

21. Cuervo SI, Bonilla DA, Murcia MI, et al. Tuberculosis of the breast. *Biomedica.* 2013;33:36–41.

22. Kumar M, Chand G, Nag VL, et al. Breast tuberculosis in immunocompetent patients at tertiary care center: a case series. *J Res Med Sci.* 2012;17: 199–202.

23. Hale JA, Peters GN, Cheek JH. Tuberculosis of the breast: rare but still extant. *Am J Surg.* 1985;150:620–624.

24. Hartstein M, Leaf HL. Tuberculosis of the breast as a presenting manifestation of AIDS. *Clin Infect Dis.* 1992;15:692–693.

25. Makanjuola D, Murshid K, Sulaimani A, et al. Mammographic features of breast tuberculosis: the skin bulge and sinus tract sign. *Clin Radiol.* 1996;51:354–358.

26. Sopeña B, Arnillas E, Garcia-Vila LM, et al. Tuberculosis of the breast: unusual clinical presentation of extrapulmonary tuberculosis. *Infection.* 1996;24:57–58.

27. Rothman GM, Kolkov Z, Meroz A, et al. Breast tuberculosis and carcinoma. *Isr J Med Sci.* 1989;25:339–340.

28. Yoo H, Choi SH, Kim YJ, et al. Recurrent bilateral breast abscess due to nontuberculous mycobacterial infection. *J Breast Cancer.* 2014;17: 295–298.

29. Mohamad B, Iqbal MN, Gopal KV, et al. MAI infection simulating metastatic breast cancer. *BMJ Case Rep.* 2012;2012. pii:bcr0120125640. doi:10.1136/bcr-01-2012-5640.

30. Lewis CG, Wells MK, Jennings WC. *Mycobacterium fortuitum* breast infection following nipple-piercing, mimicking carcinoma. *Breast J.* 2004;10:363–365.

31. Trupiano JK, Sebek BA, Goldfarb J, et al. Mastitis due to *Mycobacterium abscessus* after body piercing. *Clin Infect Dis.* 2001;33:131–134.

32. Haiavy J, Tobin H. *Mycobacterium fortuitum* infection in prosthetic breast implants. *Plast Reconstr Surg.* 2002;109:2124–2128.

33. Lacambra M, Thai TA, Lam CC, et al. Granulomatous mastitis: the histological differentials. *J Clin Pathol.* 2011;64:405–411.

34. Ang LM, Brown H. *Corynebacterium accolens* isolated from breast abscess: possible association with granulomatous mastitis. *J Clin Microbiol.* 2007;45:1666–1668.

35. Renshaw AA, Derhagopian RP, Gould EW. Cystic neutrophilic granulomatous mastitis: an underappreciated pattern strongly associated with gram-positive bacilli. *Am J Clin Pathol.* 2011;136:424–427.

36. Stary CM, Lee YS, Balfour J. Idiopathic granulomatous mastitis associated with *Corynebacterium sp.* infection. *Hawaii Med J.* 2011;70:99–101.

37. Salfelder K, Schwarz J. Mycotic 'pseudotumors' of the breast. *Arch Surg.* 1975;110:751–754.

38. Osborne BM. Granulomatous mastitis caused by *Histoplasma* and mimicking inflammatory breast carcinoma. *Hum Pathol.* 1989;20: 47–52.

39. Payne S, Kim S, Das K, et al. A 36-year-old woman with a unilateral breast mass: necrotizing granulomatous mastitis secondary to budding yeast forms morphologically consistent with *Histoplasma capsulatum*. *Arch Pathol Lab Med.* 2006;130:e1–e2.

40. Ramos-Barbosa S, Guazzelli LS, Severo LC. Cryptococcal mastitis after corticosteroid therapy. *Rev Soc Bras Med Trop.* 2004;37:65–66.

41. Haddow LJ, Sahid F, Moosa M-YS. Cryptocoal breast abscess in an HIV-positive patient: arguments for reviewing the definition of immune reconstitution inflammatory syndrome. *J Infect.* 2008;57:82–84.

42. Giovindarajan M, Verghese S, Kuruvilla S. Primary aspergillosis of the breast: report of a case with fine needle aspiration cytology. *Acta Cytol.* 1993;37:234–236.

43. Bocian JJ, Fahmy RN, Michas CA. A rare case of 'coccidioidoma' of the breast. *Arch Pathol Lab Med.* 1991;115:1064–1067.

44. Propeck PA, Scanlan KA. Blastomycosis of the breast. *AJR Am J Roentgenol.* 1996;166:726.

45. Williams K, Walton RL, Bunkis I. Aspergillus colonization associated with bilateral silicone mammary implants. *J Surg Pathol.* 1982;71:260–261.

46. Hooper JE, Lu Q, Pepkowitz SH. Disseminated coccidioidomycosis in pregnancy. *Arch Pathol Lab Med.* 2007;131:652–655.

47. Babycos PB, Hoda SA. A fatal case of disseminated coccidioidomycosis in Louisiana. *J La State Med Soc.* 1990;142:24–27.

48. Choudhury M. Bancroftian microfilaria in the breast clinically mimicking malignancy. *Cytopathology.* 1995;6:132–133.

49. Dreyer G, Brandão AC, Amaral F, et al. Detection by ultrasound of living adult *Wuchereria bancrofti* in the female breast. *Mem Inst Oswaldo Cruz.* 1996;91:95–96.

50. Chow CK, McCarthy JS, Neafie R, et al. Mammography of lymphatic filariasis. *AJR Am J Roentgenol.* 1996;167:1425–1426.

51. Mondal SK. Incidental detection of filaria in fine-needle aspirates: a cytologic study of 14 clinically unsuspected cases at different sites. *Diagn Cytopathol.* 2012;40:292–296.

52. Parida G, Rout N, Samantaray S, et al. Filariasis of breast simulating carcinoma. *Breast J.* 2008;14:598–599.

53. Chen YH, Qun X. Filarial granuloma of the female breast: a histopathologic study of 131 cases. *Am J Trop Med Hyg.* 1981;30:1206–1210.

54. Conde DM, Kashimoto E, Carvalho LE, et al. Cysticercosis of the breast: an uncommon cause of lumps. *Breast J.* 2006;12:179.

55. Karthikeyan TM, Manimaran D, Mrinalini VR. Cysticercus of the breast which mimicked a fibroadenoma: a rare presentation. *J Clin Diagn Res.* 2012;6:1555–1556.

56. Bhattacharjee HK, Ramman TR, Agarwal L, et al. Isolated cysticercosis of the breast masquerading as a breast tumor: report of a case and review of literature. *Ann Trop Med Parasitol.* 2011;105:455–461.

57. Lobaz J, Millican-Slater R, Rengabashyam B, et al. Parasitic infection of the male breast. *BMJ Case Rep.* 2014;2014. pii:bcr2013202493.

58. Alamer A, Aldhilan A, Makanjuola D, et al. Preoperative diagnosis of hydatid cyst of the breast: a case report. *Pan Afr Med J.* 2013;14:99.

59. Vega A, Ortega E, Cavada A, et al. Hydatid cyst of the breast: mammographic findings. *AJR Am J Roentgenol.* 1994;162:825–826.

60. Lucarelli AP, Martins MM, de Oliviera VM, et al. A short report: cysticercosis of the breast. *Am J Trop Med Hyg.* 2008;279:864–865.

61. Haholy A, Sonmez G, Karaman M, et al. Unilocular cystic hydatidosis in breast. *Breast J.* 2008;14:393–394.

62. Sagin HB, Kiroglu Y, Aksoy F. Hydatid cyst of the breast diagnosed by fine needle aspiration biopsy: a case report. *Acta Cytol.* 1994;38:965–967.

63. Chan ABW, Wan SK, Leung S-L, et al. Sparganosis of the breast. *Histopathology.* 2004;44:510–511.

64. Koo M, Kim JH, Kim JS, et al. Cases and literature review of breast sparganosis. *World J Surg.* 2011;35:573–579.

65. Min KW, Kim DY, Kim HJ, et al. Sparganosis infection presenting as a palpable mass in male breast. *Int J Infect Dis.* 2013;17:e663–e664.

66. Sloan BS, Rickman LS, Blau EM, et al. Schistosomiasis masquerading as carcinoma of the breast. *South Med J.* 1996;89:345–347.

67. Elma CA, Cavalcanti AC, Lima MM, et al. Pseudoneoplastic lesion of the breast caused by *Schistosoma mansoni*. *Rev Soc Bras Med Trop.* 2004;37:63–64.

68. Valdes PV, Prieto A, Diaz A, et al. Microcalcifications of pectoral muscle in trichinosis. *Breast J.* 2005;11:150.

69. de Barros N, D'Avila MS, de Pace Bauab S, et al. Cutaneous myiasis of the breast: mammographic and US features-report of five cases. *Radiology.* 2001;218:517–520.

70. Ugwu BT, Nwadiaro PO. *Cordylobia anthropophaga* mastitis mimicking breast cancer: a case report. *East Afr Med J.* 1999;76:115–116.

71. Adisa CA, Mbanaso A. Furuncular myiasis of the breast caused by the larvae of the Tumbu fly (*Cordylobia anthropophaga*). *BMC Surg.* 2004;4:5.

72. Konstantinopoulos PA, Dezube BJ, March D, et al. HIV-associated intra-mammary lymphadenopathy. *Breast J.* 2007;13:192–195.

73. Das DK, Rifaat AA, George SS, et al. Morphologic changes in fibroadenoma of breast due to chickenpox: a case report with suspicious cytology in fine needle aspiration smears. *Acta Cytol.* 2008;52:337–343.

4

Benign Papillary Tumors

FREDERICK C. KOERNER

INTRADUCTAL PAPILLOMA

A papilloma is a discrete benign tumor of the epithelium of mammary ducts. Papillomas most often arise from lactiferous ducts in the central part of the breast, but they can occur peripherally and in any quadrant. *Intracystic papilloma* is the designation applied to a papilloma protruding into a large, cystic cavity. Large, complex papillomas that have a cystic component have sometimes been referred to as *papillary cystadenomas,* whereas solid, noncystic papillomas have been variously classified as *ductal adenomas* or *solid papillomas.* An *adenomyoepithelioma* is a form of solid papilloma.

A *solitary papilloma* is a single discrete papillary tumor in one duct, whereas *multiple papillomas* grow as independent tumors and often occupy contiguous branches of the ductal system. Solitary papillomas are more common than multiple papillomas. The term *papillomatosis* has been used to refer to the presence of multiple papillomas as well as for the epithelial proliferation commonly known as usual ductal hyperplasia. Because of the possibility of confusion, one would do well to avoid the diagnosis of *papillomatosis* in most circumstances.

Clinical Presentation

Solitary papillomas occur at any age from infancy to the ninth decade, but they are most frequent in the sixth and seventh decades of life. Women with multiple papillomas tend to be younger than women with solitary papillomas, and the former most often present in their 40s and early 50s. Males with papillomas span the same age range as women (1,2). Papillomas may occur more frequently in African-American women than in women of other ethnicities (3).

Papillomas have developed in unusual settings. One report (4) documented the growth of a papilloma in residual breast tissue following a TRAM flap reconstruction. Three publications (5–7) describe the presence of papillomas in ectopic breast tissue in axillary lymph nodes of women with intramammary papillomas.

Central papillomas often provoke a discharge from the nipple. A bloody discharge occurs more commonly with papillary carcinomas than with papillomas, but degenerative changes in a papilloma can give rise to bleeding and a blood-stained discharge. A subareolar mass may be palpable. A papilloma in a 44-year-old man produced a hard, lobulated mass fixed to the chest wall (8). Multiple papillomas develop peripherally more often than centrally and typically present as palpable lesions.

Imaging Studies

Cystic, solitary papillary tumors may appear well circumscribed on mammography (9), but the presence of a cystic component is best appreciated by ultrasonography. The latter technique seems more sensitive than mammography for the detection of papillomas (10). Ductography may demonstrate the presence of a central papilloma, and MRI typically reveals duct dilation and the presence of small, oval, smoothly contoured, enhancing intraductal masses; however, papillomas do not always display these characteristic features. After a detailed mammographic and sonographic study of 40 papillary tumors, Lam et al. (11) concluded that "radiologic features are not sufficiently sensitive or specific to differentiate benign from malignant papillary lesions." By using a combination of both imaging modalities, the authors achieved a sensitivity of 61%, a specificity of 33%, a positive predictive value (PPV) of 85%, and a negative predictive value (NPV) of 13%.

Gross Pathology

Solitary papillomas may form clinically symptomatic tumors 1 cm or less in diameter, but the average size is 2 to 3 cm. Papillomas with a dominant cystic component may be as large as 20 cm (12).

In certain cases, a cyst formed by the dilated duct in which the papilloma arose accounts for a noticeable portion of the mass produced by a solitary papilloma. The cyst may contain clear fluid, bloody fluid, or clotted blood. The papilloma usually forms a single mural nodule protruding into the lumen, but multiple, separate or aggregated nodules are present occasionally. The papilloma grows as a bosselated, soft-to-firm, gray-to-reddish brown mass. Papillomas are well circumscribed, and they appear enclosed by a capsule formed by the duct wall and reactive changes in the surrounding tissue. The presence of multiple papillomas can sometimes be appreciated grossly when they form small, warty, gray-to-tan nodules in contiguous dilated ducts.

Microscopic Pathology

The basic microscopic structure of a papilloma consists of a layer of mammary epithelium supported by branching stromal fronds, which are attached to the duct wall at one or more points (**Figs. 4.1 and 4.2**). Epithelium lining the nonpapillary portion of the duct usually appears unremarkable or slightly hyperplastic (**Fig. 4.3**).

39

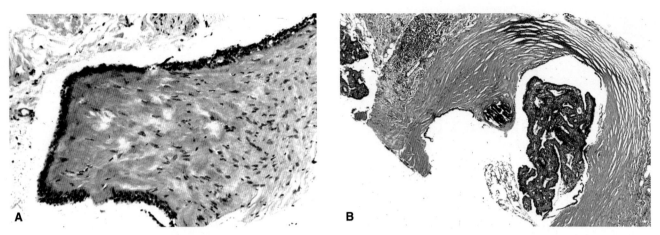

FIGURE 4.1 Intracystic Papilloma. A: This is a fragment of cyst wall surrounded a papilloma in a needle core biopsy specimen. **B:** The sample displays a portion of an intracystic papilloma and the surrounding cyst wall. Note the calcification in the cyst wall at the center of the image.

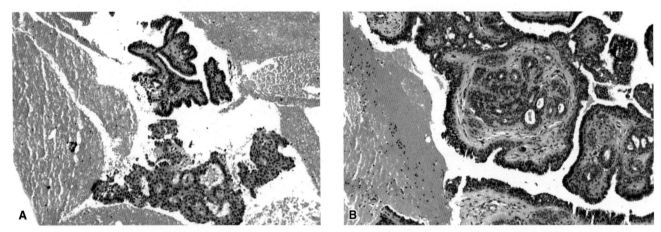

FIGURE 4.2 Papilloma. A, B: One can see detached papillary epithelial fragments in this needle core biopsy specimen. Samples such as this one are usually obtained from a cystic papilloma. Note the simple surface epithelium showing minimal hyperplasia and the distinct fibrovascular stroma.

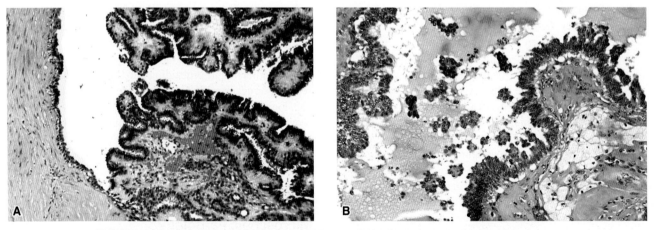

FIGURE 4.3 Papilloma. A: This needle core biopsy sample shows a cyst wall and papillary fronds extending into the lumen. The epithelium lining the cyst between the papillary fronds is not hyperplastic. **B:** The epithelium of this papilloma demonstrates slight micropapillary hyperplasia. The stroma of the papilloma contains histiocytes with clear cytoplasm.

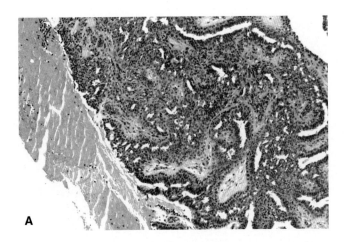

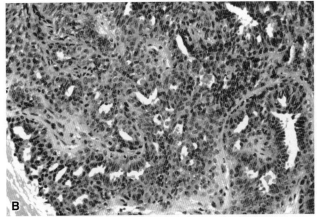

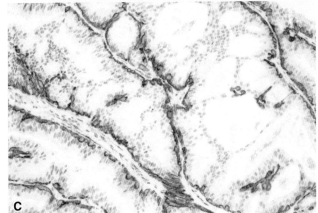

FIGURE 4.4 Papilloma with Ductal Hyperplasia.
A, B: Hyperplasia in a needle core biopsy sample is manifested by increased thickness of the epithelial layer and bridging of the epithelium across the spaces between fronds resulting in the formation of microlumina. **C:** Myoepithelium is demonstrated by reactivity for SMA.

Superimposed secondary processes such as ductal epithelial hyperplasia and stromal overgrowth can mask the underlying papillary architecture of a papilloma and thereby impede recognition of its presence. Secondary microlumina can develop within the hyperplastic epithelium, and micropapillary ductal hyperplasia may be present **(Fig. 4.4)**. Proliferation of glands within the fibrovascular cores results in a pattern resembling sclerosing adenosis **(Figs. 4.5–4.7)**. When glandular proliferation and ductal hyperplasia occur in concert, the hyperplastic ductal cells fill virtually all the space between stromal stalks, and the papilloma takes on a solid appearance **(Fig. 4.8)**.

The epithelium of the typical papilloma consists of both luminal and myoepithelial cells. The luminal cells are cuboidal to columnar, and they display little pleomorphism, nuclear hyperchromasia, or mitotic activity. Apocrine metaplasia occurs in many papillomas **(Fig. 4.9)**, and rarely nearly all or all the epithelium is of the apocrine type (13). In most papillomas, the apocrine cells appear bland, but occasionally atypical

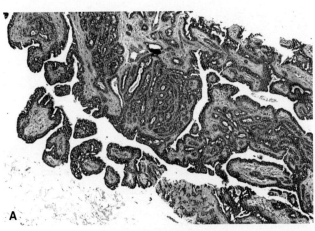

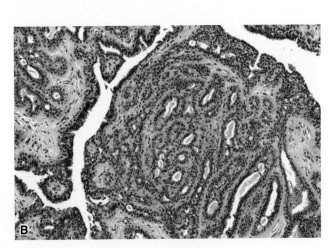

FIGURE 4.5 Papilloma with Adenosis. **A, B:** Hyperplasia in this needle core sample takes the form of nodular adenosis within the fibrovascular stroma. The surface epithelium is focally hyperplastic.

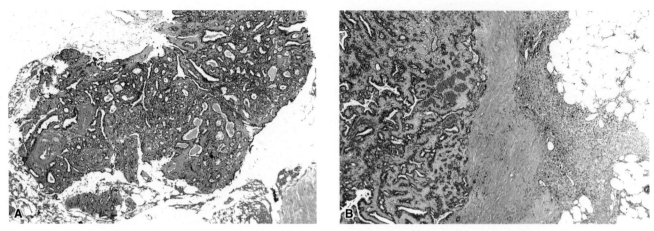

FIGURE 4.6 Papilloma with Adenosis. A: This needle core biopsy sample was obtained from a mammographically detected circumscribed papillary tumor. The mass consists almost entirely of small adenosis-type glands embedded in stroma. **B:** The excision specimen is shown. The scarring around the papilloma is attributable to the needle core biopsy.

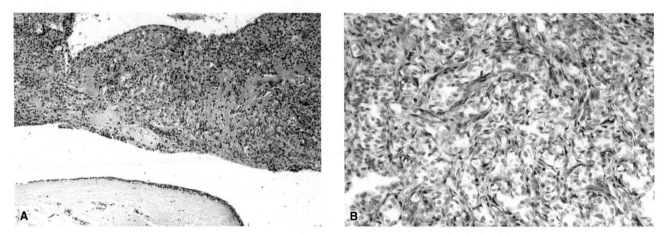

FIGURE 4.7 Cystic Papilloma with Florid Adenosis. A: This needle core biopsy sample contains a compact proliferation of adenosis in which the glands lack lumina. Part of the cyst wall is shown at the lower border. **B:** The immunostain for SMA highlights myoepithelial cells around the glands.

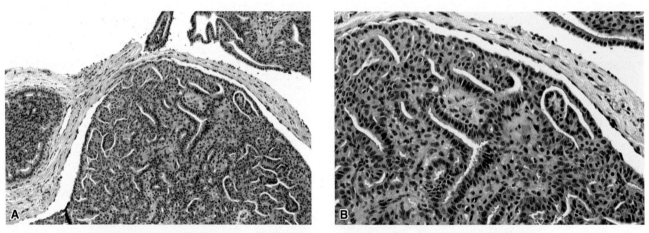

FIGURE 4.8 Solid Papilloma. A, B: The papilloma in this needle core biopsy sample displays a multinodular circumscribed architecture. Epithelial hyperplasia fills the spaces between the fibrovascular cores. **C:** An area in another biopsy sample shows solid epithelial hyperplasia and inconspicuous fibrovascular cores. **D:** Florid epithelial hyperplasia masks the underlying papillary architecture of this solid papilloma. Histiocytes help to identify the fibrovascular stromal cores.

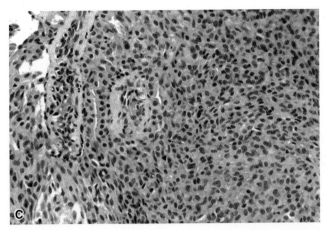
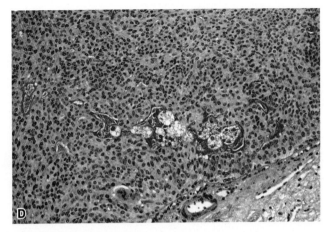

FIGURE 4.8 (continued)

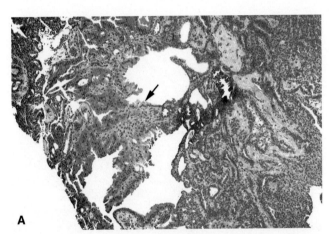
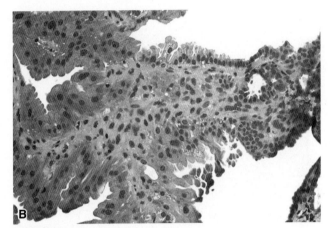

FIGURE 4.9 Papilloma with Apocrine Metaplasia. A, B: Metaplastic apocrine cells mingle with hyperplastic ductal cells in this needle core biopsy sample of a papilloma. The junction of the two types of epithelium is shown by the arrow in **(A)** and at higher magnification in **(B)**.

apocrine cells can be seen showing nuclear pleomorphism or cytoplasmic clearing can be seen. These atypical apocrine cells often occur in the sclerosing papillary tumors and in areas of sclerosing adenosis incorporated into papillomas (14). The presence of cytologically bland or mildly atypical apocrine epithelium almost always indicates that a papillary tumor is benign. Sebaceous metaplasia of the luminal cells of a papilloma has been reported (15).

The myoepithelial cells vary in their appearance and their distribution. Quiescent myoepithelial cells usually number only a few and appear flattened along the basement membrane, whereas hyperplastic myoepithelial cells form a prominent layer of cuboidal cells possessing clear cytoplasm **(Fig. 4.10)**. Certain papillomas have markedly hyperplastic myoepithelial cells that assume an epithelioid appearance **(Figs. 4.11 and 4.12)**. In this setting, the differential diagnosis includes adenomyoepithelioma. Myoepithelial cells are not equally apparent in all portions of a papilloma. They may become noticeably attenuated and focally undetectable even with the use of immunostains in sclerotic regions of a papilloma. The focal absence of myoepithelium, by itself, does not establish the diagnosis of carcinoma.

The appearance of the fibrovascular stroma varies considerably among papillomas. In some lesions, slender inconspicuous strands consisting of thin-walled capillaries, sparse fibroblasts, collagen, and mononuclear cells form the stromal network. The architecture and distribution of the stroma stands out especially clearly in sections stained for reticulin, vimentin, basement membrane proteins, or vascular markers such as CD34 and CD31. Expansion of the fibrovascular stroma by accumulated histiocytes occurs in papillomas but occurs only exceedingly rarely in papillary carcinomas (see **Figs. 4.3B and 4.8D**).

Collagenization of the fibrovascular stroma occurs in some papillomas. The papillary architecture is accentuated when this process is limited to the intrinsic papillary structure. If myofibroblastic proliferation accompanies collagenization of the stroma, the papillary arrangement is likely to become distorted **(Fig. 4.13)**. Epithelial elements entrapped in this stroma within or at the periphery of the lesion may simulate invasive carcinoma **(Fig. 4.14)**. In the most extreme situations, fibrous sclerosis is so severe as to virtually obliterate the papilloma, reducing it to a nodular scar containing sparse benign glandular elements. Such a lesion may be difficult to distinguish from a fibroadenoma.

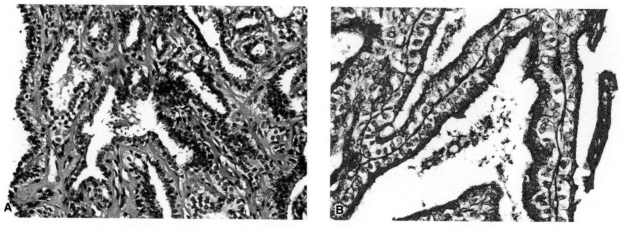

FIGURE 4.10 **Papillomas with Prominent Myoepithelial Cells.** **A, B:** Myoepithelial cells with clear cytoplasm outline glands in these needle core biopsy samples from two papillomas.

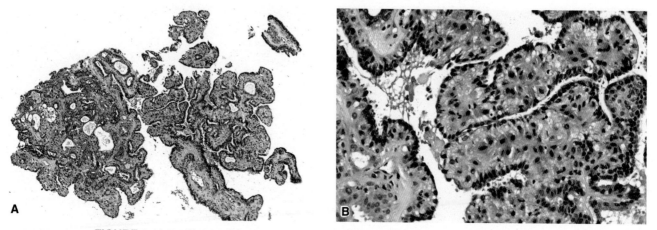

FIGURE 4.11 **Papilloma with Hyperplastic Myoepithelial Cells.** **A, B:** Clusters of myoepithelial cells with epithelioid and myoid appearances fill the subepithelial space in this needle core biopsy sample.

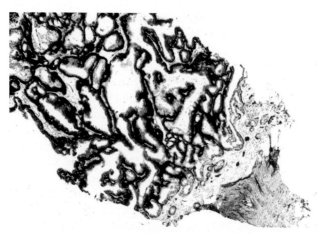

FIGURE 4.12 **Papilloma with Myoepithelial Cell Hyperplasia.** An actin stain highlights the hyperplastic myoepithelial cells in this sample.

Infarction occurs in solitary and multiple papillomas (**Fig. 4.15**). It can occur as a result of a biopsy; however, in most cases, one cannot identify a specific cause for the phenomenon. The presence of chronic inflammation and hemosiderin in

and around many papillomas suggests that these lesions are prone to transient bleeding. Spontaneous infarction usually involves superficial portions of a papilloma. Rarely, the entire lesion is infarcted. The underlying structure of a fully infarcted papilloma can be demonstrated with a reticulin stain. Sometimes immunoreactivity for cytokeratin or p63 is preserved in infarcted portions of a papilloma (16). There is no procedure for reliably distinguishing a completely infarcted papilloma from a papillary carcinoma; however, if one can demonstrate myoepithelium in the infarcted tissue, the tumor is more likely to be a papilloma than a papillary carcinoma. Cytologic atypia manifested by nuclear hyperchromasia and pleomorphism in the partially degenerated epithelium adjacent to infarcts can be commonly observed. These cytologic abnormalities may lead to an erroneous diagnosis of carcinoma in an FNA sample or a needle core biopsy (NCB) specimen.

Squamous metaplasia can occur in the epithelium of a papilloma (**Fig. 4.16**). It is more likely to be found when there is infarction. In this setting, the phenomenon probably represents a reactive or reparative process (17). Rarely, squamous metaplasia constitutes a conspicuous component of the papilloma or of the epithelium lining the cystic portion of the

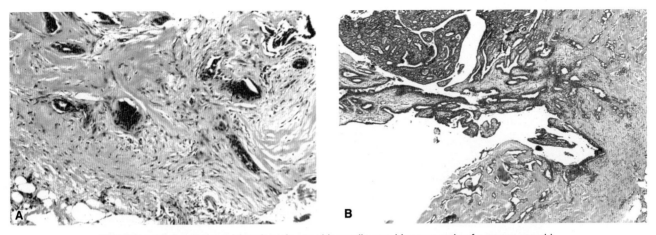

FIGURE 4.13 Papilloma with Sclerosis. A: This needle core biopsy sample of a mammographically detected circumscribed mass shows small nests of epithelial cells in collagenized stroma. This pattern can easily be mistaken for invasive carcinoma. **B:** The subsequent excision revealed a partly cystic papilloma. One can see that the epithelial clusters seen in **(A)** represent benign glands trapped within the mural sclerosis.

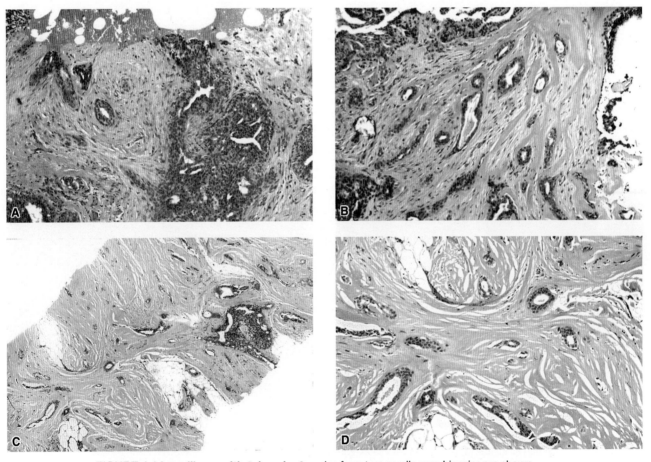

FIGURE 4.14 Papilloma with Sclerosis. Samples from two needle core biopsies are shown. **A:** This tissue has an area of papillary hyperplasia in sclerotic stroma. Note the epithelium cut tangentially as it protrudes into the stroma. This appearance should not be interpreted as invasive carcinoma. **B:** The cords of cells mostly appear distributed in parallel arrays between bands of collagenized stroma. The glands with angular contours resemble tubular carcinoma. Myoepithelial cells are inconspicuous. **C, D:** These needle core biopsy samples from a markedly sclerotic papillary lesion were mistaken for tubular carcinoma. Immunostains (not shown) revealed myoepithelium around the glandular elements.

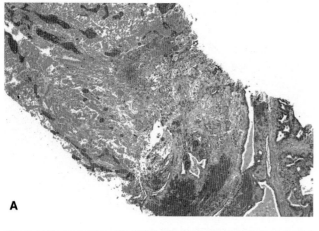

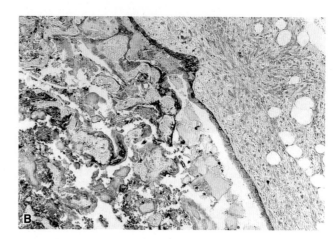

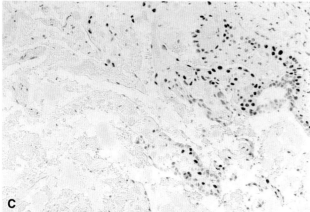

FIGURE 4.15 Papilloma with Infarction. This needle core biopsy sample was obtained from a patient with bloody nipple discharge and a mammographically detected nonpalpable mass. A needling procedure was not performed before the needle core biopsy. **A:** The ghost architecture of a papillary lesion is evident in this almost completely infarcted sample. **B:** A stain for CD10 reveals myoepithelial cells abutting the fibrovascular stroma of the papillary tumor and along the wall of the dilated duct. **C:** Myoepithelial cell nuclei are reactive for p63 in part of the infarcted lesion.

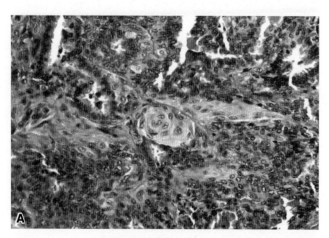

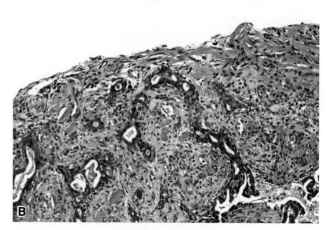

FIGURE 4.16 Papilloma with Squamous Metaplasia. A: A nest of squamous cells is present among the hyperplastic cells of the papillary glandular epithelium. **B–D:** This needle core biopsy sample from a sclerosing papilloma has focal squamous metaplasia **(D)**. The biopsy was misinterpreted as infiltrating carcinoma with squamous differentiation.

lesion. Extension of squamous metaplasia to the epithelium of adjacent ducts is an uncommon finding. Metaplastic epithelium entrapped in the stromal reaction may simulate metaplastic squamous carcinoma, and in some instances the distinction between metaplastic and neoplastic lesions is very difficult.

Like mammary epithelial cells in other locations, those within papillomas can give rise to neoplastic populations. As a rule,

the diagnostic criteria and analytic reasoning used for ductal and lobular proliferations arising in the usual settings apply when evaluating those involving a papilloma. The diagnosis of atypical ductal hyperplasia is appropriate for small collections of atypical ductal cells **(Fig. 4. 17)**. Expansive collections of atypical ductal cells and those with marked cytologic atypia merit the diagnosis of DCIS **(Fig. 4.18A)**. Chapter 11 discusses

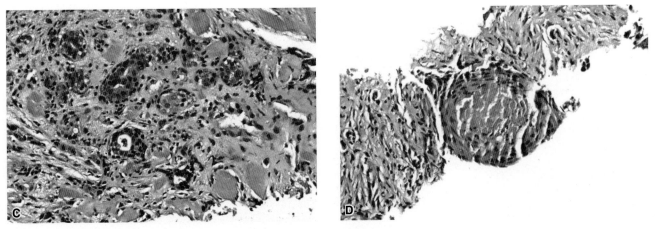

FIGURE 4.16 (*continued*)

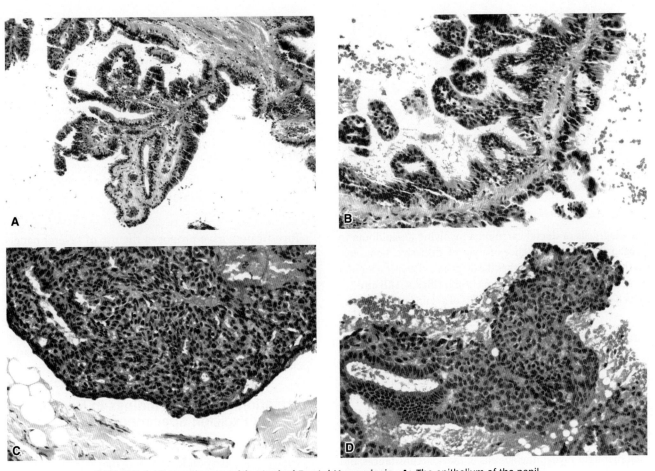

FIGURE 4.17 **Papillomas with Atypical Ductal Hyperplasia. A:** The epithelium of the papillary fronds in this part of the needle core biopsy sample consists of an orderly layer of columnar cells. **B:** This frond from the same biopsy sample exhibits atypical micropapillary hyperplasia. **C, D:** This needle core biopsy specimen contains detached epithelial fragments. Note the polarization of the cells forming the microlumina.

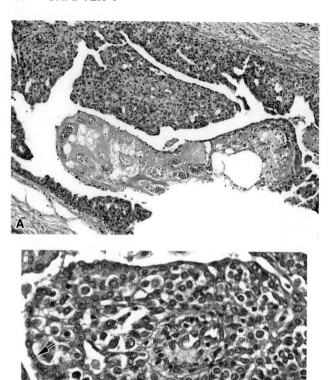

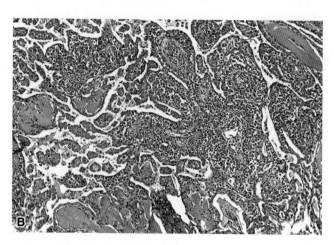

FIGURE 4.18 Papillomas with Carcinoma In Situ. A: The cells of intermediate-grade DCIS have completely overrun two fronds in this papilloma (**upper center and upper left**), and they focally involve the frond in the center of the field. Note the micropapillary DCIS in the lower left. Histiocytes in the stroma of the papillary frond in the center attest to the presence of the underlying benign papilloma. **B:** Neoplastic lobular cells mingle with the preexisting normal and hyperplastic ductal cells of this papilloma. **C:** This magnified view of an area in the upper right of (**B**) illustrates the dishesion and lack of polarization characteristic of neoplastic lobular cells, which form pagetoid nests in the epithelium of this papilloma. Attenuated remnants of the benign papillary epithelium are present (*arrows*).

the diagnosis of ductal carcinoma involving a papilloma in greater detail. The presence of atypical, dishesive, nonpolarized epithelial cells establishes the diagnosis of atypical lobular hyperplasia or lobular carcinoma in situ (**Figs. 4.18B and C**), which can be confirmed by the results of a stain for E-cadherin.

Immunohistochemistry

Immunohistochemical staining of papillomas reveals the results expected for mammary epithelial, myoepithelial, and stromal cells present apart from papillomas. The epithelial cells exhibit nuclear immunoreactivity for ER, which can appear either scattered or diffuse. Stains for actin (see **Fig. 4.12**), calponin, smooth muscle myosin heavy chain, CD10, p63, and CK5/6 will highlight myoepithelial cells in most circumstances, but the staining reactions differ somewhat depending on the choice of antibody. The transcription factor p63 resides in the nuclei of the myoepithelial cells, whereas the other proteins are found in the myoepithelial cytoplasm. Because these cytoplasmic proteins also occur in stromal and vascular cells to varying degrees, one could have difficulty distinguishing such cells from myoepithelial cells. To minimize this problem, it is advisable to include a stain for p63 among those chosen to detect myoepithelial cells. One must also remember that the p63 immunostain can stain the nuclei in a minor fraction of the neoplastic cells in a papillary carcinoma (18) and the nuclei of squamous cells.

Investigators have proposed the use of several panels of immunostains to aid in the distinction of papillomas from papillary carcinomas. These studies are summarized in Chapter 11. When using staining for CK5/6 to identify a neoplastic population in the setting of a papillary tumor, one must remember that conventional apocrine cells do not express this type of cytokeratin. The lack of CK5/6 staining can lead observers to misclassify apocrine cells as neoplastic ductal cells (13,19).

Correlation between Findings in Needle Core and Excision Specimens

The correlation between the findings in NCB and excision specimens of papillary tumors has been the subject of extensive investigation. Several recent publications tabulate data from many reports (20–22). A meta-analysis (23) using 34 relevant studies published between 1999 and 2012 revealed that 36.9% of papillomas with atypia demonstrated carcinoma in an excision specimen, whereas only 7.0% of papillomas lacking atypical cells did so.

Attempts to improve the predictive values of the findings present in NCB specimens by incorporating clinical or radiologic features in the analysis have not met with success. Several studies detected a higher likelihood of upgrade to carcinoma in older patients, but investigators have not discovered an age below which an excision would seem unnecessary. The size of the lesion has influenced the likelihood of detecting atypical cells in an excision specimen in certain studies but not in others. Many authors stress the need for careful correlation of the radiologic and pathologic findings, yet Bernik et al. (24) found that 9 of 17 benign papillomas with concordant radiologic studies proved to have ADH in the excision specimen and that 2 of the 17 contained carcinomas. Other authors report similar results.

Pathologists have searched for ways to improve their diagnostic abilities, and both the use of immunohistochemical stains and the expertise of pathologists have come under study. Shah et al. (25) reported that the use of immunohistochemical staining for calponin, CK5/6, and p63 allowed pathologists to recognize foci of ADH associated with papillomas. This technique improved the accuracy of all four participating pathologists to the point that the authors concluded that papillomas lacking atypia "do not require excision in the absence of suspicious clinical/radiological findings." Using a mixture of antisera to CK5, p63, and CK8/18 to stain NCB specimens and comparing the resulting diagnoses with those made on corresponding excision specimens, Reisenbichler et al. (19) correctly identified all 19 papillary carcinomas in their study group of 58 papillary tumors. Grin et al. (26) employed staining for CK5 and ER to identify the presence of atypical cells in NCB specimens of papillary tumors. This approach allowed the authors to classify NCB specimens of 15 of 15 papillomas and 14 of 15 papillary tumors containing atypical or malignant cells correctly when compared with the findings of excision specimens. Tse et al. (27) employed staining for ER, CK14, and p63 in an attempt to resolve discrepancies encountered in 15 NCB specimens. Although the use of these stains reduced the rate of discordance by 69%, the staining results did not eliminate either false-positive or false-negative cases.

The expertise of the pathologist influences the correlation between findings of NCB and excision specimens, but even experienced breast pathologists cannot exclude the presence of atypical cells in an excision specimen when examining a NCB specimen. In the study of Jakate et al. (28), diagnoses made by pathologists with fellowship training in breast pathology were less likely to differ from the diagnoses of the subsequent excision specimen than were diagnoses made by general pathologists; nevertheless, a substantial number of discrepancies remained. An upgrade rate of 26.3% was observed for diagnoses made by general pathologists, whereas a rate of 16.3% was observed for breast pathologists. Of the 86 cases in which breast pathologists made a diagnosis of benign papilloma on a NCB specimen, 10 excision specimens displayed atypia, and 3 showed carcinoma.

Prognosis

Papillomas do not recur except when incompletely excised. The development of subsequent papillomas is thought to represent the formation of independent, unrelated tumors.

Follow-up studies of patients with excised papillomas show that their presence indicates a slightly increased risk for the development of breast carcinoma. Moon et al. (29)

found that 4.3% of women with papillomas lacking atypia developed breast carcinoma. The relative risk (compared to women lacking suspicious findings on ultrasonography) was 4.8. When stratified by age, the relative risk for women older than 40 years was 5.1, whereas in women younger than 40 years, the presence of a papilloma without atypia did not increase the risk for breast carcinoma. The carcinomas arose in both breasts with equal frequency. MacGrogan and Tavassoli (30) studied the follow-up of 119 patients who underwent excisions of papillary breast tumors. Approximately 5% of women with benign papillomas or papillomas with "focal atypia" developed breast carcinoma at intervals between 3 and 14 years. Approximately 10% of women whose papillomas showed significant atypia developed breast carcinoma during the same span. The authors noted that the atypical cells in most cases were confined to the papilloma and that the excision seemed to have removed the entire proliferative population. The study by Cuneo et al. (31) demonstrated similar outcomes: the 5-year risk for the development of noninvasive or invasive carcinoma in either breast was 4.6% for patients with a papilloma without atypia and 13% for patients with a papilloma with atypia.

It is important to note that in all three foregoing studies, the carcinomas arose in the breasts contralateral to the ones harboring the papillomas as frequently as they did in the ipsilateral breasts. These findings would seem to indicate that the presence of a solitary papilloma poses only a very low risk for the development of an ipsilateral carcinoma and that papillomas do not give rise to carcinomas very often. The presence of a solitary papilloma may foretell a slightly heightened propensity for the entirety of the mammary tissue to develop neoplastic proliferations, but the papilloma itself does not represent a clinically significant premalignant lesion.

A greater risk for concurrent (32) or subsequent carcinoma has been demonstrated in women with multiple papillomas compared to women with solitary papillomas (33), and women with multiple papillomas are at risk to develop carcinoma in the contralateral breast (32). Lewis et al. (34) examined the follow-up of patients with solitary and multiple papillomas treated at the Mayo Clinic and determined the risk for developing breast carcinoma by comparison with an age- and calendar-period-matched cohort from the SEER database. The authors reported standardized incidence rates for breast carcinoma for women with solitary or multiple papillomas without atypia of 2.04 and 3.01, respectively. For women with solitary or multiple papillomas with atypia, the corresponding values were 5.11 and 7.01, respectively. In the study by Moon et al. (29), the relative risks posed by peripheral and central papillomas (5.2 and 4.8, respectively) did not differ across the entire cohort, but they did differ in younger women. In women younger than 40 years, the presence of a peripheral papilloma indicated a relative risk for developing breast carcinoma of 13.2 compared to a relative risk of 2.1 associated with a central papilloma. The corresponding relative risks for women older than 40 years are 4.0 and 5.8.

Treatment

Data from the foregoing studies do not provide definitive guidelines for the management of a papilloma without atypia diagnosed by NCB. A decision regarding the need for surgical excision will be influenced by factors such as the size of the lesion, techniques used during the NCB, evidence of residual tumor following the biopsy, the ease of mammographic follow-up, family history of breast carcinoma, and patient concerns, among others. For example, Jaffer et al. (35) did not detect atypia in excision specimens from 14 women in whom NCB specimens demonstrated papillomas lacking atypia spanning 0.2 cm or small and not representing the abnormality targeted by the radiologists. The authors concluded that such papillomas do not require excision. It has also been suggested that the vacuum-assisted biopsy technique provides sufficient sampling of a lesion that an excision is unnecessary in certain circumstances (36,37). In most studies, excisions have been carried out as surgical procedures, but several researchers (38–40) report results that raise the possibility that one can use the vacuum-assisted technique rather than a surgical excision to remove the entire abnormality.

Many published reports include follow-up data of patients who did not undergo an excision following the diagnosis of benign papilloma on a NCB specimen. Most studies involve small numbers of patients, but in several recent ones (21,36,37,41,42) the study groups contain 50 or more patients. Among this aggregate of more than 1,000 women, approximately 2% developed carcinoma. Follow-up periods ranged from 2 to 5 years, and the nature of the follow-up varied. These variations, among many other aspects of the studies, make it impossible to draw secure conclusions about the safety of careful clinical surveillance as an alternative to excision of papillomas diagnosed by means of a NCB. A conservative approach may prove safe, but investigators have not formulated the criteria to identify either the appropriate patients or the details of the program of surveillance.

Among women recommended for follow-up without an initial surgical excision, some will require surgical biopsy at a later date. In a series studied by Sexton et al. (43), 59 of 78 (75%) patients with a papilloma diagnosed by NCB did not undergo surgical biopsy and were followed up for 3 to 5 years. Subsequent interval mammographic changes necessitated surgical excision in 10 of the 59 (17%), and 2 (3%) had a subsequent NCB. All subsequent biopsies were reportedly "benign." This study suggests that up to 20% of patients enrolled in follow-up after a NCB diagnosis of papilloma will undergo another biopsy within 5 years of the initial procedure. The long-term risk for the development of carcinoma at the site of an incompletely excised papilloma that was sampled by NCB has not been determined.

COLLAGENOUS SPHERULOSIS

This structural alteration of unknown histogenesis represents an incidental microscopic finding. It occurs as a component of another benign breast lesion such as a papilloma, adenomyoepithelioma, fibroadenoma, or sclerosing adenosis (44–48). Rarely, the collagenous spherulosis constitutes the dominant alteration (49,50).

First described by Clement et al. in 1987 (51), this lesion features nodules of eosinophilic or basophilic basement membrane material enclosed in round spaces. Because of a superficial resemblance to adenoid cystic carcinoma, the term *adenoid cystic hyperplasia* was previously used for this condition (52). Resetkova et al. (45) summarized the clinical and morphologic features of 59 cases identified at a single institution and tabulated data from 61 cases reported prior to 2005.

Clinical Presentation

One has difficulty determining the frequency of collagenous spherulosis, because the lesion often goes unrecognized or is misinterpreted (53). Estimates place the frequency of the lesion at less than 1% of excision specimens (54). Collagenous spherulosis affects women throughout adulthood; the ages of patients in reported cases range from 19 years (55) to 90 years (45). The literature does not contain reports of collagenous spherulosis in men.

The clinical presentation of collagenous spherulosis depends upon the nature of the underlying lesion. Patients may complain of a mass, but more often the underlying lesion is detected by imaging studies.

Imaging Studies

Radiologic imaging of collagenous spherulosis may demonstrate either calcifications or a mass, but the images do not have distinctive features.

Gross Pathology

The small size of most examples of collagenous spherulosis precludes macroscopic recognition of the foci. In one case (49), the authors described a nodule formed by collagenous spherulosis as a ". . . ovoid, well-circumscribed, unencapsulated, pale tan solid mass measuring 1.0 cm × 0.9 cm." In this instance, the underlying mass was nodular adenosis.

Microscopic Pathology

Spherules composed of acellular material surrounded by epithelial cells constitute the defining features of collagenous spherulosis (**Figs. 4.19 and 4.20**). The spherules, which measure 20 to 100 μm in diameter, may be eosinophilic, amphophilic, or nearly transparent. Certain spherules appear as dense as the cylindromatous deposits in adenoid cystic carcinoma. On the other hand, the centers of the spherules sometimes look nearly transparent, and stellate fibrils may be seen radiating from a central nidus to the periphery. Degenerative changes in the spherules can result in the loss of the radial structure and create a lumen-like space; however, at least a thin rim of basement membrane material encompassed by a ring of myoepithelial cells always remains. At times, this layer

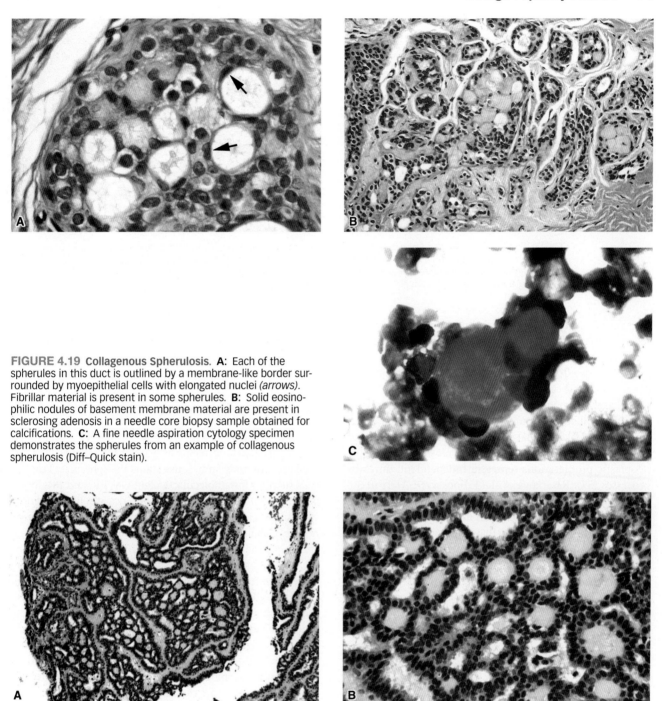

FIGURE 4.19 Collagenous Spherulosis. **A:** Each of the spherules in this duct is outlined by a membrane-like border surrounded by myoepithelial cells with elongated nuclei *(arrows)*. Fibrillar material is present in some spherules. **B:** Solid eosinophilic nodules of basement membrane material are present in sclerosing adenosis in a needle core biopsy sample obtained for calcifications. **C:** A fine needle aspiration cytology specimen demonstrates the spherules from an example of collagenous spherulosis (Diff–Quick stain).

FIGURE 4.20 Collagenous Spherulosis in a Papilloma. **A, B:** The spherules are round, weakly eosinophilic bodies in the epithelium. Myoepithelial cells are, for the most part, inconspicuous, but they can be seen rimming spherules in the lower right corner of **(B)**. The true empty glandular lumina have irregular contours.

collapses into the cystic spherule **(Fig. 4.21)**. Constituents of the spherules include components of basement membranes: elastin, PAS-positive polysaccharides, type IV collagen, and laminin (49,54,56).

Myoepithelial cells and luminal cells contribute to the formation of collagenous spherulosis, and these cells give rise to two types of spaces. Myoepithelial cells constitute the dominant population. They have long spindly shapes, flattened oval hyperchromatic nuclei, and attenuated eosinophilic cytoplasm that is sometimes referred to as a "cuticle." The myoepithelial cells create the nearly round spaces that enclose the spherules. The attenuated myoepithelial cells may be difficult to identify in H&E sections, but immunostains will highlight them. Collections of cuboidal luminal cells containing bland nuclei, inconspicuous nucleoli, and dense eosinophilic cytoplasm form glands interspersed among the myoepithelial cells and

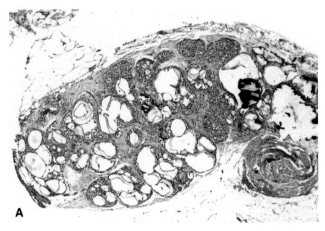
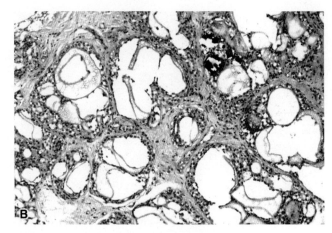

FIGURE 4.21 Collagenous Spherulosis with Degenerative Changes. A, B: The spherules in this case of collagenous spherulosis have undergone cystic degeneration. Detached strips of basement membrane material have collapsed into the cystic spherules. The biopsy was performed for mammographically detected calcifications, some of which are shown.

the spherules. These glands sometimes contain eosinophilic secretory material. This pattern of growth creates an adenoid cystic structural arrangement; however, the lumina of the glandular spaces tend to have more irregular shapes than those of adenoid cystic carcinoma.

Collagenous spherulosis usually occurs as a multifocal process, and papillomas account for the majority of the underlying lesions. Atypical epithelial proliferations and carcinomas can supervene in foci of collagenous spherulosis, but coexisting neoplastic proliferations represent independent, unrelated processes (57). Resetkova et al. (45) observed ADH in 3 of 59 (5%) cases and LCIS in 15 of 59 (25%) cases. When LCIS colonizes collagenous spherulosis and replaces the luminal cells, an appearance similar to that of low-grade DCIS results (45,58,59) **(Fig. 4.22)**.

With experience, the recognition of collagenous spherulosis does not pose problems, but the presence of two types of cells and spherules of basement membrane material can bring to

mind the diagnosis of adenoid cystic carcinoma. Immunohistochemical staining will distinguish these two entities. It will also allow one to differentiate collagenous spherulosis overrun by LCIS from low-grade DCIS.

Immunohistochemistry

The two types of cells stain in the expected ways. The myoepithelial cells stain for proteins such as SMA, p63, and CD10, and the latter antibody sometimes stains the spherules. Luminal cells stain for low-molecular-weight CK, ER, and PR. By using a panel of these markers and others, cases of collagenous spherulosis can be distinguished from adenoid cystic carcinomas. Cabibi et al. (60) found that the cells of collagenous spherulosis stained intensely for CD10, HHF35 actin, ER, and PR, whereas those of adenoid cystic carcinoma did not. Conversely, the cells of adenoid cystic carcinoma stained intensely for c-Kit (CD117), but the cells of collagenous spherulosis did so only weakly. Rabban et al. (61) pointed out that both lesions can express SMA, S-100, and p63 and suggested the use of staining for other myoepithelial proteins. These authors found that the cells of collagenous spherulosis stain intensely for calponin and smooth muscle myosin heavy chain and that those of adenoid cystic carcinoma do not.

Prognosis and Treatment

There is no evidence to indicate that the presence of collagenous spherulosis is associated with precancerous lesions (51,52), or that it is associated with adenoid cystic carcinoma. The prognosis and treatment of a patient with collagenous spherulosis depends on the nature of the associated lesion.

FIGURE 4.22 Collagenous Spherulosis with In Situ Carcinoma. Lobular carcinoma *in situ* has filled and expanded the epithelium between spherules. Note the loss of cohesion between the neoplastic cells and the fine filamentous material in some spherules.

RADIAL SCLEROSING LESION

Radial sclerosing lesions (RSLs) are proliferative abnormalities that have a stellate configuration radiologically and histologically.

Clinical interest in RSLs derives from the realization that these abnormalities may be difficult to distinguish from carcinoma by mammography and the concern that they are precursors for the development of carcinoma.

RSLs have been described by a variety of names introduced since the 1970s. Sclerosing papillary proliferation, complex sclerosing lesion, nonencapsulated sclerosing lesion, infiltrating epitheliosis, and indurative mastopathy represent just a few of the proposed terms. *Radial scar*, a widely used designation for this lesion, is a translation of "strahlige Narben," the term Hamperl (62) introduced in 1975. This name makes reference to the stellate shape of the typical example; it is short; and it avoids terminology that suggests an association with particular proliferative ductal lesions. However, inclusion of the word, "scar," in the diagnosis implies that the changes represent a reparative process. Although the stellate configuration has a cicatrix-like appearance, it is possible that the stromal change is an integral part of the proliferative lesion rather than a reparative process. The term used here, *radial sclerosing lesion*, is preferable because it describes the mammographic and histologic appearance of the process without implying a histogenesis; furthermore, this designation is sufficiently general that it encompasses the many histologic variants included in this category. RSLs are discussed in this chapter devoted to benign papillary tumors because many include a papillary component.

Clinical Presentation

Most RSLs are microscopic lesions not detectable by palpation or mammography. They are usually discovered during examination of specimens resected for unrelated indications. Consequently, the distribution of the ages of women with RSLs parallels that of women undergoing breast surgery. RSLs are uncommon before the age of 30 years and most frequent between the ages of 40 and 60 years. The reported frequency of incidental lesions varies depending upon the groups of patients studied and the diagnostic criteria. RSLs have been detected in 1.7% (63) to 28% (64) of benign breast specimens and in 4% (65) to 26% (66) of mastectomy specimens from patients with carcinomas. These data suggest that RSLs occur in women without carcinoma as frequently as they do in women with carcinomas. Multiple microscopic RSLs are not uncommon (67), and both breasts can be affected (64). A paper by Anderson and Battersby (68) describes a woman with 80 RSLs in her right breast and 46 in her left breast. RSLs virtually never affect men. One report (69) mentions in passing the presence of a RSL in the breast of a man with breast carcinoma.

Imaging Studies

Most RSLs are smaller than 2 cm when detected radiologically. Typical lesions are characterized by a lucent or dense center, radiating slender strands of tissue, and changes in appearance in different imaging projections. Microcalcifications are detected in some but not all RSLs. When evident using sonography, RSLs form an irregular hypoechogenic mass with ill-defined borders and diminished posterior acoustic transmission. Tomosynthesis may offer an especially sensitive technique for the detection of RSLs (70). Certain radiologic features favor the diagnosis of a RSL over a stellate carcinoma, but these are not sufficiently distinctive to serve as the basis for a specific diagnosis. MRI findings may help to differentiate RSLs from invasive carcinomas (71).

Gross Pathology

The typical RSL demonstrates macroscopic characteristics similar to those of a small invasive carcinoma. The nodule feels firm, and it contains a pale, retracted center in which white streaks may be seen. Slender radial bands of pale stroma extend from the core into the fat. Small cysts can be appreciated in some lesions. A minority of RSLs lacks a distinct stellate configuration; instead, they present as ill-defined firm areas or circumscribed nodules.

Microscopic Pathology

Andersen et al. (72) described the histologic appearance of the RSL as "a distinct histologic structure, characterized by a sclerotic center with a central core containing obliterated duct(s), elastin deposits, and mostly infiltrating tubules and the center is surrounded by a corona of contracted ducts and lobules, which may show different types of proliferative lesions." Dense collagen, elastic tissue, and sparse stromal cells make up the nidus of the usual, well-established scar **(Fig. 4.23)**. The elastic tissue, which one can highlight with an elastic stain, consists of dense, sometimes granular, weakly eosinophilic material in the walls of ducts and the stroma. The fibroelastotic stroma typically entraps distorted small glands. A corona of ducts, terminal duct–lobular units, and cysts arrayed in a radial orientation around the nidus is created by incorporation of these structures from the surrounding tissue. The glandular tissue displays varying degrees of usual ductal hyperplasia, sclerosing adenosis, and cyst formation, and small papillomas are frequently present **(Fig. 4.24)**. The peripheral zone can also include nonproliferative ducts and lobules, and cysts occasionally make up most or all of the corona. The proliferative zone sometimes appears asymmetrical because of off-center planes of sectioning or intrinsic differences among lesions **(Fig. 4.25)**, and occasional RSLs lack a corona entirely.

The epithelium within a RSL can exhibit a range of changes. Apocrine metaplasia frequently occurs in the cysts of RSLs, and occasionally it may be present more widely in the proliferative component, especially in areas of sclerosing adenosis. Clear cell change and nuclear atypia are not uncommon in apocrine epithelium. Squamous metaplasia occurs infrequently in RSLs. Examples with squamous metaplasia may resemble metaplastic carcinoma, especially low-grade adenosquamous carcinoma.

The fibrous reaction associated with RSLs typically entraps small ductules. Similar to nests of epithelium trapped in the stroma at the peripheries of sclerosing papillomas, those in a RSL simulate invasive carcinoma. This is an important consideration when examining NCB samples. The presence of a

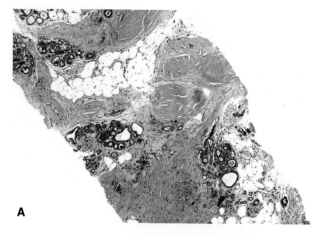

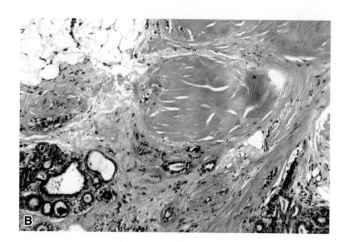

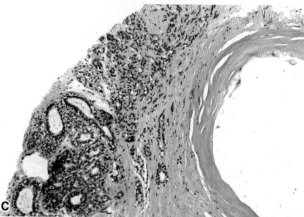

FIGURE 4.23 Radial Sclerosing Lesion. A, B: This needle core biopsy sample has a central sclerotic zone consisting of dense collagenous tissue surrounded by microcysts with calcifications. **C:** A peripheral portion of the same lesion displays prominent sclerosing adenosis and a cyst devoid of epithelium. Portions of the adenosis are attenuated and resemble infiltrating lobular carcinoma.

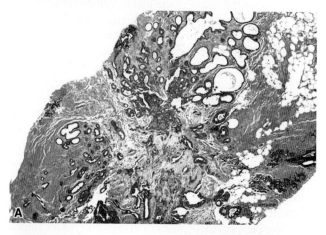

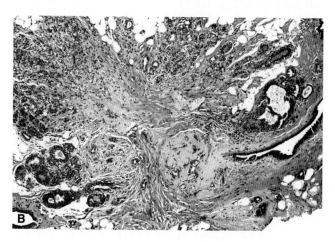

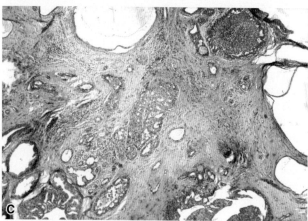

FIGURE 4.24 Radial Sclerosing Lesions. A, B: These small radial sclerosing lesions were entirely removed in the needle core biopsy samples. **C:** Cyst formation and papillary ductal hyperplasia contribute to the proliferative zone of this radial sclerosing lesion.

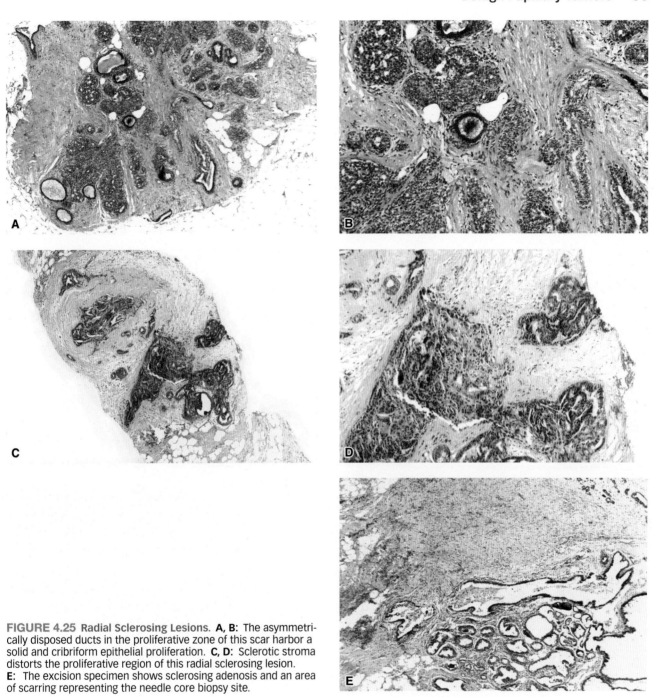

FIGURE 4.25 Radial Sclerosing Lesions. A, B: The asymmetrically disposed ducts in the proliferative zone of this scar harbor a solid and cribriform epithelial proliferation. **C, D:** Sclerotic stroma distorts the proliferative region of this radial sclerosing lesion. **E:** The excision specimen shows sclerosing adenosis and an area of scarring representing the needle core biopsy site.

myoepithelial cell layer characterizes epithelial entrapment within a RSL and thereby helps to avoid an erroneous diagnosis of invasive carcinoma. Ductules in the center of a RSL may lack myoepithelial cells; consequently, this finding does not establish the diagnosis of invasive carcinoma. Less than approximately 5% of RSLs demonstrate entrapment of small nerves (73). They are probably incorporated into RSLs by the same mechanism that is responsible for this phenomenon in other sclerosing lesions.

Sections of a RSL in a relatively early phase of development reveal branching and budding ductal structures in the core. The ductal epithelial proliferation in the proliferative zone can appear especially florid and can display necrosis. The stroma appears cellular, and the extracellular matrix appears myxoid rather than collagenous. Many of the stromal cells are myofibroblasts. They surround the ductal structures and extend in radiating bands toward the periphery. Small collections of lymphocytes and plasma cells often sit at the junction of the fat and the fibrous connective tissue. Conspicuous lymphocytic aggregates are uncommon in typical RSLs, and their presence may indicate a low-grade adenosquamous carcinoma.

RSLs usually occur as isolated, separate lesions, but occasionally, contiguous foci may be joined to form a larger complex and palpable mass in a fashion analogous to the formation of an adenosis tumor.

Ductal Hyperplasia and Carcinoma in Radial Sclerosing Lesions

Ductal proliferations in RSLs can take the form of florid and atypical hyperplasia as well as DCIS. Duct hyperplasia in a RSL may be solid, cribriform, micropapillary, or a combination of these structures (**Fig. 4.26**). Focal necrosis occurs in the hyperplastic duct epithelium of about 10% of

RSLs. The epithelial cells within these comedo-like foci are usually indistinguishable from those in hyperplastic foci lacking necrosis in the same RSL. Foci of ADH or ALH have been observed in 21% (74) to 51% (75) of RSLs. Often, the atypical cells are distributed in multiple tissue fragments in a NCB specimen. This disruption of the architecture of the lesion makes it difficult to determine the distribution and structural characteristics of the atypical population, and caution is warranted when considering a diagnosis of DCIS or invasive carcinoma in the setting of a sclerosing lesion in a NCB specimen (**Fig. 4.27**).

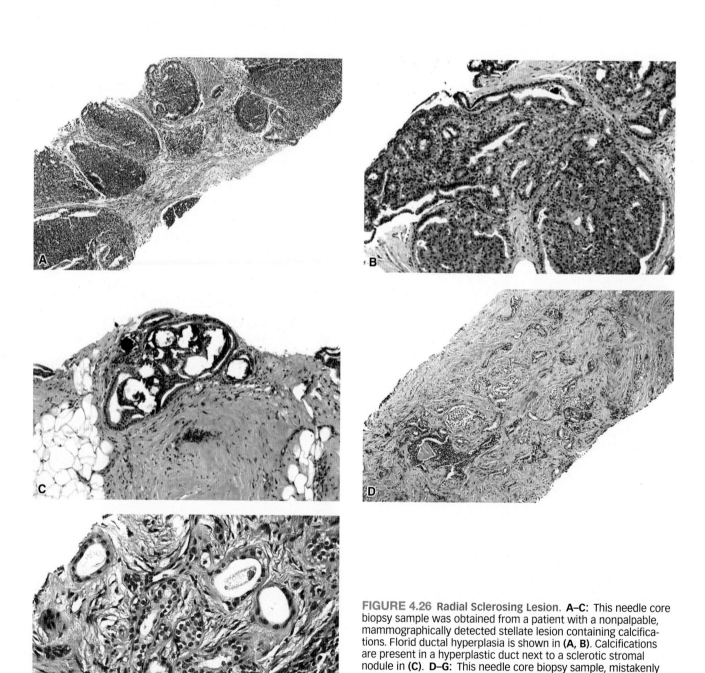

FIGURE 4.26 Radial Sclerosing Lesion. A–C: This needle core biopsy sample was obtained from a patient with a nonpalpable, mammographically detected stellate lesion containing calcifications. Florid ductal hyperplasia is shown in (**A, B**). Calcifications are present in a hyperplastic duct next to a sclerotic stromal nodule in (**C**). **D–G:** This needle core biopsy sample, mistakenly interpreted as invasive ductal carcinoma, was obtained from a radial sclerosing lesion with duct hyperplasia and adenosis. The adenosis architecture simulates the appearance of invasive ductal carcinoma (**D, E**). Myoepithelial cells highlighted by myosin (**F**) and p63 (**G**) immunostains surround the benign glands.

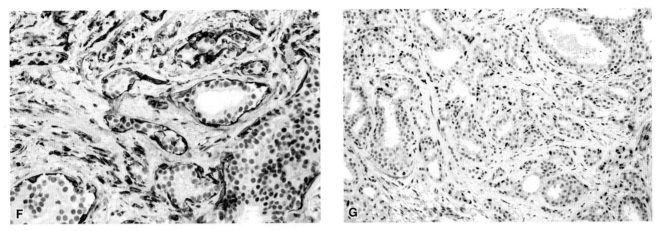

FIGURE 4.26 *(continued)*

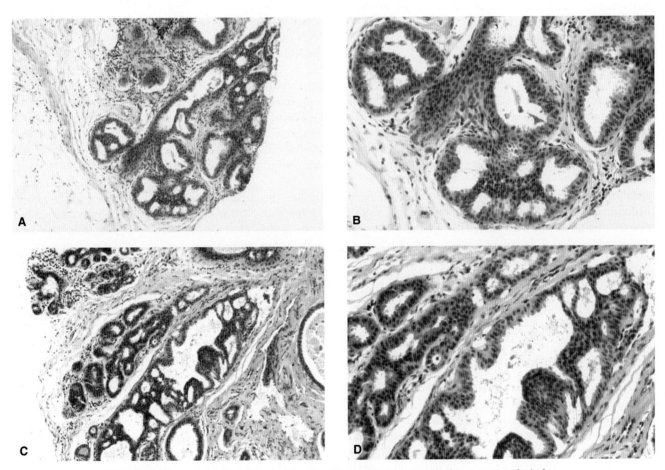

FIGURE 4.27 Radial Sclerosing Lesion with Atypical Duct Hyperplasia. **A–D:** Two foci of atypical micropapillary hyperplasia in peripheral portions of a radial sclerosing lesion are seen in these needle core biopsy samples. Note the radiating arrangement of the glands and the microcyst at the right border in **(C)**. These findings suggest the presence of an underlying radial sclerosing lesion. An excision showed only reactive changes at the biopsy site.

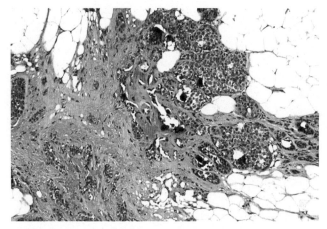

FIGURE 4.28 Radial Sclerosing Lesion with Carcinoma In Situ. A mammographically detected stellate mass with calcifications led to a needle core biopsy. Lobular carcinoma in situ fills glands with an adenosis pattern in sclerotic tissue in the right portion of the image.

The presence of carcinomas, including tubular carcinomas, in RSLs has been well documented (76), but the literature does not provide a coherent set of estimates of the frequency of this association. Values as high as 31% and 32% have been reported (74,77), and in one series, 28% of mammographically detected RSLs larger than 1 cm had foci of carcinoma (78). One finds carcinoma most frequently in RSLs larger than 0.6 cm (79) and in women older than 50 years (79,80). Both ductal and lobular carcinomas (**Fig. 4.28**) occur in RSLs, and the frequency of noninvasive carcinomas outweighs that of invasive carcinomas (73,74,79,80). The carcinomas usually involve only a small region of the RSL, sometimes as little as 5%, and they more frequently occupy the periphery rather than the center (73,79,80). Commonplace varieties of ductal and lobular carcinomas account for most malignancies seen in RSLs, but low-grade adenosquamous carcinomas sometimes develop in the setting of a RSL (81).

Immunohistochemistry

Myoepithelial cells can be demonstrated around the perimeter of most hyperplastic ducts in RSLs by means of immunostaining for p63, CD10, smooth muscle myosin heavy chain, or actin; however, in the central part of the lesion, myoepithelium may be substantially attenuated and even undetectable. The epithelial cells within RSLs and the proliferations derived from these cells display the staining characteristics seen in mammary epithelial cells in other locations. Stains for CK5/6, ER, and E-cadherin will usually allow one to classify epithelial proliferations involving RSLs.

Differential Diagnosis

A NCB usually provides a tissue sample that allows one to establish the diagnosis of a RSL, but one can misinterpret the distorted small glands or foci of sclerosing adenosis trapped in the stroma of a RSL as invasive carcinoma. The major consideration in the differential diagnosis of RSLs is tubular carcinoma. The glands in tubular carcinoma have round or distinctive angular shapes not ordinarily found in RSLs. The epithelium in tubular carcinomas lacks the myoepithelial layer usually present in the glands within RSLs. Because benign glands entrapped within the nidus of a RSL sometimes lack myoepithelial cells, one cannot rely solely on the absence of myoepithelium to distinguish a RSL from an invasive carcinoma. Permeation of the suspicious glands beyond the confines of the nidus and especially around ducts, within lobules, and into fat and the presence of cytologic atypia represent secure evidence of malignancy. The cystic and apocrine components of RSLs are absent from tubular carcinomas.

Correlation with Excision Specimens

Many studies have compared the pathologic findings in NCB specimens with those in subsequent excision samples. Bianchi et al. (82) tabulated the results of 21 studies reporting the frequency of carcinoma in excision specimens from patients in whom a NCB specimen demonstrated a RSL. The frequencies range from 0% to 40%, and the mean rate is 8.3%. DCIS accounts for 60% of the undetected carcinomas, IDC of no special type for 15%, tubular carcinoma for 10%, invasive lobular carcinoma for 5%, and other types of invasive and unclassified carcinomas for the remaining 10%.

When Conlon et al. (83) pooled data from 20 published studies, the authors calculated an average upgrade rate of 7.5% when a NCB specimen shows a RSL without atypia and a rate of 26% when the RSL harbors atypical cells. The same investigators studied 53 women with RSLs evaluated at their institution during a 17-year period. Excision of the RSLs was performed in 48 patients. Carcinoma, which took the form of DCIS, was present in just 1 (2%) of the 48 excision specimens. Twelve of the 48 (25%) excision specimens revealed epithelial atypia (flat epithelial atypia, atypical apocrine adenosis, ADH, or ALH) or LCIS. The authors noted that the upgrade rate of 2% in their study group falls well below the value of 7.5% derived from their analysis of 20 published studies. The writers attribute this low value to the detailed radiologic-pathologic correlation that they carried out. Other factors such as the technique used for the NCB and the extent of the sampling influence the likelihood of detecting carcinoma in the excision specimen, but neither clinical characteristics nor radiologic features has shown consistent predictive relationships.

Most published reports have centered on examples in which the RSLs represent the targeted abnormalities, but RSLs also occur as microscopic lesions seemingly entirely removed during the biopsy or in specimens sampled for unrelated indications. In one study (84) of 18 patients with microscopic RSLs without atypia mostly detected using a vacuum-assisted method, surgical excision did not disclose carcinoma in any; however, the excision specimens did contain ADH in 6 patients (33%) and atypical apocrine adenosis in another 6%. The study of Conlon et al. (83) included 18 RSLs not believed to represent the abnormalities targeted by the radiologists. The investigators identified epithelial atypia in 4 (22%) of the NCB specimens. The excision specimens did not disclose carcinoma in any of the 18 cases, nor did any of the patients develop carcinoma at the sites of the RSLs.

Treatment

Excision of a targeted RSL lacking an atypical epithelial proliferation diagnosed by NCB provides adequate treatment. Radiologists have used the vacuum-assisted technique in an effort to remove RSLs without atypia completely (85,86). This approach may prove a satisfactory alternative to surgical excision, but extended clinical follow-up and study of a large number of patients are required before reaching that conclusion.

It has been suggested that mammographic follow-up rather than surgical or radiologic excision can be recommended if the RSL in a NCB specimen from a mammographically detected incidental RSL does not contain atypical hyperplasia or in situ carcinoma (83,87). Certain authors recommend that at least 12 needle core samples be obtained (75,88), and many writers stress that the radiologic and pathologic findings must be concordant. Prospective long-term follow-up studies for women with RSLs diagnosed by NCB and not excised are not available, but several publications (70,83,87–89) report follow-up data of 123 such patients followed up for average periods of 29 to 49 months. No patient developed an invasive carcinoma at the site of the RSL.

Women with "incidental" RSLs detected in NCB samples may constitute an especially favorable group for radiologic follow-up rather than excision, but the literature contains only scanty data regarding the clinical significance of "incidental" RSLs detected by NCB. In two pertinent studies (83,84) comprising 36 patients, excisions did not disclose carcinoma in any of the cases. The excision samples did demonstrate epithelial atypia in approximately 20% to 40% of the cases.

Based on the current data, excision would be prudent for RSLs displaying epithelial atypia. If the RSL does not have an atypical component and there are no coexisting atypical proliferative lesions, the decision whether to recommend excision or follow-up should be made on a case-by-case basis. Factors to consider include prior biopsy findings, other factors predisposing to increased cancer risk such as family history, ease of clinical or radiologic follow-up, and the extent of removal of the targeted lesion by the NCB.

Prognosis

The presence of carcinoma or atypical hyperplasia in some RSLs and the architectural similarities between RSLs and invasive carcinomas led certain early observers to believe that RSLs represent a stage in the formation of invasive carcinomas. Subsequent morphologic and follow-up studies have not supported this belief. For example, two studies did not find significant differences in the number or frequency of RSLs in the breasts of women with and without carcinoma (68,90), and the morphologic features of RSLs from the breasts of women with carcinoma do not differ appreciably from comparable lesions not associated with carcinoma (68).

Other investigators have suggested that the presence of a RSL indicates a generalized heightened risk for the development of breast carcinoma, but the data relating to this notion are conflicting. One prospective investigation of 1,396 women with "radial scars" in excision specimens followed for a median of 12 years discovered a relative risk of 1.8 for the development of subsequent carcinoma for women with a "radial scar" compared to those not having a "radial scar" (91). The carcinomas arose in both breasts with equal frequency; so the authors concluded that "scars" constitute indicators of an increased risk for the development of breast carcinoma rather than direct precursors to carcinomas in most cases. An update of this study reaffirmed these findings (92). Several other studies (63,69,93–95), including one (94) involving 439 women followed up for a mean interval of 17 years, did not detect an increased risk for subsequent carcinomas for women with RSLs, nor did a meta-analysis (96) conducted using eligible studies published since 2000. RSLs frequently coexist with proliferative breast disease, including forms of atypical hyperplasia. The presence of ADH increases the risk for the development of carcinoma, but the presence of a coexisting RSL does not seem to increase this risk further (92–94,96). Data regarding the risk posed by a RSL in the setting of proliferative disease without atypia are conflicting. Two studies (92,96) suggest that the presence of a RSL indicates a heightened risk in this circumstance, whereas two others do not (93,94).

SUBAREOLAR SCLEROSING DUCTAL HYPERPLASIA

Subareolar sclerosing duct hyperplasia is a form of RSL that occurs immediately below the nipple (97). The lesion produces a tumor of the central or subareolar breast parenchyma without involving the substance of the nipple. The term subareolar sclerosing duct hyperplasia should be reserved for those lesions that constitute a clinicopathologic entity distinct from florid papillomatosis of the nipple.

Clinical Presentation

The age at diagnosis ranges from 26 to 73 years, averaging about 50 years. The left and right breasts are affected with equal frequency. The literature does not contain reports of bilateral subareolar sclerosing ductal hyperplasia.

The presenting symptom is a mass beneath the nipple or the areola, or both, or in the breast close to the areola. None of the lesions has been within the nipple. Erosion or ulceration of the nipple is absent. Nipple retraction may occur, and several patients have experienced bloody discharge. The mammographic findings have appeared nonspecific, and they may suggest carcinoma.

Gross Pathology

The excised lesion is a firm-to-hard, round or oval tumor with indistinct borders and measuring as much as 2.0 cm (average 1.2 cm). Yellow streaks may be noted in some examples. Because the lesion is located in the underlying mammary parenchyma, excisions typically have been performed using a periareolar incision without incising or removing the nipple. This aspect of the surgical approach is useful in the differential diagnosis of subareolar sclerosing duct hyperplasia and florid papillomatosis of the nipple.

Microscopic Pathology

The histologic structure of subareolar sclerosing duct hyperplasia is similar to that of RSLs in other parts of the breast. Sclerosis and elastosis are more marked toward the center of the tumor, whereas ductal hyperplasia is most prominent at the periphery (**Fig. 4.29**). Cartilaginous metaplasia, a rare occurrence in these lesions, typically occurs in the sclerotic core. In some cases, small hyperplastic ducts are seen at the margin, resulting in irregular borders. More often, much of the tumor has a rounded border created by the nodular expansion of confluent large ducts. Scattered mitotic figures may be encountered in the florid hyperplastic epithelium or in hyperplastic myoepithelial cells, which are found throughout much of the lesion. Rarely, focal comedonecrosis is found in the hyperplastic epithelium. In contrast to RSLs that occur elsewhere in the breast, subareolar sclerosing duct hyperplasia generally lacks cysts, cystic and papillary apocrine change, and squamous metaplasia. Carcinoma rarely arises in subareolar sclerosing duct hyperplasia.

Treatment and Prognosis

The tumors should be treated by excision, which can usually be performed through a circumareolar incision and spares the nipple. Recurrence may occur after incomplete excision, but most patients have remained well for as many as 4 years after the initial treatment. Total mastectomy has been performed when

DCIS was present in subareolar sclerosing duct hyperplasia or because the lesion was mistakenly diagnosed as carcinoma. At present, there is no evidence that this condition is a risk factor for carcinoma elsewhere in the breast, but longer follow-up will be necessary to evaluate the question fully.

CYSTIC AND PAPILLARY APOCRINE METAPLASIA

The breasts develop from anlage that give rise to apocrine glands, but apocrine cells do not constitute a component of the normal mammary gland. Any benign proliferative lesion including sclerosing adenosis, complex fibroadenomas, papillomas, RSLs, and gynecomastia to name just a few, may contain apocrine cells. In their most banal form, metaplastic apocrine cells appear identical to the cells that comprise cutaneous apocrine glands. Apocrine cells possess abundant, pink, finely granular cytoplasm, which forms apical tufts or blebs at the luminal surface, and round, regular nuclei containing small to medium size nucleoli situated near the bases of the cells.

Clinical Presentation

There are no clinical features specifically attributable to cystic and papillary apocrine metaplasia. Apocrine metaplasia is frequently present in the epithelial lining of cysts in gross cystic disease. Haagensen et al. (98) reported finding apocrine metaplasia in 78% of 1,169 biopsies performed for gross cystic disease. One group of investigators reported that apocrine cysts were significantly more numerous in the lower quadrants of the breasts than in the upper quadrants (99).

Palpable benign tumors composed of apocrine epithelium are generally divided into two groups: adenomas and papillomas. The distinction between these categories is not clear, because illustrations of some lesions reported to be apocrine adenomas have shown conspicuous papillary components. These lesions present as firm, mobile circumscribed tumors that are clinically indistinguishable from their nonapocrine counterparts.

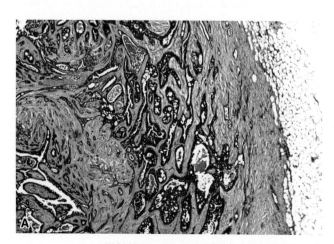
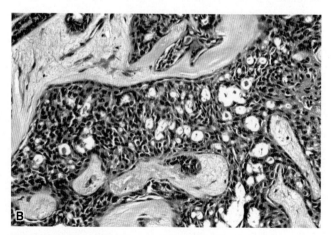

FIGURE 4.29 Subareolar Sclerosing Duct Hyperplasia. A: The border of the lesion is well circumscribed. **B:** Florid duct hyperplasia with a fenestrated pattern is evident.

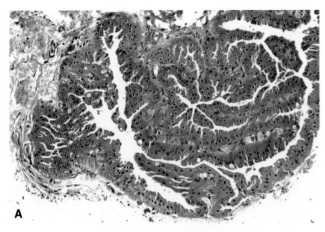
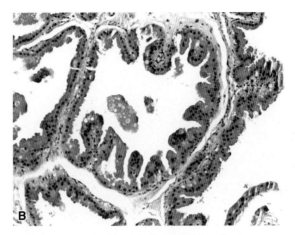

FIGURE 4.30 Cystic and Papillary Apocrine Metaplasia. A, B: Note the evenly spaced, basally oriented nuclei and blunt papillae.

Microscopic foci of apocrine metaplasia are common in the female breast after 30 years of age, and they may be found in younger women occasionally (99,100). The frequency of microscopic apocrine change plateaus in the fifth decade, possibly reflecting physiologic alterations associated with menopause; however, there is no consistent increase or decrease in the presence of apocrine metaplasia with advancing age beyond 50 years (99,100). Apocrine cysts and hyperplasia with apocrine metaplasia are more common in the breasts of American women in New York than in Japanese women in Tokyo (101).

Gross Pathology

There are no specific gross features associated with apocrine metaplasia. Apocrine foci sometimes exhibit a brown color in the unfixed state.

Microscopic Pathology

Apocrine metaplasia is most frequently observed in the epithelium of simple cysts. Cystic apocrine metaplasia consists of flat and cuboidal cells, which form either a single layer or isolated blunt papillae **(Fig. 4.30)**. The cells are usually evenly spaced, and they contain round nuclei with homogeneous, moderately dense chromatin. The nuclei typically contain a single, central nucleolus of a modest size. Metaplastic apocrine epithelium in cysts is prone to regressive changes that may lead to complete disappearance of these cells. This phenomenon is marked by conversion of columnar and cuboidal apocrine epithelium to a layer of flattened cells, which may ultimately be shed into the cyst leaving only a fibrous shell. The proliferative capacity of ordinary apocrine metaplasia is uncertain. Mitotic figures are almost never seen in ordinary apocrine metaplasia (102).

A myoepithelial cell layer is usually readily apparent beneath the apocrine luminal cells; however, the myoepithelial cells may be inconspicuous, and large gaps between them may be observed. Rarely, the myoepithelium may be focally absent in otherwise ordinary, benign apocrine cysts (103). The significance of this finding is not known. A network of congested capillaries typically underlies the basement membrane in foci of apocrine metaplasia.

Robust proliferation of apocrine cells can produce elaborate patterns of hyperplasia with micropapillary or papillary architectures. In regions of proliferation, cellular crowding first gives rise to a palisade arrangement and then to stratification of the epithelial cells. Exuberant growth can create a nodule composed of confluent glands lined by proliferative apocrine epithelium **(Fig. 4.31)**. The apocrine cells have cuboidal to tall columnar shapes, and tufts or snouts of epithelium protrude

FIGURE 4.31 Cystic and Papillary Apocrine Metaplasia. A–C: Apocrine metaplasia is present throughout this complex cystic and papillary lesion. The hyperplastic epithelium has micropapillae and cribriform areas. Complex branching papillary fronds and cysts with hyperplastic apocrine epithelium are shown in this needle core biopsy sample.

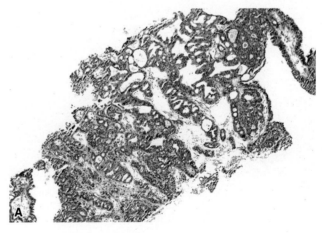

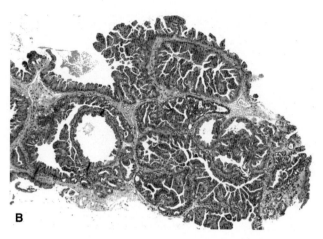

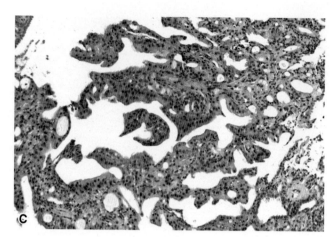

FIGURE 4.31 *(continued)*

from the apical surfaces of the cells into the glandular lumen. The cytoplasm typically is finely granular and uniformly stained, but in rare instances associated with inflammation, coarse granules are conspicuous. They may reflect a degenerative phenomenon.

Papillary apocrine change most frequently occurs associated with other proliferative fibrocystic changes. The apocrine epithelium is usually arranged in a micropapillary pattern composed of regularly spaced, cytologically benign cells. Fibrovascular stroma appears scant or is entirely absent from these fronds. Foci of papillary apocrine metaplasia sometimes coexist with columnar cell lesions, and the two conditions may merge (104).

Calcifications associated with cystic and papillary apocrine metaplasia may be coarse, basophilic, easily fractured particles of calcium hydroxyapatite or birefringent crystals of calcium oxalate **(Fig. 4.32)**.

Atypical changes can be encountered in apocrine metaplasia in virtually any proliferative configuration (14). Architectural atypia consists of irregular papillary fronds with little or no stromal support in which the apocrine cells are diagnosed

in a disordered fashion **(Fig. 4.33)**. Epithelial bridges and cribriform areas may be present.

Apocrine cells with mild cytologic atypia retain abundant granular eosinophilic cytoplasm and exhibit characteristic decapitation secretion. Small cytoplasmic vacuoles may be found, especially in the suprabasal region of the cell. In comparison with conventional apocrine metaplasia, the nuclei in mild apocrine atypia appear irregularly placed, and they may not be basally oriented. Nucleoli appear slightly pleomorphic, and occasionally, a nucleus has more than one nucleolus. With the development of more severe atypia, the cytoplasm of individual cells becomes increasingly vacuolated or clear, and the decapitation of cytoplasm at the luminal border becomes unapparent **(Fig. 4.34)**. Nuclear pleomorphism and hyperchromasia may be striking. Prominent pleomorphic nucleoli characterize the most atypical lesions. The nuclear-to-cytoplasmic ratio increases as apocrine metaplasia becomes more atypical, but the cells generally retain relatively abundant cytoplasm when compared to those of nonapocrine epithelium.

Cytologic atypia tends to be more severe in the apocrine epithelium of sclerosing lesions such as sclerosing adenosis and

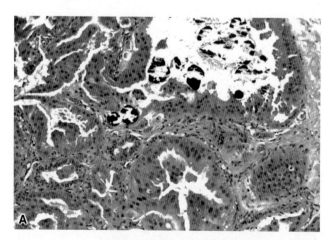

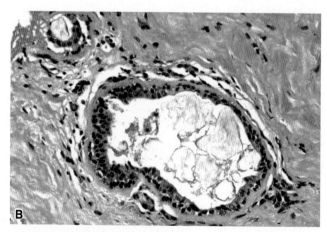

FIGURE 4.32 **Cystic and Papillary Apocrine Metaplasia with Calcifications.** **A:** Round basophilic calcifications can be seen in a lesion composed of papillary apocrine epithelium. **B:** Plate-like, transparent calcium oxalate crystals occupy the lumen of a small apocrine cyst.

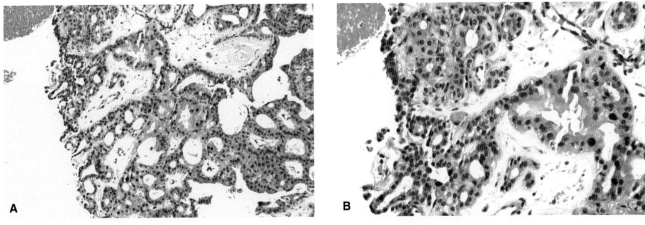

FIGURE 4.33 **Cystic and Papillary Apocrine Metaplasia with Atypia. A, B:** The epithelium has focal cribriform microlumina and isolated hyperchromatic enlarged nuclei in these needle core biopsy specimens.

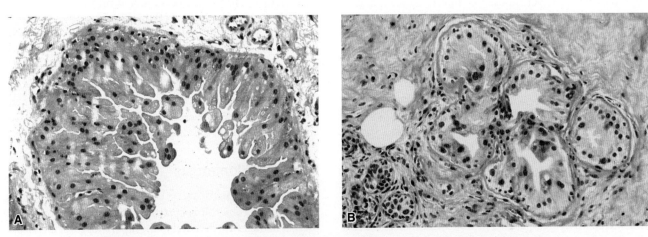

FIGURE 4.34 **Papillary Apocrine Metaplasia with Atypia. A:** The small, round nuclei are distributed in a disorderly fashion in these fused papillary fronds. The abundant cytoplasm in some cells contains vacuoles. **B:** Apocrine cells with pale cytoplasm and pleomorphic nuclei are shown. Note the presence of relatively large nuclei near the tips of papillary mounds.

RSLs, but it may be found in apocrine foci in fibroadenomas, cysts, and papillomas. Atypical cytologic features were present in 71% of adenosis tumors with apocrine metaplasia reported by Nielsen (105).

When atypical apocrine metaplasia is present, the severity of the change is usually not homogeneous in a given lesion. Cysts and papillary ductal hyperplasia, partly or entirely occupied by bland metaplastic apocrine epithelium, are usually found in the vicinity of atypical apocrine metaplasia. The distinction between atypical apocrine metaplasia and apocrine carcinoma is usually not difficult, but it may be a challenge in a NCB sample. In this situation, cytologic features may be less important than the growth pattern, especially in sclerosing lesions. A diagnosis of carcinoma is warranted in a sclerosing lesion when the atypical apocrine proliferation has the configuration of one of the conventional forms of DCIS (14). Because myoepithelial cells may not be detectable in benign apocrine lesions, the diagnosis of in situ or invasive apocrine carcinoma depends on the cytologic and architectural characteristics of the proliferative cells.

The results of stains for myoepithelial markers can provide confirmatory evidence.

Immunohistochemistry

The apical cytoplasm of apocrine cells is immunoreactive for EMA. The cytoplasm shows diffuse reactivity for GCDFP-15. A proportion of normal mammary cells also stain for this protein; so a positive reaction for GCDFP-15 does not establish the apocrine nature of a cell.

Apocrine cells typically do not stain for ER or PR, but they consistently stain for AR. Two reports (106,107) described staining for HER2 along the basal and lateral cell membranes. The granules present in apocrine cells sometimes stain for HER2. One must not misinterpret this finding as evidence of HER2 overexpression.

The myoepithelial cells in apocrine lesions vary in their reactivity for myoepithelial markers such as calponin, smooth muscle myosin heavy chain, CD10, and p63. Tramm et al. (103) observed a substantial number of cases showing large gaps between p63-positive myoepithelial cells, although staining for calponin demonstrated a continuous layer of myoepithelium. The authors also observed rare instances in which large gaps were evident between calponin-immunoreactive myoepithelial cells but not between p63-immunoreactive myoepithelial cells. These data indicate that any effort to investigate the extent of myoepithelium in apocrine lesions must include not only p63 staining but also staining with at least one cytoplasmic maker, an admonition that applies equally to breast tissues generally.

Prognosis

The relationship of apocrine metaplasia to the development of mammary carcinoma is uncertain. In most instances, apocrine metaplasia appears to be part of the fibrocystic complex manifested by cysts with simple or papillary epithelium or ductal hyperplasia with superimposed or intermingled apocrine change. Comparison of the frequencies of apocrine metaplasia in breast with and without carcinoma has not disclosed differences (105,108,109). Although the foregoing anatomic studies of apocrine metaplasia have not shown an association between the frequency of apocrine metaplasia and concurrent carcinoma, the findings of certain follow-up studies suggest that apocrine metaplasia may be a predictor for the development of carcinoma. Haagensen et al. (98) reported a 10-fold greater frequency of carcinoma in women who had apocrine metaplasia in a prior biopsy when compared to those in whom apocrine change was absent. The majority of the subsequent carcinomas had "apocrine features," but origin in apocrine metaplasia was rarely traceable. When compared to Connecticut state incidence figures, patients with apocrine metaplasia had 3.5-times the expected frequency of carcinoma, whereas the risk was only 0.3-times expected when apocrine metaplasia was absent. Page et al. (110) observed a slight overall increase in the number of subsequent carcinomas in women with papillary apocrine change in an antecedent biopsy when compared to the expected number of carcinomas based on an age-matched comparison with the Third National Cancer survey. The difference was statistically significant only in women who were older than 45 years when the apocrine lesion was detected.

Histologic evidence of transitions from apocrine metaplasia to apocrine carcinoma has been reported. Yates and Ahmed (111) recounted a case in which a biopsy that disclosed "florid apocrine metaplasia intermingled with atypical apocrine cells" was followed by the detection of a 2.5-cm tumor composed of apocrine carcinoma 19 months later. Haagensen et al. (98) reported that he had "traced the transformation of benign apocrine metaplasia into apocrine carcinoma in a considerable number of cases." Florid apocrine metaplasia with atypia often coexists with apocrine carcinoma (112), but very few examples of apocrine carcinoma have been traced to atypical apocrine lesions, and most patients with atypical apocrine hyperplasia have remained well with short-term follow-up (14).

When carcinoma arises in the opposite breast of a patient with apocrine atypia or apocrine carcinoma, the contralateral carcinoma is not necessarily apocrine.

Treatment

Specific treatment is not indicated for proliferative lesions with apocrine metaplasia. Most cysts with metaplastic apocrine epithelium collapse and do not re-form after aspiration. The shed epithelium is readily recognized in a cytologic preparation of the fluid. Surgical excision of apocrine cysts is not indicated unless the fluid is bloody, the cysts re-form, or a cytologic specimen contains atypical cells. The need for follow-up of women with breast biopsies that reveal apocrine metaplasia depends on the overall findings in the specimen and the clinical circumstances. Patients with atypical apocrine metaplasia require clinical evaluation comparable to that of women with other atypical proliferative lesions. The precancerous significance of atypical apocrine metaplasia remains undetermined.

FLORID PAPILLOMATOSIS AND SYRINGOMATOUS ADENOMA OF THE NIPPLE

Because of their superficial location in the nipple, these lesions are ordinarily not subjected to NCB; nevertheless, pathologists do receive specimens from this location obtained by punch biopsy or small wedge excision. Brief discussions of these entities are provided for reference.

Florid Papillomatosis

Clinical Presentation

Approximately one-third of patients with florid papillomatosis present in their fifth decade, but the reported ages at diagnosis range from birth to 89 years (113). Approximately 15% of patients are younger than 35 years, and an equal proportion are older than 65 years. Adolescents and infants account for just a small percent of the cases. Fewer than 5% of the reported examples of florid papillomatosis have involved men (114). Bilateral florid papillomatosis is extremely uncommon (115). Several examples of florid papillomatosis involving ectopic breast tissue have been reported (116,117).

In most cases of florid papillomatosis, the nodules have been present for no more than a few months before the patients seek medical attention. The most frequent presenting symptom is discharge, often described as bloody. Pain, itching, or burning sensations are not unusual. In many instances, the nipple appears enlarged, and a mass can be palpated. The surface of the nipple may appear granular, ulcerated, reddened, warty, or crusted. Often these symptoms and clinical findings are mistaken for Paget disease, or the patient is thought to have a papilloma.

Imaging Studies

Radiologic studies usually reveal the presence of a mass, although its small size and its location within the nipple often make it difficult to detect by mammography. The nodules typically appear well defined and smoothly contoured. Unusual cases can present mammographic or sonographic features that suggest malignancy (118). Increased flow associated with the nodule can be seen with Doppler studies (119).

Gross and Microscopic Pathology

The lesions can be grouped into four categories according to histologic growth pattern. In three subtypes, one structural feature dominates or is present exclusively, whereas the fourth group consists of tumors with mixed patterns. No prognostic significance can be attached to these subtypes, and there is no evidence that they differ in pathogenesis. Some clinicopathologic correlations have been noted with these categories, and it may be helpful to keep these correlations in mind when faced with a proliferative lesion of the nipple.

Florid papillomatosis with the *sclerosing papillomatosis* pattern typically presents as a discrete tumor. Scaling of the nipple skin may occur, but redness, ulceration, and inflammation are rarely present. The nipple contains a firm tumor, although the margins may not seem well defined. The histologic features resemble those of a sclerosing papilloma. Exuberant papillary hyperplasia of ductal epithelium is distorted by an accompanying stromal proliferation within and around the affected ducts (**Fig. 4.35**). The complex proliferative process is arranged in papillary, solid, tubular, and glandular structures. Foci of myoepithelial hyperplasia can usually be identified, but as is generally the case with sclerosing papillary lesions, myoepithelial cells may also appear inconspicuous or absent in parts of the tumor. Squamous cysts are commonly formed in the terminal portions of lactiferous ducts. Focal, comedo-type necrosis may be found in the hyperplastic duct epithelium, sometimes associated with infrequent mitoses in epithelial cells. Apocrine metaplasia and extension of glandular epithelium to the nipple surface are uncommon and not prominent when present.

Lesions with the *papillomatosis pattern* usually present as an area of induration rather than a mass. Microscopic examination reveals florid papillary hyperplasia of ductal epithelium causing expansion and crowding of the affected ducts (**Fig. 4.36**). Focal epithelial necrosis and scattered mitotic figures may be found. These tumors lack the stromal proliferation that characterizes the sclerosing papillomatosis type of lesion. Hyperplastic glandular tissue may replace the overlying squamous epithelium over part or all the apical skin of the nipple. Squamous-lined cysts and apocrine metaplasia are not prominent in this variety.

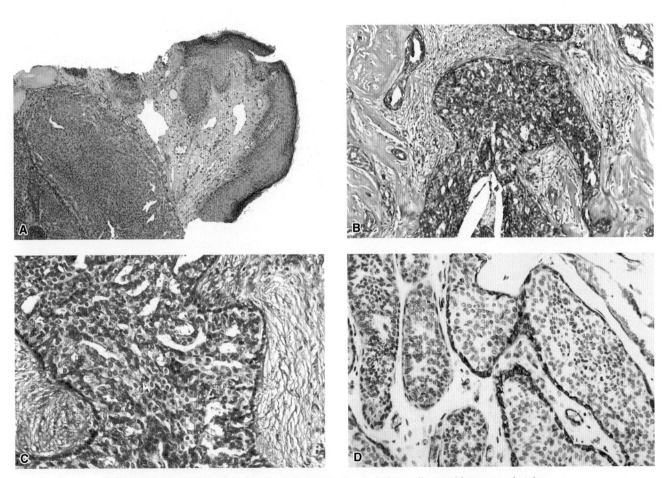

FIGURE 4.35 Florid Papillomatosis of the Nipple. A: This needle core biopsy sample taken from a nodule in the nipple shows florid ductal hyperplasia just beneath the epidermis.
B: Hyperplastic epithelium with a fenestrated pattern in sclerotic stroma is commonly present in the sclerosing type of florid papillomatosis. **C:** Myoepithelial cells outline the hyperplastic epithelium. **D:** Myoepithelial cells are accentuated by the immunostain for actin.

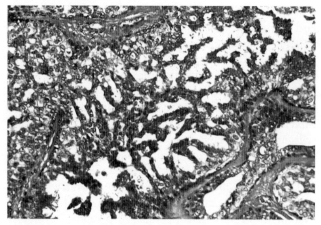

FIGURE 4.36 Florid Papillomatosis of the Nipple. Micropapillary hyperplasia occupies this duct in a papillomatosis-type lesion.

Florid papillomatosis with the *adenosis pattern* forms a discrete nodule in the nipple. Microscopically, the lesion consists of crowded, orderly glands arranged in a pattern indistinguishable from that of florid sclerosing adenosis or an adenosis tumor. Myoepithelial hyperplasia accompanies the epithelial proliferation. Prominent apocrine metaplasia, hyperplasia of the squamous epithelium, and the formation of superficial squamous cysts may be encountered. Mitotic figures and focal necrosis are uncommon.

Examples showing the *mixed proliferative pattern* contain different combinations of the other three patterns. Prominent features present in most cases include superficial squamous metaplasia of ducts with cyst formation, apocrine metaplasia, and acanthosis of the overlying epithelium. Hyperplastic duct epithelium may extend to the nipple surface, accounting for the impression of ulceration. Cystic dilation of ducts is not uncommon near the deep margin of the lesion, where this feature is interspersed with foci of duct hyperplasia. Focal necrosis may be found in duct epithelium. Mitotic activity is minimal. Adenosis occurs in about one-third of these lesions, and a syringomatous pattern may be found at the edges of rare cases.

Immunohistochemistry

The cells lining the glands stain for molecules characteristic of luminal cells such as EMA, CK18 (CAM5.2), and MUC1, whereas the cells at the periphery of the glands contain proteins found in myoepithelial cells such as SMA, calponin, and p63. One must keep in mind that one may not detect myoepithelial cells around glands within the center of a benign sclerosing lesion; consequently, one must interpret the apparent absence of myoepithelium in this light. Staining for CK7, keratin AE1/3, S-100, GCDFP-15, and CEA has yielded variable results.

Differential Diagnosis

On rare occasions, carcinoma can arise within a focus of florid papillomatosis (113). It can be difficult to detect a carcinoma arising in florid papillomatosis of the nipple (120) because the hyperplastic areas seen in many examples of florid papillomatosis exhibit atypical features such as comedonecrosis,

cribriform and micropapillary growth patterns, division figures, and cytologic atypia. In the absence of definitive evidence of invasion, Paget disease of the nipple is the most reliable evidence for a diagnosis of DCIS arising in florid papillomatosis. The CAM5.2 and CK7 immunostains for the cytokeratin are helpful for detecting Paget cells, which are selectively immunoreactive for these markers. When Paget disease is found, underlying areas of DCIS, which differ in their pattern of growth from the rest of the tumor, are usually readily identifiable. In the absence of invasive carcinoma or Paget disease, a diagnosis of DCIS arising in florid papillomatosis is difficult to substantiate in routine H&E sections, whatever the degree of cytologic atypia is. A conservative approach to the diagnosis of florid papillomatosis is recommended.

Prognosis and Treatment

Incisional biopsy and NCB do not yield sufficient tissue to exclude the presence of carcinoma arising in the lesion. Complete excision, which is recommended as definitive treatment, usually requires removal of the nipple. Local recurrence of florid papillomatosis may occur following subtotal excision, but a number of patients have reportedly remained asymptomatic after incomplete excision when a minimal amount of lesional tissue was left in the nipple, and the margins of the excision specimen were involved in only microscopic foci.

Syringomatous Adenoma of the Nipple

Syringomatous adenoma of the nipple is a benign, locally infiltrating neoplasm that has a close histopathologic resemblance to syringomatous tumors commonly found in the skin of the face and other anatomic sites (121,122). The anatomic source of the breast lesion is uncertain. The absence of epithelial proliferation in the mammary ducts and the lack of connection with the epidermis in most cases suggest an origin from other structures. Because random sections of nipples taken from breasts removed for mammary carcinoma sometimes reveal sweat ducts, it is possible that these structures give rise to syringomatous adenomas.

Clinical Presentation

The patients range from 11 to 76 years of age at diagnosis. The median and mean ages at diagnosis of females are approximately 40 years (121,123). A 76-year-old man presented with a syringomatous adenoma (121).

Typical syringomatous adenomas are unilateral lesions that affect both breasts with approximately equal frequency. In one case, tumors appeared in both breasts synchronously (124), and another woman presented with a 4.2-cm fungating syringomatous adenoma in the left breast and a mammographically detected syringomatous adenoma in subareolar region of the right breast (125). The patients usually reported that signs and symptoms began within the year prior to diagnosis, but durations of symptoms of several years have been recorded. The initial symptom is a mass in the nipple or subareolar region. A few patients have described pain, tenderness, redness, itching, discharge, or nipple inversion. Crusting of the nipple surface caused by hyperkeratosis has been reported, but ulceration and erosion are not features of syringomatous adenoma. Page et al. (126) reported the occurrence of a syringomatous adenoma in a supernumerary nipple.

Imaging Studies
Mammography in certain cases demonstrates a dense stellate tumor, calcifications, or both (124,127–129). Sonography sometimes shows an irregular mass that may be accompanied by dilated ducts or calcifications (123,124,127,128).

Gross Pathology
The excised tumors measured 1.0 to 3.5 cm, with an average size of 1.5 cm. Most consisted of an ill-defined mass of firm-to-hard, gray, tan, or white tissue. Discrete nodules and microcysts have been noted rarely.

Microscopic Pathology
The lesion consists of tubules, ductules, and strands composed of small, uniform cells infiltrating the dermis and the stroma of the nipple. The neoplastic glands sometimes seem to connect with the basal layer of the epidermis. Hyperplasia of the epidermis is slight in most cases, but occasionally pseudoepitheliomatous hyperplasia may be encountered.

The ducts, lined by one or more layers of cells, have teardrop, comma-like, and branching shapes and lumina that appear either open and round or filled with small uniform cells (**Fig. 4.37**). Some cells may exhibit cytoplasmic clearing. Mitoses are virtually absent, and the nuclei lack prominent nucleoli and pleomorphism. Flattening of cells around the lumina constitutes evidence of early squamous differentiation, which in a fully developed form results in keratotic cysts. A foreign body giant cell reaction may be elicited in the vicinity of ruptured squamous cysts. Calcification is rarely seen in the keratinized epithelium. The lumina of the ducts either appear empty, or they contain deeply eosinophilic, retracted secretion. The secretion is PAS-positive and sometimes weakly mucicarmine-positive (121).

The adenomatous tubules diffusely infiltrate the periductal stroma of nipple and may extend into the subareolar breast parenchyma in larger lesions. Invasion into the smooth muscle bundles of the nipple is very common, and occasionally perineural invasion is observed. The stroma appears altered in the vicinity of the infiltrating tubules. The collagen and fibroblasts tend to be concentrically oriented around the epithelial structures.

Syringomatous glands may be found in proximity to and, rarely, in direct contact with the epithelium of nipple ducts, ductules, and mammary lobules and with the epidermis of the nipple. This continuity probably results from the infiltrative growth of the neoplasm, and one should not misinterpret the finding as conclusive evidence of origin from any of these structures. Coincidental epithelial hyperplasia of lactiferous ducts or the underlying breast tissue may occasionally be seen, but this is not an intrinsic component of syringomatous adenoma. Paget disease, a manifestation of ductal carcinoma, is not a feature of syringomatous adenoma, either.

Immunohistochemistry
The literature contains only limited secure information regarding the immunohistochemical characteristics of syringomatous adenoma. CEA has been found in the secretion and in the cytoplasm of periluminal cells. The inner cells also express keratin. In one report (125), the outer cells stained strongly for smooth muscle myosin heavy chain, 34βE12, and CK5/6. The outer cells and others showing squamous features stained for p63.

Differential Diagnosis
Several lesions should be considered in the differential diagnosis of syringomatous adenoma of the nipple. Florid papillomatosis is predominantly a hyperplastic epithelial proliferation of the major lactiferous ducts. Patients with florid papillomatosis tend to be older, they are more likely to have erosion of the nipple with bleeding, and the duration of complaints is usually brief compared to that of syringomatous adenoma. Syringomatous

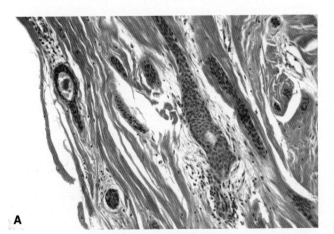
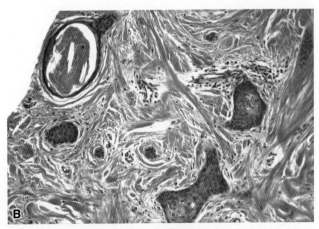

FIGURE 4.37 Syringomatous Adenoma of the Nipple. A: This area from a needle core biopsy specimen shows elongated, duct-like structures, one of which has an open lumen containing secretion. Squamoid differentiation can be seen in the center. **B:** An area with cystic dilatation and prominent squamous differentiation is evident.

foci are occasionally encountered as a minor component of florid papillomatosis.

Tubular carcinoma sometimes arises in the subareolar region and nipple, where it displays an infiltrative growth pattern that may be difficult to distinguish from syringomatous adenoma. Both invade smooth muscle and nerves. Features of tubular carcinoma in the nipple that are not seen in syringomatous adenoma include DCIS, Paget disease of the epidermis, and angular glands. Squamous metaplasia and the formation of round glands by ductules that often have a branching pattern, findings seen in syringomatous adenoma, are not features of tubular carcinoma.

Syringomatous adenoma and certain variants of low-grade adenosquamous carcinoma share certain structural characteristics (130); however, the two lesions do not represent two manifestations of a single type of neoplasm. Syringomatous adenoma arises in the nipple and secondarily involves the breast parenchyma underlying the nipple in almost all cases. Low-grade adenosquamous carcinoma usually develops peripherally, sparing the nipple, although very infrequently it can arise in the subareolar region and involve the nipple.

Treatment and Prognosis

Most patients have been treated by local excision, which required removing the entire nipple in some instances. Local recurrence, sometimes with invasive growth, after incomplete excision has occurred in approximately 30% of cases reported since 1983 (121,123,127,131,132); consequently, re-excision should be considered if the tumor involves the margin of the specimen. The time to recurrence has varied from less than 1 year to 8 years. In one case (121), the lesion slowly enlarged for 22 years after initial biopsy, at which time a partial mastectomy was performed for a 3-cm tumor that invaded the breast parenchyma. One patient experienced 3 recurrences over a 4-year period (132). None of the patients with lesions correctly diagnosed as syringomatous adenoma has developed metastases in regional lymph nodes or at distant sites. There is no evidence of an association of syringomatous adenoma and mammary adenocarcinoma.

REFERENCES

1. Volmer J. Intraduktales (intrazystisches) Papillom der männlichen Brustdrüse. *Zentralbl Allg Pathol.* 1984;129:513–519.
2. Yamamoto H, Okada Y, Taniguchi H, et al. Intracystic papilloma in the breast of a male given long-term phenothiazine therapy: a case report. *Breast Cancer.* 2006;13:84–88.
3. Rizzo M, Lund MJ, Oprea G, et al. Surgical follow-up and clinical presentation of 142 breast papillary lesions diagnosed by ultrasound-guided core-needle biopsy. *Ann Surg Oncol.* 2008;15:1040–1047.
4. Mesurolle B, Kethani K, El-Khoury M, et al. Intraductal papilloma in a reconstructed breast: mammographic and sonographic appearance with pathologic correlation. *Breast.* 2006;15:680–682.
5. Dzodic R, Stanojevic B, Saenko V, et al. Intraductal papilloma of ectopic breast tissue in axillary lymph node of a patient with a previous intraductal papilloma of ipsilateral breast: a case report and review of the literature. *Diagn Pathol.* 2010;5:17.
6. Ichihara S, Ikeda T, Kimura K, et al. Coincidence of mammary and sentinel lymph node papilloma. *Am J Surg Pathol.* 2008;32:784–792.
7. Cottom H, Rengabashyam B, Turton PE, et al. Intraductal papilloma in an axillary lymph node of a patient with human immunodeficiency virus: a case report and review of the literature. *J Med Case Rep.* 2014;8:162.
8. Shim JH, Son EJ, Kim EK, et al. Benign intracystic papilloma of the male breast. *J Ultrasound Med.* 2008;27:1397–1400.
9. Cardenosa G, Eklund GW. Benign papillary neoplasms of the breast: mammographic findings. *Radiology.* 1991;181:751–755.
10. Francis A, England D, Rowlands D, et al. Breast papilloma: mammogram, ultrasound and MRI appearances. *Breast.* 2002;11:394–397.
11. Lam WW, Chu WC, Tang AP, et al. Role of radiologic features in the management of papillary lesions of the breast. *AJR Am J Roentgenol.* 2006;186:1322–1327.
12. Fatemi Y, Hurley R, Grant C, et al. Challenges in the management of giant intraductal breast papilloma. *Clin Case Rep.* 2015;3:7–10.
13. Hayashi H, Ohtani H, Yamaguchi J, et al. A case of intracystic apocrine papillary tumor: diagnostic pitfalls for malignancy. *Pathol Res Pract.* 2013;209:808–811.
14. Carter DJ, Rosen PP. Atypical apocrine metaplasia in sclerosing lesions of the breast: a study of 51 patients. *Mod Pathol.* 1991;4:1–5.
15. Jiao YF, Nakamura S, Oikawa T, et al. Sebaceous gland metaplasia in intraductal papilloma of the breast. *Virchows Arch.* 2001;438:505–508.
16. Judkins AR, Montone KT, LiVolsi VA, et al. Sensitivity and specificity of antibodies on necrotic tumor tissue. *Am J Clin Pathol.* 1998;110:641–646.
17. Ginter PS, Hoda SA, Ozerdem U. Exuberant squamous metaplasia in an intraductal papilloma of breast. *Int J Surg Pathol.* 2015;23:125–126.
18. Stefanou D, Batistatou A, Nonni A, et al. p63 expression in benign and malignant breast lesions. *Histol Histopathol.* 2004;19:465–471.
19. Reisenbichler ES, Adams AL, Hameed O. The predictive ability of a CK5/p63/CK8/18 antibody cocktail in stratifying breast papillary lesions on needle biopsy: an algorithmic approach works best. *Am J Clin Pathol.* 2013;140:767–779.
20. Brennan SB, Corben A, Liberman L, et al. Papilloma diagnosed at MRI-guided vacuum-assisted breast biopsy: is surgical excision still warranted? *AJR Am J Roentgenol.* 2012;199:W512–W519.
21. Hawley JR, Lawther H, Erdal BS, et al. Outcomes of benign breast papillomas diagnosed at image-guided vacuum-assisted core needle biopsy. *Clin Imaging.* 2015;39(4):576–581.
22. Nayak A, Carkaci S, Gilcrease MZ, et al. Benign papillomas without atypia diagnosed on core needle biopsy: experience from a single institution and proposed criteria for excision. *Clin Breast Cancer.* 2013;13:439–449.
23. Wen X, Cheng W. Nonmalignant breast papillary lesions at core-needle biopsy: a meta-analysis of underestimation and influencing factors. *Ann Surg Oncol.* 2013;20:94–101.
24. Bernik SF, Troob S, Ying BL, et al. Papillary lesions of the breast diagnosed by core needle biopsy: 71 cases with surgical follow-up. *Am J Surg.* 2009;197:473–478.
25. Shah VI, Flowers CI, Douglas-Jones AG, et al. Immunohistochemistry increases the accuracy of diagnosis of benign papillary lesions in breast core needle biopsy specimens. *Histopathology.* 2006;48:683–691.
26. Grin A, O'Malley FP, Mulligan AM. Cytokeratin 5 and estrogen receptor immunohistochemistry as a useful adjunct in identifying atypical papillary lesions on breast needle core biopsy. *Am J Surg Pathol.* 2009;33:1615–1623.
27. Tse GM, Tan PH, Lacambra MD, et al. Papillary lesions of the breast—accuracy of core biopsy. *Histopathology.* 2010;56:481–488.
28. Jakate K, De Brot M, Goldberg F, et al. Papillary lesions of the breast: impact of breast pathology subspecialization on core biopsy and excision diagnoses. *Am J Surg Pathol.* 2012;36:544–551.
29. Moon HJ, Jung I, Kim MJ, et al. Breast papilloma without atypia and risk of breast carcinoma. *Breast J.* 2014;20:525–533.
30. MacGrogan G, Tavassoli FA. Central atypical papillomas of the breast: a clinicopathological study of 119 cases. *Virchows Arch.* 2003;443:609–617.
31. Cuneo KC, Dash RC, Wilke LG, et al. Risk of invasive breast cancer and ductal carcinoma in situ in women with atypical papillary lesions of the breast. *Breast J.* 2012;18:475–478.
32. Ali-Fehmi R, Carolin K, Wallis T, et al. Clinicopathologic analysis of breast lesions associated with multiple papillomas. *Hum Pathol.* 2003;34:234–239.
33. Estabrook A. Are patients with solitary or multiple intraductal papillomas at a higher risk of developing breast cancer? *Surg Oncol Clin North Am.* 1993;2:45–56.
34. Lewis JT, Hartmann LC, Vierkant RA, et al. An analysis of breast cancer risk in women with single, multiple, and atypical papilloma. *Am J Surg Pathol.* 2006;30:665–672.

35. Jaffer S, Bleiweiss IJ, Nagi C. Incidental intraductal papillomas (<2 mm) of the breast diagnosed on needle core biopsy do not need to be excised. *Breast J.* 2013;19:130–133.

36. Yamaguchi R, Tanaka M, Tse GM, et al. Management of breast papillary lesions diagnosed in ultrasound-guided vacuum-assisted and core needle biopsies. *Histopathology.* 2015;66:565–576.

37. Mosier AD, Keylock J, Smith DV. Benign papillomas diagnosed on large-gauge vacuum-assisted core needle biopsy which span <1.5 cm do not need surgical excision. *Breast J.* 2013;19:611–617.

38. Youk JH, Kim MJ, Son EJ, et al. US-guided vacuum-assisted percutaneous excision for management of benign papilloma without atypia diagnosed at US-guided 14-gauge core needle biopsy. *Ann Surg Oncol.* 2012;19:922–928.

39. Kibil W, Hodorowicz-Zaniewska D, Popiela TJ, et al. Vacuum-assisted core biopsy in diagnosis and treatment of intraductal papillomas. *Clin Breast Cancer.* 2013;13:129–132.

40. Carder PJ, Khan T, Burrows P, et al. Large volume "mammotome" biopsy may reduce the need for diagnostic surgery in papillary lesions of the breast. *J Clin Pathol.* 2008;61:928–933.

41. Wyss P, Varga Z, Rossle M, et al. Papillary lesions of the breast: outcomes of 156 patients managed without excisional biopsy. *Breast J.* 2014;20:394–401.

42. Swapp RE, Glazebrook KN, Jones KN, et al. Management of benign intraductal solitary papilloma diagnosed on core needle biopsy. *Ann Surg Oncol.* 2013;20:1900–1905.

43. Sexton K, Brill YM, Atkins L, et al. Outcome of benign papillary lesions of the breast diagnosed by needle core and mammotome biopsies with 3 to 5 year follow up. *Mod Pathol.* 2006;19(suppl):42A.

44. Guarino M, Tricomi P, Cristofori E. Collagenous spherulosis of the breast with atypical epithelial hyperplasia. *Pathologica.* 1993;85:123–127.

45. Resetkova E, Albarracin C, Sneige N. Collagenous spherulosis of breast: morphologic study of 59 cases and review of the literature. *Am J Surg Pathol.* 2006;30:20–27.

46. Gangane N, Joshi D, Shivkumar VB. Cytological diagnosis of collagenous spherulosis of breast associated with fibroadenoma: report of a case with review of literature. *Diagn Cytopathol.* 2007;35:366–369.

47. Ohta M, Mori M, Kawada T, et al. Collagenous spherulosis associated with adenomyoepithelioma of the breast: a case report. *Acta Cytol.* 2010;54:314–318.

48. Reis-Filho JS, Fulford LG, Crebassa B, et al. Collagenous spherulosis in an adenomyoepithelioma of the breast. *J Clin Pathol.* 2004;57:83–86.

49. Divaris DX, Smith S, Leask D, et al. Complex collagenous spherulosis of the breast presenting as a palpable mass: a case report with immunohistochemical and ultrastructural studies. *Breast J.* 2000;6:199–203.

50. Hill P, Cawson J. Collagenous spherulosis presenting as a mass lesion on imaging. *Breast J.* 2008;14:301–303.

51. Clement PB, Young RH, Azzopardi JG. Collagenous spherulosis of the breast. *Am J Surg Pathol.* 1987;11:411–417.

52. Rosen PP. Adenoid cystic carcinoma of the breast: a morphologically heterogeneous neoplasm. *Pathol Annu.* 1989;24(pt 2):237–254.

53. Mooney EE, Kayani N, Tavassoli FA. Spherulosis of the breast: a spectrum of municous and collagenous lesions. *Arch Pathol Lab Med.* 1999;123:626–630.

54. Wells CA, Wells CW, Yeomans P, et al. Spherical connective tissue inclusions in epithelial hyperplasia of the breast ("collagenous spherulosis"). *J Clin Pathol.* 1990;43:905–908.

55. Highland KE, Finley JL, Neill JS, et al. Collagenous spherulosis: report of a case with diagnosis by fine needle aspiration biopsy with immunocytochemical and ultrastructural observations. *Acta Cytol.* 1993;37:3–9.

56. Grignon DJ, Ro JY, Mackay BN, et al. Collagenous spherulosis of the breast: immunohistochemical and ultrastructural studies. *Am J Clin Pathol.* 1989;91:386–392.

57. Stephenson TJ, Hird PM, Laing RW, et al. Nodular basement membrane deposits in breast carcinoma and atypical ductal hyperplasia: mimics of collagenous spherulosis. *Pathologica.* 1994;86:234–239.

58. Hill P, Cawson J. Collagenous spherulosis with lobular carcinoma in situ: a potential diagnostic pitfall. *Pathology.* 2007;39:361–363.

59. Sgroi D, Koerner FC. Involvement of collagenous spherulosis by lobular carcinoma in situ: potential confusion with cribriform ductal carcinoma in situ. *Am J Surg Pathol.* 1995;19:1366–1370.

60. Cabibi D, Giannone AG, Belmonte B, et al. CD10 and HHF35 actin in the differential diagnosis between collagenous spherulosis and adenoid-cystic carcinoma of the breast. *Pathol Res Pract.* 2012;208:405–409.

61. Rabban JT, Swain RS, Zaloudek CJ, et al. Immunophenotypic overlap between adenoid cystic carcinoma and collagenous spherulosis of the breast: potential diagnostic pitfalls using myoepithelial markers. *Mod Pathol.* 2006;19:1351–1357.

62. Hamperl H. Strahlige narben und obliterierende mastopathie bëitrage zur pathologischen histologie der mamma XI. *Virchows Arch A Pathol Anat Histol.* 1975;369:55–68.

63. Andersen JA, Gram JB. Radial scar in the female breast: a long-term follow-up study of 32 cases. *Cancer.* 1984;53:2557–2560.

64. Nielsen M, Jensen J, Andersen JA. An autopsy study of radial scar in the female breast. *Histopathology.* 1985;9:287–295.

65. Fisher ER, Palekar AS, Kotwal N, et al. A nonencapsulated sclerosing lesion of the breast. *Am J Clin Pathol.* 1979;71:240–246.

66. Wellings SR, Alpers CE. Subgross pathologic features and incidence of radial scars in the breast. *Hum Pathol.* 1984;15:475–479.

67. Linell F, Ljungberg O, Anderson I. Breast carcinoma: aspects of early stage, progression and related problems. *Acta Pathol Microbiol Scand (Suppl).* 1980;272:1–233.

68. Anderson TJ, Battersby S. Radial scars of benign and malignant breasts: comparative features and significance. *J Pathol.* 1985;147:23–32.

69. Patterson JA, Scott M, Anderson N, et al. Radial scar, complex sclerosing lesion and risk of breast cancer: analysis of 175 cases in Northern Ireland. *Eur J Surg Oncol.* 2004;30:1065–1068.

70. Dominguez A, Durando M, Mariscotti G, et al. Breast cancer risk associated with the diagnosis of a microhistological radial scar (RS): retrospective analysis in 10 years of experience. *Radiol Med.* 2015;120:377–385.

71. Pediconi F, Occhiato R, Venditti F, et al. Radial scars of the breast: contrast-enhanced magnetic resonance mammography appearance. *Breast J.* 2005;11:23–28.

72. Andersen JA, Carter D, Linell F. A symposium on sclerosing duct lesions of the breast. *Pathol Annu.* 1986;21(pt 2):145–179.

73. Doyle EM, Banville N, Quinn CM, et al. Radial scars/complex sclerosing lesions and malignancy in a screening program: incidence and histological features revisited. *Histopathology.* 2007;50:607–614.

74. Manfrin E, Remo A, Falsirollo F, et al. Risk of neoplastic transformation in asymptomatic radial scar: analysis of 117 cases. *Breast Cancer Res Treat.* 2008;107:371–377.

75. Cawson JN, Malara F, Kavanagh A, et al. Fourteen-gauge needle core biopsy of mammographically evident radial scars: is excision necessary? *Cancer.* 2003;97:345–351.

76. Alvarado-Cabrero I, Tavassoli FA. Neoplastic and malignant lesions involving or arising in a radial scar: a clinicopathologic analysis of 17 cases. *Breast J.* 2000;6:96–102.

77. Mokbel K, Price RK, Mostafa A, et al. Radial scar and carcinoma of the breast: microscopic findings in 32 cases. *Breast.* 1999;8:339–342.

78. Caneva A, Bonetti F, Manfrin E, et al. Is a radial scar of the breast a premalignant lesion *Mod Pathol (Suppl).* 1997;10:17A.

79. Sloane JP, Mayers MM. Carcinoma and atypical hyperplasia in radial scars and complex sclerosing lesions: importance of lesion size and patient age. *Histopathology.* 1993;23:225–231.

80. Farshid G, Rush G. Assessment of 142 stellate lesions with imaging features suggestive of radial scar discovered during population-based screening for breast cancer. *Am J Surg Pathol.* 2004;28:1626–1631.

81. Denley H, Pinder SE, Tan PH, et al. Metaplastic carcinoma of the breast arising within complex sclerosing lesion: a report of five cases. *Histopathology.* 2000;36:203–209.

82. Bianchi S, Giannotti E, Vanzi E, et al. Radial scar without associated atypical epithelial proliferation on image-guided 14-gauge needle core biopsy: analysis of 49 cases from a single-center and review of the literature. *Breast.* 2012;21:159–164.

83. Conlon N, D'Arcy C, Kaplan JB, et al. Radial scar at image-guided needle biopsy: is excision necessary? *Am J Surg Pathol.* 2015;39:779–785.

84. Lee KA, Zuley ML, Chivukula M, et al. Risk of malignancy when microscopic radial scars and microscopic papillomas are found at percutaneous biopsy. *AJR Am J Roentgenol.* 2012;198:W141–W145.

85. Rajan S, Wason AM, Carder PJ. Conservative management of screen-detected radial scars: role of mammotome excision. *J Clin Pathol.* 2011;64:65–68.

86. Tennant SL, Evans A, Hamilton LJ, et al. Vacuum-assisted excision of breast lesions of uncertain malignant potential (B3)—an alternative to surgery in selected cases. *Breast.* 2008;17:546–549.

87. Resetkova E, Edelweiss M, Albarracin CT, et al. Management of radial sclerosing lesions of the breast diagnosed using percutaneous vacuum-assisted core needle biopsy: recommendations for excision based on seven years' of experience at a single institution. *Breast Cancer Res Treat.* 2011;127:335–343.

88. Brenner RJ, Jackman RJ, Parker SH, et al. Percutaneous core needle biopsy of radial scars of the breast: when is excision necessary? *AJR Am J Roentgenol.* 2002;179:1179–1184.

89. Sohn VY, Causey MW, Steele SR, et al. The treatment of radial scars in the modern era—surgical excision is not required. *Am Surg.* 2010;76:522–525.

90. Nielsen M, Christensen L, Andersen J. Radial scars in women with breast cancer. *Cancer.* 1987;59:1019–1025.

91. Jacobs TW, Byrne C, Colditz G, et al. Radial scars in benign breast-biopsy specimens and the risk of breast cancer. *N Engl J Med.* 1999;340:430–436.

92. Aroner SA, Collins LC, Connolly JL, et al. Radial scars and subsequent breast cancer risk: results from the Nurses' Health Studies. *Breast Cancer Res Treat.* 2013;139:277–285.

93. Sanders ME, Page DL, Simpson JF, et al. Interdependence of radial scar and proliferative disease with respect to invasive breast carcinoma risk in patients with benign breast biopsies. *Cancer.* 2006;106:1453–1461.

94. Berg JC, Visscher DW, Vierkant RA, et al. Breast cancer risk in women with radial scars in benign breast biopsies. *Breast Cancer Res Treat.* 2008;108:167–174.

95. Bunting DM, Steel JR, Holgate CS, et al. Long-term follow-up and risk of breast cancer after a radial scar or complex sclerosing lesion has been identified in a benign open breast biopsy. *Eur J Surg Oncol.* 2011;37:709–713.

96. Lv M, Zhu X, Zhong S, et al. Radial scars and subsequent breast cancer risk: a meta-analysis. *PLoS One.* 2014;9:e102503.

97. Rosen PP. Subareolar sclerosing duct hyperplasia of the breast. *Cancer.* 1987;59:1927–1930.

98. Haagensen CD, Bodian C, Haagensen DE. Apocrine epithelium: In: *Breast Carcinoma: Risk and Detection.* Philadelphia, PA: W.B. Saunders; 1981:83–105.

99. Benigni G, Squartini F. Uneven distribution and significant concentration of apocrine metaplasia in lower breast quadrants. *Tumori.* 1986;72:179–182.

100. Wellings SR, Alpers CE. Apocrine cystic metaplasia: subgross pathology and prevalence in cancer-associated versus random autopsy breasts. *Hum Pathol.* 1987;18:381–386.

101. Schuerch C III, Rosen PP, Hirota T, et al. A pathologic study of benign breast diseases in Tokyo and New York. *Cancer.* 1982;50:1899–1903.

102. Bussolati G, Cattani MG, Gugliotta P, et al. Morphologic and functional aspects of apocrine metaplasia in dysplastic and neoplastic breast tissue. *Ann N Y Acad Sci.* 1986;464:262–274.

103. Tramm T, Kim JY, Tavassoli FA. Diminished number or complete loss of myoepithelial cells associated with metaplastic and neoplastic apocrine lesions of the breast. *Am J Surg Pathol.* 2011;35:202–211.

104. Kosemehmetoglu K, Guler G. Papillary apocrine metaplasia and columnar cell lesion with atypia: is there a shared common pathway? *Ann Diagn Pathol.* 2010;14:425–431.

105. Nielsen BB. Adenosis tumor of the breast—a clinicopathological investigation of 27 cases. *Histopathology.* 1987;11:1259–1275.

106. Feuerhake F, Unterberger P, Höfter EA. Cell turnover in apocrine metaplasia of the human mammary gland epithelium: apoptosis, proliferation, and immunohistochemical detection of Bcl-2, Bax, EGFR, and c-erbB2 gene products. *Acta Histochem.* 2001;103:53–65.

107. Selim AG, El-Ayat G, Wells CA. Expression of c-erbB2, p53, Bcl-2, Bax, c-myc and Ki-67 in apocrine metaplasia and apocrine change within sclerosing adenosis of the breast. *Virchows Arch.* 2002;441:449–455.

108. Foote FW, Stewart FW. Comparative studies of cancerous versus noncancerous breasts. *Ann Surg.* 1945;121:6–53.

109. McCarty KS Jr, Kesterson GH, Wilkinson WE, et al. Histopathologic study of subcutaneous mastectomy specimens from patients with carcinoma of the contralateral breast. *Surg Gynecol Obstet.* 1978;147:682–688.

110. Page DL, Vander Zwaag R, Rogers LW, et al. Relation between component parts of fibrocystic disease complex and breast cancer. *J Natl Cancer Inst.* 1978;61:1055–1063.

111. Yates AJ, Ahmed A. Apocrine carcinoma and apocrine metaplasia. *Histopathology.* 1988;13:228–231.

112. Abati AD, Kimmel M, Rosen PP. Apocrine mammary carcinoma: a clinicopathologic study of 72 cases. *Am J Clin Pathol.* 1990;94:371–377.

113. Rosen PP, Caicco JA. Florid papillomatosis of the nipple: a study of 51 patients, including nine with mammary carcinoma. *Am J Surg Pathol.* 1986;10:87–101.

114. Fernandez-Flores A, Suarez-Peñaranda JM. Immunophenotype of nipple adenoma in a male patient. *Appl Immunohistochem Mol Morphol.* 2011;19:190–194.

115. Sasi W, Banerjee D, Mokbel K, et al. Bilateral florid papillomatosis of the nipple: an unusual indicator for metachronous breast cancer development—a case report. *Case Rep Oncol Med.* 2014;2014:432609.

116. Shioi Y, Nakamura SI, Kawamura S, et al. Nipple adenoma arising from axillary accessory breast: a case report. *Diagn Pathol.* 2012;7:162.

117. Shinn L, Woodward C, Boddu S, et al. Nipple adenoma arising in a supernumerary mammary gland: a case report. *Tumori.* 2011;97:812–814.

118. Fornage BD, Faroux MJ, Pluot M, et al. Nipple adenoma simulating carcinoma: misleading clinical, mammographic, sonographic, and cytologic findings. *J Ultrasound Med.* 1991;10:55–57.

119. Parajuly SS, Peng YL, Zhu M, et al. Nipple adenoma of the breast: sonographic imaging findings. *South Med J.* 2010;103:1280–1281.

120. Diaz NM, Palmer JO, Wick MR. Erosive adenomatosis of the nipple: histology, immunohistology, and differential diagnosis. *Mod Pathol.* 1992;5:179–184.

121. Rosen PP. Syringomatous adenoma of the nipple. *Am J Surg Pathol.* 1983;7:739–745.

122. Ward BE, Cooper PH, Subramony C. Syringomatous tumor of the nipple. *Am J Clin Pathol.* 1989;92:692–696.

123. Kubo M, Tsuji H, Kunitomo T, et al. Syringomatous adenoma of the nipple: a case report. *Breast Cancer.* 2004;11:214–216.

124. Mrklić I, Bezić J, Pogorelić Z, et al. Synchronous bilateral infiltrating syringomatous adenoma of the breast. *Scott Med J.* 2012;57:121.

125. Montgomery ND, Bianchi GD, Klauber-Demore N, et al. Bilateral syringomatous adenomas of the nipple: case report with immunohistochemical characterization of a rare tumor mimicking malignancy. *Am J Clin Pathol.* 2014;141:727–731.

126. Page RN, Dittrich L, King R, et al. Syringomatous adenoma of the nipple occurring within a supernumerary breast: a case report. *J Cutan Pathol.* 2009;36:1206–1209.

127. Slaughter MS, Pomerantz RA, Murad T, et al. Infiltrating syringomatous adenoma of the nipple. *Surgery.* 1992;111:711–713.

128. Toyoshima O, Kanou M, Kintaka N, et al. Syringomatous adenoma of the nipple: report of a case. *Surg Today.* 1998;28:1196–1199.

129. AlSharif S, Tremblay F, Omeroglu A, et al. Infiltrating syringomatous adenoma of the nipple: sonographic and mammographic features with pathologic correlation. *J Clin Ultrasound.* 2014;42:427–429.

130. Rosen PP, Ernsberger D. Low-grade adenosquamous carcinoma: a variant of metaplastic mammary carcinoma. *Am J Surg Pathol.* 1987;11:351–358.

131. Carter E, Dyess DL. Infiltrating syringomatous adenoma of the nipple: a case report and 20-year retrospective review. *Breast J.* 2004;10:443–447.

132. Jones MW, Norris HJ, Snyder RC. Infiltrating syringomatous adenoma of the nipple: a clinical and pathological study of 11 cases. *Am J Surg Pathol.* 1989;13:197–201.

Myoepithelial Lesions

EDI BROGI

Myoepithelial cells (MECs) are located between the glandular epithelium and the basement membrane of normal mammary ducts and lobules. They are hormone-dependent contractile cells, have "tumor-suppressor" properties (1), and are often reduced or absent around ducts involved by ductal carcinoma in situ (DCIS). Most MECs have spindle cell morphology. MECs with globoid morphology and abundant clear cytoplasm with pseudovacuoles occur physiologically during the luteal phase of the menstrual cycle, and are also common in sclerosing lesions and in myoepithelial tumors. Clear cell change and hyperplasia of the MECs are also common in irradiated breast. Rarely, myoid transformation of MECs can occur, especially in the context of sclerosing lesions. The pseudovacuoles of MECs do not stain with mucicarmine, Alcian-blue, and periodic acid–Schiff (PAS) stains. The immunoprofile of MECs is summarized in Table 5.1.

Hyperplastic MECs may occasionally mimic atypical lobular hyperplasia (ALH) and classic lobular carcinoma in situ (LCIS) with Pagetoid growth, especially in a needle core biopsy (NCB) sample. The evenly circumferential distribution along the periphery of the acini is usually sufficient for correct identification of the MECs. E-cadherin staining of MECs yields a pattern of linear but discontinuous ("dot-like") membranous reactivity, weaker in intensity than seen in the ductal cells. The pattern of E-cadherin staining in MECs should not be misdiagnosed as aberrant expression of E-Cadherin in ALH/classic LCIS. Immunoperoxidase stains for MEC markers, especially p63 and/or calponin, can be used to resolve problematic cases.

Neoplasms composed of MECs include adenomyoepithelioma, myoepithelioma, and myoepithelial carcinoma.

ADENOMYOEPITHELIOMA

Adenomyoepithelioma (AME) is a rare benign biphasic mammary neoplasm composed of epithelium and myoepithelium (2). With the exception of few small series (3–6), most reports of AME are case studies. Some AME have atypical features (atypical AME). Rarely carcinoma can arise in an AME.

TABLE 5.1

Immunophenotype of Myoepithelial Cells

	Cytoplasm	Nucleus	Membrane
p63	Negative	Positive	Negative
SMA	Positive	Negative	Negative
SMM-HC	Positive	Negative	Negative
Calponin	Positive	Negative	Negative
CD10	Positive	Negative	Negative
S100	Positive	Usually positive	Negative
Maspin	Positive	Usually positive	Negative
P75	Positive	Negative	Positive
Basal cytokeratins (5, 6, 14, 17, 34βE12)	Positive	Negative	Negative
Luminal keratins (CK 8, 18)	Negative	Negative	Negative
E-Cadherin	Negative	Negative	Granular ("dot-like") discontinuous linear staining
Keratin AE1	Negative	Negative	Negative
Keratin AE3	Positive in MECs in ducts; Negative in MECs in acini	Negative	Negative
EMA and CEA	Negative	Negative	Negative

Age and Gender

AMEs tend to occur in postmenopausal women, seldom in young women (3,4). Rare examples of AME are described in men (7,8); none had a carcinomatous (epithelial and/or myoepithelial) component.

Genetic Predisposition

AME has no documented genetic and/or familial association. A 41-year-old woman with neurofibromatosis type 1 and multiple gastrointestinal stromal tumors had a "malignant myoepithelioma" (=myoepithelial carcinoma) arising in an AME, but no other family member was affected (9).

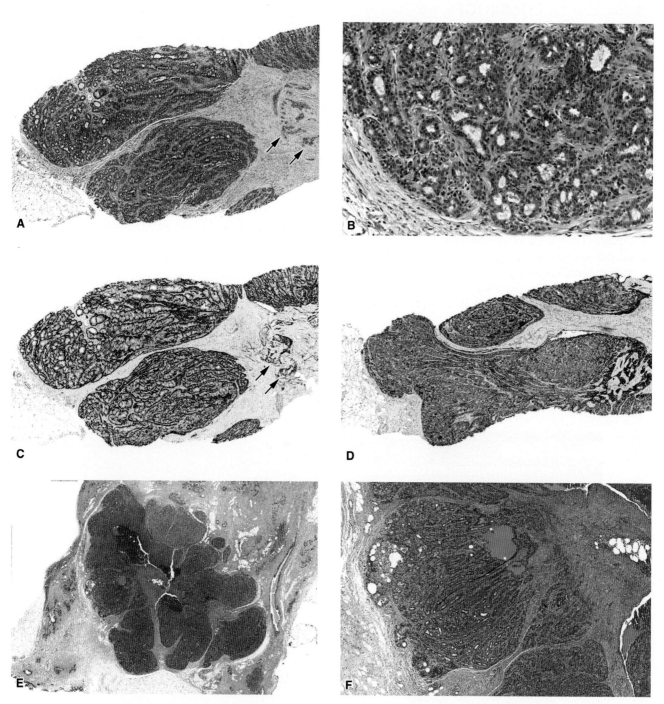

FIGURE 5.1 Adenomyoepithelioma. A: A needle core biopsy specimen. The adenomyoepithelioma consists of a few nodules. Distorted glands in the sclerotic center of the adenomyoepithelioma mimic a focus of invasive carcinoma *(arrows)*. **B:** Cuboidal epithelium lines the glands and tubules. **C, D:** The myoepithelial cells in this adenomyoepithelioma are strongly immunoreactive for smooth muscle myosin-heavy chain **(C)** and calponin **(D)**. The identification of a myoepithelial layer **(C)** around the distorted glands in the sclerotic center of the lesion **(A)** rules out stromal invasion *(arrows)*. **E, F:** Surgical excision specimen of the adenomyoepithelioma shown in **A–D**. The lesion has a well-circumscribed border.

Clinical Presentation

AME typically presents as a solitary and painless mass. The tumor commonly arises in the periphery of the breast; central or retroareolar location is rare. Nipple discharge is uncommon. Patients with carcinoma (epithelial and/or myoepithelial) in an AME may describe recent onset or report rapid growth of a long-standing lesion.

Imaging

Mammographically, AME usually appears as a single mass with well-circumscribed to microlobulated border. The mammographic appearance often suggests a fibroadenoma (FA) (10–13). Mammographic calcifications are rare (12,14–16). Sonographically (10,14), AME appears as a solid, round, or oval mass with hypo- or complex echogenic texture. The margin is typically smooth or lobulated, and rarely irregular (10,14). Posterior acoustic enhancement may be present (10,14). Hypervascularity in the vicinity of an AME has been reported (17). Adjacent ectatic ducts are also common. Mammographically inapparent AMEs can be detected by sonography (11,14). Information on the MRI features of AME is limited. Homogenous to heterogenous enhancement

with a delayed washout pattern after gadolinium injection is reported (10,14).

Size and Macroscopic Feature

AME has an average and median size of about 2.5 cm (range, 0.5–8.0), although contemporary cases tend to be smaller. Most AMEs are solid, well-circumscribed, and firm or hard. Some AMEs are cystic (4,5,18) or predominantly intracystic (14,19).

Microscopic Pathology

Adenomyoepithelioma

AME is a circumscribed tumor devoid of a fibrous capsule. Most lesions consist of an aggregate of solid or papillary nodules surrounding a slightly sclerotic center (**Fig. 5.1**). AME bears some morphologic resemblance to papilloma and ductal/tubular adenoma (18,20,21). A few AMEs appear to arise from a lobular proliferation or areas of adenomyoepithelial hyperplasia in adenosis (**Fig. 5.2**). An AME consists of closely juxtaposed small glands and tubules composed of cuboidal epithelial cells and MECs. The MECs of an AME are often polygonal or spindle-shaped with eosinophilic

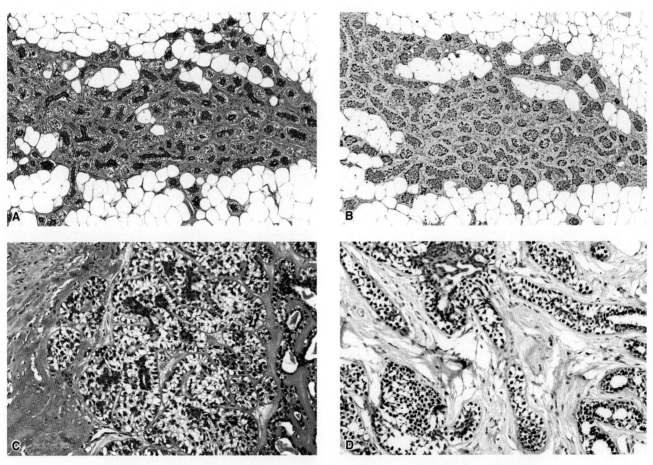

FIGURE 5.2 Adenomyoepithelial Hyperplasia in Adenosis. A: Myoepithelial cell hyperplasia is manifested by clear cells around the adenosis glands shown in fat. **B:** Myoepithelial cell nuclei are immunoreactive for p63 in the lesion shown in **A**. **C:** Clear myoepithelial cell hyperplasia around adenosis glands. **D:** Nuclear p63 reactivity in clear cell myoepithelial hyperplasia.

or clear cytoplasm. The juxtaposition of the dark-staining cytoplasm of the glandular cells and the pale or pink cytoplasm of MECs is a helpful clue to the diagnosis (**Fig. 5.3**). Apocrine metaplasia of the glandular epithelium is common, particularly in papillary areas. Squamous metaplasia can be florid, especially in areas of infarction, and can raise the differential diagnosis of squamous carcinoma (**Fig. 5.4**). Sebaceous (**Fig. 5.5**), or mucoepidermoid metaplasia can

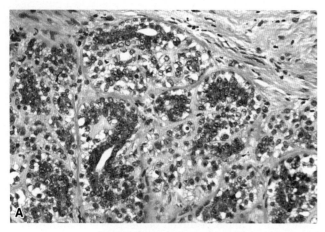
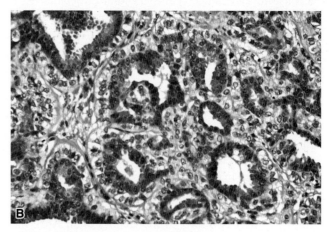

FIGURE 5.3 Adenomyoepithelioma. A: This tumor has prominent myoepithelial cells with clear cytoplasm that provide a striking contrast to the epithelial cells. **B:** Epithelioid myoepithelial cells form bands between glands composed of hyperplastic epithelial cells. The epithelioid myoepithelial cells mimic pagetoid spread of classic LCIS. Slender strands of basement membrane and fibrovascular stroma are evident.

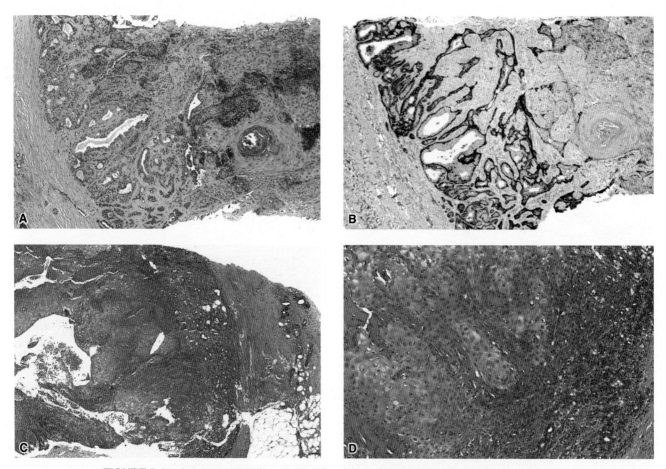

FIGURE 5.4 Adenomyoepithelioma with Infarction and Squamous Metaplasia. A: Most of the tumor in this needle core biopsy specimen is infarcted. **B:** Myoepithelium is highlighted in non-infarcted areas by reactivity for CD10. **C, D:** Another example of a partially infarcted adenomyo-epithelioma with squamous metaplasia in the infarcted area (**left**). The needle core biopsy material had been originally interpreted as diagnostic of metaplastic squamous cell carcinoma.

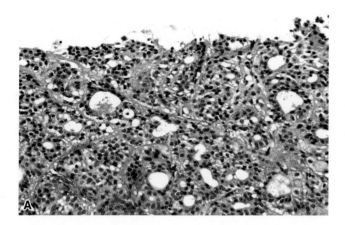

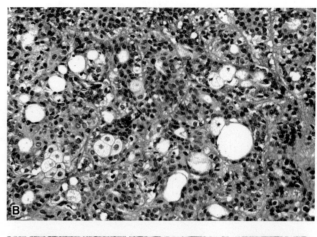

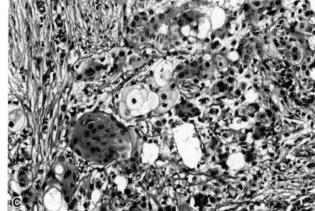

FIGURE 5.5 Adenomyoepithelioma with Sebaceous and Squamous Differentiation. A, B: In this needle core biopsy sample, the myoepithelial cells with vacuolated cytoplasm have largely overgrown the epithelial cells. Focal sebaceous differentiation is shown in **B**. **C:** Squamous and sebaceous metaplasia in another adenomyoepithelioma.

also occur. In some AMEs, MECs with clear cytoplasm are numerous and compress the tubular lumina, resulting in zones virtually devoid of glandular lumina (**Fig. 5.6**). The MECs can undergo myoid metaplasia (**Fig. 5.7**). Palisading of spindle cells and alveolar clustering of polygonal MECs are common myoid patterns. The glandular elements may be intermixed with myoid areas or overgrown by the myoepithelial proliferation (**Fig. 5.6**). Myoid hyperplasia may give rise to areas with leiomyomatous features or a storiform growth pattern (17). Stromal and myoepithelial elements may have an adenoid cystic pattern. Collagenous spherulosis (22) (**Fig. 5.8**) and cartilaginous metaplasia are rarely encountered. Occasional calcifications are present in glandular spaces (**Fig. 5.9**). Foci of stromal fibrosis or ischemic necrosis are rarely associated with coarse calcification.

Mixed Tumor (Pleomorphic Adenoma)

Mixed tumor (MT) (pleomorphic adenoma) of the breast (23,24) is a variant of AME. It occurs more frequently in the subareolar region and probably arises from large lactiferous ducts (25,26). Most MTs are solid and circumscribed tumors. Remnants of the underlying epithelial lesion, usually with myoepithelial cell hyperplasia, can be found in almost all cases (25,27). The matrix of a mammary MT can be loosely myxoid (**Fig. 5.10**) or collagenized and occasionally

shows chondroid or osseous metaplasia. Calcification and ossification can occur. Foci resembling cellular MT of the salivary glands and areas with a distinct papillary component can occur. Squamous and/or sebaceous metaplasia is not infrequent.

Atypical Adenomyoepithelioma

Atypical features in an AME include mitotic activity (4–5 mitoses/10 high power fields (HPFs)) in the epithelium and/or myoepithelium (6), focal nuclear pleomorphism, hyperchromasia, and occasional multinucleated cells. Apocrine atypia is a common finding in an atypical AME. Cytologic atypia is more common in AMEs in which MECs have a predominantly spindle cell morphology and distinctly myoid appearance or abundant clear cytoplasm and nuclear enlargement.

Carcinoma (Epithelial and/or Myoepithelial) Arising in AME

Carcinomatous transformation in an AME can be limited to either the epithelial or myoepithelial component, or can involve both elements. The diagnosis of adenocarcinoma arising in an AME applies when only the epithelium is malignant. When only the myoepithelium is malignant, the diagnosis of

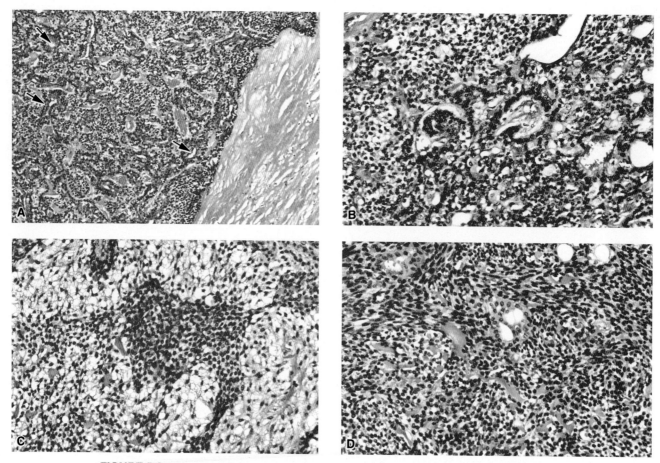

FIGURE 5.6 Adenomyoepithelioma with Myoepithelial Cell Hyperplasia. A, B: Epithelial cells are distributed in bands and nests with inconspicuous glandular lumina *(arrows)*. The myo-epithelial cells that have small, punctate nuclei and sparse clear cytoplasm tend to aggregate in poorly defined alveolar groups. **C:** This part of the tumor shown in **A** is composed entirely of myoepithelial cells. The combination of small, compact cells and cells with extremely vacuolated cytoplasm resembles a pattern seen in cellular pleomorphic adenoma (mixed tumor) of salivary gland origin. **D:** Spindle cell myoid differentiation of myoepithelial cells is shown surrounding in-conspicuous glands.

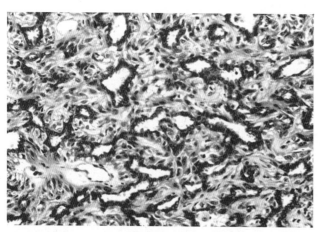

FIGURE 5.7 Adenomyoepithelioma with Myoid Differentiation. The spindly myoepithelial cells in this lesion have a myoid phenotype with eosinophilic cytoplasm.

myoepithelial carcinoma in an AME is appropriate. (Note: A malignant neoplasm with myoepithelial differentiation *not* arising in an AME is classified as metaplastic carcinoma [see Chapter 13].) The term malignant AME is reserved for exceedingly rare biphasic neoplasms in which both epithelial and myoepithelial components are carcinomatous.

High mitotic activity, necrosis, cellular pleomorphism, overgrowth of myoepithelium or epithelium, and invasion at the periphery of the tumor are features of a malignant AME. Carcinomatous AMEs with a biphasic growth pattern in the breast and at metastatic sites have also been reported (28–32).

Various morphologic types of carcinoma associated with AME are described, including adenoid cystic carcinoma (33), low-grade adenosquamous carcinoma (34,35), acantholytic squamous carcinoma (35), undifferentiated carcinoma (36),

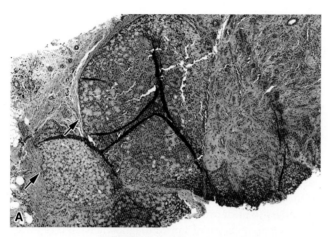 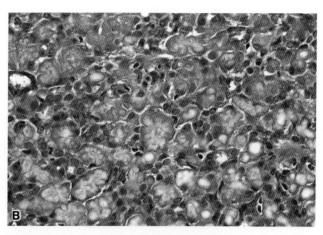

FIGURE 5.8 Adenomyoepithelioma with Collagenous Spherulosis. A: The nodules of adenomyoepithelioma in this needle core biopsy show extensive collagenous spherulosis *(arrows)*. **B:** In this unusual case, the deposits of basement membrane material comprising collagenous spherulosis have an unusual "flower-like" appearance.

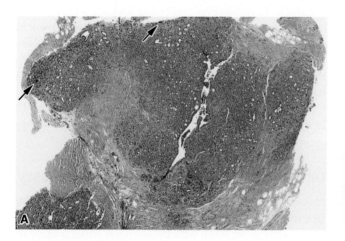 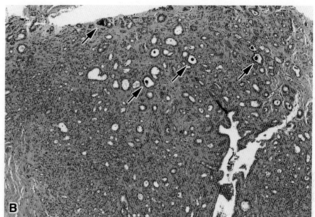

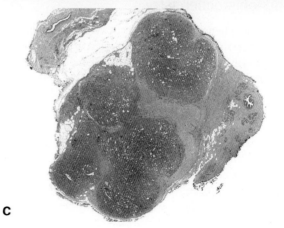

FIGURE 5.9 Adenomyoepithelioma with Calcifications.
A, B: The adenomyoepithelioma in this needle core biopsy material has scattered, minute intraluminal calcifications *(arrows)*.
C: The multinodular structure is apparent in the excised tumor.

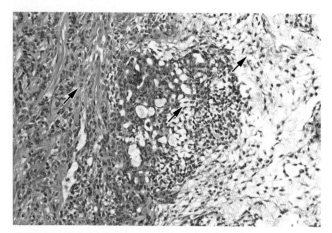

FIGURE 5.10 Mixed Tumor (Pleomorphic Adenoma) of the Breast. This mixed tumor consists of epithelial and myoepithelial cells with no evidence of cytologic atypia. The myoepithelial cells have predominantly spindle shape *(arrows)*, and some are admixed with myxoid matrix **(right)**. Fine needle aspiration material of this mixed tumor had been misdiagnosed as mucinous carcinoma.

sarcomatoid carcinoma (35), invasive ductal carcinoma (37), undifferentiated carcinoma with heterologous (osteogenic and spindle cell) differentiation (38), and myoepithelial carcinoma (39–41).

Myoepithelial Carcinoma

Myoepithelial carcinoma **Fig. 5.11** is an overgrowth of the carcinomatous myoepithelial component of an AME. It consists of spindle and/or epithelioid cells with high mitotic activity and cytologic atypia (39–42). Necrosis is common **(Fig. 5.11)**.

Immunohistochemistry

The immunophenotype of neoplastic MECs is sometimes different from that of their normal counterparts, and they are not necessarily reactive for all markers. Therefore, a panel of immunostains should be used to maximize the detection of MECs (see Table 5.1); it is recommended to include calponin and p63 stains in the diagnostic panel.

The epithelium of a benign AME usually displays some nuclear reactivity for estrogen receptor (ER), whereas progesterone receptor (PR) is typically absent. The MECs of an AME do not express ER and PR. Carcinomas arising in AMEs, whether consisting of only epithelial or myoepithelial carcinoma or of the combination of the two, are usually negative for ER and PR (31,32,43), and for HER2 (32,43).

Treatment and Prognosis

Adenomyoepithelioma

Most AMEs are benign tumors that can be treated by local excision (4). Local recurrence has been reported, usually more than 2 years after the initial excision (3,5,44). In some cases, recurrence of AME (4,44) could be attributed to incomplete excision, possibly related to multinodularity and

peripheral intraductal extension of the lesion (4). There is no evidence that cytologic atypia or the proportions of spindle and polygonal MECs are related to the risk for local recurrence. Carcinoma may be detected as a separate lesion coincidentally or subsequent to excision of an AME (5). Mastectomy, breast irradiation, and axillary dissection are not appropriate treatment for morphologically benign or atypical AME. Nadelman et al. (45) reported two morphologically "benign" AMEs that developed lung metastases with the same histologic appearance as the primary tumors. These two cases are extremely unusual. One of the mammary AMEs had been sampled by NCB, and the possibility of dissemination secondary to prior procedure cannot entirely be ruled out in this case; no mention of a prior diagnostic NCB is reported for the other mammary AME.

Carcinoma (Epithelial and/or Myoepithelial) Arising in AME

Carcinoma arising in AMEs is treated as any other type of breast carcinoma of similar grade and stage. Some morphologically carcinomatous tumors recurred locally (3,29,36–38,43,46), or resulted in distant metastases and a fatal outcome (30–32,36–40). Metastatic sites include lung (31,38), liver (40), bone (39), thyroid gland (30), brain (37), and kidney (32). Some patients had distant metastases few months after primary diagnosis (31,36,39), whereas others developed metastatic disease 12 (30) and 15 years (37) after diagnosis of the primary tumor.

Differential Diagnosis at Needle Core Biopsy

Invasive Carcinoma

In a small biopsy sample, clear cell epithelioid myoepithelial hyperplasia in an AME with the adenosis pattern could be mistaken for invasive carcinoma **(Fig. 5.12)**. Benign AME in which glandular elements are dispersed amid spindly MECs can also be mistaken for invasive carcinoma (47). Occasionally, small glandular lumina formed within the epithelial areas may have a pattern reminiscent of an endocrine neoplasm.

Metaplastic Carcinoma

The differential diagnosis of a mammary mixed tumor (pleomorphic adenoma) includes metaplastic carcinoma with myxoid/chondroid matrix (48). Metaplastic carcinoma shows cytologic atypia, increased cellularity, areas of necrosis, mitotic activity including atypical mitoses, and abnormal expansion of the neoplastic epithelial or myoepithelial component. The definitive diagnosis of mammary mixed tumor (pleomorphic adenoma) in a NCB sample is not possible, and follow-up surgical excision of the lesion is required to rule out metaplastic carcinoma.

Mucinous Carcinoma

The myxoid matrix of a mammary mixed tumor (pleomorphic adenoma) can occasionally simulate mucin, raising the differential diagnosis of mucinous carcinoma (27,49).

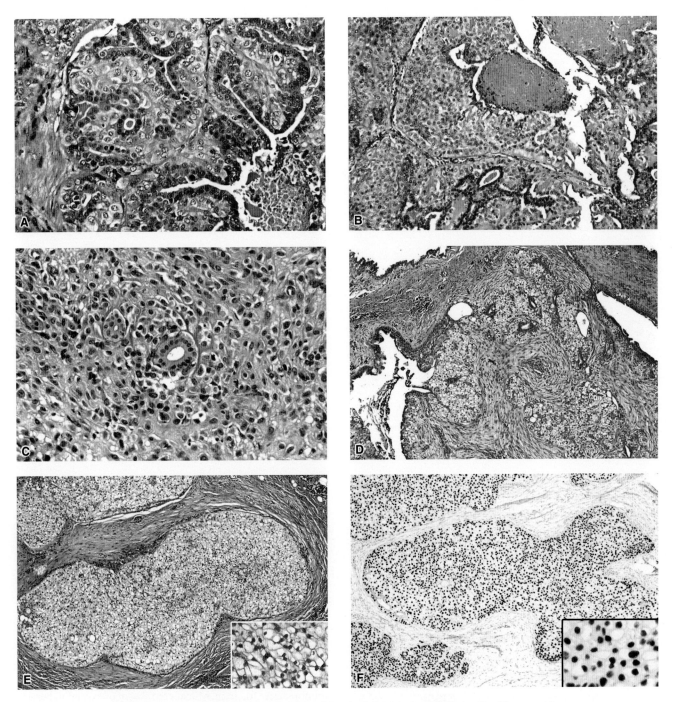

FIGURE 5.11 Myoepithelial Carcinoma Arising in Adenomyoepithelioma, Papilloma, and Adenosis. A: Epithelioid myoepithelial cells with large vesicular nuclei are indicative of an atypical proliferation in this adenomyoepithelioma. The epithelial cells are also hyperplastic. Focal necrosis is shown in the lower right corner. **B:** Sheets of neoplastic myoepithelial cells surround a focus of comedo-type necrosis. Residual glands are present. **C:** Infiltrating myoepithelial carcinoma surrounds two non-neoplastic glands. The tumor cells have eosinophilic or vacuolated cytoplasm. The needle core biopsy of this tumor had been diagnosed as suggestive of phyllodes tumor at another center. **D, E:** Intraductal myoepithelial carcinoma in a sclerosing papilloma **(D)** and in adjacent ducts **(E)**. *Inset* in **E** shows the clear cytoplasm in myoepithelial carcinoma cells. **F:** Nuclear p63 immunoreactivity in the myoepithelial intraductal carcinoma. **G–I:** Myoepithelial intraductal carcinoma arising in apocrine adenosis. Focal atypia of the apocrine epithelium is present **(H)**. Nuclear p63 is shown in the myoepithelial cells **(I)**.

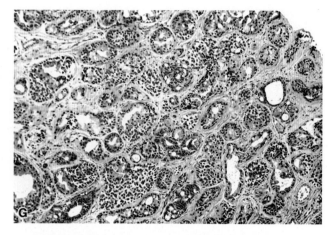

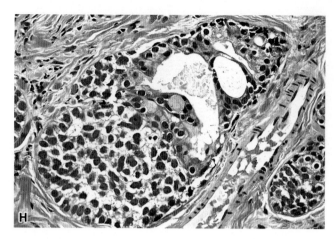

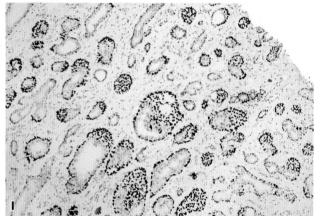

FIGURE 5.11 (*continued*)

Phyllodes Tumor

The spindle cell component of an AME or myoepithelial carcinoma arising in an AME can simulate a phyllodes tumor. AME has no frond-like architecture. The glands admixed with the spindled MECs of an AME or myoepithelial carcinoma arising in an AME are scattered throughout the lesion and have round to oval outline (**Fig. 5.11C**). Staining for MEC antigens is usually helpful to resolve the differential diagnosis.

Syringomatous Adenoma of the Nipple

Syringomatous adenoma of the nipple with myxochondroid stroma may raise the differential diagnosis of a mammary mixed tumor. Usually, syringomatous adenoma is based in the skin dermis and does arise primarily in the breast parenchyma.

MYOEPITHELIOMA

Myoepithelioma is an extremely rare tumor comprising almost exclusively benign MECs. Tumors referred to as muscular (50,51) and myoid hamartomas (52) probably arise from myoepithelial hyperplasia with myoid transformation.

Age and Gender

Most myoepitheliomas (including myoid hamartomas) are reported in peri- and postmenopausal women (50–57). Men are not affected.

Microscopic Pathology

A myoepithelioma consists of bundles of benign spindle cells sometimes arranged in a storiform pattern. The cytoplasm tends to be eosinophilic or sometimes clear. The spindle cells are immunoreactive for actin. Mitoses are absent or exceedingly rare.

Differential Diagnosis at Needle Core Biopsy

Pure spindle cell myoepithelial tumors may be difficult to distinguish by light microscopy from other spindle cell mammary neoplasms. The differential diagnosis includes myofibroblastoma, metaplastic carcinoma, and primary spindle cell sarcomas (especially leiomyosarcoma or fibrous histiocytoma). Some lesions reported in the past as myoepithelioma with peripheral infiltration into the surrounding fat might have been unrecognized examples of "low-grade" "fibromatosis-like" metaplastic spindle cell carcinoma (see also Chapter 13). Follow-up surgical excision is required for any neoplasm that yields a bland, spindle cell proliferation with myoepithelial differentiation in NCB material.

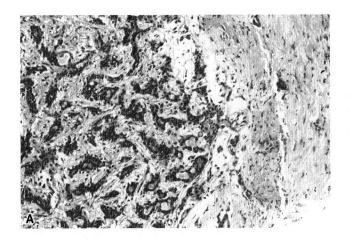

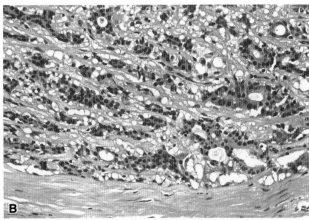

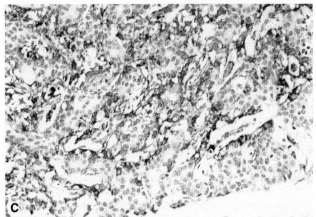

FIGURE 5.12 Adenomyoepithelioma Mistaken for Carcinoma. A: This needle core biopsy sample from an adenomyoepithelioma was interpreted as infiltrating duct carcinoma. The markedly vacuolated myoepithelial cells are difficult to recognize between the unevenly shaped glands, resulting in an appearance that simulates infiltrating carcinoma. **B:** The excisional biopsy specimen contained a well-circumscribed adenomyoepithelioma, part of which is shown here. **C:** Myoepithelial cells are highlighted in this immunostain for smooth muscle actin.

REFERENCES

1. Pandey PR, Saidou J, Watabe K. Role of myoepithelial cells in breast tumor progression. *Front Biosci.* 2010;15:226–236.

2. Hamperl H. The myothelia (myoepithelial cells): normal state; regressive changes; hyperplasia; tumors. *Curr Top Pathol.* 1970;53:161–220.

3. Loose JH, Patchefsky AS, Hollander IJ, et al. Adenomyoepithelioma of the breast: a spectrum of biologic behavior. *Am J Surg Pathol.* 1992;16:868–876.

4. Rosen PP. Adenomyoepithelioma of the breast. *Hum Pathol.* 1987;18:1232–1237.

5. Tavassoli FA. Myoepithelial lesions of the breast: myoepitheliosis, adenomyoepithelioma, and myoepithelial carcinoma. *Am J Surg Pathol.* 1991;15:554–568.

6. McLaren BK, Smith J, Schuyler PA, et al. Adenomyoepithelioma: clinical, histologic, and immunohistologic evaluation of a series of related lesions. *Am J Surg Pathol.* 2005;29:1294–1299.

7. Tamura G, Monma N, Suzuki Y, et al. Adenomyoepithelioma (myoepithelioma) of the breast in a male. *Hum Pathol.* 1993;24:678–681.

8. Berna JD, Arcas I, Ballester A, et al. Adenomyoepithelioma of the breast in a male. *AJR Am J Roentgenol.* 1997;169:917–918.

9. Hegyi L, Thway K, Newton R, et al. Malignant myoepithelioma arising in adenomyoepithelioma of the breast and coincident multiple gastrointestinal stromal tumours in a patient with neurofibromatosis type 1. *J Clin Pathol.* 2009;62:653–655.

10. Adejolu M, Wu Y, Santiago L, et al. Adenomyoepithelial tumors of the breast: imaging findings with histopathologic correlation. *AJR Am J Roentgenol.* 2011;197:W184–W190.

11. Chang A, Bassett L, Bose S. Adenomyoepithelioma of the breast: a cytologic dilemma: report of a case and review of the literature. *Diagn Cytopathol.* 2002;26:191–196.

12. Iyengar P, Ali SZ, Brogi E. Fine-needle aspiration cytology of mammary adenomyoepithelioma: a study of 12 patients. *Cancer.* 2006;108:250–256.

13. Mercado CL, Toth HK, Axelrod D, et al. Fine-needle aspiration biopsy of benign adenomyoepithelioma of the breast: radiologic and pathologic correlation in four cases. *Diagn Cytopathol.* 2007;35:690–694.

14. Lee JH, Kim SH, Kang BJ, et al. Ultrasonographic features of benign adenomyoepithelioma of the breast. *Korean J Radiol.* 2010;11:522–527.

15. Han JS, Peng Y. Multicentric adenomyoepithelioma of the breast with atypia and associated ductal carcinoma in situ. *Breast J.* 2010;16:547–549.

16. Howlett DC, Mason CH, Biswas S, et al. Adenomyoepithelioma of the breast: spectrum of disease with associated imaging and pathology. *AJR Am J Roentgenol.* 2003;180:799–803.

17. Park YM, Park JS, Jung HS, et al. Imaging features of benign adenomyoepithelioma of the breast. *J Clin Ultrasound.* 2013;41:218–223.

18. Gusterson BA, Sloane JP, Middwood C, et al. Ductal adenoma of the breast—a lesion exhibiting a myoepithelial/epithelial phenotype. *Histopathology.* 1987;11:103–110.

19. Hikino H, Kodama K, Yasui K, et al. Intracystic adenomyoepithelioma of the breast—case report and review. *Breast Cancer.* 2007;14:429–433.

20. Guarino M, Reale D, Squillaci S, et al. Ductal adenoma of the breast: an immunohistochemical study of five cases. *Pathol Res Pract.* 1993;189:515–520.

21. Jensen ML, Johansen P, Noer H, et al. Ductal adenoma of the breast: the cytological features of six cases. *Diagn Cytopathol.* 1994;10:143–145.

22. Reis-Filho JS, Fulford LG, Crebassa B, et al. Collagenous spherulosis in an adenomyoepithelioma of the breast. *J Clin Pathol.* 2004;57:83–86.

23. Chen KT. Pleomorphic adenoma of the breast. *Am J Clin Pathol.* 1990;93:792–794.

24. Diaz NM, McDivitt RW, Wick MR. Pleomorphic adenoma of the breast: a clinicopathologic and immunohistochemical study of 10 cases. *Hum Pathol.* 1991;22:1206–1214.

25. Narita T, Matsuda K. Pleomorphic adenoma of the breast: case report and review of the literature. *Pathol Int.* 1995;45:441–447.

26. Nevado M, Lopez JI, Dominguez MP, et al. Pleomorphic adenoma of the breast: case report. *APMIS.* 1991;99:866–868.

27. Reid-Nicholson M, Bleiweiss I, Pace B, et al. Pleomorphic adenoma of the breast: a case report and distinction from mucinous carcinoma. *Arch Pathol Lab Med.* 2003;127:474–477.

28. Trojani M, Guiu M, Trouette H, et al. Malignant adenomyoepithelioma of the breast: an immunohistochemical, cytophotometric, and ultrastructural study of a case with lung metastases. *Am J Clin Pathol.* 1992;98:598–602.

29. Qureshi A, Kayani N, Gulzar R. Malignant adenomyoepithelioma of the breast: a case report with review of literature. *BMJ Case Rep.* 2009;2009. pii:bcr01.2009.1442.

30. Bult P, Verwiel JM, Wobbes T, et al. Malignant adenomyoepithelioma of the breast with metastasis in the thyroid gland 12 years after excision of the primary tumor: case report and review of the literature. *Virchows Arch.* 2000;436:158–66.

31. Kihara M, Yokomise H, Irie A, et al. Malignant adenomyoepithelioma of the breast with lung metastases: report of a case. *Surg Today.* 2001;31:899–903.

32. Honda Y, Iyama K. Malignant adenomyoepithelioma of the breast combined with invasive lobular carcinoma. *Pathol Int.* 2009;59:179–184.

33. Van Dorpe J, De Pauw A, Moerman P. Adenoid cystic carcinoma arising in an adenomyoepithelioma of the breast. *Virchows Arch.* 1998;432:119–122.

34. Van Hoeven KH, Drudis T, Cranor ML, et al. Low-grade adenosquamous carcinoma of the breast: a clinicopathologic study of 32 cases with ultrastructural analysis. *Am J Surg Pathol.* 1993;17:248–258.

35. Foschini MP, Pizzicannella G, Peterse JL, et al. Adenomyoepithelioma of the breast associated with low-grade adenosquamous and sarcomatoid carcinomas. *Virchows Arch.* 1995;427:243–250.

36. Michal M, Baumruk L, Burger J, et al. Adenomyoepithelioma of the breast with undifferentiated carcinoma component. *Histopathology.* 1994;24:274–276.

37. Rasbridge SA, Millis RR. Adenomyoepithelioma of the breast with malignant features. *Virchows Arch.* 1998;432:123–130.

38. Simpson RH, Cope N, Skalova A, et al. Malignant adenomyoepithelioma of the breast with mixed osteogenic, spindle cell, and carcinomatous differentiation. *Am J Surg Pathol.* 1998;22:631–636.

39. Chen PC, Chen CK, Nicastri AD, et al. Myoepithelial carcinoma of the breast with distant metastasis and accompanied by adenomyoepitheliomas. *Histopathology.* 1994;24:543–548.

40. Jones C, Tooze R, Lakhani SR. Malignant adenomyoepithelioma of the breast metastasizing to the liver. *Virchows Arch.* 2003;442:504–506.

41. Buza N, Zekry N, Charpin C, et al. Myoepithelial carcinoma of the breast: a clinicopathological and immunohistochemical study of 15 diagnostically challenging cases. *Virchows Arch.* 2010;457:337–345.

42. Hungermann D, Buerger H, Oehlschlegel C, et al. Adenomyoepithelial tumours and myoepithelial carcinomas of the breast—a spectrum of monophasic and biphasic tumours dominated by immature myoepithelial cells. *BMC Cancer.* 2005;5:92.

43. Oka K, Sando N, Moriya T, et al. Malignant adenomyoepithelioma of the breast with matrix production may be compatible with one variant form of matrix-producing carcinoma: a case report. *Pathol Res Pract.* 2007;203:599–604.

44. Young RH, Clement PB. Adenomyoepithelioma of the breast: a report of three cases and review of the literature. *Am J Clin Pathol.* 1988;89:308–314.

45. Nadelman CM, Leslie KO, Fishbein MC. "Benign," metastasizing adenomyoepithelioma of the breast: a report of 2 cases. *Arch Pathol Lab Med.* 2006;130:1349–1353.

46. Pauwels C, De Potter C. Adenomyoepithelioma of the breast with features of malignancy. *Histopathology.* 1994;24:94–96.

47. Zhang C, Quddus MR, Sung CJ. Atypical adenomyoepithelioma of the breast: diagnostic problems and practical approaches in core needle biopsy. *Breast J.* 2004;10:154–155.

48. Djakovic A, Engel JB, Geisinger E, et al. Pleomorphic adenoma of the breast initially misdiagnosed as metaplastic carcinoma in preoperative stereotactic biopsy: a case report and review of the literature. *Eur J Gynaecol Oncol.* 2011;32:427–430.

49. Iyengar P, Cody HS III, Brogi E. Pleomorphic adenoma of the breast: case report and review of the literature. *Diagn Cytopathol.* 2005;33:416–420.

50. Davies JD, Riddell RH. Muscular hamartomas of the breast. *J Pathol.* 1973;111:209–211.

51. Eusebi V, Cunsolo A, Fedeli F, et al. Benign smooth muscle cell metaplasia in breast. *Tumori.* 1980;66:643–653.

52. Daroca PJ Jr, Reed RJ, Love GL, et al. Myoid hamartomas of the breast. *Hum Pathol.* 1985;16:212–219.

53. Erlandson RA, Rosen PP. Infiltrating myoepithelioma of the breast. *Am J Surg Pathol.* 1982;6:785–793.

54. Bigotti G, Di Giorgio CG. Myoepithelioma of the breast: histologic, immunologic, and electromicroscopic appearance. *J Surg Oncol.* 1986;32:58–64.

55. Rode L, Nesland JM, Johannessen JV. A spindle cell breast lesion in a 54-year-old woman. *Ultrastruct Pathol.* 1986;10:421–425.

56. Schurch W, Potvin C, Seemayer TA. Malignant myoepithelioma (myoepithelial carcinoma) of the breast: an ultrastructural and immunocytochemical study. *Ultrastruct Pathol.* 1985;8:1–11.

57. Thorner PS, Kahn HJ, Baumal R, et al. Malignant myoepithelioma of the breast: an immunohistochemical study by light and electron microscopy. *Cancer.* 1986;57:745–750.

Adenosis and Microglandular Adenosis

EDI BROGI

ADENOSIS

All forms of adenosis except microglandular adenosis (see section on Microglandular Adenosis in this chapter) are lobulocentric proliferations of small ducts and glands lined by epithelium and myoepithelium, and surrounded by basement membrane. Stromal sclerosis is commonly associated with adenosis, resulting in "sclerosing adenosis" (SA) (1). Coalescent areas of adenosis can form a mass (adenosis tumor).

Clinical Presentation

Age and Incidence

Adenosis is usually included in the spectrum of fibrocystic change (FCC). The mean age at diagnosis of adenosis tumor in a series of 15 cases (2) was 37 years (range, 21–68); 12 women were premenopausal. There were 88 cases with diagnosis of SA out of a total of 1,166 consecutive needle core biopsies (NCBs) (7.5%) performed over 5 years at one center (3). The mean age of women with NCB diagnosis of SA not associated with carcinoma or atypia was 48 years (range, 35–72); 23 (70%) women were younger than 50 years, and 19 (58%) were 45 to 54 years old. In another series (4), SA was present in 37 breast NCBs as either a minor (20 cases) or major (17 cases) component. Adenosis is exceedingly rare in men.

Presenting Symptoms

Adenosis consisting of closely adjacent or merging lobules can form a palpable and/or radiographically detectable mass (adenosis tumor) (2) that can mimic a fibroadenoma. The mean size of 15 adenosis tumors in one study (2) was 1.9 cm. Patients rarely report pain or tenderness (2,4,5). A 37-year-old woman with bilateral adenosis tumors had bilateral palpable and tender masses with indistinct margins (5). Calcifications are common in adenosis, and tend to be small and clustered, especially in SA.

Radiology
Mass

An adenosis tumor can appear as a lobulated solid mass mammographically and by ultrasound examination (2), closely mimicking a fibroadenoma. A patient with bilateral adenosis tumors (5) had multiple oval masses with angulated margins, complex posterior acoustic shadowing, and orientation parallel to the skin by ultrasound examination. Mild vascularity was detected on color Doppler-ultrasound. On MRI, the masses were ovoid with indistinct borders, had intermediate enhancement on T1-weighted and T2-weighted images, and had a homogeneous signal.

Calcifications

Nonpalpable adenosis is usually detected mammographically because of associated calcifications. Gill et al. (3) studied the radiologic findings of 44 lesions that yielded SA as the major component in a NCB sample, including 4/44 with ductal carcinoma in situ (DCIS), and 7/44 with atypical ductal hyperplasia (ADH). DCIS in SA was associated with pleomorphic calcifications, and ADH with amorphous calcifications. The 33 NCBs that yielded SA without carcinoma or atypia targeted clustered calcifications (16 cases), mass (15 cases), one circumscribed mass with calcifications, and one spiculated mass.

Microscopic Pathology

An *adenosis tumor* is a mass lesion formed by closely juxtaposed and/or coalescent foci of adenosis (**Figs. 6.1–6.3**).

Sclerosing Adenosis

SA is the most common form of adenosis. It shows variable attenuation of the glandular epithelium, preservation of the myoepithelium, and lobular fibrosis. The glands are arranged in a swirling lobulocentric pattern, and the glandular lumina are compressed and often inapparent (**Fig. 6.4**). The myoepithelium can undergo myoid metaplasia (**Fig. 6.5**). In some cases, fibrosis separates the glands, resulting in a dispersed pattern that can mimic tubular carcinoma (**Fig. 6.6**). SA tends to have a more glandular pattern in premenopausal women, but sclerosis and epithelial atrophy are common after menopause (**Fig. 6.7**). Multiple minute calcifications are common (**Fig. 6.8**).

Florid Adenosis

Florid adenosis is the most cellular form of adenosis with hyperplasia of epithelial and myoepithelial cells (**Fig. 6.9**). Pregnancy-associated mass-forming florid adenosis can sometimes exhibit apoptosis and mitotic activity (**Fig. 6.10**). Geographic necrosis is very rare. Calcifications are less common and extensive than in SA.

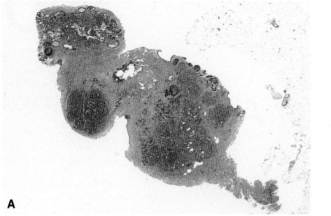

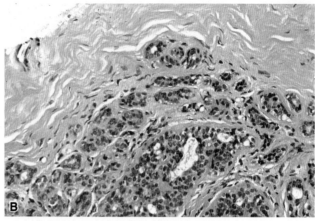

FIGURE 6.1 Adenosis Tumor. A, B: Multiple nodules of adenosis are shown in this needle core biopsy specimen. Larger nodules are the result of coalescent lobules, such as the one shown in **B**.

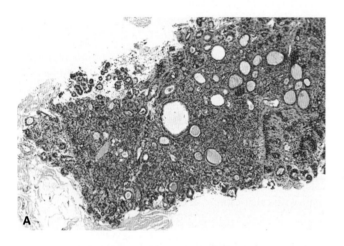

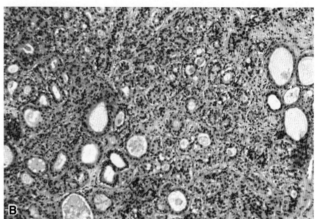

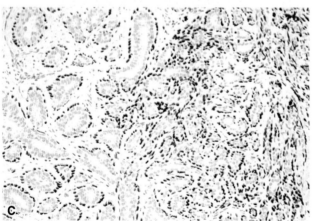

FIGURE 6.2 Adenosis Tumor. A, B: A very dense proliferation of hyperplastic epithelial and myoepithelial cells characterizes this lesion. Note the distinct border on the left **(A)** and numerous microcysts. **C:** Myoepithelial hyperplasia is highlighted by nuclear reactivity for p63.

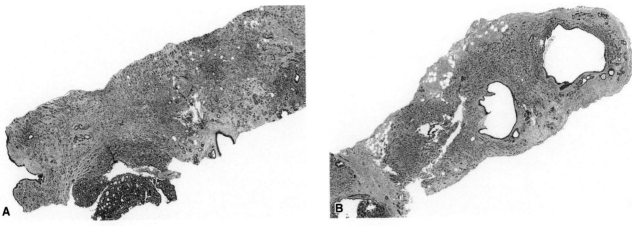

FIGURE 6.3 Adenosis Tumor. A, B: Multiple foci of adenosis are present in the tissue cores obtained from the same mass lesion. Two cysts are present in **B**.

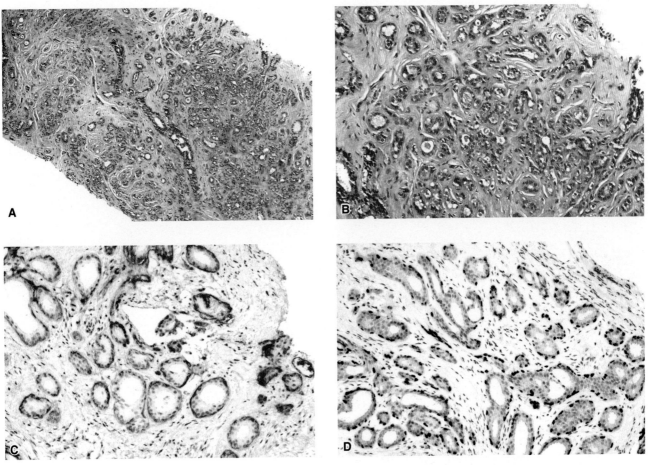

FIGURE 6.4 Sclerosing Adenosis. A, B: A needle core biopsy specimen from a confluent lesion showing stromal fibrosis, thickened periglandular basement membranes, and atrophy of some glands. **C:** Myoepithelium is highlighted by cytoplasmic reactivity for CD10. **D:** Myoepithelium around adenosis glands is identified by nuclear p63 reactivity.

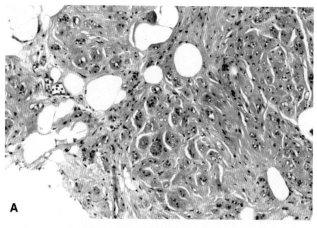

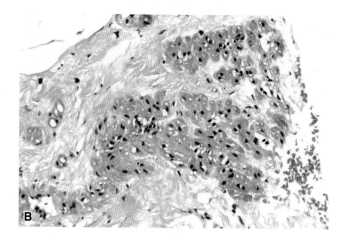

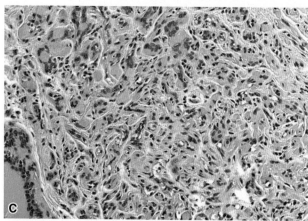

FIGURE 6.5 Sclerosing Adenosis with Myoid Metaplasia.
A, B: Well-developed myoid metaplasia of myoepithelial cells is
shown in this needle core biopsy specimen. Epithelial cells are
almost absent, and the myoepithelial cells have the eosinophilic
cytoplasm of smooth muscle. **C:** Epithelioid myoid metaplasia of
myoepithelium in sclerosing adenosis.

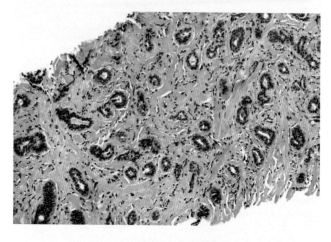

FIGURE 6.6 Adenosis with a Dispersed Pattern. Glands with
round, angular, and tubular shapes are dispersed in collagenous
stroma that exhibits pseudoangiomatous hyperplasia. This type of
adenosis resembles tubular carcinoma.

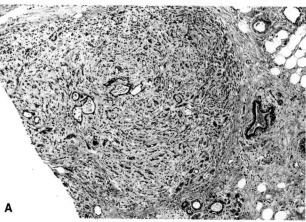

FIGURE 6.7 Sclerosing Adenosis with Atrophy. A, B: This
needle core biopsy sample shows nodular, atrophic sclerosing
adenosis that resembles invasive lobular carcinoma. **C:** Severe
atrophy of glandular cells, leaving swirling elongated myoepithelial
cells, characterizes this lesion.

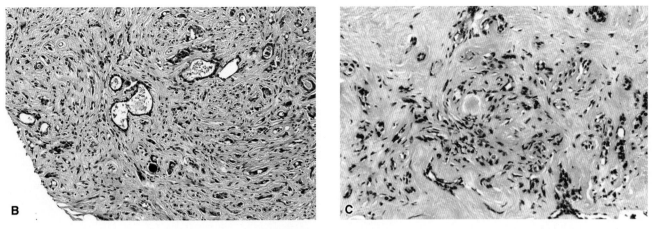

FIGURE 6.7 (*continued*)

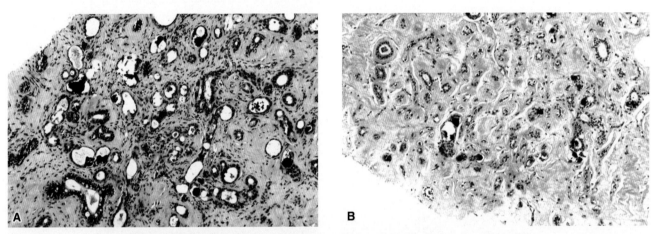

FIGURE 6.8 Sclerosing Adenosis with Calcifications. A: A lesion with abundant calcifications. **B:** A focus of sclerosing adenosis with epithelial atrophy and calcifications.

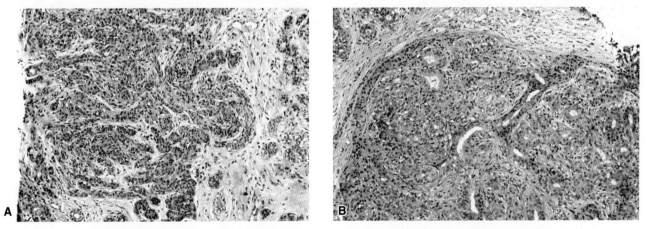

FIGURE 6.9 Florid Adenosis. A, B: Elongated, hyperplastic, entwined adenosis glands and myo-epithelium are shown in a needle core biopsy specimen. The epithelium in **B** has apocrine features.

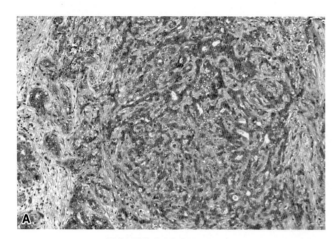
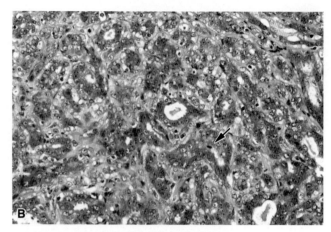

FIGURE 6.10 Florid Adenosis in Pregnancy. This needle core biopsy sample was obtained from a palpable tumor in a 35-year-old woman who was 9 weeks pregnant. **A, B:** There is marked hyperplasia of epithelial and myoepithelial cells in this example of florid adenosis. An epithelial mitosis is evident *(arrow)*.

Tubular Adenosis

Tubular adenosis (TA) consists of proliferating, elongated ductules. Most ductules are cut longitudinally and appear as tubules **(Fig. 6.11)**. TA lacks the lobulocentric distribution of florid or sclerosing adenosis, and the ductules often extend in a seemingly haphazard pattern into fibrous mammary stroma and fat **(Fig. 6.11)**. Intraluminal secretion may undergo calcification. The presence of basement membranes and an outer myoepithelial cell layer (6) are useful in separating TA and tubular carcinoma.

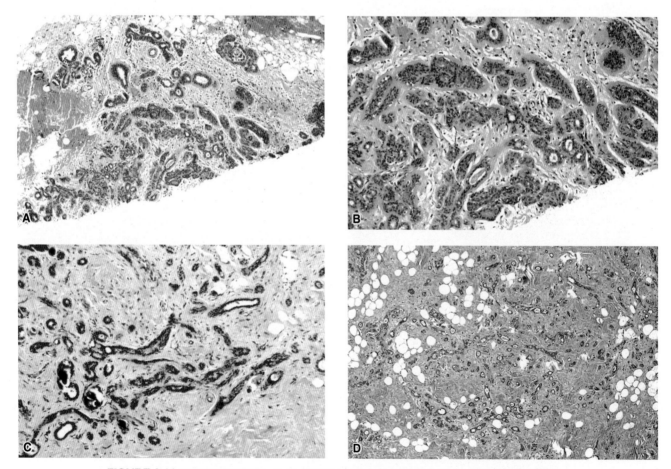

FIGURE 6.11 Tubular Adenosis. A, B: Elongated adenosis glands that resemble tubules with epithelial hyperplasia and thick basement membranes are present in this needle core biopsy sample from a premenopausal woman. **C:** Epithelial atrophy, calcifications, and stromal fibrosis in a biopsy specimen from a postmenopausal patient. **D:** An example of tubular adenosis in an excision specimen demonstrates the infiltrative nature of this lesion that closely mimics invasive carcinoma.

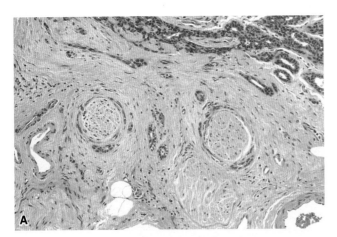

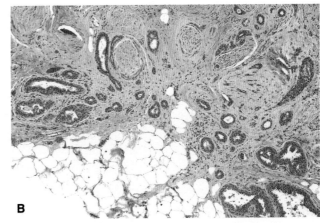

FIGURE 6.12 Adenosis with Perineural Invasion. A: Two nerves are shown surrounded circumferentially by adenosis glands. **B:** Adenosis glands encircle nerves at the perimeter of a radial sclerosing lesion in this needle core biopsy specimen.

In all aforementioned forms of adenosis, the distorted ductules and glands can closely mimic invasive carcinoma. Cystic dilation of ductules or glands is uncommon, but TA tends to have more open lumina. The epithelium lining the tubules and glands is usually inconspicuous, slightly columnar to flat. Signet ring cell morphology or intracytoplasmic vacuoles are exceedingly rare in adenosis. Apocrine metaplasia can involve all aforementioned forms of adenosis (see also section on Apocrine Adenosis and Atypical Apocrine Adenosis in this chapter). Epithelial mitoses are rare to absent but can occur in pregnancy. The myoepithelial cells can be spindled or cuboidal, with conspicuous clear cytoplasm, or attenuated. Perineural invasion may occur (**Fig. 6.12**). Invasion of the wall of blood vessels by florid adenosis was documented in 10% of cases in one study (7). Necrosis and/or infarction occasionally occur in adenosis tumor, usually during pregnancy or lactation.

Blunt Duct Adenosis

Blunt duct adenosis (BDA) is a form of terminal duct hyperplasia characterized by abortive lobule formation (1). The proliferating epithelium forms solid or microcystic aggregates of round or angulated glands (**Fig. 6.13**). The myoepithelium in cystic BDA tends to have abundant clear cytoplasm. The stroma surrounding BDA glands is slightly expanded and more cellular than usual intralobular stroma and contains scattered inflammatory cells. BDA sometimes exhibits apocrine metaplasia.

Apocrine Adenosis and Atypical Apocrine Adenosis

Apocrine adenosis (AA) designates a focus of adenosis with apocrine metaplasia (8,9) (**Fig. 6.14**). It is a common alteration, especially in the context of SA. It is readily detected at low-power examination, because the apocrine cells have more abundant apocrine-type cytoplasm than the cuboidal to flat epithelium typically found in adenosis. The cytoplasm is finely granular and eosinophilic, but can be gray to amphophilic. The nuclei are round with prominent nucleoli and show no atypical features. No mitoses are present.

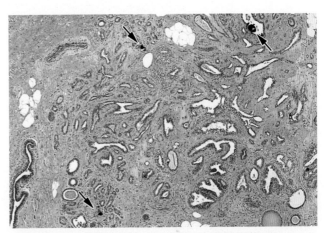

FIGURE 6.13 Blunt Duct Adenosis. An example of blunt duct adenosis in an excision specimen. A few small calcifications are present *(arrows).*

Atypical apocrine adenosis (AAA) consists of apocrine cells with cytoplasmic clearing or vacuolization and anisonucleosis. The nuclei have irregular nuclear membranes, as much as threefold variation in size, and nuclear pleomorphism (**Fig. 6.15**). Nuclear hyperchromasia and prominent nucleoli are found in the most extreme examples of AAA. Mitotic figures are uncommon, and their identification raises the differential diagnosis of apocrine DCIS (10,11). The diagnosis of DCIS with apocrine morphology is reserved for cases with substantial cytologic atypia *and/or* mitotic activity *and/or* fully developed architectural patterns characteristic of DCIS, such as solid growth, cribriform, or papillary architecture.

It is unclear whether AAA is a morphologic precursor of DCIS with apocrine features.

One study (12) found that the median Ki67 proliferation rate of AA was significantly higher than that of normal mammary epithelium but did not differ significantly from that of AAA (3.7% vs. 4.8%). Calhoun and Booth (13) reported a retrospective series including 22 NCBs with diagnosis of AA and 12 with diagnosis of AAA. The mean and median

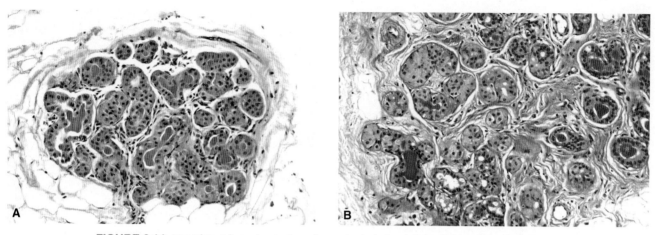

FIGURE 6.14 Apocrine Adenosis. A: Apocrine metaplasia in a lobule. **B:** Apocrine metaplasia in adenosis.

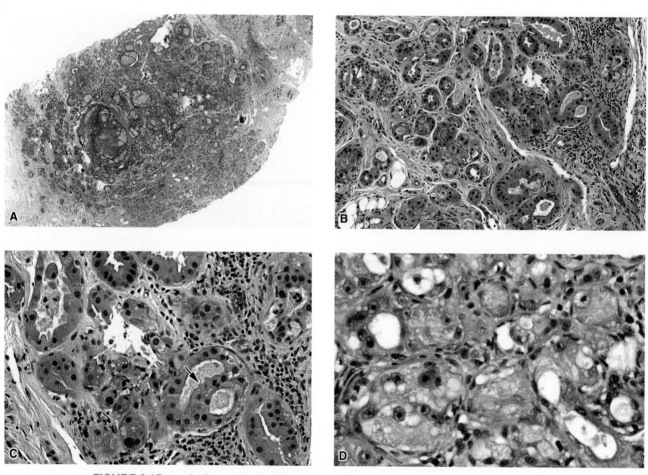

FIGURE 6.15 Atypical Apocrine Adenosis. A–D: A needle core biopsy with atypical apocrine adenosis. **A:** The epithelium in a focus of sclerosing adenosis is expanded. At low-power magnification, the apocrine epithelial cells have abundant cytoplasm. **B:** On closer examination, the apocrine cells are enlarged, and a few have hyperchromatic nuclei. **C:** Nuclear hyperchromasia and anisonucleosis are evident. The epithelium in one gland forms a small arch *(arrow)*. **D:** The cytoplasm of the atypical apocrine cells is vacuolated. The nuclei are enlarged, and nucleoli are prominent.

age at diagnosis was 60 and 58 years, respectively. The NCBs sampled calcifications (11 cases), a mass or density (18 cases), and a mass or density with calcifications (3 cases). Two NCBs sampled a focus of MRI enhancement. Seven NCBs with AA also contained atypia and/or carcinoma (one invasive carcinoma, one DCIS, and five atypical hyperplasia). Five NCBs with AAA also contained other forms of atypia or carcinoma (two atypical hyperplasia and three DCIS). No carcinoma was found in subsequent excisional biopsy specimens in patients who had only AA or AAA in the index NCB material. No long-term follow-up information was provided in this report.

Carcinoma and Atypia in Adenosis

ADH, atypical lobular hyperplasia (ALH), lobular carcinoma in situ (LCIS), and DCIS can arise in adenosis. Adenosis can also be secondarily involved by carcinoma in situ (CIS) established in the surrounding tissue.

LCIS and ALH in Adenosis

Classic LCIS is the most common form of CIS in adenosis **(Figs. 6.16–6.18)**. LCIS causes an expansion of the epithelium in a focus of adenosis, and focal cell dyshesion is usually evident. Signet ring cell morphology is seen in LCIS, but it is not a feature

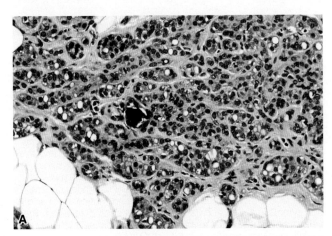
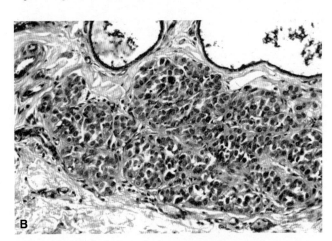

FIGURE 6.16 Sclerosing Adenosis with Lobular Carcinoma In Situ. A, B: Signet ring cell lobular carcinoma in situ with intracytoplasmic mucin demonstrated with the mucicarmine stain **(B)**.

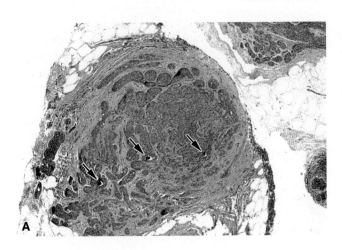
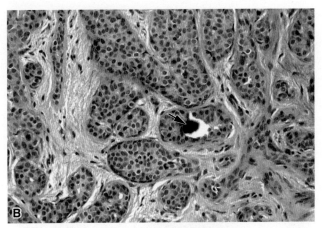
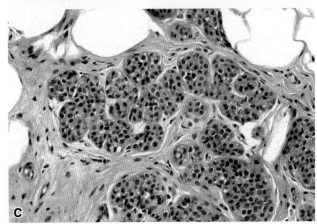

FIGURE 6.17 Tubular Adenosis with Lobular Carcinoma In Situ. A, B: Swirling tubular adenosis glands are expanded by LCIS. The needle core biopsy was performed for mammographically detected microcalcifications *(arrows)*. **C:** LCIS in adenosis from the same specimen with less architectural distortion.

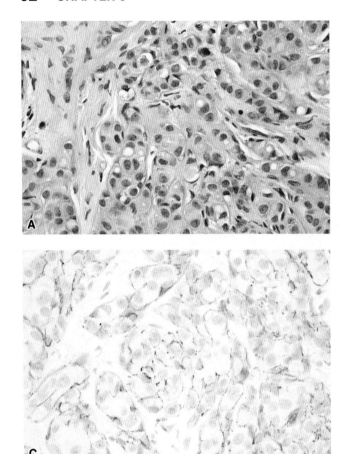

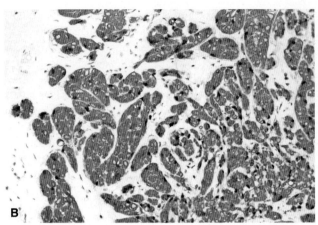

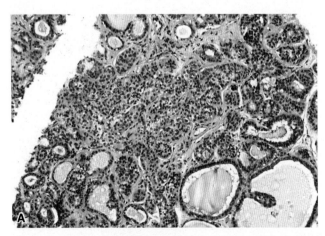

FIGURE 6.18 Sclerosing Adenosis with Lobular Carcinoma In Situ. A: Sclerosing adenosis involved by LCIS mimics invasive carcinoma. The LCIS cells have intracytoplasmic vacuoles and signet ring morphology. Basement membranes outline many of the lobular glands. **B:** Staining with the ADH5 antibody cocktail highlights the myoepithelial layer (brown chromogen: nuclear p63 and cytoplasmic CK5 and CK14), ruling out stromal invasion. The cells of LCIS show cytoplasmic reactivity for luminal cytokeratins (red chromogen: cytoplasmic CK7 and CK18). **C:** Weak membranous E-cadherin reactivity highlights myoepithelial cells. There is no reactivity around LCIS cells.

of benign epithelium in adenosis. ALH involving adenosis can be a subtle finding **(Fig. 6.19)**. The diagnosis of LCIS and ALH in adenosis is supported by negative membranous reactivity for E-cadherin **(Fig. 6.18)** and diffuse cytoplasmic staining for p120.

DCIS in Adenosis

DCIS in adenosis is less common than LCIS. The diagnosis of DCIS in adenosis needs to fulfill the same criteria required for

the diagnosis of DCIS outside of adenosis, and it is appropriate when an atypical epithelial proliferation shows solid, cribriform, or papillary architecture *and/or* substantial cytologic atypia, *and/or* comedo necrosis **(Fig. 6.20)**. The distinction between AAA and apocrine DCIS in adenosis can be especially difficult (10,11,14) **(Fig. 6.21)**. Cytoplasmic clearing or vacuolization can occur in atypical sclerosing apocrine lesions as well as in DCIS with apocrine features (see Chapter 15—Apocrine Carcinoma).

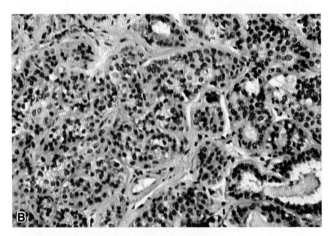

FIGURE 6.19 Adenosis with Atypical Lobular Hyperplasia. A, B: The small monomorphic cells of atypical lobular hyperplasia are apparent in some adenosis glands in this needle core biopsy specimen. The biopsy was performed for nonpalpable, mammographically detected calcifications. Note the microcystic dilatation of some glands and a small calcification right of center **(B)**.

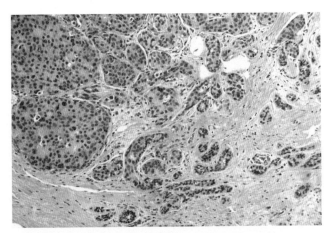

FIGURE 6.20 Sclerosing Adenosis with Intraductal Carcinoma. The glands on the left are markedly enlarged by intraductal carcinoma that has a solid growth pattern. Remnants of adenosis are evident on the right. The ductal carcinoma in situ has apocrine features with amphophilic cytoplasm.

Adenosis in Fibroepithelial Lesions

A fibroadenoma with SA is a "complex fibroadenoma" (see Chapter 7—Fibroepithelial Neoplasms). SA may be limited to a part of a fibroadinoma (FA) **(Fig. 6.22)**, or it may be diffuse, obscuring the underlying fibroepithelial structure. A NCB sample of a complex FA can simulate the appearance of invasive carcinoma. Phyllodes tumors can also have areas of adenosis.

Immunohistochemistry

Adenosis can closely mimic invasive carcinoma, especially when the glands and tubules are very compact, or appear to infiltrate the adjacent fat and breast parenchyma, or are markedly distorted by extensive sclerosis, and/or CIS is present. These scenarios often require immunohistochemical studies using a panel of myoepithelial markers (6,15). In a study (16) evaluating the reactivity of myoepithelial markers in SA, calponin was negative in 1/22 (4.5%) cases, myosin in 3/21 (14.3%), and CK5/6 in 4/20 (20%), whereas SMA, CD10, p63, and p75 stained the myoepithelium in all cases tested for these markers.

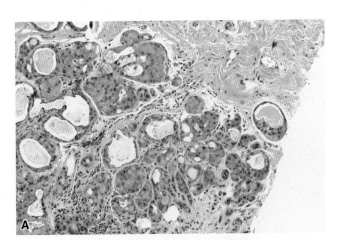

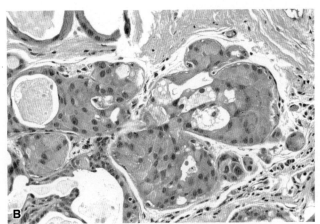

FIGURE 6.21 Sclerosing Adenosis with Apocrine Intraductal Carcinoma. A, B: The adenosis glands in this needle core biopsy specimen are expanded by apocrine carcinoma composed of cells with abundant eosinophilic cytoplasm and pleomorphic nuclei.

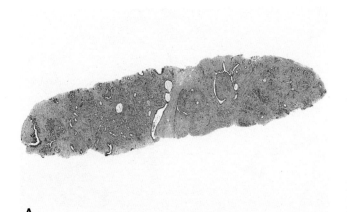

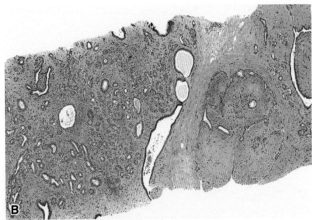

FIGURE 6.22 Sclerosing Adenosis in a Fibroadenoma. A, B: This needle core biopsy specimen of a fibroadenoma with adenosis (complex fibroadenoma) shows adenosis glands concentrated in one part of the lesion **(left)**, whereas a few elongated ducts and lobules with fibroadenomatoid changes are seen in another part of the lesion **(right)**.

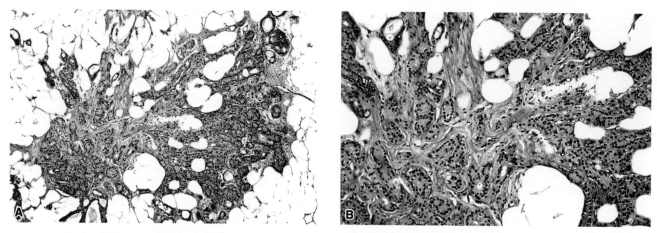

FIGURE 6.23 Adenosis Mimics Invasive Carcinoma. A, B: This needle core biopsy specimen shows sclerosing adenosis in fat, simulating invasive carcinoma.

Differential Diagnosis

Invasive Carcinoma

Adenosis can mimic invasive carcinoma, especially when the glands and tubules are very compact, or appear to infiltrate the adjacent fat (**Figs. 6.23 and 6.24**) and breast parenchyma, or are markedly distorted by extensive sclerosis (**Fig. 6.25**), and/or involved by CIS. Conversely, it is difficult to diagnose stromal invasion within foci of adenosis. The most convincing evidence for a diagnosis of invasive carcinoma arising in adenosis is the presence of invasive foci extending *beyond* the adenosis lesion. Careful evaluation of

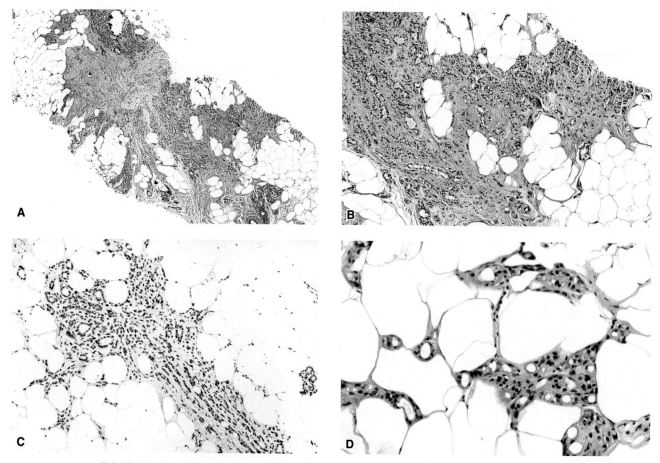

FIGURE 6.24 Sclerosing Adenosis with an Invasive Pattern. A, B: Sclerosing adenosis in this needle core biopsy specimen extends into fat in a pattern that resembles invasive carcinoma. Note the fibrous stroma that uniformly surrounds the adenosis glands. **C:** Nuclear p63 staining decorates myoepithelial cells. **D:** Another needle core biopsy sample in which fat cells are surrounded by sclerosing adenosis, and isolated glands are present in the fat.

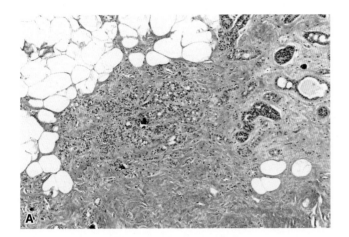

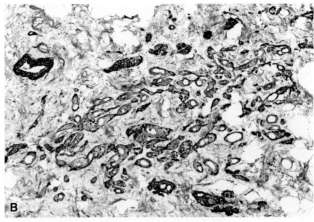

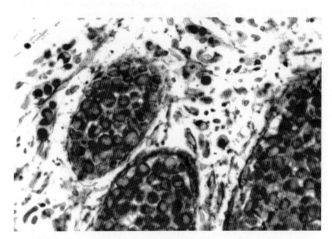

FIGURE 6.25 Sclerosing Adenosis with an Invasive Pattern. A: Sclerosing adenosis in this needle core biopsy specimen simulates tubular carcinoma. **B:** Staining of the focus in **A** with the ADH5 antibody cocktail highlights the myoepithelial cells (brown chromogen: nuclear p63 and cytoplasmic CK5 and CK14). The cytoplasm of the epithelial cells is positive for luminal cytokeratins (red chromogen: CK7 and CK18). **C:** Another needle core biopsy sample in which sclerosing adenosis mimics invasive carcinoma.

the interface of the lesion with the surrounding uninvolved breast parenchyma is most informative, although the latter is often only minimally represented in a NCB sample. The absence of nonlesional tissue in a NCB sample occasionally precludes excluding stromal invasion based on evaluation of H&E-stained sections, and requires the use of immunohistochemical stains for a panel of myoepithelial markers. A focal inflammatory cell infiltrate and reactive stromal changes separating the glands often accompany stromal (micro)invasion (**Fig. 6.26**).

Invasive Ductal Carcinoma, Well Differentiated

TA and SA can mimic well-differentiated carcinoma (**Figs. 6.11, 6.24, 6.25,** and **6.27**) and tubular carcinoma. Basement membrane and myoepithelium are usually visible around the pseudoinfiltrating glands in H&E-stained slides. Immunoperoxidase stains for myoepithelial markers can be used in problematic cases.

Invasive Lobular or Ductal Carcinoma

LCIS or DCIS involving adenosis can mimic invasive carcinoma, but the underlying adenosis tends to retain a lobulocentric arrangement (**Fig. 6.17**).

LCIS and ALH

The solid type of BDA can occasionally resemble ALH or classic LCIS. Immunohistochemical stains for E-cadherin and p120 can be used in difficult cases.

FIGURE 6.26 Sclerosing Adenosis with In Situ and Microinvasive Lobular Carcinoma. Double immunolabeling has been used to detect microinvasive lobular carcinoma in this specimen in which in situ lobular carcinoma involves sclerosing adenosis. Scattered AE1:AE3-positive epithelial cells (red chromogen) devoid of myoepithelium are evident in the stroma outside glands bounded by myoepithelial cells positive for smooth muscle actin (brown chromogen).

Treatment and Prognosis

Surgical Excision

Radiologic–pathologic correlation needs to be assessed whenever adenosis is present in a NCB specimen. Surgical excision

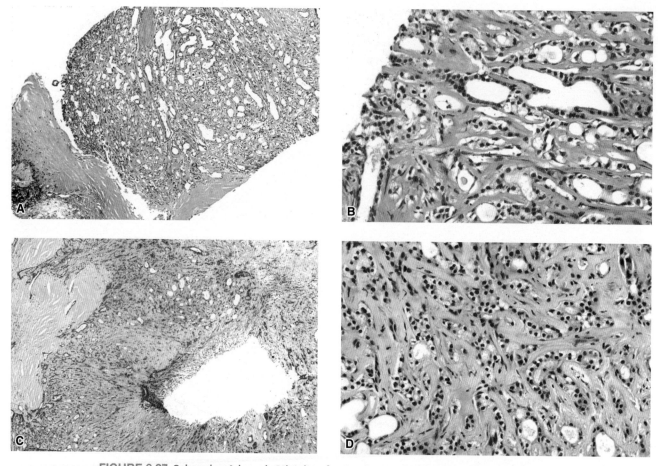

FIGURE 6.27 Sclerosing Adenosis Mistaken for Carcinoma. A, B: This needle core biopsy sample of a palpable adenosis tumor was interpreted as invasive, well-differentiated duct carcinoma. The lesion has a well-circumscribed border and lacks lobulocentric architecture. Myoepithelial cells with clear cytoplasm are evident at high magnification. **C, D:** The subsequent excisional biopsy specimen revealed a circumscribed focus of sclerosing adenosis with a defect in the center at the site of the previous needle core biopsy. The glands are outlined by thin basement membranes and myoepithelial cells with clear cytoplasm.

is recommended if the lesion has a spiculated contour, harbors suspicious calcifications, is associated with a complex (radial) sclerosing lesion, or atypical epithelial hyperplasia is present (3). In the absence of one or more of the aforementioned features, clinical follow-up of a circumscribed tumor, or of a "nonpalpable indistinctly marginated mass" that yields microscopic SA at NCB is a reasonable option (3) if the radiologic and pathologic findings are concordant. Excisional biopsy is often pursued for adenosis tumor. Gill et al. (3) reported follow-up information on a series of 33 NCBs with a major component of SA and no atypia and/or carcinoma. In one case, the radiologic target was a suspicious mass, and the NCB radiologic–pathologic findings were deemed discordant. Follow-up surgical excision yielded invasive carcinoma. The remaining 32 cases had concordant radiologic–pathologic findings: one lesion was excised as part of a mastectomy for ipsilateral invasive carcinoma, and 24 of the remaining 31 lesions were benign on radiologic follow-up.

Calhoun and Booth (13) reported the findings in the surgical excision specimens of patients with NCB diagnosis of AA or AAA. Excision of four lesions with NCB diagnosis of AA without associated atypia/carcinoma yielded AA and

columnar cell change with atypia/flat epithelial atypia (FEA) in two cases, and benign breast parenchyma in the other two. One of the four patients had prior history of AAA.

Excision of seven lesions with NCB diagnosis of AAA yielded AAA (five cases), AA (one case), and atypical hyperplasia (one case).

The treatment of carcinoma arising in adenosis depends on the stage and extent of the lesion. In many of these cases, carcinoma is also present in breast tissue outside the area of adenosis (17–19).

Risk of Subsequent Carcinoma

Foote and Stewart (1) reported that adenosis was not a precursor lesion or risk factor for carcinoma. Page et al. (20) did not detect a significantly increased risk of subsequent carcinoma associated with SA in a retrospective study of women with FCCs, but reported increased relative risk (RR) in two subsequent studies (21,22), amounting to a 2.1 RR in women with SA with atypia, and 1.7 RR in women with SA without atypia (22). The RR was not significantly affected by a family history of breast carcinoma, but the risk was 6.7-fold when SA was accompanied by atypical hyperplasia, often of the lobular type. Others have also reported an increased risk of subsequent carcinoma after a diagnosis of SA (23–27). At a median follow-up of 15.7 years, the RR of carcinoma for 3,733 women with SA in the Mayo Benign Breast Disease Cohort (28) was 2.1 (95% CI: 1.9–2.3) versus 1.52 (95% CI: 1.42–1.63) in 9,701 women without SA. Overall, the RR associated with SA without atypia is so small that no intervention is required beyond clinical surveillance.

The precancerous significance of AAA has also been evaluated. In a study by Carter and Rosen (10), none of the 51 patients with sclerosing proliferative lesions with AAA developed carcinoma after a mean follow-up of 35 months. Seidman et al. (11) reported that at a mean follow-up of 8.7 years, 4/37 (10.8%) patients with AAA developed invasive ductal carcinoma (three ipsilateral and one contralateral), but the authors did not mention whether the carcinoma had apocrine features. All carcinomas occurred more than 3 years after the index diagnosis of AAA, with a mean interval of 5.6 years. The RR of carcinoma was 5.5 [95% CI, 1.9–16] when compared to age-specific incidence rates. All patients who developed carcinoma were older than 60 years of age when AAA was diagnosed, and patients in this age group had a RR of 14 for carcinoma (95% CI: 4.1–48). AAA was present in only 37/9,340 excisional biopsy specimens from patients in the Mayo Clinic Benign Breast Disease Cohort (29). The mean age at diagnosis of AAA was 59.3 years, versus 51.4 years for all women in the cohort. Only three women (8%) with AAA developed subsequent carcinoma, a rate comparable to that of 7.8% for all women in the cohort. Two ipsilateral invasive carcinomas developed 4 years and 18 years after the index biopsy. The third patient developed contralateral DCIS 12 years after the index biopsy. None of the carcinomas had apocrine morphology, and no AAA was present in the background breast parenchyma.

MICROGLANDULAR ADENOSIS

Microglandular adenosis (MGA) is a proliferative glandular lesion that mimics carcinoma clinically and pathologically. It differs substantially from all other forms of adenosis, as the glands do not have a myoepithelial layer. MGA was characterized as a distinct clinicopathologic entity in 1983 (30–32), and there are only a few reports of MGA without atypia or associated carcinoma in recent publications (33–35). MGA often has areas of atypia (atypical MGA). Carcinoma can arise in MGA, and either it retains the distribution of MGA ("CIS arising in MGA"), or it can be frankly invasive.

Clinical Presentation

MGA, Atypical MGA, and Carcinoma Arising in MGA

Age

All reported patients with MGA are women, ranging from 28 to 82 years of age; most patients are 45 to 55 years old. Atypical MGA and carcinoma arising in MGA have an age distribution

similar to MGA (33,36–42). The median age of patients with MGA-associated carcinoma was 47 years (range, 26–68) in a series from Memorial Hospital in New York City (42), and 46 years (range, 31–61) in a series from China (43).

Presenting Symptoms

In most instances, MGA is detected as a mass (33,35), but can be an incidental finding near another lesion (33). In two separate series, all patients with MGA-associated invasive carcinoma presented with a mass lesion (33,42,43).

Family History and Genetic Association

In one series (42), six patients with MGA-associated carcinoma had family history of breast carcinoma. A 22-year-old woman with MGA had a BRCA1 germline mutation (5625G>T mutation in exon 24) (44). Another patient with MGA had neurofibromatosis (45).

Radiology

MGA and MGA-associated lesions typically present as breast masses. Mammography of MGA may reveal increased density and is sometimes reported as "suspicious" (46), but no specific radiologic changes have been described, and some lesions may not be apparent radiologically (44). None of the three cases of MGA reported by Khalifeh et al. (33) was detected mammographically. One case appeared as an ill-defined hypoechoic mass by ultrasound examination, and a mammogram showed only dense breast tissue (35). Another case appeared as a hypoechoic mass with well-defined, but irregular borders, microlobulations, and angular margins. The mass was wider than tall, had an antiparallel orientation, and was suspicious sonographically (44). On MRI, the lesion consisted of a noncircumscribed mass with moderate early and delayed enhancement, and hyperintense T2-weighted images. The radiologic differential diagnosis included FA. Atypical MGA and carcinoma arising in MGA tend to appear mammographically as infiltrative masses (33), but no radiologic abnormality was detected in the breast of a 74-year-old woman with a palpable breast mass consisting of invasive carcinoma arising in MGA (40).

Microscopic Pathology

MGA

MGA is an infiltrative proliferation of small glands in fibrous or fatty mammary stroma. At low magnification, the glands have haphazard distribution (**Fig. 6.28**), but smaller lesions sometimes have a somewhat lobular arrangement (**Figs. 6.29–6.30**). The glands of MGA are small, and round to oval; tubule formation is rare. The glands can be crowded, but gland fusion is uncommon. The epithelium consists of a monolayer of flat-to-cuboidal cells (**Fig. 6.30**), with small round nuclei and inconspicuous or absent nucleoli. The cytoplasm is clear or amphophilic; rarely, eosinophilic, and granular cytoplasm can occur. Intraluminal homogeneous eosinophilic secretions are common, and they occasionally undergo calcification (**Fig. 6.30**). The secretion is usually periodic acid–Schiff (PAS)-positive, diastase-resistant, and

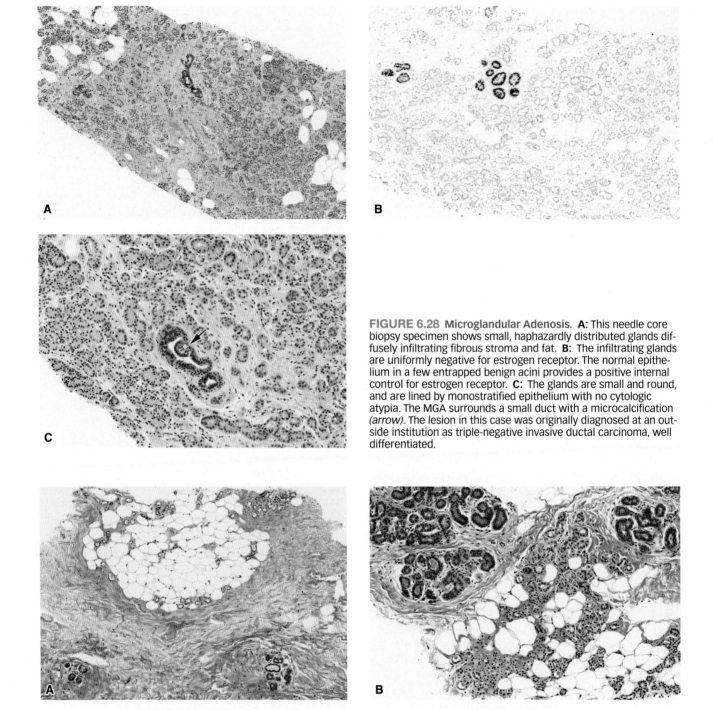

FIGURE 6.28 Microglandular Adenosis. A: This needle core biopsy specimen shows small, haphazardly distributed glands diffusely infiltrating fibrous stroma and fat. **B:** The infiltrating glands are uniformly negative for estrogen receptor. The normal epithelium in a few entrapped benign acini provides a positive internal control for estrogen receptor. **C:** The glands are small and round, and are lined by monostratified epithelium with no cytologic atypia. The MGA surrounds a small duct with a microcalcification *(arrow)*. The lesion in this case was originally diagnosed at an outside institution as triple-negative invasive ductal carcinoma, well differentiated.

FIGURE 6.29 Microglandular Adenosis, Small Foci. A: This needle core biopsy specimen shows small, haphazardly distributed glands admixed with fat. **B:** Another needle core biopsy specimen with a pseudolobulated example of MGA.

mucicarmine-positive. The glands of MGA lack a myoepithelial layer but are surrounded by basement membrane that can be highlighted using a reticulin stain or immunoperoxidase stains for laminin and collagen IV.

Atypical MGA

Atypical MGA **(Fig. 6.31)** is MGA with one or more of the following features: large and/or merging glands, focal solid growth, enlarged nuclei, nuclear hyperchromasia, focal apoptosis, and mitotic activity. The atypical epithelium has hyperchromatic and focally pleomorphic nuclei, and varying amounts of clear-to-amphophilic cytoplasm. Cytoplasmic eosinophilic granules are rare.

Carcinoma Arising in MGA

Carcinoma arising in MGA has been reported (32–34,36–42,46,47).

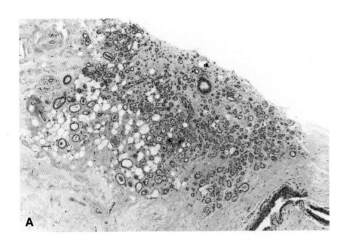

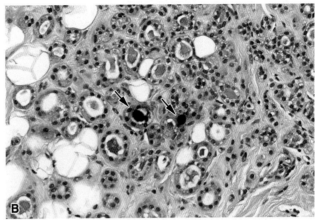

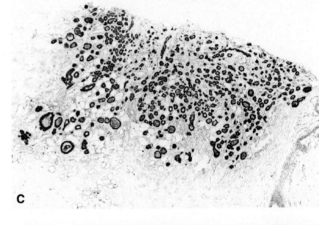

FIGURE 6.30 Microglandular Adenosis. A: This needle core biopsy specimen shows a small focus of MGA that closely resembles adenosis with myoepithelium. **B:** The glandular epithelium is cytologically bland. Basement membrane is evident around the glands. Two minute small intraluminal calcifications are present *(arrows)*. **C:** The glandular proliferation is strongly and uniformly positive for S-100 but lacks myoepithelium (not shown).

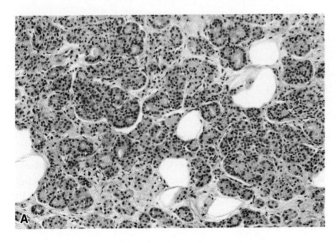

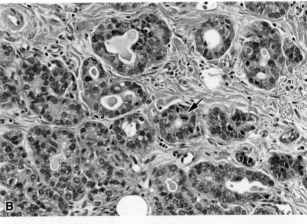

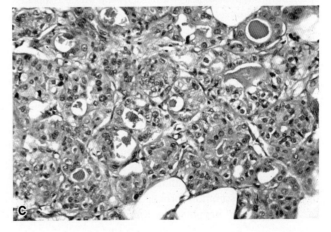

FIGURE 6.31 Atypical Microglandular Adenosis. Three examples of microglandular adenosis with atypia in needle core biopsy specimens. **A:** In this case, few glands appear to be interconnected. **B:** In another case, the glands have a more solid growth, nuclear hyperchromasia, and rare mitoses *(arrow)*. **C:** Marked cellular crowding and overgrowth obscure most of the gland lumina in this atypical lesion. Cytoplasmic vacuolization is evident.

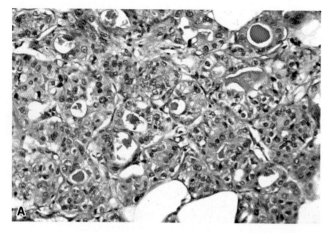

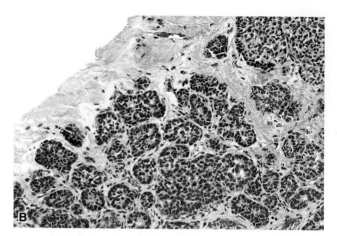

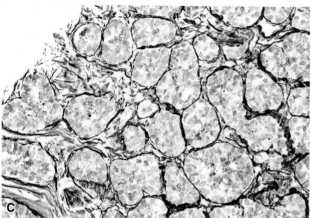

FIGURE 6.32 Carcinoma In Situ in Microglandular Adenosis. A, B: A needle core biopsy specimen with intraductal carcinoma in MGA. Basement membranes are highlighted by the reticulin stain **(B)**.

CIS in MGA

The term "CIS in MGA" is used for an epithelial proliferation that consists of basaloid epithelial cells with solid growth, cytologic atypia, and mitotic activity, but is surrounded by basement membrane, retains the growth pattern of MGA, and is not associated with stromal desmoplasia and lymphoplasmacytic infiltrate **(Figs. 6.32 and 6.33)**. Necrosis within the solid epithelial nests is common. Extensive sampling is often necessary to identify residual foci of MGA without atypia, and the latter may be not present in the limited samples obtained by NCB.

In rare cases, ordinary DCIS or LCIS (31) coexists with MGA or atypical MGA. Ordinary DCIS surrounded by myoepithelium was present in a case of MGA and MGA-associated invasive carcinoma (34).

Invasive Carcinoma Arising in MGA

Invasive carcinoma arising in MGA usually forms microscopic solid tumor nodules substantially larger than the MGA glands filled by CIS. The invasive foci are associated with stromal desmoplasia and enveloped by a conspicuous lymphocytic reaction. Necrosis may be present. Mitoses are readily apparent in these regions. Basement membranes are disrupted around invasive nests, but this finding can be difficult to evaluate, especially in the limited material obtained by NCB. Poorly differentiated carcinoma with high-grade basaloid morphology is the most common form of MGA-associated invasive carcinoma. Other morphologies include invasive carcinoma

with matrix production or squamous metaplasia (33,34,39,43). Some cases of MGA-associated acinic cell carcinoma have been reported (33,43). The two lesions show some overlapping features (48,49).

Immunohistochemistry

The glands of MGA are devoid of myoepithelium but are surrounded by basement membrane. The latter is usually visible in H&E-stained sections and can be highlighted with immunohistochemical stains for laminin and type IV collagen. Silver impregnation and PAS stains also highlight the basement membrane around MGA glands (42,50), but these stains can all be difficult to interpret and should be used with caution, especially when evaluating a limited tissue sample obtained by NCB. Some low-grade invasive carcinomas can have focal basement membrane (51).

The cells forming MGA are strongly immunoreactive for S-100 **(Fig. 6.30)** and negative for ER **(Fig. 6.28)**, PR, and HER2/neu (42), GCDFP-15, and EMA (50). P53 is absent (42) or minimally expressed (<3% of cells) (33,37) in MGA. Ki67-positive cells tend to be sparse (<3%) (33).

Atypical MGA and MGA-associated carcinoma are S-100-positive, but the staining tends to be more focal and has reduced intensity with increasing severity of the lesion (33,36,37). P53 was detected in 5% to 10% of atypical MGA cells and in

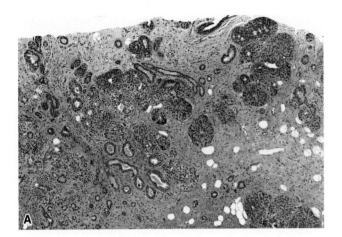

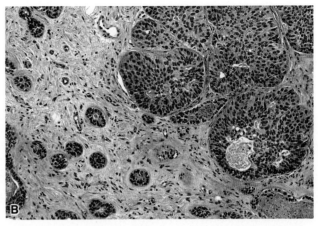

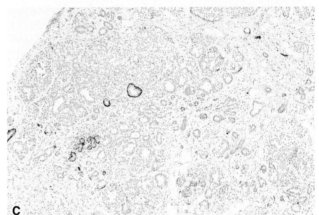

FIGURE 6.33 Carcinoma In Situ in Microglandular Adenosis. A, B: A needle core biopsy specimen with intraductal carcinoma in MGA. **C:** An immunohistochemical stain for calponin shows absence of myoepithelium around CIS in MGA and MGA glands. Reactivity for calponin is present around entrapped normal glands.

more than 30% of the cells of MGA-associated carcinoma in one series (33), but another study found no difference in the percentage of p53-positive cells in MGA-associated lesions (37). Increase in the percentage of Ki67-positive cells with increasing severity of the lesions has been reported (33,36,37). Together with recent molecular evidence (34,37), these data suggest that MGA is a nonobligate morphologic precursor of MGA-associated invasive breast carcinoma.

Although MGA is reported as EMA-negative in most series, 8/15 cases of atypical MGA, 3/9 of MGA-associated CIS, and 4/6 MGA-associated invasive carcinomas were EMA-positive in one study (36). All atypical MGA cases in one series were CK7-positive and CK20-negative (36). CK5/6 (33) and 34βE12 (36) were negative in all cases of atypical MGA, CIS in MGA, and MGA-associated invasive carcinoma in two separate studies. CK5/6 was negative in 3/3 cases of MGA in one series (33). The luminal keratins CK8/18 were positive in MGA and MGA-related lesions in two studies (33,34). EGFR, another basal marker, decorated 11/11 MGA-related lesions in one series (33) and 13/14 cases in another (34). EGFR expression was also detected in a MGA-associated invasive carcinoma (41). Focal positivity for c-kit was detected in 3/6 cases of MGA-associated invasive carcinoma, two of which were matrix-producing and one acinic-like (33).

MGA-associated invasive carcinomas are consistently negative for ER, PR, and HER2 (33,34,36,43), but one case reportedly showed focal ER positivity (36).

Differential Diagnosis of MGA at NCB

Invasive Ductal Carcinoma, Well-differentiated and Tubular Carcinoma

Tubular carcinoma is composed of angular glands of varying size, arranged in a stellate or radial configuration. The neoplastic glands are lined by predominantly columnar-to-cuboidal epithelium, which tends to have amphophilic cytoplasm. Desmoplasia and stromal elastosis are common. The glands composing well-differentiated invasive ductal carcinoma and tubular carcinoma are devoid of myoepithelium and basement membrane, and are usually strongly and diffusely positive for ER and PR but negative for S100. Tubular carcinoma is positive for EMA, whereas MGA is usually regarded as EMA-negative (50), although few cases of MGA and MGA-associated lesions were reported as EMA-positive in one series (36). In general, one or more lesions of the morphologic spectrum of low-grade mammary neoplasia (low-grade DCIS, ADH, columnar cell change with atypia/FEA, classical LCIS, and ALH) is present near well-differentiated invasive ductal carcinoma and tubular carcinoma, at least focally (see also Chapter 10).

Adenosis (with a Myoepithelial Layer)

Areas that resemble MGA can be found in adenosis. SA is usually distinctly lobulocentric, and the compressed glands tend to be arranged in a whorled or laminated fashion within the lobular nodules. TA consists predominantly of elongated glands and tubules, whereas most MGA glands are round to oval. Immunohistochemical stains for p63, calponin, and other myoepithelial markers highlight the myoepithelial cells in all forms of adenosis, except MGA. Khalifeh et al. (33) reported the histologic findings in 54 cases that had initially been misdiagnosed as MGA. The revised diagnosis included 48 cases of adenosis (21 ordinary adenosis, 17 infiltrating adenosis, 9 adenosis with clear cell changes, and 1 BDA), 2 cases of AAA, and 4 cases with no obvious pathologic abnormality. All glands present in these cases had a complete myoepithelial cell layer, as demonstrated by immunoperoxidase stains for myoepithelial markers.

Atypical MGA and CIS Arising in MGA

The differential diagnosis of atypical MGA and CIS in MGA includes invasive carcinoma. In the absence of MGA, it is extremely difficult to separate atypical MGA and CIS arising in MGA from invasive carcinoma based on review of the limited material obtained by NCB. The absence of stromal desmoplasia and of a stromal inflammatory infiltrate associated with a high-grade infiltrative epithelial proliferation with triple-negative profile should raise the differential diagnosis of atypical MGA and CIS in MGA. In these cases, positivity for S-100 further increases the suspicion of MGA-associated carcinoma, but it is insufficient for an unequivocal diagnosis. Surgical excision of the lesion is required for its definitive classification.

Acinic Cell Carcinoma

MGA and atypical MGA can show some morphologic overlap with acinic cell carcinoma, and these two lesions may be related.

Prognosis and Treatment

Even though MGA is regarded as a benign lesion, excisional biopsy is *always* recommended when a NCB sample contains MGA.

MGA is a morphologically benign proliferative lesion, and it is treated by local excision. Re-excision should be considered if MGA involves the surgical margins microscopically, because little is known about the long-term course of incompletely excised MGA. In one case, MGA involved the final margins of a lumpectomy specimen with MGA-associated in situ and invasive carcinoma (41). No radiotherapy was administered, and the patient did not undergo chemotherapy. Ten years later, a mass lesion consisting of MGA-associated CIS developed in the same region of the breast.

Patients with atypical MGA should undergo wide excision of the lesion to achieve histologically negative margins. Further excision is strongly recommended if the margins are involved. Carcinoma is reported in association with MGA and atypical MGA in most published series (33,34,36,37,42,46), and in almost all cases the carcinoma arose within the MGA lesion. One unusual patient had concurrent but separate foci of MGA and carcinoma in one breast (32). A patient with MGA in one breast developed invasive ductal carcinoma not associated with MGA in the contralateral breast (42).

In one study (42), lymph node metastases were documented in 3 of 11 patients with MGA-associated invasive carcinoma who underwent axillary dissection. Ten patients treated by mastectomy were recurrence-free with median follow-up of 57 months (range, 3–108). Two of three patients treated by excisional surgery were recurrence-free 12 and 105 months later. The third woman developed bone metastases at 51 months and was alive at 98 months posttreatment. Khalifeh et al. (33) reported that two of six patients with MGA-associated carcinoma presented with distant metastases. One patient had only bone metastases, whereas the other had widespread systemic disease, including metastases to lymph nodes, brain, bone, and spinal cord. The metastases were morphologically similar to the primary carcinoma. In a recent series (43), 7 of 11 women with MGA-associated carcinoma (1 DCIS and 10 invasive carcinomas) underwent mastectomy, and 4 were treated with lumpectomy and adjuvant radiotherapy. None of the patients had lymph node metastases at presentation. One patient received neoadjuvant chemotherapy, and all others received adjuvant chemotherapy, including the patient with MGA-associated DCIS. A patient developed lung metastases 24 months after initial diagnosis and was alive with disease at 34 months' follow-up.

Based on published reports with limited data and a median follow-up of nearly 5 years, patients with MGA-associated carcinomas appear to have a relatively favorable outcome, even though MGA-associated carcinoma has histopathologic and immunohistochemical features of basal-like carcinoma that is usually associated with a poor prognosis. The treatment of MGA-associated carcinoma should be based on the stage of disease in the individual patient. In cases of MGA-associated DCIS and MGA-associated invasive carcinoma, breast-conserving surgery should always be combined with radiotherapy. Adjuvant chemotherapy is recommended for patients with axillary lymph node metastases or with invasive tumors larger than 1 cm in the absence of nodal metastases.

Extreme caution is recommended in the diagnostic evaluation of NCB material that contains a triple-negative small glandular proliferation devoid of myoepithelium, and immunohistochemical staining for S-100 should be performed to rule out the possibility of MGA. In the current era of neoadjuvant treatment, it is imperative to remember that well-differentiated invasive ductal carcinoma with triple-negative profile is *exceedingly* rare and can be confidently diagnosed only upon review of the morphology of the entire tumor.

REFERENCES

Adenosis

1. Foote FW, Stewart FW. Comparative studies of cancerous versus noncancerous breasts. *Ann Surg.* 1945;121:197–222.
2. Markopoulos C, Kouskos E, Phillipidis T, et al. Adenosis tumor of the breast. *Breast J.* 2003;9:255–256.
3. Gill HK, Ioffe OB, Berg WA. When is a diagnosis of sclerosing adenosis acceptable at core biopsy? *Radiology.* 2003;228:50–57.
4. Taskin F, Koseoglu K, Unsal A, et al. Sclerosing adenosis of the breast: radiologic appearance and efficiency of core needle biopsy. *Diagn Interv Radiol.* 2011;17:311–316.

5. Oztekin PS, Tuncbilek I, Kosar P, et al. Nodular sclerosing adenosis mimicking malignancy in the breast: Magnetic Resonance Imaging findings. *Breast J.* 2011;17:95–97.

6. Lee KC, Chan JK, Gwi E. Tubular adenosis of the breast: a distinctive benign lesion mimicking invasive carcinoma. *Am J Surg Pathol.* 1996;20:46–54.

7. Eusebi V, Azzopardi JG. Vascular infiltration in benign breast disease. *J Pathol.* 1976;118:9–16.

8. Nielsen BB. Adenosis tumour of the breast—a clinicopathological investigation of 27 cases. *Histopathology.* 1987;11:1259–1275.

9. Simpson JF, Page DL, Dupont WD. Apocrine adenosis—a mimic of mammary carcinoma. *Surg Pathol.* 1990:289–299.

10. Carter DJ, Rosen PP. Atypical apocrine metaplasia in sclerosing lesions of the breast: a study of 51 patients. *Mod Pathol.* 1991;4:1–5.

11. Seidman JD, Ashton M, Lefkowitz M. Atypical apocrine adenosis of the breast: a clinicopathologic study of 37 patients with 8.7-year follow-up. *Cancer.* 1996;77:2529–2537.

12. Elayat G, Selim AG, Wells CA. Cell cycle alterations and their relationship to proliferation in apocrine adenosis of the breast. *Histopathology.* 2009;54:348–354.

13. Calhoun BC, Booth CN. Atypical apocrine adenosis diagnosed on breast core biopsy: implications for management. *Hum Pathol.* 2014;45:2130–2135.

14. Abati AD, Kimmel M, Rosen PP. Apocrine mammary carcinoma: a clinicopathologic study of 72 cases. *Am J Clin Pathol.* 1990;94:371–377.

15. Eusebi V, Collina G, Bussolati G. Carcinoma in situ in sclerosing adenosis of the breast: an immunocytochemical study. *Semin Diagn Pathol.* 1989;6:146–152.

16. Hilson JB, Schnitt SJ, Collins LC. Phenotypic alterations in myoepithelial cells associated with benign sclerosing lesions of the breast. *Am J Surg Pathol.* 2010;34:896–900.

17. Moritani S, Ichihara S, Hasegawa M, et al. Topographical, morphological and immunohistochemical characteristics of carcinoma in situ of the breast involving sclerosing adenosis: two distinct topographical patterns and histological types of carcinoma in situ. *Histopathology.* 2011;58:835–846.

18. Oberman HA, Markey BA. Noninvasive carcinoma of the breast presenting in adenosis. *Mod Pathol.* 1991;4:31–35.

19. Fechner RE. Lobular carcinoma in situ in sclerosing adenosis: a potential source of confusion with invasive carcinoma. *Am J Surg Pathol.* 1981;5:233–239.

20. Page DL, Vander Zwaag R, Rogers LW, et al. Relation between component parts of fibrocystic disease complex and breast cancer. *J Natl Cancer Inst.* 1978;61:1055–1063.

21. Dupont WD, Page DL. Risk factors for breast cancer in women with proliferative breast disease. *N Engl J Med.* 1985;312:146–151.

22. Jensen RA, Page DL, Dupont WD, et al. Invasive breast cancer risk in women with sclerosing adenosis. *Cancer.* 1989;64:1977–1983.

23. Bodian CA, Perzin KH, Lattes R, et al. Prognostic significance of benign proliferative breast disease. *Cancer.* 1993;71:3896–3907.

24. Carter CL, Corle DK, Micozzi MS, et al. A prospective study of the development of breast cancer in 16,692 women with benign breast disease. *Am J Epidemiol.* 1988;128:467–477.

25. Hutchinson WB, Thomas DB, Hamlin WB, et al. Risk of breast cancer in women with benign breast disease. *J Natl Cancer Inst.* 1980;65:13–20.

26. Kodlin D, Winger EE, Morgenstern NL, et al. Chronic mastopathy and breast cancer: a follow-up study. *Cancer.* 1977;39:2603–2607.

27. Krieger N, Hiatt RA. Risk of breast cancer after benign breast diseases: variation by histologic type, degree of atypia, age at biopsy, and length of follow-up. *Am J Epidemiol.* 1992;135:619–631.

28. Visscher DW, Nassar A, Degnim AC, et al. Sclerosing adenosis and risk of breast cancer. *Breast Cancer Res Treat.* 2014;144:205–212.

29. Fuehrer N, Hartmann L, Degnim A, et al. Atypical apocrine adenosis of the breast: long-term follow-up in 37 patients. *Arch Pathol Lab Med.* 2012;136:179–182.

Microglandular Adenosis

30. Clement PB, Azzopardi JG. Microglandular adenosis of the breast—a lesion simulating tubular carcinoma. *Histopathology.* 1983;7:169–180.

31. Rosen PP. Microglandular adenosis: a benign lesion simulating invasive mammary carcinoma. *Am J Surg Pathol.* 1983;7:137–144.

32. Tavassoli FA, Norris HJ. Microglandular adenosis of the breast: a clinicopathologic study of 11 cases with ultrastructural observations. *Am J Surg Pathol.* 1983;7:731–737.

33. Khalifeh IM, Albarracin C, Diaz LK, et al. Clinical, histopathologic, and immunohistochemical features of microglandular adenosis and transition into in situ and invasive carcinoma. *Am J Surg Pathol.* 2008;32:544–552.

34. Geyer FC, Lacroix-Triki M, Colombo PE, et al. Molecular evidence in support of the neoplastic and precursor nature of microglandular adenosis. *Histopathology.* 2012;60:E115–E130.

35. Kim DJ, Sun WY, Ryu DH, et al. Microglandular adenosis. *J Breast Cancer.* 2011;14:72–75.

36. Koenig C, Dadmanesh F, Bratthauer GL, et al. Carcinoma arising in microglandular adenosis: an immunohistochemical analysis of 20 intraepithelial and invasive neoplasms. *Int J Surg Pathol.* 2000;8:303–315.

37. Shin SJ, Simpson PT, Da Silva L, et al. Molecular evidence for progression of microglandular adenosis (MGA) to invasive carcinoma. *Am J Surg Pathol.* 2009;33:496–504.

38. Shui R, Yang W. Invasive breast carcinoma arising in microglandular adenosis: a case report and review of the literature. *Breast J.* 2009;15:653–656.

39. Shui R, Bi R, Cheng Y, et al. Matrix-producing carcinoma of the breast in the Chinese population: a clinicopathological study of 13 cases. *Pathol Int.* 2011;61:415–422.

40. Geyer FC, Kushner YB, Lambros MB, et al. Microglandular adenosis or microglandular adenoma? A molecular genetic analysis of a case associated with atypia and invasive carcinoma. *Histopathology.* 2009;55:732–743.

41. Resetkova E, Flanders DJ, Rosen PP. Ten-year follow-up of mammary carcinoma arising in microglandular adenosis treated with breast conservation. *Arch Pathol Lab Med.* 2003;127:77–80.

42. James BA, Cranor ML, Rosen PP. Carcinoma of the breast arising in microglandular adenosis. *Am J Clin Pathol.* 1993;100:507–513.

43. Zhong F, Bi R, Yu B, et al. Carcinoma arising in microglandular adenosis of the breast: triple negative phenotype with variable morphology. *Int J Clin Exp Pathol.* 2014;7:6149–6156.

44. Sabate JM, Gomez A, Torrubia S, et al. Microglandular adenosis of the breast in a BRCA1 mutation carrier: radiological features. *Eur Radiol.* 2002;12:1479–1482.

45. Kay S. Microglandular adenosis of the female mammary gland: study of a case with ultrastructural observations. *Hum Pathol.* 1985;16:637–641.

46. Rosenblum MK, Purrazzella R, Rosen PP. Is microglandular adenosis a precancerous disease? A study of carcinoma arising therein. *Am J Surg Pathol.* 1986;10:237–245.

47. Lin L, Pathmanathan N. Microglandular adenosis with transition to breast carcinoma: a series of three cases. *Pathology.* 2011;43:498–503.

48. Damiani S, Pasquinelli G, Lamovec J, et al. Acinic cell carcinoma of the breast: an immunohistochemical and ultrastructural study. *Virchows Arch.* 2000;437:74–81.

49. Coyne JD, Dervan PA. Primary acinic cell carcinoma of the breast. *J Clin Pathol.* 2002;55:545–547.

50. Eusebi V, Foschini MP, Betts CM, et al. Microglandular adenosis, apocrine adenosis, and tubular carcinoma of the breast: an immunohistochemical comparison. *Am J Surg Pathol.* 1993;17:99–109.

51. Cserni G. Presence of basement membrane material around the tubules of tubulolobular carcinoma. *Breast Care (Basel).* 2008;3:423–425.

7

Fibroepithelial Neoplasms

EDI BROGI

SCLEROSING LOBULAR HYPERPLASIA (FIBROADENOMATOID MASTOPATHY)

Clinical Presentation

Sclerosing lobular hyperplasia (SLH) occasionally forms a localized tumor (1,2) and may be associated with tenderness.

Age

Patient age ranges from 12 (3) to 46 (4) years, with a mean age of about 32 years. There is no significant association with oral contraceptive use.

Radiology

The imaging findings closely resemble those of fibroadenoma (FA). Calcifications may be present.

Microscopic Pathology

The lobules are enlarged, with an increased number of acini. The intralobular stroma is collagenized, with variable levels of sclerosis (**Fig. 7.1**). Adjacent lobules appear as minute FAs with a prominent glandular component (**Fig. 7.2**). The acini are lined by monostratified epithelium, and myoepithelial cells are evident. Secretory activity may be present. Calcifications are uncommon. SLH can occur near FAs and phyllodes tumors (PTs) (1,5).

Treatment and Prognosis

SLH is a benign alteration of the breast parenchyma and does not require any specific treatment. Surgical excision might be considered if the needle core biopsy (NCB) sampling from a breast mass yields only SLH to rule out peripheral/inadequate sampling of a PT. Clinical and radiological correlation is necessary.

FIBROADENOMA

Clinical Presentation

Age

FAs with usual/adult-type morphology can occur at any age, but the median age at diagnosis ranges from 30 to 40 years, approximately 10 to 20 years lower than the median age of patients with PTs. Juvenile FAs tend to occur in girls younger than 20 years old and are the most common fibroepithelial lesions in pediatric patients (6,7). Fibroepithelial lesions with the histologic features of juvenile FA also occur in adult women (8). Complex FAs tend to occur at an older age than adult FAs. The mean age at diagnosis was 34.5 years in one study (9). In another series (10), the median age of patients with complex FA was significantly higher than the median age of patients with noncomplex FAs (47 years vs. 28.5 years, respectively).

Risk Factors

Some studies have suggested a relationship with hormonal treatment. Some FAs develop during puberty after menarche (6). The familial occurrence of multiple successive FAs has been observed. Rare examples of FAs are reported in men (11–15), usually in the context of gynecomastia.

Women treated with cyclosporin A for immunosuppression may develop large, multiple, and bilateral FAs (16,17). The duration of cyclosporin A treatment prior to the detection of a FA is generally more than a year (17). Some FAs regressed completely after cyclosporin was replaced with another immunosuppressive drug, whereas other FAs remained stable or decreased in size (18).

Women with Carney syndrome may develop myxoid FAs (19). The percentage of women with myxoid FA who have Carney syndrome is unknown.

Presenting Symptoms

A FA usually presents as a painless, firm or rubbery, well-circumscribed, solitary mass. Some patients have multiple and/or bilateral synchronous or metachronous FAs. FAs can undergo infarction during pregnancy, following trauma, or for no apparent reason. The infarcted FA may be tender or painful. A FA in axillary breast tissue can mimic neoplastic lymphadenopathy clinically.

Radiology

An increasing percentage of FAs are nonpalpable tumors detected by mammography as discrete nodular densities. Mammographic calcifications in the stroma of adult FAs are common in postmenopausal women. By ultrasound examination, most FAs are nodular, iso- or hypo-echoic solid masses with circumscribed borders. In one study (20), myxoid FAs showed significantly greater depth-to-width ratio than usual FAs, and some were suspicious for mucinous carcinoma. The MRI appearance of FAs is variable and influenced by the structure and relative proportions of epithelial and stromal

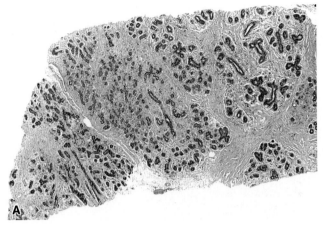
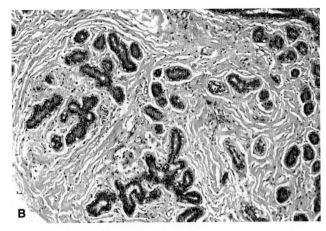

FIGURE 7.1 Fibroadenomatoid Mastopathy. A, B: This needle core biopsy specimen was obtained from one of multiple bilateral breast nodules in a 16-year-old girl. The biopsy specimen shows enlarged lobules with sclerotic stroma.

components. In an MRI study of 81 FAs (21), 70.4% had well-defined margins, 90.1% were round or lobulated, 49.4% had heterogeneous internal structure, and 27.2% displayed nonenhancing internal septations. After contrast injection, 22.2% of FAs had a suspicious signal intensity–time course.

Size

Most FAs are smaller than 3 cm. FAs larger than 4 cm are more frequent in patients under 20 years of age (22), and usually have morphology of juvenile FA. The so-called "giant" FA (a descriptive term that we do not endorse) in the breast of adolescent girls often has the morphology of juvenile FA. The mean size of 23 juvenile FAs in women 18-years-old or younger studied by Ross et al. (6) was 3.1 cm (range 0.5–7). In one series (10), the average size of complex FAs (1.3 ± 0.57 cm) was about half the size of usual FAs in the same study (2.5 ± 1.44 cm).

Microscopic Pathology

FA is a tumor of the specialized mammary stroma, associated with a secondary proliferation of the glandular elements. The stroma shows either intra- or pericanalicular growth pattern

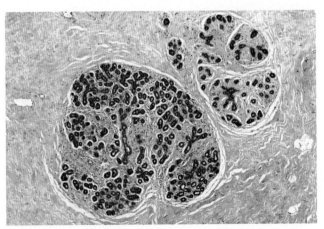

FIGURE 7.2 Fibroadenomatoid Mastopathy. The lobules resemble small fibroadenomas.

(**Fig. 7.3**). FAs with a prominent intracanalicular pattern can mimic benign PTs, especially in NCB samples. Within any given FA, the stroma has homogeneous cellularity, and the epithelium-to-stroma ratio is similar throughout the tumor (**Fig. 7.3**). In contrast, PTs have an uneven distribution of glands and heterogeneous stromal cellularity, including foci indistinguishable from a FA. Adipocytic differentiation does not occur in FAs, but it may occur in PTs.

Multinucleated stromal giant cells can be found in FAs (23) and PTs (23), in some benign breast tumors (24), as well as in nonlesional mammary stroma. The nuclei may be pleomorphic and hyperchromatic, or have a florette-like pattern. The presence of multinucleated stromal cells does not appear to influence the clinical course of the lesion. FAs with focal multinucleated stromal giant cells should not be misclassified as PTs, even if the cells are focally p53- and Ki67-positive (24).

The usual (adult-type) FA is the most common type of FA (**Fig. 7.4**). Usual FAs in postmenopausal women tend to be hypocellular and hyalinized, and they may harbor coarse dystrophic stromal calcifications (**Fig. 7.5**). FAs from women younger than 20 years of age usually have more cellular stroma. Epithelial hyperplasia is usually absent; focal secretory changes may be present (**Fig. 7.6**). Mitotic figures are uncommon in usual FAs, but scattered mitoses may be observed in usual FAs in adolescent girls (6,7).

A *tubular adenoma* is a variant of pericanalicular FA with adenosis (**Fig. 7.7**). It consists of closely approximated round or oval glandular structures lined by monostratified glandular epithelium and myoepithelium.

An adult-type FA with cellular stroma but no cytologic atypia is often referred to as cellular FA, but this diagnosis has low interobserver reproducibility. The differential diagnosis between cellular FA and benign PT can be problematic, especially if only NCB material is available for review (**Figs. 7.8 and 7.9**); surgical excision of the lesion is warranted for its definitive classification. Usual FAs rarely pose a diagnostic challenge in NCB material. A hyalinized FA with conspicuous epithelium may occasionally raise the differential diagnosis of a sclerosed papilloma, but the pseudopapillary fronds lack true fibrovascular cores.

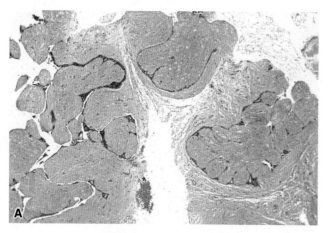
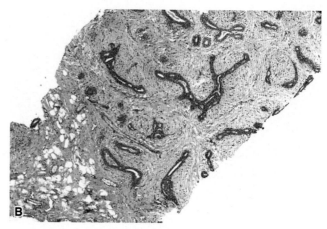

FIGURE 7.3 Fibroadenomatous Growth Patterns. **A:** The intracanalicular growth pattern is formed by compressed epithelial lined spaces. **B:** A pericanalicular lesion in which the stroma is arranged in a circumferential nodular pattern around ductules with focal epithelial hyperplasia.

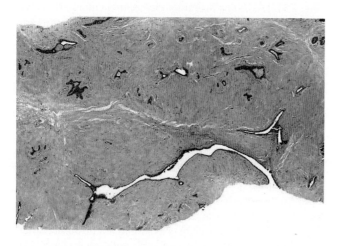

FIGURE 7.4 Fibroadenoma, Usual Type. This needle core biopsy specimen is from a palpable lesion in a 37-year-old woman.

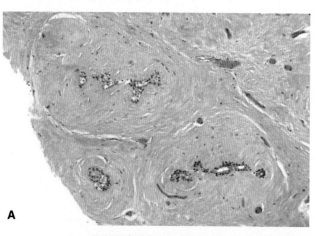
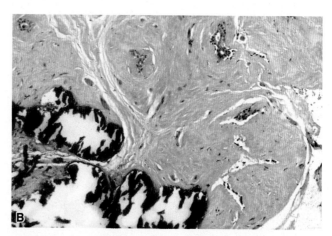

FIGURE 7.5 Fibroadenoma, Usual Type with Sclerosis and Calcification. **A, B:** This needle core biopsy specimen is from a nonpalpable, calcified lesion in a 74-year-old woman.

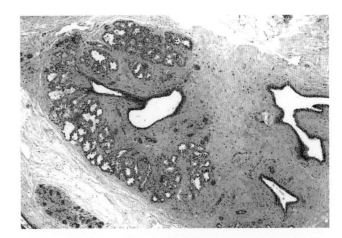

FIGURE 7.6 Fibroadenoma, Usual Type with Secretory Changes. This needle core biopsy specimen is from a palpable lesion in a 32-year-old woman. The patient is a BRCA1 germline mutation carrier, and the lesion was suspicious clinically.

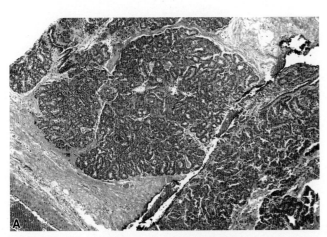

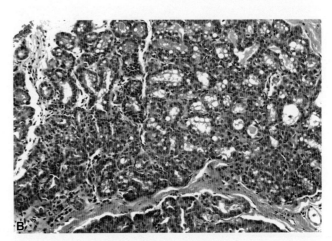

FIGURE 7.7 Lactating Adenoma. A, B: Enlarged lobules with lactational secretory hyperplasia in needle core biopsy samples from a breast tumor in a 37-year-old pregnant woman.

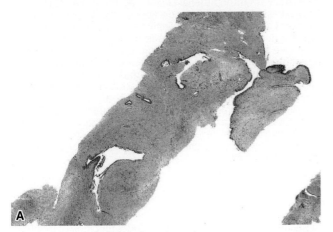

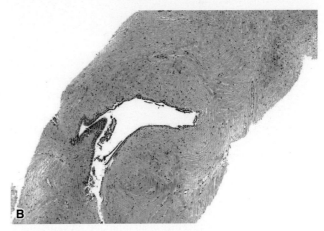

FIGURE 7.8 Fibroepithelial Lesion. A, B: The stroma of the fibroepithelial lesion in this needle core biopsy sample shows minimally increased cellularity with no evidence of cytologic atypia. The ducts are open and have a clefted outline, but no epithelial hyperplasia is present. Some of the features (cellularity and clefts) raise the differential diagnosis of benign PT. Surgical excision of the lesion yielded a fibroadenoma.

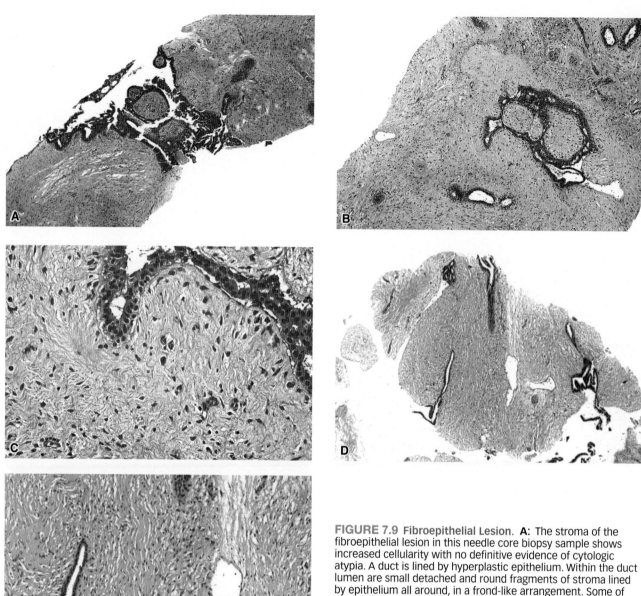

FIGURE 7.9 Fibroepithelial Lesion. A: The stroma of the fibroepithelial lesion in this needle core biopsy sample shows increased cellularity with no definitive evidence of cytologic atypia. A duct is lined by hyperplastic epithelium. Within the duct lumen are small detached and round fragments of stroma lined by epithelium all around, in a frond-like arrangement. Some of the features (cellularity, epithelial hyperplasia, and small fronds) raise the possibility of benign PT. Surgical excision of the lesion confirmed the latter diagnosis. **B, C:** This needle core biopsy sample shows a fibroepithelial tumor with moderately cellular stroma that proved to be a benign phyllodes tumor. **D, E:** These needle core biopsy samples are from a benign phyllodes tumor, a diagnosis suggested by the moderately cellular stroma and epithelium-lined clefts.

The underlying architecture of an infarcted FA can usually be identified in H&E-stained sections and can be highlighted with CK stains **(Fig. 7.10)**.

Myxoid FAs are characterized by diffuse and homogenous myxoid change of the stroma **(Fig. 7.11)**. Myxoid FAs can occur in patients with Carney syndrome (19), but most patients with a myxoid FA do not have a known systemic abnormality. Myxoid FAs have uniformly hypocellular stroma with evident vascularity, whereas myxoid change in a PT tends to be less homogeneous, and stromal cellularity is increased. The differential diagnosis of myxoid FA in NCB specimens includes mucinous carcinoma **(Fig. 7.12)** and PT with focal myxoid stroma.

Complex FAs are FAs with at least one of the following histologic features: sclerosing adenosis (SA), papillary apocrine hyperplasia, cysts (≥3 mm), and epithelial calcifications **(Fig. 7.13)** (9,25). In a series of 63 complex FAs (10), 57% had SA, 8% had apocrine metaplasia, and 1.6% had cysts. Calcifications in SA were found in 9.5% of the cases. Fibrocystic changes (FCCs) such as papillary epithelial hyperplasia and SA can mask the basic fibroadenomatous nature of a complex

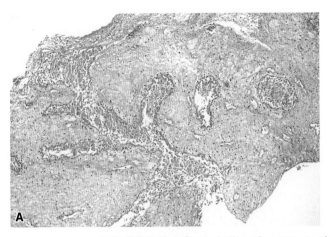
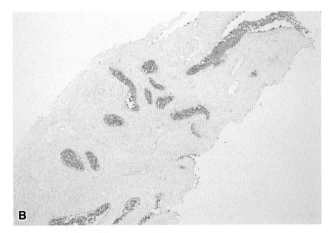

FIGURE 7.10 Infarcted Fibroadenoma. A: This needle core biopsy of a palpable lesion in the breast of a 15-year-old girl had been initially interpreted as a vascular lesion, but the ghostly outline of the tissue suggests an infarcted fibroadenoma. **B:** A cytokeratin 7 stain highlights the necrotic epithelium, confirming that the lesion is an infarcted fibroadenoma, not a hemangioma.

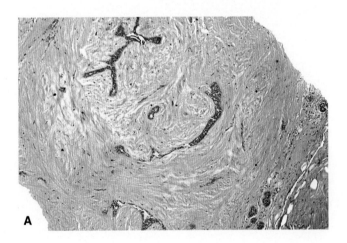
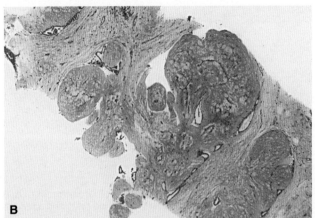
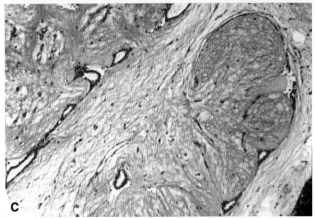

FIGURE 7.11 Fibroadenomas with Myxoid Stroma.
A: A needle core biopsy sample showing myxoid stroma in a fibroadenoma. **B, C:** Needle core biopsy specimens in which the epithelium is compressed into slender cords and small glands by myxoid stroma.

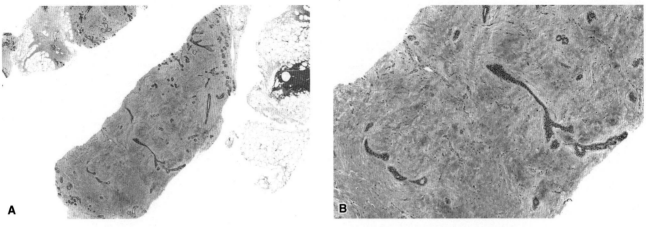

FIGURE 7.12 Fibroadenoma with Myxoid Stroma. A, B: A needle core biopsy sample showing myxoid stroma in a fibroadenoma. This lesion had been misinterpreted as mucinous carcinoma.

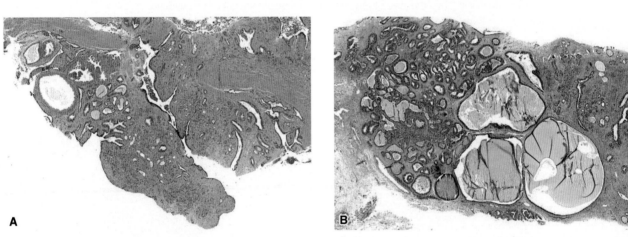

FIGURE 7.13 Complex Fibroadenoma. A, B: A needle core biopsy sample showing a complex fibroadenoma with apocrine cysts and adenosis.

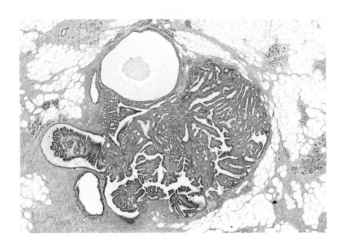

FIGURE 7.14 Complex Fibroadenoma. This complex fibroadenoma has foci with a papillary appearance that could raise the differential diagnosis of papilloma in a needle core biopsy sample.

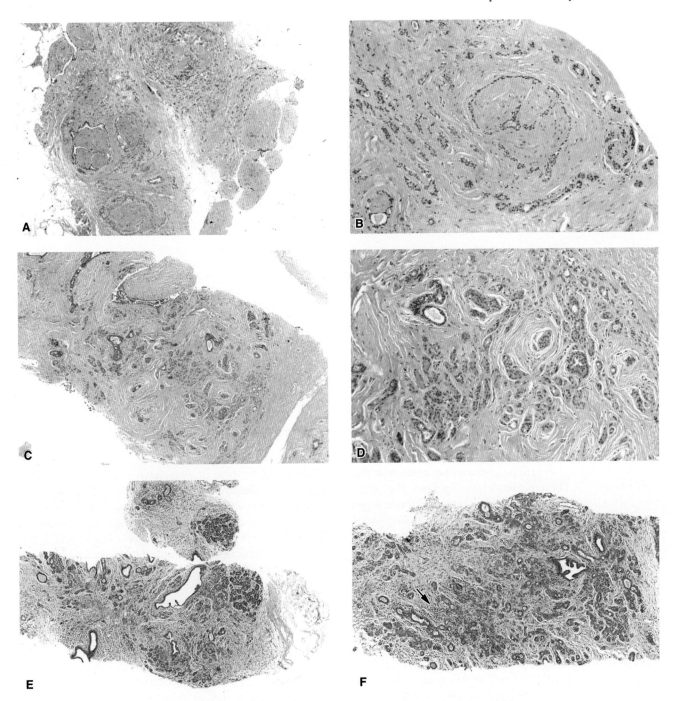

FIGURE 7.15 Complex Fibroadenomas with Sclerosing Adenosis Misinterpreted as Carcinoma. A, B: A needle core biopsy specimen showing sclerosing adenosis in a fibroadenoma. This specimen was erroneously interpreted as infiltrating lobular carcinoma. **C, D:** This needle core biopsy specimen with sclerosing adenosis in a fibroadenoma was diagnosed as invasive tubular carcinoma. **E, F:** The needle core biopsy of this complex fibroadenoma with adenosis raises the differential diagnosis of invasive carcinoma. A stromal lymphocytic infiltrate is also noted *(arrow in F).*

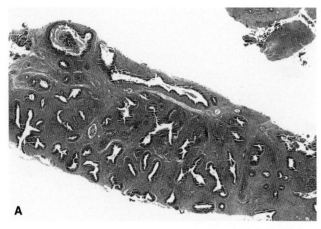
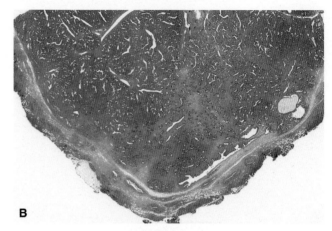

FIGURE 7.16 Juvenile Fibroadenoma. **A:** The needle core biopsy of a large palpable mass in the breast of a 15-year-old girl shows a fibroepithelial lesion with slightly increased stromal cellularity, adenosis, and mild epithelial hyperplasia. **B:** Surgical excision of the mass yielded a juvenile fibroadenoma.

FA, especially in the limited sample of a NCB, and raise the differential diagnosis of FCCs (**Fig. 7.13**), juvenile papillomatosis, and papilloma (**Fig. 7.14**). The differential diagnosis of complex FAs with extensive SA also includes invasive carcinoma (**Fig. 7.15**). Surgical excision of a complex FA is not necessary, unless the epithelium shows evidence of atypia or the diagnosis is uncertain.

A *juvenile fibroadenoma* is characterized microscopically by increased stromal cellularity and epithelial hyperplasia. Pericanalicular architecture is more common than intracanalicular architecture (6,7). The tumor border is well defined. The stroma tends to be uniformly cellular, with scant separation between intralobular/periglandular stroma and interlobular stroma (6). The glandular element tends to be uniformly distributed, but some juvenile FAs can show slight stromal expansion as well as gland-rich areas (6), creating an overall impression of intratumoral heterogeneity that might raise the differential diagnosis of PT, especially on review of NCB material. The uniform quality of the stromal proliferation and lack of nuclear stromal atypia are features that support the diagnosis of FA. Epithelial hyperplasia is common in juvenile FAs and can be conspicuous, raising the differential diagnosis of atypical ductal hyperplasia (ADH) or cribriform ductal carcinoma in situ (DCIS), which are exceedingly rare in this setting. Necrosis and/or calcifications are uncommon. A definitive diagnosis of juvenile FA cannot be rendered based on review of NCB material alone (**Fig. 7.16**). Evaluation of the entire lesion is necessary. The differential diagnosis usually includes benign PT and papilloma. The epithelial hyperplasia in a juvenile FA may raise the differential diagnosis of ADH if the presence of the underlying stromal lesion is not appreciated, especially in NCB material.

Fibroadenoma with Carcinoma In Situ or Epithelial Atypia

LCIS and DCIS can arise within or secondarily involve FAs. Classic LCIS and ALH (**Fig. 7.17**) are the most common atypical epithelial proliferations found in FAs; pleomorphic LCIS

is exceedingly rare. Occasionally, ADH and DCIS (**Fig. 7.17**) are identified (26,27). The differential diagnosis of ADH in FA includes artifactual telescoping of the benign epithelium in the FA (**Fig. 7.18**). A FA may be involved by invasive carcinoma arising in the adjacent breast parenchyma.

Immunohistochemistry

The epithelium and stroma of FAs show some positivity for ER and PR, but these findings have no specific diagnostic applications. The stromal cells of FAs are CD34-positive and show immunoreactivity for actin in cases with myofibroblastic proliferation. Moderate-to-strong nuclear staining for β-catenin has been documented in the stroma cells of FAs (28). A few investigators have reported significant differences in the Ki67 indices of FAs and benign PTs in NCB (29,30), but substantial overlap exists, limiting the practical utility of this marker in the evaluation of NCB specimens.

Treatment and Prognosis

Recent molecular studies suggest that some PTs might develop from FAs (31–33), but this occurrence is exceedingly rare. Correlation of the clinical, radiologic, and pathologic findings of the lesion is of foremost importance. In the absence of atypical findings, surgical excision is not warranted for radiologic–pathologic concordant lesions yielding the diagnosis of FA at NCB.

Ultrasound-guided Vacuum-assisted Percutaneous Excision

Small (≤1.5 cm) FAs can be completely excised in the course of vacuum-assisted, ultrasound-guided biopsy (34,35). In a series of 52 FAs (35) removed percutaneously under sonographic guidance, and followed up with clinical and sonographic examination every 6 months, the recurrence rate was 15% at a median follow-up of 22 months (range 7–59), with an actuarial recurrence rate of 33% at 59 months. None of the recurrent lesions

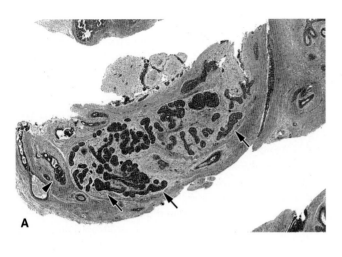

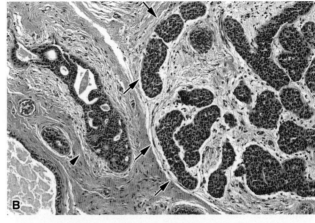

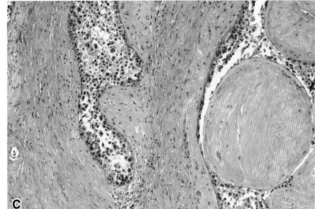

FIGURE 7.17 **Fibroadenomas with Epithelial Atypia or Carcinoma In Situ. A, B:** The complex fibroadenoma in this needle core biopsy sample has an area of lobular carcinoma in situ *(arrows)* and a minute focus of atypical ductal hyperplasia *(arrowhead).* **C:** Intraductal carcinoma is present in this sclerotic fibroadenoma.

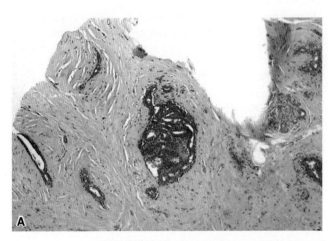

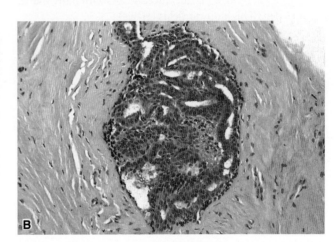

FIGURE 7.18 **Fibroadenoma with Telescoping of the Epithelium. A, B:** The ductal epithelium in this fibroadenoma is detached from the duct wall and shows "telescoping" within the ductal lumen, in a pattern that simulates atypical ductal hyperplasia.

was symptomatic, and only three were palpable. All recurrences pertained to FAs ≥2 cm at initial diagnosis (range 2.1–2.8).

Cryoablation

Cryoablation has been used for treating FAs (36–38). The mean pretreatment tumor diameter of 444 FAs treated with cryoablation was 1.8 cm (37). A palpable abnormality was present in 46% of patients at 6 months' follow-up and in 35%

at 12 months. In two other series (37,38), a persistent palpable abnormality was more common if the index FA was ≥2 cm. The residual lesion consisted of shrunken hyaline matrix in two cases with tissue evaluation (38).

Surgical Excision

Most solitary FAs are treated by local excision. Excision of juvenile FAs in adolescent patients is usually carried out to preserve as much breast tissue as possible. The risk of upgrade to carcinoma (DCIS and/or invasive carcinoma) at surgical excision following radiologic–pathologic concordant NCB diagnosis of FA with any morphology is negligible.

Follow-up without Excision

Some patients with radiologic–pathologic concordant NCB diagnosis of FA do not undergo surgical excision of the radiologic target. Semiannual clinical and mammographic follow-up to document stability of the lesion is usually recommended. Features that raise concern for PT include increasing size of the tumor, size larger than 3 cm in a patient older than 35 years, lobulated mammographic contour, and ultrasonographic examination showing attenuation or cystic areas in a solid mass (39).

Relative Risk of Subsequent Carcinoma

The Relative Risk (RR) of subsequent carcinoma in women with FA is minimally increased, even in patients with proliferative changes in the FA or in the surrounding breast, as well as a family history of breast carcinoma (25). Proliferative FCCs are more common within/near complex FAs than noncomplex FAs. In one study (25), the RR of invasive carcinoma for women with any type of FAs was 1.6, but it was 2.4 for women with complex FA, and 3.72 for women with a complex FA and a family history of breast carcinoma. Follow-up information of patients with juvenile FAs is limited but does not reveal predisposition to develop carcinoma (6,7). Some FAs may recur after excision, especially juvenile FAs with more than 2 mitoses per 10 high power fields (HPFs) (7).

PHYLLODES TUMOR

PTs are rare fibroepithelial lesions characterized by increased cellularity and heterogeneity of the stromal component. The epithelium-to-stroma ratio varies within the tumor, and some areas may resemble FAs. PTs are further classified as *benign, borderline, or malignant* based on the histologic characteristics of the lesion, a classification which is predictive of the probable clinical course.

Clinical Presentation

A PT usually presents as a firm-to-hard discrete palpable mass. Large tumors may invade and ulcerate the skin or extend into the chest wall. Rarely, a PT was associated with bloody nipple discharge (40). Clinically, size larger than 4 cm and/or rapid growth favor PT over FA, but no clinical features can reliably distinguish among the different types of PTs, or between a cellular FA and benign PT. Enlargement of a preexisting tumor stable for a number of years suggests malignant transformation of a benign PT or PT arising in a FA. Recent genetic evidence raises the possibility that some PTs might develop from FAs (32,33), but given the relative frequencies of these tumors this is an exceedingly uncommon event.

Multifocal ipsilateral or bilateral PTs are rare (5,41–44). There are reports of malignant PTs with paraneoplastic production of human chorionic gonadotropin (HCG) (45), and of insulin-like growth factor II, which resulted in hypoglycemia (46–48).

Age

The median age at diagnosis of PT is about 45 to 50 years. PTs are rare in women younger than 30 years of age, and exceedingly uncommon before menarche, but rare cases have been reported (40,49–51). Most PTs in girls under age 18 years are benign (6,7). Malignant PTs are very rare in pediatric patients and during pregnancy (44,52–54). A benign PT that developed in a 31-weeks pregnant woman did not recur in a subsequent pregnancy (53). A PT may have developed from a preexisting FA during hormonal treatment for in vitro fertilization (55).

Ethnicity

The annual age-adjusted incidence of malignant PT in a population-based study in Los Angeles county was 2.1 per 1 million women (56). The risk of malignant PT was three- to four-folds higher for foreign-born than US-born Latina women. Another study (57) found a higher percentage of borderline and malignant PTs in Hispanic patients. Asian ethnicity also appears associated with a higher risk of PTs. In a study conducted in Australia (58), 31% of 65 women with PTs and 6/9 (67%) women with recurrent PTs were of Asian descent. Furthermore, 32% of the Asian patients developed recurrent disease versus only 7% of non-Asian patients.

Genetic Predisposition

Women with *P53* germline mutation (Li-Fraumeni syndrome) have a significantly increased risk of developing a malignant PT ($p = 0.0003$) (59).

Male Gender

PTs are exceedingly rare in men. A 70-year-old man with gynecomastia and a breast tumor slowly growing over 50 years reportedly had a focally malignant PT in a 30 cm FA (60).

Size

The mean tumor size in a study of 605 PTs was 5.2 cm (range 0.3–25) (41). Malignant PTs tend to be larger than benign PTs, but there are exceptions. In a study of 293 PTs (5), the size was ≤3 cm in 54% of cases: 66% of benign PTs measured ≤3 cm, whereas 67% of borderline and malignant PTs were >3 cm.

Radiology

Mammography reveals a rounded or lobulated, sharply defined opaque mass (61,62). Sonographically, most PTs appear well circumscribed, but they are structurally inhomogeneous owing to cysts and epithelium-lined clefts (61). Calcifications are uncommon. Neither mammography nor ultrasonography can reliably classify PTs, or distinguish benign PTs from cellular FAs. MRI of benign PTs reveals an oval or lobulated shape with internal septations (21), but the MRI characteristics do not permit a definitive separation from cellular FA. A study of 30 PTs (63) found no significant differences in the MRI characteristics of benign and malignant PTs. Dynamic enhancement is observed after administration of contrast material (21).

Microscopic Pathology

PTs are fibroepithelial tumors characterized by increased cellularity and expansion of the stromal component. Further classification of PTs takes into account multiple histologic parameters, including stromal cellularity, atypia, and mitotic activity, the microscopic character of the tumor border, stromal overgrowth, and presence of heterologous elements. Stromal cellularity, atypia, and mitotic activity in the NCB specimen of a PT tend to be good indicators of the PT grade. Because of the intratumoral heterogeneity characteristic of PTs, it is usually not possible to definitively classify a large fibroepithelial tumor based on evaluation of NCB material alone. The diagnostic interpretation should convey the possibility that the lesion may be of higher grade than seen in the NCB material.

Stromal cellularity within a PT tends to be heterogeneous, with more cellular regions adjacent to less cellular foci, some of which might be indistinguishable from FA. Varied stromal cellularity in a NCB sample suggests a PT (**Fig. 7.19**). Because of the intratumoral heterogeneity characteristic of PTs, it is usually not possible to definitively classify a large fibroepithelial tumor based on evaluation of only NCB material alone. The diagnostic interpretation should convey the possibility that the lesion may be of higher grade than that seen in the NCB material.

Elongated and dilated ducts with cleft-like appearance are one of the characteristic morphologic features of PTs. The stromal fronds protruding into the ducts usually do not mold to one another. In NCB material, the frond-like architecture of PTs correlates with fragmentation of the tissue cores, and the presence of detached, round-to-oval stromal fragments of different diameter that are completely lined by epithelium (**Fig. 7.19**). FAs with an intracanalicular structure can bear a superficial resemblance to benign PTs, but the fronds tend to completely fill the duct lumina and fit in to one another like pieces of a jigsaw puzzle. The stroma of intracanalicular FAs also tends to be uniform and hypocellular. In NCB samples of some benign or borderline PTs, the intracanalicular pattern of clefts sometimes may be obscured by ductal epithelial hyperplasia, or by a focally conspicuous glandular component.

Stromal myxoid change is common in PT, but it tends to be patchy, and areas of pseudoangiomatous stromal hyperplasia (PASH) are also frequent (64) (**Fig. 7.20**). Multinucleated stromal giant cells (**Fig. 7.21**) occur in about 10% of the cases (64), especially in higher-grade PTs. Stromal metaplasia is not characteristic of benign PTs, but it can occur in borderline PTs, and especially in malignant PTs. The most frequent stromal change consists of liposarcoma-like areas with lipoblasts-like cells, but rhabdomyosarcoma-, angiosarcoma-, and osteosarcoma-like foci can also occur.

Stromal overgrowth (65) (defined as absence of an epithelial component in at least one microscopic field at 40X total magnification in sections from the surgical excision specimen) is associated with an increased risk of distant metastases. This

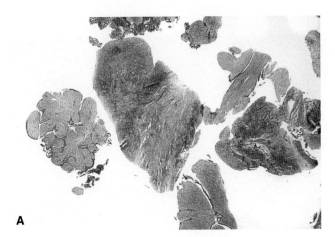

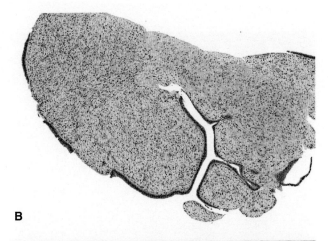

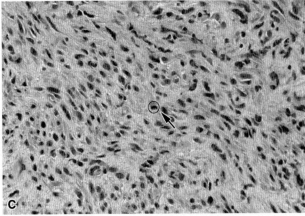

FIGURE 7.19 Morphologic Features of Phyllodes Tumors. A: Fragmentation of the tissue cores, relative paucity of the epithelial component, expansion of the stroma, and varied stromal cellularity are features of phyllodes tumors. **B:** In this needle core biopsy of a benign phyllodes tumor, the stroma is cellular and forms small fronds lined by epithelium. **C:** A stromal mitosis (*arrow*) in the same tumor shown in **B**.

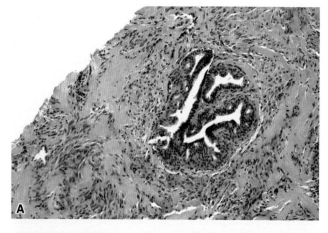

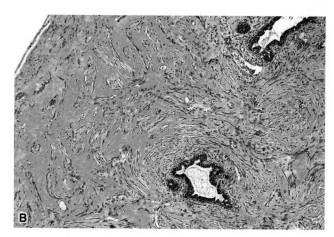

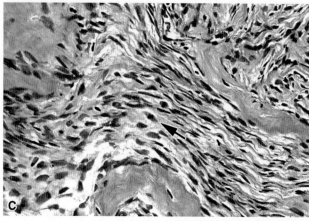

FIGURE 7.20 **Phyllodes Tumor with Pseudoangiomatous Stromal Hyperplasia. A:** This benign phyllodes tumor has a prominent fascicular stromal pattern composed of bundles of myofibroblasts. The patient was a 75-year-old woman with a recently detected 1.5-cm tumor. **B, C:** Fascicular pseudoangiomatous stroma in a benign phyllodes tumor from a 15-year-old girl. A mitosis *(arrow)* is shown in a fascicular region **(C)**.

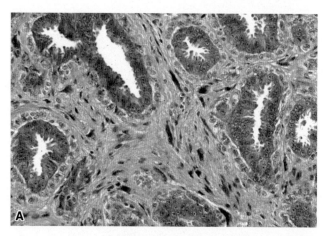

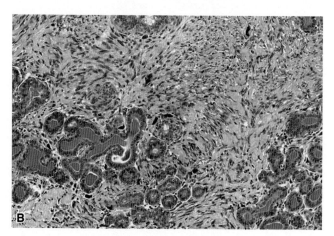

FIGURE 7.21 **Phyllodes Tumor with Stromal Giant Cells. A:** Multinucleated giant cells are present in the stroma of this benign phyllodes tumor. **B:** A borderline phyllodes tumor with numerous multinucleated stromal cells in PASH.

feature is more common in malignant PTs, but it can also occur in borderline PTs. Stromal overgrowth cannot be definitively assessed in NCB samples, but lack of epithelium at 40×(29) or 10×(68) final magnification in NCB material is regarded as an indicator. Stromal mitotic activity is also an important parameter of the grade of a PT.

A benign phyllodes tumor has minimal-to-mild stromal atypia, and stromal cellularity and mitotic activity are more pronounced around the ducts. Epithelial hyperplasia can be prominent. The tumor border has focal peripheral infiltration **(Fig. 7.22)**, but this feature is not always present in NCB material. Multinucleated cells with hyperchromatic nuclei may be present in the stroma **(Fig. 7.21A)**. Focal stromal myxoid change is not uncommon in a benign PT, but usually it does not involve the entire tumor. Necrotic foci are infrequent.

The most common differential diagnosis of a benign PT in NCB material is with cellular FA **(Figs. 7.8, 7.9, 7.19, and 7.22)**. Many studies have tried to identify clinical and

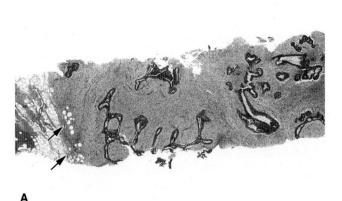
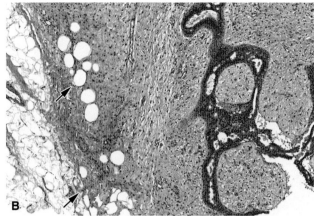

FIGURE 7.22 Benign Phyllodes Tumor. A, B: The stroma is cellular and slightly expanded. Infiltration into the adjacent fat at the periphery of the lesion *(arrows)*. Surgical excision of this lesion yielded a benign phyllodes tumor.

morphologic features predictive of PT in the surgical excision specimen, but no single morphologic feature, or any combination thereof, is absolutely reliable. Findings in the NCB material that correlate with the diagnosis of PT in the follow-up surgical excision specimen include at least 2 (29,30,66) or 3 (67) stromal mitoses per 10 HPF, increased stromal cellularity (29,66), stromal overgrowth (defined as absence of epithelial elements in at least one microscopic field at 10×(68) or 40×(29) final magnification), invasive margins (defined as microscopic extension of the tumor into the adjacent tissue), fragmentation of the tissue cores (defined as detached stromal fragments entirely surrounded by epithelium) (66,68), presence of adipose tissue admixed with stroma (68), and nuclear atypia. Patient age higher than 50 to 55 years favors a diagnosis of PT in some studies (66,69) but not in others (67,68). In a study evaluating morphologic parameters predictive of PT versus cellular FA, 74% of PTs had at least 3 stromal mitoses per 10 HPFs in the NCB material, and 11% had one or two mitoses per 10 HPFs, whereas the NCB samples of cellular FAs showed 3 or more stromal mitoses in 11% of cases, 1 to 2 mitoses per 10 HPFs in 30% of cases, and no mitotic activity in the remaining 60% (67).

All of the aforementioned features can be difficult to assess in NCB material. A study (70) found that even after a training period, interobserver agreement was poor for mitotic count and stromal cellularity, and it was only fair for all the other features. In our opinion, if review of NCB material raises the differential diagnosis of benign PT, surgical excision of the lesion is required to fully evaluate the tumor, and excision should include a rim of the surrounding tissue.

The differential diagnosis of benign PT sometimes includes other low-grade mammary spindle cell proliferations, such as PASH, myofibroblastoma, fibromatosis, and metaplastic "low-grade" spindle cell carcinoma, especially when a NCB sample consists largely or entirely of stromal tissue (see discussion in the corresponding chapters).

A *borderline phyllodes tumor* has moderately cellular stroma with a heterogeneous distribution. Invasion into the adjacent tissue may be present in the form of spindle cells surrounding adjacent adipocytes. Focal atypical adipose metaplasia with lipoblast-like cells as well as chondroid and osseous metaplasia can be encountered **(Fig. 7.23)**. Focal necrosis may be present. Stromal mitoses are usually evident **(Fig. 7.23)**. In most cases the epithelial component of a borderline PT is at least focally present in NCB material, enabling the diagnosis of a fibroepithelial tumor. However, the grade of the fibroepithelial tumor is difficult to assess because of intratumoral heterogeneity. Nuclear pleomorphism and ≥2 mitoses in 10 HPFs in a NCB sample usually correlate with the finding of at least borderline PT in the surgical excision specimen.

The differential diagnosis of a borderline PT in NCB material includes benign PT and malignant PT. In some cases, the differential diagnosis may include PASH, fibromatosis, and low-grade fibrosarcoma (see also discussions in the corresponding chapters).

A *malignant phyllodes tumor* is characterized by hypercellular stroma with high-grade nuclei and conspicuous mitotic activity **(Fig. 7.24)**; areas of necrosis are common. The relative paucity of the epithelial component within a malignant PT correlates with limited and widely spaced epithelial elements in NCB material. Lack of epithelium in a 40X final magnification field of view is an indicator of stromal overgrowth in the surgical excision specimen. Areas of sarcomatous metaplasia are common, especially liposarcoma-like areas, whereas epithelial hyperplasia is uncommon in malignant PTs, and most ducts are lined by flattened epithelium. Squamous metaplasia can be present. Rarely, carcinoma can develop (71).

The NCB of a malignant PT usually yields only a minimal amount of epithelium, often times limited to a monostratified and flat layer lining a stretched out duct. In some cases, no duct/glandular elements are present in the NCB material. In the latter scenario, the differential diagnosis of a high-grade spindle cell lesion involving the breast, in addition to malignant PT, includes metaplastic spindle cell carcinoma with high-grade morphology, high-grade angiosarcoma, other sarcomas, either primary or metastatic, and melanoma with spindle cell morphology. In these cases, the use of a panel of immunohistochemical markers, such as CK 34βE12, CK14,

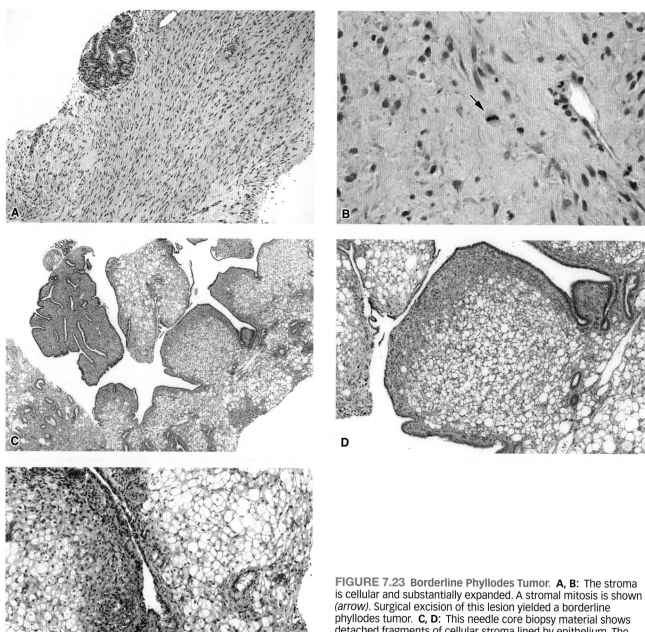

FIGURE 7.23 Borderline Phyllodes Tumor. A, B: The stroma is cellular and substantially expanded. A stromal mitosis is shown *(arrow)*. Surgical excision of this lesion yielded a borderline phyllodes tumor. **C, D:** This needle core biopsy material shows detached fragments of cellular stroma lined by epithelium. The stroma shows extensive atypical adipose differentiation, and the stromal cells tend to be denser in subepithelial location. **E:** Another borderline phyllodes tumor with liposarcoma-like component.

CK5/6, MNF116, p63, CD34, CD31, ERG, S-100, and HMB45, is helpful in sorting out the differential diagnosis. In the absence of staining for any of the aforementioned antigens, the report should indicate diagnostic uncertainty and the need for complete evaluation of the lesion for a more definitive classification.

Epithelium in Phyllodes Tumors

Many PTs exhibit epithelial hyperplasia, which tends to be more frequent and pronounced in borderline and benign PTs, and less common in malignant lesions. Most malignant PTs have inconspicuous, flattened epithelium. Myoepithelial hyperplasia

can occur focally. Squamous metaplasia of the ductal epithelium occurs in 3.6% (64) to 10% of PTs (72,73), whereas it is not reported in FA. The identification of a cyst lined by squamous epithelium within a cellular fibroepithelial lesion favors the diagnosis of PT. Apocrine metaplasia can occur in PTs, but it is also encountered in FAs, especially in complex FAs. Mammary lobules and foci of adenosis can also be present within a PT. In rare instances, adenosis and/or papillary hyperplasia can obscure the underlying architecture of a PT, mimicking mass-forming adenosis, adenomyoepithelioma, or a papillary neoplasm.

ALH, LCIS, ADH, and DCIS are uncommon in PTs (58,64). In particular, the diagnosis of DCIS should be rendered with

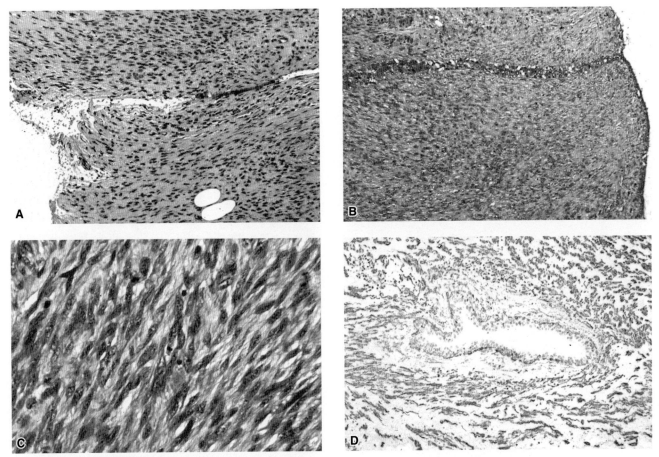

FIGURE 7.24 Malignant Phyllodes Tumor. A: This needle core biopsy specimen is from a fibrosarcomatous phyllodes tumor. **B–D:** The epithelial-lined cleft in **B** is virtually obliterated in this needle core biopsy specimen from a tumor with leiomyosarcomatous differentiation. The tumor cells are immunoreactive for smooth muscle actin in **D**.

extreme caution on examination of limited NCB material if an underlying fibroepithelial lesion is recognized. On the other hand, the identification of DCIS in a spindle cell tumor resembling a PT supports the diagnosis of metaplastic spindle cell carcinoma. Invasive carcinoma is even less frequent in PTs (58,64,74–81). An invasive carcinoma with squamous differentiation arising in a high-grade malignant PT has been reported (82).

Morphology of Recurrent/Metastatic Phyllodes Tumor

Ductal elements may be present in locally recurrent PTs in the breast. The morphology of recurrent tumors is usually similar to that of the primary PT; occasionally, the recurrent PT differs from the primary and usually is of higher grade (5,64).

Metastatic PTs at distant sites consist entirely of the stromal component, and only one case with concomitant glandular component has been reported (83). The most common appearance encountered in metastatic lesions is that of a high-grade spindle cell tumor with a fibrosarcomatous pattern. Rarely, locally recurrent or metastatic lesions exhibit heterologous differentiation that was not apparent in the primary malignant PT.

Immunohistochemistry

Immunohistochemical stains are not useful in the subclassification of PTs but play a role in the differential diagnosis with other spindle cell lesions occurring in the breast.

CD34
CD34 is expressed in the stroma of most PTs (84–86). A study (87) reported CD34 staining in 72.5% of benign PTs, 66.7% of borderline PTs, and 44.4% of (high-grade) malignant PTs.

Keratins and p63
Keratins and p63 are useful in the differential diagnosis of PTs, especially malignant PT and metaplastic spindle cell carcinoma, with the caveat that the latter may show only very focal or even no staining for CKs. Furthermore, a study of 109 PTs (87) identified focal patchy stromal staining for CK7 in 28.4% of cases, for 34βE12 in 22%, for MNF116 in 11.9%, for AE1:AE3 in 8.3%, and for CAM5.2 and CK14 in 1.8% of cases each. MNF116 and 34βE12 staining in the stromal cells decreased significantly with increasing PT grade. In one series, no p63 staining was identified in the neoplastic stromal

cells (87). Another group (88) reported p63 and p40 staining in the stromal cells of malignant PTs but not in benign and borderline PTs. A subsequent study of six malignant PTs did not confirm these findings, although it documented focal p63 staining in a spindle cell sarcoma (89). Based on these observations, cautious interpretation of focal CK or p63 positivity in the NCB material of spindle cell lesions occurring in the breast is recommended, particularly in the absence of the morphologic findings characteristic of metaplastic carcinoma or PT (**Fig. 7.25**).

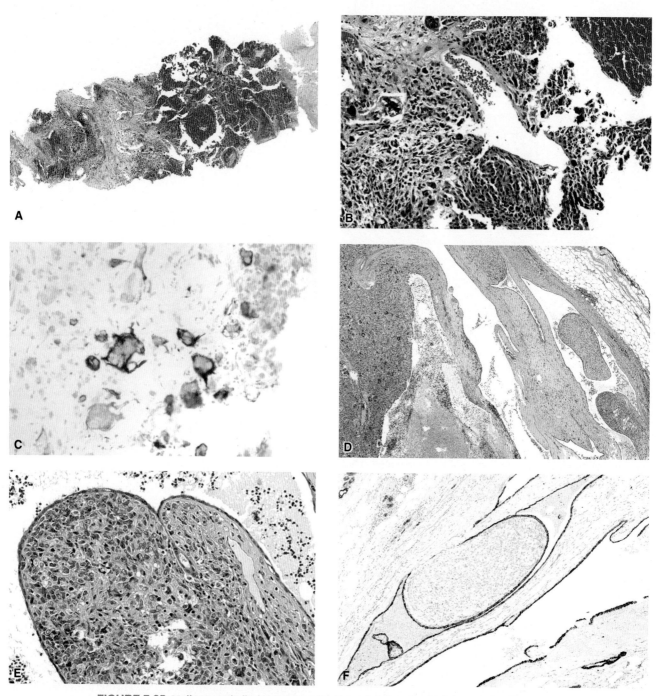

FIGURE 7.25 Malignant Phyllodes Tumor with Focal Cytokeratin Staining. A, B: This needle core biopsy specimen from a 3-cm solid and cystic mass shows necrosis and few viable tumor cells. **C**: Focal CAM5.2 staining was identified. No reactivity for other epithelial markers, as well as for vascular and melanocytic antigens was documented (not shown), and a diagnosis of poorly differentiated carcinoma was rendered. **D, E**: The tumor in the surgical excision specimen consisted of epithelium-lined fronds. **F**: The immunohistochemical stain for CAM5.2 highlights the epithelium lining the neoplastic fronds but not the neoplastic spindle cells. The final interpretation was malignant phyllodes tumor with focal aberrant CAM5.2 staining.

ER, PR, AR, and HER2

The expression of ER and PR in the epithelium of PTs appears inversely correlated with increasing grade of the PT. AR occurs in less than 5% of the epithelium and stroma of all PTs (90). Focal membranous reactivity for HER2 is detected in the epithelium but not in the stroma of PTs, and does not correlate with tumor prognosis (91). None of these markers has practical diagnostic utility in the evaluation of mammary fibroepithelial lesions.

Nuclear β-catenin diffusely stains 80% to 100% of cases of primary mammary fibromatosis (92,93) and also decorates the stromal cells of approximately three-fourths of PTs (93–95), including 94% of the stromal cells of benign PTs, mostly in periductal distribution. Staining for nuclear β-catenin is weaker in borderline and malignant PTs compared to benign PTs. Nuclear β-catenin is also detected in 23% of metaplastic mammary carcinomas (93). In the absence of the diffuse nuclear positivity typical of fibromatosis, the finding of focal nuclear β-catenin staining in the NCB material from a spindle cell lesion involving the breast should be interpreted cautiously.

CD117/c-kit

A few studies (84,96–100) have reported staining for c-kit in PTs. One group (101) attributed the staining for c-kit to infiltrating mast cells and reported focal expression in the stromal cells of only two PTs.

p53

p53 is present in the nucleus of the neoplastic stromal cells, and its expression correlates with higher grade (91,99,100,102–107), with the greatest reactivity in the periepithelial stroma of malignant PTs (108). P53 reactivity in PTs correlated with reduced survival (106,109), but it was not predictive of tumor recurrence in other series (91,99,102).

Ki67

Ki67 immunoreactivity also correlates with tumor grade (102,104,105,107).

CD10

CD10 is expressed in the stromal cells of fibroepithelial lesions, including FAs. Some studies (110,111) report higher CD10 expression in malignant PTs, including 6 of 10 PTs that developed distant metastases (111), but another group found no difference in the expression of CD10 in FAs and PTs (112).

Immunoperoxidase studies have been applied to the diagnosis of fibroepithelial tumors in NCB samples. Ki67 and topoisomerase II immunoreactivity showed a statistically significant correlation with PT diagnosis in two studies (29,30). However, some overlap exists between the results in FAs and PTs using both markers (Ki67 index: 1.6, range 0.4–4 in FAs vs. 6.0, range 0–18 in PTs; topoisomerase II index: 2.8, range 0–10 in FAs vs. 7.0, range 1.2–29 in PTs), even though the results were statistically significant, especially for Ki67 ($p = 0.002$) (30). In another study (29), Ki67 and topoisomerase II indexes greater or equal to 5% and reduced or patchy CD34 staining in lesional stromal cells in NCB material correlated with the diagnosis of PT in the surgical excision specimen. The specificity of these markers has not been validated prospectively, and neither is routinely used in diagnostic practice.

Treatment and Prognosis

Surgical Excision

The treatment of PT involves complete excision to prevent local recurrence (5,41,52,64,113–116). Most studies recommend a margin clearance of at least 1.0 cm (52,115,117,118), although the need for such a wide margin is not supported by definitive evidence. Higher rates of local recurrence are reported if the final margin is diffusely rather than focally involved (64), but local recurrences also occur in approximately 10% patients with negative excision margins. Mastectomy might be indicated if a large malignant PT cannot be encompassed with a cosmetically acceptable excision.

The risk of LN metastases is extremely low (52,115), and sentinel LN biopsy is not indicated in the absence of a coexisting ipsilateral invasive carcinoma or clinical nodal enlargement.

Local Recurrence

Benign PTs will not metastasize, but historically they recur locally in 11% to 17% of cases (5,41,64,119). The recurrent tumor has higher-grade morphology than the index PT in more than one-third of cases (5,41). Recently, some groups (113,120–124) have reported less than 10% rate of local recurrence for benign PTs, and suggested a wait-and-see approach instead of re-excision of benign PTs with positive excision margins, particularly for small benign PTs. In recent series (123,124), most of the locally recurrent benign PT also had benign PT morphology, and none was morphologically malignant. Historically, borderline PTs recur locally in 14% to 25% of cases (41,64,125); the recurrence may have malignant morphology.

About one-third of patients with malignant PT (41) develop a local recurrence that tends to occur earlier than for benign or borderline PTs.

Distant Metastases

Distant metastases of PTs are rare and occur almost exclusively in patients with malignant tumors (5,41), usually within 3 years of primary treatment (5,52,64,117,126). In a recent study (41), nuclear atypia, stromal overgrowth, and surgical margin status were significant predictors of local and/or distant recurrence free survival (RFS) in multivariate analysis, whereas mitotic rate approached statistical significance. A nomogram that estimates the RFS of patients with PTs based on the aforementioned parameters is available, but it has not been validated in a non-Asian patient population (41).

It has been suggested that radiotherapy may be beneficial in preventing local recurrence of borderline and malignant PTs, but two studies evaluating this approach had limited numbers of cases and lacked study control groups, limiting the interpretation of the findings (118,127). At present, radiotherapy is not part of the standard treatment of PT managed with breast-conserving surgery, especially if the PT was excised with negative margins. Radiotherapy is usually part of the management of a primary or recurrent PT invading the chest wall.

The RFS in a series of patients with primary malignant PTs who received chemotherapy was not significantly improved (128).

Survival

Analysis of 821 patients with malignant PTs recorded in the SEER program with median follow-up of 5.7 years revealed disease free survival (DFS) of 91%, 89%, and 89% at 5, 10, and 15 years, respectively (129), with no statistically significant difference in disease-specific survival between patients treated with surgical excision versus mastectomy. The most common sites of metastatic disease are the lungs and bone. Most deaths occur within 5 years of primary PT diagnosis (5,41,64,117), and nearly all fatalities occur in patients who presented with malignant PTs or developed malignant recurrences. Stromal overgrowth, invasive borders, cellular pleomorphism, and frequent mitoses are factors significantly associated with distant metastases (5,64,65). In the largest series published to date (41), margin involvement, atypia, and stromal overgrowth were statistically significant predictors of disease recurrence (41), and mitotic rate was nearly statistically significant.

REFERENCES

1. Kovi J, Chu HB, Leffall LD Jr. Sclerosing lobular hyperplasia manifesting as a palpable mass of the breast in young black women. *Hum Pathol.* 1984;15:336–340.
2. Poulton TB, de Paredes ES, Baldwin M. Sclerosing lobular hyperplasia of the breast: imaging features in 15 cases. *AJR Am J Roentgenol.* 1995;165:291–294.
3. Kapur P, Rakheja D, Cavuoti DC, et al. Sclerosing lobular hyperplasia of breast: cytomorphologic and histomorphologic features: a case report. *Cytojournal.* 2006;3:8.
4. Panikar N, Agarwal S. Sclerosing lobular hyperplasia of the breast: fine-needle aspiration cytology findings—a case report. *Diagn Cytopathol.* 2004;31:340–341.
5. Barrio AV, Clark BD, Goldberg JI, et al. Clinicopathologic features and long-term outcomes of 293 phyllodes tumors of the breast. *Ann Surg Oncol.* 2007;14:2961–2970.
6. Ross DS, Giri D, Akram M, et al. Fibroepithelial lesions in the breast of adolescent females: a clinicopathological study of 54 cases [published online ahead of print]. *Breast J.*
7. Tay TK, Chang KT, Thike AA, et al. Paediatric fibroepithelial lesions revisited: pathological insights. *J Clin Pathol.* 2015;68:633–641.
8. Mies C, Rosen PP. Juvenile fibroadenoma with atypical epithelial hyperplasia. *Am J Surg Pathol.* 1987;11:184–190.
9. Kuijper A, Mommers EC, van der Wall E, et al. Histopathology of fibroadenoma of the breast. *Am J Clin Pathol.* 2001;115:736–742.
10. Sklair-Levy M, Sella T, Alweiss T, et al. Incidence and management of complex fibroadenomas. *AJR Am J Roentgenol.* 2008;190:214–218.
11. Ansah-Boateng Y, Tavassoli FA. Fibroadenoma and cystosarcoma phyllodes of the male breast. *Mod Pathol.* 1992;5:114–116.
12. Gupta P, Foshee S, Garcia-Morales F, et al. Fibroadenoma in male breast: case report and literature review. *Breast Dis.* 2011;33:45–48.
13. Uchida T, Ishii M, Motomiya Y. Fibroadenoma associated with gynaecomastia in an adult man: case report. *Scand J Plast Reconstr Surg Hand Surg.* 1993;27:327–329.
14. Kanhai RC, Hage JJ, Bloemena E, et al. Mammary fibroadenoma in a male-to-female transsexual. *Histopathology.* 1999;35:183–185.
15. Lemmo G, Garcea N, Corsello S, et al. Breast fibroadenoma in a male-to-female transsexual patient after hormonal treatment. *Eur J Surg Suppl.* 2003;(588):69–71.
16. Weinstein SP, Orel SG, Collazzo L, et al. Cyclosporin A-induced fibroadenomas of the breast: report of five cases. *Radiology.* 2001;220:465–468.
17. Son EJ, Oh KK, Kim EK, et al. Characteristic imaging features of breast fibroadenomas in women given cyclosporin A after renal transplantation. *J Clin Ultrasound.* 2004;32:69–77.
18. Iaria G, Pisani F, De Luca L, et al. Prospective study of switch from cyclosporine to tacrolimus for fibroadenomas of the breast in kidney transplantation. *Transplant Proc.* 2010;42:1169–1170.
19. Carney JA, Toorkey BC. Myxoid fibroadenoma and allied conditions (myxomatosis) of the breast: a heritable disorder with special associations including cardiac and cutaneous myxomas. *Am J Surg Pathol.* 1991;15:713–721.
20. Yamaguchi R, Tanaka M, Mizushima Y, et al. Myxomatous fibroadenoma of the breast: correlation with clinicopathologic and radiologic features. *Hum Pathol.* 2011;42:419–423.
21. Wurdinger S, Herzog AB, Fischer DR, et al. Differentiation of phyllodes breast tumors from fibroadenomas on MRI. *AJR Am J Roentgenol.* 2005;185:1317–1321.
22. Foster ME, Garrahan N, Williams S. Fibroadenoma of the breast: a clinical and pathological study. *J R Coll Surg Edinb.* 1988;33:16–19.
23. Powell CM, Cranor ML, Rosen PP. Multinucleated stromal giant cells in mammary fibroepithelial neoplasms: a study of 11 patients. *Arch Pathol Lab Med.* 1994;118:912–916.
24. Ryska A, Reynolds C, Keeney GL. Benign tumors of the breast with multinucleated stromal giant cells: immunohistochemical analysis of six cases and review of the literature. *Virchows Arch.* 2001;439:768–775.
25. Dupont WD, Page DL, Parl FF, et al. Long-term risk of breast cancer in women with fibroadenoma. *N Engl J Med.* 1994;331:10–15.
26. Ben Hassouna J, Damak T, Ben Slama A, et al. Breast carcinoma arising within fibroadenomas: report of four observations. *Tunis Med.* 2007;85:891–895.
27. Petersson F, Tan PH, Putti TC. Low-grade ductal carcinoma in situ and invasive mammary carcinoma with columnar cell morphology arising in a complex fibroadenoma in continuity with columnar cell change and flat epithelial atypia. *Int J Surg Pathol.* 2010;18:352–357.
28. Sawyer EJ, Hanby AM, Poulsom R, et al. Beta-catenin abnormalities and associated insulin-like growth factor overexpression are important in phyllodes tumours and fibroadenomas of the breast. *J Pathol.* 2003;200:627–632.
29. Jara-Lazaro AR, Akhilesh M, Thike AA, et al. Predictors of phyllodes tumours on core biopsy specimens of fibroepithelial neoplasms. *Histopathology.* 2010;57:220–232.
30. Jacobs TW, Chen YY, Guinee DG Jr, et al. Fibroepithelial lesions with cellular stroma on breast core needle biopsy: are there predictors of outcome on surgical excision? *Am J Clin Pathol.* 2005;124:342–354.
31. Piscuoglio S, Murray M, Fusco N, et al. MED12 somatic mutations in fibroadenomas and phyllodes tumours of the breast. *Histopathology.* 2015;67:719–729.
32. Yoshida M, Ogawa R, Yoshida H, et al. TERT promoter mutations are frequent and show association with MED12 mutations in phyllodes tumors of the breast. *Br J Cancer.* 2015;113:1244–1248.
33. Piscuoglio S, Ng CK, Murray M, et al. Massively parallel sequencing of phyllodes tumours of the breast reveals actionable mutations, and TERT promoter hotspot mutations and TERT gene amplification as likely drivers of progression. *J Pathol.* 2016;238:508–518.
34. Sperber F, Blank A, Metser U, et al. Diagnosis and treatment of breast fibroadenomas by ultrasound-guided vacuum-assisted biopsy. *Arch Surg.* 2003;138:796–800.
35. Grady I, Gorsuch H, Wilburn-Bailey S. Long-term outcome of benign fibroadenomas treated by ultrasound-guided percutaneous excision. *Breast J.* 2008;14:275–278.
36. Littrup PJ, Freeman-Gibb L, Andea A, et al. Cryotherapy for breast fibroadenomas. *Radiology.* 2005;234:63–72.
37. Nurko J, Mabry CD, Whitworth P, et al. Interim results from the FibroAdenoma Cryoablation Treatment Registry. *Am J Surg.* 2005;190:647–651; discussion 51–52.
38. Kaufman CS, Littrup PJ, Freeman-Gibb LA, et al. Office-based cryoablation of breast fibroadenomas with long-term follow-up. *Breast J.* 2005;11:344–350.

39. Jacklin RK, Ridgway PF, Ziprin P, et al. Optimising preoperative diagnosis in phyllodes tumour of the breast. *J Clin Pathol.* 2006;59:454–459.

40. Tagaya N, Kodaira H, Kogure H, et al. A case of phyllodes tumor with bloody nipple discharge in juvenile patient. *Breast Cancer.* 1999;6:207–210.

41. Tan PH, Thike AA, Tan WJ, et al. Predicting clinical behaviour of breast phyllodes tumours: a nomogram based on histological criteria and surgical margins. *J Clin Pathol.* 2012;65(1):69–76.

42. Mallory MA, Chikarmane SA, Raza S, et al. Bilateral synchronous benign phyllodes tumors. *Am Surg.* 2015;81:E192–E194.

43. Seal SK, Kuusk U, Lennox PA. Bilateral and multifocal phyllodes tumours of the breast: a case report. *Can J Plast Surg.* 2010;18:145–146.

44. Mrad K, Driss M, Maalej M, et al. Bilateral cystosarcoma phyllodes of the breast: a case report of malignant form with contralateral benign form. *Ann Diagn Pathol.* 2000;4:370–372.

45. Reisenbichler ES, Krontiras H, Hameed O. Beta-human chorionic gonadotropin production associated with phyllodes tumor of the breast: an unusual paraneoplastic phenomenon. *Breast J.* 2009;15:527–530.

46. Kataoka T, Haruta R, Goto T, et al. Malignant phyllodes tumor of the breast with hypoglycemia: report of a case. *Jpn J Clin Oncol.* 1998;28:276–280.

47. Hino N, Nakagawa Y, Ikushima Y, et al. A case of a giant phyllodes tumor of the breast with hypoglycemia caused by high-molecular-weight insulin-like growth factor II. *Breast Cancer.* 2010;17:142–145.

48. Aguiar Bujanda D, Rivero Vera JC, Cabrera Suarez MA, et al. Hypoglycemic coma secondary to big insulin-like growth factor II secretion by a giant phyllodes tumor of the breast. *Breast J.* 2007;13:189–191.

49. Selamzade M, Gidener C, Koyuncuoglu M, et al. Borderline phylloides tumor in an 11-year-old girl. *Pediatr Surg Int.* 1999;15:427–428.

50. Inder M, Vaishnav K, Mathur DR. Benign breast lesions in prepubertal female children—a study of 20 years. *J Indian Med Assoc.* 2001;99:619–620.

51. Sorelli PG, Thomas D, Moore A, et al. Malignant phyllodes tumor in an 11-year-old premenarchal girl. *J Pediatr Surg.* 2010;45:e17–e20.

52. Guillot E, Couturaud B, Reyal F, et al. Management of phyllodes breast tumors. *Breast J.* 2011;17:129–137.

53. Way JC, Culham BA. Phyllodes tumour in pregnancy: a case report. *Can J Surg.* 1998;41:407–409.

54. Blaker KM, Sahoo S, Schweichler MR, et al. Malignant phylloides tumor in pregnancy. *Am Surg.* 2010;76:302–305.

55. Pacchiarotti A, Frati P, Caserta D, et al. First case of transformation for breast fibroadenoma to high-grade malignant cystosarcoma in an in vitro fertilization patient. *Fertil Steril.* 2011;96:1126–1127.

56. Bernstein L, Deapen D, Ross RK. The descriptive epidemiology of malignant cystosarcoma phyllodes tumors of the breast. *Cancer.* 1993;71:3020–3024.

57. Pimiento JM, Gadgil PV, Santillan AA, et al. Phyllodes tumors: race-related differences. *J Am Coll Surg.* 2011;213:537–542.

58. Karim RZ, Gerega SK, Yang YH, et al. Phyllodes tumours of the breast: a clinicopathological analysis of 65 cases from a single institution. *Breast.* 2009;18:165–170.

59. Birch JM, Alston RD, McNally RJ, et al. Relative frequency and morphology of cancers in carriers of germline TP53 mutations. *Oncogene.* 2001;20:4621–4628.

60. Pantoja E, Llobet RE, Lopez E. Gigantic cystosarcoma phyllodes in a man with gynecomastia. *Arch Surg.* 1976;111:611.

61. Buchberger W, Strasser K, Heim K, et al. Phylloides tumor: findings on mammography, sonography, and aspiration cytology in 10 cases. *AJR Am J Roentgenol.* 1991;157:715–719.

62. Cosmacini P, Zurrida S, Veronesi P, et al. Phyllode tumor of the breast: mammographic experience in 99 cases. *Eur J Radiol.* 1992;15:11–14.

63. Yabuuchi H, Soeda H, Matsuo Y, et al. Phyllodes tumor of the breast: correlation between MR findings and histologic grade. *Radiology.* 2006;241:702–709.

64. Tan PH, Jayabaskar T, Chuah KL, et al. Phyllodes tumors of the breast: the role of pathologic parameters. *Am J Clin Pathol.* 2005;123:529–540.

65. Hawkins RE, Schofield JB, Fisher C, et al. The clinical and histologic criteria that predict metastases from cystosarcoma phyllodes. *Cancer.* 1992;69:141–147.

66. Tsang AK, Chan SK, Lam CC, et al. Phyllodes tumours of the breast—differentiating features in core needle biopsy. *Histopathology.* 2011;59:600–608.

67. Yasir S, Gamez R, Jenkins S, et al. Significant histologic features differentiating cellular fibroadenoma from phyllodes tumor on core needle biopsy specimens. *Am J Clin Pathol.* 2014;142:362–369.

68. Lee AH, Hodi Z, Ellis IO, et al. Histological features useful in the distinction of phyllodes tumour and fibroadenoma on needle core biopsy of the breast. *Histopathology.* 2007;51:336–344.

69. Morgan JM, Douglas-Jones AG, Gupta SK. Analysis of histological features in needle core biopsy of breast useful in preoperative distinction between fibroadenoma and phyllodes tumour. *Histopathology.* 2010;56:489–500.

70. Bandyopadhyay S, Barak S, Hayek K, et al. Can problematic fibroepithelial lesions be accurately classified on core needle biopsies? *Hum Pathol.* 2016;47:38–44.

71. Sin EI, Wong CY, Yong WS, et al. Breast carcinoma and phyllodes tumour: a case series. *J Clin Pathol.* 2016;69:364–369.

72. Grimes MM. Cystosarcoma phyllodes of the breast: histologic features, flow cytometric analysis, and clinical correlations. *Mod Pathol.* 1992;5:232–239.

73. Norris HJ, Taylor HB. Relationship of histologic features to behavior of cystosarcoma phyllodes: analysis of ninety-four cases. *Cancer.* 1967;20:2090–2099.

74. Grove A, Deibjerg Kristensen L. Intraductal carcinoma within a phyllodes tumor of the breast: a case report. *Tumori.* 1986;72:187–190.

75. Knudsen PJ, Ostergaard J. Cystosarcoma phylloides with lobular and ductal carcinoma in situ. *Arch Pathol Lab Med.* 1987;111:873–875.

76. Yamaguchi R, Tanaka M, Kishimoto Y, et al. Ductal carcinoma in situ arising in a benign phyllodes tumor: report of a case. *Surg Today.* 2008;38:42–45.

77. Korula A, Varghese J, Thomas M, et al. Malignant phyllodes tumour with intraductal and invasive carcinoma and lymph node metastasis. *Singapore Med J.* 2008;49:e318–e321.

78. Nomura M, Inoue Y, Fujita S, et al. A case of noninvasive ductal carcinoma arising in malignant phyllodes tumor. *Breast Cancer.* 2006;13:89–94.

79. Kodama T, Kameyama K, Mukai M, et al. Invasive lobular carcinoma arising in phyllodes tumor of the breast. *Virchows Arch.* 2003;442:614–616.

80. Quinlan-Davidson S, Hodgson N, Elavathil L, et al. Borderline phyllodes tumor with an incidental invasive tubular carcinoma and lobular carcinoma in situ component: a case report. *J Breast Cancer.* 2011;14:237–240.

81. Choi Y, Lee KY, Jang MH, et al. Invasive cribriform carcinoma arising in malignant phyllodes tumor of breast: a case report. *Korean J Pathol.* 2012;46:205–209.

82. Sugie T, Takeuchi E, Kunishima F, et al. A case of ductal carcinoma with squamous differentiation in malignant phyllodes tumor. *Breast Cancer.* 2007;14:327–332.

83. Kracht J, Sapino A, Bussolati G. Malignant phyllodes tumor of breast with lung metastases mimicking the primary. *Am J Surg Pathol.* 1998;22:1284–1290.

84. Noronha Y, Raza A, Hutchins B, et al. CD34, CD117, and Ki-67 expression in phyllodes tumor of the breast: an immunohistochemical study of 33 cases. *Int J Surg Pathol.* 2011;19:152–158.

85. Chen CM, Chen CJ, Chang CL, et al. CD34, CD117, and actin expression in phyllodes tumor of the breast. *J Surg Res.* 2000;94:84–91.

86. Moore T, Lee AH. Expression of CD34 and bcl-2 in phyllodes tumours, fibroadenomas and spindle cell lesions of the breast. *Histopathology.* 2001;38:62–67.

87. Chia Y, Thike AA, Cheok PY, et al. Stromal keratin expression in phyllodes tumours of the breast: a comparison with other spindle cell breast lesions. *J Clin Pathol.* 2012;65:339–347.

88. Cimino-Mathews A, Sharma R, Illei PB, et al. A subset of malignant phyllodes tumors express p63 and p40: a diagnostic pitfall in breast core needle biopsies. *Am J Surg Pathol.* 2014;38(12):1689–1696.

89. D'Alfonso TM, Ross DS, Liu YF, et al. Expression of p40 and laminin 332 in metaplastic spindle cell carcinoma of the breast compared with other malignant spindle cell tumours. *J Clin Pathol.* 2015;68:516–521.

90. Tse GM, Lee CS, Kung FY, et al. Hormonal receptors expression in epithelial cells of mammary phyllodes tumors correlates with pathologic grade of the tumor: a multicenter study of 143 cases. *Am J Clin Pathol.* 2002;118:522–526.

91. Shpitz B, Bomstein Y, Sternberg A, et al. Immunoreactivity of p53, Ki-67, and c-erbB-2 in phyllodes tumors of the breast in correlation with clinical and morphologic features. *J Surg Oncol.* 2002;79:86–92.

92. Abraham SC, Reynolds C, Lee JH, et al. Fibromatosis of the breast and mutations involving the APC/beta-catenin pathway. *Hum Pathol.* 2002;33:39–46.

93. Lacroix-Triki M, Geyer FC, Lambros MB, et al. beta-catenin/Wnt signalling pathway in fibromatosis, metaplastic carcinomas and phyllodes tumours of the breast. *Mod Pathol.* 2010;23:1438–1448.

94. Sawyer EJ, Hanby AM, Rowan AJ, et al. The Wnt pathway, epithelial-stromal interactions, and malignant progression in phyllodes tumours. *J Pathol.* 2002;196:437–444.

95. Karim RZ, Gerega SK, Yang YH, et al. Proteins from the Wnt pathway are involved in the pathogenesis and progression of mammary phyllodes tumours. *J Clin Pathol.* 2009;62:1016–1020.

96. Tse GM, Putti TC, Lui PC, et al. Increased c-kit (CD117) expression in malignant mammary phyllodes tumors. *Mod Pathol.* 2004;17:827–831.

97. Carvalho S, de Silva AO, Milanezi F, et al. c-KIT and PDGFRA in breast phyllodes tumours: overexpression without mutations? *J Clin Pathol.* 2004;57:1075–1079.

98. Sawyer EJ, Poulsom R, Hunt FT, et al. Malignant phyllodes tumours show stromal overexpression of c-myc and c-kit. *J Pathol.* 2003;200:59–64.

99. Tan PH, Jayabaskar T, Yip G, et al. p53 and c-kit (CD117) protein expression as prognostic indicators in breast phyllodes tumors: a tissue microarray study. *Mod Pathol.* 2005;18:1527–1534.

100. Korcheva VB, Levine J, Beadling C, et al. Immunohistochemical and molecular markers in breast phyllodes tumors. *Appl Immunohistochem Mol Morphol.* 2011;19:119–125.

101. Djordjevic B, Hanna WM. Expression of c-kit in fibroepithelial lesions of the breast is a mast cell phenomenon. *Mod Pathol.* 2008;21:1238–1245.

102. Kleer CG, Giordano TJ, Braun T, et al. Pathologic, immunohistochemical, and molecular features of benign and malignant phyllodes tumors of the breast. *Mod Pathol.* 2001;14:185–190.

103. Tse GM, Lui PC, Scolyer RA, et al. Tumour angiogenesis and p53 protein expression in mammary phyllodes tumors. *Mod Pathol.* 2003;16:1007–1013.

104. Erhan Y, Zekioglu O, Ersoy O, et al. p53 and Ki-67 expression as prognostic factors in cystosarcoma phyllodes. *Breast J.* 2002;8:38–44.

105. Esposito NN, Mohan D, Brufsky A, et al. Phyllodes tumor: a clinicopathologic and immunohistochemical study of 30 cases. *Arch Pathol Lab Med.* 2006;130:1516–1521.

106. Kuijper A, de Vos RA, Lagendijk JH, et al. Progressive deregulation of the cell cycle with higher tumor grade in the stroma of breast phyllodes tumors. *Am J Clin Pathol.* 2005;123:690–698.

107. Gatalica Z, Finkelstein S, Lucio E, et al. p53 protein expression and gene mutation in phyllodes tumors of the breast. *Pathol Res Pract.* 2001;197:183–187.

108. Millar EK, Beretov J, Marr P, et al. Malignant phyllodes tumours of the breast display increased stromal p53 protein expression. *Histopathology.* 1999;34:491–496.

109. Yonemori K, Hasegawa T, Shimizu C, et al. Correlation of p53 and MIB-1 expression with both the systemic recurrence and survival in cases of phyllodes tumors of the breast. *Pathol Res Pract.* 2006;202:705–712.

110. Tse GM, Tsang AK, Putti TC, et al. Stromal CD10 expression in mammary fibroadenomas and phyllodes tumours. *J Clin Pathol.* 2005;58:185–189.

111. Al-Masri M, Darwazeh G, Sawalhi S, et al. Phyllodes tumor of the breast: role of CD10 in predicting metastasis. *Ann Surg Oncol.* 2012;19(4):1181–1184.

112. Zamecnik M, Kinkor Z, Chlumska A. CD10+ stromal cells in fibroadenomas and phyllodes tumors of the breast. *Virchows Arch.* 2006;448:871–872.

113. Bartoli C, Zurrida S, Veronesi P, et al. Small sized phyllodes tumor of the breast. *Eur J Surg Oncol.* 1990;16:215–219.

114. Salvadori B, Cusumano F, Del Bo R, et al. Surgical treatment of phyllodes tumors of the breast. *Cancer.* 1989;63:2532–2536.

115. Ben Hassouna J, Damak T, Gamoudi A, et al. Phyllodes tumors of the breast: a case series of 106 patients. *Am J Surg.* 2006;192:141–147.

116. Asoglu O, Ugurlu MM, Blanchard K, et al. Risk factors for recurrence and death after primary surgical treatment of malignant phyllodes tumors. *Ann Surg Oncol.* 2004;11:1011–1017.

117. Chaney AW, Pollack A, McNeese MD, et al. Primary treatment of cystosarcoma phyllodes of the breast. *Cancer.* 2000;89:1502–1511.

118. Belkacemi Y, Bousquet G, Marsiglia H, et al. Phyllodes tumor of the breast. *Int J Radiat Oncol Biol Phys.* 2008;70:492–500.

119. Barth RJ Jr. Histologic features predict local recurrence after breast conserving therapy of phyllodes tumors. *Breast Cancer Res Treat.* 1999;57:291-5.

120. Zurrida S, Bartoli C, Galimberti V, et al. Which therapy for unexpected phyllode tumour of the breast? *Eur J Cancer.* 1992;28:654-7.

121. Teo JY, Cheong CS, Wong CY. Low local recurrence rates in young Asian patients with phyllodes tumours: less is more. *ANZ J Surg.* 2012;82:325–328.

122. Park HL, Kwon SH, Chang SY, et al. Long-term follow-up result of benign phyllodes tumor of the breast diagnosed and excised by ultrasound-guided vacuum-assisted breast biopsy. *J Breast Cancer.* 2012;15:224–229.

123. Borhani-Khomani K, Talman ML, Kroman N, et al. Risk of Local Recurrence of Benign and Borderline Phyllodes Tumors: A Danish Population-Based Retrospective Study. *Ann Surg Oncol.* 2016;23:1543–15438.

124. Kim S, Kim JY, Kim do H, et al. Analysis of phyllodes tumor recurrence according to the histologic grade. *Breast Cancer Res Treat.* 2013;141:353–363.

125. Reinfuss M, Mitus J, Duda K, et al. The treatment and prognosis of patients with phyllodes tumor of the breast: an analysis of 170 cases. *Cancer.* 1996;77:910–916.

126. Tan EY, Tan PH, Yong WS, et al. Recurrent phyllodes tumours of the breast: pathological features and clinical implications. *ANZ J Surg.* 2006;76:476–480.

127. Barth RJ Jr, Wells WA, Mitchell SE, et al. A prospective, multi-institutional study of adjuvant radiotherapy after resection of malignant phyllodes tumors. *Ann Surg Oncol.* 2009;16:2288–2294.

128. Morales-Vasquez F, Gonzalez-Angulo AM, Broglio K, et al. Adjuvant chemotherapy with doxorubicin and dacarbazine has no effect in recurrence-free survival of malignant phyllodes tumors of the breast. *Breast J.* 2007;13:551–556.

129. Macdonald OK, Lee CM, Tward JD, et al. Malignant phyllodes tumor of the female breast: association of primary therapy with cause-specific survival from the Surveillance, Epidemiology, and End Results (SEER) program. *Cancer.* 2006;107:2127–2133.

8

Ductal Hyperplasia, Atypical Ductal Hyperplasia, and Ductal Carcinoma In Situ

SYED A. HODA

DUCTAL HYPERPLASIA AND ATYPICAL DUCTAL HYPERPLASIA

The distinction between ductal hyperplasia (DH), atypical ductal hyperplasia (ADH), and ductal carcinoma in situ (DCIS) is important for the appropriate management of patients, because these lesions are "associated with an increased risk, albeit of different magnitudes, for the development of invasive carcinoma" (1,2). In most instances, ductal epithelial proliferations are readily classified by pathologists on the basis of generally accepted histopathological features as either hyperplasia or DCIS (3). There exists a subset of lesions for which assignment to either of these categories is less certain. These "borderline" lesions may be diagnosed as either ADH or DCIS (synonym: intraductal carcinoma) or even DH by different pathologists depending on the criteria employed. Studies of interobserver differences in the interpretation of highly selected examples of these lesions with "blurry boundaries" (4) have focused attention on this troublesome diagnostic problem that applies to a relatively small percentage of proliferative epithelial lesions (5–7).

Clinical Features

There are no clinical features specifically associated with DH. The alterations caused by epithelial proliferation in individual ducts or in groups of ducts are almost always microscopic in dimension. DH of various degrees is a common constituent of "fibrocystic changes." The latter may be either detected on imaging studies or can form a palpable mass. The lesion complex can include fibrosis, pseudoangiomatous stromal hyperplasia (PASH), duct ectasia, sclerosing adenosis, cystic papillary apocrine hyperplasia, and lobular hyperplasia.

An important corollary to the lack of clinical indicators of DH is the inability to determine the duration of these lesions. The date on which DH was first diagnosed is customarily used as if it were the date of "onset." This practice, which is a consequence of inability to determine the preclinical duration of hyperplastic ductal lesions, could be a source of bias in assessing the precancerous significance of proliferative lesions.

Imaging

The mammographic manifestations of DH, usually in the context of fibrocystic changes, include altered density, parenchymal distortion, nonpalpable mass formation, and calcifications. The latter are the most frequent, specific mammographic indication of DH, ADH, and DCIS in the absence of a palpable abnormality (8–10). Lesions described on mammography as radial scars (that is, radial sclerosing lesions) often have a component of DH. Some, but not all, radial scars contain calcifications. Before the widespread use of mammography, DH was found in about 25% of biopsies performed for a palpable abnormality (11,12). No more than 5% of these biopsies showed ADH. The frequency of these atypical abnormalities is higher (approximately 15%) among mammographically directed biopsies including excisional biopsies and needle core biopsies (NCBs) (13–17). The yield of ADH in MRI-directed vacuum-assisted NCB ranged from 3% to 8% in several studies (18–20).

DH can be found in adult women at any age. In younger patients (age: <30 years), most examples of DH occur either as juvenile papillomatosis (21) or as one of the group of lesions referred to as papillary DH in teenage girls and young women (22). The majority of women with DH are between 35 and 60 years of age. After age 60, DH becomes relatively infrequent, and when present it is relatively less florid than in younger women. Occasionally, an older woman (age: >60 years) may have extensive proliferative changes with florid DH. Use of exogenous estrogens can be documented in some, but not all, of these cases.

Pathology of Ductal Hyperplasia

DH describes a proliferative epithelial process that is manifested histologically by an increase in the number of epithelial cells within ducts. Because the normal resting ductal epithelium consists of a continuous monolayer of cuboidal-to-columnar epithelial cells supported by a layer of myoepithelial cells, an increase in the cellularity of this two-layer composition constitutes hyperplasia. The increased thickness of the epithelial layer may result in partial or complete obstruction of ductal lumen.

If DH is traced in serial sections, it is often possible to observe its discontinuous and multifocal nature. Various distortions of the basic ductal architecture occur when hyperplastic ducts become more serpiginous or are incorporated into complex proliferative lesions, such as papillomas or radial sclerosing lesions. DH can extend into smaller ductules and may involve the terminal duct–lobular unit (TDLU).

The histologic criteria for DH are the same for NCB and excisional biopsies. However, more often than not, disconnected and fragmented portions of the lesional tissue appear in NCB. This lesional disintegration disrupts the helpful topographical information provided by the larger intact samples of an excisional biopsy. This circumstance can lead to overinterpretation of individual isolated ductal proliferative processes in NCB or failure to recognize the presence of a significant abnormality.

Usual Ductal Hyperplasia

When individual cell borders are inconspicuous, the epithelial proliferation in DH (also referred to as *usual ductal hyperplasia*) often has a syncytial appearance. Intracytoplasmic vacuolization may occur. True cytoplasmic microlumina that contain secretions positive for mucicarmine or alcian blue–PAS (periodic acid–Schiff) stains are extremely uncommon in hyperplastic ductal epithelia (23). The presence of intracytoplasmic, mucin-containing microlumina is an atypical feature that should result in careful consideration of the diagnosis of DCIS or of pagetoid lobular carcinoma in situ (LCIS). In DH, nuclear spacing is uneven so that in some foci the cells are crowded and nuclei overlap. Depending upon the plane of section, nuclei in DH are either round, ovoid, elliptical, or kidney-shaped. Nucleoli are typically inconspicuous—unless there is apocrine metaplasia. Mitotic figures are infrequent.

DH has been subdivided on the basis of qualitative and quantitative criteria, into the categories of mild, moderate, and florid (or marked). The application of this classification is limited by the fact that disordered epithelial growth with varied structural patterns is a characteristic feature of DH.

As a consequence, hyperplastic epithelium is not uniformly distributed in a stratified fashion that permits ready determination of the number of cell layers. Also, epithelial thickness is difficult to appraise in tangentially sectioned glands. Furthermore, the criteria for making these distinctions based on number of epithelial layers are difficult to apply to ductules and TDLUs. In these structures, the lumen is minuscule, and it can be filled even when there is a minimal increase in epithelial layers. Degrees of hyperplasia based on epithelial layers are meaningful only when applied to selected nontangential sections of glandular structures of sufficient dimension to manifest diagnostic features. Thus, the classification of DH based on epithelial thickness alone has significant limitations.

Mild hyperplasia may affect the entire epithelium circumferentially in a ductal cross section or only a segment of the duct. It occurs as an increase in the amount of epithelium, which rarely exceeds three cell layers in thickness. The epithelium may assume a papillary configuration (**Fig. 8.1**).

In *moderate hyperplasia,* the epithelium tends to be more than three cell layers in thickness. The epithelial proliferation is more pronounced relative to that in mild hyperplasia, and secondary glandular lumina may form (**Fig. 8.2**). Parts of the ductal lumen may persist as crescentic spaces at the perimeter of the duct or as intraductal cribriform spaces (**Fig. 8.3**). Micropapillary hyperplasia is part of the spectrum of mild and moderate DH (**Fig. 8.4**). The papillae appear as slender, irregular fronds of hyperplastic epithelium in which the apical cells are smaller and have more condensed nuclei relative to those in the underlying epithelia.

The nuclei in moderate hyperplasia are often irregularly spaced, frequently overlap, and may be distributed in a streaming manner (**Fig. 8.5**). Streaming refers to a growth pattern in which the nuclei of hyperplastic epithelial cells are oriented parallel to the long axes of the cells (**Fig. 8.6**). Because the cytoplasmic borders of these cells are often indistinct, streaming is usually detected as a parallel orientation of oval or spindle-shaped nuclei (that is, resembling a "school of fish"). Streaming occurs in most structural patterns of DH

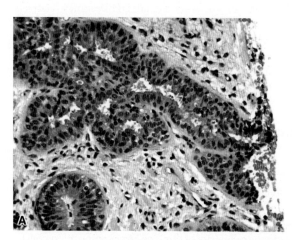
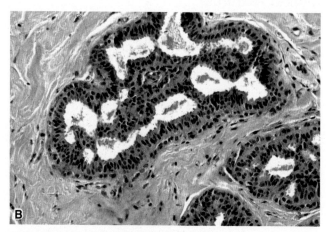

FIGURE 8.1 Ductal Hyperplasia, Mild. A: The ducts in this needle core biopsy specimen are lined by epithelium that is one or two cells in thickness. **B:** Minimal papillary hyperplasia is shown in another needle core biopsy specimen. Hyperplasia of myoepithelial cells is also evident.

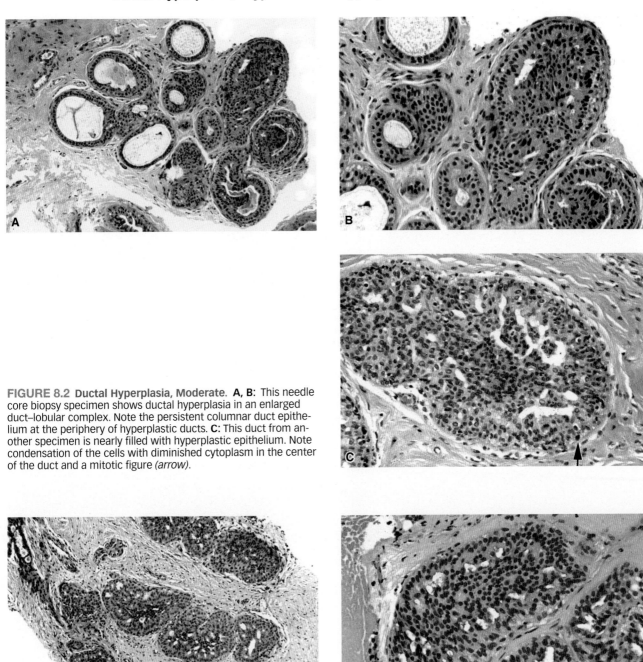

FIGURE 8.2 Ductal Hyperplasia, Moderate. A, B: This needle core biopsy specimen shows ductal hyperplasia in an enlarged duct–lobular complex. Note the persistent columnar duct epithelium at the periphery of hyperplastic ducts. **C:** This duct from another specimen is nearly filled with hyperplastic epithelium. Note condensation of the cells with diminished cytoplasm in the center of the duct and a mitotic figure *(arrow)*.

FIGURE 8.3 Ductal Hyperplasia, Moderate. A, B: Hyperplastic epithelium fills the ducts in this needle core biopsy specimen forming a cribriform pattern. Cells in the center of the duct have small, condensed nuclei and scant cytoplasm. Columnar epithelium is present at the periphery of the affected duct **(B)**.

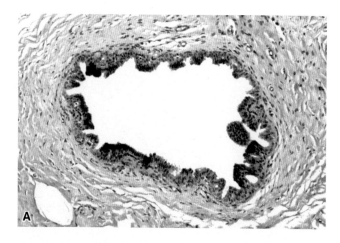

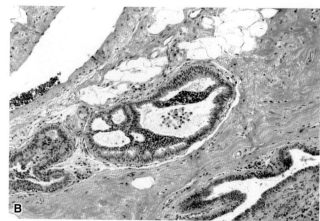

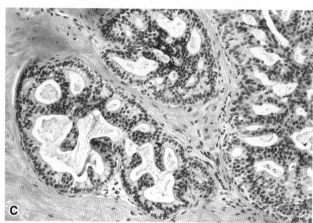

FIGURE 8.4 Ductal Hyperplasia, Micropapillary. A: The micropapillary epithelium consists of columnar cells with dark, condensed nuclei and scant cytoplasm. **B:** Well-preserved columnar ductal epithelium is present at the periphery of this duct, with a more complex mildly atypical micropapillary proliferation in the lumen. **C:** Mixed moderately atypical micropapillary and cribriform hyperplasia.

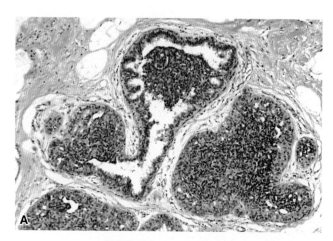

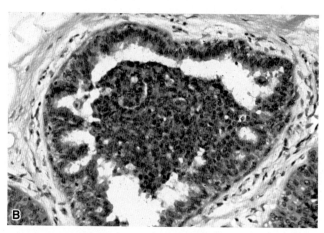

FIGURE 8.5 Ductal Hyperplasia, Florid. A, B: In this needle core biopsy specimen, the dense, overlapping cellular proliferation has solid and papillary patterns. Columnar cell and micropapillary hyperplasia are shown in **(B)** at the periphery of the duct. **C, D:** Solid and cribriform florid hyperplasia is seen in these lesions. The epithelium in the duct in **(D)** has a streaming pattern. Note the loss of cytoplasm and nuclear condensation in cells in the centers of the ducts. **E:** Cribriform florid hyperplasia, involving multiple duct profiles, is seen in this biopsy. **F:** The cribriform florid hyperplasia in this biopsy involves an intraductal papilloma.

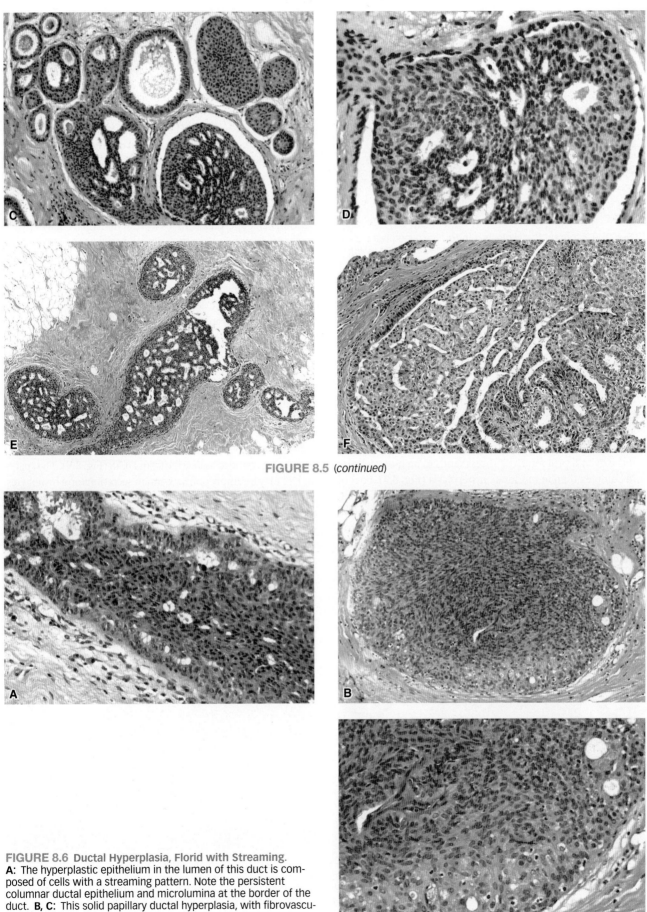

FIGURE 8.5 (*continued*)

FIGURE 8.6 Ductal Hyperplasia, Florid with Streaming.
A: The hyperplastic epithelium in the lumen of this duct is composed of cells with a streaming pattern. Note the persistent columnar ductal epithelium and microlumina at the border of the duct. **B, C:** This solid papillary ductal hyperplasia, with fibrovascular stroma, is composed of spindle cells with a streaming pattern. Microlumina are present at the perimeter of the duct.

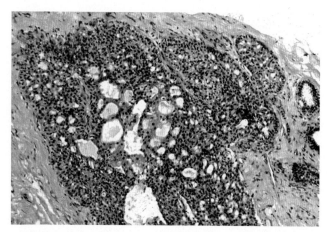

FIGURE 8.7 Ductal Hyperplasia, Florid. The hyperplastic duct in this needle core biopsy specimen is enlarged and filled by epithelium with solid and cribriform areas. Apocrine metaplasia is present in the center of the duct.

and ADH. The association of the streaming pattern with DH has been confirmed by computerized morphometric analysis of the orientation of nuclei in proliferative ductal lesions (24).

The distinction between moderate and *florid hyperplasia* is not sharp, but lesions are generally placed in the latter category when the affected ducts are appreciably expanded and filled with proliferative epithelium in comparison with nonhyperplastic counterparts. Florid hyperplasia has the papillary and bridging growth patterns that are encountered in moderate hyperplasia, but the overall proliferative process tends to be more cellular and complex than in moderate hyperplasia (**Fig. 8.7**). Foci of florid hyperplasia are more likely to fill the entire ductal lumen in a solid or cribriform (fenestrated) manner.

Necrotic cellular debris is rarely present in hyperplastic ducts. Necrosis may be present in association with florid papillary hyperplasia (**Fig. 8.8**), sclerosing papillary lesions, subareolar sclerosing DH, and florid papillomatosis of the nipple. In these lesions, the hyperplastic ducts with necrosis

are cytologically and architecturally indistinguishable from adjacent ducts with hyperplastic epithelium without necrosis. Histiocytes ("foam" cells) are relatively common in the lumina of hyperplastic ducts. Degenerating histiocytes should not be mistaken for necrotic debris.

The cribriform (fenestrated) growth pattern that occurs in moderate and florid DH results from the formation of epithelial bridges that are joined as they traverse the ductal lumen. The cribriform spaces represent portions of original ductal lumen that have been subdivided by the complex arborizing epithelial proliferation. Using a serial section, three-dimensional reconstruction method, Ohuchi et al. (25) demonstrated that the lumina that appear separate in a two-dimensional histologic section of a hyperplastic focus were actually part of a network of channels representing the original ductal lumen surrounded by hyperplastic epithelium. By contrast, three-dimensional reconstruction of DCIS revealed that the fenestrations in these lesions were newly formed disconnected spaces bounded by polarized neoplastic cells.

The spaces that are found in histologic sections of cribriform DH have distinctive features. The secondary lumina tend to be larger and more numerous at the periphery of the duct than centrally, but the reverse distribution may be encountered. Cells outlining these spaces are distributed in a haphazard fashion except at the edge of the duct, where residual columnar or cuboidal epithelium composed of cells with more regularly oriented nuclei may persist. The spaces in a given hyperplastic duct usually have varied shapes (ovoid, crescentic, irregular, or serpiginous) rather than being rounded as in cribriform DCIS (**Fig. 8.9**). The spaces in DH may be empty or may contain secretions and histiocytes. Fine calcifications can develop in the glandular lumina of DH.

A layer of myoepithelial cells may be evident at the edge of a hyperplastic duct on H&E sections (**Fig. 8.10**). These cells may accompany the proliferative process into the ductal lumen when the fibrovascular stromal framework of papillary hyperplasia is present. Immunostains readily highlight the myoepithelium in DH, ADH, and DCIS. Experience has led

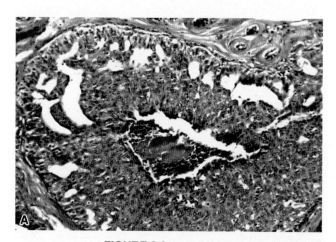

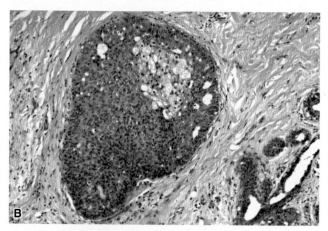

FIGURE 8.8 Ductal Hyperplasia, Florid with Necrosis and Histiocytes. A: Necrosis is present in the center of this hyperplastic duct that was part of sclerosing papillary duct hyperplasia. Columnar epithelium can be seen at the periphery of the duct, where there are microlumina of various sizes and shapes. **B:** The epithelial proliferation in this enlarged duct is solid with peripheral fenestrations. Histiocytes are present in the duct.

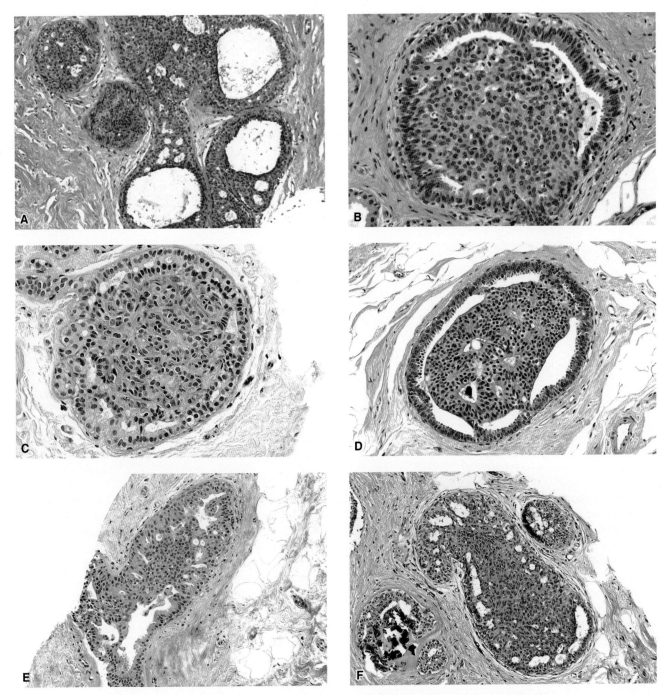

FIGURE 8.9 Ductal Hyperplasia, Florid. A–F: Microlumina are present at the periphery of multiple ducts in six different needle core biopsies. Polypoid florid duct hyperplasia in **(B–D)** is anchored focally to the persisting columnar cell epithelium at the perimeter of the duct.

to the conclusion that the reactivity of individual markers is unpredictable in a given case and that it is advantageous to employ at least three myoepithelial markers.

p63 and p40 are the only immunostains currently available that are localized in the nuclei of myoepithelial cells (26,27). Neither marker is reactive with myofibroblasts or blood vessels. Nuclear staining with p63 and p40 produces a "string of dots" between the epithelium and the basement membrane in benign ducts and lobules. Rarely, p63 and p40 may be positive in scattered epithelial cell nuclei in papillary lesions, and less

often in DH. These epithelial cells can be distinguished from myoepithelial cells by the cytologic appearance and position thereof.

Several cytoplasmic markers are available for highlighting the myoepithelium including smooth muscle actin (SMA), smooth muscle myosin-heavy chain (SMM-HC), calponin, CD10, and maspin. These markers exhibit variable degrees and extent of cross-reactivity with myofibroblasts and blood vessels (27–30). Because of the variable reactivity of these reagents with myoepithelial cells, it is prudent to employ two

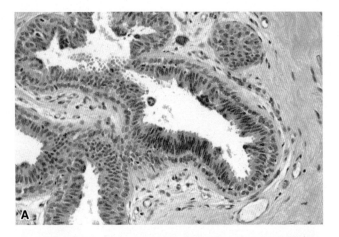

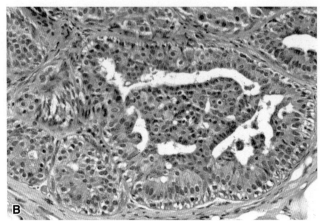

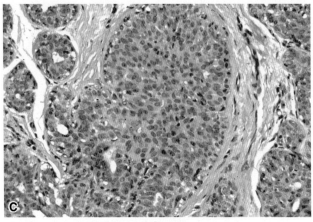

FIGURE 8.10 Ductal Hyperplasia with Myoepithelial Cells.
Three different samples with progressively more florid epithelial
hyperplasia and diminishing myoepithelial cell hyperplasia.
A: Columnar cell hyperplasia with prominent myoepithelium.
B: Papillary hyperplasia with persisting myoepithelium. **C:** Solid
hyperplasia with inconspicuous myoepithelium.

or more cytoplasmic markers as well as either p63 or p40 for
the evaluation of myoepithelium in each case.

The myoepithelium is usually uniformly present in ducts with
proliferative fibrocystic changes, such as adenosis and various
degrees of DH. Attenuation of myoepithelial cells that occurs in
some forms of epithelial hyperplasia, especially sclerosing papillary lesions and ADH, results in increased space between p63
or p40 reactive nuclei relative to the staining pattern observed
in inactive glands. In this situation, myoepithelial integrity can
usually be demonstrated with one of the immunostains that show
cytoplasmic reactivity. Because stromal proliferation accompanies
many of these proliferative lesions, care must be taken not to
mistake myofibroblastic reactivity for myoepithelial positivity.
The demonstration of a myoepithelial cell layer is not helpful
in distinguishing DH and DCIS because myoepithelial cells are
present to varying degrees at the perimeter of some examples
of DCIS. An intraductal proliferative lesion that is devoid of
myoepithelium (within the duct and its perimeter) is almost
certainly DCIS—with the exception of some densely sclerosing
papillary proliferations and certain types of apocrine lesions (31).

The cells of DH show variable positivity, often in a "mosaic
pattern," for high-molecular-weight cytokeratins (HMW-CK:
e.g., CK 5/6 and CK-K903) and variable reactivity for ER. In
contrast, the epithelial cells that comprise ADH (and DCIS) are
negative for HMW-CK and are typically diffusely positive for
ER **(Fig. 8.11)**. Notably, some high-grade DCIS can be positive for HMW-CK (and also for p63 and p40). It must also be

remembered that *columnar cell lesions* (CCLs, including FEA)
and apocrine metaplastic cells are generally negative for HMW-
CK (32,33). A commercially available immunohistochemical
cocktail (ADH5, Biocare, Concord, CA) that combines low-
molecular-weight CK (CK7/CK18, using Fast Red chromogen),
HMW-CK (CK5/CK14 utilizing brown DAB chromogen),
and p63 (also using DAB) is of potential use in distinguishing
DH from ADH. ADH is negative for CK5/14 and positive for
CK7/18 (34). ADH5 can also identify myoepithelial cells with
cytoplasmic CK5/14 and nuclear p63 reactivities.

Collagenous Spherulosis

Collagenous spherulosis is a special form of DH wherein
myoepithelial cells contribute to the formation of nodular
subepithelial deposits of basement membrane material similar
to those found in adenoid cystic carcinoma **(Fig. 8.12)**. The
center of the spherule can undergo degeneration and resemble a
glandular lumen. Immunostains can demonstrate myoepithelial
cells around these spherules and distinguish these structures
from true glandular lumina in cribriform spaces that form in
DH and cribriform type of DCIS.

Atypical Ductal Hyperplasia

There is broad agreement on the general definition of ADH
as a proliferative epithelial lesion that fulfills some but not

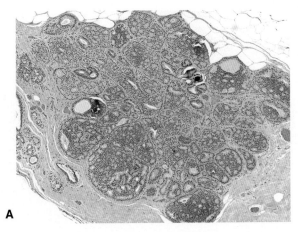

A

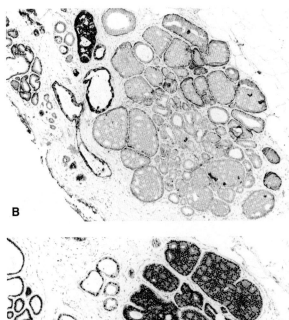

B

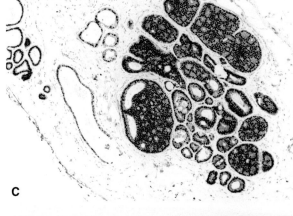

C

FIGURE 8.11 Limited Value of Cytokeratin (CK)5/6 and Estrogen Receptor (ER) in Differential Diagnosis of Atypical Ductal Hyperplasia (ADH) versus Low-Grade Ductal Carcinoma In Situ (DCIS). **A:** DCIS of cribriform type is shown, in which ADH was a consideration in the differential diagnosis. Note relatively expanded ducts, uniform cribriform spaces, and monotonous epithelial cells. **B:** CK5/6 shows absence of staining in lesional cells. This staining result does not help in distinguishing ADH from DCIS. Both processes are typically negative for CK5/6. Usual ductal hyperplasia shows a "mosaic" pattern of staining with CK5/6. **C:** ER shows strong uniform staining in DCIS cells. This staining pattern also does not help in distinguishing ADH from DCIS as both processes can be strongly positive for ER. However, strong uniform staining supports the interpretation of DCIS because usual ductal hyperplasia typically displays patchy, weak-to-moderate staining for ER. This case exemplifies the importance of morphologic features, and limitations of immunohistochemistry, in establishing the diagnosis in such borderline (ADH vs. DCIS) cases.

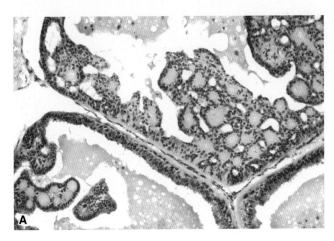

A

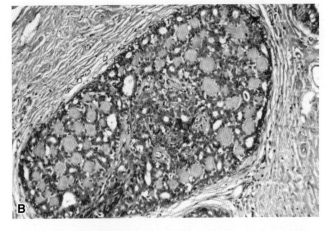

B

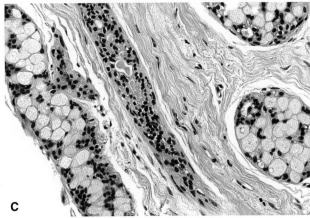

C

FIGURE 8.12 Ductal Hyperplasia with Collagenous Spherulosis that Mimics Cribriform Architecture. Three patterns of hyperplasia with collagenous spherulosis. **A:** Papillary growth with prominent eosinophilic spherules. **B:** Solid papillary hyperplasia with prominent spherules. **C–H:** Cribriform hyperplasia where microspherules are present amid the microlumina in these cases. The collagenous spherules are well-formed in **(A–E).** Degenerative changes are present in the collagenous spherules (in **F** and **G**). Detail of the degenerative change in **(G)** is shown in **(H).**

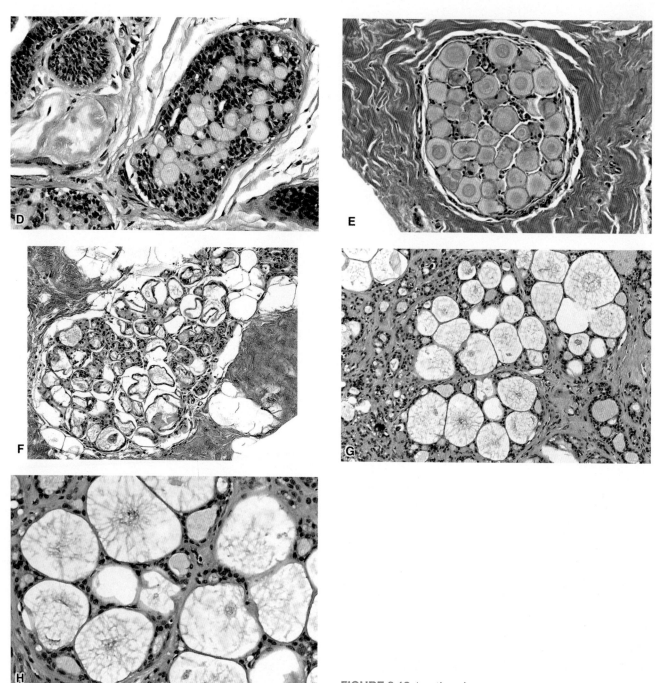

FIGURE 8.12 (continued)

all criteria for the diagnosis of DCIS. The most recent WHO classification defines ADH as "proliferation of monomorphic, evenly placed epithelial cells involving TDLUs" (2). This definition could also easily be applied to low-grade DCIS. The difficulty in arriving at a more crisp definition of ADH lies in the specifics of the atypical hyperplastic process. In general, these specifics can be considered under two headings: quantitative and qualitative. The former refers to the amount and extent of the proliferative abnormality while the latter is concerned with architectural and cytologic details.

Quantitative criteria for distinguishing between DH and DCIS based on the number of duct cross sections that exhibit the abnormality or the dimension of the affected area have been proposed. Some investigators have classified proliferative lesions

limited to a single duct as ADH, even if the abnormality is qualitatively consistent with DCIS (12). On the basis of a criterion requiring at least two fully involved duct cross sections for a diagnosis of DCIS, cases are arbitrarily assigned to the category of ADH when only one qualitatively diagnostic duct is present.

Another scheme emphasizes the histologic extent of a lesion as the basis for the diagnosis of ADH (35). According to this criterion, foci spanning <2 mm are diagnosed as ADH, regardless of the number of duct cross sections, even if the individual ducts qualify as DCIS. The 2-mm criterion was selected because ". . .it was at the level of one or more small ducts or ductules measuring around 2 mm in aggregate cross-sectional diameter that most pathologists felt hesitant in diagnosing a lesion as intraductal carcinoma" (36). Another explanation offered by the proponents of this criterion was that "questions about quantity are raised generally when dispersed lesions add up to from 1.6 to 2.7 mm in aggregate size. Therefore, we arbitrarily chose 2 mm as a cutoff point" (35).

As yet, no scientific study has compared the clinical significance of different quantitative criteria for diagnosing ADH. There is no *a priori* reason for choosing two duct cross sections or 2 mm as the critical "tipping points" in relation to risk stratification. For example, no data exist for the risk to develop subsequent carcinoma in patients whose biopsies contained epithelial proliferative lesions qualitatively consistent with DCIS limited to one, two, or three duct cross sections, respectively. Regarding the dimensions of these lesions, no analysis comparing foci measuring 1.5 mm, 2.0 mm, 2.5 mm, or larger has been reported.

A number of technical issues hinder the application of quantitative criteria, especially in the diagnosis of findings in NCB. What appear to be two contiguous cross sections may prove in serial sections to be part of a single duct, or deeper sections of what appears to be a single duct lesion may uncover additional involved cross sections of the duct. How close must two duct cross sections be to be considered contiguous? Is the stroma between duct cross sections included in the measurement? Quantitative criteria assume that the ducts in question have been sectioned perpendicular to their long axis. How to assess ducts cut longitudinally has not been adequately addressed. If the longitudinal dimension of a duct in a section exceeds 2 mm but the transverse diameter is 1 mm, should this focus be considered DCIS when employing the 2-mm criterion?

Others have also rejected utilizing quantitative factors in the diagnosis of ADH. This position was elaborated by Fisher et al. (37) who stated that "our definition of ADH consists of a ductal epithelial alteration approximating but not unequivocally satisfying the criteria for a diagnosis of DCIS. It does not include arbitrarily established quantities of unequivocal DCIS (less than 2.0 mm or 2 'spaces')." In their study of the prognostic significance of proliferative breast "disease," Bodian et al. (11) reported that "during the course of many years, intraductal carcinoma has been diagnosed if the characteristic features are present in only one ductal space."

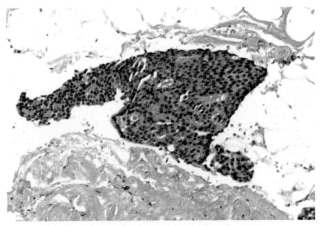

FIGURE 8.13 Atypical Ductal Hyperplasia. This needle core biopsy specimen included a detached fragment of nearly solid proliferative duct epithelium.

The role of quantitative factors in the diagnosis of proliferative ductal lesions seems to lie between these extremes. The use of rigid criteria such as two ductal cross sections or 2 mm can be justified in a research setting to ensure a homogeneous study group or to assess a particular criterion, but the strict application of these arbitrary rules in a clinical setting is difficult for the technical reasons stated earlier and is poorly substantiated by existing data. Given the limitations of current methods for diagnosing ductal lesions, quantitative factors sometimes play a role in the assessment of a particular lesion in material obtained in a NCB. This situation arises when the biopsy specimen contains detached fragments of cytologically atypical epithelium **(Fig. 8.13)**, or when only part of one duct with changes suggestive of DCIS is represented **(Figs. 8.14–8.17)**. The same issue arises when a process that suggests lobular extension of DCIS is present **(Fig. 8.18)**.

In many instances, the diagnosis of ADH depends upon the presence of structural elements of DCIS mingling with hyperplasia. Architecturally, this may be manifested by a cribriform pattern partially involving a duct **(Figs. 8.19 and 8.20)**.

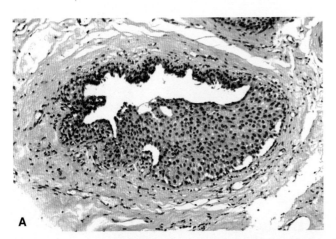

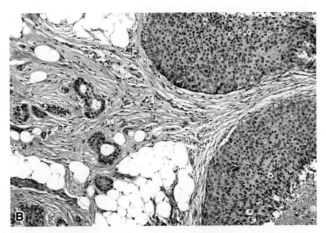

FIGURE 8.14 Atypical Ductal Hyperplasia. A: The needle core biopsy specimen from this patient contained this duct that is partly occupied by a solid epithelial proliferation of monomorphic cells. Myoepithelial cells are apparent around the upper perimeter of the duct. This partially involved duct is insufficient evidence for a diagnosis of DCIS in a needle core biopsy specimen. **B:** The excisional biopsy specimen revealed intraductal and infiltrating duct carcinoma. The area of DCIS shown here has a denser and cytologically more atypical cellular population with necrosis than does the duct in **(A)**.

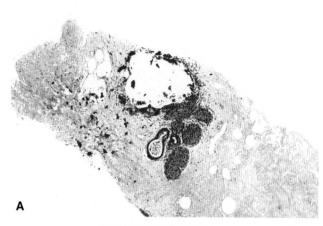

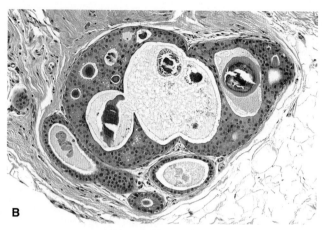

FIGURE 8.15 Atypical Ductal Hyperplasia. **A:** This needle core biopsy specimen of mammographically detected calcifications shows solid atypical duct hyperplasia with calcification. A large intraductal calcification was fractured in preparing the slide causing blue-stained fragments to be deposited on the adjacent breast stroma. **B:** Cribriform atypical duct hyperplasia with concentrically laminated (psammoma body–like) calcifications. The hyperplastic epithelial cells display apocrine cytoplasmic traits. Note the orderly distribution of nuclei at the perimeter of the duct.

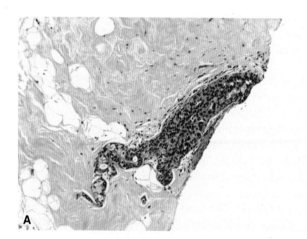

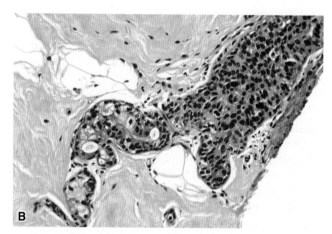

FIGURE 8.16 Atypical Ductal Hyperplasia. **A, B:** The duct at the edge of this specimen was the only significant abnormality in this needle core biopsy specimen. Note the overlapping, hyperchromatic, pleomorphic nuclei, and transition to clear cell apocrine change in the narrowest part of the duct. Excisional biopsy yielded a 3-mm focus of atypical duct hyperplasia similar to this duct.

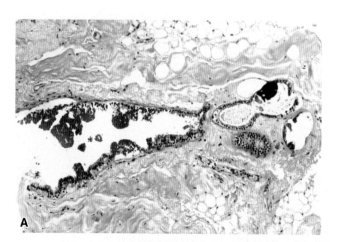

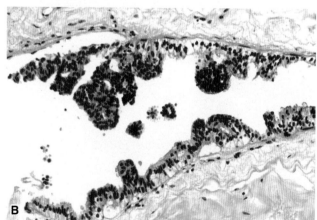

FIGURE 8.17 Atypical Ductal Hyperplasia, Micropapillary. **A, B:** Mammographically detected calcifications led to this needle core biopsy specimen. The micropapillae are composed of cells with small, overlapping, hyperchromatic nuclei. **C, D:** Two other examples of atypical micropapillary hyperplasia with condensation of nuclei in the micropapillae.

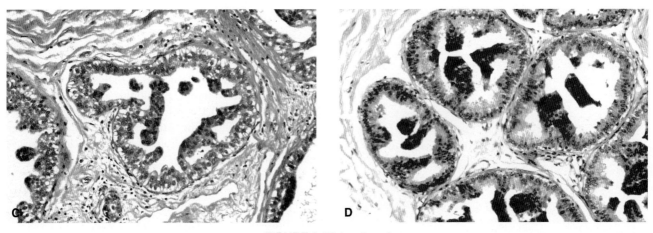

FIGURE 8.17 (*continued*)

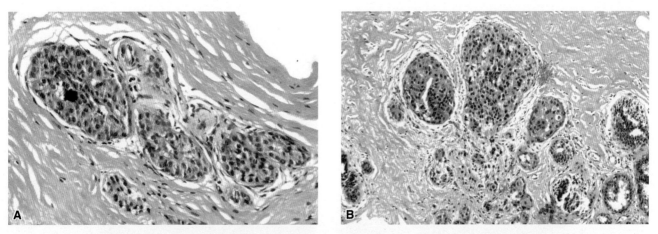

FIGURE 8.18 **Atypical Ductal Hyperplasia, Lobular Extension.** Shown are two foci of intra-lobular proliferation that raise concern about lobular extension of DCIS. **A:** A thin layer of persistent glandular epithelium outlines a narrow, slit-shaped lumen next to a calcification in the largest lobular gland. Solid DCIS was found in the excisional biopsy specimen. **B:** An irregular proliferation of cells with apocrine differentiation fills three lobular glands in this needle core biopsy specimen. Excisional biopsy revealed foci of atypical apocrine ductal hyperplasia.

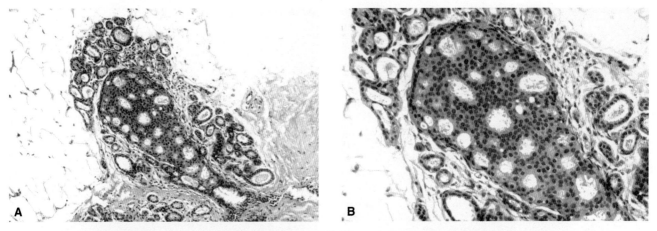

FIGURE 8.19 **Atypical Ductal Hyperplasia, Cribriform. A, B:** The only proliferative abnormality in the needle core biopsy specimen in this case was one focus of cribriform proliferation in an intralobular duct shown in two views from the specimen. Part of the duct in **(A)** is not involved by the hyperplasia **(lower right)**, and it does not extend into lobular glands. Sclerosing adenosis with calcifications was found in the excisional biopsy specimen. **C:** Atypical cribriform hyperplasia with calcifications in another case.

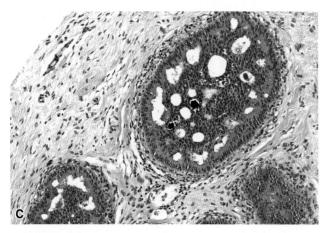

FIGURE 8.19 (continued)

These foci feature sharply defined round-to-ovoid spaces outlined by cells with distinct borders and a rigid arrangement. Rarely, ADH can have a solid growth pattern. Cribriform, micropapillary, and true papillary foci involving hyperplastic ducts constitute other architectural manifestations of ADH (**Fig. 8.21**). ADH can be encountered in ducts exhibiting apocrine metaplasia (**Figs. 8.21 and 8.22**). Cytologic atypia may involve individual cells, groups of cells, or the entire population of a proliferative epithelial lesion. Atypical features include nuclear enlargement with an increased nuclear-to-cytoplasmic ratio, nuclear hyperchromasia, an irregular chromatin pattern, mitoses, and the presence of enlarged, pleomorphic nucleoli (**Fig. 8.23**).

The most challenging atypical ductal proliferations, sometimes referred to as "borderline" lesions, feature marked cytologic and architectural atypia. Most of these foci retain a

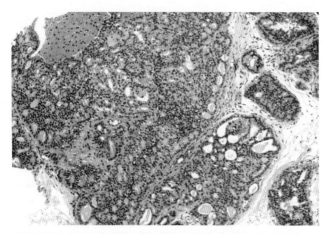

FIGURE 8.20 **Atypical Ductal Hyperplasia, Cribriform.** The florid atypical hyperplasia in this needle core biopsy specimen from a solid papillary lesion has areas of cribriform microlumen formation.

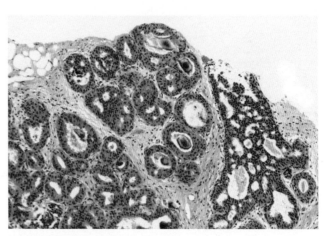

FIGURE 8.22 **Atypical Columnar Cell Ductal Hyperplasia.** This needle core biopsy procedure was performed for mammographically detected clustered calcifications. The atypical ductal hyperplasia with a columnar cell–cribriform pattern and hyperplastic epithelium in lobular glands shows apocrine differentiation. There are calcifications in some lobular glands.

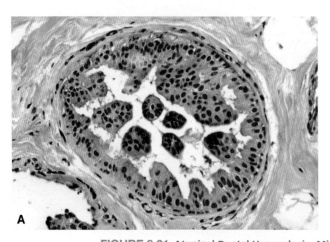

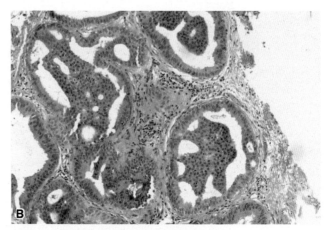

FIGURE 8.21 **Atypical Ductal Hyperplasia, Micropapillary, and Cribriform. A:** Crowded, multilayered cells in atypical columnar cell duct hyperplasia. Crowding and hyperchromasia of shrunken nuclei at the tips of some micropapillae is apparent in this duct. The cells have apocrine cytoplasm, and there is a ring of evenly spaced ductal cell nuclei at the periphery of the duct. **B:** A monomorphic population of cells forms bridges across these ducts, creating irregularly shaped microlumina. Epithelium at the perimeter of each duct consists of cuboidal or low columnar cells with evenly spaced, basally oriented nuclei.

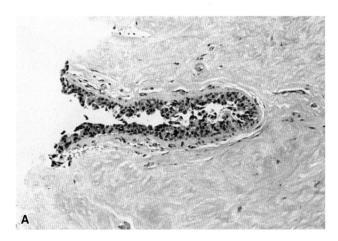

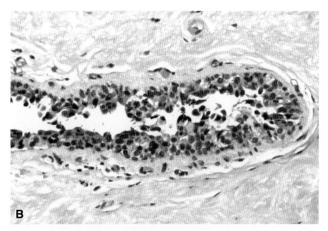

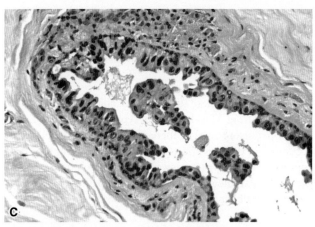

FIGURE 8.23 Atypical Ductal Hyperplasia with Severe Cytologic Atypia. A, B: The only proliferative abnormality in this needle core biopsy specimen was this duct at the edge of one tissue sample. The epithelial layer is thickened and composed of cells distributed in a disordered pattern. Many nuclei are hyperchromatic, especially at the luminal border, and there is some nuclear overlap. The proliferation has micropapillary traits. **C:** The subsequent excisional biopsy revealed micropapillary DCIS with marked nuclear pleomorphism. Periductal reactive changes and vascularity are more pronounced than around the duct in **(B)**, and there is a fully developed micropapillary structure. Note the persistent myoepithelium at the perimeter of the DCIS.

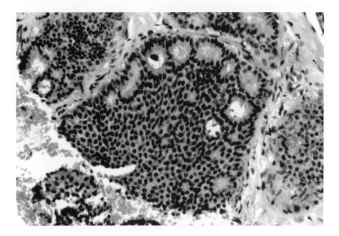

FIGURE 8.24 Atypical Ductal Hyperplasia, Borderline. The ducts in this needle core biopsy specimen have a solid central population of small, monomorphic cells. Microlumina outlined by cells oriented around the rounded fenestrations are present at the periphery of some ducts.

minor characteristic of hyperplasia, such as epithelial overlapping, with a structure that is otherwise typical of DCIS **(Figs. 8.23–8.25)**. These slight variations will be disregarded by observers who classify the lesions as DCIS, whereas others may diagnose ADH. Similarly, those who place credence in quantitative criteria will diagnose ADH because the extent of a lesion is not sufficient, while others, not adhering to these rules, will diagnose DCIS.

Insufficient emphasis has been placed on diagnosing specific proliferative lesions in the context of the overall spectrum of histologic changes in NCB. In a research setting, a pathologist can be required to make a diagnosis that is based only on one focus or selected foci on a single slide. This situation, duplicated to a large extent in assessing NCB, is different from the circumstances

under which the various diagnostic criteria were originally developed by the review of multiple histologic sections (12,35,37).

When faced with an atypical ductal proliferative lesion in a NCB, slides from previous biopsy samples diagnosed as ADH or DCIS should be reviewed whenever possible. A focus of concern in a NCB may be found to be substantially more atypical than the previously diagnosed ADH, or it may be as atypical, or it may be less so. The first situation would tend to support a diagnosis of DCIS, whereas the second would suggest ADH, and third should prompt re-evaluation of the diagnosis of ADH.

Obtaining H&E-stained serial sections, levels, or deepers from the corresponding tissue block can be useful in most, if not all, of the cases. Immunohistochemical evaluation, with either various cytokeratins or hormonal receptors, is seldom helpful

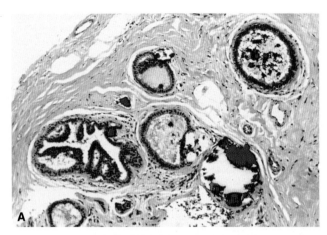
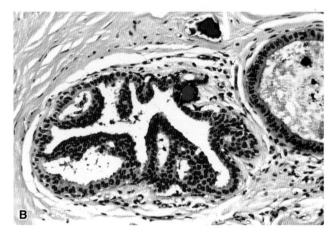

FIGURE 8.25 Atypical Ductal Hyperplasia, Borderline. A, B: The needle core biopsy that yielded the specimen containing this lesion was performed for clustered microcalcifications. Calcifications are present in microcysts and the stroma. The proliferation has a micropapillary structure and is composed of cells with condensed, hyperchromatic nuclei. The nonpapillary peripheral epithelium consists of regular cuboidal cells that are indistinguishable from cells lining the adjacent nonproliferative cysts. The micropapillary abnormality was limited to this site.

in this regard—as these stains may be able to separate usual hyperplasia from ADH but cannot separate ADH from DCIS.

It must also be remembered that the "highest level of accuracy" of diagnosis in NCB is achieved "using the triple approach, combining imaging and clinical examination assessment with pathological results" and that pathologic findings "should not be reported in isolation" (38).

Columnar Cell Lesions

CCLs, often considered to be part of the spectrum of DH, have come under enhanced scrutiny as a result of being increasingly detected on mammography and sampled via NCB. Lubelsky et al. (39) reported that 21% of NCB obtained for calcifications in mammographically screened women had CCLs. These abnormalities have been referred by terms such as *columnar cell change* (CCC) *or columnar cell hyperplasia* (CCH) (40,41) and *flat epithelial atypia* (FEA) (42). Other more cumbersome names that have been offered include *atypical cystic lobules* (43), *cancerization of*

lobules and ADH adjacent to DCIS (44), and *columnar alteration with prominent apical snouts and secretions* (CAPSS) (45).

The fundamental lesion, *CCC,* is localized in a TDLU that becomes enlarged as a result of cystic dilatation due to accumulation of distinctly eosinophilic secretions. The simplest form of this process features a thin, flat epithelial layer composed of cuboidal-to-tall columnar cells distributed in a relatively uniform pattern. Because the nuclei tend to be relatively large, the cells appear crowded and dark. The apical cell surface usually has an apocrine-type cytoplasmic protrusion ("snout"), and in some cases this is an unusually prominent feature. In the plainest form of CCL, the epithelium is one to two cells deep, and there is minimal nuclear pleomorphism **(Fig. 8.26)**. Nucleoli are uncommon, and mitotic figures are rare. When present, calcification is in the form of amorphous granular material or discrete basophilic deposits **(Fig. 8.27)**. Notably, the lesional cells in CCC (typically tall with apical snouts) can resemble those of tubular carcinoma. The cytologic features of CCLs can suggest apocrine differentiation. The cells often express

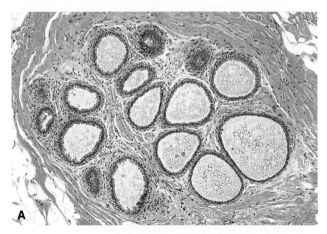
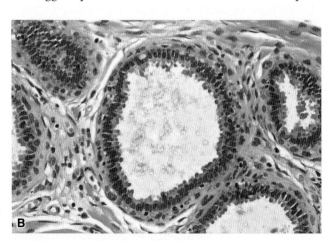

FIGURE 8.26 Columnar Cell Change. A: Cystic dilatation of lobular ductules lined by cuboidal and columnar cells with closely approximated, basally oriented nuclei and luminal cytoplasmic tufts ("snouts"). The dilated structures are embedded in loose, vascularized intralobular stroma. **B:** A magnified view showing the crowded epithelial cells, myoepithelium, and stroma. **C:** Microcystic columnar cell change with luminal cytoplasmic tufts and calcifications.

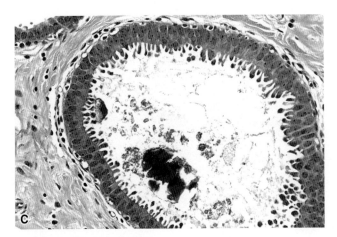

FIGURE 8.26 *(continued)*

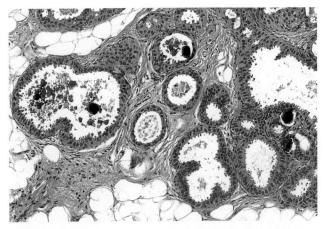

FIGURE 8.27 Columnar Cell Change with Calcifications. Granular and punctate basophilic calcifications are shown.

GCDFP-15 (BRST-2), an apocrine marker. The proliferation rate is low, even in hyperplastic foci (46). The epithelium in CCL is almost always ER-positive, whereas apocrine change is typically ER-negative (46).

CCH is a multifocal process that may also be bilateral. CCH is most often encountered in women aged 35 to 50 years, but it can also be present after menopause. CCH rarely produces a palpable abnormality, and it is usually detected on mammogram because calcifications are frequently formed. CCH is present when the epithelium is more than two cells thick. This is most readily apparent when cellular crowding becomes

pronounced, and nuclei are not distributed in a single plane relative to the basement membrane. This tendency toward "stacking" of nuclei is usually accompanied by nuclear hyperchromasia, and diminutive epithelial mounds may be formed in the cellular regions **(Fig. 8.28)**.

More complex columnar cell-proliferative foci comprise lesions described as *atypical columnar cell hyperplasia* (ACCH). Mild ACCH is usually manifested by the presence of minute and often isolated foci of micropapillary growth in a background of otherwise usual CCH **(Fig. 8.29)**. The presence of more elaborate growth patterns as well as cytologic atypia characterize

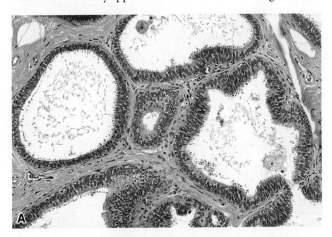

FIGURE 8.28 Columnar Cell Hyperplasia. A, B: The thickened epithelium is composed of crowded, columnar cells with overlapping nuclei.

FIGURE 8.29 Columnar Cell Hyperplasia, Mild Atypia. A, B: Small mounds are formed in the epithelium and there is mild cytological atypia. **C:** Focal blunt micropapillary proliferation of the hyperplastic columnar cell epithelium. Histiocytes are present in some lumina.

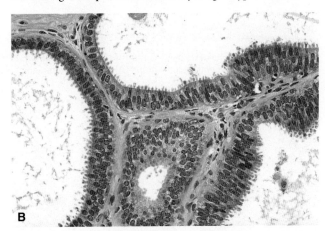

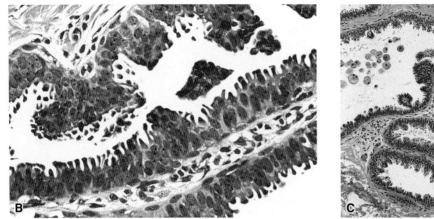

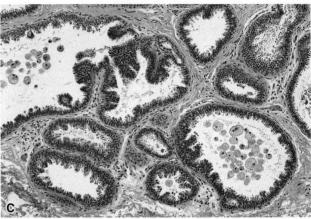

FIGURE 8.29 (*continued*)

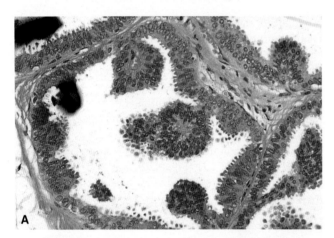

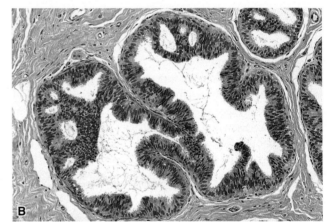

FIGURE 8.30 Columnar Cell Hyperplasia, Moderate Atypia. Atypical micropapillary hyperplasia with calcifications **(A)**, and without calcifications **(B)**.

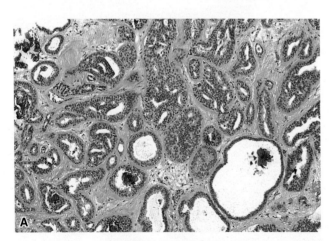

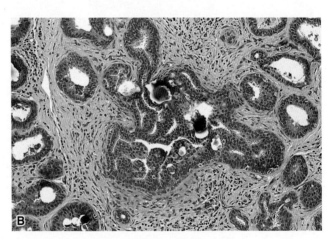

FIGURE 8.31 Columnar Cell Hyperplasia, Moderate Atypia. A: Cribriform epithelium in ducts surrounded by glands with columnar cell hyperplasia and calcifications. **B:** Papillary hyperplasia in a duct with punctate calcifications.

CCH with moderate-to-marked atypia that in its most severe form approaches the appearance of DCIS (**Figs. 8.30 and 8.31**). In most instances of ACCH, the cytologic atypia is more pronounced than the architectural abnormality (**Fig. 8.32**). When carcinoma arises in the setting of CCH, the growth pattern is usually one of the characteristic forms of DCIS (**Figs. 8.33 and 8.34**). Flat micropapillary (so-called "clinging") DCIS with minimal epithelial complexity is rarely encountered in this setting (**Fig. 8.35**). ALH and LCIS frequently accompanies CCL, and tubular carcinoma may also be present (**Fig. 8.36**).

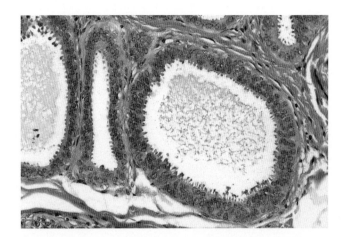

FIGURE 8.32 Columnar Cell Hyperplasia with Cytologic Atypia. The epithelial cells display cytologic atypia. There are no structural abnormalities and no mitoses.

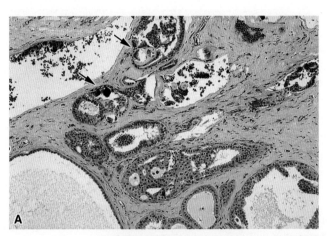
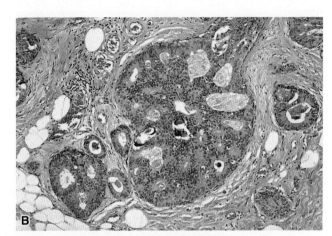

FIGURE 8.33 Ductal Carcinoma In Situ and Atypical Columnar Cell Hyperplasia, and Columnar Cell Change with Ossifying-Type Calcifications. This needle core biopsy specimen was obtained from a focus of nonpalpable mammographically detected calcifications. **A:** Basophilic and ossifying-type calcifications *(arrows)* are associated with atypical hyperplasia (hematoxylin–phloxine–safranin). **B:** Cribriform DCIS with calcifications was present in the subsequent excisional biopsy specimen.

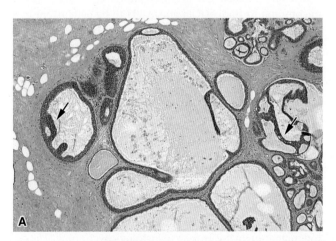
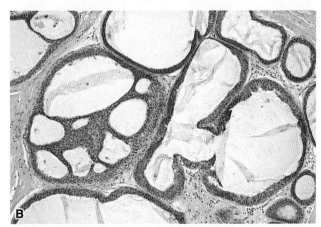

FIGURE 8.34. Ductal Carcinoma In Situ Following Atypical Columnar Cell Duct Hyperplasia. **A:** An excisional biopsy revealed multifocal, predominantly cystic columnar cell hyperplasia with focal atypia, shown here with micropapillary architecture *(arrows)*. **B, C:** Four years later, repeat biopsy of the same breast performed for calcifications revealed columnar cell hyperplasia with severe atypia **(B)** and a focus of cribriform DCIS **(C)**.

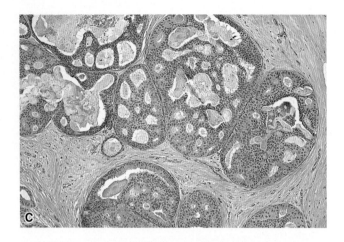

FIGURE 8.34 *(continued)*

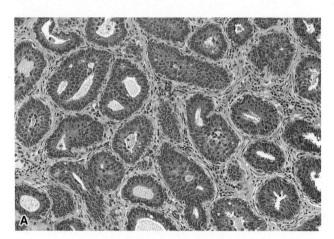

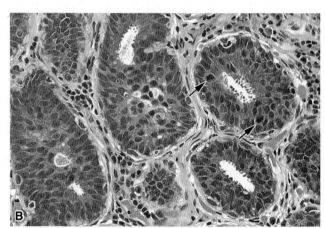

FIGURE 8.35 **Ductal Carcinoma In Situ (DCIS) Associated with Columnar Cell Duct Hyperplasia.** **A, B:** Flat and cribriform DCIS with mitoses *(arrows)*.

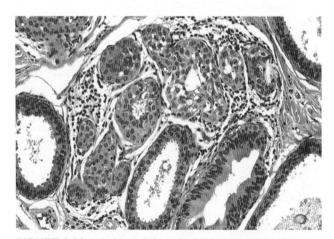

FIGURE 8.36 **Lobular Carcinoma In Situ (LCIS) Associated with Columnar Cell Change.** LCIS is surrounded by cystic columnar cell change.

CCLs are part of a triad that includes LCIS and tubular carcinoma ("The Rosen triad") (47).

The term FEA has been used as a synonym for the lesion described as ACCH (please see foregoing section). The term "flat" implies simple (that is, noncomplex) architecture—mainly represented by epithelium of a single layer or few layers at worst (hence the term "flat"). By contrast, the term ADH should be restricted to lesions that show *complex* architecture. It is not uncommon to find ACCH and ADH to be concurrent in a biopsy, and can be occasionally seen to merge. Whether or not ACCH and ADH are biologically equivalent is uncertain at this time. Nevertheless, the rate of upgrade of FEA found on NCB to either DCIS or invasive carcinoma on subsequent excision has been reported to be 3.2% in two series (48,49), 9.5% (50), 9.6% (51), 15% (52), 19% (53), and 33% (54). This wide range in the frequency of upgrade rate is most likely attributable to variations in the diagnostic threshold of "atypia" in CCLs.

CCLs develop *calcifications* that are formed in multiple glands in many of the proliferative sites. Two types of calcifications are encountered: crystalline and ossifying. The crystalline type, usually associated with lesions with less atypia, is deeply basophilic, opaque, round, or angular and is prone to fragmentation in the process of histologic sectioning. The ossifying type of calcification usually has a rounded, well-defined contour and an internal structure that resembles an ossifying nodule in which basophilic granular calcific deposits are embedded in lacunar-like spaces within an eosinophilic matrix **(Fig. 8.37)**. Ossifying type calcifications occur throughout the range of CCLs, and they appear to develop in the proliferative epithelium, whereas basophilic crystalline deposits are

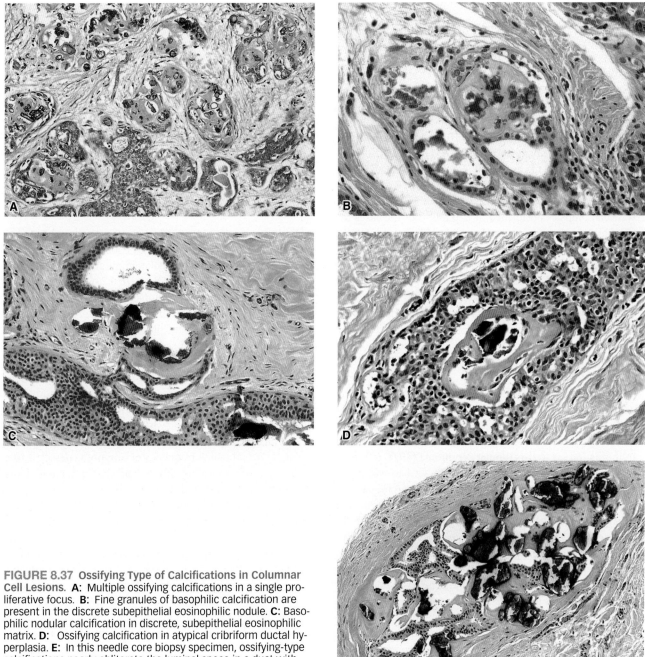

FIGURE 8.37 Ossifying Type of Calcifications in Columnar Cell Lesions. A: Multiple ossifying calcifications in a single proliferative focus. **B:** Fine granules of basophilic calcification are present in the discrete subepithelial eosinophilic nodule. **C:** Basophilic nodular calcification in discrete, subepithelial eosinophilic matrix. **D:** Ossifying calcification in atypical cribriform ductal hyperplasia. **E:** In this needle core biopsy specimen, ossifying-type calcifications nearly obliterate the luminal space in a duct with columnar cell change.

predominantly intraluminal. Both types of calcification can be found in one specimen, and they may occur together in a single proliferative focus.

The proliferative activity of CCLs has been evaluated by Ki-67 reactivity (55). The Ki-67 index was significantly lower in CCC (mean 0.1%) and CCH without atypia (mean 0.76%) than in normal TDLU (mean 2.4%). The Ki-67 indices of CCH with flat atypia (mean 8.2%) and low-grade DCIS (8.9%) were not significantly different. The highest Ki-67 index was found in intermediate to high-grade DCIS (mean 25.5%). If confirmed in a substantially larger series of cases, the Ki-67 index could be a helpful adjunctive tool for distinguishing CCH with atypia from some forms of low-grade DCIS that arise in CCLs.

Dabbs et al. (56) studied molecular changes in selected microdissected CCLs and found "a gradient of progressive mutational change" between CCC and invasive carcinoma arising in a background of CCLs. Mutational changes manifested as loss of heterozygosity (LOH) at selected loci were absent from CCC and only rarely found in CCH. Increasing LOH was detected across the spectrum of ACCH, DCIS, and invasive carcinoma. These results parallel those obtained in noncolumnar cell-proliferative lesions (57) and appear to support the concept that ADH may, in situations yet to be defined, be a precursor to DCIS and invasive ductal carcinoma.

Although there is cumulative evidence to support the position that follow-up with imaging is a "reasonable" option for nonatypical CCLs diagnosed on NCB (58), and that patients with a diagnosis of ACCH on NCB should undergo excision of the lesional area (59), the management of CCLs found in NCB obtained for mammographically detected calcifications remains contentious (60). In this regard, two issues need to be considered. The first concern is the likelihood that the NCB is not fully representative of abnormalities that are present. Guerra-Wallace et al. (61) evaluated patients who underwent excisional biopsy after a CCL was found in a NCB specimen. They reported finding carcinoma in 10 of 135 (7.4%) women with CCH without atypia and in 11 of 60 (18.3%) with coexisting ADH. Chivukula et al. (62), who referred to ACCH as "flat epithelial atypia" (FEA), reported that FEA was detected in 301 of 8,054 (3.7%) of NCB obtained in a 2-year period. Excisional biopsies performed in 270 (90%) of the cases revealed invasive carcinoma in 18 patients (7%) and DCIS in 23 (8.5%) patients. Piubello et al. (63) reported that 2 of 10 (20%) excisional biopsies from patients with FEA and ADH in a NCB obtained for calcifications yielded DCIS and that invasive carcinoma was found in one-third (10%) of the patients. In this study, no carcinoma was detected in excisional biopsies from 20 women who had FEA without ADH in a prior NCB. DCIS was found in 1 of 51 (2%) of excisional biopsies performed after a NCB diagnosis of CCH or FEA without ADH reported by Senetta et al. (64).

DCIS associated with CCH and ACCH tend to have low-grade nuclei, micropapillary, and cribriform architecture, and to lack necrosis (65). ACCH is significantly related to ALH and LCIS (40,65), and it has been associated with invasive lobular carcinoma (66) as well as tubular carcinoma (40,66,67).

The second issue is the long-term risk for CCL to evolve into carcinoma. The role of CCL as precursors to carcinoma was reviewed by Turashvili et al. (68), who concluded that "the natural history of CCLs is currently uncertain in any given patient." In a long-term follow-up study of a large series of patients with CCL, Boulos et al. (69) reported a slight, statistically significant increased relative risk (RR) for developing breast carcinoma (1.47) when compared with controls with neither proliferative fibrocystic changes nor CCLs. In this study, the RR was not significantly affected by the presence or absence of ACCH.

With respect to immediate clinical management, the foregoing data support a recommendation to perform an excisional biopsy in a patient found to have ACCH in a NCB. An excisional biopsy would also be prudent if a NCB reveals LCIS or ALH coexisting with CCL without ADH. Clinical circumstances such as the extent and character of mammographically detected calcifications, the presence of a palpable lesion, or a family history of breast carcinoma may also play a role in deciding whether an excisional biopsy should follow the diagnosis of CCL without ADH on NCB.

The long-term significance of CCLs with or without ADH for the later development of DCIS or invasive carcinoma remains to be determined. Unfortunately, most studies of the cancer risk attributable to ADH discussed later in this chapter did not distinguish between ADH with and without CCLs. Hence, it is not certain that the elevated cancer risk associated with ADH generally applies equally to CCLs with and without atypical hyperplasia. If the results presented by Boulos et al. (69) are

confirmed by other investigators, CCLs may prove to be in a relatively low-risk category.

Presently, clinical follow-up with no other intervention is appropriate for the patient whose only abnormality is a nonatypical CCL diagnosed by a NCB and confirmed by an excisional biopsy or if a nonatypical CCL is found in a NCB and there are no indications to perform an excisional biopsy. If the NCB and/or excisional biopsy show ADH or LCIS in conjunction with a CCL, treatment with selective estrogen receptor modulators (SERMs) may be considered as part of the management.

Diagnosis of ADH by Needle Core Biopsy

ADH has been diagnosed in <10% of patients subjected to NCB (9,10,70–73). In four studies consisting of 323 to 900 patients who underwent NCB of mammographically detected lesions, the frequencies of ADH were 6.7%, 4.7%, 4.5%, and 4.3% (74–77). Follow-up excisional biopsies were performed on most women with ADH in these reports. Among women who underwent an excisional biopsy, the reported frequencies of DCIS in the excisional specimen were 27%, 12.5%, 33%, and 36%, respectively. Invasive carcinoma was found in 14%, 12.5%, 0%, and 11% of patients, respectively. In these reports, approximately 25% of excisional biopsies revealed additional foci of ADH. The yield of significant lesions in the excisional biopsy specimen may be somewhat lower after a NCB diagnosis of ADH if the entire radiologically detected lesion was removed by NCB (78). The high frequency of carcinoma detected after a diagnosis of ADH in a NCB dictates that excisional biopsy should be performed in this setting (10,79).

The reported frequency of ADH in vacuum-assisted MRI-directed NCB ranges from 3% to 8% (18–20). Among patients with ADH detected in vacuum-assisted NCB who undergo excisional biopsy, the yield of carcinoma has averaged 34% (20). The higher yield of subsequent carcinoma, sometimes termed *underestimation of ADH*, found in MRI-detected lesions than in mammographically directed biopsies probably reflects the tendency to employ MRI predominantly in women at higher risk for carcinoma. Almost all of the carcinomas found after detecting ADH by MRI-directed NCB have been DCIS.

Because of the limited and often-fragmented nature of NCB, added consideration is given to quantitative issues in assessing these specimens. Pathologists should avoid overinterpretation of findings in NCB because of the expectation that more lesional tissue remains at the biopsy site. In the evaluation of NCB of breast lesions, especially those that are only evident by mammography, it must be anticipated that the material seen in NCB may be the most extreme and potentially the only abnormality present. ADH may be diagnosed if detached fragments of abnormal epithelium suggest carcinoma, or if only part of a duct with features of carcinoma is contained in the sample. The importance of quantitative issues and adequate sampling was documented by Jackman et al. (9) who "progressively increased the average number of NCB samples obtained per lesion and have found a decrease in both the number of ADH lesions and the discordance of ADH lesion." The greater success in diagnosis was attributable to more lesions being diagnosed as DCIS rather than as ADH as a result of more complete sampling (9). Wagoner et al. (79) reported that the following features of ADH in NCB were predictive of finding DCIS in the subsequent excision: micropapillary ADH, more than two foci of ADH, ADH in multiple samples, and residual mammographic calcifications.

ADH and Breast Carcinoma Risk

The major clinical concern related to usual form of DH and ADH is the risk for the subsequent development of carcinoma. In a minority of women with biopsy findings classified as nonproliferative or proliferative, carcinoma subsequently develops in either breast. The overall proportion of women in whom carcinoma later develops rarely exceeds 10%, even with follow-up of two decades or more. Bodian et al. (11) detected subsequent breast carcinoma in 139 of 1,521 patients (9.1%) with biopsy-proven proliferative changes, and in 18 of 278 (6.5%) with nonproliferative biopsies within a follow-up period of 21 years. Overall, 8.7% of the patients developed breast carcinoma. In other reports involving at least 1,000 patients, the proportions of women in whom carcinoma developed were 2.2% (80), 4.1% (81), and 4.9% (82). The proportion of patients with subsequent carcinoma tends to increase with the length of follow-up, being highest after follow-up of more than a decade (81,82). This observation is consistent with the rising risk for developing breast carcinoma with advancing age.

The risk for the development of carcinoma subsequent to unilateral biopsy-proven proliferative changes affects both breasts. The bilaterality of risk was noted by Davis et al. (83) in a review of 297 patients with "cystic disease." These authors also tabulated data from 11 articles with at least 100 patients, to show that carcinoma subsequently developed in 0.7% to 4.9% of patients, with 50% of the carcinomas in the contralateral breast.

Krieger and Hiatt (82) found that only 56% of subsequent carcinomas occurred in the previously sampled breast with benign proliferative changes (82). Laterality of subsequent carcinoma was not significantly influenced by the type of antecedent proliferative change or the age at biopsy. The mean interval to subsequent ipsilateral carcinomas (11.2 years) was less than that for contralateral carcinomas (14 years). Page et al. (84) reported that 8/18 (44%) carcinomas subsequent to ADH occurred in the contralateral breast. Involvement of the contralateral breast in a similar proportion of patients was also described by Connolly et al. (85).

The chances for the development of breast carcinoma are influenced by factors that can modify the level of risk associated with benign proliferative changes. Age at diagnosis is inversely related to subsequent risk. Carter et al. (86) found that the rate of subsequent breast carcinoma, when compared with that of normal women, was increased 3.7-fold in women with ADH who were 46 to 55 years of age and 2.3-fold in women older than 55 years. London et al. (87) also observed an inverse relationship of age and risk, in which the RR increased 2.6-fold among premenopausal women who had biopsy-proven atypia in comparison with postmenopausal subjects.

A history of breast carcinoma among first-degree female relatives is a particularly strong additive factor in women who have ADH. Page et al. (84) and Dupont and Page (88) found that the risk associated with ADH in women with a positive family history was more than double that of women without this factor. London et al. (87) also reported that the increased risk associated with family history was strongest in patients with ADH. The RR was not increased by a positive family history in women with nonproliferative biopsies.

Among women who have had a benign result on breast biopsy, the risk for developing subsequent carcinoma is related to the histologic components of the antecedent biopsy. When assessed independently, sclerosing adenosis has been associated with an increased risk in several studies (80,88,89). Some of these investigators reported a greater increase in risk for relatively small groups of women who had ADH coexisting with sclerosing adenosis (88,90).

The proportion of patients who develop carcinoma is highest in the group of women with ADH, intermediate in those with proliferative ductal changes without atypia, and least when there are no proliferative changes. Proliferative changes were identified in 152 (85%) of 1,799 biopsies studied by Bodian et al. (11). Moderate-to-severe atypia was present in 70 specimens, representing 3.8% of all cases and 4.6% of specimens with proliferative changes. Follow-up revealed that the RR for the development of carcinoma (in comparison with the general population, represented by the Connecticut Tumor Registry) was higher in women with any proliferative changes (RR of 2.2) than in those with nonproliferative findings on biopsy (RR of 1.6). The RR associated with severe ductal atypia was 3.9. Page et al. (84) found the RR to be 4.7 for women with ADH in comparison with women who had nonproliferative biopsy results. The RR for women with ADH and a family history of breast carcinoma was increased further in comparison with women with nonproliferative biopsies and a positive family history (84). Ma and Boyd (89) undertook a meta-analysis of studies that investigated the association between ADH and breast cancer risk. Fifteen reports between 1960 and 1992 fulfilled the authors' requirements for inclusion in the study, resulting in a total sample size of 182,980 women. The overall odds ratio in comparison with controls for the development of carcinoma in women with ADH was 3.67 (95% CI: 3.16–4.26).

Needle Core Biopsy of ADH and the Need for Subsequent Excision

ADH, rarely encountered in the premammographic period, was reportedly present in about 4% of benign biopsies in that era. This lesion has become relatively more common in the current mammographic era and is diagnosed in 10% to 20% of benign biopsies (84,91). Until recently, the need for an excisional biopsy following the diagnosis of ADH was unquestioned. Such automatic triggering of excision was based on the reportedly high rate of "upgrade"—ranging from 11.5% to 62% (15,92–94). The term "upgrade" implies the finding of a more significant lesion, DCIS or invasive carcinoma, in the subsequent excision, and has varied somewhat with the radiologic method used to guide NCBs. For instance, ADH diagnosed on sonographically guided NCB shows higher underestimation rate, which was as high as 56% in one series (95). Notably, no significant difference has been reported in upgrade rate of stereotactic vacuum-assisted NCB using 11-gauge (11.9%) versus 8-gauge (14.3%) needles (93).

When the number of foci of involvement by ADH on NCB (based on a mean of about 12 cores per case) was correlated with excisional biopsy results by Ely et al. (96), all cases of ADH in two or less than two foci had no worse lesion on excision, whereas ADH present in four or more than four foci was found to be statistically predictive of a worse lesion on excision.

It should be realized that some, if not all, "upgraded" lesions either represent cases of ADH associated with DCIS that were minimally sampled, or represent cases of DCIS that were underdiagnosed. Hence, removal of the entire "target" could leave no residual lesional tissue.

Recent reports have indicated that correlation of the histologic findings in a NCB with pre- and postprocedure mammograms could spare excision in at least some patients. Studies by de Mascarel et al. (97) and Villa et al. (15) showed that patients without residual calcification after a diagnosis of ADH on a vacuum-assisted breast biopsy could possibly be managed with mammographic follow-up alone. McGhan et al. (92) reported that patients <50 years of age with focal atypia only and no residual calcifications post biopsy may represent a low-risk group who could potentially avoid excisional biopsy. Nguyen et al. (16) concluded that ADH without "significant cytologic atypia and/or necrosis," regardless of extent, and with >95% removal of the targeted calcifications, is associated with a minimal risk (<3%) of carcinoma and may undergo mammographic follow-up only.

Nomograms devised to calculate the likelihood of upgrade for ADH may facilitate decision-making in selected cases. A nomogram developed by Khoury et al. (98) includes age, menopausal status, hormonal receptor status, personal history of breast carcinoma, number of involved cores, solid growth pattern, extent of largest focus, and presentation (mass vs. calcification.

At the present time, the need for excisional biopsy following the diagnosis of ADH on NCB should be determined on an individualized basis after clinical and radiologic correlation is performed. This process may also help in determining the extent of excision.

Chemoprevention of ADH

ER is strongly expressed in more than 90% of breast carcinomas that develop in women with ADH (99). This finding provides a rationale for the use of SERMs and aromatase inhibitors (AIs) to prevent breast carcinoma in women with ADH. Results of several large breast chemoprevention trials, as well as subgroup analyses, have shown RR reductions ranging from 41% to 79% (100) The use of a chemopreventive agent should be considered in at least a proportion of women with ADH and who are otherwise considered to be at a higher risk. However, such chemoprevention is "infrequently prescribed and infrequently used" at the present time (100).

DUCTAL CARCINOMA IN SITU

Frequency of DCIS

The incidence of DCIS in the United States increased from around 5/100,000 women in the 1970s to more than 30/100,000 women in recent years (101). Currently, approximately 25% of breast carcinomas are DCIS, and more than 60,000 American women will be diagnosed to have DCIS in 2016 (out of 246,660 cases of breast carcinoma) (102). DCIS is uncommon in women younger than 30 years of age, and the risk of DCIS increases with age. The rate of DCIS increases with age from 0.6/1,000 screening examinations in women aged 40 to 49 years to 1.3/1,000 screening examinations in women aged 70 to 84 years (103). Risk of development of metastases and/or death in a patient diagnosed with pure DCIS is rare (<1%) (104). The beneficial effects of mammography as a diagnostic or screening modality and of improved systemic therapy are reflected in these trends (105).

Imaging

Currently, DCIS is most commonly detected on screening mammography. Mammography is a sensitive diagnostic procedure for detecting DCIS. Among nonpalpable carcinomas detected by mammography, approximately 25% were DCIS (106–108). Mammographically detected calcifications are found in 80% to 85% of DCIS (107,108). Other radiologic findings that lead to the "incidental" detection of a lesser proportion (about 5%) of DCIS are densities and asymmetric soft tissue changes, sometimes with calcifications. Calcifications alone are more likely to be the mammographic indicator of DCIS in women younger than 50 years, whereas coexistent soft tissue abnormalities are evident more often in women older than 50 years—a distinction that probably results from differences in breast density between these age groups rather than from intrinsic differences in the malignancy (108).

Mammographic calcifications associated with DCIS are generally large and pleomorphic, and either linear and cast-like or vermicular and branching (follow the distribution of the disease in the ductal system (109)). Round or oval, well-circumscribed calcifications are less common in DCIS. The majority of DCIS have five or more calcifications (109). The mammographic distribution of calcifications has been used as a guide to assess the extent of DCIS. However, these measurements may underestimate the size of the lesion when compared with careful histologic sampling (110). When the extent of lesions was measured both mammographically and pathologically, discrepancies were found more often between the interpretations for cases that are predominantly cribriform or micropapillary than for high-grade solid DCIS with prominent necrosis (so-called "comedo" type of DCIS). A discrepancy of more than 20 mm was found in 44% of pure cribriform-micropapillary lesions, in 12% of pure "comedo" carcinomas, and in 50% of cases with both patterns (110). The likelihood of detecting multifocal DCIS (that is, multiple foci of DCIS in one quadrant) radiologically and pathologically is related to the size of the lesion as determined by either procedure. Multifocality is appreciably more frequent in lesions larger than 2.0 to 2.5 cm than in smaller foci of DCIS (111).

The mammographic appearance of calcifications bears some relationship to the histologic type of DCIS. In general, mammographic calcifications that are "highly suspicious for malignancy" are associated with high-grade DCIS (112); however, as noted by Stomper and Connolly (113), "there is considerable overlap, and the predominant histological subtype cannot be predicted on the basis of the microcalcification type with a high degree of accuracy." Predominantly linear or "casting-type" calcifications are found significantly more often in "comedo" carcinomas than in cribriform, papillary, or solid types, which typically contain granular calcifications (110,113). Nonetheless, 22% of linear calcifications were associated with non-"comedo" carcinomas, and 47% of granular calcifications occurred in "comedo" DCIS in one series (113). The presence of extensive casting-type calcifications occupying more than one quadrant in a mammogram was associated with high-grade DCIS, multifocal invasive ductal carcinoma, and axillary nodal metastases in 33% of 12 patients who had lymph node examined (114).

Abnormal mammographic findings without calcifications are more likely to call attention to DCIS of the small cell type than of the large cell type, regardless of the growth pattern (solid, cribriform, or mixed) of the lesion (115). Linear calcifications are a marker of necrosis, and small punctate or granular calcifications are associated with DCIS without necrosis (115). DCIS that overexpress HER2 are more likely to have calcifications detected by mammography than are HER2-negative carcinomas (116).

Although DCIS can occur in adult women of any age, the mean age of patients at diagnosis in multiple studies is between 50 and 59 years. The age factor assumes considerable significance in determining screening guidelines. There are no significant differences in the age distribution of structural subtypes of DCIS (117). Extreme "density" of breast on mammography has been reported to be a risk factor for multicentricity (118).

Sonography is of limited value in the detection, or determination of extent, of DCIS. Scoggins et al. (119) reported sonographic visibility of DCIS in 362/691 (52%) of pure DCIS lesions. Lesion visibility was most commonly due to the presence of a "mass" and was unrelated to nuclear grade or necrosis.

MRI is an effective method for detecting DCIS of all grades (120). The technique is relatively more sensitive for the diagnosis of invasive carcinoma, and the rate of false-negatives is higher for DCIS (121). Menell et al. (122) found that MRI was overall more sensitive than mammography for detecting DCIS and for detecting multifocal DCIS. Manion et al. (123) found that the most common types of carcinoma identified by MRI screening were ER-positive invasive carcinomas (mean size: 0.7 cm) and high-grade DCIS. Detection of lesions is based on the finding of contrast enhancement in breast parenchyma after injection of a gadolinium contrast agent when compared with the preinjection image (124–126). Orel et al. (127) described three patterns of enhancement associated with DCIS: ductal, regional, and a peripherally enhancing mass. The mean size of MRI-detected DCIS was 10 mm. Correlation of immunohistochemical studies for vascularity and MRI characteristics of the lesions suggested that tumor angiogenesis contributed to MRI enhancement in one series (124). Contrast-enhanced MRI has proven to be an effective method for the detection of concurrent, unsuspected contralateral carcinoma in women with ipsilateral DCIS (128).

Intraoperative Consultation (Frozen Section) Diagnosis of DCIS

DCIS can be recognized in frozen sections prepared from an excisional biopsy, but if any difficulty is encountered, the decision should be immediately deferred to permanent sections because there is a significant risk of trimming away the lesional area as more sections are made **(Fig. 8.38)**. In one study of DCIS, 50% of the lesions were diagnosed at the time of frozen section examinations, 36% were reported to be benign, 8%

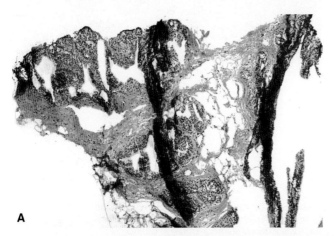
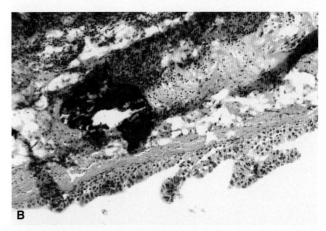

FIGURE 8.38 Ductal Carcinoma In Situ (DCIS), Frozen Section. The patient had a needle core biopsy procedure for nonpalpable calcifications, and the needle core biopsy sample was submitted for frozen section. **A:** The frozen section slide has folds and tears. **B:** A displaced calcification is present near the center, and a band of atypical cells is present at the lower border of the tissue in the frozen section. The diagnosis was deferred. **C:** Solid DCIS with frozen section artifact in a slide from the permanent-embedded tissue after examination by frozen section.

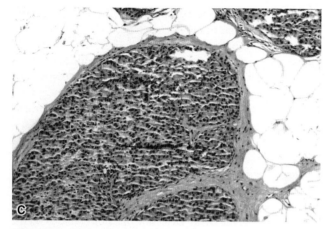

FIGURE 8.38 (continued)

were deferred, 5% were diagnosed as ADH, and one case was diagnosed as invasive carcinoma (129). Approximately 3% of biopsies reported to be benign at frozen section examination prove to contain carcinoma when permanent sections are examined (130). Because the limited amount of tissue can be examined by frozen sections during an intraoperative consultation, approximately 20% of patients with a frozen section diagnosis of DCIS prove to have invasive carcinoma when it is possible to examine multiple permanent sections of the same biopsy specimen (131). Presently, frozen section is not recommended for the diagnosis of NCB or excisional biopsies of mammographically detected, nonpalpable lesions, unless there are exceptional clinical circumstances.

Pathology of DCIS

The anatomic site of origin of many examples of DCIS appears to be in the TDLU. Evidence for this conclusion originally came from the subgross microdissection studies of Wellings et al. (132). Recently characterized CCLs, described earlier in this chapter, lend support to this conclusion with respect to low-grade, micropapillary DCIS but not high-grade DCIS. However, a substantial but undetermined proportion of DCIS lesions arise from primary or segmental ducts or their branches. This is evidenced by DCIS involving major, central lactiferous ducts, sometimes with Paget disease, and multifocal DCIS with papillary architecture. Both sites of origin are compatible with the presence of DCIS involving the epithelium of lobules, which is referred to as "lobular cancerization" **(Fig. 8.39)**. Because greatly enlarged TDLU involved by DCIS are very difficult to distinguish from primary or segmental ducts expanded by DCIS, the relative frequency of origin from TDLU and from larger ductal structures, and the clinical significance of this distinction, remains to be determined.

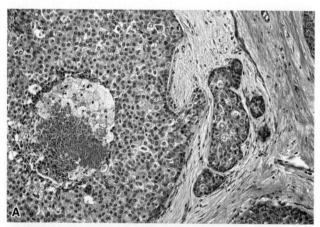

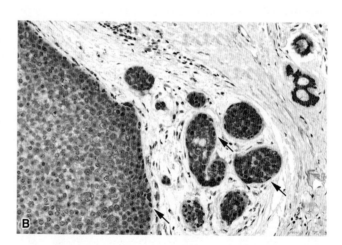

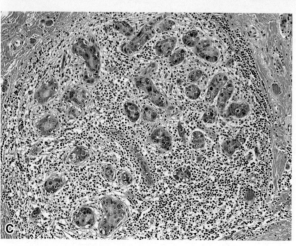

FIGURE 8.39 Ductal Carcinoma In Situ (DCIS), Lobular Extension (Lobular Cancerization). A, B: DCIS with central necrosis extending into a lobule in periductal fibrosis. This pattern can be mistaken for microinvasion. Myoepithelial cells at the perimeter of the lobular glands are highlighted by the p63 (brown nuclear immunostain, *arrows*). Epithelial cells are decorated by cytokeratin (red cytoplasmic immunostain). **C:** In another case, this enlarged lobular complex is involved by DCIS with high-grade nuclei. There is a prominent intralobular lymphocytic infiltrate.

In standard histologic sections, DCIS appears confined within the lumina of ducts and lobules involved in the process. When studied by immunohistochemistry, basement membranes in DCIS are intact or only focally discontinuous and often reduplicated in high-grade DCIS (133). The diagnosis of DCIS alone does not apply to lesions in which invasive foci are also present, even if the later comprise a minimal portion of the lesion.

The presence or absence of mitotic figures is not a definitive feature in the diagnosis of DCIS, because mitoses may also be found in normal lobules and in DH or ADH, albeit infrequently. The finding of numerous mitoses, such as one or more per high-power field strongly suggests DCIS. Myoepithelial cells are variably retained but attenuated and occasionally hyperplastic at the periphery of a duct involved by DCIS **(Fig. 8.40)**. Carcinoma cells at the periphery of the duct exhibit loss of basal polarity as a manifestation of cellular crowding. Rarely, remnants of non-neoplastic normal or hyperplastic duct epithelium persist in ducts involved by DCIS **(Fig. 8.41)**.

A range of cell types are found in DCIS. Certain distinct variants have been identified and described by specific names. *Signet ring cells*, usually associated with lobular carcinoma, also occur in DCIS, most often in the papillary and cribriform types **(Fig. 8.42)**. Signet ring cells have eccentric nuclei that may be often indented by a cytoplasmic mucin vacuole. A minute droplet of secretion may be apparent in the vacuole. Intracytoplasmic mucin sometimes imparts a diffuse pale

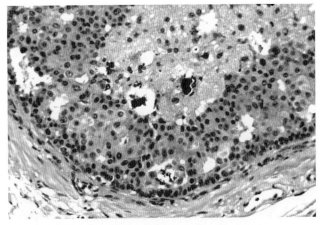

FIGURE 8.41 Ductal Carcinoma In Situ. Microlumina are present at the perimeter of the duct with central necrosis and calcifications.

blue color to the cytoplasm without forming distinct vacuoles **(Fig. 8.43)**. Clear holes in the cytoplasm can be mistaken for signet ring vacuoles. These cytoplasmic defects, sometimes the site of glycogen accumulation, are not reactive with the mucicarmine stain, they do not indent the nucleus, and there is ordinarily no secretion evident in the lumen.

Clear cell DCIS is a poorly defined variant typically encountered with solid and "comedo" patterns. Some clear cell DCIS are composed of cells with an arrangement described as *mosaic*

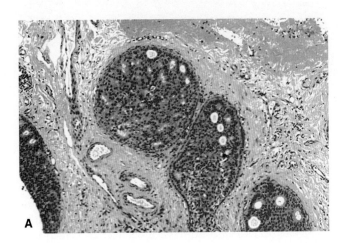

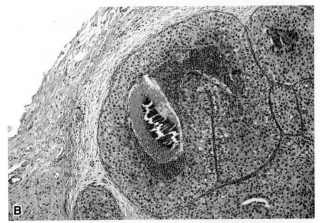

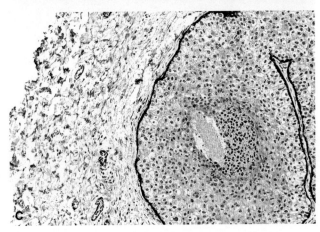

FIGURE 8.40 Ductal Carcinoma In Situ (DCIS) and Myoepithelial Cells. A: Myoepithelial cells are evident at the perimeter of the flask-shaped duct cross section involved by cribriform DCIS. **B, C:** In this needle core biopsy specimen, "comedo" DCIS is encircled by myosin-positive myoepithelial cells **(C)**.

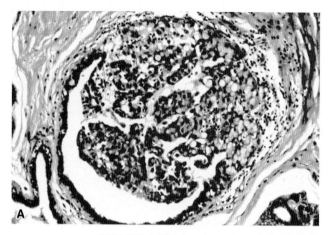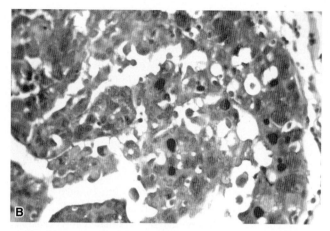

FIGURE 8.42 Ductal Carcinoma In Situ, Signet Ring Cells. A: Papillary DCIS with signet ring cells. **B:** The intracytoplasmic mucin is stained magenta with the mucicarmine stain.

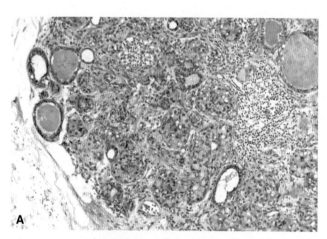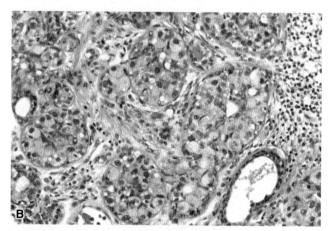

FIGURE 8.43 Ductal Carcinoma In Situ (DCIS), Intracytoplasmic Mucin. A, B: DCIS in sclerosing adenosis in a needle core biopsy specimen. The cells have pale blue cytoplasm that was reactive with the mucicarmine stain.

because of the appearance created by sharply defined cell borders **(Fig. 8.44)**. A large subset of lesions that are classified under this heading are a form of apocrine carcinoma. Occasionally, clear cell DCIS has strongly mucicarmine-positive cytoplasm. The presence of a monomorphic clear cell population in a ductal proliferative

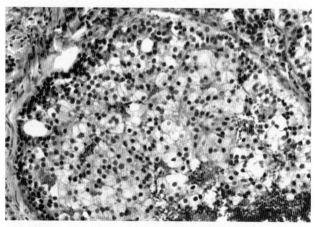

FIGURE 8.44 Ductal Carcinoma In Situ, Clear Cell Type. The cells have sharply defined borders and low-grade nuclei.

lesion is highly suggestive of intraducal carcinoma. Other clear cell lesions are the in situ forms of lipid-rich or glycogen-rich carcinomas discussed in Chapter 20. Apocrine cytology is encountered in all of the structural types of DCIS **(Fig. 8.45)**. These cells have abundant cytoplasm that ranges from granular and eosinophilic to vacuolated or clear. There is variable nuclear pleomorphism, sometimes manifested by prominent nucleoli.

Spindle cell DCIS may express neuroendocrine markers such as chromogranin, synaptophysin, CD56, and neuron-specific enolase (134) **(Fig. 8.46)**. The swirling growth pattern of cells in spindle cell DCIS mimics "streaming" that is characteristically found in usual DH. Spindle cell DCIS often coexists with cribriform DCIS.

The expression of *neuroendocrine markers* can be found in DCIS with non–spindle cell cytology and with various growth patterns. Kawasaki et al. (135) found neuroendocrine marker expression in 20 of 294 (6.8%) DCIS. The diagnosis of neuroendocrine DCIS was made when at least 50% of the tumor cells expressed chromogranin A and/or synaptophysin. Neuroendocrine DCIS had a significantly higher frequency of presentation with bloody nipple discharge (72%) than non-neuroendocrine DCIS (5%). Most of the lesions had solid

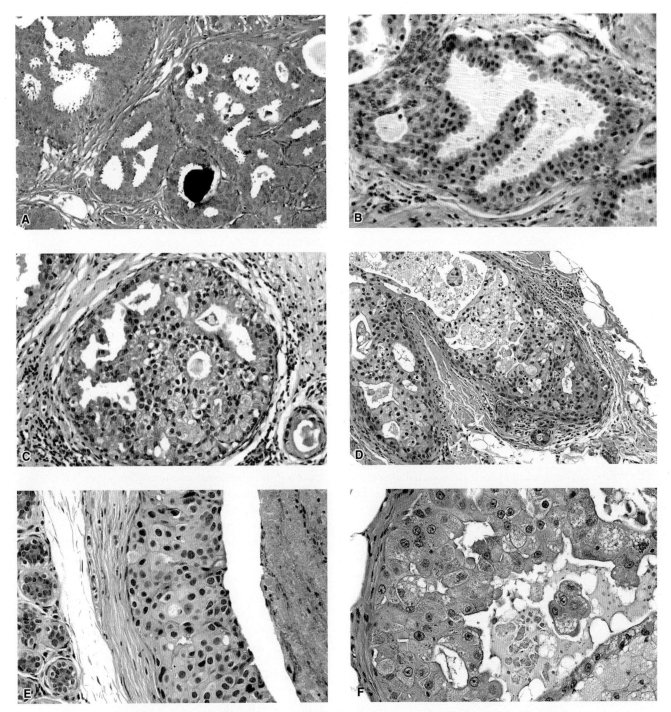

FIGURE 8.45 Ductal Carcinoma In Situ (DCIS), Apocrine Type. A: Cribriform DCIS with apocrine cytology and calcifications. **B:** Micropapillary apocrine DCIS with intermediate nuclear grade. **C:** Cribriform apocrine DCIS with low nuclear grade and cytoplasmic granularity. **D:** Apocrine intraductal carcinoma with clear cell change and lobular extension. **E, F:** Two additional cases of apocrine DCIS are shown. Note luminal necrosis in **(E)**. Pink granular cytoplasm of the apocrine type is shown in **(F)**.

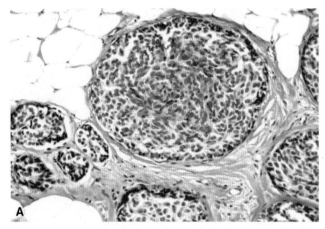
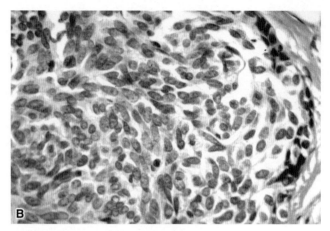

FIGURE 8.46 Ductal Carcinoma In Situ, Spindle Cell Type. **A, B:** The swirling spindle cell proliferation mimics the streaming pattern of ductal hyperplasia. The monomorphic spindle cells extend to the perimeter of the duct in this needle core biopsy specimen.

papillary or papillary architecture with low nuclear grade in 90% and an absence of calcifications in 75%. Neuroendocrine DCIS tended to express estrogen and progesterone receptors and not to overexpress HER2.

Primary neuroendocrine carcinomas of the gastrointestinal tract and lung metastatic to the breast can architecturally and cytologically mimic primary in situ carcinoma of the breast, and in this context, "clinical history is paramount for optimal diagnosis" (136).

Small cell DCIS is extremely uncommon **(Fig. 8.47)**. The growth patterns are typically cribriform and solid or a mixture of these forms. When present by itself, the solid pattern can be distinguished from LCIS with the E-cadherin immunostain. Membrane reactivity will be present in DCIS and absent or fragmented and weak in the lobular lesion.

The cellular composition of DCIS is usually described as *monomorphic,* a term applied especially to cribriform, solid,

and micropapillary carcinomas. In this context, monomorphic means that there is overall homogeneity in the cytologic appearance of the lesion, although the cells are not always similar in such features as the amount of cytoplasm or nuclear size. Cell and nuclear shape may be altered by the presence or absence of crowding in one or another part of the duct. The presence of a myoepithelial cell layer is not a consideration in judging whether a ductal proliferation is monomorphic. Dimorphic variants of DCIS, consisting of two distinctly different populations of cells, are unusual **(Fig. 8.47)**.

DCIS in a particular case can have multiple cytologic, structural, or immunohistochemical phenotypes (117). Mixed histologic patterns are found in 30% to 40% of cases. Although some structural combinations such as micropapillary-cribriform and papillary-cribriform occur relatively more often than others, there is considerable heterogeneity with respect to growth patterns (137). The probability of structural variability

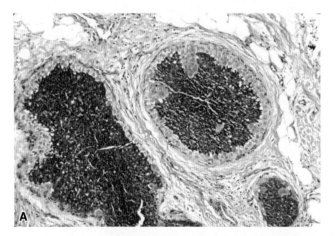
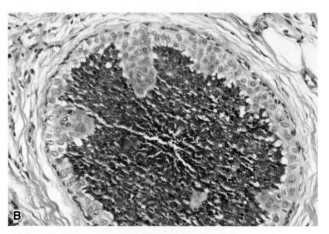

FIGURE 8.47 Ductal Carcinoma In Situ, Small Cell Type. **A, B:** This extraordinary lesion consists of a central nearly syncytial mass of small undifferentiated carcinoma cells and an outer zone of larger polygonal cells. Two protruding mounds of large cells show apical traces of squamous differentiation, a feature that was more pronounced in other ducts. Persistent myoepithelial cells that were immunoreactive for actin are represented by the small dark elongated nuclei at the outer border of the duct. **C, D:** Solid, small cell DCIS with cribriform microlumina. This architectural and cytologic appearance of the lesion could be mistaken for pagetoid spread of LCIS in a duct. All cells were strongly E-cadherin positive **(D)**. **E, F:** Small cell DCIS in a lobule **(E)**. The in situ carcinoma is E-cadherin positive.

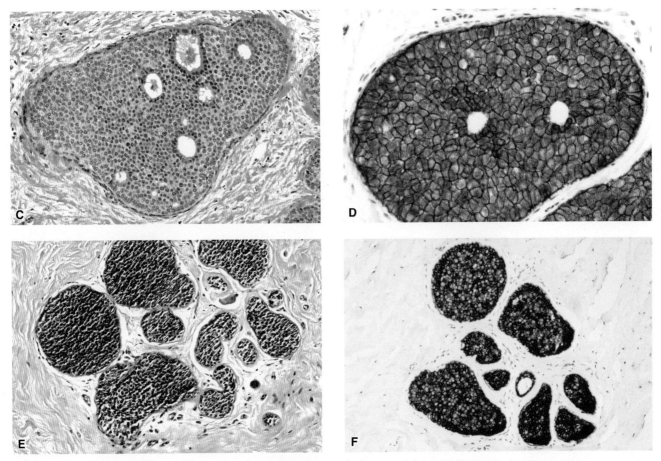

FIGURE 8.47 (continued)

increases with the extent of the lesion, a phenomenon that must be considered in using NCB for the subclassification of a mammographically detected DCIS.

Cytologic features, especially at the nuclear level, tend to be more homogeneous than the growth pattern in a given case. Some combinations of growth patterns and cytologic appearances occur more frequently, such as classic "comedo" DCIS, composed of pleomorphic cells with high-grade nuclei and necrosis, or the low nuclear grade typically present in micropapillary DCIS. However, the considerable range of heterogeneity is illustrated by lesions composed of small, cytologically low-grade nuclei growing in a solid pattern with central "comedo" necrosis, and others having a micropapillary pattern composed of cells with high-grade nuclei found in some examples of flat micropapillary/clinging DCIS.

Micropapillary DCIS consists of ducts lined by a layer of neoplastic cells that intermittently give rise to slender papillary fronds or arcuate formations that protrude into the ductal lumen **(Fig. 8.48)**. The papillae are variable in appearance, ranging from blunt bumps or mounds to pronounced, slender, elongated processes. The latter almost always lack a fibrovascular core and are lined by cytologically homogenous carcinoma cells. Arcuate structures, commonly referred to as "Roman bridge arches," occur when microlumina are formed beneath adjacent coalescent fronds or within a mound of neoplastic cells. These fenestrations resemble the lumina formed in cribriform

DCIS. In conjunction with micropapillae, they are a feature of micropapillary DCIS.

The appearance of the micropapillary fronds varies somewhat with the plane of individual histologic sections. While some micropapillae are cut perpendicular to their long axis, others are sectioned tangentially or transversely, resulting in irregular nests of seemingly detached cell clusters in the ductal lumen **(Fig. 8.48)**. Apart from the epithelial proliferation, ducts with low nuclear grade micropapillary DCIS are usually relatively free of cellular debris or inflammatory cells, but they may contain calcifications.

Micropapillary DCIS is usually composed of cytologically low-grade, small homogeneous cells with a high nuclear-to-cytoplasmic ratio and dark nuclei **(Fig. 8.48)**. The nuclei typically vary little in size and chromatin density between cells at the base and tip of micropapillae. They may be slightly smaller and darker at the surface, but marked disparity in these characteristics is a feature of micropapillary hyperplasia. At the margin of the duct, between papillary and arcuate structures, the neoplastic cells typically form a thin layer one to not more than three or four cells deep. Persistent non-neoplastic epithelium between micropapillae is a feature of micropapillary hyperplasia rather than micropapillary carcinoma. Mitoses are rarely evident in low-grade micropapillary DCIS. In most instances, the cells are so crowded that their individual borders and cytoplasm cannot be identified. Occasionally, the cells have

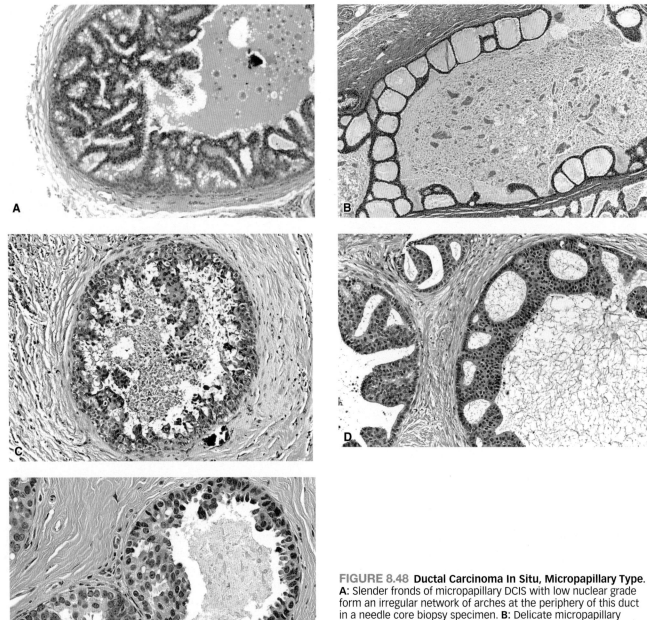

FIGURE 8.48 Ductal Carcinoma In Situ, Micropapillary Type.
A: Slender fronds of micropapillary DCIS with low nuclear grade form an irregular network of arches at the periphery of this duct in a needle core biopsy specimen. **B:** Delicate micropapillary bands of monomorphic cells with low-grade nuclei outline microlumina in this duct (in the pattern of "Roman bridges"). **C:** Micropapillary DCIS in a needle core biopsy specimen with apocrine cytology and high nuclear grade. **D:** Relatively "rigid" arches characterize this example of micropapillary DCIS. **E:** Another example of micropapillary DCIS with features similar to those seen in (**C**).

slightly more abundant cytoplasm, with apocrine-type protrusions at the luminal border. In one variant of this cell type, the nuclei of the tumor cells are contained in cytoplasmic blebs that are extruded into the ductal lumen. Clear cell change and squamous metaplasia are rarely seen in micropapillary DCIS.

A minority of DCIS with a micropapillary structural phenotype are composed of cells with intermediate- or high-grade nuclei (**Fig. 8.48**). This type of micropapillary carcinoma tends to occur in women between 35 and 50 years of age, to be multifocal, and sometimes bilateral. Cells forming this type of carcinoma, which is mainly localized in TDLU, differ from those in conventional micropapillary lesions in that they are larger,

with more abundant cytoplasm. Nuclei are also correspondingly larger, and nucleoli are usually apparent. Mitoses can be seen in this epithelium, and the cells often have a distinctly apocrine appearance. This cytologically high-grade form of micropapillary DCIS is more likely to have calcifications than the low-grade variant, and necrotic cellular debris may be found in the ductal lumen. Florid micropapillary proliferation tends to result in fusion of the epithelial fronds and the formation of cribriform microlumina. It is not unusual to find DCIS with a combination of micropapillary and cribriform features.

The term *flat micropapillary (clinging) carcinoma* refers to DCIS with the cytologic appearance of the micropapillary lesion that is lacking in fully developed epithelial fronds (**Fig. 8.48**). Lesions composed entirely of flat micropapillary DCIS are uncommon, and more often one or more epithelial fronds or bridges are present. In the absence of calcification or necrosis, flat micropapillary DCIS is easily overlooked. This type of DCIS is most often found in a background of CCH. The lesions are typically multifocal or multicentric and can be bilateral. Calcifications with distinctive crystalline, ossifying, and laminated appearances tend to occur in CCH, leading to mammographic detection. Patients with CCH may have tubular carcinoma and LCIS ("the Rosen triad"), as well as invasive lobular carcinoma, and micropapillary DCIS.

Cribriform DCIS is a fenestrated epithelial proliferation in which microlumina are formed in the malignant epithelium that bridges most or all of the ductal lumen (**Fig. 8.49**). Extension into lobular epithelium (so-called lobular cancerization) or into the lactiferous ducts of the nipple is uncommon. Dilated ducts with cribriform DCIS can be mistaken for adenoid cystic carcinoma or a complex papilloma.

Collagenous spherulosis, which is usually associated with hyperplastic ductal lesions that may be secondarily involved by LCIS, can also be mistaken for cribriform DCIS. The presence of collagenous spherulosis can be confirmed with myoepithelial immunostains. The latter will highlight myoepithelial cells at

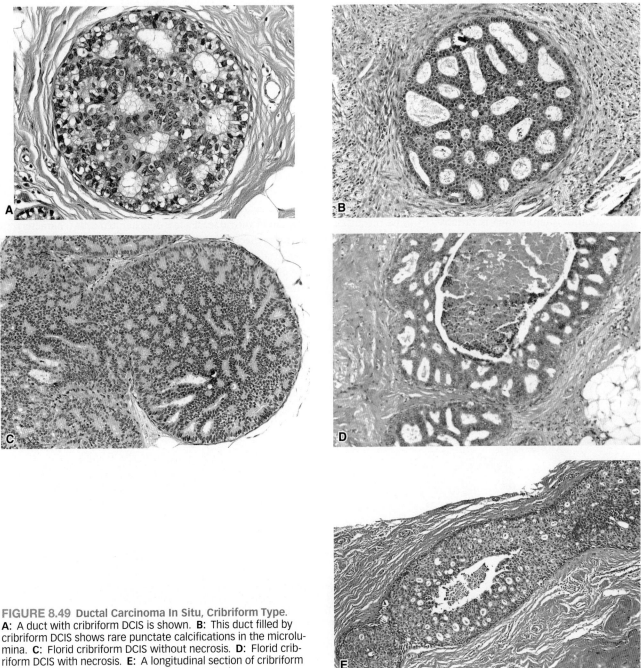

FIGURE 8.49 Ductal Carcinoma In Situ, Cribriform Type.
A: A duct with cribriform DCIS is shown. **B:** This duct filled by cribriform DCIS shows rare punctate calcifications in the microlumina. **C:** Florid cribriform DCIS without necrosis. **D:** Florid cribriform DCIS with necrosis. **E:** A longitudinal section of cribriform DCIS with necrosis in a needle core biopsy sample.

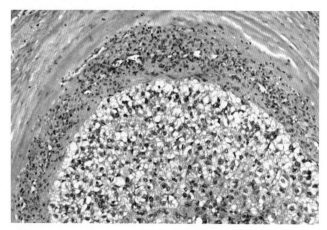

FIGURE 8.50 Ductal Carcinoma In Situ, Solid Type. An un-usual example of solid, clear cell DCIS with marked periductal angiogenesis.

throughout the duct are the hallmark of cribriform DCIS. The microlumina may contain secretions, rare degenerated or necrotic cells, and punctate calcifications.

Bands of neoplastic cells between and around the microlumina are described as rigid, a term that refers to the uniform, not overlapping distribution of polygonal cells, in contrast to the streaming pattern of overlapping, frequently oval cells in DH. Polarization of the cells in a radial fashion around the microlumina contributes to the rigid appearance. The most orderly type of low-grade cribriform DCIS is composed of monomorphic cuboidal-to-low columnar cells. Nucleoli are inconspicuous or absent, and mitoses are rarely encountered. The cells usually have sparse cytoplasm. Cribriform DCIS can be composed of cells with intermediate to high-grade nuclei. Necrosis may be present in such foci.

Solid DCIS is formed by neoplastic cells that fill most or all of the duct space **(Fig. 8.50)**. Microlumina and papillary structures are absent, but calcifications may be present. Patients with "comedo" DCIS often have coexistent foci of non-necrotic solid DCIS. The polygonal cells are typically of a single type with low-to-intermediate nuclear grade. The cytoplasm has a spectrum of cytologic appearances including clear, granular, amphophilic, and apocrine.

"Comedo" DCIS is composed of carcinoma cells with mitotically active high-grade nuclei and "comedo"-type necrosis **(Fig. 8.51)**. The term "comedo" necrosis should be used only when there is DCIS with high-grade nuclei and prominent necrotic debris centrally in the duct—a finding that is typically associated with at least a few degenerated cells (characterized by karyorrhectic or pyknotic nuclei with loss of nuclear detail).

The aforementioned architectural patterns of DCIS may coexist in a particular case; however, typically one pattern is either predominant or the only one present **(Fig. 8.51)**. In a

the perimeter of spherules. Laminin and collagen IV immunostains can highlight the basement membrane components in the "spherules." The distinction between DCIS and LCIS in collagenous spherulosis depends on cytologic features of the lesion and can be confirmed with E-cadherin or p120 immunostains. The appearance of coexisting in situ carcinoma in the immediate vicinity of collagenous spherulosis can also be helpful.

The *secondary lumina* in cribriform DCIS tend to be round or oval, with smooth edges bordered by cuboidal cells. The distribution of microlumina is variable. In some instances, the spaces are spread across the entire duct, but in others they are concentrated toward the center or rarely in a zone largely at the periphery of the duct. Microlumina surrounded by a homogeneous cell population that is uniformly distributed

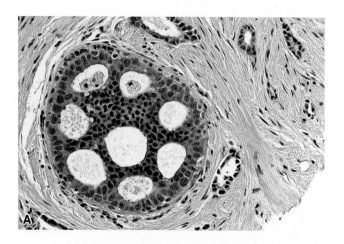

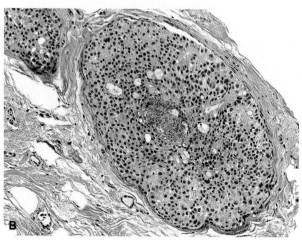

FIGURE 8.51 Ductal Carcinoma In Situ, Various Architectural Types. A: Cribriform DCIS, without necrosis in tubular carcinoma. **B:** Cribriform DCIS, with punctate necrosis. **C:** Micropapillary DCIS with luminal secretions (without necrosis). **D:** Flat micropapillary ("clinging") DCIS with high-grade nuclei and central necrosis. Note a focal deposit of stromal calcification. **E:** Solid DCIS with high-grade nuclei is present at the perimeter of a duct with "comedo"-type necrosis. Angiogenesis is evident in the periductal tissue. **F:** "Comedo" necrosis with dystrophic calcification is apparent in this duct with solid DCIS. **G, H:** Two examples of "colliding" architectural types with differing cytology are shown. DCIS of micropapillary and cribriform types **(G)**. Cribriform DCIS and small cell DCIS with necrosis **(H)**.

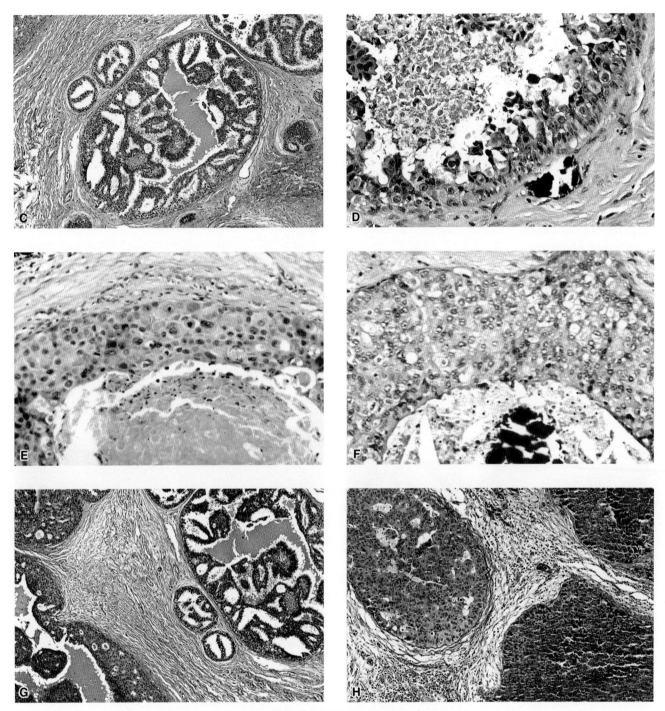

FIGURE 8.51 (*continued*)

1997 consensus report (138), *nuclear grade* was stratified into three categories (**Table 8.1**). Pleomorphic nuclei of similar size were not consistent with low nuclear grade. The pathology report should reflect the highest nuclear grade but may indicate the relative proportions of grade when there is heterogeneity (**Fig. 8.52**). *Necrosis* was defined as the "presence of ghost cells and karyorrhectic debris" (**Table 8.2**). Five architectural patterns were identified as follows: micropapillary, cribriform, solid, "comedo," and papillary. It was specified that "comedo" referred "to solid intraepithelial growth within the basement

membrane with central (zonal) necrosis. Such lesions are often but not invariably high nuclear grade."

The *myoepithelial cell layer* is sometimes obscured and rarely eliminated (exhibiting "necrosis to the wall" pattern) by the carcinomatous proliferation, but in other instances it may be hyperplastic and produce a distinct ring around the afflicted gland. The latter configuration is usually accompanied by accentuation of the basement membrane itself, as well as a circumferential periductal collar of desmoplastic stroma. A "cocktail" of antibodies to SMM-HC and p63 is especially

TABLE 8.1

Consensus Committee Recommendation for Grading Nuclei in Ductal Carcinoma In Situ

Low-grade nuclei

Monomorphic (monotonous) appearance
Size of ductal epithelial nuclei or 1.5–2.0X normal red blood cells
Chromatin diffuse, finely dispersed
"Occasional nucleoli and mitoses"
Cells usually polarized

High-grade nuclei

"Markedly pleomorphic"
Size: usually more than 2.5X that of ductal epithelial nuclei
Chromatin: vesicular with irregular distribution
"Prominent, often multiple, nucleoli"
"Mitoses may be conspicuous"

Intermediate-grade nuclei

"Nuclei that are neither low-grade nor high-grade"

Based on The Consensus Conference Committee. Consensus Conference on the classification of ductal carcinoma in situ. *Cancer.* 1997;80:1798–1802.

sensitive for detecting myoepithelium in high-grade DCIS (139). Neovascularity in many instances is represented by proliferation of capillaries immediately external to the basement membrane (140). A variable inflammatory infiltrate is present in the periductal stroma, with a granulomatous reaction in foci where the ductal wall is partially disrupted, and it appears that necrotic contents of the duct have been discharged into the stroma. Calcification can also be found in the stroma.

It is important to distinguish between "comedo" necrosis and the accumulation of secretions accompanied by an inflammatory reaction that occurs in ductal stasis. Both conditions are prone to the formation of calcifications. Cellular necrosis is rarely seen in ductal stasis, and when present, the degenerated cells are usually histiocytes. The ductal contents in "comedo" DCIS consist of necrotic carcinoma cells represented by "ghost" outlines thereof and karyorrhectic debris associated with minimal, if any, inflammation **(Fig. 8.53)**. There is typically a sharp demarcation between viable carcinoma cells and the necrotic center. A space may be formed between the viable and necrotic elements. Dying cells at the inner edge of the viable zone have pyknotic nuclei and frayed cytoplasmic borders. The outlines of necrotic ("ghost") cells may be visible in the center of the duct.

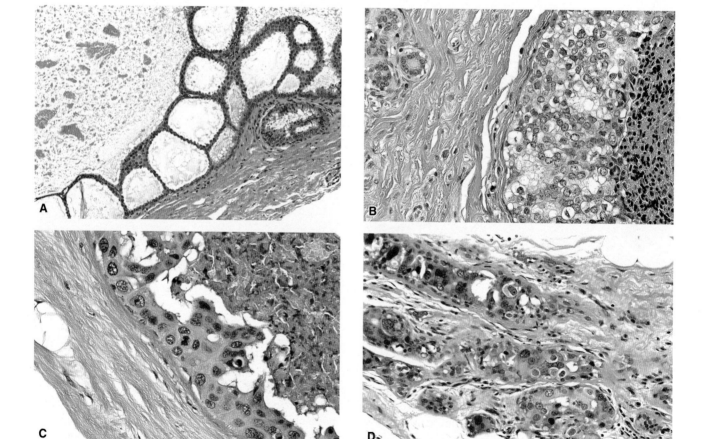

FIGURE 8.52 Ductal Carcinoma In Situ (DCIS), Various Nuclear Grades. A: DCIS, micropapillary type with low-grade nuclei. **B:** DCIS, cribriform type with intermediate-grade nuclei. **C:** DCIS, flat micropapillary ("clinging") type with high-grade nuclei. **D:** DCIS in terminal ducts, status-post chemotherapy with highly pleomorphic cells and scattered high-grade nuclei.

TABLE 8.2

Consensus Committee Recommendation for Defining Necrosis in Ductal Carcinoma In Situ

"Comedo" necrosis

"Central zone necrosis within a duct, usually exhibiting a linear pattern within ducts if sectioned longitudinally"

Punctate necrosis

"Nonzonal type necrosis (foci of necrosis that do not exhibit a linear pattern if longitudinally sectioned)"

Based on The Consensus Conference Committee. Consensus Conference on the classification of ductal carcinoma in situ. *Cancer* 1997;80:1798–1802.

Calcification develops in the necrotic center when there is "comedo" necrosis. The calcification can be finely granular and mixed with cellular debris in some instances or, it forms more solid irregular masses that correspond to casting calcifications on mammography. Calcifications in "comedo" DCIS almost always consist of calcium salts, mainly calcium phosphate, rather than crystalline calcium oxalate, which is typically found in benign apocrine lesions. In routine H&E-stained sections, calcium phosphate calcifications are magenta to purple, both in "comedo" carcinoma or other varieties of DCIS. Calcifications and necrotic debris may become dislodged in NCB, and rarely this material is the only component of the lesion found in the specimen. When dislodged calcifications are present in a NCB, serial sections of the biopsy specimen should be prepared. An excisional biopsy is indicated even if no epithelial elements are found in the NCB that contains dislodged calcifications or crystalloids (**Fig. 8.54**). If a dislodged fragment of carcinoma becomes embedded in stroma or fat in a NCB, the resulting appearance can be mistaken for invasive carcinoma (**Fig. 8.55**).

Occasionally, marked periductal fibrosis can be associated with extensive obliteration of ducts that contain "comedo" DCIS, a process referred to as *healing* by Muir and Aitkenhead (141) or as "regressive change" by Wasserman et al. (142). Prominent necrosis can contribute to this process. The residual structures typically consist of round-to-oval scars composed of

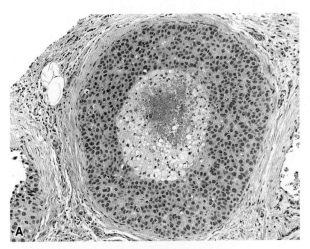
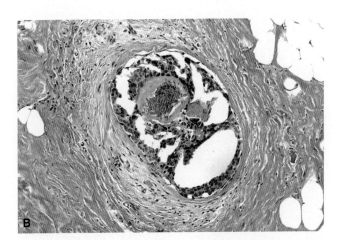
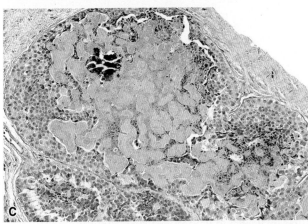
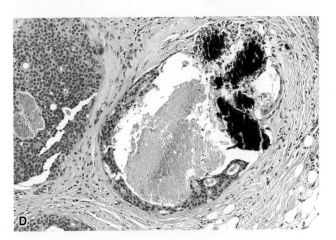

FIGURE 8.53 Ductal Carcinoma In Situ (DCIS), with Varying Degrees of Necrosis and Calcification. A: Cribriform DCIS with central punctate necrosis and faint calcifications in the midst of histiocytes. **B:** Micropapillary DCIS with punctate necrosis. **C:** Micropapillary DCIS with abundant necrosis and focal calcification. **D:** Micropapillary DCIS with necrosis and dense calcifications. **E:** Micropapillary DCIS with mainly granular calcifications obscuring necrosis. **F:** Micropapillary DCIS with necrosis and dense calcification.

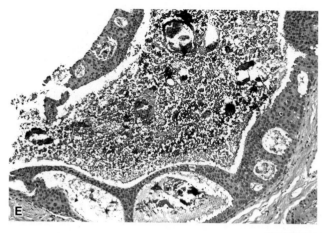

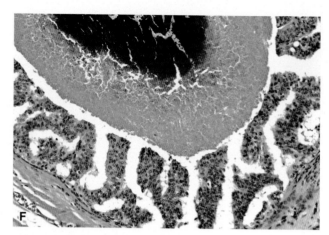

FIGURE 8.53 (continued)

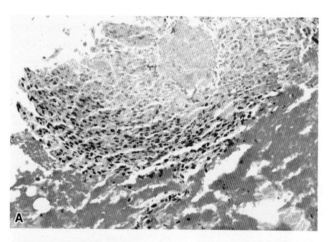

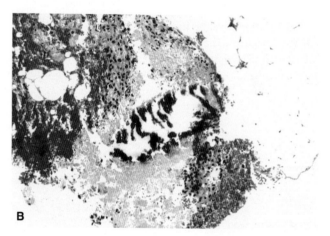

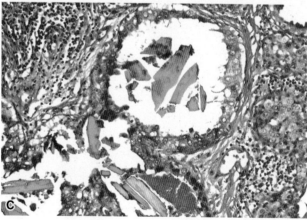

FIGURE 8.54 Probable Intraductal Carcinoma, Solid "Comedo" Type. A, B: The needle core biopsy specimen had these fragments of calcification, "comedo"-type necrosis, and atypical cells. A needle core biopsy specimen such as this is an indication for prompt excisional biopsy to determine if "comedo" carcinoma is present. **C:** Crystalloids in DCIS. These protein precipitates are often associated with DCIS.

circumferential layers of collagen and elastic tissue **(Fig. 8.56)**. The center of the scar, representing the remnants of the duct, is often less dense, and it may contain a few residual carcinoma cells, histiocytes, fragments of calcification, and granulation tissue. End-stage scars of periductal mastitis are not distinguishable from those of obliterated "comedo" carcinoma (143). When this type of scar is found in a NCB, serial sections should be obtained because minute foci of carcinoma cells may be detected in the scar. The very limited histologic evidence

for carcinoma found in some of these cases may result in a diagnosis of ADH.

It is notable that "distorting" periductal sclerosis around DCIS in a NCB, defined as "irregular angulation of gland" that "may be related to regressive change," has been shown to be predictive of upstaging to invasive carcinoma on subsequent excisional biopsy (144).

Triple-negative basal-like DCIS has the triple-negative basal-like immunophenotype (negative for ER, PR, and HER2). This form

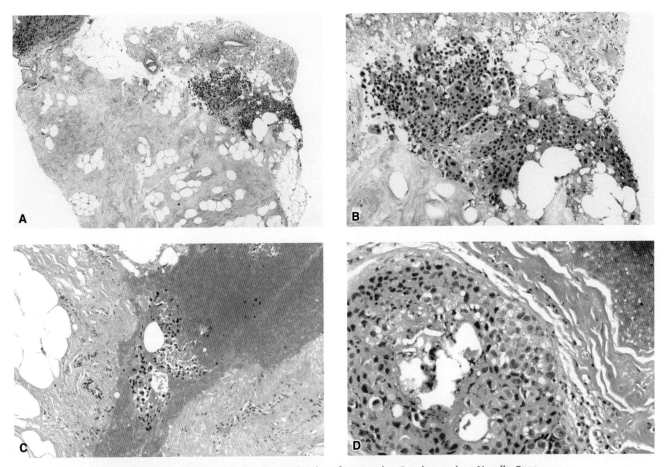

FIGURE 8.55 Displaced Epithelium Mistaken for Invasive Carcinoma in a Needle Core Biopsy Sample. A, B: This fragment of carcinoma displaced in fibrofatty tissue was interpreted as invasive carcinoma. **C:** The subsequent excisional biopsy specimen had similar fragments of displaced carcinoma such as the one shown here in an area of hemorrhage caused by the needle core biopsy procedure. **D:** The excisional biopsy specimen contained intraductal "comedo" carcinoma with no intrinsic invasion. Note hemorrhage caused by the needle core biopsy procedure in the upper right corner.

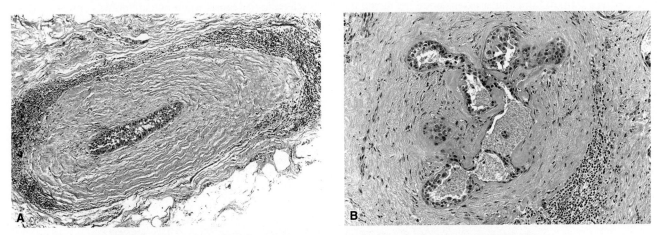

FIGURE 8.56 Intraductal Carcinoma, with Obliterative Sclerosis. A–D: Four different biopsies arranged in a sequence that suggests the progressive replacement of degenerating and necrotic DCIS by circumferential sclerosis of the ducts and calcifications. In **(D)**, there is minimal evidence of DCIS (arrowheads), but foci of lymphovascular channel involvement by carcinoma cells (arrows) are evident around the sclerotic duct.

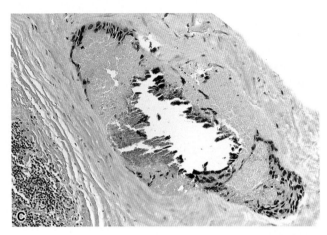
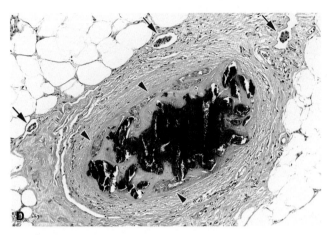

FIGURE 8.56 (*continued*)

of DCIS is the putative precursor to invasive basal-like ductal carcinoma (145–147). Bryan et al. (146) found the basal-like immunophenotype in 4/55 (6%) DCIS with high-grade nuclei. This form of DCIS typically expresses basal cytokeratins and epidermal growth factor receptor (EGFR) significantly more often than high-grade DCIS, which did not have basal-like immunophenotype, and may display either solid, flat, or micropapillary architectural features (147).

Papillary DCIS is distinguished by the presence of prominent papillary fibrovascular stromal architecture and is discussed in Chapter 11. Spindle cell DCIS is sometimes a variant of papillary DCIS, but spindle cell growth also occurs in nonpapillary types of DCIS.

DCIS in sclerosing adenosis assumes the structural configuration of the underlying adenosis, and may be mistaken for invasive carcinoma (148–150). Because sclerosing adenosis is fundamentally a lesion formed by altered lobules, this presentation can be viewed as either DCIS that arose in TDLU units or as a form of intralobular extension of the ductal lesion **(Fig. 8.57)**. The condition usually occurs focally, but it can be diffuse. The growth patterns of DCIS are usually solid

and cribriform. An organoid appearance can be formed when there is alveolar expansion of lobular structures in the adenosis. Calcifications may be present in the underlying adenosis or as part of the DCIS. DCIS can be limited to the sclerosing adenosis, or there may be additional foci thereof in the vicinity (149). In particular, atypical apocrine adenosis (that is, sclerosing adenosis with atypical apocrine metaplasia) can mimic invasive apocrine carcinoma (151). Features that distinguish atypical from malignant apocrine epithelia include marked variation in nuclear size, prominence of nucleoli, mitoses, and presence of necrosis. The underlying architecture of sclerosing adenosis can be appreciated with stains for basement membranes (e.g., reticulin, laminin, etc.) and myoepithelial cells (e.g., myosin, calponin, etc.) (149). Invasive carcinoma arising in sclerosing adenosis is difficult to detect unless the invasive component has clearly grown beyond the area of adenosis and has an architectural pattern that differs from that of adenosis.

Neural entrapment occurs when nerves are incorporated in sclerosing adenosis when no carcinoma is present (152). The presence of this unusual finding coexisting with DCIS in adenosis is not indicative of invasion. Neural entrapment has

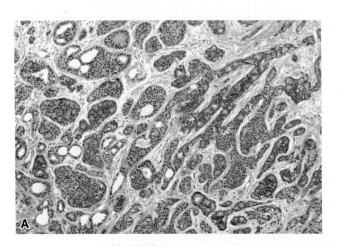
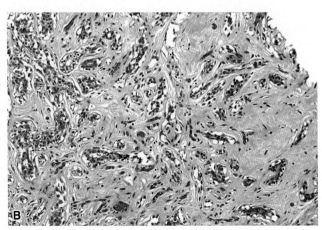

FIGURE 8.57 **Ductal Carcinoma In Situ in Sclerosing Adenosis. A:** The carcinoma has solid and cribriform growth patterns with low nuclear grade. Some of the underlying architecture is tubular adenosis. **B–D:** A needle core biopsy specimen showing sclerosing adenosis **(B)** that was involved by DCIS **(C, D)**.

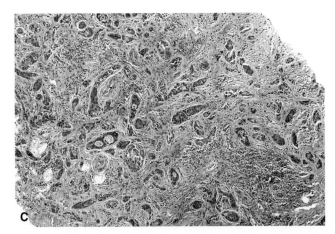

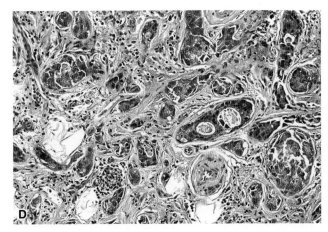

FIGURE 8.57 (*continued*)

also been observed in areas of sclerosing papillary DCIS not associated with sclerosing adenosis (153).

DCIS in radial sclerosing lesions may be difficult to distinguish from ADH. The presence of an underlying radial scar is indicated by the overall configuration of the lesion and association with cysts, sclerosing adenosis, and apocrine metaplasia **(Fig. 8.58)**. Fragmented portions of radial scars obtained in a NCB are difficult to assess for the presence of DCIS or for invasion, and they are likely to be reported as ADH.

Concurrent DCIS and LCIS are present when there are separate foci of in situ carcinoma with the characteristic histologic features of these lesions. This is illustrated by instances in which the lobular lesion with the classical small cell phenotype of lobular carcinoma is limited to TDLU units that are separate from ducts with the classical features of "comedo," cribriform, or micropapillary DCIS.

In some instances, the distinction is less clear, especially when the proliferation in the ducts and lobules is composed of uniform cells with low-to-intermediate-grade nuclei. The difficulty presented by these lesions is whether they should be classified as DCIS with "lobular cancerization," or as LCIS with "pagetoid type" of ductal extension. The E-cadherin and p120 stains will display strong membrane reactivity if the lesion is DCIS. E-cadherin staining will be either attenuated, fragmented, or absent, and p120 reactivity will be localized in the cytoplasm, in LCIS. The presence of the cribriform pattern is suggestive, but not diagnostic, of DCIS with lobular extension. Cells with apocrine differentiation are more consistent with DCIS, although pleomorphic form of LCIS is in the differential diagnosis. Ultimately, some cases defy classification even after careful consideration of all features. The definitive classification of the in situ carcinoma in such cases should be deferred to examination of the excisional biopsy specimen.

Coexistent DCIS and LCIS in a single duct–lobular unit constitutes one of the most unusual microscopic patterns of noninvasive carcinoma (154). This diagnosis depends on finding carcinoma with two distinctly different cytologic and architectural patterns in a single duct **(Fig. 8.59)**. In these combined lesions, LCIS with the conventional small cell cytology is typically present within lobular glands as well as in a pagetoid distribution in the ductal epithelium. The ductal lumen contains a cribriform, micropapillary, or solid proliferation composed

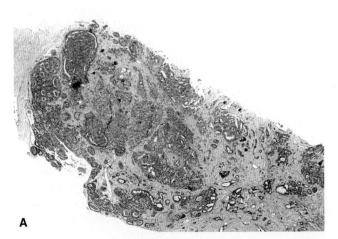

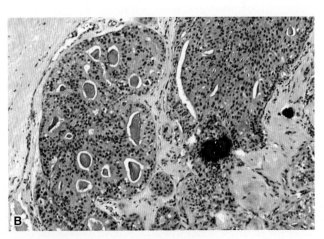

FIGURE 8.58 Ductal Carcinoma In Situ in a Radial Sclerosing Lesion. A: Cribriform DCIS is present in the upper left portion of this needle core biopsy specimen. Atypical duct hyperplasia occupies the mid-portion, and sclerosing adenosis is present on the lower right. **B:** The area of cribriform DCIS.

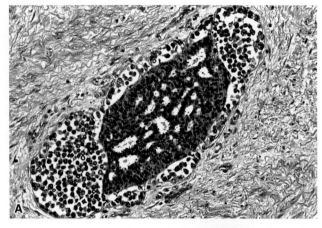

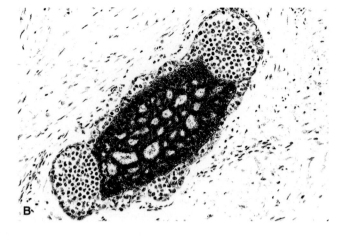

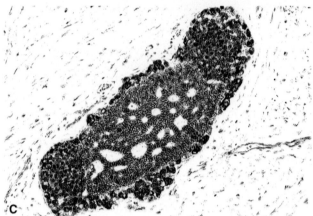

FIGURE 8.59 Coexistent DCIS and LCIS in a Single Duct–Lobular Unit. A: DCIS of the cribriform type is present centrally, and LCIS of classic type is present at either end of the duct. Note the uniform cell population that inhabits the cribriform structure of DCIS. The LCIS is represented by uniform but noncohesive cells (that are cytologically different from the DCIS cells). **B:** An E-cadherin immunostain shows negative reaction in the LCIS, and strong cytoplasmic membrane staining in the DCIS cells. Note weaker staining of the myoepithelial cells at the perimeter of the duct. **C:** A p120 immunostain shows *cytoplasmic staining* in the LCIS cells, and strong *cytoplasmic membrane staining* in the DCIS cells (similar to that seen with E-cadherin, in **B**). The difference in staining in subtle and may be difficult to appreciate at low-magnification microscopy.

of more pleomorphic cells typically found in DCIS. Coexistent DCIS and LCIS have been found in association with invasive ductal and invasive lobular carcinoma. With lobular extension of DCIS, so-called "lobular cancerization," the non-neoplastic lobular epithelium is displaced by carcinoma cells with the same cytologic appearance as the DCIS. E-cadherin and p120 stains can be used to identify LCIS and DCIS in combined lesions.

Some types of DCIS, including *cystic hypersecretory carcinoma in situ* (discussed elsewhere in this book, please check index) and *noninvasive adenoid cystic carcinoma* (155,156) are exceptionally uncommon.

Distinct genetic abnormalities have been documented in DCIS (157). In general, loss of 16q occurs almost exclusively in lower-grade DCIS. Intermediate-grade DCIS shows frequent gains of 1q and loss of 11q. High-grade DCIS shows high frequency of amplifications at 17q12 and 11q13, and a higher rate of genetic imbalances.

Grading of DCIS

The purpose of grading DCIS is to predict its biologic behavior. Over the years, multiple grading systems for DCIS have been proposed; however, no system has found universal acceptance.

When an invasive element is associated with DCIS, both components tend to have similar nuclear grades (158). Grading schemes consisting of two categories (high-grade and other grades) and three categories (high-, intermediate-, and

low-grade) have been devised. The determination of grade is based largely upon nuclear cytology. Nuclear grade tends to be relatively constant in a given patient, even when substantial variation in architectural pattern is noted (159). The presence or absence of necrosis and the architecture of DCIS are also considerations in grading.

By definition, "comedo" DCIS is a noninvasive carcinoma with solid architectural pattern and high-grade nuclei accompanied by prominent necrosis. High-grade nuclei and necrosis are infrequently encountered in papillary, micropapillary, and cribriform forms of DCIS (158). DCIS is considered to be in the intermediate-grade category when it has a cribriform, solid, or papillary pattern with necrosis but lacks the marked nuclear atypia of "comedo" DCIS, or if one of these growth patterns is composed of high-grade carcinoma cells in the absence of necrosis. Any pattern of DCIS composed of uniform cells without atypia or necrosis is classified as low grade. A case is usually classified on the basis of the highest nuclear grade present (138).

Grading has been a component of most attempts to develop classification schemes for assessing the effectiveness of breast conservation therapy in the treatment of DCIS. Several classifications have been proposed (79,159). These have been based on some or all of the following features: architecture, nuclear grade, presence or absence of necrosis, lesion size, and cell polarity. Most classifications have emphasized nuclear grade, necrosis, and architecture. There is a significant correlation between the grade of DCIS and that of the corresponding invasive carcinoma (159). The grading categories also have significant associations with biologic characteristics of DCIS, especially lesions classified as high- and low-grade. High-grade DCIS typically exhibits the following features: negativity for ER and PR, HER2 expression, p53-positivity, high proliferation rate, and increased periductal angiogenesis **(Fig. 8.59)**. Low-grade DCIS are characterized by the following: positivity for ER and PR, negativity for HER2 and p53, low proliferation rate, and minimal periductal angiogenesis. Intermediate-grade DCIS tend to have mixed patterns of biologic marker expression.

The *Holland* classification system of DCIS is three-tiered (160). The system primarily utilizes nuclear grading and secondarily uses cellular polarization. The term "comedo-necrosis" is not a criterion in this system. The *Lagios* system (161) stratifies DCIS into high-grade (high-grade nuclei and extensive necrosis), intermediate-grade (intermediate-grade nuclei with focal or absent necrosis), and low-grade (low-grade nuclei without necrosis). The *Van Nuys* scale of DCIS (162) uses nuclear grade and necrosis to classify DCIS into three groups. Group 3 includes DCIS cases with high-grade nuclei (with or without necrosis). Group 2 DCIS cases are represented by those that are not high-grade but show necrosis. Group 1 DCIS are not high-grade and show no necrosis. The Van Nuys system has been shown to be most reproducible *vis a vis* Holland and Lagios systems (163).

An image analysis-based "automated proliferation index" utilizing nuclear grade and proliferation index (using Ki67 immunostain) offers the promise of a less-subjective approach to grading DCIS (164).

No single grading system for DCIS has been demonstrated to be superior for anticipating successful breast conservation, and none has gained universal acceptance. A consensus conference convened in 1997 did not endorse any single system of classification but recommended that a pathology report for DCIS provides information about the descriptive characteristics considered to be necessary in most grading schemes (138). The three essential elements noted were: nuclear grade, necrosis, and architectural pattern(s). It was observed that the pathology report should reflect the highest nuclear grade but may indicate the relative proportions of grade when there is heterogeneity. Necrosis was defined as the "presence of ghost cells and karyorrhectic debris." Five architectural patterns were identified—"comedo," cribriform, papillary, micropapillary, and solid. It was specified that "comedo" referred "to solid intraepithelial growth within the basement membrane with central (zonal) necrosis. Such lesions are often but not invariably of high nuclear grade." Other elements recommended for inclusion in the diagnosis were lesion "size (extent, distribution)" and margin status. No particular methods for assessing size or margins were suggested.

Extent of DCIS

Extent of DCIS is difficult to determine in most cases. This difficulty is because of the (a) complex three-dimensional nature of the disease, (b) multifocality and multicentricity in some cases, (c) compressibility of breast tissue, (d) inherent

limitations of sampling on NCB specimens, and (e) the presence of DCIS in the initial NCB and in the subsequent excisional biopsy specimen (165,166).

It may be possible to obtain an accurate measurement of DCIS size when DCIS is limited to a single core biopsy. Determination of size of DCIS when it is distributed in multiple, widely separated foci within a NCB or when it involves multiple foci in more than one NCB is imprecise. Kestin et al. (167) were unable to determine tumor size in 58% of the cases they analyzed. For this and other reasons summarized by Schnitt et al. (168), classifications for assessing the prognosis of DCIS that depend on and offer precise size categories may be viewed, at best, as general guidelines rather than as strict criteria for making therapeutic decisions.

It is exceedingly unusual for DCIS to be limited to NCB. This material is not optimal for determining the size of DCIS even if the procedure is performed for calcifications alone and calcifications are no longer present in a follow-up mammogram. NCB cannot provide a single intact sample of DCIS, and it is not feasible to reassemble the foci from multiple NCB to obtain a single measurement.

ANCILLARY STUDIES

Approximately 75% of DCIS lesions express ER. PR expression in DCIS is "somewhat lower" (2). Tamoxifen has been used in receptor-positive disease since NSABP-17and B-24 trials demonstrated reduced ipsilateral breast tumor recurrence as well as reduced development of contralateral primary tumors. It is likely that other SERMs, including anastrozole, will replace tamoxifen for adjuvant endocrine therapy in postmenopausal women with DCIS (169,170).

Forty percent of DCIS lesions demonstrate HER2 positivity—a finding that has therapeutic implications and promise as a treatment option in this set of DCIS, which is typically high-grade and hormone receptor–negative (169,171).

A high rate of concordance in the status of ER, PR, and HER2 between DCIS and subsequent invasive carcinoma (172,173) demonstrates the importance of chemoprevention in patients with hormone-positive and HER2-positive cases of DCIS.

DCIS AND INVASIVE CARCINOMA

The diagnosis of DCIS by NCB cannot be relied upon to exclude the concurrent presence of invasive carcinoma in the affected breast. Several studies have reported the frequency of invasive carcinoma detected by excisional biopsy after a NCB diagnosis of DCIS to be in the range of 15% to 27% (9,77,174–176). In one study, the diagnosis of DCIS was reported to be more reliable with a directional vacuum-assisted biopsy procedure than with an automated NCB system (77).

Ultrastructural studies have detected foci of discontinuity in the basement membranes of ducts with DCIS (177), and similar observations have been reported in tissues studied by immunohistochemistry (178). Breaks in the basement

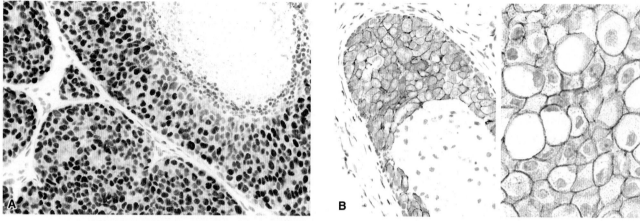

FIGURE 8.60 Ductal Carcinoma In Situ, Biologic Markers. **A:** Nuclear immunoreactivity for estrogen receptor (ER) in cribriform DCIS with intermediate-grade nuclei. Note absence of immunoreactivity in necrotic and degenerating cells. **B:** Strong circumferential membrane immunoreactivity for HER2 in cribriform DCIS with "comedo" necrosis and high-grade nuclei.

membrane are more common when DCIS is of the "comedo" type, that is, it is of a higher grade with central necrosis. In such foci, the neoplastic epithelium appears to protrude from the duct, coming in contact with the stroma while it remains connected to the DCIS (179). This finding often elicits diagnostic uncertainty, reflected in such caveats as "microinvasive carcinoma is suspected" or "microinvasion cannot be ruled out."

Microinvasive Ductal Carcinoma and DCIS

Microinvasive ductal carcinoma is most commonly encountered in association with DCIS and is only rarely detected in the absence of ADH or DCIS in its vicinity (180). When microinvasive ductal carcinoma is present, the carcinoma cells are distributed singly or in small groups that have irregular shapes, with no particular orientation relative to the DCIS, in the periductal stroma **(Fig. 8.60)**. The stroma sometimes appears relatively less dense, and occasionally edematous, at the sites of microinvasion. The detection of microinvasive ductal carcinoma can be difficult when there is a marked inflammatory cell reaction in the periductal region; however, microinvasive ductal carcinoma is typically associated with an inflammatory cell, mainly lymphocytic, reaction. A granulomatous reaction may be elicited at foci of microinvasive ductal carcinoma (181). In this setting, tumor cells can resemble histiocytes, and it may require immunostains for cytokeratin to confirm their presence outside the ducts **(Fig. 8.60)**. Carcinomatous epithelium displaced by needling procedures should not be misinterpreted as intrinsic invasive carcinoma **(Fig. 8.55)**. Hemorrhage, granulation tissue, reactive fibrosis, and hemosiderin deposition typically accompany artifactually displaced epithelia.

Microinvasive ductal carcinoma is more often associated with high-grade DCIS, but it may occur in other types as well (117). There have been several studies that identified features of DCIS in NCB specimens that were predictive of detecting invasive carcinoma in the subsequent lumpectomy. Renshaw (175) reported that invasive carcinoma in the excisional biopsy specimen was significantly associated with cribriform/papillary

architecture and necrosis in DCIS and more than 4 mm of lobular extension. Hou et al. (182) also found lobular extension to be predictive of invasion. Other features of DCIS in a NCB that have been cited as predictive of invasion include the presence of a mass lesion on the imaging study (182–184), high-grade nuclei (185–187), extensive calcifications (185,186), and palpability of the lesion (187). In general, the diagnosis of microinvasive ductal carcinoma carries an excellent prognosis (188,189). It is staged as T1*mic* in the TNM/UICC/AJCC classification system.

Lee et al. (190) developed a nomogram to predict invasive carcinoma in the subsequent excision for DCIS cases diagnosed on NCB. The nomogram included five factors: hormone receptor expression, nuclear grade, extent, structure (cribriform or not), and type of biopsy (vacuum assisted or not). This nomogram could potentially be useful in deciding on axillary sampling.

In light of the foregoing discussion, it is evident that there are instances in which the presence or absence of microinvasion can be difficult to determine with certainty, even with the immunohistochemical reagents currently available. Some guidelines can be suggested—based on experience examining numerous specimens in which microinvasion was a concern.

1. The presence of myoepithelial cells at the perimeter of the lesional glands is the most convincing evidence of noninvasive carcinoma, especially if demonstrated with p63 or p40 immunostain. It is essential to use more than one immunostain, because reactivity is not equally evident with all reagents (191).
2. Absence of demonstrable immunoreactivity with an appropriate marker implies that myoepithelial cells are not present, although they can be severely attenuated and difficult to recognize in some cases. Loss of the myoepithelial cell layer can occur in some DCIS cases. By itself, the absence of myoepithelial cells is not indicative of invasive carcinoma, and the interpretation of this finding depends on the histologic appearance of the lesion in the corresponding H&E section(s).
3. A new "contemporaneous" H&E-stained section must be prepared whenever immunostains are performed for

suspected microinvasive carcinoma (192). This is necessary because the structure of the lesional tissue invariably changes as additional "levels" or "deeper" slides are prepared (193).

4. Cytokeratin immunostains are essential for the evaluation of any focus suspected to be the site of microinvasive carcinoma. It is recommended that at least two different immunostains be used (e.g., CK7, AE1/3) because of the variable reactivity of carcinoma cells with various cytokeratins. Cytokeratin highlights the distribution of epithelial cells, helps in determining extent of invasive carcinoma, and also prevents misinterpretation of histiocytes and endothelial cells.

5. Immunostains for basement membrane components laminin and collagen type IV are occasionally helpful. Absence of reactivity for both components indicates a strong likelihood of invasive carcinoma, especially when coupled with absence of myoepithelial cells.

6. The immunohistochemical demonstration of basal lamina in the absence of myoepithelial cells can rarely present a difficult diagnostic situation. The presence of laminin and collagen type IV favors a diagnosis of in situ carcinoma. However, consideration must be given to the possibility of microglandular adenosis (a lesion in which myoepithelial cells are absent but basement membrane is present) and of the prospect that basal lamina is rarely formed by certain invasive carcinomas (including adenoid cystic carcinoma).

It is essential to use the term *microinvasion* for lesions wherein no single focus of invasive carcinoma exceeds 1 mm in greatest dimension. This definition has been adopted by the TNM staging system with the rubric T1*mic*. When multiple foci of microinvasive carcinoma are present, there is no precise method for estimating their aggregate dimension, and these cases qualify as multifocal microinvasive carcinoma. Invasive foci larger than 1 mm are diagnosed as invasive ductal carcinoma and reported on the basis of their measured size extent (**Figs. 8.61 and 8.62**).

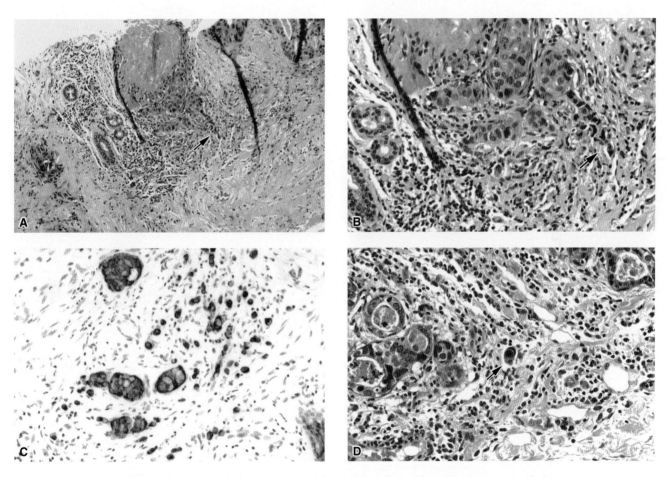

FIGURE 8.61 Ductal Carcinoma In Situ with Microinvasion. Three different patterns of microinvasion found in needle core biopsy specimens are shown. **A–C:** Microinvasion (**A, B**) consists of a linear strand of tumor cells *(arrows)* extending into the stroma surrounded by a lymphocytic reaction. Carcinoma cells in the stroma are highlighted here by the CAM 5.2 cytokeratin immunostain. **D, E:** Another needle core biopsy specimen in which there is an isolated carcinoma cell *(arrow)* in the perilobular stroma (**D**). Invasive carcinoma cells *(arrows)* are highlighted by an immunostain for CAM 5.2 cytokeratin (**E**). **F:** Well-differentiated infiltrating duct carcinoma is present in the stroma *(arrows)* to the left of a large duct with DCIS. **G, H:** Microinvasive carcinoma *(arrow)* surrounded by lymphocytes next to DCIS in a needle core biopsy sample (**G**). Myoepithelium around the DCIS stains brown and the carcinoma cells are red (**H**). The microinvasive carcinoma lacks myoepithelium that is stained brown around the DCIS (triple immunostain).

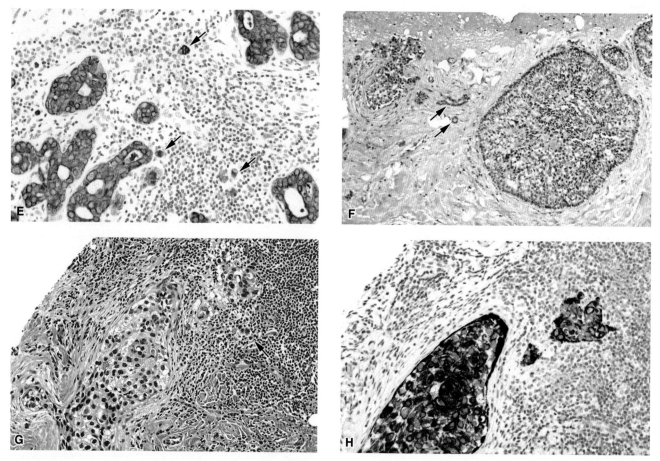

FIGURE 8.61 *(continued)*

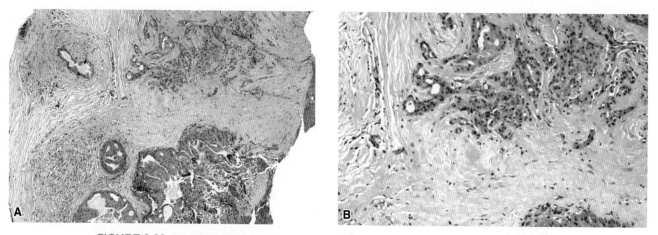

FIGURE 8.62 Ductal Carcinoma In Situ with Invasive Carcinoma. A, B: A 1-mm focus of orderly invasive ductal carcinoma is present in the upper half of this needle core biopsy specimen. DCIS is apparent below the invasive area. **C:** Another specimen that consisted of multiple needle core biopsy samples with extensive DCIS. **D:** The specimen shown in **(C)** contained these areas of solid high-grade DCIS and a 2-mm focus of invasive ductal carcinoma in a marked lymphocytic reaction *(arrow)*. **E:** A magnified view of the invasive ductal carcinoma *(arrows)*. **F:** Groups of invasive carcinoma cells are highlighted by the CAM 5.2 cytokeratin immunostain.

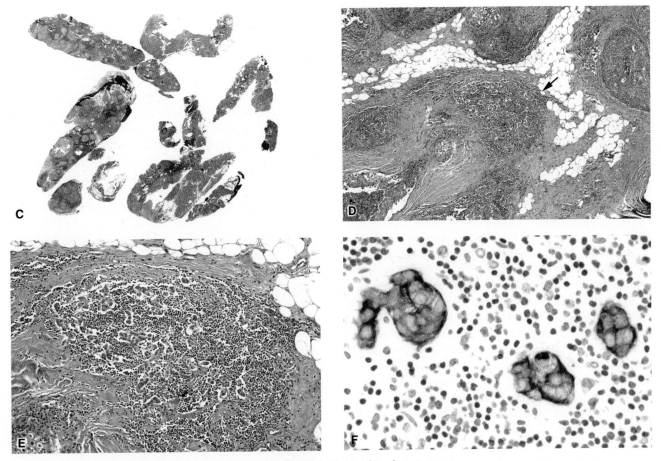

FIGURE 8.62 *(continued)*

de Mascarel et al. (194) subclassified microinvasive ductal carcinoma into type 1 (single tumor cells) and type 2 (clusters of tumor cells). None of the 59 type 1 patients who had axillary lymph nodes removed had nodal metastases. On the other hand, there were nodal metastases in 14 (10%) of the 139 patients with type 2 microinvasive carcinoma who had axillary lymph nodes examined. Distant metastases were reported in 2 (3%) of the 72 patients with type 1 microinvasion and in 12 (7%) of 171 with type 2 microinvasion. The survival of patients with type 1 microinvasive carcinoma was similar to that of women with pure DCIS and significantly better than that of patients with type 2 microinvasion.

Reporting of DCIS on NCB

DCIS is the stage of carcinoma at its most curable stage. The NCB pathology report of DCIS should include the following: nuclear grade (that is, low, intermediate, or high), architectural pattern (that is, cribriform, micropapillary, flat micropapillary/ clinging, papillary, or solid), necrosis (that is, incipient/punctate or "comedo"), and an estimation of extent (195).

Given the increasing body of evidence indicating a therapeutic benefit for chemoprevention, ER, PR, and HER2 testing of DCIS in NCB has assumed considerable clinical importance (196). Results of ER and PR testing should record the proportion (between 0% and 100%) and intensity (weak, moderate, or strong) of reactivity.

Immunohistochemical testing for HER2 should be reported on a scale of 0 to 3+, as per ASCO-CAP guidelines (197).

The results of other biologic markers including those related to cell cycle regulation, apoptosis, and angiogenesis are novel in the context of DCIS and are currently of investigational interest (198).

Genetics of Ductal Proliferative Lesions and Ductal Carcinoma In Situ

Consistent chromosomal aberrations have not been found in the usual type of DH. The characteristic genetic alterations in ADH and low-grade DCIS have not been found in UDH. Thus, at least from the molecular level perspective, UDH could be regarded as a "dead end" process—or a marker of, but not a direct precursor, of more significant lesions (199). Cumulative evidence suggests that the spectrum of CCLs (including FEA) are putative precursors of ADH and low-grade DCIS, because loss of 16q is common in CCLs as well as in ADH in low-grade DCIS (200). DCIS and the associated invasive carcinomas, of all grades, can be similar in their respective genetic makeups, although considerable intratumoral genetic heterogeneity is present in some DCIS. It has been speculated that "the process of progression to invasive disease may constitute an 'evolutionary bottleneck,' resulting in the selection of subsets of tumor cells with specific genetic and/or epigenetic aberrations" (201).

A comprehensive description of the cytogenetic and molecular genetic aspects of DCIS appears in *Rosen's Breast Pathology,* fourth edition (202), and elsewhere (157).

Principles of Management of DCIS

A detailed discussion of controversies surrounding the management of DCIS appears in the Introduction to this book. A synopsis of the principles for the management of DCIS appears below; nevertheless, it should be noted that final management decisions on DCIS cases ought not to be made on the basis of results of the NCB but should await pathologic findings in the subsequently performed excisional biopsy or mastectomy.

In current clinical practice, the great majority of DCIS is diagnosed on NCB performed to evaluate mammographically detected calcifications and/or other abnormality, and its management is optimally planned after an excisional biopsy of the lesional area is subsequently performed. The management options are optimally offered by a team of specialists, and final decision is rendered after consultation with the patient. The management team includes the medical oncologist, surgeon, radiation oncologist, and pathologist. In some cases, reconstructive surgeons and genetic counselors are included in the team. The treatment plan is ideally "personalized," that is, based on specific clinical and pathologic findings. Important considerations include the manner of clinical presentation (e.g., palpable or imaging abnormality), extent on imaging and as measured macroscopically or microscopically (when possible), margin status, and histologic features of the DCIS including nuclear grade, growth pattern (e.g., solid, cribriform, micropapillary, solid papillary, etc.), and the presence or absence of necrosis. Ancillary studies, ranging from ER testing to genomic assays, play an increasingly important role in customizing management.

Numerous studies cited indicate that margin status and the biologic characteristics of DCIS represented histologically by nuclear grade and the presence or absence of necrosis are the most important predictors of local recurrence after breast conservation with or without radiotherapy. Although the definitions of "negative" or "close" margins may vary among experts, most would agree that the goal of a lumpectomy is to resect all of the DCIS (that is, evident either clinically or on imaging) with no overt involvement of the margin ("no tumor at ink"). Biologic characteristics, at least partially reflected in the histologic appearance of DCIS, have a complex influence on the success of treatment by affecting the rate of growth (and to some extent the time to detection of clinical recurrences) and radiosensitivity of residual DCIS after lumpectomy. Consequently, it is possible for patients with comparable amounts of incompletely excised residual high-grade ("comedo") and low-grade (cribriform) DCIS who receive the same treatment to have similar absolute risks for breast recurrence, but they may differ in time to clinical detection of recurrence, especially of invasive lesions, and in responsiveness to radiotherapy or to a SERM, such as tamoxifen, raloxifen, or toremifene.

Risk factors for noninvasive and invasive local recurrence may differ. The former has been associated with symptomatic presentation, and the latter has been shown to be associated with larger extent, margin status, and African–American race (203).

Retrospective and prospective randomized studies have demonstrated that radiotherapy after excisional surgery reduces the chance of recurrence in the breast by about 50%. The degree to which a reduced frequency of breast recurrence contributes to overall survival remains to be determined for patients with DCIS. The possibility that there could be a survival advantage conferred by reducing breast recurrences is suggested by a meta-analysis of randomized studies of radiotherapy and breast conservation in women with invasive breast carcinoma that detected this beneficial effect. The addition of SERM to breast conservation therapy reduces breast recurrences in women with ER-positive DCIS.

Radiotherapy is usually indicated for any of the following circumstances: high-grade DCIS, close margins (variously described as 10 mm or less), and younger (<50 years) patients. SERM therapy can be considered for ER-positive DCIS. Omitting radiotherapy is an option for some women older than 50 years with a widely clear margin (variously defined as more than 10 mm) and with low-grade histology. This type of DCIS is likely to be ER-positive and therefore amenable to adjuvant use of SERM.

Various imaging techniques, including MRI, are an essential component in the clinical follow-up of women treated by breast conservation with or without radiotherapy and/or SERMs. Attention should be paid to the follow-up of the contralateral breast, especially in women with ADH or LCIS coexisting with DCIS.

Some patients may choose mastectomy even if they are candidates for breast conservation. Typically, a mastectomy is preferable for patients with such widespread DCIS that negative margins cannot be achieved with cosmetically acceptable results. Many of these patients have widely dispersed "suspicious" calcifications on mammography. Bilateral mastectomy is an option that is increasingly being exercised in younger women who have high-grade DCIS (204) or bilateral widespread (multifocal or multicentric) disease, or those who are regarded as "high risk" (especially those are genetically predisposed to breast carcinoma or have a strong family history).

In general, a lumpectomy with or without radiation will suffice for most women with DCIS limited to a single focus, and if the margins are negative, and if the lesion is not of the "comedo" type (with high-grade nuclei and necrosis), and it is small (variously defined as less than 1.0 cm or less than 2.5 cm). Radiation after lumpectomy is recommended regardless of size when the DCIS is of high-grade nuclei with necrosis, or is widespread multifocal or multicentric), or is margin-positive.

As discussed earlier in this chapter, the management of ADH and low-grade DCIS is evolving. Although most would continue to recommend excision for ADH (205), some have questioned the "necessity and benefit" of surgery for low-grade DCIS (206).

Axillary lymph node dissection is not indicated in most of the patients with DCIS. A sentinel lymph node biopsy or "low" axillary lymph node dissection may be performed in the course of a lumpectomy or mastectomy for high-grade and/or palpable DCIS (207).

Treatment for the majority of patients with microinvasive ductal carcinoma, previously described in the literature, has been mastectomy. The overall outcome was relatively favorable after mastectomy, but the studies were not directly comparable because of differing criteria for defining microinvasion. Patients treated by breast conservation were described in several reports with results indicating that this was equally effective as mastectomy. These and other published reports indicate that the presence of microinvasion, as variously defined in the past or as currently described in the TNM staging system (T1*mic*), probably has minimal independent impact on the effectiveness of conservation therapy for local control. The characteristics of the DCIS that are associated with microinvasive carcinoma, such as formation of a palpable mass, high-grade nuclei, and necrosis are crucial determinants for appropriate treatment. The significance of multiple foci of microinvasive carcinoma is yet to be determined. The finding of microinvasive carcinoma usually leads to sentinel lymph node biopsy prior to consideration of systemic therapy.

The *University of Southern California/Van Nuys Prognostic Index* (USC/VNPI) is a theoretically simple scoring method that can be used to stratify patients with regards to risk of local recurrence. The USC/VNPI uses age, grade, extent, margin width, and necrosis—as evaluated in lumpectomy specimens (208,209). It should be noted that the scheme now referred to as the USC/NPI Index has undergone revisions involving inclusions and/or exclusions of various parameters or combinations of parameters since its initial presentation more than 20 years ago as the Van Nuys Prognostic Index (210,211). As a consequence, the validity and usefulness of various versions of this scheme, including that currently proposed (209) for recommending treatment is questionable, as evidenced by the authors' 2010 admonition that the recommendations in this article represent substantial changes from those previously published" (208). The authors also noted more recently that there is no difference in mortality rate regardless of which treatment is chosen" (209).

Rudloff et al. (212) developed the Memorial Sloan-Kettering Cancer Center's Nomogram, to predict ipsilateral local recurrence in DCIS cases. Ten independent predictive factors were identified: age, personal/family history, presentation (clinical vs. imaging), nuclear grade, necrosis, margins, adjuvant endocrine treatment, adjuvant radiotherapy, number of excisions, and duration of treatment period. The nomogram was internally validated, but Yi et al. (213) evaluated Rudloff et al.'s nomogram in a cohort of 794 DCIS patients at M.D. Anderson Cancer Center and found that the 5- and 10-year prediction for recurrence was "imperfect" and "limited."

The quest to reliably identify a subgroup of DCIS patients who could benefit from less-aggressive management has brought about the development of the molecular-based *Oncotype® DCIS score*. Using a validated technique, the 12-gene signature score independently predicts the risk of ipsilateral recurrence of DCIS or invasive carcinoma. The 12 genes include 5 that are related to proliferation: Ki67, STK15, survivin, cyclin B1, and MYBL2. The other seven include PR and GSTM1 genes as well as five reference genes. Solin (214) reported that for patients with a low, intermediate, and high DCIS score, the 10-year risk of developing either an ipsilateral carcinoma (DCIS or invasive carcinoma) were 10.6%, 26.7%, and 25.9%, respectively; and for invasive carcinoma were 3.7%, 12.3%, and 19.2%, respectively. The Oncotype DCIS score provides additional "personalized" information on DCIS that can affect management (215), and it has also been shown to provide independent information on the risk of local recurrence beyond those clinicopathological variables that are usually assessed, such as size, age, grade, necrosis, multifocality, and subtype (216).

The declining rate of recurrence of DCIS after breast-conserving surgery over the last 30 years can be attributed not only to earlier detection, attainment of negative margins, and use of adjuvant therapies but also due to improved pathologic assessment (217).

REFERENCES

1. Connolly JL, Schnitt SJ. Benign breast disease: resolved and unresolved issues. *Cancer*. 1993;71:1187–1189.
2. Lakhani SR, Ellis IO, Schnitt SR, et al., eds. *WHO/IARC Classification of Tumours of the Breast*. Vol 4. 4 ed. Lyon, France: World Health Organization; 2012.
3. Bodian CA, Perzin KH, Lattes R, et al. Reproducibility and validity of pathologic classifications of benign breast disease and implications for clinical applications. *Cancer*. 1993;71:3908–3913.
4. Choi DX, Eaton AA, Olcese C, et al. Blurry boundaries: do epithelial borderline lesions of the breast and ductal carcinoma in situ have similar rates of subsequent invasive cancer? *Ann Surg Oncol*. 2013;20:1302–1310.
5. Rosai J. Borderline epithelial lesions of the breast. *Am J Surg Pathol*. 1991;15:209–221.
6. Schnitt SJ, Connolly JL, Tavassoli FA, et al. Interobserver reproducibility in the diagnosis of ductal proliferative breast lesions using standardized criteria. *Am J Surg Pathol*. 1992;16:1133–1143.
7. Palli D, Galli M, Bianchi S, et al. Reproducibility of histological diagnosis of breast lesions: results of a panel in Italy. *Eur J Cancer*. 1996;32A:603–607.
8. Helvie MA, Hessler C, Frank TS, et al. Atypical hyperplasia of the breast: mammographic appearance and histologic correlation. *Radiology*. 1991;179:759–764.
9. Jackman RJ, Nowels KW, Shepard MJ, et al. Stereotaxic large-core needle biopsy of 450 nonpalpable breast lesions with surgical correlation in lesions with cancer or atypical hyperplasia. *Radiology*. 1994;193:91–95.
10. Liberman L, Cohen MA, Abramson AF, et al. Atypical ductal hyperplasia diagnosed at stereotaxic core biopsy of breast lesions: an indication for surgical biopsy. *AJR Am J Roentgenol*. 1995;164:1111–1113.
11. Bodian CA, Perzin KH, Lattes R, et al. Prognostic significance of benign proliferative breast disease. *Cancer*. 1993;71:3896–3907.
12. Page DL, Rogers LW. Combined histologic and cytologic criteria for the diagnosis of mammary atypical ductal hyperplasia. *Hum Pathol*. 1992;23:1095–1097.
13. Rubin E, Visscher DW, Alexander RW, et al. Proliferative disease and atypia in biopsies performed for nonpalpable lesions detected mammographically. *Cancer*. 1988;61:2077–2082.
14. Stomper PC, Cholewinski SP, Penetrante RB, et al. Atypical hyperplasia, frequency and mammographic and pathologic relationships in excisional biopsies guided by mammography and clinical examination. *Radiology*. 1993;189:667–671.
15. Villa A, Tagliafico A, Chiesa F, et al. Atypical ductal hyperplasia diagnosed at 11-gauge vacuum-assisted breast biopsy performed on suspicious clustered microcalcifications: could patients without residual microcalcifications be managed conservatively? *AJR Am J Roentgenol*. 2011;197:1012–1018.
16. Nguyen CV, Albarracin CT, Whitman GJ, et al. Atypical ductal hyperplasia in directional vacuum-assisted biopsy of breast microcalcifications: considerations for surgical excision. *Ann Surg Oncol*. 2011;18:752–761.

17. Calhoun BC, Collins LC. Recommendations for excision following core needle biopsy of the breast: a contemporary evaluation of the literature. *Histopathology*. 2016;68:138–151.

18. Orel SG, Rosen M, Miles C, et al. MR imaging guided 9-gauge vacuum assisted core needle breast biopsy: initial experience. *Radiology*. 2006;238:54–61.

19. Perlet C, Heywang-Kobrunner SH, Heinig A, et al. Magnetic resonance-guided, vacuum-assisted breast biopsy: results from a European multicentre study of 538 lesions. *Cancer*. 2006;106:982–990.

20. Liberman L, Holland AE, Marjan D, et al. Underestimation of atypical ductal hyperpasia at MRI-guided 9-gauge vacuum-assisted breast biopsy. *AJR Am J Roentgenol*. 2007;188:684–690.

21. Rosen PP, Cantrell B, Mullen DL, et al. Juvenile papillomatosis (Swiss cheese disease) of the breast. *Am J Surg Pathol*. 1980;4:3–12.

22. Wilson M, Cranor ML, Rosen PP. Papillary duct hyperpasia of the breast in children and young women. *Mod Pathol*. 1993;6:570–574.

23. Arapantoni-Dadioti P, Panayiotides J, Georgakila H, et al. Significance of intracytoplasmic lumina in the differential diagnosis between epithelial hyperplasia and carcinoma in situ of the breast. *Breast Dis*. 1996;9:277–282.

24. Ozaki D, Kondo Y. Comparative morphometric studies of benign and malignant intraductal proliferative lesions of the breast by computerized image analysis. *Hum Pathol*. 1995;26:1109–1113.

25. Ohuchi N, Abe R, Takahashi T, et al. Three-dimensional atypical structure in intraductal carcinoma differentiating from papilloma and papillomatosis of the breast. *Breast Cancer Res Treat*. 1985;5:57–65.

26. Kővári B, Szász AM, Kulka J, et al. Evaluation of p40 as a myoepithelial marker in different breast lesions. *Pathobiology*. 2015;82:166–171.

27. Barbareschi M, Pecciarini L, Gangi MG, et al. p63, a p53 homologue, is a selective nuclear marker of myoepithelial cells of the human breast. *Am J Surg Pathol*. 2001;25:1054–1060.

28. Kalof AN, Tam D, Beatty B, et al. Immunostaining patterns of myoepithelial cells in breast lesions: a comparison of CD10 and smooth muscle myosin heavy chain. *J Clin Pathol*. 2004;57:625–629.

29. Moritani S, Kushima R, Sugihara H, et al. Availability of CD10 immunohistochemistry as a marker of breast myoepithelial cells on paraffin sections. *Mod Pathol*. 2002;15:397–405.

30. Lerwill M. Current practical applications of diagnostic immunohistochemistry in breast pathology. *Am J Surg Pathol*. 2004;28:1076–1091.

31. Tramm T, Kim JY, Tavassoli FA. Diminished number or complete loss of myoepithelial cells associated with metaplastic and neoplastic apocrine lesions of the breast. *Am J Surg Pathol*. 2011;35:202–211.

32. Liu H. Application of immunohistochemistry in breast pathology: a review and update. *Arch Pathol Lab Med*. 2014;138:1629–1642.

33. Lee AH. Use of immunohistochemistry in the diagnosis of problematic breast lesions. *J Clin Pathol*. 2013;66:471–477.

34. Reisenbichler ES, Ross JR, Hameed O. The clinical use of a p63/cytokeratin7/18/cytokeratin 5/14 antibody cocktail in diagnostic breast pathology. *Ann Diagn Pathol*. 2014;18:313–318.

35. Tavassoli FA, Norris HJ. A comparison of the results of long-term follow-up for atypical intraductal carcinoma of the breast. *Cancer*. 1990;65:518–529.

36. Tavassoli FA. Intraductal hyperplasias, ordinary and atypical. In: Tavassoli FA, ed. *Pathology of the Breast*. New York, NY: Elsevier Science Publishing; 1992:155–191.

37. Fisher ER, Costantino J, Fisher B, et al. Pathologic findings from the National Surgical Adjuvant Breast Project (NSABP) Protocol B-17: intraductal carcinoma (ductal carcinoma in situ). *Cancer*. 1995;75:1310–1319.

38. Pinder SE, Reis-Filho JS. Non-operative breast pathology. *J Clin Pathol*. 2007;60:1297–1299.

39. Lubelsky SM, Bane AL, Shin V, et al. Columnar cell lesions and flat epithelial atypia: incidence and significance in a mammographically screened population. *Mod Pathol*. 2005;18(suppl):41A.

40. Rosen PP. Columnar cell hyperplasia is associated with lobular carcinoma in situ and tubular carcinoma. *Am J Surg Pathol*. 1999;23:1561.

41. Rosen PP. Ductal hyperplasia: ordinary and atypical. In: Rosen PP, ed. *Breast Pathology*. 2nd ed. Philadelphia, PA: Lippincott Williams & Wilkins; 2001:215–223.

42. Tavassoli FA, Hoefler H, Rosai J, et al. Intraductal proliferative lesions. In: Tavassoli FA, Devilee P, eds. *Pathology and Genetics of Tumours of the Breast and Female Genital Organs*. Lyon, France: IARC Press; 2003:63–67.

43. Oyama T, Maluf H, Koerner F. Atypical cystic lobules: an early stage in the formation of low-grade ductal carcinoma in situ. *Virchows Arch*. 1999;435:413–421.

44. Goldstein NS, Lacerna M, Vicini F. Cancerization of lobules and atypical ductal hyperplasia adjacent to ductal carcinoma in situ of the breast. *Am J Clin Pathol*. 1998;110:357–367.

45. Fraser JL, Raza S, Chorny K, et al. Columnar alteration with prominent apical snouts and secretions: a spectrum of changes frequently present in breast biopsies performed for microcalcifications. *Am J Surg Pathol*. 1998;22:1521–1527.

46. Fraser JL, Pliss N, Connolly JL, et al. Immunophenotype of columnar alteration with prominent apical snouts and secretions (CAPSS). *Mod Pathol*. 2000;13:21A.

47. Brandt SM, Young GQ, Hoda SA. The "Rosen Triad": tubular carcinoma, lobular carcinoma in situ, and columnar cell lesions. *Adv Anat Pathol*. 2008;15:140–146.

48. Prowler VL, Joh JE, Acs G, et al. Surgical excision of pure flat epithelial atypia identified on core needle breast biopsy. *Breast*. 2014;23:352–356.

49. Uzoaru I, Morgan BR, Liu ZG, et al. Flat epithelial atypia with and without atypical ductal hyperplasia: to re-excise or not: results of a 5-year prospective study. *Virchows Arch*. 2012;461:419–423.

50. Bianchi S, Bendinelli B, Castellano I, et al. Morphological parameters of flat epithelial atypia (FEA) in stereotactic vacuum-assisted needle core biopsies do not predict the presence of malignancy on subsequent surgical excision. *Virchows Arch*. 2012;461:405–417.

51. Khoumais NA, Scaranelo AM, Moshonov H, et al. Incidence of breast cancer in patients with pure flat epithelial atypia diagnosed at core-needle biopsy of the breast. *Ann Surg Oncol*. 2013;20:133–138.

52. Peres A, Barranger E, Becette V, et al. Rates of upgrade to malignancy for 271 cases of flat epithelial atypia (FEA) diagnosed by breast core biopsy. *Breast Cancer Res Treat*. 2012;133:659–666.

53. Rajan S, Sharma N, Dall BJ, et al. What is the significance of flat epithelial atypia and what are the management implications? *J Clin Pathol*. 2011;64:1001–1004.

54. Biggar MA, Kerr KM, Erzetich LM, et al. Columnar cell change with atypia (flat epithelial atypia) on breast core biopsy-outcomes following open excision. *Breast J*. 2012;18:578–581.

55. Noel J-C, Fayt I, Fernandes-Aguillar S, et al. Proliferating activity in columnar cell lesions of the breast. *Virchows Arch*. 2006;449:617–621.

56. Dabbs DJ, Carter G, Fudge M, et al. Molecular alterations in columnar cell lesions of the breast. *Mod Pathol*. 2006;19:344–349.

57. Kaneko M, Arihiro K, Takeshima Y, et al. Loss of heterozygosity and microsatellite instability in epithelial hyperplasia of the breast. *J Exp Ther Oncol*. 2002;2:9–18.

58. Seo M, Chang JM, Kim WH, et al. Columnar cell lesions without atypia initially diagnosed on breast needle biopsies: is imaging follow-up enough? *AJR Am J Roentgenol*. 2013;201:928–934.

59. Verschuur-Maes AH, van Deurzen CH, Monninkhof EM, et al. Columnar cell lesions on breast needle biopsies: is surgical excision necessary? A systematic review. *Ann Surg*. 2012;255:259–265.

60. Schnitt SJ, Vincent-Salomon A. Columnar cell lesions of the breast. *Adv Anat Pathol*. 2003;10:113–124.

61. Guerra-Wallace MM, Christensen WN, White RL. A retrospective study of columnar alteration with prominent apical snouts and secretions and the association with cancer. *Am J Surg*. 2004;188:395–398.

62. Chivukula M, Bhargava R, Tseng G, et al. Clinicopathologic implications of 'flat epithelial atypia' in core needle biopsy specimens of the breast. *Am J Clin Pathol*. 2009;131:802–808.

63. Piubello Q, Parisi A, Eccher A, et al. Flat epithelial atypia on core needle biopsy: which is the right management? *Am J Surg Pathol*. 2009;33:1078–1084.

64. Senetta R, Campanino PP, Mariscotti G, et al. Columnar cell lesions associated with breast calcifications on vacuum-assisted core biopsies: clinical, radiographic, and histological correlations. *Mod Pathol*. 2009;22:762–769.

65. Collins LC, Achacoso NA, Nekhlyudov L, et al. Clinical and pathologic features of ductal carcinoma in situ associated with the presence of flat epithelial atypia: an analysis of 543 patients. *Mod Pathol.* 2007;20:1149–1155.

66. Abdel-Fatah TM, Powe DG, Hodi Z, et al. High frequency of coexistence of columnar cell lesions, lobular neoplasia, and low grade ductal carcinoma in situ with invasive tubular carcinoma and invasive lobular carcinoma. *Am J Surg Pathol.* 2007;31:416–426.

67. Sahoo S, Recant WM. Triad of columnar cell alteration, lobular carcinoma in situ, and tubular carcinoma of the breast. *Breast J.* 2005;11:140–142.

68. Turashvili G, Hayes M, Gilks B, et al. Are columnar cell lesions the earliest histologically detectable non-obligate precursor of breast cancer? *Virchows Arch.* 2008;452:589–598.

69. Boulos FI, Dupont WD, Simpson JF, et al. Histologic associations and long-term cancer risk in columnar cell lesions of the breast: a retrospective cohort and a nested core-control study. *Cancer.* 2008;113:2415–2421.

70. Tocino I, Garcia BM, Carter D. Surgical biopsy findings in patients with atypical hyperplasia diagnosed by stereotaxic core needle biopsy. *Ann Surg Oncol.* 1996;3:483–488.

71. Jackman RJ, Birdwell RL, Ikeda DM. Atypical ductal hyperplasia: can some lesions be defined as probably benign after stereotactic 11-gauge vacuum-assisted biopsy, eliminating the recommendation for surgical excision? *Radiology.* 2002;224:548–554.

72. Maganini RO, Klem DA, Huston BJ, et al. Upgrade rate of core biopsy-determined atypical ductal hyperplasia by open excisional biopsy. *Am J Surg.* 2001;182:355–358.

73. Winchester DJ, Bernstein JR, Jeske JM, et al. Upstaging of atypical ductal hyperplasia after vacuum-assisted 11-gauge stereotactic core needle biopsy. *Arch Surg.* 2003;138:619–623.

74. Brem RF, Behrndt VS, Sanow L, et al. Atypical ductal hyperplasia: histologic underestimation of carcinoma in tissue harvested from impalpable breast lesions using 11-gauge stereotactically guided directional vacuum-assisted biopsy. *AJR Am J Roentgenol.* 1999;172:1405–1407.

75. Moore MM, Hargett CW, Hanks JB, et al. Association of breast cancer with the finding of atypical ductal hyperplasia at core breast biopsy. *Ann Surg.* 1997;225:726–731.

76. Gadzala DE, Cederbom GJ, Bolton JS, et al. Appropriate management of atypical ductal hyperplasia diagnosed by stereotactic core needle breast biopsy. *Ann Surg Oncol.* 1977;4:283–286.

77. Burbank F. Stereotactic breast biopsy of atypical ductal hyperplasia and ductal carcinoma in situ lesions: improved accuracy with directional, vacuum-assisted biopsy. *Radiology.* 1997;202:843–847.

78. Renshaw AA, Cartagena N, Schenkman RH, et al. Atypical ductal hyperplasia in breast core needle biopsies. *Am J Clin Pathol.* 2001;116:92–96.

79. Wagoner MJ, Laronga C, Acs G. Extent and histologic pattern of atypical ductal hyperplasia present on needle core biopsy specimens of the breast can predict ductal carcinoma in situ in subsequent excision. *Am J Clin Pathol.* 2009;131:112–121.

80. Kodlin D, Winger EE, Morgenstern NL, et al. Chronic mastopathy and breast cancer: a follow-up study. *Cancer.* 1977;39:2603–2607.

81. Dupont WD, Page DL. Breast cancer risk associated with proliferative disease, age at first birth, and family history of breast cancer. *Am J Epidemiol.* 1987;1225:769–779.

82. Krieger N, Hiatt RA. Risk of breast cancer after benign breast diseases: variation by histologic type, degree of atypia, age at biopsy, and length of follow-up. *Am J Epidemiol.* 1992;135:619–631.

83. Davis HH, Simons M, Davis JB. Cystic disease of the breast: relationship to carcinoma. *Cancer.* 1964;17:957–978.

84. Page DL, DuPont WD, Rogers LW, et al. Atypical hyperplastic lesions of the female breast: a long-term follow-up study. *Cancer.* 1985;55:2698–2708.

85. Connolly J, Schnitt S, London S, et al. Both atypical lobular hyperplasia (ALH) and atypical ductal hyperplasia (ADH) predict for bilateral breast cancer risk. *Lab Invest.* 1992;66:13A.

86. Carter CL, Corle DK, Micozzi MS, et al. A prospective study of the development of breast cancer in 16,692 women with benign breast disease. *Am J Epidemiol.* 1988;128:467–477.

87. London SJ, Connolly JL, Schnitt SJ, et al. A prospective study of benign breast disease and the risk of breast cancer. *JAMA.* 1992;267:941–944.

88. Dupont WD, Page DL. Risk factors for breast cancer in women with proliferative breast disease. *N Engl J Med.* 1985;312:146–151.

89. Ma L, Boyd NF. Atypical hyperplasia and breast cancer risk: a critique. *Cancer Causes Control.* 1992;3:517–525.

90. Jensen RA, Page DL, Dupont WD, et al. Invasive breast cancer risk in women with sclerosing adenosis. *Cancer.* 1989;64:1977–1983.

91. Bernstein L, Patel AV, Ursin G, et al. Lifetime recreational exercise activity and breast cancer risk among black women and white women. *J Natl Cancer Inst.* 2005;97:1671–1679.

92. McGhan LJ, Pockaj BA, Wasif N, et al. Atypical ductal hyperplasia on core biopsy: an automatic trigger for excisional biopsy? *Ann Surg Oncol.* 2012;19:3264–3269.

93. McLaughlin CT, Neal CH, Helvie MA. Is the upgrade rate of atypical ductal hyperplasia diagnosed by core needle biopsy of calcifications different for digital and film-screen mammography? *AJR Am J Roentgenol.* 2014;203:917–922.

94. Neal L, Sandhu NP, Hieken TJ, et al. Diagnosis and management of benign, atypical, and indeterminate breast lesions detected on core needle biopsy. *Mayo Clin Proc.* 2014;89:536–547.

95. Mesurolle B, Perez JCH, Azzumea F, et al. Atypical ductal hyperplasia diagnosed at sonographically guided core needle biopsy: frequency, final surgical outcome, and factors associated with underestimation. *AJR Am J Roentgenol.* 2014;202:1389–1394.

96. Ely KA, Carter BA, Jensen RA, et al. Core biopsy of the breast with atypical ductal hyperplasia: a probabilistic approach to reporting. *Am J Surg Pathol.* 2001;25:1017–1021.

97. de Mascarel I, Brouste V, Asad-Syed M, et al. All atypia diagnosed at stereotactic vacuum-assisted breast biopsy do not need surgical excision. *Mod Pathol.* 2011;24:1198–1206.

98. Khoury T, Chen X, Wang D, et al. Nomogram to predict the likelihood of upgrade of atypical ductal hyperplasia diagnosed on a core needle biopsy in mammographically detected lesions. *Histopathology.* 2015;67:106–120.

99. Visscher DW, Frost MH, Hartmann LC, et al. Clinicopathologic features of breast cancers that develop in women with previous benign breast disease. *Cancer.* 2016;122:378–385.

100. Hartmann LC, Degnim AC, Santen RJ, et al: Atypical hyperplasia of the breast—risk assessment and management options. *N Engl J Med.* 2015;372:78–89.

101. U.S. Department of Health & Human Services; National Institutes of Health. National Institutes of Health State-of-the-Science Conference Statement: diagnosis and management of ductal carcinoma in situ (DCIS). https://consensus.nih.gov/.

102. Siegel RL, Miller KD, Jemal A. Cancer statistics, 2016. *CA Cancer J Clin.* 2016;66:7–30.

103. Kerlikowske K. Epidemiology of ductal carcinoma in situ. *J Natl Cancer Inst Monogr.* 2010;2010(41):139–141.

104. Roses RE, Arun BK, Lari SA, et al. Ductal carcinoma-in-situ of the breast with subsequent distant metastasis and death. *Ann Surg Oncol.* 2011;18:2873–2878.

105. Verbeek ALM, Hendriks JHCL, Holland R, et al. Reduction of breast cancer mortality through mass screening with modern mammography: first results of the Nijmegen Project 1975–1981. *Lancet.* 1984;1:1222–1224.

106. Ciatto S, Cataliotti L, Distante V. Nonpalpable lesions detected with mam-mography: review of 512 consecutive cases. *Radiology.* 1987;165:99–102.

107. Dershaw DD, Abramson A, Kinne DW. Ductal carcinoma in situ: mammo-graphic findings and clinical implications. *Radiology.* 1989;170:411–415.

108. Stomper PC, Connolly JL, Meyer JE, et al. Clinically occult ductal carcinoma in situ detected with mammography: analysis of 100 cases with radiologic-pathologic correlation. *Radiology.* 1989;172:235–241.

109. Tse GM, Tan PH, Pang AL, et al. Calcification in breast lesions: pathologists' perspective. *J Clin Pathol.* 2008;61:145–151.

110. Holland R, Hendriks JHCL, Verbeek ALM, et al. Extent, distribution, and mammographic/histological correlations of breast ductal carcinoma in situ. *Lancet.* 1990;335:519–522.

111. Lagios MD. Multicentricity of breast carcinoma demonstrated by routine correlated subgross and radiographic examination. *Cancer.* 1977;40:1726–1734.

112. Hayes BD, Brodie C, O'Doherty A, et al. High-grade histologic features of DCIS are associated with R5 rather than R3 calcifications in breast screening mammography. *Breast J.* 2013;19:319–324.

113. Stomper PC, Connolly JL. Ductal carcinoma in situ of the breast: correlation between mammographic calcification and tumor subtype. *AJR Am J Roentgenol.* 1992;159:483–485.

114. Zunzunegui R, Chung MA, Oruwari J, et al. Casting-type calcifications with invasion and high-grade ductal carcinoma in situ: a more aggressive disease? *Arch Surg.* 2003;138:537–540.

115. Evans A, Pinder S, Wilson R, et al. Ductal carcinoma in situ of the breast: correlation between mammographic and pathologic findings. *AJR Am J Roentgenol.* 1994;162:1307–1311.

116. Evans AJ, Pinder SE, Ellis IO, et al. Correlations between the mammographic features of ductal carcinoma in situ (DCIS) and c-erb-s oncogene expression. *Clin Radiol.* 1994;49:559–562.

117. Patchefsky AS, Schwartz GF, Finkelstein SD, et al. Heterogeneity of intraductal carcinoma of the breast. *Cancer.* 1989;63:731–741.

118. Rauch GM, Kuerer HM, Scoggins ME, et al. Clinicopathologic, mammographic, and sonographic features in 1,187 patients with pure ductal carcinoma in situ of the breast by estrogen receptor status. *Breast Cancer Res Treat.* 2013;139:639–647.

119. Scoggins ME, Fox PS, Kuerer HM, et al. Correlation between sonographic findings and clinicopathologic and biologic features of pure ductal carcinoma in situ in 691 patients. *AJR Am J Roentgenol.* 2015;204:878–888.

120. Baur A, Bahrs SD, Speck S, et al. Breast MRI of pure ductal carcinoma in situ: sensitivity of diagnosis and influence of lesion characteristics. *Eur J Radiol.* 2013;82:1731–1737.

121. Pilewskie M, Morrow M. Applications for breast magnetic resonance imaging. *Surg Oncol Clin N Am.* 2014;23:431–449.

122. Menell JH, Morris EA, Dershaw DD, et al. Determination of the presence and extent of pure ductal carcinoma in situ by mammography and magnetic resonance imaging. *Breast J.* 2005;11:382–390.

123. Manion E, Brock JE, Raza S, et al. MRI-guided breast needle core biopsies: pathologic features of newly diagnosed malignancies. *Breast J.* 2014;20:453–460.

124. Gilles R, Zafrani B, Guinebretiere J-M, et al. Ductal carcinoma in situ: MR imaging-histopathologic correlation. *Radiology.* 1995;196:415–419.

125. Orel S, Schnall M, Livolsi V, et al. Suspicious breast lesions: MR imaging with radiologic-pathologic correlation. *Radiology.* 1994;190:485–493.

126. Heywang-Kobrunner S. Contrast-enhanced magnetic resonance imaging of the breast. *Invest Radiol.* 1994;29:94–104.

127. Orel SG, Mendonca MH, Reynolds C, et al. MR imaging of ductal carcinoma in situ. *Radiology.* 1997;202:413–420.

128. Pediconi F, Catalano C, Roselli A, et al. Contrast-enhanced MR mammography for evaluation of the contralateral breast in patients with diagnosed unilateral breast cancer or high risk lesions. *Radiology.* 2007;243:670–680.

129. Cheng L, Al-Kaisi NK, Liu AY, et al. The results of intraoperative consultations in 181 ductal carcinomas in situ of the breast. *Cancer.* 1997;80:75–79.

130. Rosen PP. Frozen section diagnosis of breast lesions: recent experience with 556 consecutive biopsies. *Ann Surg.* 1978;187:17–19.

131. Rosen PP, Senie R, Schottenfeld D, et al. Noninvasive breast carcinoma: frequency of unsuspected invasion and implication for treatment. *Ann Surg.* 1979;189:98–103.

132. Wellings SR, Jensen HM, Marcum RG. An atlas of subgross pathology of the human breast with special reference to possible precancerous lesions. *J Natl Cancer Inst.* 1975;55:231–273.

133. Barsky SH, Siegal GP, Jannotta F, et al. Loss of basement membrane components by invasive tumors but not by their benign counterparts. *Lab Invest.* 1983;49:140–147.

134. Farshid G, Moinfar F, Meredith DJ, et al. Spindle cell ductal carcinoma in situ: an unusual variant of ductal intraepithelial neoplasia that stimulates ductal hyperplasia or a myoepithelial proliferation. *Virchows Arch.* 2001;439:70–77.

135. Kawasaki, T, Nakamura S, Sakamoto G, et al. Neuroendocrine ductal carcinoma in situ (NE-DCIS) of the breast-comparative clinicopathologic study of 20 NE-DCIS cases and 274 non-NE-DCIS cases. *Histopathology.* 2008;53:288–298.

136. Perry KD, Reynolds C, Rosen DG, et al. Metastatic neuroendocrine tumour in the breast: a potential mimic of in-situ and invasive mammary carcinoma. *Histopathology.* 2011;59:619–630.

137. Lennington WJ, Jensen RA, Dalton LW, et al. Ductal carcinoma in situ of the breast: heterogeneity of individual lesions. *Cancer.* 1994;73:118–124.

138. Consensus Conference Committee. Consensus conference on the classification of ductal carcinoma in situ. *Cancer.* 1997;80:1798–1802.

139. Wen P, Marsh WL. SMMHC-p63 cocktail improves detection of myoepithelial layer in high-grade ductal carcinoma in-situ. *Mod Pathol.* 2005;18(suppl):54a–55a.

140. Bose S, Lesser ML, Norton L, et al. Immunophenotype of intraductal carcinoma. *Arch Pathol Lab Med.* 1996;100:81–85.

141. Muir R, Aitkenhead AC. The healing of intraduct carcinoma of the mamma. *J Pathol Bacteriol.* 1934;38:117–127.

142. Wasserman JK, Parra-Herran C. Regressive change in high-grade ductal carcinoma in situ of the breast: histopathologic spectrum and biologic importance. *Am J Clin Pathol.* 2015;144:503–510.

143. Davies JD. Hyperelastosis, obliteration and fibrous plaques in major ducts of the human breast. *J Pathol.* 1973;110:13–26.

144. Walters LL, Pang JC, Zhao L, et al. Ductal carcinoma in situ with distorting sclerosis on core biopsy may be predictive of upstaging on excision. *Histopathology.* 2015;66:577–586.

145. Thike AA, Iqbal J, Cheok PY, et al. Ductal carcinoma in situ associated with triple negative invasive breast cancer: evidence for a precursor-product relationship. *J Clin Pathol.* 2013;66:665–670.

146. Bryan BA, Schnitt SJ, Collins LC. Ductal carcinoma in situ with basal-like phenotype: a possible precursor to invasive basal-like breast cancer. *Mod Pathol.* 2006;19:617–621.

147. Dabbs DJ, Chivukula M, Carter G, et al. Basal phenotype of ductal carcinoma in situ: recognition and immunohistologic profile. *Mod Pathol.* 2006;19:1506–1511.

148. Chan JKC, Ng WF. Sclerosing adenosis cancerized by intraductal carcinoma. *Pathology.* 1987;19:425–428.

149. Eusebi V, Collina G, Bussolati G. Carinoma in situ in sclerosing adenosis of the breast: an immunocytochemical study. *Semin Diagn Pathol.* 1989;6:146–152.

150. Oberman HA, Markey BA. Non-invasive carcinoma of the breast presenting in adenosis. *Mod Pathol.* 1991;4:31–35.

151. Calhoun BC, Booth CN. Atypical apocrine adenosis diagnosed on breast core biopsy: implications for management. *Hum Pathol.* 2014;45:2130–2135.

152. Taylor HB, Norris HJ. Epithelial invasion of nerves in benign diseases of the breast. *Cancer.* 1967;20:2245–2249.

153. Tsang WYW, Chan JKC. Neural invasion in intraductal carcinoma of the breast. *Hum Pathol.* 1992;23:202–204.

154. Rosen PP. Coexistant lobular carcinoma in situ and intraductal carcinoma in a single lobular-duct unit. *Am J Surg Pathol.* 1980;4:241–246.

155. Wells J, Ozerdem U, Scognamiglio T, et al. Invasive mammary adenoid cystic carcinoma with an intraductal component. *Breast J.* 2016;22(2):233–234. doi:10.1111/tbj.12558. 26662616.

156. Fusco N, Guerini-Rocco E, Schultheis AM, et al. The birth of an adenoid cystic carcinoma. *Int J Surg Pathol.* 2015;23:26-27.

157. Ross DS, Wen YH, Brogi E. Ductal carcinoma in situ: morphology-based knowledge and molecular advances. *Adv Anat Pathol.* 2013;20:205–216.

158. Goldstein NS, Murphy T. Intraductal carcinoma associated with invasive carcinoma of the breast: a comparison of the two lesions with implications for intraductal carcinoma classification systems. *Am J Clin Pathol.* 1996;106:312–318.

159. Douglas-Jones AG, Gupta SK, Attanoos RL, et al. A critical appraisal of six modern classifications of ductal carcinoma in situ of the breast (DCIS): correlation with grade of associated invasive carcinoma. *Histopathology.* 1996;29:397–409.

160. Holland R, Peterse JL, Millis RR, et al. Ductal carcinoma in situ: a proposal for a new classification. *Semin Diagn Pathol.* 1994;11:167–180.

161. Scott MA, Lagios MD, Axelsson K, et al. Ductal carcinoma in situ of the breast: reproducibility of histological subtype analysis. *Hum Pathol.* 1997;28:967–973.

162. Consensus conference on the classification of ductal carcinoma in situ. *Hum Pathol.* 1997;28:1221–1225.

163. Schuh F, Biazús JV, Resetkova E, et al. Reproducibility of three classification systems of ductal carcinoma in situ of the breast using a web-based survey. *Pathol Res Pract.* 2010;206:705–711.

164. Stasik CJ, Davis M, Kimler BF, et al. Grading ductal carcinoma in situ of the breast using an automated proliferation index. *Ann Clin Lab Sci.* 2011;41:122–130.

165. Saqi A, Osborne MP, Rosenblatt R, et al. Quantifying mammary duct carcinoma in situ: a wild-goose chase? *Am J Clin Pathol.* 2000;113(5, suppl 1):S30–S537.

166. Lester SC, Bose S, Chen YY, et al. Protocol for the examination of specimens from patients with ductal carcinoma in situ of the breast. *Arch Pathol Lab Med.* 2009;133:15–25.

167. Kestin I, Goldstein NS, Lacerna MD, et al. Factors associated with local recurrence of mammographically detected ductal carcinoma in situ in patients given breast conserving therapy. *Cancer.* 2000;88:596–607.

168. Schnitt SJ, Connolly JL. Classification of ductal carcinoma in situ: striving for clinical relevance in the era of breast conserving therapy. *Hum Pathol.* 1997;28:887–880.

169. Mitchell KB, Kuerer H. Ductal carcinoma in situ: treatment update and current trends. *Curr Oncol Rep.* 2015;17:48.

170. Wapnir IL, Dignam JJ, Fisher B, et al. Long-term outcomes of invasive ipsilateral breast tumor recurrences after lumpectomy in NSABP B-17 and B-24 randomized clinical trials for DCIS. *J Natl Cancer Inst.* 2011;103(6):478–488.

171. Siziopikou KP, Anderson SJ, Cobleigh MA, et al. Preliminary results of centralized HER2 testing in ductal carcinoma in situ (DCIS): NSABP B-43. *Breast Cancer Res Treat.* 2013;142:415–421.

172. King TA, Sakr RA, Muhsen S, et al. Is there a low-grade precursor pathway in breast cancer? *Ann Surg Oncol.* 2012;19:1115–1121.

173. Arvold ND, Punglia RS, Hughes ME, et al. Pathologic characteristics of second breast cancers after breast conservation for ductal carcinoma in situ. *Cancer.* 2012;118:6022–6030.

174. Liberman L, Dershaw DD, Rosen PP, et al. Stereotaxic core biopsy of breast carcinoma: accuracy at predicting invasion. *Radiology.* 1995;194:379–381.

175. Renshaw AA. Predicting invasion in the excision specimen from breast core needle biopsy specimens with only ductal carcinoma in situ. *Arch Pathol Lab Med.* 2002;126:39–41.

176. Mendez I, Andreu FJ, Saez E, et al. Ductal carcinoma in situ and atypical ductal hyperplasia of the breast diagnosed at stereotactic core biopsy. *Breast J.* 2001;7:14–18.

177. Ozzello L. Ultrastructure of intraepithelial carcinomas of the breast. *Cancer.* 1971;28:1508–1515.

178. Rajan PB, Perry RH. A quantitative study of patterns of basement membrane in ductal carcinoma in situ (DCIS) of the breast. *Breast J.* 1995;1:315–321.

179. Ozello L. The behaviour of basement membranes in intraductal carcinoma of the breast. *Am J Pathol.* 1959;35:887–899.

180. Prasad ML, Osborne MP, Giri DD, et al. Microinvasive carcinoma (T1mic) of the breast: clinicopathologic profile of 21 cases. *Am J Surg Pathol.* 2000;24:422–428.

181. Coyne J, Haboubi NY. Microinvasive breast carcinoma with granulomatous stromal response. *Histopathology.* 1992;20:184–185.

182. Hou L, Sneige N, Hunt KK, et al. Predictors of invasion in patients with core-needle biopsy-diagnosed ductal carcinoma in situ and recommendations for a selective approach to sentinel lymph node biopsy in ductal carcinoma in situ. *Cancer.* 2006;107:1760–1768.

183. Jackman RJ, Burbank F, Parker SH, et al. Stereotactic breast biopsy of non-palpable lesions: determinants of ductal carcinoma in situ underestimation rates. *Radiology.* 2001;218:497–502.

184. King TA, Farr Jr GH, Cederblom GI, et al. A mass on breast imaging predicts coexisting invasive carcinoma in patients with a core biopsy diagnosis of ductal carcinoma in situ. *Am Surg.* 2001;67:907–912.

185. Bagnall MJ, Evans AJ, Wilson AR, et al. Predicting invasion in mammographically detected microcalcification. *Clin Radiol.* 2001;56:828–832.

186. Hoorntje LE, Schipper ME, Peeters PH, et al. The finding of invasive cancer after a preoperative diagnosis of ductal carcinoma in situ: causes of ductal carcinoma in situ underestimates with stereotactic 14-gauge needle biopsy. *Ann Surg Oncol.* 2003;10:748–753.

187. Yen TW, Hunt KK, Rose MI, et al. Predictors of invasive breast cancer in patients with an initial diagnosis of ductal carcinoma in situ: a guide to selective use of sentinel lymph node biopsy in management of ductal carcinoma in situ. *J Am Coll Surg.* 2005;200:516–526.

188. Lee SK, Yang JH, Woo SY, et al. Nomogram for predicting invasion in patients with a preoperative diagnosis of ductal carcinoma in situ of the breast. *Br J Surg.* 2013;100:1756–1763.

189. Matsen CB, Hirsch A, Eaton A, et al. Extent of microinvasion in ductal carcinoma in situ is not associated with sentinel lymph node metastases. *Ann Surg Oncol.* 2014;21:3330–3335.

190. Shatat L, Gloyeske N, Madan R, et al. Microinvasive breast carcinoma carries an excellent prognosis regardless of the tumor characteristics. *Hum Pathol.* 2013;44:2684–2689.

191. Hilson JB, Schnitt SJ, Collins LC. Phenotypic alterations in ductal carcinoma in situ-associated myoepithelial cells: biologic and diagnostic implication. *Am J Surg Pathol.* 2009;33:227–232.

192. Hoda SA, Rosen PP. Contemporaneous H&E sections should be standard practice in diagnostic immunopathology. *Am J Surg Pathol.* 2007;31:1627.

193. Lee AH, Villena Salinas NM, Hodi Z, et al. The value of examination of multiple levels of mammary needle core biopsy specimens taken for investigation of lesions other than calcification. *J Clin Pathol.* 2012;65:1097–1099.

194. de Mascarel I, MacGrogan G, Mathoulin-Pelissier S, et al. Breast ductal carcinoma in situ with microinvasion: a definition supported by a long-term study of 1248 serially sectioned ductal carcinomas. *Cancer.* 2002;94:2134–2142.

195. Provenzano E, Brown JP, Pinder SE. Pathological controversies in breast cancer: classification of ductal carcinoma in situ, sentinel lymph nodes and low volume metastatic disease and reporting of neoadjuvant chemotherapy specimens. *Clin Oncol (R Coll Radiol).* 2013;25:80–92.

196. Walker RA, Hanby A, Pinder SE, et al. Current issues in diagnostic breast pathology. *J Clin Pathol.* 2012;65:771–785.

197. Wolff AC, Hammond ME, Hicks DG, et al. Recommendations for human epidermal growth factor receptor 2 testing in breast cancer: American Society of Clinical Oncology/College of American Pathologists clinical practice guideline update. *J Clin Oncol.* 2013;31:3997–4013.

198. Lari SA, Kuerer HM. Biological markers in DCIS and risk of breast recurrence: a systematic review. *J Cancer.* 2011;2:232–261.

199. Boecker W, Moll R, Dervan P, et al. Usual ductal hyperplasia of the breast is a committed stem (progenitor) cell lesion distinct from atypical ductal hyperplasia and ductal carcinoma in situ. *J Pathol.* 2002;198:458–467.

200. Simpson PT, Gale T, Reis-Filho JS, et al. Columnar cell lesions of the breast: the missing link in breast cancer progression? A morphological and molecular analysis. *Am J Surg Pathol.* 2005;29:734–746.

201. Cowell CF, Weigelt B, Sakr RA, et al. Progression from ductal carcinoma in situ to invasive breast cancer: revisited. *Mol Oncol.* 2013;7:859–869.

202. Hoda SA. In: Hoda SA, Brogi E, Koerner F, et al, eds. *Rosen's Breast Pathology.* Philadelphia, PA: Wolters Kluwer/Lippincott Williams Wilkins; 2013:271–272, 377–378.

203. Collins LC, Achacoso N, Haque R, et al. Risk factors for non-invasive and invasive local recurrence in patients with ductal carcinoma in situ. *Breast Cancer Res Treat.* 2013;139:453–460.

204. Sue GR, Lannin DR, Au AF, et al. Factors associated with decision to pursue mastectomy and breast reconstruction for treatment of ductal carcinoma in situ of the breast. *Am J Surg.* 2013;206:682–685.

205. VandenBussche CJ, Khouri N, Sbaity E, et al. Borderline atypical ductal hyperplasia/low-grade ductal carcinoma in situ on breast needle core biopsy should be managed conservatively. *Am J Surg Pathol.* 2013;37:913–923.

206. Sagara Y, Mallory MA, Wong S, et al. Survival benefit of breast surgery for low-grade ductal carcinoma in situ: a population-based cohort study. *JAMA Surg.* 2015;150:739–745.

207. Shah DR, Canter RJ, Khatri VP, et al. Utilization of sentinel lymph node biopsy in patients with ductal carcinoma in situ undergoing mastectomy. *Ann Surg Oncol.* 2013;20:24–30.

208. Silverstein MJ, Lagios MD. Choosing treatment for patients with ductal carcinoma in situ: fine tuning the University of Southern California/Van Nuys Prognostic Index. *J Natl Cancer Inst Monogr.* 2010;2010(41):193–196.

209. Silverstein MJ, Lagios MD. Treatment selection for patients with ductal carcinoma in situ (DCIS) of the breast using the University of Southern California/Van Nuys (USC/VNPI) prognostic index. *Breast J.* 2015;21:127–132.

210. Silverstein MJ, Poller DN, Waisman JR, et al. Prognostic classification of breast ductal carcinoma-in-situ. *Lancet.* 1995;345:1154–1157.

211. Silverstein MJ, Lagios MD, Craig PH, et al. A prognostic index for ductal carcinoma in situ of the breast. *Cancer.* 1996;77:2267–2274.

212. Rudloff U, Jacks LM, Goldberg JI, et al. Nomogram for predicting the risk of local recurrence after breast-conserving surgery for ductal carcinoma in situ. *J Clin Oncol.* 2010;28:3762–3769.

213. Yi M, Meric-Bernstam F, Kuerer HM, et al. Evaluation of a breast cancer nomogram for predicting risk of ipsilateral breast tumor recurrences in patients with ductal carcinoma in situ after local excision. *J Clin Oncol.* 2012;30:600–607.

214. Solin LJ, Gray R, Baehner FL, et al. A multigene expression assay to predict local recurrence risk for ductal carcinoma in situ of the breast. *J Natl Cancer Inst.* 2013;105:701–710.

215. Alvarado M, Carter DL, Guenther JM, et al. The impact of genomic testing on the recommendation for radiation therapy in patients with ductal carcinoma in situ: a prospective clinical utility assessment of the 12-gene DCIS score™ result. *J Surg Oncol.* 2015;111:935–940.

216. Rakovitch E, Nofech-Mozes S, Hanna W, et al. A population-based validation study of the DCIS score predicting recurrence risk in individuals treated by breast-conserving surgery alone. *Breast Cancer Res Treat.* 2015;152:389–398.

217. Subhedar P, Olcese C, Patil S, et al. Decreasing recurrence rates for ductal carcinoma in situ: analysis of 2996 women treated with breast-conserving surgery over 30 years. *Ann Surg Oncol.* 2015;22:3273–3281.

Invasive Ductal Carcinoma

SYED A. HODA

NOMENCLATURE

Invasive ductal carcinoma constitutes approximately 75% of mammary carcinomas. A generic term sometimes employed for this type of neoplasm is invasive ductal carcinoma, not otherwise specified (NOS). This is a useful designation that recognizes the distinction between the majority of invasive ductal carcinomas and other specific forms of ductal carcinoma, such as tubular, medullary, and mucinous carcinoma.

Invasive ductal carcinoma was rebranded as "invasive carcinoma of no special type" in the 2012 WHO Classification System (1). It was the opinion of the authors of the WHO Classification that "the use of the term 'ductal' perpetuates the traditional but incorrect concept that these tumors are derived exclusively from mammary ductal epithelium in distinction from lobular carcinomas, which were deemed to have arisen from within lobules, for which there is also no evidence." This is a meaningless amendment to a well-established term, for which no convincing data are presented. The ludicrous nature of this proposal is highlighted by the fact that the aforementioned Classification System has retained terms such as atypical ductal hyperplasia, ductal carcinoma in situ, etc. Until a sound basis for a change in nomenclature is provided, we recommend the continued use of the term "invasive ductal carcinoma" where appropriate.

Invasive ductal carcinoma includes a subset of tumors that express, at least in part, characteristics of one of the specific types of breast carcinoma but does not constitute pure examples of the individual tumors. One example of this phenomenon is invasive ductal carcinoma with architectural and cytologic features of invasive lobular carcinoma (**Figs. 9.1 and 9.2**). Foci of tubular, mucinous, or papillary differentiation can be found in invasive ductal carcinomas. The presence of a mixed growth pattern in needle core biopsy (NCB) sampling should be reported descriptively, with final classification deferred until the excisional biopsy specimen is examined. The relatively favorable prognosis associated with some specific histologic types of invasive carcinoma (e.g., tubular) has been found to apply to those tumors that are composed entirely, or in a large part (approximately 90%), of the designated pattern.

Notably, invasive tubulolobular carcinoma, a relatively uncommon type of carcinoma that displays features of tubular carcinoma as well as invasive lobular carcinoma, should be regarded as a variant of invasive ductal carcinoma—a categorization supported by immunoreactivity for E-cadherin in both components (tubular as well as the seemingly lobular one) of the neoplasm (2).

The specimens obtained in a NCB typically include multiple samples of neoplastic tissue. Occasionally, only a minuscule portion of the neoplasm may be present (**Fig. 9.3**). All tissue on each slide must be carefully examined to ensure that no material is overlooked. In the most extreme circumstance, the evidence for carcinoma is so scant that a definitive diagnosis cannot be rendered with confidence. In these cases, excisional biopsy is necessary to confirm carcinoma.

FROZEN SECTION AND IMMEDIATE CYTOLOGIC EVALUATION

In a series of 59 ultrasound-guided NCBs subjected to frozen section evaluation, Brunner et al. (3) reported no false-positive case, a false-negative rate of 3.3% (n:2), and an unsatisfactory rate of 3.3% (n:2). Despite the obvious technical feasibility of this technique, the evaluation of NCB specimens by frozen section is certainly not standard practice and should only be performed in exceptional situations—such as when there is strong clinical evidence of carcinoma, and immediate intervention is planned in the event that a malignant diagnosis is rendered (**Fig. 9.4**). Major reasons for avoiding frozen section diagnosis of NCB samples include the invariable loss of some tissue from these limited specimens during slide preparation and the potential for misdiagnosis of various benign, pseudoinfiltrative lesions (e.g., sclerosing adenosis, radial scar, etc.) that can mimic invasive ductal carcinoma. The concern over interpretive issues that apply to such possibly deceptive lesions when they are excised intact is compounded in the disrupted material of NCB samples—especially when examined by frozen section.

Touch imprint cytology of NCB specimens of breast can be a useful option to provide on-site assessment of adequacy, and diagnosis, in appropriate clinical settings (4). The technique of core wash cytology has the potential for a relatively rapid diagnosis as well (5,6).

PRESENTATION

There are no specific clinical or radiologic features that distinguish invasive ductal carcinoma from other types of invasive carcinoma and some benign mass-forming lesions such as radial sclerosing lesions. Invasive ductal carcinomas typically occur throughout the age range of adult women, either form

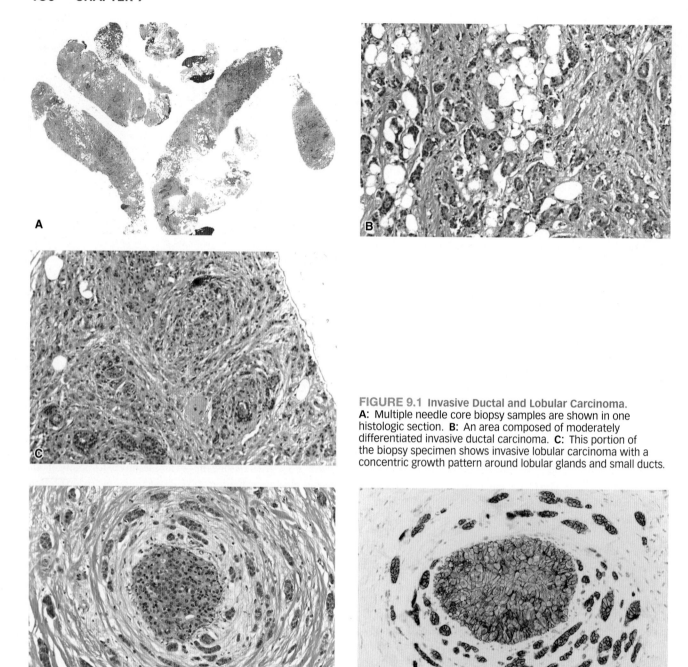

FIGURE 9.1 Invasive Ductal and Lobular Carcinoma.
A: Multiple needle core biopsy samples are shown in one histologic section. **B:** An area composed of moderately differentiated invasive ductal carcinoma. **C:** This portion of the biopsy specimen shows invasive lobular carcinoma with a concentric growth pattern around lobular glands and small ducts.

FIGURE 9.2 Ductal Carcinoma Simulating Lobular Carcinoma. **A:** An invasive ductal carcinoma with circumferential growth around DCIS mimicking invasive lobular carcinoma. **B:** An E-cadherin immunostain shows the characteristic "chicken-wire" membrane reactivity in the tumor cells—a result that supports ductal differentiation.

a palpable mass or produce a radiologic abnormality. Various imaging techniques including digital mammography, ultrasonography, magnetic resonance imaging (MRI), and positron emission tomography (PET) can detect nonpalpable invasive ductal carcinomas early in their evolution.

MRI is an increasingly utilized screening tool in women who are considered "high-risk" or those who have dense breasts. The great majority of breast lesions (up to 79%) detected by MRI are benign (7), and the most common benign lesion is cystic apocrine hyperplasia (8). Carcinomas detected by MRI

screening are typically better differentiated invasive ductal tumors that span <1 cm and are ER-positive and HER2-negative (7).

It is uncommon for invasive ductal carcinomas to present as cyst, which is typically a manifestation of central necrosis in a high-grade carcinoma. The uncommon presence of central fibrosis, that is, scarring following degeneration, is also usually indicative of a poorly differentiated carcinoma—and about one-quarter of the latter carcinomas are found to be "triple-negative," that is, negative for ER, PR, and HER2. Carcinomas with large central acellular zones (LCAZ) can be

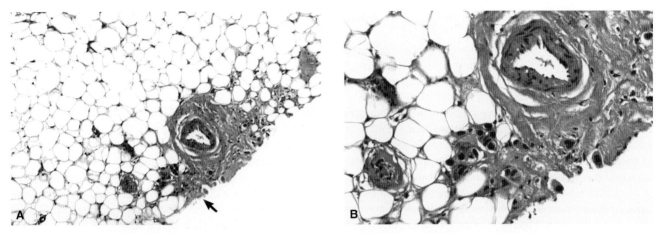

FIGURE 9.3 **Invasive Ductal Carcinoma.** **A, B:** A minuscule group of atypical epithelial cells in fat *(arrow)* around a blood vessel in this needle core biopsy specimen was the only evidence of carcinoma. The material was not considered diagnostic. Excisional biopsy of an 8-mm circumscribed tumor revealed invasive poorly differentiated ductal carcinoma.

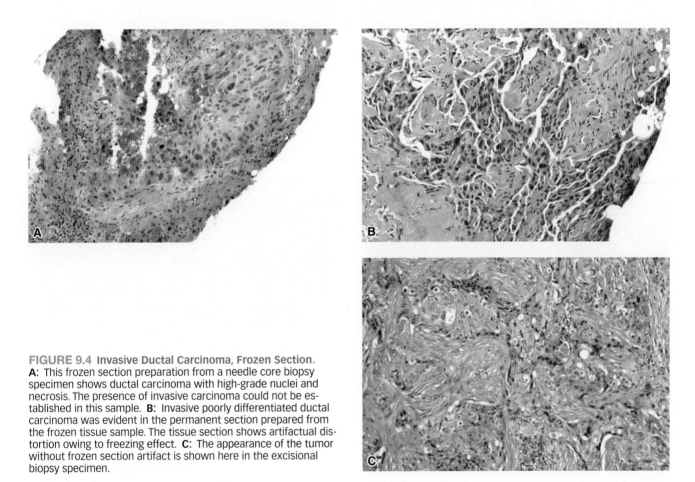

FIGURE 9.4 **Invasive Ductal Carcinoma, Frozen Section.** **A:** This frozen section preparation from a needle core biopsy specimen shows ductal carcinoma with high-grade nuclei and necrosis. The presence of invasive carcinoma could not be established in this sample. **B:** Invasive poorly differentiated ductal carcinoma was evident in the permanent section prepared from the frozen tissue sample. The tissue section shows artifactual distortion owing to freezing effect. **C:** The appearance of the tumor without frozen section artifact is shown here in the excisional biopsy specimen.

identified on imaging studies, including ultrasonography and MRI scans, because of their characteristic appearance (9,10).

SIZE

Tumor volume rather than its one-dimensional size equates with tumor burden; however, at the present time, practical limitations inherent in pathologic evaluation techniques

preclude the reliable calculation of tumor volume because of the highly asymmetric shapes of most of these neoplasms. It must also be realized that although breast tumors can be well visualized via various three-dimensional radiologic techniques, these methods cannot reliably differentiate between malignant and nonmalignant tissues, much less between invasive and intraductal carcinoma. Thus, currently the size, that is greatest dimension (in centimeters), of an invasive carcinoma is used to record its extent. The size of an invasive carcinoma, the

"T" in the TNM Staging system, is one of its most significant prognostic variables.

The gross measurement of the size of a carcinoma is only an approximation of the actual amount of invasive tumor present (11,12). In some tumors, a considerable part of the mass is composed of invasive carcinoma, whereas other lesions of comparable size may have a substantial component of intraductal carcinoma, resulting in a lesser volume of invasive carcinoma. Measurement of the invasive component exclusive of peripheral extensions of intraductal carcinoma is recommended when it is practical on the basis of histologic sections.

Survival decreases with increasing size of invasive ductal carcinoma and most other subtypes of breast carcinoma, and there is a coincidental increase in the frequency of axillary nodal metastases (13–15). This phenomenon applies not only to the overall spectrum of primary tumor size but also within subsets such as those defined by TNM (tumor-node-metastasis) staging. For example, among T_1 breast carcinomas ($\leq$2 cm in diameter), there is a significant relationship between size, the frequency of nodal metastases, and prognosis when the tumors are stratified in 5-mm groups (16,17).

Concerted breast screening efforts have resulted in a progressive increase in the proportion of smaller tumors over recent decades. This is reflected in SEER registry data, which show that the proportion of carcinomas that measured <1 cm rose from <10% in the period 1975 to 1979 to about 25% in 1995 to 1999 among node-negative patients (18).

SIZE AND NEEDLE CORE BIOPSY SAMPLES

It is rarely possible to accurately measure the size of an invasive ductal carcinoma in a NCB specimen, because it is difficult to ensure that the sample represents its largest dimension (19). The only focus of a microinvasive ductal carcinoma in a case may be limited to one of multiple slides prepared from a case (**Fig. 9.5**). It is more likely that a larger invasive carcinoma will be found upon excision in cases wherein a NCB specimen suggests that a smaller tumor is present.

Charles et al. (20) did not find that NCBs affected the final staging of invasive ductal carcinoma except in 1/61 cases wherein there was no residual carcinoma identified on subsequent excision. In a much larger study, Rakha et al. (21) reported that NCB resulted in complete removal of the tumor in 165/40,395 (0.43%) of malignant NCBs. The median mammographic size of the tumor in this set was 0.6 cm. Complete removal of the tumor by NCB

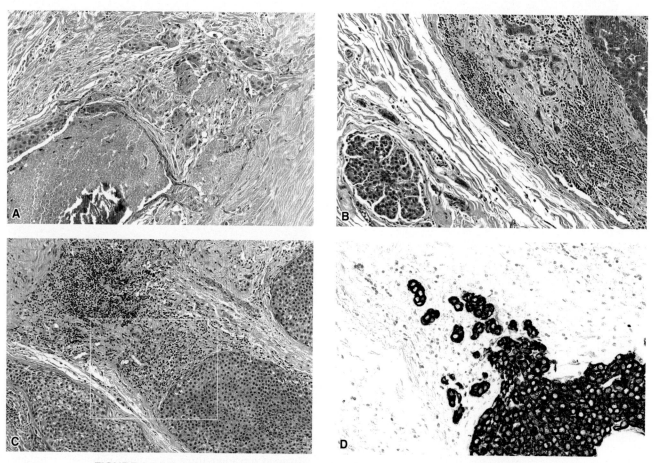

FIGURE 9.5 Microinvasive Ductal Carcinoma. A: Microinvasive carcinoma (invasive carcinoma spanning <0.1 cm) associated with high-grade ductal carcinoma in situ (DCIS). Luminal necrosis and calcification is evident in the DCIS. **B:** Microinvasive carcinoma associated with high-grade DCIS. Note lobular carcinoma in situ of the classic type (lower left). **C, D:** Microinvasive carcinoma–associated DCIS of solid type with intermediate grade nuclei (box). A cytokeratin AE1/3 immunostain highlights the microinvasive carcinoma (**D**). The microinvasive carcinoma has elicited a modest lymphocytic response in (**B**) and (**C**).

was associated with vacuum-assisted procedure using a wide-bore needle. Edwards et al. (22) showed that the size of invasive carcinoma on NCB was greater than the size of residual invasive carcinoma on excisional biopsy in 24/222 (12%) cases. In 15 of these 24 cases (7.5% of all cases), the "T" was upstaged because a larger invasive carcinoma was present in the initial NCB than on the subsequent excisional biopsy. These data suggest that correlation of the extent of invasive ductal or other type of carcinoma in the initial NCB with that in the subsequent excisional biopsy specimen is crucial in determining "T." The extent of the radiologically evident tumor mass must also be a consideration in this regard.

SIZE AND MULTIFOCAL CARCINOMA

A minority of patients have multifocal invasive ductal carcinoma (multiple foci of invasive carcinoma in the same quadrant), or multicentric invasive ductal carcinoma (multiple foci of invasive ductal carcinoma in more than one quadrant). When clinically apparent, multiple nodules may be sampled by NCBs to confirm this impression. The latest edition of the *American Joint Committee on Cancer Staging Manual* (AJCC) (23) refers to tumor size (the "T" in the TNM system) as the maximum dimension of the largest focus of invasive carcinoma—even when multiple separate invasive carcinomas are present with one caveat: macroscopic foci of "apparently distinct tumors" that lie "very close (e.g., <5 mm)" should be regarded as a single mass, and in such cases, the "T" should be reported with the combined dimension of such foci.

The pathology reports of excisional biopsies or mastectomies in cases of multifocal or multicentric invasive ductal carcinomas and other types of carcinoma should not only provide the maximum dimension of the single largest focus of invasive carcinoma but also the aggregate extent of the largest dimensions of all measurable foci of invasive carcinoma. This information can be provided separately for multiple grossly evident foci of invasive carcinoma and for additional foci that are only histologically identified. The data elements that could be used to compute the tumor volume in a NCB specimen, if estimation of volume in such specimens ever assumes clinical significance, would be total aggregate length of invasive carcinoma in NCBs and the diameter of the needles used in the core biopsy (24).

As noted previously, needle core biopsy samples are not a reliable basis for reporting maximum dimension of invasive carcinoma in many cases, and these samples cannot be relied upon to determine multifocality.

SIZE AND MAGNETIC RESONANCE IMAGING

MRI offers an objective method for determining the maximum dimension of a mammary tumor. Measurements of tumor extent obtained on MRI correlate more closely with pathologic tumor size than those obtained by mammography, ultrasound, or clinical examination (25,26). MRI has also proven to be the most accurate method for measuring tumor size during, and after, neoadjuvant chemotherapy (27), and has been shown to

correlate better than mammography in cases of invasive ductal carcinoma with an extensive intraductal component (28); however, it must be realized that no radiologic technique can reliably distinguish between invasive and noninvasive carcinoma.

The complexities and challenges in assessing the extent of invasive carcinoma have been detailed by Varma et al. (29).

GRADING

Grading of invasive ductal carcinomas provides an estimation of how closely an invasive carcinoma resembles normal breast glands, and it is regarded as one of its most important prognostic features. The most widely used histologic grading schema is the Nottingham Grading System (NGS), which is based on criteria established by Bloom and Richardson (30), and Elston and Ellis (31). The parameters measured are the extent of gland formation, nuclear characteristics, and mitotic rate (32). Each of the three elements is assigned a score on a scale of 1 to 3, and the final grade is determined by the sum of the scores. Histologic grade is usually expressed in three categories: scores 3 to 5, well differentiated or grade 1; scores 6 to 7, intermediate or grade 2; scores 8 to 9, poorly differentiated or grade 3. The NGS is outlined in Table 9.1. In invasive

TABLE 9.1
Nottingham Grading System for Invasive Carcinoma

Gland formation

Score 1: >75% of the invasive carcinoma shows gland formation
Score 2: 10%–75% of the invasive carcinoma shows gland formation
Score 3: <10% of the invasive carcinoma shows gland formation

Nuclear features

Score 1: Nuclei of invasive carcinoma cells are similar to nuclei of normal ductal cells (2–3X RBC size) with regular nuclear outlines and uniform chromatin
Score 2: Nuclei of invasive carcinoma cells are of intermediate-size with open vesicular nuclei, visible nucleoli, and moderate variability in both size and shape
Score 3: Nuclei of invasive carcinoma cells are large, with prominent nucleoli, marked variation in size and shape

Mitotic count

On the basis of 10 high power fields (40X objective, 400X magnification, field area 0.196 mm^2)
Score 1: 0–7 mitoses
Score 2: 8–14 mitoses
Score 3: ≥15 mitoses

Modified from Robbins P, Pinder S, de Klerk N, et al. Histological grading of breast carcinomas: a study of interobserver agreement. *Hum Pathol.* 1995;26:873–879.

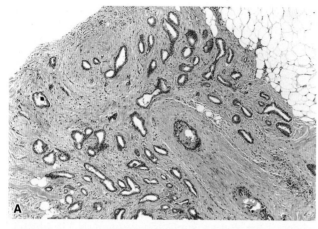

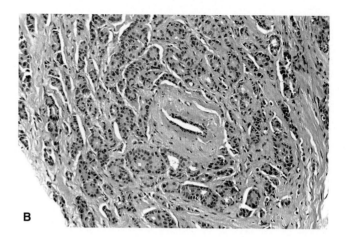

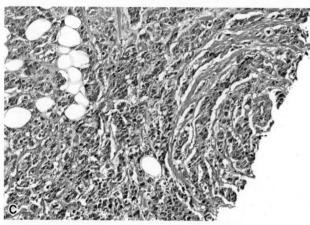

FIGURE 9.6 Invasive Ductal Carcinoma, Architectural (Histologic) Grade. **A:** The needle core biopsy specimen of an invasive, well-differentiated ductal (tubular) carcinomas characterized by glands with distinct lumina (gland formation: score 1). **B:** In this sampling, this invasive, moderately differentiated ductal carcinoma shows less than 10% of glands with distinctly open lumina (gland formation: score 2). **C:** No gland formation is present in this invasive, poorly differentiated ductal carcinoma (gland formation: score 3).

ductal carcinomas that display morphologic heterogeneity, final grade of the tumor should be based on its most poorly differentiated portion.

Glandular differentiation assesses the formation of clear-cut glands by an invasive carcinoma. A true glandular structure is one with central luminal space lined by "polarized" tumor cells. This factor is best assessed on low-power examination of the entire tissue section (19). The proportion occupied by true glands is assessed (**Fig. 9.6**).

Nuclear pleomorphism is a reflection of grading at the cytopathologic level. The appearance of normal breast epithelial cells in the vicinity of an invasive carcinoma should be used as a standard for a nuclear score of 1 (**Fig. 9.7**). Lymphocytes (or even endothelial cells) can be used as a substitute in the event that normal breast tissue is absent in a NCB. Assignment of nuclear score of 1 is uncommon in invasive ductal carcinoma. The most common type of invasive carcinoma cells to be assigned a nuclear score of 1 are those of the classic form of invasive lobular carcinoma. As much as possible, in a NCB sampling, nuclear grading should be performed at the advancing edge of an invasive carcinoma or in the least differentiated (with the highest nuclear grade) portion of the tumor. Notably, nuclear grading is subject to a high degree of interobserver variation.

Mitotic count is a reflection of the proliferation activity in an invasive carcinoma. Only cells that are unequivocally undergoing mitoses are counted. Most commonly, apoptotic carcinoma cells or intratumoral lymphocytes are mistaken for a mitotic figure. Absence of a nuclear membrane and the presence of at least one separate chromosome supports a mitotic over an apoptotic figure (**Fig. 9.8**). Apoptotic cells commonly possess denser, more eosinophilic, cytoplasm. As with nuclear grade, mitotic activity should also be assessed at the advancing edge of an invasive carcinoma, or in its least differentiated (that is, most mitotically active) focus. Fibrotic and necrotic foci need not be evaluated. Mitotic figures are scored on the number of mitoses per 10 high-power fields. The latter can vary up to six-fold between different makes and models of microscopes, and this factor should be taken into consideration. The field with the highest count, not the mean count, should be recorded.

Mitotic activity can be under-assessed in NCB specimens because of the limited nature of the specimen. In this regard, two studies seeking to (hypothetically) remedy this concern are notable. Firstly, it has been shown that use of MIB-1 proliferation marker and PPH3 mitotic marker correlates better with mitotic count in the excisional biopsy than counting in routine H&E sections (33). Secondly, it has been suggested that

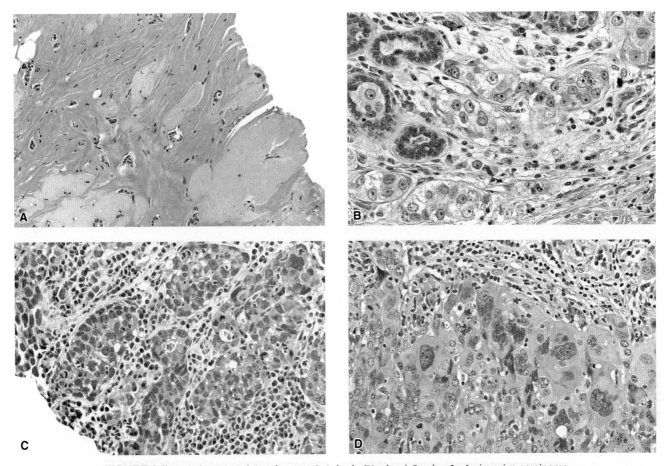

FIGURE 9.7 Invasive Ductal Carcinoma, Cytologic (Nuclear) Grade. A: An invasive carcinoma with low-grade nuclei (nuclear score: 1) and tubulolobular architectural features. A myoepithelial layer was absent around the infiltrating glands (not shown). **B:** Intermediate-grade nuclei (nuclear score: 2) in this invasive carcinoma are characterized by modest nuclear pleomorphism and enlargement. The nuclei are slightly hyperchromatic. **C:** High-grade nuclei (nuclear score: 3) feature marked nuclear pleomorphism and enlargement with hyperchromasia. **D:** Overtly pleomorphic nuclei are evident in the constituent cells of this invasive, poorly differentiated carcinoma.

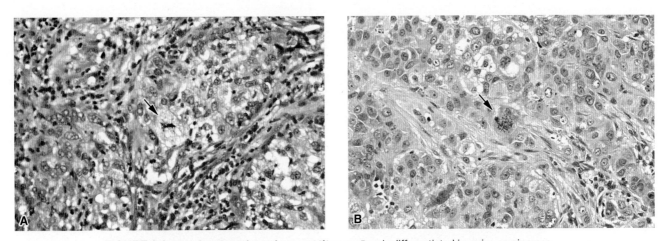

FIGURE 9.8 Invasive Ductal Carcinoma, Mitoses. Poorly differentiated invasive carcinomas with mitotic figures in prophase **(A)** is shown. An abnormal mitotic figure is shown in **(B).** Arrows point to the mitotic figures.

lowering the threshold for a mitotic score of 2 from 11 mitoses in 10 high-power fields to 6 mitoses in 10 high-power fields for invasive carcinomas in NCB specimens (particularly those with a gland formation score of 3 and nuclear grade score of 3) would improve agreement in the grading of invasive ductal carcinoma vis a vis excisional biopsy specimen (34).

Several studies have investigated the accuracy of histologic grading based on NCB specimens when compared with the final grade determined from the excised tumor. The reported concordance rates ranged from 59% to 86% (35–40). In the same studies, concordance with respect to tumor type ranged from 66.6% to 81%. These data suggest that classification and grading of invasive ductal carcinomas based on the NCB sample should be regarded as provisional. This consideration should be borne in mind when neoadjuvant chemotherapy is administered on the basis of a diagnosis made with a NCB sample. Tumor heterogeneity is the most common source of discordant classification and grading, but interobserver and intraobserver variation are also factors.

Tumor grade have been shown to be useful predictors of prognosis for patients stratified by stage of disease, especially those without axillary lymph node metastases (41,42). Increasing tumor grade has been associated with several factors that are related to an increased risk for breast recurrence after conservation therapy, including greater tumor size, diagnosis at a relatively young age, and absence of estrogen receptor (ER) expression. Although some investigators found a significant relationship between grade and local recurrence (43), others concluded that grade was not a significant predictor of local recurrence (44).

Women with *BRCA1* mutations have a significantly higher frequency of invasive, poorly differentiated ductal carcinomas when compared with individuals not carrying this mutation. *BRCA1* mutations occurring in sporadic and familial breast

carcinomas have been associated with similar patterns of poorly differentiated growth. This is manifested by a higher nuclear grade, lower frequency of ER-positivity, and high histologic grade (45). Women with *BRCA2* mutations generally develop invasive ductal carcinomas of a higher grade than those that occur in sporadic age-matched controls but have a different histologic and immunohistichemical profile from that of *BRCA1* patients. Data from 4,325 *BRCA1* and 2,568 *BRCA2* mutation carriers showed strong evidence that the proportion of ER-negative breast tumors decreased with age at diagnosis among *BRCA1* but increased with age at diagnosis among *BRCA2* carriers. The proportion of "triple-negative" tumors decreased with age at diagnosis in *BRCA1* carriers but increased with age at diagnosis of *BRCA2* carriers (46).

LYMPHOVASCULAR INVOLVEMENT

Lymphatics are defined as vascular channels lined by endothelium without supporting smooth muscle or elastica. Most lymphatics do not contain red blood cells, but undoubtedly some blood capillaries are included in this definition, and for practical purposes the terms lymphatic involvement (LI) and lymphovascular involvement (LVI) are synonymous terms.

The presence of LVI (**Figs. 9.9 and 9.10**) in the breast is an unfavorable prognostic finding. LVI can be simulated when artifactual spaces are formed around nests of invasive and in situ carcinoma as a result of tissue retraction during specimen processing. It can be difficult to distinguish such retraction artifacts from true lymphatic spaces (47). Assessment for LVI is more reliably accomplished in breast tissue beyond the edges of the invasive carcinoma (48). An unusual pattern of necrosis in carcinoma that involves pseudoangiomatous

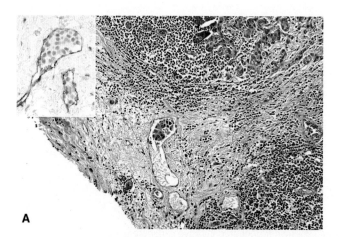
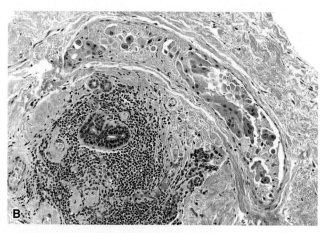

FIGURE 9.9 **Invasive Ductal Carcinoma with Lymphovascular Channel Involvement.** **A:** This needle core biopsy specimen shows a cluster of carcinoma cells in a dilated lymphovascular channel adjacent to an invasive ductal carcinoma. Inset shows CD31 immunoreactivity in the endothelial cells. **B:** Lymphovascular channel involvement in a case of invasive apocrine-type of ductal carcinoma. This may be the only finding in a needle core biopsy in a case of an invasive apocrine carcinoma that presents with axillary nodal metastases and vague nodularity of the breast.

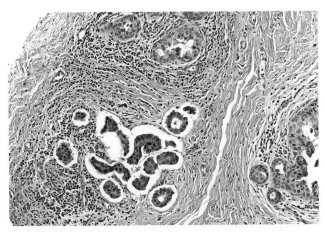

FIGURE 9.10 Invasive Micropapillary Carcinoma Resembling Lymphovascular Channel Involvement. A minute focus of invasive micropapillary carcinoma simulating lymphovascular channel involvement by carcinoma cells. Micropapillary DCIS is present in adjacent ducts.

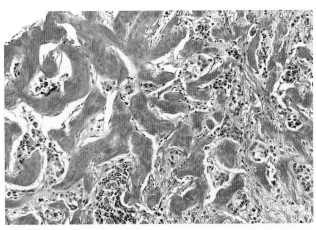

FIGURE 9.11 Invasive Ductal Carcinoma Amid Pseudoangiomatous Stroma. The invasive carcinoma infiltrates pseudoangiomatous stromal hyperplasia with dense collagenized stroma.

stromal hyperplasia (PASH) can simulate LVI by carcinoma **(Fig. 9.11)**.

Retraction artifact is more commonly found in ductal than in lobular carcinomas. Carcinomas with retraction artifact tend to exhibit high histologic and nuclear grade. Acs et al. (49) found that there was a significant direct correlation between retraction artifact and LVI in node-negative patients. Furthermore, node-negative patients with retraction artifact had a significantly higher frequency of distant metastases than those without—suggesting that retraction artifact could reflect aspects of tumoral–stromal interaction, possibly related to the formation of lymphatic channels and not simply a passive phenomenon related to tissue fixation. The presence of micropapillary features, possibly a special type of retraction artifact, in invasive ductal carcinomas also appears to predispose to axillary nodal metastases (50).

NCBs of breast can cause mechanically induced displacement of neoplastic and non-neoplastic epithelium—a finding that is commonly evident on the subsequently performed excisional biopsies. Rarely, epithelial displacement can be found in the initial NCB itself—a finding that can occasionally be diagnostically confounding. Koo et al. (51) found epithelial displacement into lymphovascular channels in 7/218 (3.2%) NCB specimens with ductal carcinoma in situ (DCIS). There was no evidence of invasive carcinoma in the initial NCB or in the subsequent excisional biopsy. This finding suggests that the presence of tumor cell clusters within lymphovascular channels in NCB specimen with DCIS may not always represent true lymphovascular involvement.

Immunostains for endothelial cells (including CD31, D2-40, ERG, FVIII, LYVE-1, VEGFR3, and WT1) can be confirmatory of LVI and can be useful to distinguish between retraction artifact and LVI (52–54). Thus far, ERG, a member of the ETS family of transcription factors, is the only nuclear marker of endothelial cells (55). D2-40 is a monoclonal antibody directed at podoplanin with a high degree of specificity for the lymphatic endothelia. A vascular channel that is D2-40(+) and CD31(−) is purportedly more likely to be a lymphatic space, whereas the reverse immunophenotype [D2-40(−), CD31(+)] is indicative of blood vessel channel. The presence of axillary nodal metastases was associated with peritumoral but not with intratumoral lymphatic tumor emboli detected by D2-40 immunostain by Van den Eynden et al. (56) and de Mascarel et al. (57).

Periductal myoepithelial cells are sometimes immunoreactive for D2-40 (58), and this is a potential source of misdiagnosis of LVI when intraductal carcinoma becomes detached from the myoepithelial layer and is displaced into the ductal lumen.

LVI is found in approximately 15% of excisional biopsy specimens with invasive ductal carcinomas. The majority of these patients also have axillary lymph node metastases, but LVI is found in 5% to 10% of patients with node-negative invasive ductal carcinomas. Several studies have shown that LVI confers unfavorable prognosis to node-negative patients treated by either mastectomy (59–62) or by breast conservation therapy (63). LVI does not predispose to local recurrence in patients treated by mastectomy (61), but they have been associated with an increased risk for recurrence in the breast after breast conservation therapy (63). Liljegren et al. (64) reported that the relative risk for recurrence in the breast after conservation therapy was 1.9% (95% CI: 1.1–3.5) in a comparison of women with or without peritumoral lymphatic tumor emboli.

The deleterious effect of LVI is most pronounced in women with $T_1N_0M_0$ disease. In a 10-year follow-up study of 378 patients treated for $T_1N_0M_0$ carcinoma, 33% of 30 women with lymphatic emboli died of the disease. Death due to breast carcinoma was observed in 20% of the 348 women who did not have lymphatic emboli (48). Another study comparing similar subsets of $T_1N_0M_0$ patients found recurrences in 32% of those with lymphatic emboli and in

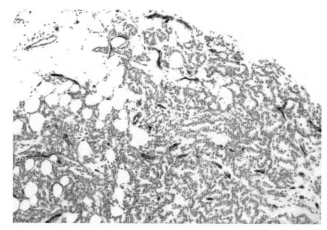

FIGURE 9.12 Invasive Ductal Carcinoma with Angiogenesis. Vascularity is demonstrated in the needle core biopsy specimen of an invasive ductal carcinoma with the immunostain for CD34. The tumor invades adipose tissue.

10% of controls (65). In stage I patients with tumors larger than 2 cm ($T_2N_0M_0$), those with lymphatic emboli also experienced a higher metastatic rate (62). Metastases that develop in node-negative patients who have peritumoral lymphatic emboli tend to occur more than 5 years after diagnosis, and they are almost always systemic.

Blood vessel invasion, defined as penetration by carcinoma into the lumen of an artery or vein, is an extremely uncommon finding in NCB specimens. These vascular structures are invariably larger than lymphatics or capillaries and can be identified by the presence of a smooth muscle wall supported by elastic fibers. It may be necessary to employ special histochemical stains (e.g., Verhoeff van Gieson stains) that highlight elastic tissue in the vessel wall. Notably, elastic fibers may also be deposited around ducts with intraductal carcinoma, and the resulting appearance on an elastic stain may be difficult to distinguish from vascular invasion. The independent prognostic significance of blood vessel invasion has not been established.

As stated earlier, various immunostains for endothelial cells can be employed in cases where there is uncertainty about the presence of LVI. Whenever such an investigation is undertaken, a contemporaneous H&E-stained slide should also be prepared to ensure correlation of the immunostained and routinely stained recut sections (66).

A variety of diagnostic issues relating to lymphovascular involvement in breast carcinoma were reviewed by Hoda et al. (67).

ANGIOGENESIS

Angiogenesis associated with breast carcinomas reflects the capacity of neoplastic tissue to induce vascular proliferation. Tumor growth is enhanced not only by increased perfusion associated with neovascularization **(Fig. 9.12)** but also by the paracrine mitogenic effects of growth factors produced by endothelial cells. Angiogenesis may have a significant role in progression of breast carcinoma (68), and anti-angiogenic therapy may have a potential role in this regard (69).

Studies of angiogenesis should take intratumoral variability into consideration, and utilization of all available tumor tissue is recommended (70). The limited tumor samples obtained on NCBs are not suitable for estimating angiogenesis by conventional techniques.

PERINEURAL INVASION

Perineural invasion can be identified in approximately 1% of invasive ductal carcinomas **(Fig. 9.13)**; thus, it is about 10% less frequent than lymphovascular involvement (71). Perineural invasion tends to occur in higher-grade carcinomas and is frequently observed in association with lymphovascular involvement; however, it has not been proven as an independent prognostic factor.

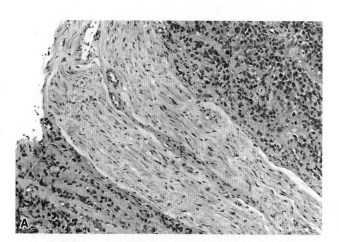
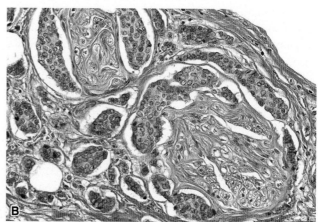

FIGURE 9.13 Invasive Ductal Carcinoma with Perineural Infiltration. A, B: Carcinoma cells are shown invading in and around nerves in biopsy specimens from two patients. Involvement of a major nerve trunk is shown in **(A)**, and a smaller nerve in **(B)**. Carcinoma surrounding a Pacinian corpuscle is shown in **(C)**.

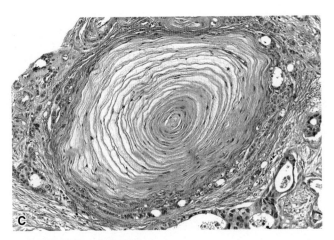

FIGURE 9.13 (continued)

STROMAL ELASTOSIS

Stromal elastosis refers to the presence of clumps of elastic fibers amid connective tissue and is usually observed in association with invasive ductal carcinomas of lower grade (**Fig. 9.14**). Stromal elastosis has been significantly associated with ER-positivity but has not been proven to be an independent prognostic factor (72,73).

ABSENCE OF MYOEPITHELIUM

Invasive ductal carcinoma lacks myoepithelium (**Figs. 9.15 and 9.16**). This characteristic helps to distinguish it from benign proliferative lesions with three notable exceptions: microglandular adenosis (discussed at length elsewhere), certain intraductal carcinomas, and some apocrine lesions. Failure to detect myoepithelium is not by itself diagnostic of invasive carcinoma, because myoepithelial cells can be markedly diminished or completely lost in some in situ carcinomas—particularly those that are of the solid type with high-grade nuclei. Myoepithelial cells can also be absent in certain forms of noninvasive papillary carcinoma (discussed at length elsewhere). The diminution and absence of myoepithelial cells, particularly as evident via p63 immunostain, in certain unequivocally benign apocrine lesions is a well-documented enigmatic phenomenon (74,75). The latter phenomenon emphasizes the need to always utilize at least two myoepithelial markers and underlines the danger of interpreting immunohistochemical findings in isolation without regard to histologic features.

Cross reactivity of stromal myofibrobasts with myoepithelial markers, particularly smooth muscle actin, can be a confounding factor by creating the false impression that myoepithelium is present especially in invasive ductal carcinoma. For this reason, the p63 or p40 immunostains are preferable because reactivity is limited to myoepithelial cell nuclei. It is

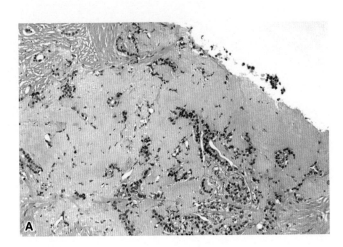

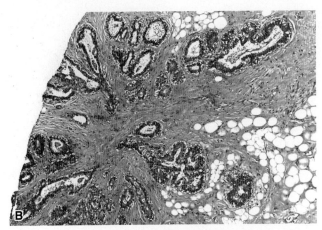

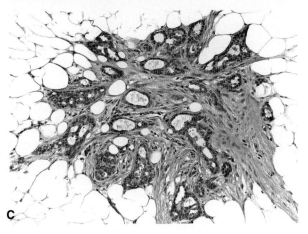

FIGURE 9.14 Invasive Ductal Carcinomas and Radial Scar Associated with Stromal Elastosis and Fibrosis. A: The stroma in this needle core biopsy specimen contains homogeneous masses of amphophilic elastin in invasive ductal carcinoma. **B:** A radial scar with characteristic spoke-like glands radiating from a fibrotic nidus is shown. **C:** An invasive ductal carcinoma with desmoplastic stroma is shown to compare with the radial scar depicted in (**B**).

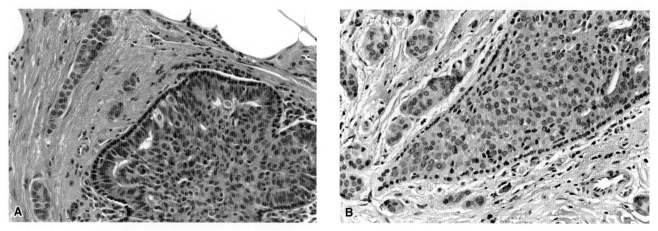

FIGURE 9.15 Invasive Ductal Carcinoma without Myoepithelial Cell Layer on Routine Staining. A, B: Two examples of invasive ductal carcinoma in needle core biopsy specimens. A hyperplastic myoepithelial cell layer is evident around the ducts with atypical hyperplasia, but not the invasive carcinoma, in each case in routine H&E-stained preparations.

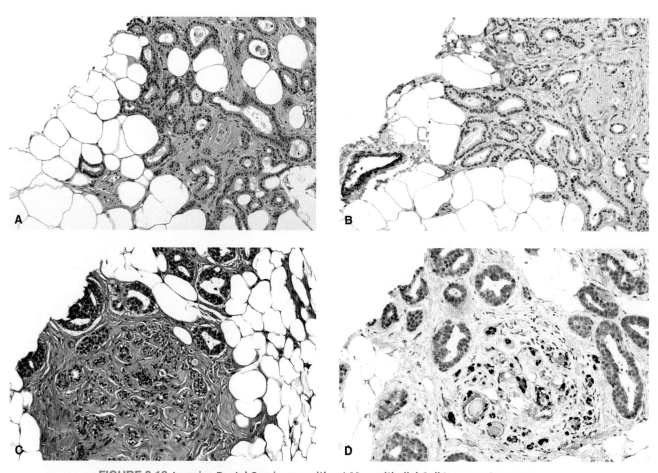

FIGURE 9.16 Invasive Ductal Carcinoma without Myoepithelial Cell Layer on Immunostaining. A, B: The heavy chain myosin immunostain shows no staining around this invasive carcinoma, indicating absence of myoepithelial cell layer. Myosin immunoreactivity is seen in a blood vessel wall **(B)**. **C, D:** In this needle core biopsy, the p63 immunostain shows no staining around the invasive carcinoma, proving absence of a myoepithelial cell layer. Reactivity for p63 is seen in the associated adenosis **(D)**. **E, F:** In this needle core biopsy sample, the smooth muscle actin (SMA) immunostain shows absence of staining around the invasive carcinoma. Faint SMA reactivity is present in scattered stromal myofibroblastic cells and in myoepithelial cells in a small duct **(D)**.

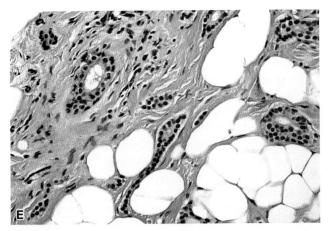
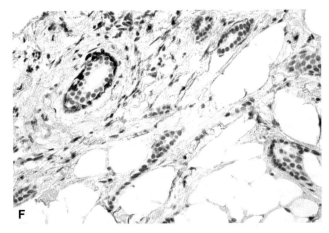

FIGURE 9.16 (continued)

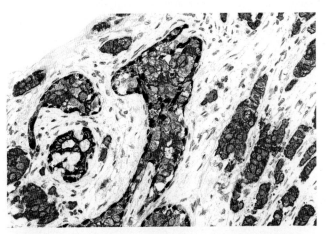

FIGURE 9.17 Invasive Ductal Carcinoma, Triple Immunostaining. This triple immunostained preparation facilitates the diagnosis of invasive carcinoma. The preparation uses a combination of cytokeratin AE1/3 (with red chromogen), and two myoepithelial markers: p63 to mark myoepithelial nuclei (with brown chromogen) and myosin (also with brown chromogen) to highlight myoepithelial cytoplasm. In this "cocktail," p63 and myosin stains decorate the entire myoepithelial cell (nucleus and cytoplasm) and in DCIS.

also useful to employ a cytokeratin stain, or double or even triple immunostains, combining cytokeratin with myoepithelial marker(s), to highlight foci of invasive carcinoma **(Fig. 9.17)**.

DUCTAL CARCINOMA IN SITU

The presence of DCIS in a NCB specimen associated with invasive ductal carcinoma should be reported. Included in the diagnostic report should be mention of the architectural pattern and nuclear grade of the DCIS, as well as the presence or absence of necrosis and calcifications therein.

Invasive ductal carcinoma arises from DCIS, and the two components usually share similar cytologic features. In situ and invasive components of single tumors typically undergo similar molecular alterations (76). Invasive ductal carcinomas vary in the relative proportions of in situ and invasive components.

As the proportion of DCIS increases, for any gross tumor size, there is a trend to decreased nodal metastases and a more favorable prognosis. The distribution of DCIS in and around the primary tumor appears to correlate with the risk for local recurrence after breast conservation (77) but has no bearing on the risk for systemic recurrence in women treated by breast conservation or mastectomy (78). Local recurrence occurs more often after lumpectomy and radiation therapy in women who have high-grade DCIS or an extensive intraductal component (EIC). The latter is defined as DCIS that comprises at least 25% of a tumor mass and extends beyond it. The increased risk for local recurrence after breast conservation attributable to EIC is probably a manifestation of a greater probability of there being carcinoma at margins of excision, and beyond. In patients with negative margins, the presence of EIC does not increase the risk for local recurrence in the breast after breast conservation therapy (79,80).

A reliable estimate of the proportion of DCIS associated with an invasive carcinoma and its extent beyond the invasive carcinoma cannot be reliably estimated in conventional NCB samples.

ROLE OF NEEDLE CORE BIOPSY SPECIMEN IN NEOADJUVANT CHEMOTHERAPY AND NOVEL TREATMENT MODALITIES

Neoadjuvant chemotherapy and emerging techniques of minimally invasive tumor ablation (such as radiofrequency ablation and cryoablation) rely on NCB for providing an unequivocal diagnosis of invasive carcinoma.

Neoadjuvant chemotherapy has not been shown to improve overall survival compared with conventional adjuvant chemotherapy; however, the possibility of "downstaging" or elimination ("complete pathologic response") of the primary invasive carcinoma using this approach potentially reduces the need for mastectomy and axillary lymph node dissection. Thus, neoadjuvant chemotherapy can decrease the morbidity of extensive surgery, without compromising outcome.

The objective of minimally invasive ablative techniques is to eradicate an invasive carcinoma by nonsurgical means. In the event that the carcinoma is entirely removed by these means, the NCB specimen may be the only diagnostic tissue that will ever be available to assess the histopathologic, immunohistochemical, and molecular pathologic characteristics of the invasive carcinoma.

At a minimum, pathologic information that must be available before the initiation of treatment includes diagnosis of invasive carcinoma and its grade and type. ER, PR, and HER2 test results must also be available. In some cases, results of genomic assay (Oncotype DX, Mammaprint, or Mammostrat) obtained on NCB specimen could influence clinical decision-making. Every effort should be made to conserve as much tissue as possible in obtaining sections for these tests in order to accommodate this array of testing. In view of the foregoing, the practice of routinely obtaining multiple H&E-stained levels without saving intervening sections should be discontinued.

Selection of cases most likely to benefit from preoperative chemotherapy, and the development of personalized approaches based on the degree of response, is critical and is the subject of ongoing clinical trials. There is evidence suggesting that neoadjuvant chemotherapy may not have significant beneficial impact on the surgical treatment of invasive lobular carcinoma (81), but this subject needs further investigation.

ER, PR, AND HER2 TESTING ON NEEDLE CORE BIOPSIES

The use of the initial NCB specimen for ER, PR, and HER2 testing vis a vis subsequent excisional biopsy specimen has been increasing in recent years (**Fig. 9.18**) (82). The use of NCB specimens for this purpose offers the advantage of better tissue fixation and lesser ischemic time. The issue of tumor heterogeneity is a legitimate consideration, but less than 3% of invasive carcinomas were heterogeneous enough to affect

testing for predictive factors in one study (83). Numerous studies comparing results of ER, PR, and HER2 testing on initial NCBs and on the subsequent excisional biopsy have shown excellent agreement between the two types of specimens (83–86).

An update of ASCO-CAP guidelines for HER2 testing states that "if the initial HER2 test result in a core needle biopsy specimen of a primary breast cancer is negative, a new HER2 test *may* (emphasis added) be ordered on the excision specimen." This statement represents a change from the previous guideline that required re-testing, and is based on the "...greater clinical experience confirming the high concordance in HER2 testing between core and excisional biopsies" (87).

NCB specimens can also be used for genomic assays, including the one most commonly utilized: Oncotype DX (88). The latter test not only provides prognostic information in terms of 10-year distant recurrence rate and predicts the likelihood of the benefit conferred by adjuvant chemotherapy in ER-positive invasive carcinomas but also provides results of ER, PR, and HER2 results. The Oncotype DX results are based on the expression of a panel of 21 genes (including 16 cancer-related and 5 reference genes) on RT-PCR (and not on in situ hybridization). HER2 results based on RT-PCR testing, as reported by Oncotype DX, have generated controversy (89,90).

TUMOR-INFILTRATING LYMPHOCYTES

Medullary carcinoma of the breast, a special type of invasive ductal carcinoma described in 1949, is characterized by prominent lymphocytic response as well as circumscription, syncytial growth, and high-grade nuclei (91). The role of "tumor-infiltrating lymphocytes" (TIL) has long been regarded as a major factor in influencing the better prognosis of medullary carcinoma (92).

Neoadjuvant chemotherapy results in complete pathologic response, that is, complete absence of carcinoma, in a minority (<25%) of cases. Pretherapy NCBs provide an excellent substrate

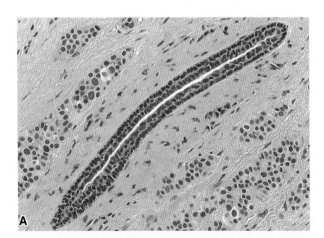
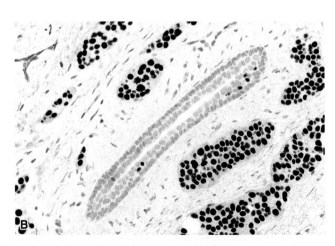

FIGURE 9.18 Invasive Ductal Carcinoma, Estrogen Receptor (ER) Immunostain. A, B: The ER stain shows strong and diffuse (approximately 100%) staining in the invasive carcinoma. The normal gland in the center shows rare, scattered reactivity in the luminal epithelial cells, and no reactivity in the abluminal myoepithelial cells **(B)**.

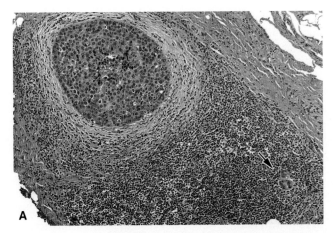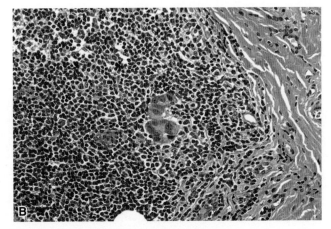

FIGURE 9.19 Microinvasive and In Situ Ductal Carcinoma with Prominent Lymphocytic Infiltration (So-called "Tumor Infiltrating Lymphocytes"). **A, B:** A needle core biopsy specimen showing a marked lymphocytic reaction around microinvasive ductal carcinoma **(B)**. The lymphocytic infiltrate is less pronounced around the DCIS.

for the assay of predictive factors that could identify patients who would benefit most from several types of neoadjuvant chemotherapy. In this context, TIL has generated considerable interest and promise based on evidence that the likelihood and degree of response is directly related to the abundance of the TIL **(Fig. 9.19)** (93–96). Recommendations for a "pragmatic starting point" for the standardized evaluation of TIL in invasive breast carcinomas appeared in 2014 (97). Further study is needed to assess the reliability of measuring TIL in a NCB sample as a predictive marker prior to neoadjuvant therapy. TIL may coexist with "tertiary lymphoid structures," which are peculiar lymph node–like structures characterized by lymphoid aggregates with venules lined by plump endothelial cells (95,98).

The presence of particularly abundant TIL has been noted in medullary carcinomas, *BRCA* mutation–associated breast carcinomas, carcinomas that are associated with better response to neoadjuvant chemotherapy, and "triple-negative" carcinomas (99). Given the potential significance of TIL, it has been suggested that ". . .pathologists should perhaps get used to reporting this parameter as a part of the standard histological description of breast cancer" (100), but no standardized reporting system is presently available.

ROLE OF NEEDLE CORE BIOPSY: STATUS POST NEOADJUVANT CHEMOTHERAPY

Neoadjuvant chemotherapy is increasingly being utilized as a treatment option for appropriately selected larger invasive ductal carcinomas. In some clinical situations, NCBs may be used to assess treatment response. The reporting of such specimens should include presence of invasive and in situ carcinoma, their type, cellularity (relative to that observed in pre-neoadjuvant chemotherapy), and the presence or absence of lymphovascular involvement (101). Neoadjuvant chemotherapy can have the following effects on invasive carcinomas: (a) some invasive ductal carcinomas can display lobular architectural

features with "single-filing" pattern; (b) some carcinomas can show increased nuclear hyperchromasia and pleomorphism (review of pre-neoadjuvant chemotherapy appearance can confirm whether this effect is treatment-related); (c) a markedly reduced mitotic rate; and (d) uncommonly, tumoral necrosis **(Fig. 9.20)**.

MOLECULAR PATHOLOGY ASPECTS

"Intrinsic subtypes" of breast carcinoma, including invasive ductal carcinoma, utilizing microarray-based gene expression profiling (102) were described in 2000. As discussed in the forthcoming, this is an unstable area of investigation as over time, criteria for subtype classification have changed and additional subtypes have been described. Four subtypes (that is, luminal, basal-like, HER2-positive, and normal-like) were initially described. Later, the luminal tumors were divided into A and B groups. The "normal-like" subtype is now considered to be the result of contamination of samples by non-neoplastic tissue rather than an authentic subtype.

Luminal A tumors are ER-positive, PR-positive, HER2-negative, and are of low grade. **Luminal B** tumors are ER-positive, PR-positive or -negative, HER2-postive or -negative, and are of a higher grade with relatively higher proliferation rate based on Ki67. A rare subset of luminal B tumors is "triple-positive" (that is, ER-positive, PR-positive, and HER2-positive). The minimum Ki67 value required by the majority of the 2015 St. Gallen panel for Luminal B categorization was at least 20 (103). The two luminal subtypes differ in their genomic makeup, genetic alterations, and prognosis. Patients with luminal A tumors have better survival rates when compared to other groups (104).

The ER-negative groups include the basal-like and HER2-positive subtypes. The **basal-like** tumors are characterized by "triple negativity" (that is, ER-negative, PR-negative, and HER2-negative) and immunoreactivity for high-molecular-weight cytokeratins as well as for EGFR. In particular, attention has

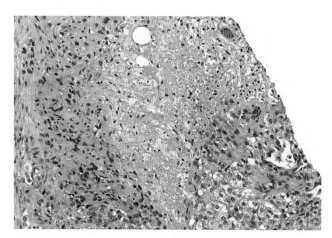

FIGURE 9.20 Invasive Ductal Carcinoma with De Novo Necrosis. A needle core biopsy specimen showing focal necrosis in a poorly differentiated invasive ductal carcinoma.

centered on CK5, CK5/6, CK14, and CK17 that have been referred to as "basal cytokeratins" because of their predominant localization in the basal (myoepithelial) layer of the bilayered (that is, epithelial and myoepithelial) normal breast epithelium. Tumors that belong to this group have a high proliferation rate, are high-grade, and not surprisingly display aggressive clinical behavior. The greatest molecular and clinical differences are between basal-like tumors and other subtypes (105,106). The **HER2** group is defined by high expression of HER2 and related genes. Several subtypes that are associated with different phenotypes as well as outcomes exist within the HER2 group. Tumors that are HER2-positive and ER-positive typically belong to the luminal B group.

Several additional subtypes (including claudin-low, molecular apocrine, and interferon-related) have been additionally described. **Claudin-low** tumors are usually also triple-negative

and may show metaplastic or "medullary-like" differentiation (107). Survival rates for this group lie between those for luminal and basal-like tumors. **Molecular apocrine** group of tumors are ER-negative and androgen receptor (AR)-positive, and their constituent cells display apocrine cytologic features (108). These tumors may be HER2-postive or HER2-negative. The **interferon-related** group shows high expression of interferon-associated genes—including *STAT1* (104). The clinical significance of these more recently described subtypes is as yet not fully established.

Gene expression profiling of breast carcinomas is mainly used in research settings. This sophisticated technique is of limited practical utility in clinical practice, because it is prohibitive in terms of time, effort, and cost. Immunohistochemical surrogates for gene expression profile–based intrinsic subtypes have been developed. ER, PR, and HER2 are critical to these surrogate profiles (**Table 9.2**). Ki67 appears to be a useful discriminator between luminal A and B groups. The addition of CK5/6 and EGFR are helpful in identifying the basal-like type of tumors (**Fig. 9.21**) (105,106).

Surrogate immunohistochemical profiling overlaps, for the most part, with gene expression profiling; however, it does not replace it. The immunohistochemically characterized triple-negative carcinomas and gene expression–profiled basal-like carcinomas have some commonality; however, the two terms cannot be regarded to be synonymous. A carcinoma cannot be identified as having the basal-like phenotype solely on the basis of the triple-negative marker status. Not all triple-negative tumors express basal cytokeratins, and a subset of basal-like carcinomas are not triple-negative (109,110). In this respect, a discordance rate of up to 30% has been reported (111,112). Nevertheless, the role of "surrogate profiling," particularly with respect to "high" proliferation rate and "low" hormone receptor status, continues to evolve with respect to implications for management (113).

TABLE 9.2
Surrogate Immunohistochemical Classification for Gene Expression Profile–Based Intrinsic Subtypes

	Luminal A	Luminal B	HER2	Basal-like[a]
ER	+	+	−	−
PR	+	+/Weak	−	−
HER2	−	+/−	+	−
Ki67	Low	High	Higher	Highest

[a]Basal-like invasive carcinomas are typically also immunoreactive for CK5/6, CK14, CK17, EGFR and p53.

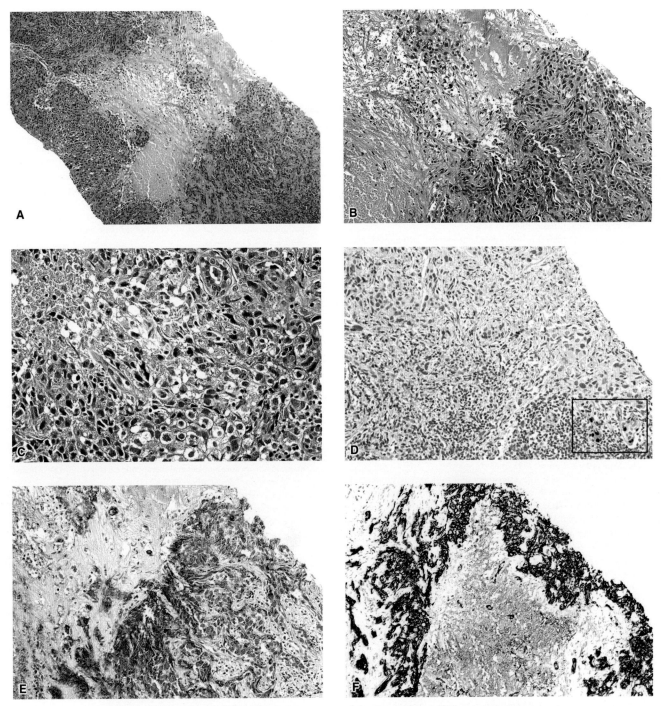

FIGURE 9.21 Invasive Ductal Carcinoma, Triple Negative and Basal-like Immunopheno-type. This needle core biopsy sample is from a 30-year-old woman. **A–C:** Invasive ductal carci-noma, poorly differentiated, with prominent lymphocytic infiltration and focal necrosis, features commonly found in triple-negative and basal-like carcinomas. **D:** The carcinoma did not express hormone receptors or HER2. Estrogen receptor reactivity is evident in the nuclei of non-neoplastic lobular cells *(box)*. **E, F:** The carcinoma was immunoreactive for CK5/6 **(E)** and EGFR **(F)**, markers of basal-like immunophenotype.

REFERENCES

1. Lakhani SR, Ellis IO, Schnitt SJ, et al. *WHO Classification of Breast Tumors.* 4th ed. Lyon, France: IARC Press; 2012:34.

2. Esposito NN, Chivukula M, Dabbs DJ. The ductal phenotypic expression of the E-cadherin/catenin complex in tubulolobular carcinoma of the breast: an immunohistochemical and clinicopathologic study. *Mod Pathol.* 2007;20:130–138.

3. Brunner AH, Sagmeister T, Kremer J, et al. The accuracy of frozen section analysis in ultrasound-guided core needle biopsy of breast lesions. *BMC Cancer.* 2009;9:341.

4. Kehl S, Mechler C, Menton S, et al. Touch imprint cytology of core needle biopsy specimens for the breast and quick stain procedure for immediate diagnosis. *Anticancer Res.* 2014;34:153–157.

5. Wauters CA, Sanders-Eras CT, Kooistra BW, et al. Modified core wash cytology procedure for the immediate diagnosis of core needle biopsies of breast lesions. *Cancer.* 2009;117:333–337.

6. Wauters CA, Sanders-Eras MC, de Kievit-van der Heijden IM, et al. Modified core wash cytology (CWC), an asset in the diagnostic work-up of breast lesions. *Eur J Surg Oncol.* 2010;36:957–962.

7. Manion E, Brock JE, Raza S, et al. MRI-guided breast needle core biopsies: pathologic features of newly diagnosed malignancies. *Breast J.* 2014;20:453–460.

8. Ginter PS, Winant AJ, Hoda SA. Cystic apocrine hyperplasia is the most common finding in MRI detected breast lesions. *J Clin Pathol.* 2014;67:182–186.

9. Sung JS, Jochelson MS, Brennan S, et al. MR imaging features of triple-negative breast cancers. *Breast J.* 2013;19:643–649.

10. Yamaguchi R, Tanaka M, Mizushima Y, et al. "High-grade" central acellular carcinoma and matrix-producing carcinoma of the breast: correlation between ultrasonographic findings and pathological features. *Med Mol Morphol.* 2011;44:151–157.

11. Seidman JD, Schnaper LA, Aisner SC. Relationship of the size of the invasive component of the primary breast carcinoma to axillary lymph node metastasis. *Cancer.* 1995;75:65–71.

12. Silverberg SG, Chitale AR. Assessment of significance of proportions of intraductal and infiltrating tumor growth in ductal carcinoma of the breast. *Cancer.* 1978;32:830–837.

13. Say CC, Donegan WL. Invasive carcinoma of the breast: prognostic significance of tumor size and involved axillary lymph nodes. *Cancer.* 1974;34:468–471.

14. Smart CR, Myers MH, Gloecker LA. Implications for SEER data on breast cancer management. *Cancer.* 1978;41:787–789.

15. Weaver DL, Rosenberg RD, Barlow WE. Pathologic findings from the breast cancer surveillance consortium: population-based outcomes in women undergoing biopsy after screening mammography. *Cancer.* 2006;106:732–742.

16. Rosen PP, Saigo PE, Braun DW Jr, et al. Predictors of recurrence in stage I ($T_1N_0M_0$) breast carcinoma. *Ann Surg.* 1981;193:15–25.

17. Rosen PP, Saigo PE, Braun DW Jr, et al. Prognosis in stage II ($T_1N_1M_0$) breast cancer. *Ann Surg.* 1981;194:576–584.

18. Elkin EB, Hudis C, Begg CB, et al. The effect of changes in tumor size on breast carcinoma survival in the U.S.: 1975–1999. *Cancer.* 2005;104:1149–1157.

19. Renshaw AA. Minimal (<0.1 cm) invasive carcinoma in breast core needle biopsies. *Arch Pathol Lab Med.* 2004;128:996–999.

20. Charles M, Edge SB, Winston JS, et al. Effect of stereotactic core needle biopsy on pathologic measurement of tumor size of T1 invasive breast carcinomas presenting as mammographic masses. *Cancer.* 2003;97:2137–2141.

21. Rakha EA, El-Sayed ME, Reed J, et al. Screen-detected breast lesions with malignant needle core biopsy diagnoses and no malignancy identified in subsequent surgical excision specimens (potential false-positive diagnosis). *Eur J Cancer.* 2009;45:1162–1167.

22. Edwards HD, Oakley F, Koyama T, et al. The impact of tumor size in breast needle biopsy material on final pathologic size and tumor stage: a detailed analysis of 222 consecutive cases. *Am J Surg Pathol.* 2013;37:739–744.

23. Edge SB, Byrd DR, Compton CC, et al, eds; for the American Joint Committee on Cancer. *AJCC Cancer Staging Manual.* 7th ed. New York, NY: Springer-Verlag; 2010.

24. Ozerdem U, Hoda SA. Correlation of maximum breast carcinoma dimension on needle core biopsy and subsequent excisional biopsy: a retrospective study of 50 nonpalpable imaging-detected cases. *Pathol Res Pract.* 2014;210:603–605.

25. Berg WA, Gutierrez L, Ness-Aiver MS, et al. Diagnostic accuracy of mammography, clinical examination, US, and MR imaging in preoperative assessment of breast cancer. *Radiology.* 2004;233:830–849.

26. Thomassin-Naggara I, Siles P, Trop I, et al. How to measure breast cancer tumoral size at MR imaging? *Eur J Radiol.* 2013;82:e790–e800.

27. Yeh E, Slantez P, Kopans SB, et al. Prospective comparison of mammography, sonography, and MRI in patients undergoing neoadjuvant chemotherapy for palpable breast cancer. *Am J Roentgenol.* 2005;184:868–877.

28. Schouten van der Velden AP, Boetes C, Bult P, et al. Magnetic resonance imaging in size assessment of invasive breast carcinoma with an extensive intraductal component. *BMC Med Imaging.* 2009;9:5.

29. Varma S, Ozerdem U, Hoda SA. Complexities and challenges in the pathologic assessment of size (T) of invasive breast carcinoma. *Adv Anat Pathol.* 2014;21:420–432.

30. Bloom HJG, Richardson WW. Histological grading and prognosis in breast cancer: a study of 1,049 cases, of which 359 have been followed 15 years. *Br J Cancer.* 1957;11:359–377.

31. Elston CW, Ellis IO. Pathological prognostic factors in breast cancer: I: the value of histological grade in breast cancer: experience from a large study with long-term follow-up. *Histopathology.* 1991;19:403–410.

32. Robbins P, Pinder S, de Klerk N, et al. Histological grading of breast carcinomas: a study of interobserver agreement. *Hum Pathol.* 1995;26:873–879.

33. Kwok TC, Rakha EA, Lee AH. Histological grading of breast cancer on needle core biopsy: the role of immunohistochemical assessment of proliferation. *Histopathology.* 2010;57:212–219.

34. O'Shea AM, Rakha EA, Hodi Z, et al. Histological grade of invasive carcinoma of the breast assessed on needle core biopsy—modifications to mitotic count assessment to improve agreement with surgical specimens. *Histopathology.* 2011;59:543–548.

35. Harris GC, Denley HE, Pinder SE, et al. Correlation of histologic prognostic factors in core biopsies and therapeutic excisions of invasive breast carcinoma. *Am J Surg Pathol.* 2003;27:11–15.

36. Sharifi S, Peterson MK, Baum JK, et al. Assessment of pathologic prognostic factors in breast core needle biopsies. *Mod Pathol.* 1999;12:941–945.

37. Andrade VP, Gobbi H. Accuracy of typing and grading invasive mammary carcinomas on core needle biopsy compared with the excisional specimen. *Virchows Arch.* 2004;445:597–602.

38. Ough M, Velasco J, Hieken TJ. A comparative analysis of core needle biopsy and final excision for breast cancer: histology and marker expression. *Am J Surg.* 2011;201:692–694.

39. Zheng J, Alsaadi T, Blaichman J, et al. Invasive ductal carcinoma of the breast: correlation between tumor grade determined by ultrasound-guided core biopsy and surgical pathology. *AJR Am J Roentgenol.* 2013;200:W71–W74.

40. Dhaliwal CA, Graham C, Loane J. Grading of breast cancer on needle core biopsy: does a reduction in mitotic count threshold improve agreement with grade on excised specimens? *J Clin Pathol.* 2014;67:1106–1108.

41. Dawson PJ, Ferguson DJ, Karrison T. The pathologic findings of breast cancer in patients surviving 25 years after radical mastectomy. *Cancer.* 1982;50:2131–2138.

42. LeDoussal V, Tubiana-Hulin M, Friedman S, et al. Prognostic value of histologic grade/nuclear components of Scarff-Bloom-Richardson (SBR): an improved score modification based on a multivariate analysis of 1262 invasive ductal carcinomas. *Cancer.* 1989;64:1914–1921.

43. Locker A, Ellis IO, Morgan DA, et al. Factors influencing local recurrence after excision and radiotherapy for primary breast cancer. *Br J Surg.* 1989;76:890–894.

44. Nixon AJ, Schnitt SJ, Gelman R, et al. Relationship of tumor grade to other pathologic features and to treatment outcome of patients with early stage breast carcinoma treated with breast-conserving therapy. *Cancer.* 1996;78:426–431.

45. Karp SE, Tonin PN, Begin LR, et al. Influence of BRCA1 mutations on nuclear grade and estrogen receptor status of breast carcinoma in Ashkenazi Jewish women. *Cancer.* 1997;80:435–441.

46. Mavaddat N, Barrowdale D, Andrulis IL, et al. Pathology of breast and ovarian cancers among BRCA1 and BRCA2 mutation carriers: results from the Consortium of Investigators of Modifiers of BRCA1/2 (CIMBA). *Cancer Epidemiol Biomarkers Prev.* 2012;21:134–147.

47. Gilchrist KW, Gould VE, Hirschl S, et al. Interobserver variation in the identification of breast carcinoma in intramammary lymphatics. *Hum Pathol.* 1982;13:170–172.

48. Rosen PP. Tumor emboli in intramammary lymphatics in breast carcinoma: pathologic criteria for diagnosis and clinical significance. *Pathol Annu.* 1983;18(pt 2):215–232.

49. Acs G, Dumoff KL, Solin LJ, et al. Extensive retraction artifact correlates with lymphatic invasion and nodal metastasis and predicts poor outcome in early stage breast carcinoma. *Am J Surg Pathol.* 2007;31:129–140.

50. Acs G, Paragh G, Chuang S-T, et al. The presence of micropapillary features and retraction artifact in needle core biopsy material predicts lymph node metastasis in breast carcinoma. *Am J Surg Pathol.* 2009;33:202–210.

51. Koo JS, Jung WH, Kim H. Epithelial displacement into the lymphovascular space can be seen in breast core needle biopsy specimens. *Am J Clin Pathol.* 2010;133:781–787.

52. Saigo PE, Rosen PP. The application of immunohistochemical stains to identify endothelial-lined channels in mammary carcinoma. *Cancer.* 1987;59:51–54.

53. Kahn HJ, Marks A. A new monoclonal antibody, D2-40, for detection of lymphatic invasion in primary tumors. *Lab Invest.* 2002;82:1255–1257.

54. Fukunaga M. Expression of D2-40 in lymphatic endothelium of normal tissues and in vascular tumors. *Histopathology.* 2005;46:396–402.

55. Miettinen M, Wang ZF, Paetau A, et al. ERG transcription factor as an immunohistochemical marker for vascular endothelial tumors and prostatic carcinoma. *Am J Surg Pathol.* 2011;35:432–441.

56. Van den Eynden GG, van der Auwera I, van Laere SJ, et al. Distinguishing blood and lymph vessel invasion in breast cancer: a prospective immunohistochemical study. *Br J Cancer.* 2006;94:1643–1649.

57. de Mascarel I, MacGrogan G, Debled M, et al. D2-40 in breast cancer: should we detect more vascular emboli? *Mod Pathol.* 2009;22:216–222.

58. Rabban JT, Chen Y-Y. D2-40 expression in breast myoepithelium: potential pitfalls in distinguishing intralymphatic carcinoma from *in situ* carcinoma. *Hum Pathol.* 2008;39:175–183.

59. Quiet CA, Ferguson DJ, Weichselbaum RR, et al. Natural history of node-positive breast cancer: the curability of small cancers with a limited number of positive nodes. *J Clin Oncol.* 1996;14:3105–3111.

60. Bettelheim R, Penman HG, Thornton-Jones H, et al. Prognostic significance of peritumoral vascular invasion in breast cancer. *Br J Cancer.* 1984;50:771–777.

61. Nime F, Rosen PP, Thaler H, et al. Prognostic significance of tumor emboli in intramammary lymphatics in patients with mammary carcinoma. *Am J Surg Pathol.* 1977;1:25–30.

62. Lauria R, Perrone F, Carlomagno C, et al. The prognostic value of lymphatic and blood vessel invasion in operable breast cancer. *Cancer.* 1995;76:1772–1778.

63. Clemente CG, Boracchi P, Andreola S, et al. Peritumoral lymphatic invasion in patients with node-negative mammary duct carcinoma. *Cancer.* 1992;69:1396–1403.

64. Liljegren G, Holmberg I, Bergh J, et al. 20-year results after sector resection with or without postoperative radiotherapy for stage I breast cancer: a randomized trial. *J Clin Oncol.* 1999;17:2326–2333.

65. Roses DF, Bell DA, Flotte TJ, et al. Pathologic predictors of recurrence in stage 1 ($T_1N_0M_0$) breast cancer. *Am J Clin Pathol.* 1982;78:817–820.

66. Hoda SA, Rosen PP. Contemporaneous H&E sections should be standard practice in diagnostic immunopathology. *Am J Surg Pathol.* 2007;31:1627.

67. Hoda SA, Hoda RS, Merlin S, et al. Issues relating to lymphovascular invasion in breast carcinoma. *Adv Anat Pathol.* 2006;13:308–315.

68. Rak JW, St. Croix BD, Kerbel RS. Consequences of angiogenesis for tumor progression, metastasis and cancer therapy. *Anticancer Drugs.* 1995;6:3–18.

69. Vasudev NS, Reynolds AR. Anti-angiogenic therapy for cancer: current progress, unresolved questions and future directions. *Angiogenesis.* 2014;17:471–494.

70. de Jong JS, van Diest PJ, Baak JPA. Methods in laboratory investigation: heterogeneity and reproducibility of microvessel counts in breast cancer. *Lab Invest.* 1995;73:922–926.

71. Karak SG, Quatrano N, Buckley J, et al. Prevalence and significance of perineural invasion in invasive breast carcinoma. *Conn Med.* 2010;74:17–21.

72. Tamura S, Enjoji M. Elastosis in neoplastic and non-neoplastic tissues from patients with mammary carcinoma. *Acta Pathol Jpn.* 1988;38:1537–1546.

73. Glaubitz LC, Bowen JH, Cox ED, et al. Elastosis in human breast cancer: correlation with sex steroid receptors and comparison with clinical outcome. *Arch Pathol Lab Med.* 1984;108:27–30.

74. Tramm T, Kim JY, Tavassoli FA. Diminished number or complete loss of myoepithelial cells associated with metaplastic and neoplastic apocrine lesions of the breast. *Am J Surg Pathol.* 2011;35:202–211.

75. Cserni G. Benign apocrine papillary lesions of the breast lacking or virtually lacking myoepithelial cells-potential pitfalls in diagnosing malignancy. *APMIS.* 2012;120:249–252.

76. Ross DS, Wen YH, Brogi E. Ductal carcinoma in situ: morphology-based knowledge and molecular advances. *Adv Anat Pathol.* 2013;20:205–216.

77. Schnitt SJ, Connolly JL, Harris JR, et al. Pathologic predictors of early local recurrences in stage I and II breast cancer treated by primary radiation therapy. *Cancer.* 1984;53:1049–1057.

78. Rosen PP, Kinne DW, Lesser ML, et al. Are prognostic factors for local control of breast cancer treated by primary radiotherapy significant for patients treated by mastectomy? *Cancer.* 1986;57:1415–1420.

79. Hurd TC, Sneige N, Allen PK, et al. Impact of extensive intraductal component on recurrence and survival in patients with stage I and II breast cancer treated with breast conservation therapy. *Ann Surg Oncol.* 1997;4:119–124.

80. Schnitt SJ, Abner A, Gelman R, et al. The relationship between microscopic margins of resection and the risk of local recurrence in patients with breast cancer treated with breast-conserving surgery and radiation therapy. *Cancer.* 1994;74:1746–1751.

81. Joh JE, Esposito NN, Kiluk JV, et al. Pathologic tumor response of invasive lobular carcinoma to neo-adjuvant chemotherapy. *Breast J.* 2012;18:569–574.

82. Hicks DG, Fitzgibbons P, Hammond E. Core vs. breast resection specimen: does it make a difference for HER2 results? *Am J Clin Pathol.* 2015;144:533–535.

83. Arnould L, Roger P, Macgrogan G, et al. Accuracy of HER2 status determination on breast core-needle biopsies (immunohistochemistry, FISH, CISH and SISH vs. FISH). *Mod Pathol.* 2012;25:675–682.

84. Petrau C, Clatot F, Cornic M, et al. Reliability of prognostic and predictive factors evaluated by needle core biopsies of large breast invasive tumors. *Am J Clin Pathol.* 2015;144:555–562.

85. Lee AH, Key HP, Bell JA, et al. Concordance of HER2 status assessed on needle core biopsy and surgical specimens of invasive carcinoma of the breast. *Histopathology.* 2012;60:880–884.

86. Chen X, Yuan Y, Gu Z, et al. Accuracy of estrogen receptor, progesterone receptor, and HER2 status between core needle and open excision biopsy in breast cancer: a meta-analysis. *Breast Cancer Res Treat.* 2012;134:957–967.

87. Hammond ME, Hicks DG. American Society of Clinical Oncology/College of American Pathologists HER2 testing clinical practice guideline upcoming modifications: proof that clinical practice guidelines are living documents. *Arch Pathol Lab Med.* 2015;139:970–971.

88. Markopoulos C. Overview of the use of Oncotype DX as an additional treatment decision tool in early breast cancer. *Expert Rev Anticancer Ther.* 2013;13:179–194.

89. Bartlett JM, Starczynski J. Quantitative reverse transcriptase polymerase chain reaction and the Oncotype DX test for assessment of human epidermal growth factor receptor 2 status: time to reflect again? *J Clin Oncol.* 2011;29:4219–4221.

90. Dabbs DJ, Klein ME, Mohsin SK, et al. High false-negative rate of HER2 quantitative reverse transcription polymerase chain reaction of the Oncotype DX test: an independent quality assurance study. *J Clin Oncol.* 2011;29:4279–4285.

91. Moore OS Jr, Foote FW Jr. The relatively favorable prognosis of medullary carcinoma of the breast. *Cancer.* 1949;2:635–642.

92. Kuroda H, Tamaru J, Sakamoto G, et al. Immunophenotype of lymphocytic infiltration in medullary carcinoma of the breast. *Virchows Arch.* 2005;446:10–14.

93. Denkert C, Loibl S, Noske A, et al. Tumor-associated lymphocytes as an independent predictor of response to neoadjuvant chemotherapy in breast cancer. *J Clin Oncol.* 2010;28:105–113.

94. Ocaña A, Diez-Gónzález L, Adrover E, et al. Tumor-infiltrating lymphocytes in breast cancer: ready for prime time? *J Clin Oncol.* 2015;33:1298–1299.

95. Lee HJ, Kim JY, Park IA, et al. Prognostic significance of tumor-infiltrating lymphocytes and the tertiary lymphoid structures in HER2-positive breast cancer treated with adjuvant trastuzumab. *Am J Clin Pathol.* 2015;144:278–288.

96. Ono M, Tsuda H, Shimizu C, et al. Tumor-infiltrating lymphocytes are correlated with response to neoadjuvant chemotherapy in triple-negative breast cancer. *Breast Cancer Res Treat.* 2012;132:793–805.

97. Salgado R, Denkert C, Demaria S, et al. The evaluation of tumor-infiltrating lymphocytes (TILs) in breast cancer: recommendations by an International TILs Working Group 2014. *Ann Oncol.* 2015;26:259–271.

98. Martinet L, Garrido I, Girard JP. Tumor high endothelial venules (HEVs) predict lymphocyte infiltration and favorable prognosis in breast cancer. *Oncoimmunology.* 2012;1:789–790.

99. Matsumoto H, Koo SL, Dent R, et al. Role of inflammatory infiltrates in triple negative breast cancer. *J Clin Pathol.* 2015;68:506–510.

100. Denkert C. Diagnostic and therapeutic implications of tumor-infiltrating lymphocytes in breast cancer. *J Clin Oncol.* 2013;31:836–837.

101. Provenzano E, Bossuyt V, Viale G, et al. Standardization of pathologic evaluation and reporting of postneoadjuvant specimens in clinical trials of breast cancer: recommendations from an international working group. *Mod Pathol.* 2015;28:1185–1201.

102. Perou CM, Sørlie T, Eisen MB, et al. Molecular portraits of human breast tumors. *Nature.* 2000;406:747–752.

103. Gnant M, Thomssen C, Harbeck N. St. Gallen/Vienna 2015: a brief summary of the consensus discussion. *Breast Care (Basel).* 2015;10:124–130.

104. Hu Z, Fan C, Oh DS, et al. The molecular portraits of breast tumors are conserved across microarray platforms. *BMC Genomics.* 2006;7:96.

105. Blows FM, Driver KE, Schmidt MK, et al. Subtyping of breast cancer by immunohistochemistry to investigate a relationship between subtype and short and long-term survival: a collaborative analysis of data for 10,159 cases from 12 studies. *PLoS Med.* 2010;7:e1000279.

106. Green AR, Powe DG, Rakha EA, et al. Identification of key clinical phenotypes of breast cancer using a reduced panel of protein biomarkers. *Br J Cancer.* 2013;109:1886–1894.

107. Prat A, Parker JS, Karginova O, et al. Phenotypic and molecular characterization of the claudin-low intrinsic subtype of breast cancer. *Breast Cancer Res.* 2010;12:R68.

108. Farmer P, Bonnefoi H, Becette V, et al. Identification of molecular apocrine breast tumors by microarray analysis. *Oncogene.* 2005;24:4660–4671.

109. Reis-Filho JS, Tutt ANJ. Triple negative tumors: a critical review. *Histopathology.* 2008;52:108–118.

110. Rakha EA, Ellis IO. Triple negative/basal-like breast cancer: a review. *Pathology.* 2009;41:40–47.

111. Oakman C, Viale G, Di Leo A. Management of triple negative breast cancer. *Breast.* 2010;19:312–321.

112. Schmadeka R, Harmon BE, Singh M. Triple-negative breast carcinoma: current and emerging concepts. *Am J Clin Pathol.* 2014;141:462–477.

113. Coates AS, Winer EP, Goldhirsch A, et al. Tailoring therapies—improving the management of early breast cancer: St. Gallen International Expert Consensus on the Primary Therapy of Early Breast Cancer 2015. *Ann Oncol.* 2015;26:1533–1546.

Tubular Carcinoma

EDI BROGI

Tubular carcinoma (TC) is a highly differentiated invasive ductal carcinoma composed of at least 90% simple monostratified neoplastic tubules with low-grade cytologic atypia (1). TC constitutes up to 2% of all breast carcinomas (2–6). It tends to have small size and is relatively more frequent among T_1 tumors (5–15) and mammographically detected carcinomas (3,7,10,11,16,17). It represents 3% to 4% of stage I and II breast carcinoma (9–11,15). TC has an excellent prognosis (5–15).

CLINICAL PRESENTATION

Symptoms

TC usually occurs in peripheral portions of the breast. It rarely arises near the major lactiferous ducts of the nipple or in the subareolar region, where it can raise the differential diagnosis of florid papillomatosis of the nipple. Nipple discharge, Paget's disease, and skin retraction are rarely associated with TC.

Imaging Studies

TC is frequently detected mammographically as a spiculated mass or an area of architectural distortion. In two recent series, TC constituted only 2% of interval carcinomas, and of carcinomas found in women not participating in a mammographic screening program (3,16) but constituted 8% (3,16) of screen-detected carcinomas. In one study, the average radiographic size of nonpalpable TC was 0.8 cm and that of palpable lesions was 1.2 cm (18). TC often harbors calcifications. The radiologic differential diagnosis of TC includes benign sclerosing lesions, such as radial sclerosing lesion (RSL) and sclerosing adenosis. In particular, TC and RSL are indistinguishable radiologically, and TC can occasionally arise in a RSL (19,20). TC has no distinctive features by ultrasonography or magnetic resonance imaging. Because most TCs are detected by imaging studies, they are often the target of needle core biopsy (NCB) sampling.

Age, Ethnicity, and Gender

TC can occur at any age, but it is more common in postmenopausal women (5,6,8–15,17). A study based on SEER data for breast carcinomas diagnosed in the USA from 1992 to 2007 found that 73.6% of 4,477 TCs occurred in women 50 to 79 years old, 17.5% in women 40 to 49 years old, 6.9% in women older than 80 years, and only 2% in women 30 to 39 years old (4). Between 80% (21) and 90% (4) of TCs occur in non-Hispanic white women. TC constitutes less than 1% of male breast carcinomas (22).

Family History

A high frequency of breast carcinoma has been reported among first-degree relatives of women with TC. A study (10) found that 45% of patients with stage I or II TC had a family history of breast carcinoma, but this finding was not statistically significant compared with the 36% rate in a woman with well-differentiated invasive ductal carcinoma (IFDC) of similar stage. Rakha et al. (11) reported a 20% rate of family history of breast carcinoma in women with TC. Family history of breast carcinoma in women with screen-detected carcinomas was associated with a relative risk of 1.71 for TC compared to 1.57 for any type of invasive carcinoma (23). Family history of breast carcinoma in a first-degree relative tripled the risk of TC in premenopausal women but was not significantly related to TC in postmenopausal patients (21). At least two studies have reported a two- to three-fold increase in the risk of TC in postmenopausal women who used hormone replacement therapy (21,24).

Size

Most TCs are 1 cm or smaller (7,9) **(Table 10.1)**, but larger tumors are encountered occasionally. In one study (11), 59% of 102 TCs measured 1 cm or less, compared to only 30% of 212 IFDC grade I/III; the median tumor size was also significantly smaller.

Multifocality

Few studies have described multifocality in the setting of TC. In one study (25), 5% of 120 patients with TC treated by mastectomy had an additional and separate invasive carcinoma, and 3.3% had multifocal ductal carcinoma in situ (DCIS). In another study (26), invasive lobular carcinoma was identified in 7% of patients with TC. In a recent series (27), 9% of patients with TC had multifocal disease. A second invasive carcinoma of higher histologic grade was present in 15% of cases and consisted of moderately or poorly differentiated IFDC in eight patients, an invasive lobular carcinoma in four patients, and a tubulolobular carcinoma in another patient.

TABLE 10.1

Differential Diagnosis

	Tubular Carcinoma	Microglandular Adenosis	Invasive Ductal Carcinoma, Grade I/III
Morphologic Features			
Glands			
% of the tumor composed of simple glands	≥90%	100%	<90%
Distribution	Haphazard, but fairly uniform within a lesion	Haphazard, but can be somewhat lobulated	Haphazard, but the glands tend to be more tightly clustered in some parts of the tumor, and sparser in other areas
Shape	Round to oval, or angulated (tear drop–shaped glands)	Round to oval	Round to oval, or angulated (tear drop–shaped glands can be present)
Complex architecture	Focal (<10%), if any	Unacceptable (complex glands are diagnostic of atypical MGA)	Present (≥10%)
Epithelium lining the glands			
Stratification	Monostratified in ≥90% of tumor	Monostratified	Focally multistratified (>10% of tumor)
Cell shape	Mostly columnar, focally cuboidal or flat	Mostly cuboidal, focally flat	Mostly columnar, focally cuboidal, or flat
Cytoplasm (volume)	Scant to abundant	Scant	Scant to abundant
Cytoplasm (staining hue)	Amphophilic, rarely eosinophilic	Pale to clear	Amphophilic or eosinophilic
Apical snouts	Common	Absent	Can be present
Nuclear atypia	Mostly low, can be focally intermediate	Absent (unacceptable)	Mostly low, but intermediate nuclear grade atypia can involve a large area
Mitoses	Absent to very rare	Absent (unacceptable)	Absent to rare
Other features			
Basement membrane	Absent (rarely present and discontinuous)	Present (usually complete)	Absent (rarely present and discontinuous)
Intraluminal secretion	Common	Common	Absent
Intraluminal secretion (staining)	Bluish tinge, if present	Densely eosinophilic	Bluish tinge, if present
Microcalcifications	Common in glands and stroma	Can be present in the glands	Common in glands and stroma
Stromal desmoplasia	Usually prominent	Absent	Usually present, but not exceedingly prominent
Stromal elastosis	Usually present, can be prominent	Absent	Usually present, can be prominent
Immunohistochemistry			
ER	Positive (usually >90% cells)	Negative	Usually positive
PR	Positive (usually >80% cells)	Negative	Usually positive
HER2	Negative	Negative	Negative
S-100	Negative	Positive	Negative
EMA	Positive along apical cytoplasmic membrane	Negative	Positive along apical cytoplasmic membrane

In another study (12), multifocal TC was identified in 9.7% of patients, including eight women with two foci each, one with four foci, and another patient with five foci. In general, it is not possible to comment on tumor multifocality when evaluating NCB material from a single radiologic target.

Contralateral Carcinoma

The reported frequency of contralateral carcinoma in contemporary patients with TC ranges from 8% to 26% (5,10,28,29). IFDC is the most common type of contralateral carcinoma. Bilateral TC is uncommon (8,30–32).

Microscopic Pathology

TC consists of a haphazard and infiltrative proliferation of small glands and tubules lined by a single layer of neoplastic ductal epithelium with low-grade nuclear atypia. The diagnosis of TC applies only to lesions in which at least 90% of the tumor mass has the aforementioned morphology (**Fig. 10.1**). Multistratification of the neoplastic epithelium and/or complex glandular architecture can be only very focal, if at all present (**Figs. 10.1 and 10.2**). An IFDC with low nuclear grade and tubular component representing less than 90% of the tumor is classified as well-differentiated (grade I/III) IFDC and does not carry the same excellent prognosis as a TC (11).

The tubules of TC have slightly angular profile (**Fig. 10.1**). Tear drop–shaped glands are common (**Fig. 10.2**). The glandular lumen usually is widely patent, a feature best appreciated at low-power examination (**Figs. 10.1 and 10.2**). The neoplastic epithelium lining the glands is cuboidal or columnar. The neoplastic cells within a given lesion are usually homogeneous, but some variation in the height of the epithelium is often present, and nearly flat epithelium can be found in continuity with columnar cells within an individual gland (**Fig. 10.2**). The cytoplasm is relatively abundant and has amphophilic quality. Cytoplasmic snouts often protrude from the apical surface of the glandular epithelium of TC (**Fig. 10.2**), but this finding is not exclusive to TC. Very uncommon variants of TC feature mucin secretion (**Fig. 10.3**) or apocrine differentiation (33). Eosinophilic cytoplasm and apical intracytoplasmic granules characteristic of apocrine differentiation usually are not present in TC. The nuclei are basally located, round to oval, and show low-grade atypia, with even chromatin and a smooth nuclear membrane. Focal intermediate grade nuclear atypia may be present. Nucleoli are inconspicuous or inapparent, and tend to be adjacent to the nuclear membrane. Mitoses are rare, and necrosis is absent.

The stroma admixed with TC is rich in myofibroblasts, abundant elastic tissue, and myxoid matrix (**Figs. 10.1, 10.2, and 10.4**). It tends to be more abundant than in well-differentiated IFDC and separates the neoplastic glands more widely. Elastosis

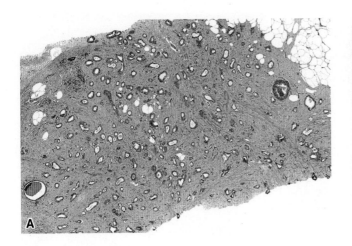

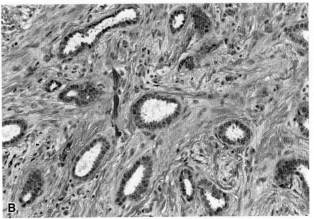

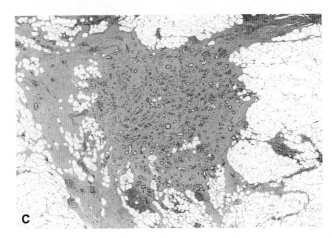

FIGURE 10.1 Tubular Carcinoma. A: A needle core biopsy sample from the tubular carcinoma (TC) shown in (**C**). **B:** The neoplastic glands are monostratified and embedded in desmoplastic stroma. **C:** Residual TC in the excisional biopsy specimen. Note hemorrhage in the surrounding tissue.

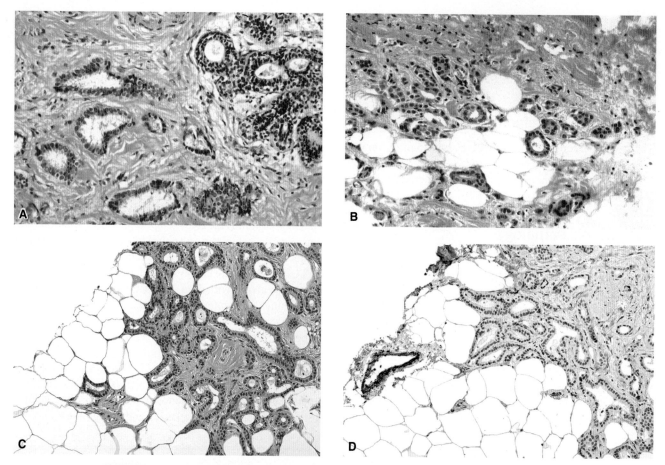

FIGURE 10.2 Tubular Carcinoma. The neoplastic ductules consist of a single layer of uniform cuboidal cells. **A:** A normal terminal duct is shown on the right for contrast with the angular carcinomatous structures. **B:** This carcinoma is composed partly of glands with rounded shapes. **C:** Tubular carcinoma composed of glands of various shapes invades fat. **D:** Absence of myoepithelium is demonstrated by the myosin immunostain. A blood vessel on the left is myosin-positive.

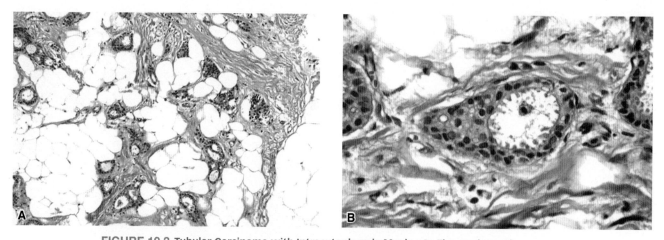

FIGURE 10.3 Tubular Carcinoma with Intracytoplasmic Mucin. **A:** The carcinoma is composed mainly of glands lined by cuboidal cells. **B:** Some cells have intracytoplasmic lumina. **C:** The lumina of some intracytoplasmic vacuoles are outlined in red with the mucicarmine stain *(arrow)*.

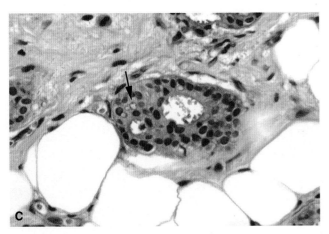

FIGURE 10.3 (continued)

has been regarded as a hallmark of TC (**Fig. 10.5**), but it is not present in all cases and can be a prominent feature also of non-TCs and in some benign lesions, especially those with the "radial scar" pattern.

Calcifications are detected microscopically in at least 50% of TC (**Fig. 10.6**). They are present in the lumen of the neoplastic glands and in the stroma admixed with TC, or are associated with DCIS, atypical ductal hyperplasia (ADH), and columnar cell change (CCC) with or without cytologic atypia. TC does not elicit a notable lymphocytic reaction. Lymphovascular involvement (LVI) is exceedingly rare (6,8,9,11). Clusters of carcinoma can occasionally be identified within vascular spaces in the surgical excision specimen after a needling procedure. Perineural invasion is extremely uncommon, especially in a NCB samples.

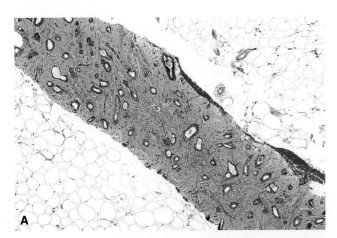
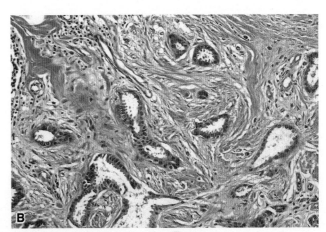

FIGURE 10.4 Tubular Carcinoma and Stromal Desmoplasia. A: The neoplastic glands of tubular carcinoma are admixed with abundant desmoplastic stroma in this needle core biopsy sample. **B:** At high-power examination, abundant desmoplastic stroma separates the neoplastic glands. Note the tear drop–shaped gland on the right and apical "snouts" around many neoplastic gland lumina.

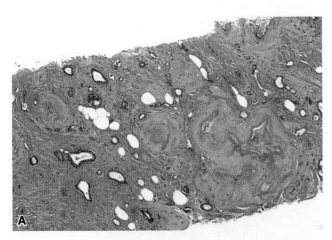
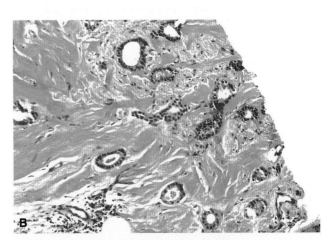

FIGURE 10.5 Tubular Carcinoma and Stromal Elastosis. A: The abundant elastotic stroma associated with this tubular carcinoma in a needle core biopsy sample simulates the elastotic core of a radial scar. The widely open lumina of the neoplastic glands are incompatible with a benign sclerosing lesion and support the diagnosis of tubular carcinoma. No myoepithelium was detected with immunoperoxidase stains for calponin and p63 (not shown). **B:** This needle core biopsy specimen from a nonpalpable tumor shows basophilic elastic tissue in the stroma of a tubular carcinoma.

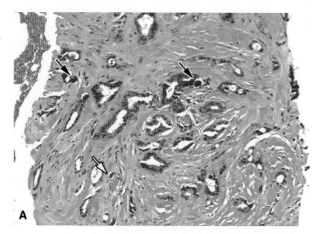
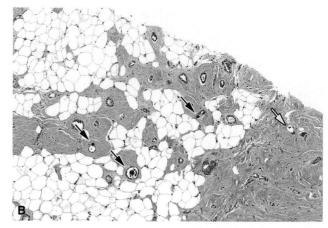

FIGURE 10.6 Tubular Carcinoma and Calcifications. A, B: These needle core biopsy specimens show small, evenly distributed glands with calcifications *(black arrows)*. A minute stromal calcification is also present *(white arrow)*.

Precursor Lesions Associated with Tubular Carcinoma

DCIS has been described in 21% to 41% of cases of TC in recent series (27,34,35). It usually has papillary, micropapillary, cribriform architecture or a mixed pattern **(Fig. 10.7)**, and low to intermediate nuclear grade. TC is frequently associated with ADH and/or CCC of the terminal duct–lobular unit (TDLU) (27,36) **(Figs. 10.8 and 10.9)**, a lesion previously designated informally as "pretubular" hyperplasia (37). The morphologic spectrum of columnar cell lesions ranges from CCC and columnar cell hyperplasia without atypia (CCH) through CCC and/or CCH with atypia, to ADH and low-grade DCIS. The term flat epithelial atypia (FEA) is also used to indicate atypical CCH (38). Apical snouts are present frequently at the luminal aspect of the epithelium showing CCC/CCH, but they are not exclusive to this alteration.

In CCH with atypia, the involved acini are cystically dilated and are lined by polarized cells showing slight nuclear enlargement, nuclear hyperchromasia, and increased nuclear-to-cytoplasmic ratio. The cytoplasm tends to be abundant and has an amphophilic quality. The cells of atypical CCH

have low-grade cytologic atypia, with round-to-oval nuclei, smooth nuclear membranes, and finely dispersed and homogeneous chromatin. The acini affected by CCC/CCH often contain dense secretions that can undergo calcification and are detected mammographically as fine punctate clustered calcifications of indeterminate significance. Blunt micropapillae, abortive cribriform spaces, and/or trabecular bars that alter the "flat" outline of the TDLUs involved by atypical CCC constitute focal ADH.

ADH and DCIS with low nuclear grade and cribriform or micropapillary architecture often arise in the background of CCH with atypia (35,39). TC and columnar cell lesions are also often associated with classical lobular carcinoma in situ (LCIS) and ALH **(Figs. 10.10 and 10.11)**. This complex has been referred to as the "Rosen triad" (27) **(Fig. 10.11)**. In a study of 14 TCs (34), 57% were associated with CCC with atypia (FEA), 50% with micropapillary ADH, 21% with low-grade DCIS, and 29% with ALH and/or classical LCIS. In a study of 102 TCs (11), TC was associated more frequently with columnar cell lesions (93%) than with usual ductal hyperplasia (UDH) (18%) or high-grade DCIS (1%). Columnar cell alterations coexisted

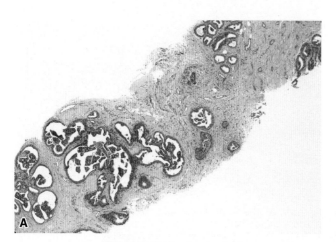
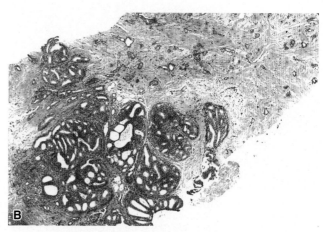

FIGURE 10.7 Tubular Carcinoma with Intraductal Carcinoma. Two needle core biopsy specimens of tubular carcinoma **(upper right)** are shown. **A:** Papillary intraductal carcinoma. **B:** Cribriform intraductal carcinoma.

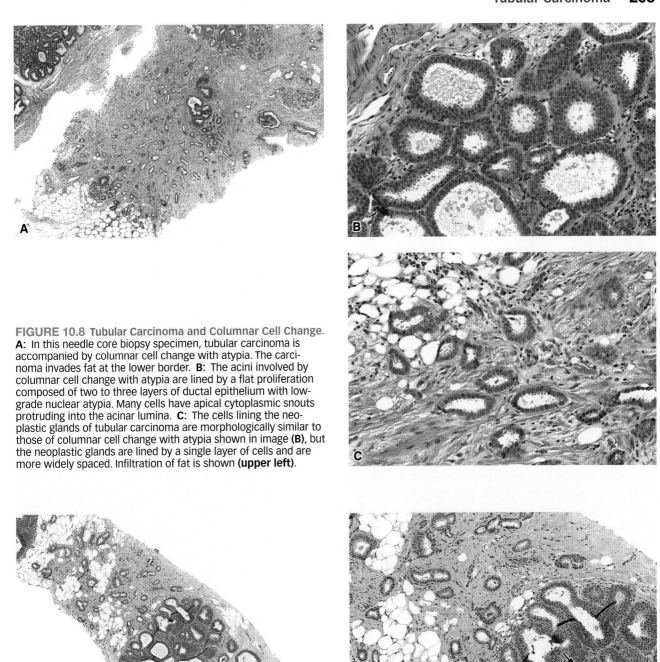

**FIGURE 10.8 Tubular Carcinoma and Columnar Cell Change.
A:** In this needle core biopsy specimen, tubular carcinoma is accompanied by columnar cell change with atypia. The carcinoma invades fat at the lower border. **B:** The acini involved by columnar cell change with atypia are lined by a flat proliferation composed of two to three layers of ductal epithelium with low-grade nuclear atypia. Many cells have apical cytoplasmic snouts protruding into the acinar lumina. **C:** The cells lining the neoplastic glands of tubular carcinoma are morphologically similar to those of columnar cell change with atypia shown in image **(B)**, but the neoplastic glands are lined by a single layer of cells and are more widely spaced. Infiltration of fat is shown **(upper left)**.

FIGURE 10.9 Tubular Carcinoma and Columnar Cell Change with Atypia. A: In this needle core biopsy specimen, tubular carcinoma is adjacent to lobules involved by columnar cell change with atypia. **B:** The haphazard and scattered distribution of the monostratified glands of the tubular carcinoma contrasts with the compact and lobulocentric arrangement of the cystic acini lined by multistratified columnar epithelium with low-grade nuclear atypia. Two glands with focal trabecular bars are diagnostic of atypical ductal hyperplasia *(arrows)*.

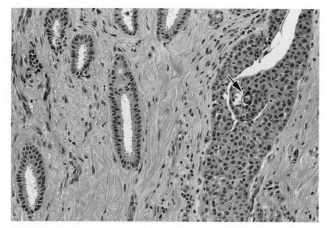

FIGURE 10.10 Tubular Carcinoma and Lobular Carcinoma In Situ, Classical Type. Tubular carcinoma glands **(left)** are adjacent to a focus of lobular carcinoma in situ, classical type in a duct **(right)**. There is a calcification in the duct *(arrow)*.

with 89% of 27 TC in another series (35) and showed atypia in 22 cases; low-grade DCIS was present in 37% of cases.

ALH and/or classical LCIS are found in 10% to 50% of cases of TC (11,27,34,35). They are usually located near TC **(Figs. 10.10 and 10.11)** but can also occur separately in the ipsilateral or contralateral breast.

The identification of any of the aforementioned noninvasive lesions in a NCB specimen mandates careful evaluation to rule out the presence of TC and other low-grade invasive carcinomas. In particular, the proliferative nature of ADH and CCH, often coupled with ALH and/or classic LCIS, sometimes diverts the eye from an inconspicuous focus of stromal invasion. In this setting, examination of the tissue cores at low-power magnification is helpful to identify foci of stromal desmoplasia containing the haphazardly distributed, widely patent and irregular glands characteristic of TC. In contrast, acini involved by CCH with atypia retain a lobulocentric

arrangement and are closely juxtaposed to one another with minimal to no intervening stroma. The acini of CCH with atypia have a cystic and open lumen, but the acinar profile has no angulated contour **(Fig. 10.9)**. At high magnification, CCC with atypia and TC show remarkable cytologic similarity, but the glands of TC have an irregular outline and are lined by epithelium of variable height, devoid of myoepithelium and basement membrane. Few clefts are usually present around the glands of TC, at least focally **(Fig. 10.12)**. This morphologic feature, likely an artifact, is commonly associated with invasive carcinoma, whereas no cleft-like spaces are usually found around normal mammary epithelial structures, including acini involved by CCH with atypia. Focal infiltration of the neoplastic glands into fat, with direct juxtaposition to adipocytes without intervening myoepithelium and basement membrane, is a feature associated with an invasive carcinoma, including TC **(Fig. 10.12)**.

TC is characterized by loss of 16q (40). This chromosomal abnormality is also present in other low-grade mammary epithelial neoplastic lesions, namely CCH with atypia/FEA, ADH, low-grade DCIS, ALH and classical LCIS, well-differentiated IFDC, and tubulolobular carcinoma (41). Rarely, TC arises in association with a benign proliferative lesion with a RSL configuration (42,43).

Immunohistochemistry

Myoepithelial Markers

Consistent with their invasive nature, the glands of TC lack a myoepithelial layer **(Figs. 10.12–10.14)**. Calponin and p63 are the most reliable myoepithelial markers for the diagnosis of stromal invasion. Staining for SMA, albeit sensitive, is difficult to interpret because of substantial reactivity in the myofibroblasts comprising the desmoplastic stroma **(Fig. 10.13D)**. A commercially available cocktail of antibodies targeting myoepithelial and epithelial antigens and optimized for dual

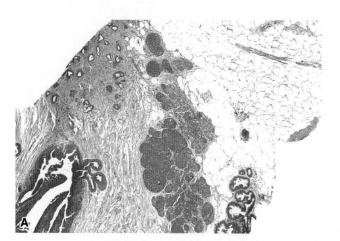

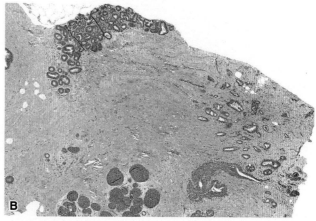

FIGURE 10.11 Tubular Carcinoma, Lobular Carcinoma In Situ, and Columnar Cell Change (Rosen's Triad) in Needle Core Biopsy Samples. A: The triad of tubular carcinoma **(upper left)**, lobular carcinoma in situ **(center)**, and atypical columnar cell duct hyperplasia **(lower left and lower right)**. **B:** Another example of the Rosen's triad in which tubular carcinoma **(right)**, lobular carcinoma in situ **(lower center)**, and columnar cell hyperplasia **(upper center)** coexist in a needle core biopsy specimen.

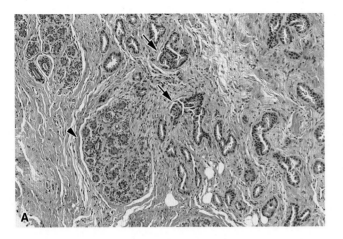

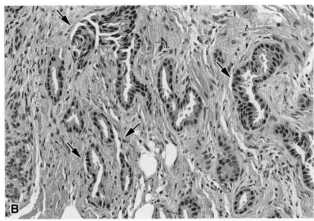

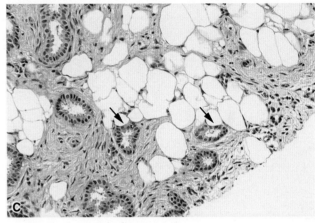

FIGURE 10.12 Tubular Carcinoma, Additional Morphologic Features of Stromal Invasion. A, B: Few cleft-like spaces adjacent to neoplastic glands, with no intervening basement membrane *(arrows)*. Cleft-like spaces are not seen near normal glands and ducts, or a layer of basement membrane is interposed between the cleft and the normal gland epithelium *(arrowhead)* **(A)**. **C:** Small neoplastic glands that abut adipocytes *(arrows)* without an intervening basement membrane are diagnostic of stromal invasion. Subtle evidence of stromal desmoplasia is also present extending into the fat.

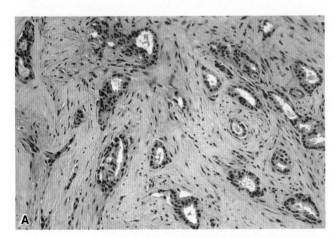

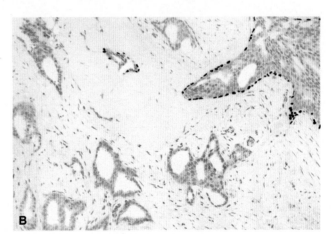

FIGURE 10.13 Tubular Carcinoma, Immunohistochemistry. A: The tumor is composed of angular glands in scleroelastotic stroma. **B:** Myoepithelial nuclei immunoreactive for p63 surround a duct with low-grade cribriform intraductal carcinoma in the upper right corner. p63 reactivity is not present around the glands of the tubular carcinoma. **C:** The CD10 immunostain shown here is difficult to interpret because of cross-reactivity with the stroma. Lack of discrete staining around the tumor glands suggests absence of myoepithelium. **D:** The SMA immunostain shows strong stromal reactivity. The presence or absence of myoepithelium cannot be determined with the SMA stain in this situation. **E:** The immunostain for type IV collagen shown here highlights the basement membranes of a duct and small blood vessels. Immunoreactivity is absent around tubular carcinoma glands in this needle core biopsy specimen.

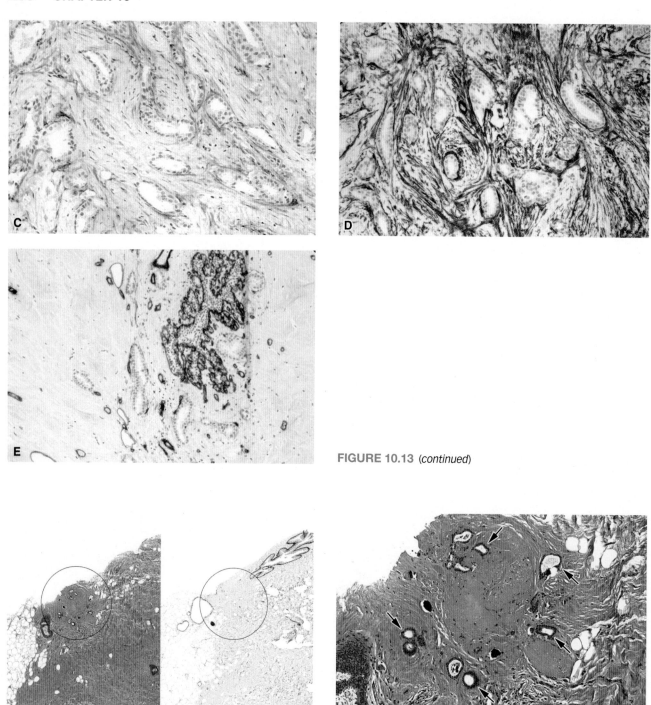

FIGURE 10.13 *(continued)*

FIGURE 10.14 Tubular Carcinoma, Immunohistochemistry. A: At low magnification view, this tubular carcinoma is barely noticeable as a few round small glands in a small focus of stromal elastosis *(circle)*. The calponin stain highlights the myoepithelium in the normal ducts **(right)**, but the tubular carcinoma shows no reactivity *(circle)*. **B:** On closer examination, the neoplastic glands are cytologically bland *(arrows)*. Stromal and glandular calcifications are present.

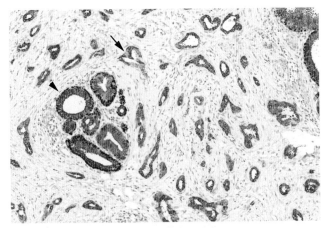

FIGURE 10.15 Tubular Carcinoma, Immunohistochemistry. This image shows the pattern of staining of tubular carcinoma with a commercially available cocktail of antibodies for detection of myoepithelial and epithelial markers in the same tissue section using two different chromogens. The brown chromogen highlights the nuclei (p63) and the cytoplasm (basal cytokeratin 5 and 14) of myoepithelial cells in normal glands *(arrowhead)*. The red-pink chromogen for luminal cytokeratins 7 and 18 decorates the cytoplasm of the epithelial cells comprising normal ducts and lobules as well as the invasive carcinoma. Focally, heterogenous staining intensity in the neoplastic glandular epithelium is evident in some of the glands *(arrow)*.

chromogenic detection (brown chromogen: nuclear p63 and basal cytokeratins CK5 and CK14; red chromogen: luminal cytokeratins CK7 and CK18) **(Fig. 10.15)** might be particularly useful when the invasive carcinoma present in the NCB material is limited, but its sensitivity for the detection of TC has not been specifically investigated. Basement membrane is usually absent around the glands of TC **(Fig. 10.13)**, but immunostaining of basement membrane components is usually not pursued/recommended owing to difficulties in interpretation.

ER, PR, and HER2
At least 90% of TC are strongly and diffusely positive for estrogen receptor (ER) (6,9–13,15,17,28,44) **(Fig. 10.16)**. Progesterone receptor (PR) is detected in 69% to 75% of TC (10,11,15,44,45). All TCs studied by Rakha et al. (11) were negative for HER2/neu and

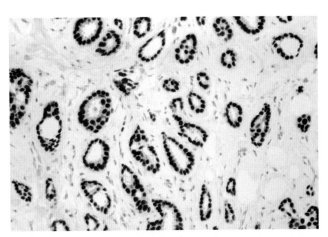

FIGURE 10.16 Tubular Carcinoma and Estrogen Receptor. Nuclei in the carcinomatous glands are strongly and diffusely immunoreactive for the estrogen receptor.

p53. Oakley et al. (46) reported that none of the 55 TCs studied by FISH exhibited *HER2/neu* gene amplification. Considering the bland histomorphology and very indolent behavior of TC, it is recommended to carefully reassess the morphologic diagnosis for any carcinoma classified as TC that is found to be HER2/neu-positive and/or amplified. TC is negative for S-100, CK5/6, and EGFR. Epithelial membrane antigen (EMA) decorates the luminal aspect of the cell membrane of the neoplastic epithelium.

Differential Diagnosis of Tubular Carcinoma

Malignant Lesions
Well-differentiated Invasive Ductal Carcinoma
IFDC (grade I/III) has complex architecture in more than 10% of the tumor and/or consists of glands with two or more cell layers **(Figs. 10.17 and 10.18)** (Table 10.1). The outline of the glands of grade I/III IFDC tends to be irregular and not as sharply defined as for a TC. The glands tend to be more clustered in some parts of the tumor and sparser in others, whereas the glands of TC are somewhat more evenly dispersed in the desmoplastic stroma, despite having a haphazard distribution. The

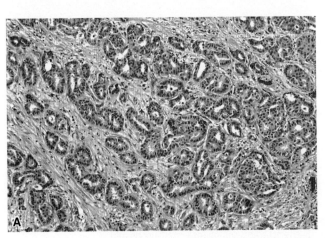
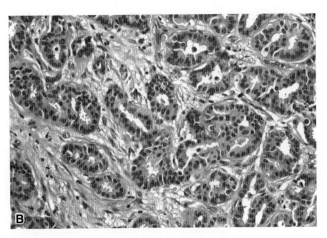

FIGURE 10.17 Well-differentiated Invasive Ductal Carcinoma. A, B: The glandular pattern is more complex than in tubular carcinoma. Intraglandular proliferation is evident.

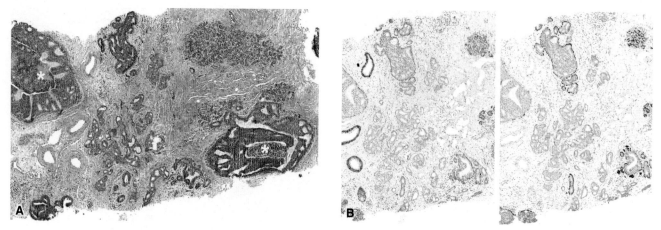

FIGURE 10.18 Well-differentiated Invasive Ductal Carcinoma. A: This well-differentiated invasive ductal carcinoma with cribriform architecture mimics lobular involvement by intraductal carcinoma. The neoplastic glands are adjacent and connected to one another without much intervening stroma. Minimal stromal desmoplasia is present. Two ducts are involved by cribriform ductal carcinoma in situ with central necrosis *(white asterisks).* **B:** Immunostaining for calponin **(left)** and p63 **(right)** demonstrate absence of myoepithelium around the glands of this well-differentiated invasive ductal carcinoma.

stroma of grade I/III IFDC is often less cellular and abundant than in TC **(Table 10.1)**. Pure tubular morphology in a NCB sample does not a guarantee that the rest of the lesion has the same morphology, and definitive diagnosis requires evaluation of the entire tumor. This limitation should be indicated in the diagnostic report.

Tubulolobular Carcinoma

A tubulolobular carcinoma is an invasive carcinoma with areas of TC and invasive lobular carcinoma **(Fig. 10.19)**. Because the percentage of tubular and lobular component necessary for this diagnosis is not defined, the term is used inconsistently. Carcinomas with tubular and invasive lobular areas are part of the spectrum of low-grade epithelial mammary neoplasia (36,41) and often associate with low-grade precursor lesions (47–49).

Invasive carcinomas reported in the literature as tubulolobular range from 0.3 cm to 2.5 cm in greatest dimension (mean size about 1.3 cm) (47–49). Multifocality was noted in 19% (48) and 29% (47) of tubulolobular carcinoma versus 10% (48) and 20% (47) of TC in two studies. Tubulolobular carcinoma is strongly immunoreactive for ER and PR (47,49). It is only very rarely HER2/neu-positive (49). Most tubulolobular carcinomas show membranous reactivity for E-cadherin (48,49), a finding supportive of ductal differentiation.

The identification of cytologically bland epithelium in linear arrays is usually sufficient to separate tubulolobular carcinoma from TC **(Fig. 10.19)**.

Benign Lesions
Microglandular Adenosis

Microglandular adenosis (MGA) (see Chapter 6) is a rare benign epithelial lesion. MGA is an infiltrative proliferation of small glands lined by cytologically benign monostratified epithelium,

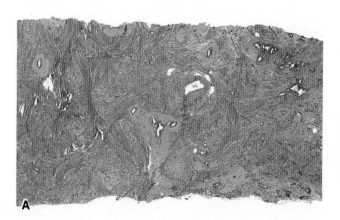
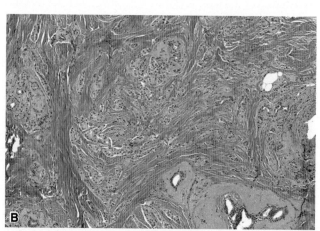

FIGURE 10.19 Tubulolobular Carcinoma. A: The invasive carcinoma in this needle core biopsy specimen consists of small individual neoplastic glands **(right)** transitioning into small cords and trabeculae with lobular features **(left)**. **B:** A higher-magnification view of the lobular-appearing component with typical tubular carcinoma glands **(right)**.

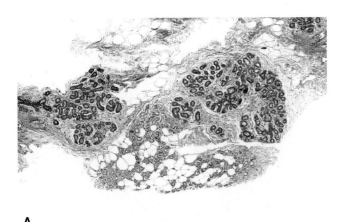
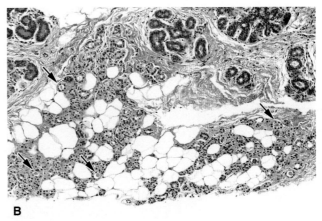

A   **B**

FIGURE 10.20 Microglandular Adenosis. A: A small glandular proliferation invasive into adipose tissue is present in this needle core biopsy. **B:** The glands are round to oval. They are lined by cuboidal monostratified epithelium with pale cytoplasm and inconspicuous nuclei. A few glands contain eosinophilic secretion *(arrows)*. This lesion was strongly S100-positive and negative for estrogen receptor (not shown). This pattern of immunoreactivity distinguishes microglandular adenosis from tubular carcinoma.

devoid of myoepithelium, but surrounded by basement membrane **(Fig. 10.20)** (Table 10.1). The glands are small, round to oval, and have a smooth contour. The epithelium is cuboidal to flat, has uniform height within each individual gland, and has pale-to-clear cytoplasm. The lumen of the glands is open and often contains dense and homogenous eosinophilic secretion that can calcify. The stroma surrounding MGA shows no desmoplasia and inflammation. Small foci of MGA often have a somewhat lobulated arrangement and/or appear confined within lobules of adipose tissue **(Fig. 10.20)**. MGA has been reported only in women. Surgical excision of a radiologic target that yields MGA at NCB is standard practice. TC can closely mimic MGA, but its glands tend to be open and angulated, and they are embedded in desmoplastic and/or elastotic stroma **(Fig. 10.21)**.

Sclerosing and/or Tubular Adenosis

Sclerosing adenosis (SA) is a lobulocentric proliferation of benign small glands and ductules in sclerotic stroma.

Although few scattered glands retain a round open lumen, most glands have a compressed or only minimally patent lumen. Tubular adenosis (TA) consists of elongated benign tubules that tend to be more infiltrating and open than those of SA. The glands and tubules of SA and/or TA are surrounded by spindly myoepithelium that can be highlighted with stains for myoepithelial markers, whereas myoepithelial cells are absent around the glands of TC. A conspicuous layer of eosinophilic basement membrane usually encircles all glands and tubules of SA and TA. The stroma admixed with SA and/or TA is not desmoplastic **(Table 10.1)** (see Chapter 6).

Radial Sclerosing Lesion—Radial Scar

A RSL is a benign sclerosing lesion composed of adenosis and duct hyperplasia or papilloma, often accompanied by cysts. Stromal elastosis is a feature of many RSLs **(Fig. 10.22)**. Compared to a RSL, TC tends to have more open glands, stromal desmoplasia, and infiltrative growth at the periphery of the lesion.

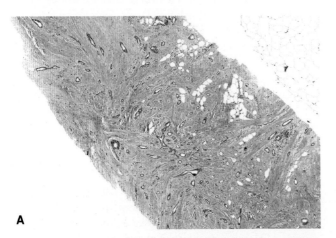
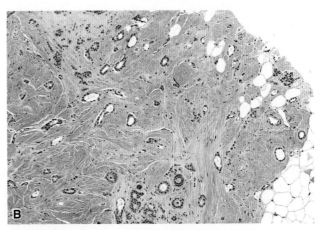

A   **B**

FIGURE 10.21 Microglandular Adenosis-like Tubular Carcinoma. A: The tubular carcinoma in this needle core biopsy sample is partly composed of small round-to-oval glands. It has elastotic stroma with only minimal desmoplasia. A few of the glands have angulated profiles. This lesion was strongly positive for estrogen receptor (not shown). **B:** Round and angular glands are shown in the tubular carcinoma surrounding an atrophic lobule **(lower center)**.

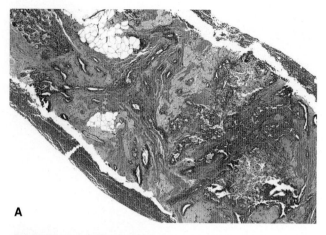

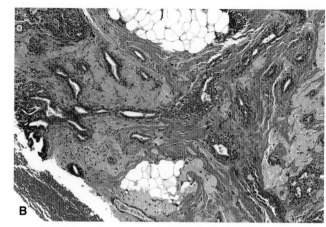

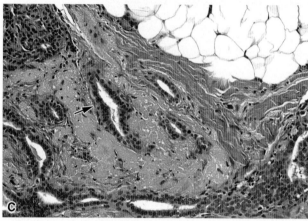

FIGURE 10.22 Radial Scar. **A, B:** The lumens of the ducts and glands in the elastotic nidus of this radial scar are compressed, consistent with a sclerosing process. **C:** A continuous layer of basement membrane is visible around the sclerotic tubules. A few myoepithelial cell nuclei are also noted *(arrow)*.

The use of a panel of myoepithelial markers inclusive of calponin and p63 is recommended for the evaluation of any problematic sclerosing lesion. The sensitivity of a commercially available antibody cocktail (p63, basal cytokeratins CK5 and CK14, luminal cytokeratins CK7 and CK18) suitable for visualization of epithelial and myoepithelial cell in the same tissue section **(Fig. 10.15)** has not been fully assessed for distinguishing between benign sclerosing lesion and TC in NCB material. Whenever immunohistochemical stains for myoepithelial markers are performed, a contemporaneous H&E-stained immuno recut slide should always be prepared (50).

Treatment and Prognosis

Contemporary patients with TC usually undergo surgical excision of the lesion to obtain clear margins; mastectomy is rarely performed. In a study based on SEER data, 82.4% of 4,477 patients with TC diagnosed between 1992 and 2007 underwent breast-conserving surgery, and only 17% had a mastectomy (4).

Most patients with TC treated with breast-conserving surgery receive adjuvant radiotherapy. In an analysis of SEER data (14), 56.1% of 6,465 patients with TC diagnosed between 1992 and 2007 were treated with breast-conserving surgery and radiation therapy, whereas 23.6% had breast-conserving surgery but did not receive radiation. The investigators reported a 5-year OS benefit associated with radiotherapy following breast-conserving surgery (95% vs. 90%, respectively), with a hazard ratio of 1.368 for patients who did not receive it. Other studies have confirmed the benefit of adjuvant radiotherapy following breast-conserving surgery in patients with TC (6–10,12–14,17,51). In particular, three of six patients (50%) with stage I TC and no histologic evidence of extensive DCIS or LVI who were prospectively treated by surgical excision with at least 1 cm wide clear margin and no adjuvant radiation or systemic therapy developed a local recurrence within 5 years after the protocol registration (52).

The frequency of axillary lymph node (ALN) metastases ranges from 5% (12,13) to 25% (5) in contemporary series. Metastatic TC usually involves only one to two LNs (11). In a retrospective analysis of sentinel lymph node (SLN) biopsy in 234 patients with TC (53), 2.5% of patients had macrometastases, and 6.4% had micrometastases. The median size of TC with SLN metastases was 12.17 mm versus 9.39 mm for TC not involving SLN(s). All patients with macrometastases had a TC greater than 1 cm in size, and the latter parameter was the only feature significantly associated with LN involvement on multivariate analysis. SLN biopsy is usually performed in patients with TC and should always be performed if the tumor is larger than 1 cm (53), or if there are other indications that suggest ALN involvement, such as multifocal TC.

According to SEER data, 90.5% of women diagnosed with TC presented at stage I, 8.9% at stage II, 0.4% at stage III, and 0.2% at stage IV (4). A compilation of Netherlands registry data found that 70% of 3,456 patients with TC presented at stage I, 26% at stage II, 2% at stage III, and 1% at stage IV (3).

Adjuvant chemotherapy is rarely administered to patients with TC, and at present no evidence indicates that it is beneficial. The percentage of patients with TC who receive adjuvant hormonal therapy ranges from 10% to 90% (6–13,15,17). Even though TC theoretically constitutes an ideal target for hormonal therapy owing to the high expression of ER, available data do not suggest a substantial benefit associated with hormonal therapy.

A review of contemporary studies with follow-up data (6–13,15,17) shows a local recurrence rate ranging from 1% (17) to 13% (9), with most large series reporting local recurrence rate of 4% to 7% (7,8,10,11).

Rakha et al. (11) compared the outcomes and local recurrence rates in 102 patients with TCs and 212 patients with grade I/III IFDCs. The median follow-up time was 127 months. Local recurrence developed in 7% of patients with TC compared to 25% of patients with grade I/III IFDC. None of the patients with TC died of disease, compared to 9% of patients with grade I/III IFDC. Even when analysis was limited to subcentimeter tumors, TC patients had a longer DFS and breast carcinoma-specific survival than patients with grade I/III IFDC (11). Liu et al. (10) also reported that patients with TC treated with breast-conservation therapy had a lower rate of distant metastases (1% vs. 13%) and breast cancer–specific death (1% vs. 10%) than patients with IFDC. A study (6) of 248 patients with unilateral and unicentric TC reported a survival rate of 96.3% at 5 years, 79.1% at 10 years, and 73.1% at 15 years. Several contemporary series with long-term follow-up report no deaths attributable to TC (7,8,10,11,44,47,54). The hazard ratio of breast cancer–specific mortality in patients aged 50 years or older with ER$^+$/PR$^+$ tumors was 0.58 for TC compared to IFDC of no special type (4).

Overall, TC has an exceedingly good prognosis, which justifies separating it from other forms of low-grade IFDCs.

REFERENCES

1. Foote FW Jr. Surgical pathology of cancer of the breast. In: Parsons W, ed. *Cancer of the Breast*. Springfield, MA: Charles C. Thomas; 1959.
2. Northridge ME, Rhoads GG, Wartenberg D, et al. The importance of histologic type on breast cancer survival. *J Clin Epidemiol*. 1997;50:283–290.
3. Louwman MW, Vriezen M, van Beek MW, et al. Uncommon breast tumors in perspective: incidence, treatment and survival in the Netherlands. *Int J Cancer*. 2007;121:127–135.
4. Li CI. Risk of mortality by histologic type of breast cancer in the United States. *Horm Cancer*. 2010;1:156–165.
5. Gunhan-Bilgen I, Oktay A. Tubular carcinoma of the breast: mammographic, sonographic, clinical and pathologic findings. *Eur J Radiol*. 2007;61:158–162.
6. Fritz P, Bendrat K, Sonnenberg M, et al. Tubular breast cancer: a retrospective study. *Anticancer Res*. 2014;34:3647–3656.
7. Livi L, Paiar F, Meldolesi E, et al. Tubular carcinoma of the breast: outcome and loco-regional recurrence in 307 patients. *Eur J Surg Oncol*. 2005;31:9–12.
8. Sullivan T, Raad RA, Goldberg S, et al. Tubular carcinoma of the breast: a retrospective analysis and review of the literature. *Breast Cancer Res Treat*. 2005;93:199–205.
9. Vo T, Xing Y, Meric-Bernstam F, et al. Long-term outcomes in patients with mucinous, medullary, tubular, and invasive ductal carcinomas after lumpectomy. *Am J Surg*. 2007;194:527–531.
10. Liu GF, Yang Q, Haffty BG, et al. Clinical-pathologic features and long-term outcomes of tubular carcinoma of the breast compared with invasive ductal carcinoma treated with breast conservation therapy. *Int J Radiat Oncol Biol Phys*. 2009;75:1304–1308.
11. Rakha EA, Lee AH, Evans AJ, et al. Tubular carcinoma of the breast: further evidence to support its excellent prognosis. *J Clin Oncol*. 2010;28:99–104.
12. Fedko MG, Scow JS, Shah SS, et al. Pure tubular carcinoma and axillary nodal metastases. *Ann Surg Oncol*. 2010;17(suppl 3):338–342.
13. Hansen CJ, Kenny L, Lakhani SR, et al. Tubular breast carcinoma: an argument against treatment de-escalation. *J Med Imaging Radiat Oncol*. 2012;56:116–122.
14. Li B, Chen M, Nori D, et al. Adjuvant radiation therapy and survival for pure tubular breast carcinoma-experience from the seer database. *Int J Radiat Oncol Biol Phys*. 2012;84(1):23–29.
15. Colleoni M, Rotmensz N, Maisonneuve P, et al. Outcome of special types of luminal breast cancer. *Ann Oncol*. 2012;23:1428–1436.
16. Nagtegaal ID, Allgood PC, Duffy SW, et al. Prognosis and pathology of screen-detected carcinomas: how different are they? *Cancer*. 2011;117:1360–1368.
17. Javid SH, Smith BL, Mayer E, et al. Tubular carcinoma of the breast: results of a large contemporary series. *Am J Surg*. 2009;197:674–677.
18. Leibman AJ, Lewis M, Kruse B. Tubular carcinoma of the breast: mammographic appearance. *AJR Am J Roentgenol*. 1993;160:263–265.
19. Vega A, Garijo F. Radial scar and tubular carcinoma: mammographic and sonographic findings. *Acta Radiol*. 1993;34:43–47.
20. Frouge C, Tristant H, Guinebretiere JM, et al. Mammographic lesions suggestive of radial scars: microscopic findings in 40 cases. *Radiology*. 1995;195:623–625.
21. Li CI, Daling JR, Malone KE, et al. Relationship between established breast cancer risk factors and risk of seven different histologic types of invasive breast cancer. *Cancer Epidemiol Biomarkers Prev*. 2006;15:946–954.
22. Burga AM, Fadare O, Lininger RA, et al. Invasive carcinomas of the male breast: a morphologic study of the distribution of histologic subtypes and metastatic patterns in 778 cases. *Virchows Arch*. 2006;449:507–512.
23. Couto E, Banks E, Reeves G, et al. Family history and breast cancer tumour characteristics in screened women. *Int J Cancer*. 2008;123:2950–2954.
24. Flesch-Janys D, Slanger T, Mutschelknauss E, et al. Risk of different histological types of postmenopausal breast cancer by type and regimen of menopausal hormone therapy. *Int J Cancer*. 2008;123:933–941.
25. McDivitt RW, Boyce W, Gersell D. Tubular carcinoma of the breast: clinical and pathological observations concerning 135 cases. *Am J Surg Pathol*. 1982;6:401–411.
26. Mitnick JS, Gianutsos R, Pollack AH, et al. Tubular carcinoma of the breast: sensitivity of diagnostic techniques and correlation with histopathology. *AJR Am J Roentgenol*. 1999;172:319–323.
27. Brandt SM, Young GQ, Hoda SA. The "Rosen Triad": tubular carcinoma, lobular carcinoma in situ, and columnar cell lesions. *Adv Anat Pathol*. 2008;15:140–146.
28. Winchester DJ, Sahin AA, Tucker SL, et al. Tubular carcinoma of the breast: predicting axillary nodal metastases and recurrence. *Ann Surg*. 1996;223:342–347.
29. Thurman SA, Schnitt SJ, Connolly JL, et al. Outcome after breast-conserving therapy for patients with stage I or II mucinous, medullary, or tubular breast carcinoma. *Int J Radiat Oncol Biol Phys*. 2004;59:152–159.
30. Peters GN, Wolff M, Haagensen CD. Tubular carcinoma of the breast: clinical pathologic correlations based on 100 cases. *Ann Surg*. 1981;193:138–149.
31. Deos PH, Norris HJ. Well-differentiated (tubular) carcinoma of the breast: a clinicopathologic study of 145 pure and mixed cases. *Am J Clin Pathol*. 1982;78:1–7.
32. Carstens PH, Huvos AG, Foote FW Jr, et al. Tubular carcinoma of the breast: a clinicopathologic study of 35 cases. *Am J Clin Pathol*. 1972;58:231–238.
33. Eusebi V, Betts CM, Bussolati G. Tubular carcinoma: a variant of secretory breast carcinoma. *Histopathology*. 1979;3:407–419.
34. Kunju LP, Ding Y, Kleer CG. Tubular carcinoma and grade 1 (well-differentiated) invasive ductal carcinoma: comparison of flat epithelial atypia and other intra-epithelial lesions. *Pathol Int*. 2008;58:620–625.

35. Aulmann S, Elsawaf Z, Penzel R, et al. Invasive tubular carcinoma of the breast frequently is clonally related to flat epithelial atypia and low-grade ductal carcinoma in situ. *Am J Surg Pathol.* 2009;33:1646–1653.

36. Abdel-Fatah TM, Powe DG, Hodi Z, et al. High frequency of coexistence of columnar cell lesions, lobular neoplasia, and low grade ductal carcinoma in situ with invasive tubular carcinoma and invasive lobular carcinoma. *Am J Surg Pathol.* 2007;31:417–426.

37. Rosen PP. Columnar cell hyperplasia is associated with lobular carcinoma in situ and tubular carcinoma. *Am J Surg Pathol.* 1999;23:1561.

38. Lakhani SR, Ellis IO, Schnitt SJ, et al. *WHO Classification of Breast Tumors.* 4th ed. Lyon, France: IARC Press; 2012.

39. Collins LC, Achacoso NA, Nekhlyudov L, et al. Clinical and pathologic features of ductal carcinoma in situ associated with the presence of flat epithelial atypia: an analysis of 543 patients. *Mod Pathol.* 2007;20:1149–1155.

40. Waldman FM, Hwang ES, Etzell J, et al. Genomic alterations in tubular breast carcinomas. *Hum Pathol.* 2001;32:222–226.

41. Abdel-Fatah TM, Powe DG, Hodi Z, et al. Morphologic and molecular evolutionary pathways of low nuclear grade invasive breast cancers and their putative precursor lesions: further evidence to support the concept of low nuclear grade breast neoplasia family. *Am J Surg Pathol.* 2008;32:513–523.

42. Linell F, Ljungberg O. Breast carcinoma: progression of tubular carcinoma and a new classification. *Acta Pathol Microbiol Scand A.* 1980;88:59–60.

43. Linell F, Ljungberg O, Andersson I. Breast carcinoma: aspects of early stages, progression and related problems. *Acta Pathol Microbiol Scand Suppl.* 1980:1–233.

44. Diab SG, Clark GM, Osborne CK, et al. Tumor characteristics and clinical outcome of tubular and mucinous breast carcinomas. *J Clin Oncol.* 1999;17:1442–1448.

45. Fasano M, Vamvakas E, Delgado Y, et al. Tubular carcinoma of the breast: immunohistochemical and DNA flow cytometric profile. *Breast J.* 1999;5:252–255.

46. Oakley GJ III, Tubbs RR, Crowe J, et al. HER-2 amplification in tubular carcinoma of the breast. *Am J Clin Pathol.* 2006;126:55–58.

47. Green I, McCormick B, Cranor M, et al. A comparative study of pure tubular and tubulolobular carcinoma of the breast. *Am J Surg Pathol.* 1997;21:653–657.

48. Wheeler DT, Tai LH, Bratthauer GL, et al. Tubulolobular carcinoma of the breast: an analysis of 27 cases of a tumor with a hybrid morphology and immunoprofile. *Am J Surg Pathol.* 2004;28:1587–1593.

49. Esposito NN, Chivukula M, Dabbs DJ. The ductal phenotypic expression of the E-cadherin/catenin complex in tubulolobular carcinoma of the breast: an immunohistochemical and clinicopathologic study. *Mod Pathol.* 2007;20:130–138.

50. Hoda SA, Rosen PP. Contemporaneous H&E sections should be standard practice in diagnostic immunopathology. *Am J Surg Pathol.* 2007;31:1627.

51. Haffty B, Perrotta P, Ward B. Conservatively treated breast cancer: outcome by histologic subtype. *Breast J.* 1997;3:7–14.

52. Lim M, Bellon JR, Gelman R, et al. A prospective study of conservative surgery without radiation therapy in select patients with stage I breast cancer. *Int J Radiat Oncol Biol Phys.* 2006;65:1149–1154.

53. Dejode M, Sagan C, Campion L, et al. Pure tubular carcinoma of the breast and sentinel lymph node biopsy: a retrospective multi-institutional study of 234 cases. *Eur J Surg Oncol.* 2013;39(3):248–254.

54. Rosen PR, Groshen S, Saigo PE, et al. A long-term follow-up study of survival in stage I ($T_1N_0M_0$) and stage II ($T_1N_1M_0$) breast carcinoma. *J Clin Oncol.* 1989;7:355–366.

11

Papillary Carcinoma

FREDERICK C. KOERNER

Papillary carcinoma represents an uncommon form of ductal carcinoma in which the neoplastic cells proliferate on an arborizing skeleton of fibrovascular fronds. Many papillary carcinomas have cystic areas, but the diagnosis of papillary carcinoma does not require the presence of such foci. In cases showing minimal cyst formation, the underlying fronds do not appear obvious; consequently, one can appreciate the papillary architecture only on the basis of the underlying fibrovascular stromal network. Papillary carcinomas of this type are referred to as *solid papillary carcinomas.*

Because of variation in the use of the term papillary, the literature contains only scant secure data concerning the frequency of genuine papillary carcinoma. It seems to account for approximately 1% to 2% of breast carcinomas in women and a slightly greater percentage in men. Like other forms of breast carcinoma, papillary carcinoma occurs in both noninvasive and invasive forms.

CLINICAL PRESENTATION

Papillary carcinomas usually occur in adults beyond the age of 50 years. On average, women with papillary carcinomas are older than women with other types of breast carcinoma; mean ages range from 63 to 71 years. Small series and case reports document the occurrence of papillary carcinomas in women as young as 29 years (1) and as old as 91 years (2). Men with papillary carcinoma span the same range of ages.

Nearly 50% of papillary carcinomas arise in the central part of the breast. The average clinically determined size of tumors is 2 to 3 cm. At least one-third of patients report a discharge from the nipple. Patients with papillary carcinomas experience bleeding from the nipple more often than do women with papillomas. Paget's disease rarely occurs in association with papillary carcinoma, but it may do so if the carcinoma involves a lactiferous duct.

IMAGING STUDIES

Imaging studies of papillary carcinomas frequently display round, oval, or lobulated masses (3–5). Irregularity of the contour suggests the presence of an invasive component. Studies may also display multinodular densities in a segmental distribution, sometimes confined to a single quadrant (4). Most papillary carcinomas do not contain abundant calcifications; however, punctate calcifications can mark the associated intraductal component (2), and coarse, irregular calcifications may develop in areas of sclerosis or resolved hemorrhage. Sonography typically demonstrates masses that appear well defined, solid or mixed solid and cystic, inhomogeneous, and hypoechogenic with posterior enhancement (3,4,6). Magnetic resonance imaging usually does not reveal distinctive findings.

GROSS PATHOLOGY

Papillary carcinomas are usually well circumscribed, and they may even appear encapsulated. An irregular or ill-defined border suggests an invasive component. The tumor is soft-to-moderately firm depending upon the extent of the fibrosis. Bleeding into the tumor can impart a dark brown or hemorrhagic appearance, but the carcinomas are usually described as tan or gray.

MICROSCOPIC PATHOLOGY

The following morphologic features characterize the histopathology of conventional papillary carcinomas and provide the basis for distinguishing papillary carcinomas from papillomas.

Types of Cells

Malignant ductal cells comprise the entire epithelial population of most papillary carcinomas, whereas benign luminal and myoepithelial cells make up the epithelium of papillomas. A mixture of benign and malignant cells may be present when a carcinoma involves a papilloma. The epithelial cells in papillary carcinomas grow in a disorderly fashion manifest by the loss of nuclear polarity with respect to the basement membrane and uneven stratification of the cells (**Fig. 11.1**). The nuclei exhibit varying degrees of atypia, and the tumor cells sometimes have cytoplasmic "snouts" at the luminal surface (**Fig. 11.2**). The cells form papillary, micropapillary, filiform, cribriform, reticular, or solid arrangements identical to those of conventional ductal carcinoma in situ (DCIS) (**Fig. 11.3**). Rare, low-grade papillary carcinomas have an orderly frond-forming structure and minimal epithelial stratification (**Fig. 11.4**). One may have difficulty distinguishing such cases from papillomas based on H&E-stained sections of needle core biopsy (NCB)

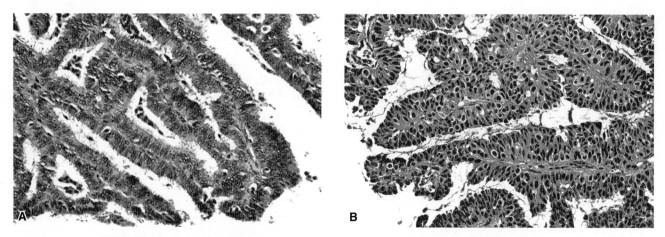

FIGURE 11.1 Papillary Carcinoma. **A:** The columnar cells in this papillary carcinoma demonstrate high nuclear-to-cytoplasmic ratios and inconsistent positioning of the nuclei with respect to the basement membrane. **B:** This needle core biopsy specimen from a 55-year-old woman shows irregular stratification of the neoplastic cells and mucin between the fronds.

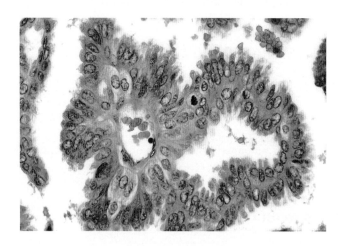

FIGURE 11.2 Papillary Carcinoma. The cytoplasm of the carcinoma cells forms apical blebs. A mitotic figure is present **(upper center)**.

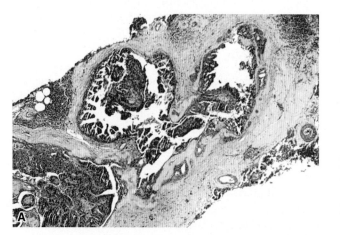

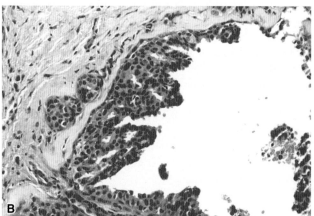

FIGURE 11.3 Papillary Carcinoma. Various growth patterns are represented in these needle core biopsy specimens. **A, B:** Papillary and micropapillary ductal carcinoma in situ (DCIS) are seen. Myoepithelial cells represented by oval nuclei arranged parallel to the basement membrane lie beneath the micropapillary carcinoma in **(B)**. **C, D:** Arborizing micropapillary DCIS with well-differentiated nuclear grade is shown. **E:** A cribriform pattern is evident. **F:** Solid architecture characterizes this region.

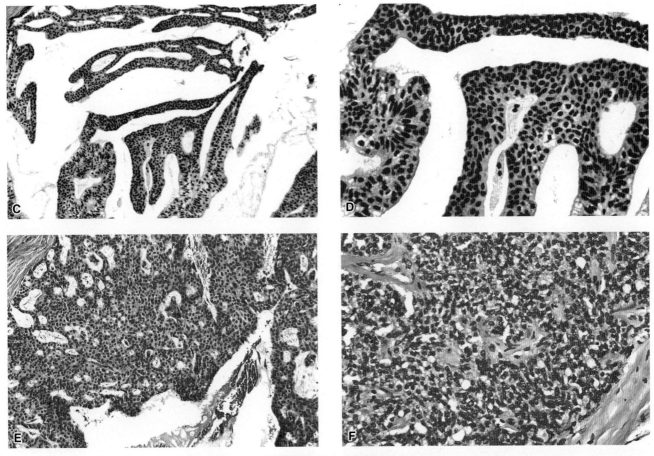

FIGURE 11.3 (continued)

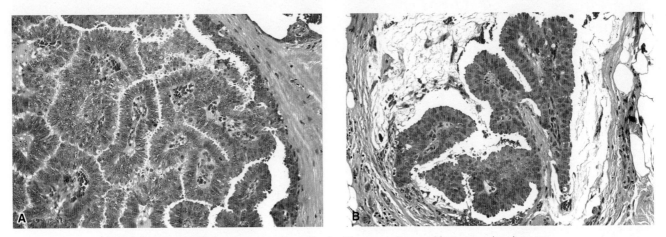

FIGURE 11.4 Papillary Carcinoma, Low Grade. These needle core biopsy samples show an orderly papillary carcinoma. Intraductal papillary carcinoma with mucin formation is shown in **(A)**. Frond-forming invasive papillary carcinoma with mucin is shown in **(B, C)**. Note the stroma in the invasive papillary fronds.

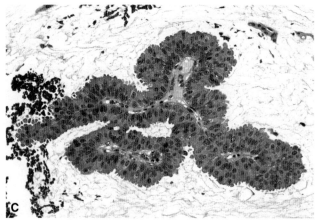

FIGURE 11.4 *(continued)*

samples, but the morphologic features of the proliferative cells identify them as malignant and thereby establish the diagnosis of papillary carcinoma.

Myoepithelial cells, which are distributed relatively uniformly and proportionately within the epithelium of papillomas, are characteristically absent from invasive papillary carcinoma. Although one can usually identify myoepithelial cells in H&E-stained sections, immunohistochemical staining provides a more reliable method for detecting them **(Fig. 11.5)**. Cytoplasmic markers of myoepithelial cells include CD10, smooth muscle actin (SMA), calponin, smooth muscle myosin heavy chain (SMMHC), and cytokeratin 5/6 (CK5/6). The markers cross react with stromal myofibroblasts and vascular structures to varying and unpredictable degrees. The transcription factor

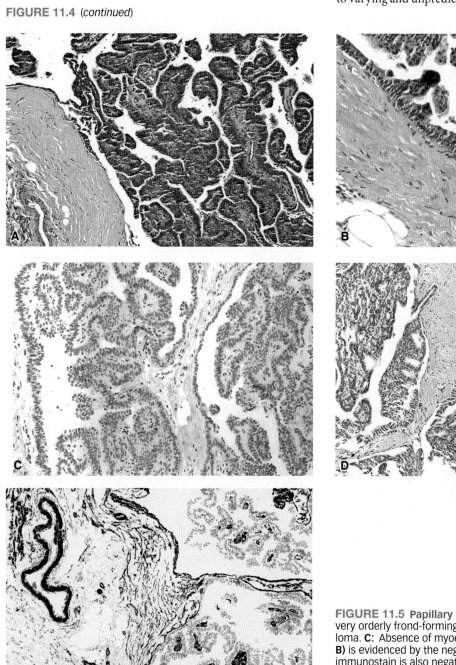

FIGURE 11.5 Papillary Carcinoma, Low Grade. A, B: This very orderly frond-forming papillary carcinoma resembles a papilloma. **C:** Absence of myoepithelium in the lesion shown in **(A, B)** is evidenced by the negative CD10 immunostain. **D:** The p63 immunostain is also negative. Note p63 reactivity around normal ducts **(upper right)**. **E:** The smooth muscle actin immunostain highlights stromal cells and vascular structures. No myoepithelial reactivity is evident.

p63 stains nuclei of myoepithelial cells but does not react with those of stromal cells; however, the marker can also stain the nuclei of occasional carcinomas (7), and it regularly stains the nuclei of squamous cells. The position of spuriously staining epithelial cells apart from the basement membrane and the round or oval shapes of their nuclei identify these cells as epithelial rather than myoepithelial. Whenever possible, it is prudent to employ a panel composed of p63 and two or more cytoplasmic markers when investigating the presence of myoepithelial cells in a papillary tumor (8–10).

The presence of myoepithelial cells in parts of a papillary lesion does not exclude the diagnosis of carcinoma (11–14). Noninvasive papillary carcinomas containing myoepithelial cells often represent papillomas overtaken by carcinoma (15). The myoepithelial cells constitute remnants of the preexisting benign epithelium. They may persist in segments of residual epithelium or as a layer beneath the carcinomatous population.

Cytologic Attributes

The malignant cells of papillary carcinomas demonstrate the cytologic features of commonplace DCIS. These features vary according to the grade of the carcinoma; however, alterations common to all grades include an increase in the size of the cells and their nuclei, hyperchromasia of the nuclei, and an increase in the nuclear-cytoplasmic ratio. In common low-grade papillary carcinomas, the cells appear uniform. Rare high-grade papillary carcinomas demonstrate conspicuous cellular pleomorphism. Mitotic figures can be seen, especially in carcinomas that exhibit severe cytologic atypia. The presence of more than an occasional mitotic figure in a papillary tumor suggests the diagnosis of papillary carcinoma.

Apocrine Cells

Although the cells of papillary carcinoma sometimes have eosinophilic cytoplasm or secretory "snouts," papillary carcinomas do not contain usual, cytologically bland apocrine cells. Uncommon papillary carcinomas consist of cells with apocrine features, but these cells also display the nuclear atypia seen in the nonapocrine portions of the carcinoma, and they do not resemble the bland apocrine cells commonly seen in papillomas. The presence of conventional apocrine cells provides strong evidence to support the diagnosis of papilloma, but their absence does not favor a diagnosis of papillary carcinoma.

Glandular Pattern

The cribriform pattern characteristic of low-grade DCIS occurs in many papillary carcinomas. One must distinguish it from the *complex glandular pattern*, a back-to-back arrangement of glands within the stalk of a papilloma. To make this distinction, one should look for stromal elements between the glands. Cribriform spaces form within aggregates of carcinoma cells unsupported by a surrounding stroma, whereas thin strands of collagen and slender capillaries encompass each of the glands that compose the complex glandular pattern.

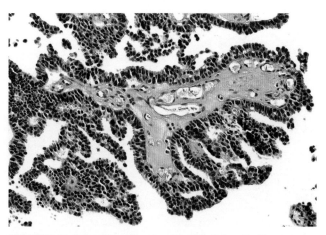

FIGURE 11.6 Papillary Carcinoma with Sclerotic Stroma. Dense collagen forms the stroma in this papillary carcinoma.

Stroma

Although all noninvasive papillary carcinomas possess fibrovascular stroma, it usually appears less conspicuous than the stroma seen in papillomas. One must take care when evaluating this feature, because one can observe inconspicuous cores of dense fibrous tissue in many papillary carcinomas (16), and occasional papillary carcinomas contain prominent stalks of sclerotic fibrous stroma (**Fig. 11.6**).

Adjacent Epithelial Proliferations

Carcinoma in situ usually involves ducts in the region of a papillary carcinoma. When one finds it difficult to diagnose an orderly papillary tumor, study of epithelial proliferations in nearby structures often helps to establish the diagnosis. The presence of papillary, cribriform, or comedocarcinoma in adjacent ducts or lobules usually indicates that the papillary lesion also contains carcinoma. Study of an epithelial proliferation situated on the wall of the duct harboring a papillary tumor can also shed light on the nature of the epithelial cells within the papillary portion.

Coexisting Sclerosing Adenosis

Sclerosing adenosis does not coexist with papillary carcinomas commonly; however, it may involve the tissue surrounding many papillomas, and it can protrude into ducts to simulate a papilloma in uncommon instances.

Intraepithelial Mucin

Many papillary carcinomas do not produce intraepithelial mucin; however, a small number contain signet ring cells, abundant intracellular mucin (**Fig. 11.7**), or mucin within the spaces between papillary fronds (**Figs. 11.8, 11.1B, and 11.4**). Alcian blue, mucicarmine, and periodic acid–Schiff stains will highlight mucin not easily seen on H&E stains. Papillomas rarely produce detectable mucin; thus, the presence of intraepithelial mucin in a papillary tumor suggests the diagnosis of papillary

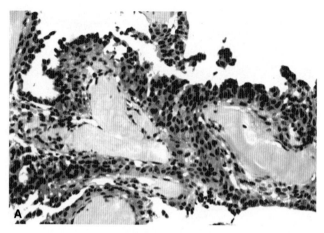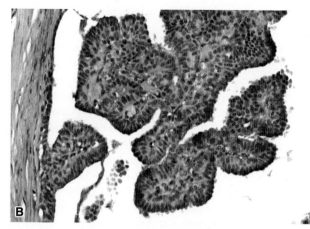

FIGURE 11.7 **Papillary Carcinoma with Intracytoplasmic Mucin.** **A:** Intracytoplasmic mucin is represented by discrete pale blue vacuoles. **B:** The mucicarmine stain colors the mucin magenta.

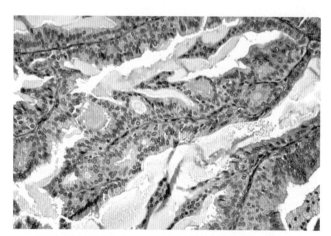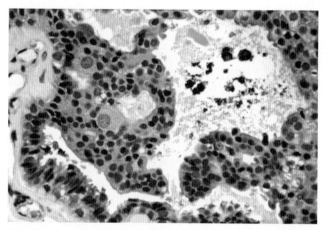

FIGURE 11.8 **Papillary Carcinoma with Extracellular Mucin.** This papillary carcinoma has a micropapillary structure and unusually abundant mucin between the papillary fronds.

FIGURE 11.9 **Papillary Carcinoma with Calcification.** Granular calcifications are present in a ductular lumen in this needle core biopsy specimen containing papillary carcinoma with a micropapillary pattern.

carcinoma. The absence of intraepithelial mucin, on the other hand, does not exclude this diagnosis.

Calcifications

When present, the calcifications in papillary carcinomas often occupy the spaces enclosed by the malignant cells (**Fig. 11.9**). Papillomas do not usually have calcifications in the lumen of the affected duct. Calcifications can form in the stromal cores of both papillary carcinomas and papillomas; so the presence of calcifications in this location does not provide reliable diagnostic information.

IMMUNOHISTOCHEMISTRY

Researchers have studied the immunohistochemical expression of several molecules to facilitate the distinction between papillary carcinomas and papillomas. For example, high-molecular-weight, or basal, cytokeratin molecules (CK5/6, CK14, and 34βE12),

present in hyperplastic ductal cells and myoepithelial cells, are absent or diminished in amount in the neoplastic cells of conventional papillary carcinomas (12,17,18). Because most normal luminal cells also lack high-molecular-weight cytokeratins, staining for these molecules finds its most reliable use in distinguishing hyperplastic ductal cells involving a papilloma from neoplastic ductal proliferations with a papillary growth pattern. Rabban et al. (17) reported the absence of reactivity for CK5/6 in the epithelium of 14 solid papillary carcinomas. CK5/6 antibodies did stain residual non-neoplastic epithelial cells and myoepithelial cells, and they also stained hyperplastic ductal cells strongly. Tan et al. (18) reported that immunostaining for CK5/6 had higher sensitivity and specificity for distinguishing papillomas from papillary carcinomas than did staining for CK14 and 34βE12. Tse et al. (12) observed that moderate to strong staining for CK14 in 50% or more of the epithelial cells resulted in 100% specificity for identifying benign epithelial proliferations involving papillomas. These results make it clear that the expression of these proteins, especially CK5/6, is greatly diminished or absent in most papillary carcinomas, but that the focal, weak presence of these molecules does not exclude the diagnosis of papillary carcinoma. If a diagnosis of papillary carcinoma is being contemplated for a papillary tumor in which there is strong epithelial expression of CK5/6, CK14, or 34βE12, the diagnosis should be reconsidered.

Coupling staining for keratin with staining for other molecules such as myoepithelial proteins, ER, and cyclin D1 offers an additional diagnostic approach. For example, by using sequential staining for 34βE12 and p63, Ichihara et al. (19) identified the neoplastic population in 8 papillomas harboring ADH or focal low-grade DCIS and in 15 papillary carcinomas. The staining results allowed the investigators to distinguish these tumors from 9 of 10 papillomas with usual ductal hyperplasia. Douglas-Jones et al. (20) stained 129 NCB samples of papillary tumors for CK5/6, calponin, and p63. By referring to the staining results, a panel of four pathologists improved their rate of agreement regarding the diagnosis from 44% to 91% and their overall weighted kappa values from 0.696 to 0.954. A prediluted cocktail of antisera to CK5, p63, and CK8/18 allowed Reisenbichler et al. (14) to distinguish 18 papillary carcinomas from 24 papillomas.

Grin et al. (21) combined staining for CK5 and estrogen receptor (ER) in an attempt to identify the presence of atypical cells in NCB specimens of papillary tumors. The investigators observed that more than 90% of the atypical cells in papillomas stained uniformly and strongly for ER, but fewer than 20% stained for CK5. Hyperplastic ductal cells involving papillomas demonstrated the opposite staining pattern. The use of this method allowed the authors to classify NCB specimens of 15 of 15 papillomas and 14 of 15 papillary tumors containing atypical or malignant cells correctly when compared with the findings of excision specimens.

Wang et al. (22) found that many cells of papillary carcinomas express cyclin D1, but only a few cells of papillomas do so. In this investigation, papillomas demonstrated high expression of CK5/6 and low expression of cyclin D1, whereas papillary carcinomas yielded the opposite results. In one study (23), 32 of 33 (97%) papillomas showed strong staining for CD133, whereas only 3 of 33 (9%) stained strongly.

Papillary carcinomas typically express ER and PR, but those composed of apocrine cells have not stained for these receptors. The carcinomas usually do not stain for HER2.

Although these special studies can help to clarify the diagnosis of papillary tumors in certain settings, the distinction between a papilloma with unusual features and a papillary carcinoma remains difficult when examining specimens obtained by NCB. Occasionally, a core biopsy will provide diagnostic tissue; however, one must note that fragments of florid ductal hyperplasia can suggest the diagnosis of DCIS when seen out of context such as in a NCB sample and that epithelial clusters entrapped in the stromal fragments of a benign sclerosing papillary lesion can mimic invasive carcinoma. Moreover, because carcinoma may only focally involve a papillary tumor, the absence of carcinoma in a NCB specimen showing a seemingly benign papilloma might simply represent incomplete sampling of a papilloma harboring carcinoma. Excision is recommended when a NCB sample reveals a papillary tumor.

CARCINOMA INVOLVING A PAPILLOMA

Certain noninvasive carcinomas displaying a papillary architecture represent papillomas overrun by DCIS rather than conventional papillary carcinomas. Papillomas harboring DCIS display remnants of the preexisting papilloma as well as malignant ductal cells. The intermingling of benign and malignant cells can make the diagnosis of this type of papillary lesion difficult even when one has the entire mass to study. This difficulty increases when faced with the small and fragmented samples provided by NCBs. Significant signs of an underlying papilloma include blunt bulky fronds composed of dense acellular collagen, collections of histiocytes within stromal cores, and segments of epithelium containing well-arranged bland luminal and myoepithelial cells. To make a diagnosis of carcinoma in the presence of an underlying papilloma, one must find a sizeable region in which the growth pattern and cytologic features constitute one of the established patterns of DCIS (**Fig. 11.10**). Some authors have illustrated focal DCIS in papillomas but classified these lesions as "papillomas with atypical ductal hyperplasia." In one of these studies (24), the relative risk for the development of "subsequent" carcinoma in women with such papillomas was more than four times the risk of women with papillomas that lacked ADH/DCIS. Underdiagnosis of such lesions is likely to result in inadequate treatment, as reflected in the outcomes of the patients in these reports.

INVASIVE PAPILLARY CARCINOMA

The growth patterns and cytologic characteristics shown by the invasive components of papillary carcinomas usually resemble those of the in situ portions of the lesions. Carcinoma cells growing on a branching framework form a more-or-less compact mass, sometimes with cystic regions, that dissects into the surrounding tissue. Cribriform, comedo, tubular, and mucinous foci may also be present in the invasive component.

Although the invasive nature of papillary carcinomas often appears obvious, the recognition of minimal invasion can be difficult. Fibrosis, hemorrhage, and chronic inflammation surround many papillary carcinomas, and similar alterations may occur within the tumors. The diagnosis of epithelial clusters within these areas presents a challenge. Groups of neoplastic cells distributed parallel to layers of reactive stroma at the border of a papillary carcinoma usually represent cells entrapped in distorted preexisting glands rather than invasive carcinoma. As a rule, extension of the suspicious cells beyond the zone of reactive changes into the mammary parenchyma and fat offers the most reliable histologic evidence of invasion. Immunohistochemical staining for myoepithelial cells can clarify uncertain cases, especially when coupled with a stain for keratin. A change in the pattern of growth also strongly suggests the presence of invasion. These observations become especially useful when examining cases of solid papillary carcinoma with endocrine differentiation because the detection of invasion typically poses problems in this lesion.

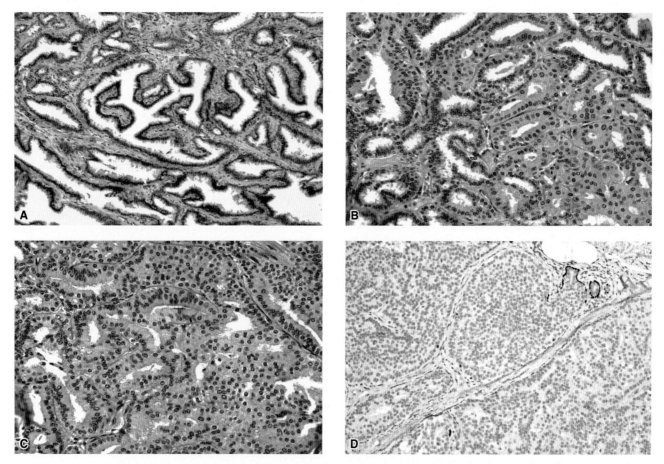

FIGURE 11.10 Papillary Carcinoma Arising in a Papilloma. Several areas in a single tumor are shown. **A:** This papilloma has a thin uniform layer of cuboidal and low-columnar cells overlying a prominent layer of myoepithelial cells and broad strands of stroma. **B:** An enlarged view from another region shows mingling of atypical ductal cells and normal luminal cells. In the region dominated by the atypical ductal cells **(right)**, one has difficulty recognizing myoepithelial cells, and the stromal strands appear more slender. **C:** The carcinoma cells form cribriform structures. Note the persisting arborizing stroma and the virtual absence of myoepithelial cells. **D:** The p63 immunostain reveals that this focus of solid ductal carcinoma in situ lacks myoepithelial cells. A few residual myoepithelial cells remain **(upper right)**.

Papillary carcinomas subjected to needle aspiration or core biopsy before excision can exhibit alterations that complicate the recognition of invasion. The best microscopic clues to such manipulation are the presence of fresh hemorrhage and acute inflammation associated with unexpected fragmentation of the lesion. One can find single tumor cells or compact cell clusters in regions of hemorrhage or granulation tissue formation along the track of the needle. In this clinical setting, one should usually regard these detached cells as an artifact produced by the earlier procedure rather than evidence of invasion. These displaced cells can make their way into capillaries and lymphatic vessels. One should report this uncommon finding because it may be misinterpreted as evidence of invasive carcinoma in some instances (25). Epithelial displacement associated with needling procedures is discussed more extensively in Chapter 25.

Clusters of invasive papillary carcinoma cells are particularly prone to shrinkage artifact, and they often seem to lie in spaces. This phenomenon creates the appearance of lymphatic tumor emboli. When one applies strict criteria for the diagnosis of lymphatic invasion, most groups like these prove to be artifactual.

INFARCTION IN PAPILLARY TUMORS

Both papillary carcinomas and papillomas can undergo complete infarction either spontaneously or after a needling procedure **(Fig. 11.11A, B)**. In many examples of this phenomenon, the structure of the lesion becomes so altered that one cannot differentiate a papillary carcinoma from a papilloma using H&E-stained sections. Immunostains can help to resolve uncertainties if the reactivity of the antigens in question remains. For example, preserved reactivity for keratin may allow one to determine the structure of the tumor **(Fig. 11.11C)**, and reactivity for p63 may reveal the presence of myoepithelial cells.

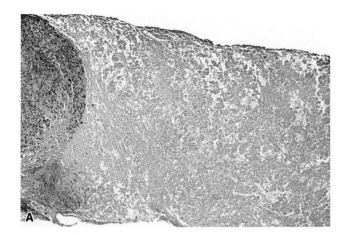

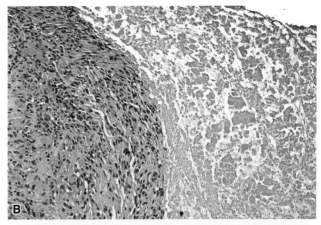

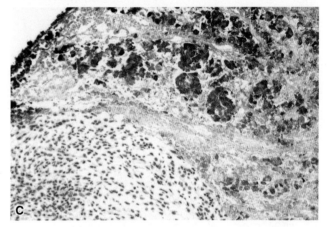

FIGURE 11.11 Infarcted Papillary Tumor, Probably Carcinoma. A, B: The needle core biopsy sample consists of infarcted tumor. Stroma with inflammatory cells is shown on the left. **C:** Papillary clusters of epithelial cells in the infarcted tissue are highlighted by the CK7 immunostain.

SOLID VARIANT OF PAPILLARY CARCINOMA

The solid variant of noninvasive papillary carcinoma has only recently become widely recognized (26). These well-circumscribed and often multinodular tumors consist of ducts nearly or completely filled by solid proliferations of neoplastic ductal cells supported by cores of fibrovascular stroma (**Figs. 11.12 and 11.13**). The solid pattern of growth sometimes gives way to cribriform or conventional papillary formations. Comedonecrosis usually does not occur. The stromal network in the cellular areas often appears so delicate that one might overlook it, but the stroma in the cribriform areas may stand out more prominently. Collagenization of the periductal stroma,

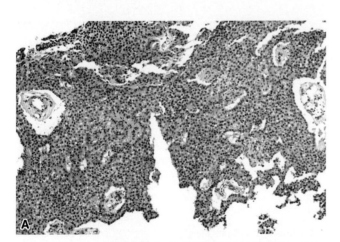

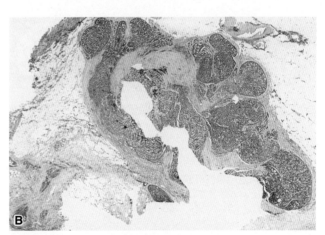

FIGURE 11.12 Solid Papillary Carcinoma. A: A needle core biopsy specimen shows solid areas of in situ carcinoma arranged around fibrovascular stromal cores. The tumor cells have vacuolated amphophilic cytoplasm and well-differentiated round nuclei. One could mistake this specimen for invasive carcinoma if one failed to appreciate the basic papillary structure. **B:** A low-magnification view illustrates the tumor in the excision specimen. **C:** An area at the periphery of the excised tumor duplicates the appearance of the carcinoma in the needle core biopsy specimen.

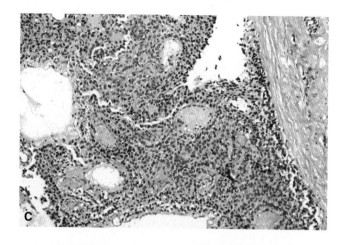

FIGURE 11.12 (*continued*)

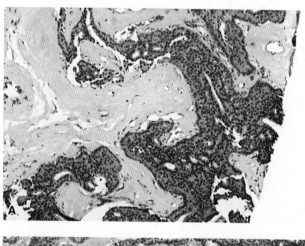

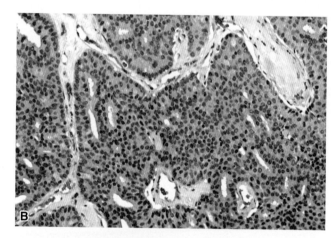

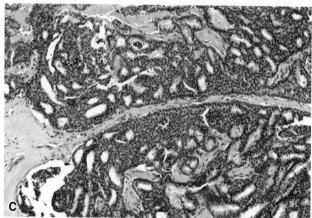

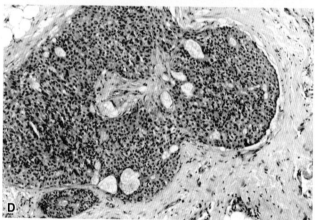

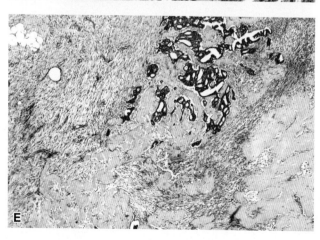

FIGURE 11.13 Solid Papillary Carcinoma. A: Collagenized stroma in this needle core biopsy specimen has distorted the structure of an in situ solid papillary carcinoma. This pattern might be mistaken for that of an invasive carcinoma with a trabecular arrangement if one failed to appreciate the papillary character of the lesion. Spaces formed by separation of the epithelium from the stroma are common in solid papillary carcinoma. **B:** This part of the lesion has a cribriform structure. **C:** Cribriform ductal carcinoma in situ is apparent in the excision specimen. **D:** Solid papillary carcinoma is present in a duct at the periphery of the excised tumor. **E:** One can see an area in the center of the excised tumor showing a reactive stromal proliferation resulting from the needle core biopsy. One has difficulty distinguishing the disrupted glands in the granulation tissue from invasive carcinoma.

present to a variable degree, can distort the entrapped ducts to form ribbons or trabeculae of neoplastic cells, which one can mistake for invasive carcinoma. Reactive stromal changes such as those consequent to a NCB or those associated with sclerosing lesions can distort the arrangement of the involved glands. The disorderly appearance of these structures evokes the pattern of an invasive carcinoma or a radial sclerosing lesion. If the neoplastic cells extend into adjacent ducts, they usually display the cytologic and architectural features seen in the dominant portion of the carcinoma.

The presence of myoepithelium around the entire circumference of a solid papillary tumor supports the diagnosis of solid papillary DCIS, but focal or even complete absence of peripheral myoepithelium does not establish the presence of invasion. The development of a focal cribriform, tubular, or mucinous pattern that extends beyond the perimeter of the tumor represents a persuasive diagnostic feature of invasion, especially when coupled with the absence of myoepithelial cells associated with the suspicious cells (**Fig. 11.14**). Cytokeratin immunostains will help to detect individual invasive carcinoma cells located beyond the perimeter of a seemingly circumscribed solid papillary carcinoma.

An unusual pattern of invasion observed in solid papillary carcinomas simulates epithelial displacement associated with needling procedures. This form of invasion gives rise to one or more irregularly shaped cohesive sheets of carcinoma cells surrounding fat or stroma without the reactive stromal changes that ordinarily accompany invasive carcinoma. These invasive foci sharply abut normal fat cells or, less commonly, fibrous stroma in a fashion superficially suggesting that they were artifactually displaced into this location (**Fig. 11.15**). Features that favor the interpretation of true invasion include the absence of tissue changes attributable to a prior procedure such as fat necrosis, hemorrhage, inflammation, granulation tissue formation, and a distinct needle track at this site. Intimate mingling of carcinoma and normal tissue occurs in these foci, especially in fat, where one can see individual adipocytes within the sheets of carcinoma cells. The malignant cells appear molded around the fat cells within or at the border of such foci.

INTRACYSTIC PAPILLARY CARCINOMA

The lesion once known as *intracystic papillary carcinoma* arises when the cystic component of a papillary carcinoma greatly overshadows the papillary component. The resulting mass consists of ". . .a large, usually solitary hemorrhagic cyst surrounded by a fibrous wall into which projects a predominantly papillary adenocarcinoma which often also lines the inner surface of the cyst" (27). Despite the distinctive macroscopic appearance of intracystic papillary carcinoma, this variant of papillary carcinoma does not exhibit consistent histologic features. A core biopsy specimen might reveal findings

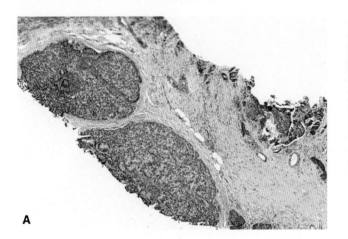

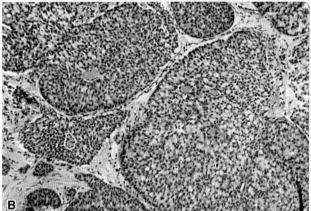

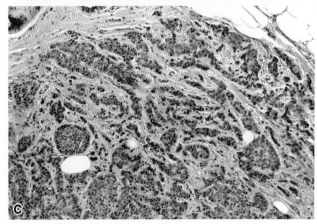

FIGURE 11.14 Solid Papillary Carcinoma with Invasion.
A, B: A needle core biopsy specimen showing solid papillary carcinoma with signet ring cells, which were positive with the mucicarmine stain. Some glandular areas in the lower left of **(B)** have uneven borders, but invasion is not evident. **C:** The excision specimen contained this area of invasive carcinoma. Note the distinctly different growth patterns of the noninvasive and invasive components.

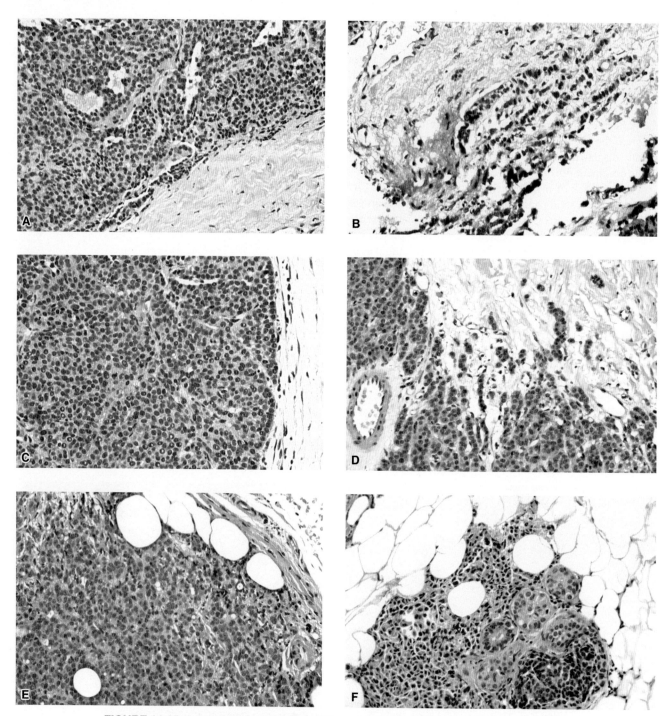

FIGURE 11.15 Solid Papillary Carcinoma with Invasion. A: This needle core biopsy specimen shows solid papillary carcinoma. **B:** Another part of the specimen contains this fragment of tissue in which one sees infiltrating carcinoma cells with a linear pattern suggestive of invasive lobular carcinoma. **C:** The excision specimen shows solid papillary carcinoma similar to that seen in **(A)**. **D:** Infiltrating carcinoma at the edge of the excised carcinoma duplicates the appearance of the region of the needle core biopsy specimen shown in **(B)**. **E:** An area of excised tumor demonstrates invasion of fat with a solid growth pattern. **F:** Carcinoma extends into fat and around a lobule in another biopsy specimen of solid papillary carcinoma. The absence of hemorrhage and fat necrosis and the delicate manner in which the carcinoma cells surround lipocytes support the interpretation of invasive carcinoma.

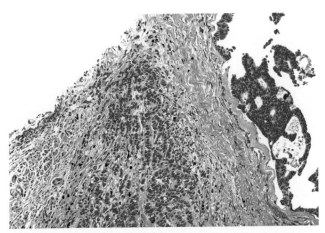

FIGURE 11.16 Intracystic Papillary Carcinoma. This needle core biopsy sample shows intracystic papillary carcinoma with cribriform architecture **(right)** and invasive carcinoma **(left)**.

suspicious of intracystic papillary carcinoma (**Fig. 11.16**), but one cannot establish this diagnosis without knowledge of the characteristics of the entire lesion.

DIMORPHIC PAPILLARY CARCINOMA

Lefkowitz et al. (28) drew attention to the presence of cuboidal cells with abundant clear or faintly eosinophilic cytoplasm in papillary carcinomas. Situated near the basement membrane, these cells occur singly, in small clusters, or in broad sheets (**Fig. 11.17**). When the cells in question become numerous, they can create solid and cribriform aggregates beneath the superficial columnar carcinoma cells. The proximity of the cuboidal cells to the basement membrane can give rise to the mistaken belief that they represent myoepithelial cells. Despite the difference in cytoplasmic features between the basal cuboidal cells and the superficial columnar cells, the two types of cells contain similar nuclei. Both types of cells are immunoreactive for cytokeratin, and the basal cells do not display reactivity for

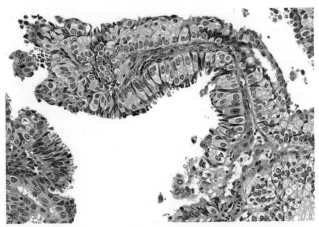

FIGURE 11.17 Dimorphic Papillary Carcinoma. Basal cells with abundant pale cytoplasm mingle with compressed columnar cells with scant eosinophilic cytoplasm. The juxtaposition is most apparent near the left border.

SMA or p63. Both types of cells are malignant, and papillary carcinomas showing this pattern are referred to as *dimorphic papillary carcinomas.*

SO-CALLED ENCAPSULATED PAPILLARY CARCINOMA

The term *encapsulated papillary carcinoma* is an alternative designation sometimes used in place of *cystic and solid papillary carcinoma.* The designation arose from immunohistochemical studies of myoepithelial markers by Hill and Yeh (8). These investigators found five papillary carcinomas with "no staining or only focal staining of a basal [myoepithelial cell] layer" for calponin, SMMHC, and p63. The absence of myoepithelial cells led the authors to propose the term, "encapsulated papillary carcinoma." Other investigations (9,29,30) yielded similar results, and the contributors to the fourth edition of the WHO classification of tumors of the breast (31) have taken up this usage. These carcinomas typically display low- or intermediate-grade cytologic features; approximately 3% of cases in one study demonstrate high-grade attributes (32).

The infiltrative nature of encapsulated papillary carcinoma remains open to controversy. For example, Rakha et al. (30) wrote ". . .most [encapsulated papillary carcinomas] are indolent invasive carcinoma, with a small proportion that may be in situ.," whereas Esposito et al. stated ". . .[encapsulated papillary carcinomas] are confined within an intact basement membrane and are thus in situ carcinomas." It is true that there are examples of this type of papillary carcinoma that elicit uncertainty regarding the presence of an invasion. However, investigators have not yet identified a subset of these uncertain tumors that have a propensity to cause metastases. Our inability to detect the presence of invasion in some papillary carcinomas reflects the limitations of our knowledge and technology. To overcome this inability, researchers must discover markers that distinguish the cells of in situ carcinoma from those of invasive carcinoma, an advance that would focus attention on the tumor cells themselves rather than on their pattern of growth. At present, it is preferable to describe a papillary carcinoma as cystic, solid, or a combination of cystic and solid and to state that invasion is present, absent, or indeterminate (e.g., "suspected"; "cannot be ruled out"). Rare instances of axillary nodal metastases have been detected in cases in which invasion was not detected (33–35). We see no advantage in the use of the term *encapsulated papillary carcinoma*, and it may be misleading by suggesting the absence of invasion in situations when invasion is actually present.

ENDOCRINE DIFFERENTIATION IN PAPILLARY CARCINOMA

Solid papillary carcinoma with endocrine differentiation represents a subtype of solid papillary carcinoma showing distinctive clinical and pathologic characteristics. With one exception (36), all patients have been women. Although the

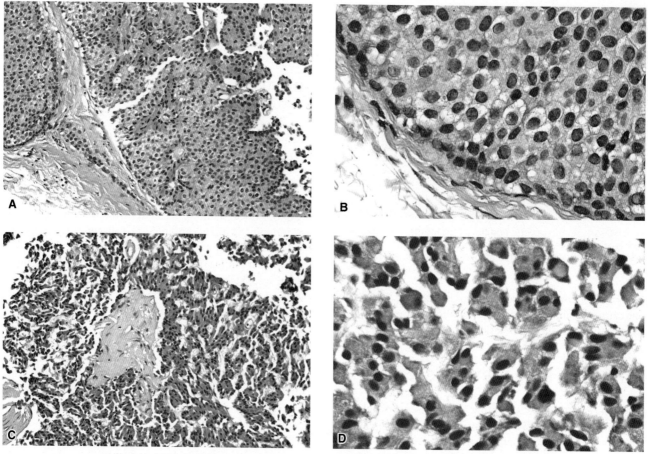

FIGURE 11.18 Solid Papillary Carcinoma with Endocrine Differentiation. A: In this needle core biopsy specimen, the in situ carcinoma contains small cords of fibrovascular stroma, which make it possible to recognize the papillary character of the tumor. The circumscribed border typifies solid papillary ductal carcinoma in situ with endocrine differentiation. **B:** This magnified view demonstrates uniform cells with mosaic-like distinct borders. **C:** Needle core biopsy samples from solid papillary carcinoma with endocrine differentiation are often fragmented, as shown here. Note the collagenized stroma. **D:** Eccentric placement of the nuclei gives the carcinoma cells a plasmacytoid appearance.

ages of patients range from 30 to 105 years, most patients presented during their seventh or eighth decade. The neoplastic cells usually demonstrate low-grade atypia **(Fig. 11.18)**, but intermediate- and high-grade cytologic features occur in a minority of cases (36). The cells have oval-to-spindle shapes, and the cytoplasmic borders sometimes stand out clearly. In uncommon cases, a spindle morphology predominates (37). The nuclei often resemble those of commonplace low-grade ductal carcinoma, but they can display irregular shapes, granular chromatin, and small nucleoli, instead. Eccentric positioning of the nuclei results in a plasmacytoid appearance **(Fig. 11.18D)**. The cytoplasm usually appears eosinophilic or amphophilic and granular. In many cases, the cytoplasm contains mucin, either in the form of miniscule droplets or large vacuoles that create signet ring cells. One sometimes observes extracellular mucin in the spaces formed by the carcinoma cells or between the neoplastic cells and the adjacent stroma **(Fig. 11.19)**. This phenomenon can occur within the tumor, adjacent to fibrovascular stalks, and at the border of tumor cell clusters. Frequent mitotic figures are characteristic, but calcifications,

cribriform spaces, and comedonecrosis are not. The supporting stroma varies from delicate strands of collagen surrounding dilated capillaries to broad, blunt fronds composed of acellular, hyalinized collagen. Cells abutting the stroma sometimes line up to form a palisade pattern.

Cellular evidence of endocrine differentiation takes the form of a positive reaction with the Grimelius stain, immunoreactivity for chromogranin, synaptophysin **(Fig. 11.20)**, or neuron specific enolase (NSE), or the detection of dense core granules. Solid papillary carcinomas with endocrine differentiation virtually always stain for ER and most stain for PR. They do not show HER2 overexpression.

Solid papillary carcinomas with endocrine differentiation frequently coexist with conventional types of invasive carcinoma. Pure or mixed mucinous carcinomas and endocrine carcinomas represent the most common coexisting carcinomas. Small pools of mucin that form between the epithelial cells and the stroma are not interpreted as invasive mucinous carcinoma unless they contain detached neoplastic cells. Larger accumulations may surround or disrupt portions of the epithelium, and

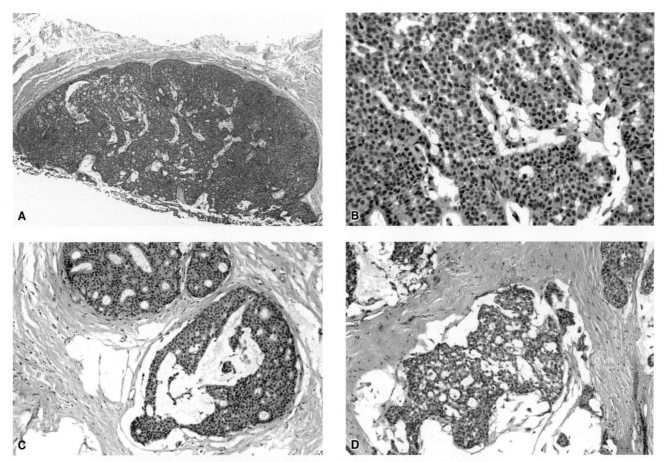

FIGURE 11.19 Solid Papillary Carcinoma with Mucinous and Endocrine Differentiation and Invasion. **A:** This needle core biopsy specimen shows a well-circumscribed nodule of solid papillary carcinoma with endocrine differentiation. **B:** Mucin accumulation is evident between the neoplastic epithelium and fibrovascular stroma. **C:** The excision specimen shown here includes cribriform ductal carcinoma in situ **(upper border)** as well as mucin in and partially around a duct **(center)**. The presence of mucin in the stroma is not diagnostic of invasive carcinoma. **D:** Invasive mucinous carcinoma consists of extracellular mucin surrounding irregular groups of carcinoma cells in the stroma.

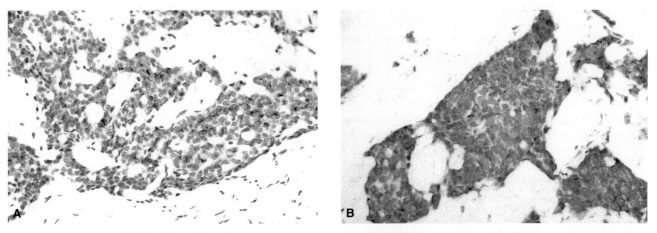

FIGURE 11.20 Solid Papillary Carcinoma with Endocrine Differentiation. **A:** Cytoplasmic immunoreactivity for chromogranin is evident. **B:** Cytoplasmic immunoreactivity for synaptophysin is depicted.

the resulting appearance is interpreted as invasive mucinous carcinoma when carcinoma cells surrounded by mucin extend into the adjacent stroma. One can also observe invasive ductal carcinoma not otherwise specified, invasive lobular carcinoma, tubular carcinoma, and small cell carcinoma in association with solid papillary carcinoma with endocrine differentiation.

TALL CELL VARIANT OF PAPILLARY CARCINOMA

A variant of papillary carcinoma termed *breast tumor resembling the tall cell variant of papillary thyroid carcinoma* has been described recently (38–40). The carcinoma cells grow in solid, papillary, and cribriform aggregates. The glands typically contain densely eosinophilic, homogeneous material with scalloped borders that resembles thyroid colloid. In this respect, the appearance of this type of papillary carcinoma bears a resemblance to cystic hypersecretory carcinoma growing in a papillary configuration. The neoplastic cells have columnar to cuboidal shapes, slightly pleomorphic oval nuclei, and eosinophilic granular cytoplasm. The nuclei usually occupy the basal aspects of the cells, but they can sit next to the luminal membranes. The nuclei have angular contours, grooves, and eosinophilic pseudoinclusions, and some appear clear. Psammoma bodies were noted in several cases. Most examples have stained for CK7, but staining for EMA, GCDFP-15, ER, and PR has yielded variable results. The carcinoma cells do not stain for TTF-1 or thyroglobulin, nor do they display mutations of the *RET* protooncogene or the *BRAF* gene.

PROGNOSIS AND TREATMENT

Patients with papillary carcinomas experience an excellent prognosis (41). Seemingly noninvasive carcinomas growing as a cystic mass spread only very rarely (29,33,42–44), and they do not recur after proper excision often (8,29,33,42,43,45). The prognosis of patients with invasive cystic papillary carcinoma is very favorable, even in women who have axillary node metastases (33,46). Grabowski et al. (47) found that the relative cumulative survival rates of patients with noninvasive cystic papillary carcinoma and invasive cystic papillary carcinoma did not differ significantly. The literature contains only a few instances of death from this tumor. A few additional patients have developed visceral metastases but remained alive at the time of publication of the reports. Like those of mucinous carcinoma, local and metastatic recurrences of invasive cystic papillary carcinoma often become clinically apparent more than 5 years after diagnosis.

The prognosis for patients with solid papillary carcinomas is relatively favorable but not to the degree observed for patients with cystic papillary carcinomas. In most cases described in the literature, the patients remained free of metastatic carcinoma, but axillary lymph node and systemic metastases developed at a noticeable rate. In about one-half of the reported cases, the axillary metastases resembled the primary solid papillary

carcinoma; in the others, coexisting invasive carcinomas gave rise to the metastatic foci. Six deaths have been attributed to solid papillary carcinomas (36).

The definitive treatment of patients with papillary carcinomas has ranged from diagnostic excision to modified radical mastectomy, and a minority of patients have received irradiation and systemic therapy. This variation in treatment coupled with uncertainties regarding the interpretation of certain histologic findings make it impossible to formulate generic, well-founded treatment recommendations. Complete excision of the carcinoma would seem prudent in all cases. For patients with invasive cystic papillary carcinoma, features such as the patient's age and the size and grade of the invasive component could help to determine the need for sampling or removal of axillary lymph nodes and for the use of irradiation and systemic therapy. Based on results presented by Nassar et al. (36), it may be advisable to offer adjuvant systemic therapy to certain patients with invasive solid papillary carcinoma.

REFERENCES

1. Baykara M, Coskun U, Demirci U, et al. Intracystic papillary carcinoma of the breast: one of the youngest patient in the literature. *Med Oncol.* 2010;27:1427–1428.
2. Soo MS, Williford ME, Walsh R, et al. Papillary carcinoma of the breast: imaging findings. *AJR Am J Roentgenol.* 1995;164:321–326.
3. McCulloch GL, Evans AJ, Yeoman L, et al. Radiological features of papillary carcinoma of the breast. *Clin Radiol.* 1997;52:865–868.
4. Schneider JA. Invasive papillary breast carcinoma: mammographic and sonographic appearance. *Radiology.* 1989;171:377–379.
5. Estabrook A, Asch T, Gump F, et al. Mammographic features of intracystic papillary lesions. *Surg Gynecol Obstet.* 1990;170:113–116.
6. Silva R, Ferrozzi F, Paties C. Invasive papillary carcinoma in elderly women: sonographic and mammographic features. *AJR Am J Roentgenol.* 1992;159:898–899.
7. Stefanou D, Batistatou A, Nonni A, et al. p63 expression in benign and malignant breast lesions. *Histol Histopathol.* 2004;19:465–471.
8. Hill CB, Yeh IT. Myoepithelial cell staining patterns of papillary breast lesions: from intraductal papillomas to invasive papillary carcinomas. *Am J Clin Pathol.* 2005;123:36–44.
9. Collins LC, Carlo VP, Hwang H, et al. Intracystic papillary carcinomas of the breast: a reevaluation using a panel of myoepithelial cell markers. *Am J Surg Pathol.* 2006;30:1002–1007.
10. Nicolas MM, Wu Y, Middleton LP, et al. Loss of myoepithelium is variable in solid papillary carcinoma of the breast. *Histopathology.* 2007;51:657–665.
11. Papotti M, Gugliotta P, Ghiringhello B, et al. Association of breast carcinoma and multiple intraductal papillomas: an histological and immunohistochemical investigation. *Histopathology.* 1984;8:963–975.
12. Tse GM, Tan PH, Lui PC, et al. The role of immunohistochemistry for smooth-muscle actin, p63, CD10 and cytokeratin 14 in the differential diagnosis of papillary lesions of the breast. *J Clin Pathol.* 2007;60:315–320.
13. Papotti M, Eusebi V, Gugliotta P, et al. Immunohistochemical analysis of benign and malignant papillary lesions of the breast. *Am J Surg Pathol.* 1983;7:451–461.
14. Reisenbichler ES, Balmer NN, Adams AL, et al. Luminal cytokeratin expression profiles of breast papillomas and papillary carcinomas and the utility of a cytokeratin 5/p63/cytokeratin 8/18 antibody cocktail in their distinction. *Mod Pathol.* 2011;24:185–193.
15. Moritani S, Ichihara S, Hasegawa M, et al. Uniqueness of ductal carcinoma in situ of the breast concurrent with papilloma: implications from a detailed topographical and histopathological study of 50 cases treated by mastectomy and wide local excision. *Histopathology.* 2013;63:407–417.
16. Yamaguchi R, Tanaka M, Tse GM, et al. Broad fibrovascular cores may not be an exclusively benign feature in papillary lesions of the breast: a cautionary note. *J Clin Pathol.* 2014;67:258–262.

17. Rabban JT, Koerner FC, Lerwill MF. Solid papillary ductal carcinoma in situ versus usual ductal hyperplasia in the breast: a potentially difficult distinction resolved by cytokeratin 5/6. *Hum Pathol.* 2006;37:787–793.

18. Tan PH, Aw MY, Yip G, et al. Cytokeratins in papillary lesions of the breast: is there a role in distinguishing intraductal papilloma from papillary ductal carcinoma in situ? *Am J Surg Pathol.* 2005;29:625–632.

19. Ichihara S, Fujimoto T, Hashimoto K, et al. Double immunostaining with p63 and high-molecular-weight cytokeratins distinguishes borderline papillary lesions of the breast. *Pathol Int.* 2007;57:126–132.

20. Douglas-Jones A, Shah V, Morgan J, et al. Observer variability in the histopathological reporting of core biopsies of papillary breast lesions is reduced by the use of immunohistochemistry for CK5/6, calponin and p63. *Histopathology.* 2005;47:202–208.

21. Grin A, O'Malley FP, Mulligan AM. Cytokeratin 5 and estrogen receptor immunohistochemistry as a useful adjunct in identifying atypical papillary lesions on breast needle core biopsy. *Am J Surg Pathol.* 2009;33:1615–1623.

22. Wang Y, Zhu JF, Liu YY, et al. An analysis of cyclin D1, cytokeratin 5/6 and cytokeratin 8/18 expression in breast papillomas and papillary carcinomas. *Diagn Pathol.* 2013;8:8.

23. Lin CH, Liu CH, Wen CH, et al. Differential CD133 expression distinguishes malignant from benign papillary lesions of the breast. *Virchows Arch.* 2015;466:177–184.

24. Page DL, Salhany KE, Jensen RA, et al. Subsequent breast carcinoma risk after biopsy with atypia in a breast papilloma. *Cancer.* 1996;78:258–266.

25. Youngson BJ, Cranor M, Rosen PP. Epithelial displacement in surgical breast specimens following needling procedures. *Am J Surg Pathol.* 1994;18:896–903.

26. Rosen P, Oberman H. Papillary carcinomas in tumors of the mammary gland. In: *Atlas of Tumor Pathology.* Washington, DC: Armed Forces Institute of Pathology; 1993.

27. Czernobilsky B. Intracystic carcinoma of the female breast. *Surg Gynecol Obstet.* 1967;124:93–98.

28. Lefkowitz M, Lefkowitz W, Wargotz ES. Intraductal (intracystic) papillary carcinoma of the breast and its variants: a clinicopathological study of 77 cases. *Hum Pathol.* 1994;25:802–809.

29. Wynveen CA, Nehhozina T, Akram M, et al. Intracystic papillary carcinoma of the breast: an in situ or invasive tumor? Results of immunohistochemical analysis and clinical follow-up. *Am J Surg Pathol.* 2011;35:1–14.

30. Rakha EA, Gandhi N, Climent F, et al. Encapsulated papillary carcinoma of the breast: an invasive tumor with excellent prognosis. *Am J Surg Pathol.* 2011;35:1093–1103.

31. Lakhani SR, Ellis IO, Schnitt SJ, et al. *WHO Classification of Breast Tumors.* 4th ed. Lyon, France: IARC Press; 2012.

32. Rakha EA, Varga Z, Elsheik S, et al. High-grade encapsulated papillary carcinoma of the breast: an under-recognized entity. *Histopathology.* 2015;66:740–746.

33. Solorzano CC, Middleton LP, Hunt KK, et al. Treatment and outcome of patients with intracystic papillary carcinoma of the breast. *Am J Surg.* 2002;184:364–368.

34. Mulligan AM, O'Malley FP. Metastatic potential of encapsulated (intracystic) papillary carcinoma of the breast: a report of 2 cases with axillary lymph node micrometastases. *Int J Surg Pathol.* 2007;15:143–147.

35. Esposito NN, Dabbs DJ, Bhargava R. Are encapsulated papillary carcinomas of the breast in situ or invasive? A basement membrane study of 27 cases. *Am J Clin Pathol.* 2009;131:228–242.

36. Nassar H, Qureshi H, Adsay NV, et al. Clinicopathologic analysis of solid papillary carcinoma of the breast and associated invasive carcinomas. *Am J Surg Pathol.* 2006;30:501–507.

37. Maluf HM, Zukerberg LR, Dickersin GR, et al. Spindle-cell argyrophilic mucin-producing carcinoma of the breast: histological, ultrastructural, and immunohistochemical studies of two cases. *Am J Surg Pathol.* 1991;15:677–686.

38. Eusebi V, Damiani S, Ellis IO, et al. Breast tumor resembling the tall cell variant of papillary thyroid carcinoma: report of 5 cases. *Am J Surg Pathol.* 2003;27:1114–1118.

39. Cameselle-Teijeiro J, Abdulkader I, Barreiro-Morandeira F, et al. Breast tumor resembling the tall cell variant of papillary thyroid carcinoma: a case report. *Int J Surg Pathol.* 2006;14:79–84.

40. Masood S, Davis C, Kubik MJ. Changing the term "breast tumor resembling the tall cell variant of papillary thyroid carcinoma" to "tall cell variant of papillary breast carcinoma". *Adv Anat Pathol.* 2012;19:108–110.

41. Liu ZY, Liu N, Wang YH, et al. Clinicopathologic characteristics and molecular subtypes of invasive papillary carcinoma of the breast: a large case study. *J Cancer Res Clin Oncol.* 2013;139:77–84.

42. Carter D, Orr SL, Merino MJ. Intracystic papillary carcinoma of the breast: after mastectomy, radiotherapy or excisional biopsy alone. *Cancer.* 1983;52:14–19.

43. Fayanju OM, Ritter J, Gillanders WE, et al. Therapeutic management of intracystic papillary carcinoma of the breast: the roles of radiation and endocrine therapy. *Am J Surg.* 2007;194:497–500.

44. Seal M, Wilson C, Naus GJ, et al. Encapsulated apocrine papillary carcinoma of the breast—a tumor of uncertain malignant potential: report of five cases. *Virchows Arch.* 2009;455:477–483.

45. Calderaro J, Espie M, Duclos J, et al. Breast intracystic papillary carcinoma: an update. *Breast J.* 2009;15:639–644.

46. Fisher ER, Palekar AS, Redmond C, et al. Pathologic findings from the National Surgical Adjuvant Breast Project (protocol no. 4): VI: invasive papillary cancer. *Am J Clin Pathol.* 1980;73:313–322.

47. Grabowski J, Salzstein SL, Sadler GR, et al. Intracystic papillary carcinoma: a review of 917 cases. *Cancer.* 2008;113:916–920.

12

Medullary Carcinoma

FREDERICK C. KOERNER

As classically described, *medullary carcinoma* is a well-circumscribed carcinoma composed of poorly differentiated cells with scant stroma and a prominent lymphoid infiltrate. The term *atypical medullary carcinoma*, introduced to describe carcinomas that have certain features of medullary carcinoma but lack one or more of the defining histologic characteristics, are now classified as *invasive ductal carcinomas with medullary features*.

The editors and contributors to the fourth edition of the *WHO Classification of Tumors of the Breast* recommend, "that classic [medullary carcinoma], atypical [medullary carcinoma] and invasive carcinoma NST with medullary features be grouped within the category of carcinomas with medullary features." (1). This movement away from classifying certain carcinomas as medullary seems regrettable and premature because well-conducted clinical follow-up studies continue to demonstrate the favorable prognosis afforded by this type of breast carcinoma. It would be a shame to abandon the diagnosis of medullary carcinoma at the moment when contemporary genomic studies offer the hope of a greater understanding of this type of tumor and improved specificity of the diagnosis. Until investigators have explored this group of tumors at the genetic level, it seems preferable to continue to classify certain carefully characterized carcinomas as medullary.

CLINICAL PRESENTATION

Medullary carcinomas constitute fewer than 5% of most series of breast carcinomas (2–5). Patients as young as 21 years (6) and as old as 95 years (7) with medullary carcinomas have been reported. This broad range of ages notwithstanding, patients with medullary carcinoma tend to be relatively young. The mean age in several series ranges from 45 to 54 years (6,8–10). Medullary carcinoma occurs in the male breast only very rarely (11).

The anatomic and size distributions of medullary carcinomas do not differ from those of commonplace breast carcinomas. Medullary carcinoma is not especially common among patients with bilateral mammary carcinoma. On the other hand, bilateral carcinomas have been found in 3% to 12% of patients with medullary carcinoma (2,7,12). Synchronous or metachronous medullary carcinoma involving both breasts is very uncommon (7,12).

Because of the presence of reactive hyperplasia, ipsilateral axillary lymph nodes tend to be enlarged in patients with medullary carcinoma even in the absence of nodal metastases. This phenomenon may complicate clinical staging (13), and the greater ease of detecting enlarged hyperplastic lymph nodes accounts for the larger number of lymph nodes retrieved from axillary dissection specimens from patients with medullary carcinoma compared with specimens from patients with conventional carcinoma (14).

IMAGING STUDIES

Radiologic images of medullary carcinomas typically demonstrate a dense, round or oval mass with indistinct or lobulated borders lacking calcifications (15). Because they have circumscribed margins, medullary carcinomas may be mistaken for fibroadenomas. Radiologic findings cannot differentiate medullary carcinoma from circumscribed nonmedullary carcinoma (16), but a mass with an irregular or jagged margin is unlikely to be a true medullary carcinoma.

GROSS PATHOLOGY

The typical intact medullary carcinoma is a moderately firm discrete tumor that one can mistake for a fibroadenoma. A distinct margin usually outlines the tumor and demarcates it from the surrounding tissue; however, an intense lymphoplasmacytic infiltrate extending beyond the immediate perimeter of a small carcinoma may blur its border. The carcinoma has a lobulated or nodular internal structure. Hemorrhage and necrosis occur at times, even in medullary carcinomas smaller than 2 cm; however, the extent of necrosis is directly related to tumor size. As the extent of necrosis increases, so, too, does the likelihood that the tumor will develop cystic foci.

MICROSCOPIC PATHOLOGY

It is necessary to adhere to established morphologic criteria strictly if the diagnosis of medullary carcinoma is to be predictive of a relatively favorable prognosis (7,8). Although researchers have proposed modified criteria, those set forth by Ridolfi et al. (8) remain the most reliable for detecting survival differences between true medullary, atypical medullary, and nonmedullary carcinomas (17).

Medullary carcinoma is defined by the following constellation of histopathologic features: prominent lymphoplasmacytic infiltrate, noninvasive microscopic circumscription, growth in sheets (syncytial pattern), poorly differentiated nuclear grade, and a high mitotic rate. A tumor must display all of these attributes to merit classification as a medullary carcinoma. When most but not all of these findings are present, the tumor may be termed an *infiltrating ductal carcinoma with medullary features*. Tumors in the latter category have a syncytial growth pattern and certain other histologic features of medullary carcinoma but deviate from the definitive appearance by demonstrating one or more of the following structural variations: invasive growth at the periphery of the tumor, sparse or diminished lymphoplasmacytic reaction, well-differentiated nuclear cytology, low mitotic rate, or conspicuous glandular, trabecular or papillary growth with fibrosis. Invasive ductal carcinomas with medullary features can display immunohistochemical findings seen in typical medullary carcinomas, but they do so less frequently. One cannot make a conclusive diagnosis of medullary carcinoma from examination of a needle core biopsy specimen because of the limited nature of such samples. In these circumstances, it is appropriate to report that the findings raise the possibility of medullary carcinoma and that the final classification depends on evaluation of the completely excised tumor.

The *lymphoplasmacytic reaction* must involve the periphery and be present diffusely in the substance of the tumor. The internal lymphoplasmacytic infiltrate tends to be limited to fibrovascular stroma between syncytial zones of tumor cells. Uncommon medullary carcinomas seem to be largely devoid of stroma, and the lymphoplasmacytic infiltrate mingles intimately with carcinoma (**Fig. 12.1**). One can find it difficult to differentiate such a tumor from metastatic carcinoma in a lymph node, especially when the mass occupies the lateral aspect of the breast. The presence of uninvolved lymph node and nearby in situ carcinoma are useful distinguishing findings.

At the periphery of the tumor, the amount of the lymphoplasmacytic infiltrate may vary, but it should appear at least moderately intense at the interface of the carcinoma with the mammary parenchyma and in the adjacent tissue. In the usual case, the lymphoplasmacytic reaction encompasses adjacent ducts and lobules occupied by in situ carcinoma. The inflammatory cells also tend to surround more distant ducts and lobules, which do not contain identifiable tumor cells. These secondary peripheral alterations are so common in medullary carcinoma that the diagnosis may be questioned in their absence.

The lymphoplasmacytic infiltrate may be composed almost entirely of either lymphocytes or plasma cells, but one most often finds a mixture of these cells. Bässler et al. (18) reported that lymphocytes predominated at the periphery of medullary carcinomas, whereas plasma cells represented the preponderant inflammatory cell in the center of the carcinoma. This phenomenon does not occur in every case. Because intense lymphocytic infiltrates can occur in nonmedullary infiltrating ductal carcinomas, this finding does not have diagnostic significance. A predominance of plasma cells, on the other hand, favors the diagnosis of medullary carcinoma. A few neutrophils, eosinophils, and monocytes can be found in a medullary carcinoma, especially in the presence of necrosis or cystic degeneration, but they never dominate. Rarely, the lymphocytic infiltrate gives rise to germinal centers within the tumor or in the surrounding tissue. Hence, one cannot rely on the presence of germinal centers as evidence that one is dealing with metastatic carcinoma in a lymph node.

Noninvasive microscopic circumscription refers to the appearance of the border of the infiltrating carcinoma rather than the periphery of the surrounding lymphoplasmacytic reaction. In medullary carcinoma, the edge of the tumor should have a smooth, rounded contour that appears to push aside the breast parenchyma rather than to infiltrate it (**Fig. 12.2**). Consequently, non-neoplastic glandular or fatty breast tissue should not be found within the body of the invasive portion of the tumor. In assessing the margin of the carcinoma, one must not confuse the extension of inflammatory cells into the surrounding parenchyma with invasion of glandular tissue or

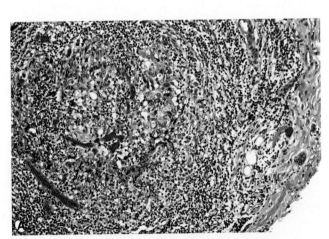 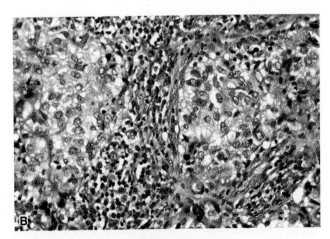

FIGURE 12.1 Medullary Carcinoma. A, B: This needle core biopsy sample shows a diffuse lymphoplasmacytic infiltrate between syncytial masses of poorly differentiated carcinoma cells. Excision revealed a typical medullary carcinoma.

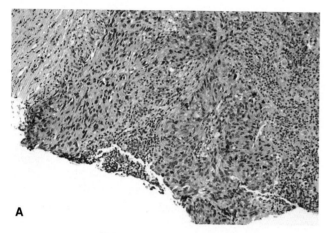
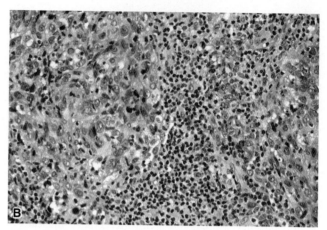

FIGURE 12.2 Medullary Carcinoma. A: This needle core biopsy sample shows the well-defined border of a medullary carcinoma. **B:** The round cell infiltrate is lymphoplasmacytic, and the tumor cells have poorly differentiated nuclei.

fat by the carcinoma cells. In the latter instance, the tumor cells tend to grow in trabecular, dendritic, or dispersed patterns, and the carcinoma typically lacks the cohesive syncytial structure of a medullary carcinoma.

A *syncytial growth pattern* refers to the formation of broad irregular sheets or islands of carcinoma cells in which the borders of individual cells are indistinct (**Figs. 12.2 and 12.3**). The appearance sometimes resembles that of a poorly differentiated squamous carcinoma. A tumor that is otherwise characteristic may be accepted as a medullary carcinoma if it has minor components of trabecular, glandular, alveolar, or papillary growth. Such regions may have a diminished lymphoplasmacytic infiltrate and fibrosis and thus appear distinct from the medullary growth pattern. It has been reported that overall survival and relapse-free survival are directly related to the extent of the syncytial component (19). Although there was not a significant difference in outcome between patients with 75% and 90% syncytial growth, survival was diminished when less than 75% of a tumor was syncytial, and the difference was most marked at and below the 50% level. These data

justify the currently employed requirement for at least a 75% syncytial component for a diagnosis of medullary carcinoma.

Poorly differentiated nuclear grade and *high mitotic rate* are related characteristics of medullary carcinoma. Typically, the tumor cells have pleomorphic nuclei with coarse chromatin and prominent nucleoli. Pyknotic nuclei of degenerating cells are easily found, as are mitotic figures.

A number of other microscopic features may be found in medullary carcinomas. The presence of one or more of these secondary histopathologic characteristics is helpful to confirm a diagnosis of medullary carcinoma, but the diagnosis does not depend on the presence of any of them. These ancillary microscopic features include: in situ carcinoma, squamous metaplasia, pseudosarcomatous metaplasia, and necrosis.

Ductal carcinoma in situ (DCIS) is found at the periphery of a substantial number of medullary carcinomas. The DCIS often has a comedo or solid growth pattern, and it only rarely contains calcifications. It is also not unusual for the carcinoma cells to involve the epithelium of lobules (lobular extension of ductal carcinoma), thereby creating foci of DCIS in lobules.

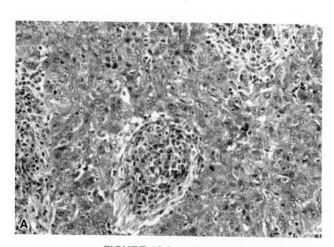
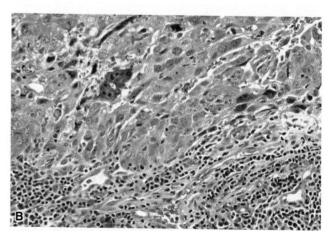

FIGURE 12.3 Medullary Carcinoma. A: The carcinoma cells form bands surrounded by a reaction predominantly composed of plasma cells. The borders of individual carcinoma cells are indistinct, and they have poorly differentiated nuclei. **B:** A multinucleated giant cell is present.

One tends to see foci of intraductal and intralobular carcinoma more frequently as the size of the tumor increases, and they are accompanied by the same prominent mononuclear cell infiltrate that occurs in the main tumor. This mononuclear infiltrate can be so intense that it obscures the presence of subtle extension of ductal carcinoma in situ into lobules. However, close inspection reveals that these lobules contain cells with the same poorly differentiated nuclei as those in the invasive portion of the medullary carcinoma.

Around the main mass, expansile growth of in situ carcinoma in ducts and lobules leads to the formation of secondary peripheral tumor nodules that have the appearance of small "satellite" medullary carcinomas (20). Fat and mammary stroma may persist between nodules at the margin of the tumor. One should not interpret the presence of these marginal foci separated by stroma as evidence of invasion. Coalescence of these nodules and their incorporation into the expanding main mass account for the nodular appearance of medullary carcinomas evident during macroscopic examination.

Rarely, one may encounter a lesion consisting only of DCIS showing the histologic features of DCIS found at the periphery of a medullary carcinoma. Such foci typically have the poorly differentiated cytologic features that characterize medullary carcinoma, a comedo growth pattern, and an intense lymphocytic reaction that can obscure the duct margin, thereby making it difficult to evaluate the lesion for invasion. There is no definite proof that these lesions constitute an in situ form of medullary carcinoma, but this possibility can be inferred from uncommon examples of medullary carcinoma composed largely of DCIS with only a minor invasive component.

Metaplastic changes occur in a minority of medullary carcinomas, and they usually involve only a part of the lesion. Squamous metaplasia has been found in 16% of medullary carcinomas (8). Osseous, cartilaginous, and spindle cell metaplasia are much less common. Bizarre epithelial giant cells can be found in otherwise typical medullary carcinomas **(Fig. 12.3)**. It is not clear whether the bizarre appearance of these cells reflects a metaplastic or degenerative phenomenon.

Necrosis initially develops in medullary carcinomas within zones of syncytial epithelial growth. Expansion of these microscopic foci leads to the formation of small clefts and eventually to cystic areas. The pattern resembles the process of cystic degeneration sometimes seen in squamous carcinomas. Necrosis is often found in conjunction with squamous metaplasia in medullary carcinomas.

IMMUNOHISTOCHEMISTRY

Most medullary carcinomas express keratin and stain with the AE1/AE3 cocktail. Investigators have tested medullary carcinomas for the presence of specific keratin molecules such as CK4, CK5/6, CK7, CK14, CK8/18, CK19, and CK20, but the studies have not yielded consistent findings. Consequently, one cannot rely on the expression of any of the types of cytokeratin to distinguish medullary carcinomas from nonmedullary carcinomas. Immunoreactivity for HLA-DR, GATA3, EMA,

and E-cadherin is frequently demonstrable in medullary carcinomas. One can observe staining for mammaglobin or GCDFP-15 in occasional cases (21,22).

Rodríguez-Pinilla et al. (23) observed that carcinomas classified as invasive ductal carcinoma with medullary features display immunohistochemical features characteristic of basal-like carcinomas more often than do high-grade conventional invasive ductal carcinomas (62.9% vs. 18.9% of cases). Jacquemier et al. (24) observed that 71% of medullary carcinomas expressed EGFR, whereas only 37% of invasive ductal carcinoma did so, and Vincent-Salomon et al. (25) reported similar results. Jacquemier et al. (24) also found that 44% of medullary carcinomas expressed S-100, but only 24% of nonmedullary high-grade ductal carcinomas did so.

Fewer than 10% of medullary carcinomas are ER- or PR-positive (24), and only a small percentage of medullary carcinoma express the HER2 (24,26–28).

The microscopic features of medullary carcinoma with an exceptionally abundant lymphoplasmacytic reaction resemble those of lymphoepithelial carcinomas that arise at other sites (29). These and other characteristics have suggested that the Epstein–Barr virus might play a role in pathogenesis of medullary carcinoma; however, a study of 10 medullary carcinomas using immunohistochemistry, in situ hybridization, and the polymerase chain reaction failed to detect evidence of EBV (30). A lymphoepithelioma-like tumor studied by Naidoo and Chetty (29) was also negative for EBV.

BRCA MUTATIONS

Medullary carcinomas constitute between 11% (31) and 19% (32) of BRCA1-associated breast carcinomas. Moreover, one can find BRCA1 mutations in patients with medullary carcinomas more frequently than in patients with other varieties of breast carcinomas. Without knowledge of family histories, Eisinger et al. (32) tested 18 medullary carcinomas selected from a hospital registry and discovered BRCA1 nonsense mutations in 2 tumors (11%), 7 times the frequency of such mutations in the general population. In neither case did the patient report a family history suggestive of heritable breast carcinoma. The 11% detection rate is higher than that encountered when using early onset as a criterion for genetic testing. This observation suggests that the diagnosis of medullary carcinoma could represent an indication for BRCA testing (33).

STAGING, PROGNOSIS, AND TREATMENT

Patients with medullary carcinoma tend to have a lower frequency of axillary lymph node metastases than patients with either invasive ductal carcinoma with medullary features or usual invasive ductal carcinoma (2,3,6,8,34,35). The prognosis of patients with small, node-negative medullary carcinoma is particularly favorable, with a disease-free survival of 90% or better (6,8). When nodal metastases are present, they typically involve 3 or fewer lymph nodes (2,6,34,36,37). The survival results for stage II, $T_1N_1M_0$ medullary carcinoma have also been exceptionally good at 10 years (5) and 20 years of follow-up. Although stage II medullary carcinoma patients have a more favorable prognosis than equivalent patients with nonmedullary carcinoma, tumor size and nodal status are still significant determinants of disease-free survival (34). Patients whose medullary carcinomas are larger than 3 cm or who have four or more involved lymph nodes have high recurrence rates that are not appreciably different from the recurrence rates of patients with usual invasive ductal carcinoma (8).

Recurrences tend to occur early in the clinical course of patients with medullary carcinoma, with very few women having recurrences or dying 5 years or more after the time of diagnosis (6,8,34,38). This phenomenon is observed equally in stage I and stage II patients. Most initial recurrences are systemic, but local recurrence has been observed even in patients treated by radical or modified radical mastectomy. Survival after systemic recurrence tends to be brief, regardless of the site of the initial metastasis (34), although an occasional patient may benefit from resection of a solitary metastasis (6).

In most reported cases of medullary carcinoma, surgical treatment consisted of a mastectomy. There is little reported experience with the use of breast-conserving surgery and radiotherapy in this setting. Combined data from two institutions included 27 women with medullary carcinoma treated by breast-conserving surgery and radiotherapy (39). The mammary recurrence rate was 4%, the 5-year overall survival was 90%, and relapse-free survival was 92% at 5 years. A series of 1,008 patients treated by breast conservation with radiotherapy at Yale University included 17 women with medullary carcinoma (40). None of the patients developed a systemic recurrence, but there were five local breast recurrences (29%) after a median follow-up of nearly 17 years. The longest interval to recurrence was 18 years.

Breast conservation with excision and irradiation seems to represent a reasonable form of therapy for patients with medullary carcinoma and especially for tumors 3 cm or smaller. Sentinel lymph node mapping is an appropriate procedure for staging the axilla. Indications for systemic adjuvant therapy are controversial. Although it has been suggested that adjuvant systemic therapy can be omitted for patients with stage $T_1N_0M_0$ true medullary carcinoma, those who question the specificity of the diagnosis (1) are likely to recommend therapy similar to that offered to patients with conventional invasive ductal carcinoma.

REFERENCES

1. Jacquemier J, Reis-Filho JS, Lakhani SR, et al. Carcinomas with medullary features. In: Lakhani SR, Ellis IO, Schnitt SJ, et al, eds. *WHO Classification of Tumors of the Breast*. 4th ed. Lyon, France: IARC Press; 2012.
2. Rapin V, Contesso G, Mouriesse H, et al. Medullary breast carcinoma: a reevaluation of 95 cases of breast cancer with inflammatory stroma. *Cancer.* 1988;61:2503–2510.
3. Li CI, Uribe DJ, Daling JR. Clinical characteristics of different histologic types of breast cancer. *Br J Cancer.* 2005;93:1046–1052.
4. Rosen PP, Saigo PE, Braun DW Jr, et al. Predictors of recurrence in stage I ($T_1N_0M_0$) breast carcinoma. *Ann Surg.* 1981;193:15–25.
5. Rosen PP, Saigo PE, Braun DW, et al. Prognosis in stage II ($T_1N_1M_0$) breast cancer. *Ann Surg.* 1981;194:576–584.
6. Wargotz ES, Silverberg SG. Medullary carcinoma of the breast: a clinicopathologic study with appraisal of current diagnostic criteria. *Hum Pathol.* 1988;19:1340–1346.
7. Maier WP, Rosemond GP, Goldman LI, et al. A ten year study of medullary carcinoma of the breast. *Surg Gynecol Obstet.* 1977;144:695–698.
8. Ridolfi RL, Rosen PP, Port A, et al. Medullary carcinoma of the breast: a clinicopathologic study with 10 year follow-up. *Cancer.* 1977;40:1365–1385.
9. Rosen PP, Lesser ML, Senie RT, et al. Epidemiology of breast carcinoma IV: age and histologic tumor type. *J Surg Oncol.* 1982;19:44–51.
10. Rosen PP, Lesser ML, Kinne DW. Breast carcinoma at the extremes of age: a comparison of patients younger than 35 years and older than 75 years. *J Surg Oncol.* 1985;28:90–96.
11. Martinez SR, Beal SH, Canter RJ, et al. Medullary carcinoma of the breast: a population-based perspective. *Med Oncol.* 2011;28:738–744.
12. Lesser ML, Rosen PP, Kinne DW. Multicentricity and bilaterality in invasive breast carcinoma. *Surgery.* 1982;91:234–240.
13. Neuman ML, Homer MJ. Association of medullary carcinoma with reactive axillary adenopathy. *AJR Am J Roentgenol.* 1996;167:185–186.
14. Rosen PP, Lesser ML, Kinne DW, et al. Discontinuous or "skip" metastases in breast carcinoma: analysis of 1228 axillary dissections. *Ann Surg.* 1983;197:276–283.
15. Jeong SJ, Lim HS, Lee JS, et al. Medullary carcinoma of the breast: MRI findings. *AJR Am J Roentgenol.* 2012;198:W482–W487.
16. Tominaga J, Hama H, Kimura N, et al. MR imaging of medullary carcinoma of the breast. *Eur J Radiol.* 2009;70:525–529.
17. Jensen ML, Kiaer H, Andersen J, et al. Prognostic comparison of three classifications for medullary carcinomas of the breast. *Histopathology.* 1997;30:523–532.
18. Bässler R, Dittmann AM, Dittrich M. Mononuclear stromal reactions in mammary carcinoma, with special reference to medullary carcinomas with a lymphoid infiltrate: analysis of 108 cases. *Virchows Arch A Pathol Anat Histol.* 1981;393:75–91.
19. Pedersen L, Schiodt T, Holck S, et al. The prognostic importance of syncytial growth pattern in medullary carcinoma of the breast. *APMIS.* 1990;98:921–926.
20. Reyes C, Nadji M. The immunophenotype of nodular variant of medullary carcinoma of the breast. *Appl Immunohistochem Mol Morphol.* 2015;23:624–627.
21. Reyes C, Gomez-Fernandez C, Nadji M. Metaplastic and medullary mammary carcinomas do not express mammaglobin. *Am J Clin Pathol.* 2012;137:747–752.
22. Wendroth SM, Mentrikoski MJ, Wick MR. GATA3 expression in morphologic subtypes of breast carcinoma: a comparison with gross cystic disease fluid protein 15 and mammaglobin. *Ann Diagn Pathol.* 2015;19:6–9.
23. Rodríguez-Pinilla SM, Rodriguez-Gil Y, Moreno-Bueno G, et al. Sporadic invasive breast carcinomas with medullary features display a basal-like phenotype: an immunohistochemical and gene amplification study. *Am J Surg Pathol.* 2007;31:501–508.
24. Jacquemier J, Padovani L, Rabayrol L, et al. Typical medullary breast carcinomas have a basal/myoepithelial phenotype. *J Pathol.* 2005;207:260–268.
25. Vincent-Salomon A, Gruel N, Lucchesi C, et al. Identification of typical medullary breast carcinoma as a genomic subgroup of basal-like carcinomas, a heterogeneous new molecular entity. *Breast Cancer Res.* 2007;9:R24.
26. Rosen PP, Lesser ML, Arroyo CD, et al. Immunohistochemical detection of HER2/neu in patients with axillary lymph node negative breast carcinoma: a study of epidemiologic risk factors, histologic features, and prognosis. *Cancer.* 1995;75:1320–1326.
27. Bertucci F, Finetti P, Cervera N, et al. Gene expression profiling shows medullary breast cancer is a subgroup of basal breast cancers. *Cancer Res.* 2006;66:4636–4644.
28. Flucke U, Flucke MT, Hoy L, et al. Distinguishing medullary carcinoma of the breast from high-grade hormone receptor-negative invasive ductal carcinoma: an immunohistochemical approach. *Histopathology.* 2010;56:852–859.

29. Naidoo P, Chetty R. Lymphoepithelioma-like carcinoma of the breast with associated sclerosing lymphocytic lobulitis. *Arch Pathol Lab Med.* 2001;125:669–672.

30. Lespagnard L, Cochaux P, Larsimont D, et al. Absence of Epstein–Barr virus in medullary carcinoma of the breast as demonstrated by immunophenotyping, in situ hybridization and polymerase chain reaction. *Am J Clin Pathol.* 1995;103:449–452.

31. Lakhani SR, Gusterson BA, Jacquemier J, et al. The pathology of familial breast cancer: histological features of cancers in families not attributable to mutations in BRCA1 or BRCA2. *Clin Cancer Res.* 2000;6:782–789.

32. Eisinger F, Jacquemier J, Charpin C, et al. Mutations at BRCA1: the medullary breast carcinoma revisited. *Cancer Res.* 1998;58:1588–1592.

33. Eisinger F, Nogues C, Birnbaum D, et al. BRCA1 and medullary breast cancer. *JAMA.* 1998;280:1227–1228.

34. Reinfuss M, Stelmach A, Mitus J, et al. Typical medullary carcinoma of the breast: a clinical and pathological analysis of 52 cases. *J Surg Oncol.* 1995;60:89–94.

35. Mitze M, Goepel E. [Prognostic factors in medullary breast cancer]. *Geburtshilfe Frauenheilkd.* 1989;49:635–641.

36. Dendale R, Vincent-Salomon A, Mouret-Fourme E, et al. Medullary breast carcinoma: prognostic implications of p53 expression. *Int J Biol Markers.* 2003;18:99–105.

37. Fisher ER, Kenny JP, Sass R, et al. Medullary cancer of the breast revisited. *Breast Cancer Res Treat.* 1990;16:215–229.

38. Bloom HJ, Richardson WW, Field JR. Host resistance and survival in carcinoma of breast: a study of 104 cases of medullary carcinoma in a series of 1,411 cases of breast cancer followed for 20 years. *Br Med J.* 1970;3:181–188.

39. Kurtz JM, Jacquemier J, Torhorst J, et al. Conservation therapy for breast cancers other than infiltrating ductal carcinoma. *Cancer.* 1989;63:1630–1635.

40. Haffty BG, Perrotta PL, Ward B, et al. Conservatively treated breast cancer: outcome by histologic subtype. *Breast J.* 1997;3:7–14.

13

Metaplastic Carcinoma Including Low-grade Adenosquamous Carcinoma

EDI BROGI

METAPLASTIC CARCINOMA

Metaplastic carcinomas are malignant tumors of epithelial origin that exhibit nonglandular morphology, such as squamous, spindle cell, chondroid, and osseous features. These phenotypic alterations are the expression of a process of genomic dedifferentiation, scientifically referred to as "epithelial to mesenchymal transition" (EMT) (1). There are no criteria regarding the extent of metaplasia required to diagnose metaplastic carcinoma, and mention of the presence and type of metaplasia(s) should always be included in the diagnostic report. Metaplastic carcinomas of the breast are usually "triple-negative" and, with very few exceptions, have a poor prognosis.

Metaplastic low-grade adenosquamous carcinoma (LGASC) has characteristic morphology and clinical behavior, and it is discussed separately at the end of this chapter.

Clinical Presentation

Incidence

Metaplastic carcinomas are rare, and the precise incidence is difficult to establish. In a study based on data from the National Cancer Database, metaplastic carcinomas constituted only 0.24% of 365,464 breast malignant tumors diagnosed between 2001 and 2003 (2).

Age, Gender, and Genetic Predisposition

Metaplastic carcinomas can occur in women of any age, but peri- or postmenopausal women are affected more commonly (2–21). In one study (2), the mean age at diagnosis was 61 years, with 13.5% of cases occurring in women older than 80 years of age, and 8% in women younger than 40 years of age. Other series report younger median age (22), or no age differences (12) compared to women with invasive ductal carcinomas of no special type. More than 70% (2,8) of metaplastic carcinomas occur in white women. Metaplastic carcinomas do not affect men. Rare cases have been reported in *BRCA1* germline mutation carriers (13,23–25).

Presenting Symptoms

Most patients present with a palpable tumor, and many report its rapid growth and short duration before diagnosis. Most tumors are unilateral; nipple discharge is uncommon. The mean and median size (3–4 cm) in various series tend to be greater than that of ordinary invasive ductal carcinomas. Large lesions can be fixed to chest wall, or infiltrate the skin, causing ulceration.

Imaging Studies

Mammographically and sonographically, metaplastic carcinomas tend to be more nodular and less infiltrative than invasive ductal carcinomas (19,22). They have fewer calcifications and less acoustic shadowing (22). Microcalcifications are present in about 20% of the cases (19), and sometimes they are found in ductal carcinoma in situ (DCIS) rather than in the metaplastic carcinoma. Rarely, calcified areas in carcinomas with chondroid and osseous metaplasia are detected mammographically (26–29). Sonographically, metaplastic carcinomas have a parallel orientation to the skin in 97% of the cases, complex echogenicity in 81%, irregular shape in 60%, posterior acoustic enhancement in 50%, and microlobulated margin in 41% of the cases (19). The most common MRI findings included an irregular heterogeneous enhancing mass, with an irregular shape (52.4%) and margin (57%). High T2-weighted signal intensity is detected in nearly 60% of the cases (19), correlating with necrosis (27) and chondroid areas (28). The tumors are highly metabolic on F^{18}–fluorodeoxyglucose PET. Cystic areas may be present, especially in tumors with squamous metaplasia. Hemorrhagic areas may occur in metaplastic carcinomas with choriocarcinomatous morphology.

Microscopic Pathology

The diagnosis of metaplastic carcinoma requires evidence of epithelial origin and/or differentiation such as identification of DCIS and/or focal invasive carcinoma with epithelial morphology, and/or positive immunoreactivity for keratin and/or (myo)epithelial markers. Metaplastic changes are more common in poorly differentiated invasive ductal carcinomas but rarely occur in other types of carcinomas, or near papillary lesions. The extent of metaplasia varies from microscopic foci to complete involvement of the tumor. Metaplastic carcinomas encompass a wide morphologic spectrum, and their precise subclassification is limited by their extreme morphologic heterogeneity and the difficulty in quantifying the metaplastic components in each tumor. In resection specimens of metaplastic carcinomas, DCIS is identified in 10% (30) to 65% (31) of the cases, and it tends to have high or intermediate nuclear grade. Rarely, only lobular carcinoma in situ (LCIS) or atypical ductal hyperplasia (ADH) is found. A papillary or sclerosing lesion sometimes is present near a metaplastic carcinoma, especially metaplastic spindle cell carcinoma (MSpCC) with "fibromatosis-like" morphology or LGASC. Chronic inflammation often occurs at the periphery and within a metaplastic carcinoma.

Histologic examination of the entire tumor is required to assess all different patterns of metaplasia present in a metaplastic carcinoma, but in some cases a definitive diagnosis of metaplastic carcinoma can be rendered on review of the morphologic features and immunoreactivity in the needle core biopsy (NCB) material. Metaplastic carcinoma is often part of the differential diagnosis of a malignant spindle cell tumor in the breast. Traditionally, metaplastic carcinomas are divided into carcinomas with squamous and/or spindle cell metaplasia, and carcinomas with heterologous component(s), such as chrondromyxoid and/or osseous matrix.

Squamous Cell Carcinoma

Morphologically, mammary squamous cell carcinomas (SCCs) resemble squamous carcinomas that arise in other sites **(Figs. 13.1 and 13.2)**. The diagnosis of SCC of the breast applies to carcinomas in which the squamous component represents at least 90% of the tumor. Consequently, this diagnosis cannot be rendered definitively on review of only NCB material. Some tumors show cytoplasmic clearing. A spindle cell component may be present, but it may be difficult to distinguish from the reactive stroma, especially in NCB material. The neoplastic spindle cells can be highlighted with immunohistochemical stains for high-molecular-weight and basal cytokeratins (CKs), such as 34βE12 (K903), CK14, CK5/6, and also for p63. An inflammatory infiltrate rich in granulocytes and lymphocytes is often present in association with SCC, especially in necrotic and/or keratinized areas **(Figs. 13.1 and 13.2)**, accounting for the common clinical impression of an abscess. DCIS of intermediate

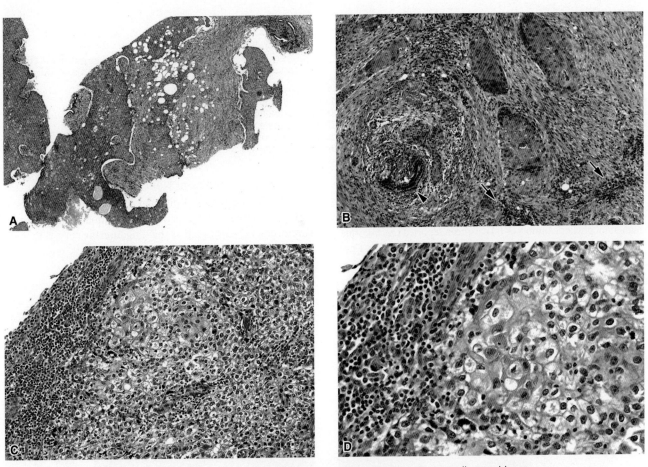

FIGURE 13.1 Invasive Carcinoma with Squamoid Morphology. A: A needle core biopsy specimen from a 3-cm mass in the breast of a 66-year-old woman shows a carcinoma with squamous morphology, well to moderately differentiated. **B:** The carcinoma consists of squamous nests with low-grade nuclear atypia, in a background of stromal desmoplasia. Lymphocytes are also noted *(arrows)*. A benign duct is present *(arrowhead)*. **C, D:** Another needle core biopsy specimen showing focal squamous differentiation in a poorly differentiated infiltrating duct carcinoma.

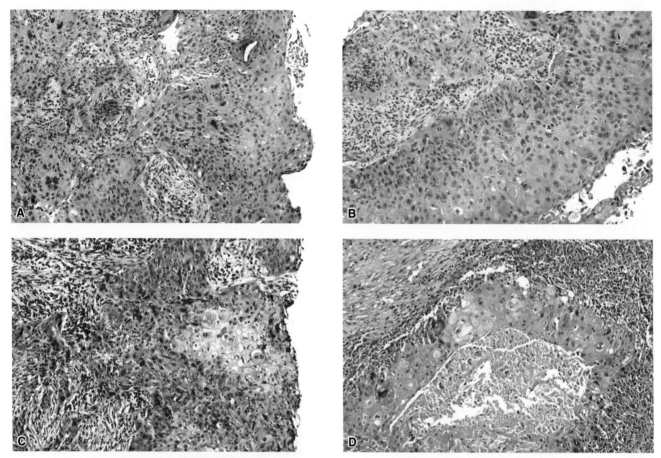

FIGURE 13.2 Invasive Squamous Carcinoma. A, B: A needle core biopsy specimen showing well to moderately differentiated invasive squamous carcinoma and invasive poorly differentiated carcinoma. **C:** A part of the same tumor with poorly differentiated squamous carcinoma. **D:** An area in the surgically excised tumor that duplicates the appearance of the needle core biopsy specimen. Note the cystic degeneration and the lymphoplasmacytic stromal infiltrate, frequent components of primary squamous carcinoma of the breast.

or high nuclear grade can be associated with mammary SCC, or very rarely it has squamous morphology **(Fig. 13.3).**

Rare cases of SCC or squamous carcinoma in situ arising in malignant phyllode tumors (PTs) have been reported (32,33). Squamous metaplasia can occur in benign mammary ducts **(Fig. 13.4).**

Differential Diagnosis at Needle Core Biopsy

A definitive diagnosis of primary SCC of the breast is possible only after a metastasis from an extramammary primary carcinoma (34–36), such as the lung, uterine cervix, urinary bladder and carcinomas of the head and neck region (37),

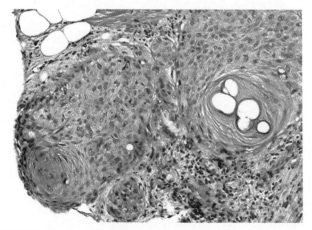

FIGURE 13.3 Intraductal Squamous Carcinoma. This needle core biopsy sample shows two contiguous ducts occupied by centrally keratinizing, well-differentiated squamous carcinoma.

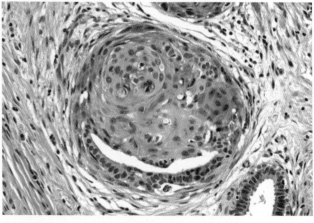

FIGURE 13.4 Squamous Metaplasia in a Hyperplastic Duct. Benign squamous metaplasia tends to be more common in ducts closer to the nipple or in the context of reactive changes.

and secondary extension into the breast of a primary SCC arising in the overlying skin have been ruled out. Clinical and radiologic correlation is required to exclude the aforementioned scenarios.

Metaplastic Spindle Cell Carcinoma (MSpCC)

MSpCCs are usually split into two groups having low-grade and intermediate- to high-grade morphology. The two different morphologies correspond to different differential diagnoses and clinical behavior.

MSpCC with Intermediate- and High-grade Morphology

Most or all of the neoplasm consists of spindle cells with moderate to marked nuclear atypia; tumor cellularity is also moderate to marked **(Fig. 13.5)**. Mitoses are easily identified and usually numerous. Necrosis is common, especially in high-grade tumors. Focal areas of squamous differentiation, DCIS, or invasive carcinoma of no special type **(Fig. 13.5)** may be identified, but most cases have no obvious epithelial component, especially in NCB material. In one study (38), DCIS was present in the surgical excision specimen only in 14% of the cases. Usual ductal hyperplasia of the gynecomastoid type is often present in the mammary ducts at the periphery of the tumor. Immunohistochemical stains for epithelial markers, such as CK 34βE12, CK14, CK 5/6, CK18, and p63 can be positive, but the expression of epithelial antigens in MSpCC with intermediate- and high-grade morphology tends to be very focal, if any, even in the main resection specimen, and a NCB sample may not show any staining for epithelial markers. Positivity for GATA3 has also been reported (39) **(Fig. 13.5)**.

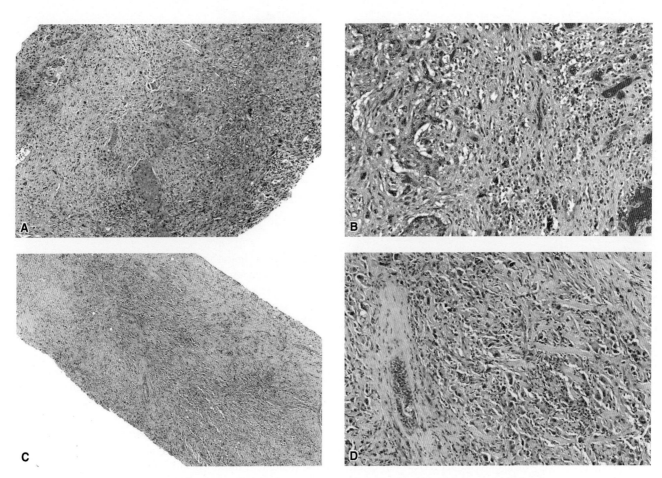

FIGURE 13.5 Metaplastic Carcinoma with High-grade Morphology. A, B: This needle core biopsy sample from a rapidly growing mass in the breast of a 34-year-old woman shows a high-grade malignant tumor composed for most part of spindle cells with a focal epithelial component. **B:** The carcinomatous component consists of few irregular clusters, whereas the sarcomatoid component is composed of large and bizarre spindle cells. **C–H:** Needle core biopsy and excision specimens of a mass in the breast of an 85-year-old woman. The needle core biopsy material shows a high-grade malignant spindle and epithelioid neoplasm **(C–D)**. Reportedly, the neoplastic cells were positive for CK7 and SOX10 (not shown). The tumor in the excision specimen has high-grade morphology **(E)**. The neoplastic cells show weak nuclear staining for GATA3. Nuclear staining in the benign epithelium of a duct is also present *(arrow)* **(F)**. The neoplastic cells show weak nuclear staining for SOX10 **(G)**. The benign epithelium of a duct *(arrow)* shows focal membranous reactivity but no nuclear staining. The neoplastic spindle cells are strongly positive for keratin 34βE12 **(H)**. This pattern of immunoreactivity supports the diagnosis of carcinoma with high-grade metaplastic spindle cell morphology.

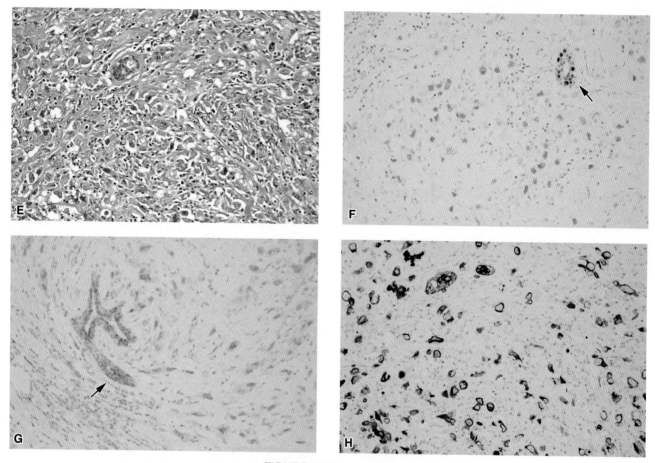

FIGURE 13.5 (continued)

Differential Diagnosis at Needle Core Biopsy

The identification of a focal attenuated epithelium lining a hyper-cellular stromal fragment is often the only evidence differentiating *high-grade malignant phyllodes tumor* from MSpCC with intermediate- or high-grade morphology (see Chapter 7). NCB sampling of areas of stromal expansion or overgrowth in a borderline or malignant PT may yield no ductal epithelial component, raising the differential diagnosis of high-grade MSpCC. It has been reported that the neoplastic cells of PTs may be focally positive for CKs (40). PTs are usually positive for CD34, whereas MSpCCs are usually CD34-negative (41). S-100 can be positive in some MSpCCs and PTs (41). A malignant tumor entirely composed of spindle cells of intermediate- and high-grade atypia and having no overt epithelial component or frond-like architecture cannot reliably be classified in a NCB, and both MSpCC and malignant PT need to be included in the differential diagnosis. Focal staining for CK favors MSpCC, but caution is recommended when the positivity is extremely focal, limited to epithelium near foci of necrosis, and limited to only one of the CKs less sensitive for the detection of MSpCC, such as CAM5.2. It is worth noting that definitive diagnosis of MSpCC, a "triple-negative" carcinoma, at the time of NCB may lead to treatment with neoadjuvant chemotherapy, which is usually not indicated for the treatment of malignant PTs. Patient prognosis also differs greatly.

Primary *sarcomas* of the breast are extremely rare, with angiosarcoma being the most common type (see Chapter 20 for detailed discussion). A clinical history of prior ipsilateral breast carcinoma treated with breast-conserving surgery and radiotherapy is often obtained in cases of radiation-induced sarcoma. Sporadic primary mammary angiosarcomas tend to occur in young women. The NCB sample of an angiosarcoma is characteristically very hemorrhagic. Most angiosarcomas are positive for CD31 and ERG, and negative for CKs and epithelial markers, but focal positivity for CKs has been reported (42), especially in epithelioid angiosarcomas. A group reported p63 positivity in angiosarcomas (43), but others have not observed this finding (44). Awareness of the patient's prior clinical history is important to rule out sarcoma metastatic from an extramammary site.

The differential diagnosis of any epithelioid and spindle cell malignant tumor includes *melanoma* and requires the appropriate immunohistochemical workup. S-100 can be positive in some MSpCC with intermediate- and high-grade morphology (41). SOX10, a Schwann cell and melanocytic marker, has been detected in some metaplastic carcinomas (45) **(Fig. 13.5)**. Rarely, p63 is focally and weakly positive in melanoma *(personal observation)*.

In the absence of definitive reactivity for vascular or melanocytic markers in NCB material of an intermediate- to high-grade malignant spindle cell tumor, the diagnosis of MSpCC is the most likely, but the need for further evaluation of the entire tumor in the surgical excision specimen should be indicated.

Low-grade Fibromatosis-like Metaplastic Spindle Cell Carcinoma

MSpCC with dense, keloid-like areas of fibrosis, storiform pattern, and minimal cytologic atypia is referred to as "fibromatosis-like" (46) or "low grade" (47) (**Figs. 13.6–13.8**). This tumor often shows heterogeneous cellularity, with closely juxtaposed hypercellular and hypocellular areas. Collagenous fibrosis can be extensive and deceivingly hypocellular to nearly acellular, especially in the center of the tumor. The neoplastic cells are haphazardly arranged in short interlacing fascicles, and tend to be inconspicuous, with

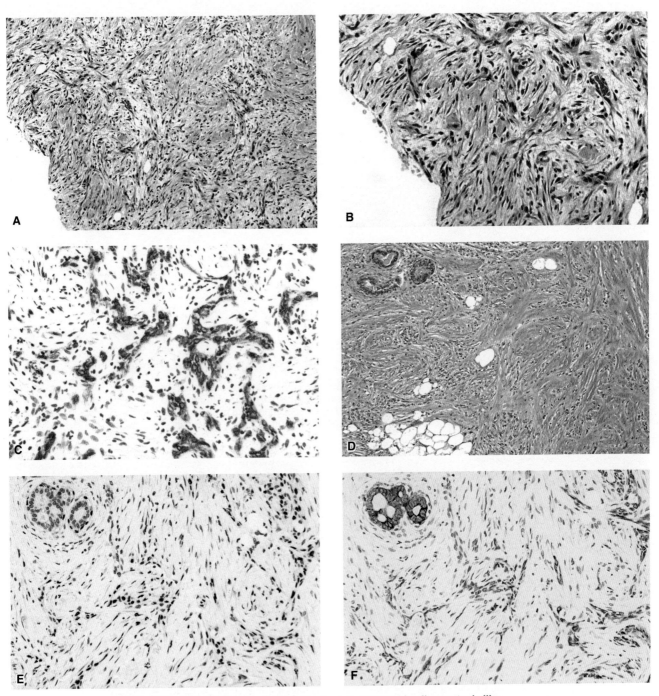

FIGURE 13.6 Metaplastic Spindle Cell Carcinoma, Low-grade Fibromatosis-like.
A, B: The bland spindle cells comprising this "low-grade" metaplastic spindle cell carcinoma are arranged in short and haphazardly fascicles. The storiform pattern is suggestive of metaplastic carcinoma. No obvious epithelial component is seen in the moderately cellular tumor tissue composed of uniform spindle cells, but some of the spindle cells have epithelioid morphology and are arranged in structures that resemble capillaries. Cytokeratin AE1/AE3 reactivity highlights the epithelioid cells **(C)**. **D–F:** A spindle cell metaplastic carcinoma with bands of keloid-like collagen **(D)**. The neoplastic spindle cells shown in **D** display nuclear reactivity for p63 **(E)** and cytoplasmic positivity for 34βE12 **(F)**. **G–H:** The spindle cell metaplastic carcinoma in this needle core biopsy sample has storiform architecture and no overt epithelial elements.

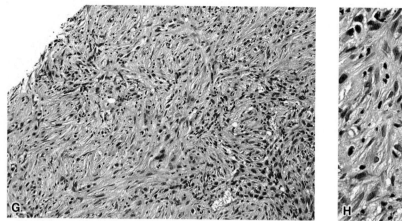
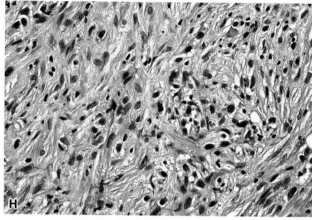

FIGURE 13.6 (*continued*)

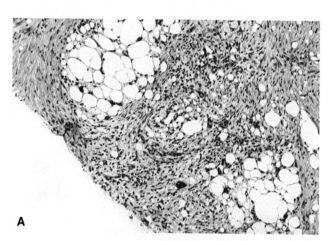
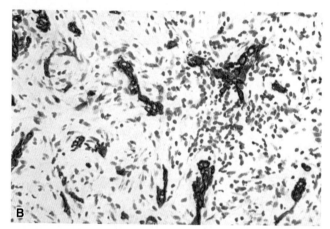

FIGURE 13.7 Metaplastic Spindle Cell Carcinoma, Low-grade Fibromatosis-like. A tumor with features that resemble an inflammatory lesion. **A:** The pattern of infiltration into fat and lymphocytic reaction shown in this needle core biopsy specimen were mistaken for fat necrosis. **B:** Cytokeratin 34βE12 expression is demonstrated in some of the spindle cells.

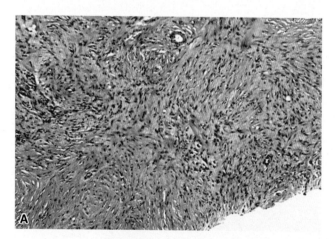
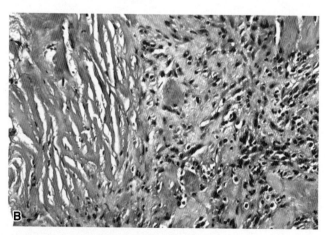

FIGURE 13.8 Metaplastic Spindle Cell Carcinoma, Low-grade Fibromatosis-like. **A:** This area in the needle core biopsy specimen has a storiform pattern. **B:** Another region with a component that resembles **(A)** on the right. A keloidal area composed of dense collagen and a pseudoangiomatous appearance is shown on the left. These findings resemble an area of scarring. **C:** A fully developed keloid-like area with prominent spaces between collagen bands. **D:** Some spindle cells among the collagen bands are immunoreactive for cytokeratin 34βE12. **E:** A densely cellular metaplastic spindle cell carcinoma. **F:** Nuclear reactivity for p63 is present in the carcinoma shown in **D**.

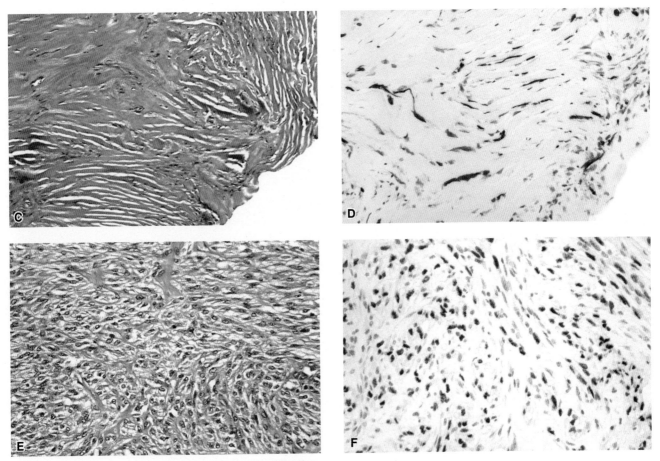

FIGURE 13.8 (continued)

ill-defined cell borders, no obvious cytoplasm, and elongated nuclei. In the more cellular areas, the spindle cells may have slightly more abundant and denser cytoplasm, and align in short files and chords that superficially resemble capillaries but are not associated with red blood cells. These epithelioid foci usually are positive for CKs with a characteristic linear and branching arrangement (**Figs. 13.6 and 13.7**). Atypical spindle cells with enlarged and hyperchromatic nuclei may be identified focally, but the nuclear atypia tends to be of low grade. Mitoses are sparse, ranging from <2 mitoses/10 HPFs to 3–5 mitoses/10HPFs (46,47). Atypia and mitoses are more common in the cellular or epithelioid areas. Chronic inflammation is scattered throughout the tumor and at its periphery; it can be substantial and raise the differential diagnosis of inflammatory PT with inflammation or nodular fasciitis (**Figs. 13.6 and 13.7**).

Invasive carcinoma with epithelial morphology and low-grade atypia can constitute up to 5% of the tumor mass in the surgical excision specimen (46,47). Invasive lobular carcinoma is extremely rare (3). Focal low-grade squamous morphology is uncommon. Low-grade DCIS (46,47), classic LCIS (47), and ADH (3,46) have been described, but usual ductal hyperplasia of gynecomastoid type is the most common intraductal epithelial alteration.

MSpCCs with "low-grade" "fibromatosis-like" morphology can arise in association with papillomas (47,48), complex sclerosing lesions, and nipple adenomas (49,50).

Differential Diagnosis at Needle Core Biopsy

Fibromatosis may arise primarily in the breast parenchyma (primary mammary fibromatosis) or extend into the breast from the chest wall. Fibromatosis tends to occur in women of reproductive age, whereas metaplastic carcinoma is most common in peri- and postmenopausal women, but there are exceptions. The myofibroblasts composing fibromatosis are arranged in broad, sweeping fascicles and show no cytologic atypia. Mitoses are extremely infrequent. Fibromatosis usually shows diffuse nuclear staining for β-catenin (**Fig. 13.9**). Focal nuclear staining for β-catenin has been documented in about 25% of metaplastic carcinomas, as well as in most PTs (51). Limited nuclear staining for β-catenin in the NCB material of a cytologically bland spindle cell lesion in the breast should thus be interpreted cautiously. In particular, the current clinical management of fibromatosis may not necessarily include surgical excision of the lesion, or excision of a local recurrence, whereas the clinical management of "fibromatosis-like" MSpCC requires complete resection of the tumor with negative margins and radiation therapy, or mastectomy. There is no definitive consensus regarding the use of adjuvant chemotherapy in patients with "fibromatosis-like" MSpCC.

Nodular fasciitis, a transient neoplasia secondary to USP6 gene rearrangement (52), and *inflammatory pseudotumor*, a benign neoplasm secondary to *ALK1* gene overexpression (53)

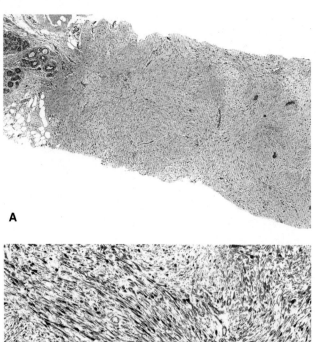

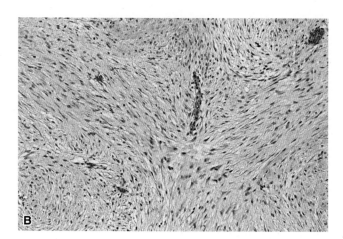

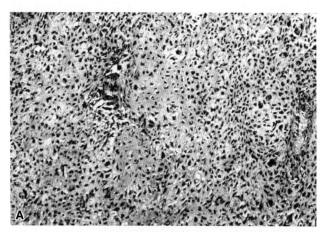

FIGURE 13.9 Primary Mammary Fibromatosis. A, B: This needle core biopsy sampled a mass in the breast of a 32-year-old woman. The spindle cell proliferation is cytologically bland and arranged in broad sweeping fascicles. Blood vessels are conspicuous. **C:** A β-catenin stain decorates the cytoplasm and the nuclei of nearly all lesional cells; p63 and cytokeratins were negative (not shown). The tumor morphology and immunoprofile support the diagnosis of fibromatosis.

are very infrequent in the breast (see Chapter 20) and usually limited in size. Prominent inflammation is present in both lesions. Both neoplasms are negative for CKs.

Myofibroblastoma (see Chapter 20) may occasionally enter the differential diagnosis of "fibromatosis-like" MSpCC when evaluating NCB material. The myofibroblasts of myofibroblastoma have no cytologic atypia, do not express CKs, but are positive for PR and ER. Epithelioid cells in a linear arrangement are absent. Scattered mast cells are common, but chronic inflammation is rare.

Metaplastic Carcinoma with Heterologous Elements

Metaplastic carcinoma with heterologous elements is traditionally defined as an "overt carcinoma with direct transition to a cartilaginous and/or osseous stromal matrix without an intervening spindle cell zone or osteoclastic cells" (54). Some carcinomas show only matrix production (**Fig. 13.10**), whereas others have foci that resemble cartilage (**Fig. 13.11**); osteosarcomatous, rhabdomyosarcomatous, liposarcomatous, and angiosarcomatous metaplasia are less common (**Fig. 13.12**).

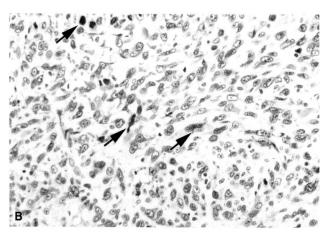

FIGURE 13.10 Metaplastic Carcinoma, Osteocartilaginous Metaplasia. A: The tumor has poorly formed osteoid and chondroid matrix. **B:** Cytokeratin CAM5.2 expression is demonstrated in spindle and round cells *(arrows)*.

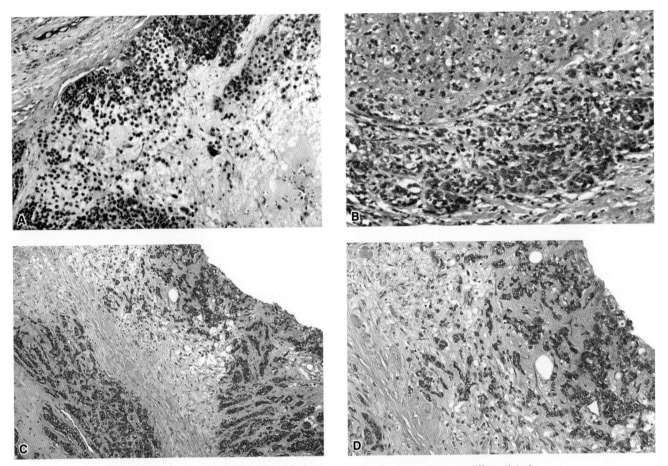

FIGURE 13.11 Metaplastic Carcinoma, Matrix-producing Type. A, B: Undifferentiated carcinoma cells are seen blending with matrix material. The lacunar structure of cartilage is not present. **C, D:** The needle core biopsy sample from a poorly differentiated invasive duct carcinoma with focal matrix production. Taken out of context, the matrix-forming component could be mistaken for mucin.

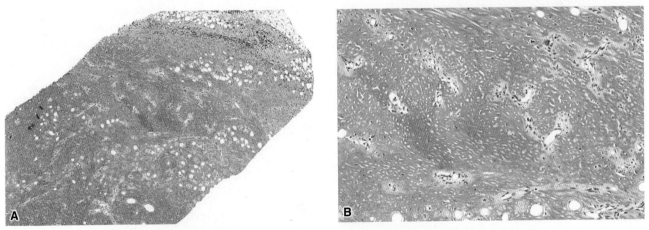

FIGURE 13.12 Metaplastic Carcinoma with Osteoid Matrix Production. A–C: This needle core biopsy specimen shows a tumor with osteoid production. The neoplastic cells in the osteoid matrix are relatively inconspicuous **(B)**, but atypia and increased cellularity are present at the periphery of the lesion **(C)**. **D:** The excision specimen shows a focus of cribriform ductal carcinoma in situ with low nuclear grade adjacent to the lesion. This finding supports the diagnosis of metaplastic carcinoma with osteoid differentiation.

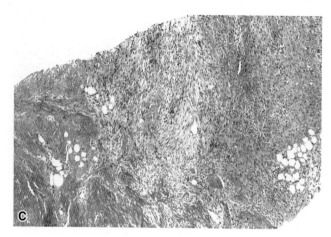

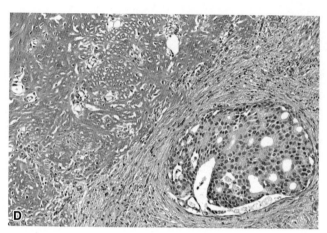

FIGURE 13.12 (*continued*)

Epithelial foci with glandular and/or squamous morphology are usually present. Myxoid areas are also common (**Fig. 13.13**).

In a series evaluating resection specimens of matrix-producing carcinomas (21), chondromyxoid or chondroid matrix constituted more than 40% of the tumor mass in nearly one-third of the cases. The neoplastic cells within the matrix had low-grade morphology in 72% of the cases, but 95% of the associated invasive carcinomas had high-grade morphology. Approximately 60% of the cases showed central necrosis, and 25% had foci of lymphovascular invasion (LVI) (21). Squamous differentiation was present in nearly 40% of the cases in another series (26). Carcinomas with central acellular necrosis/fibrosis occupying at least 30% of the tumor mass (55,56) are also best regarded as metaplastic carcinomas (**Fig. 13.14**). The associated epithelial component usually consists of moderately to poorly differentiated carcinoma.

Nearly, all matrix-producing metaplastic carcinomas are triple-negative (26,57). They are positive for S-100, p63, and calponin (26,57). Lymph node (LN) metastases occur in 20% to 45% of the cases (21,26,58), and can be matrix-producing (26). Distant metastases can also show matrix production.

The DCIS associated with matrix-producing metaplastic carcinomas has solid, cribriform or micropapillary architecture, intermediate or high nuclear grade, and areas of comedo necrosis (26). Matrix-producing DCIS is exceedingly rare. Some matrix-producing metaplastic carcinomas arise in association with microglandular adenosis (57,59,60).

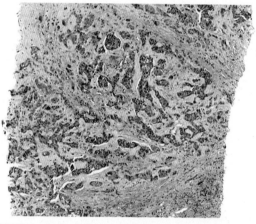

FIGURE 13.13 Metaplastic Carcinoma with Matrix Production. This needle core biopsy specimen shows a matrix-producing carcinoma. The matrix has a homogenous, hypocellular bluish quality and may raise the differential diagnosis of stromal mucin.

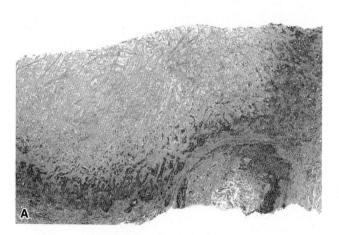

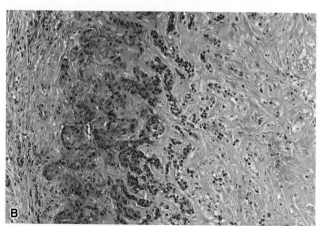

FIGURE 13.14 Metaplastic Matrix-producing Carcinoma with Large Acellular Zone of Necrosis. A, B: This needle core biopsy specimen shows a high-grade carcinoma with a large central area of necrosis. Viable carcinoma has a ring-like distribution at the periphery of the tumor **(B)**. Focal stromal matrix is present between the neoplastic cells.

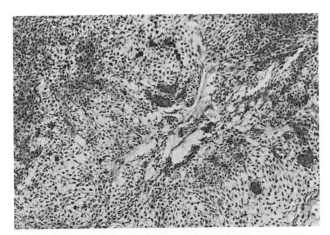

FIGURE 13.15 Mixed Tumor (Pleomorphic Adenoma). This primary epithelial neoplasm of the breast closely resembles a mixed tumor (pleomorphic adenoma) in the salivary glands. It consists of cytologically benign myoepithelial cells with spindle cell morphology in a background of delicate pale matrix, and a few epithelial clusters or glands. A definitive diagnosis of pleomorphic adenoma of the breast cannot be rendered on review of needle core biopsy material. Examination of the entire tumor is necessary to rule out metaplastic carcinoma.

Differential Diagnosis at Needle Core Biopsy

The matrix present in some metaplastic carcinoma may focally resemble mucin and raise the differential diagnosis of *mucinous carcinoma*, especially if only NCB material is available for review (**Fig. 13.13**). Although sometimes mucin positivity can be demonstrated in the stroma, the matrix-producing tumor cells do not contain intracellular mucin. Metaplastic matrix-producing carcinomas are generally strongly and diffusely positive for S-100, and ER- and PR-negative, whereas most mucinous carcinomas are strongly and diffusely positive for ER and PR, but negative for S-100.

Pleomorphic adenoma of the breast is an extremely rare benign biphasic (epithelial and myoepithelial) neoplasm

morphologically similar to its counterpart in the salivary glands (**Fig. 13.15**). The cells composing the lesion are cytologically bland, and no necrosis is present. Mitoses are very sparse, if any. A definitive diagnosis of pleomorphic adenoma can be rendered only upon histologic examination of the entire tumor. Given the rarity of this lesion and its similarities to metaplastic matrix-producing carcinoma, pleomorphic adenoma of the breast is sometimes confused with the latter, especially based on review of only limited material (61). Examples of matrix-producing metaplastic carcinoma arising from a pleomorphic adenoma have been reported (62). Complete excision of any lesion with the morphology of pleomorphic adenoma in core biopsy material is required.

Metastatic chondrosarcoma and osteosarcoma may rarely involve the breast parenchyma but do not show positivity for epithelial markers, and no DCIS is present. Awareness of the patient's clinical history is very important.

Some carcinomas with acantholytic pattern, which is usually secondary to incomplete tissue fixation, may simulate *pseudoangiomatous stromal hyperplasia (PASH) or angiosarcoma*. Immunohistochemical stains for CKs are positive in the carcinoma cells (**Fig. 13.16**).

Metaplastic Carcinoma with Choriocarcinomatous Morphology

Metaplastic carcinomas with choriocarcinomatous areas are extremely rare. They can occur at any age, have no specific presenting features (63–67), and tend to be hemorrhagic microscopically. The choriocarcinomatous component consists of large, multinucleated, pleomorphic cells that express β-HCG. A cytotrophoblastic component may be present, but it tends to be less conspicuous. The identification of invasive carcinoma of no special type, of metaplastic carcinoma with nonchoriocarcinomatous morphology, or of mammary carcinoma in situ supports primary mammary origin of the tumor. These rare carcinomas tend to have an aggressive clinical course.

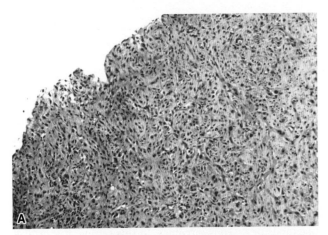 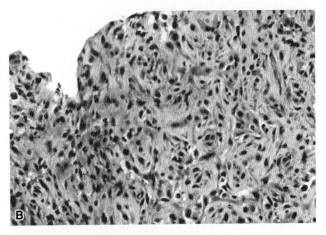

FIGURE 13.16 Metaplastic Carcinoma, Acantholytic (Pseudoangiosarcomatous) Type. Needle core biopsy specimens from several tumors are shown. **A, B:** Epithelial elements form slender, serpiginous strands in basophilic stroma. **C:** Cytokeratin AE1/AE3 immunoreactivity is present. **D:** Spaces have been formed between the spindle cells in this tumor. **E:** There is strong immunoreactivity for cytokeratin CK7 in the tumor shown in **D**. **F:** The fully developed acantholytic pattern. This lesion could be mistaken for pseudoangiomatous stromal hyperplasia. **G:** Pronounced cytokeratin 34βE12 reactivity in the tumor shown in **F**.

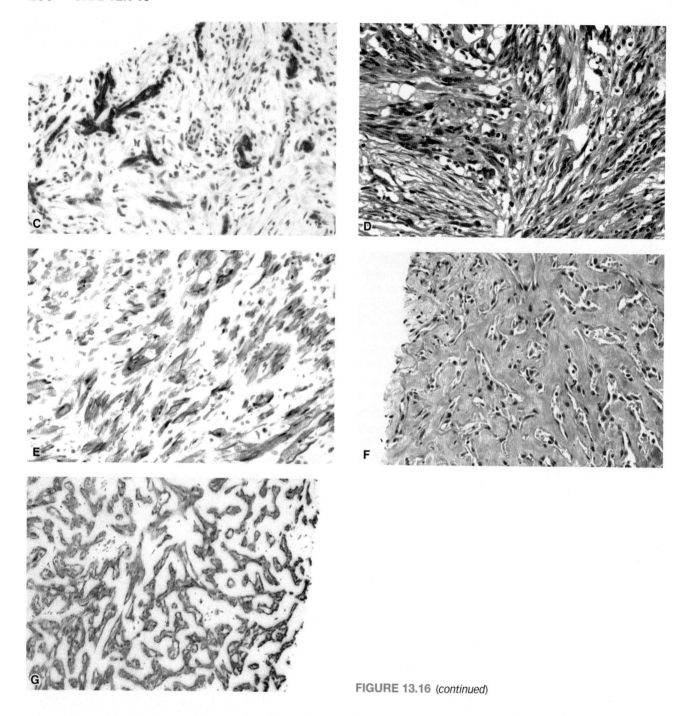

FIGURE 13.16 (continued)

The differential diagnosis of this rare form of metaplastic carcinoma includes metastatic choriocarcinoma. Clinical information about a recent pregnancy, and possible prior history of hydatiform mole or choriocarcinoma should be obtained. Choriocarcinoma, although aggressive, usually has an excellent response to combined chemotherapy, and its prompt diagnosis is critical to avoid unnecessary surgery and to ensure appropriate and timely treatment.

Metaplastic Breast Carcinoma Metastatic to Extramammary Sites

Metaplastic mammary carcinomas tend to have an aggressive course and develop distant metastases, especially to lung and bone. The metastases can consist entirely of carcinoma, of metaplastic elements, or of both components. Separate metastases of the same metaplastic carcinoma may show different morphologies (30) or contain heterologous elements not identified in the index lesion (68). Skeletal metastases of metaplastic carcinoma with chondroid or osseous metaplasia can be especially difficult to differentiate from primary cartilaginous or osseous sarcomas. In this setting, it is critical that the pathologist be informed of the patient's prior history of metaplastic breast carcinoma, so that appropriate immunohistochemical evaluation of the biopsy material obtained from the bone tumor can be performed. Knowledge of the prior history of metaplastic breast carcinoma is fundamental to avoid possible misdiagnosis. Morphologic comparison with the prior tumor, if it is available, and immunohistochemical workup for a panel of epithelial antigens are recommended. GATA3 is reportedly useful to document mammary origin of a metastatic metaplastic carcinoma (39).

Immunohistochemistry

Cytokeratins

The expression of CKs in metaplastic carcinomas varies among different tumors and can be very heterogeneous within a lesion. Thus, the diagnostic workup needs to include a broad panel of CKs (38,69). Keratin MNF116, 34βE12 (K903), CK5/6, CK14, and CK17 are among the CKs most useful to document epithelial differentiation.

MSpCCs with intermediate- and high-grade morphology are the type of metaplastic carcinomas least positive for CKs; the reactivity for CKs may be very focal or even absent, especially in NCB material. Conversely, "fibromatosis-like" MSpCC is usually positive for CKs, especially CK5/6, CK14, and 34βE12, with a characteristic linear and reticular pattern. A study detected MNF116 in 93% of all MSpCC (38). CK14 is positive in 30% (41) to 90% of MSpCCs (38,70). Other CKs expressed in sarcomatous areas include 34βE12 (41,71), CK5 (41), and CK5/6 (70,71). Keratin AE1:AE3 stained only 28% (41) to 41% (38) of MSpCCs. Similarly, CAM5.2 decorated only 30% (41) to 40% (38) of the cases. EMA was positive in 43% of MSpCCs (38). CK7 and CK19 are positive less frequently (41). AE1:AE3 decorated 38% of 21 matrix-producing metaplastic carcinomas (26).

Myoepithelial Antigens

Most metaplastic carcinomas are positive for p63 (38,71,72). In particular, p63 is expressed in 60% to 90% of MSpCCs (38,71–73). In one study (72), the sensitivity and specificity of p63 for the diagnosis of metaplastic carcinoma was 86.7% and 99.4%, respectively.

Most PTs and primary mammary sarcomas are negative for p63 (72), but reactivity for p63 has been documented in some malignant PTs (74). The expression of p63 in nonmammary soft tissue tumors is very limited (44). Focal p63 staining has been detected in osteoblastic tumors, including osteosarcomas (75), and in rare hemangioendotheliomas and angiosarcomas (43). Focal CK and/or EMA expression sometimes occurs in vascular tumors, particularly in epithelioid angiosarcomas and hemangioendotheliomas (42), as well as in other sarcomas. Therefore, the use of vascular markers, such as ERG, FLI1, and CD31 should be included in the diagnostic workup of p63-positive spindle cell lesions of the breast suspected to be MSpCC, especially if the tumor is hemorrhagic. In general, metaplastic carcinomas show stronger and more diffuse positivity for p63 and CKs than sarcomas. Nonetheless, tumors with ambiguous morphology and sparse staining for p63 require thorough analysis of all histologic and immunohistochemical features to distinguish between metaplastic carcinoma and sarcoma. CD10, myosin, maspin, and smooth muscle actin (SMA) are often expressed in the sarcomatoid areas of some

metaplastic carcinomas, although less consistently than p63 (41,73,76). CD10 is detected in 50% of malignant PTs (77). A CD10-positive variant of mammary sarcoma has also been described (78). Focal CD10 positivity has also been detected in vascular tumors (79).

ER, PR, and HER2

Metaplastic carcinomas usually are triple-negative carcinomas. Focal positivity for ER and/or HER2 is usually confined to the neoplastic epithelial component (18,70,71,80).

Epidermal Growth Factor Receptor

Epidermal Growth Factor Receptor (EGFR) is detected in some metaplastic carcinomas, especially carcinomas with squamous morphology. At present, this finding has no specific diagnostic or therapeutic applications. A study (81) identified no EGFR-activating mutations in 303 triple-negative breast carcinomas, including 4 metaplastic carcinomas.

GATA3

GATA3 was detected in 54% of metaplastic carcinomas in one study (39), and can be useful to document mammary origin of distant metastases of metaplastic carcinomas (39). GATA3 is also expressed in 86% of urothelial carcinomas, in 2% of endometrial adenocarcinomas (82), and in many other epithelial and nonepithelial tumors (83).

Snail and Other EMT-related Proteins

Snail (SNAI1) and other EMT-related proteins are expressed in metaplastic carcinomas. In one study (10), the sensitivity of Snail for the diagnosis of metaplastic carcinoma was 100%, but its specificity was only 3.8%, as Snail was positive in myofibroblastomas, in PTs, and in PASH.

Matrix Components

Laminin 5 β3 and χ2 chains decorated 80% to 95% cases of metaplastic carcinoma in two series, but also few PTs (71,84). These markers were less useful than p63 in the diagnosis of metaplastic carcinoma (84). *αβ-crystallin* was detected in 86% of 29 metaplastic carcinomas (85), predominantly in the carcinomatous component. Another study (86) found positive αβ-crystallin only in 20% of metaplastic carcinomas. The sensitivity of these markers in NCB material has not been studied.

SOX10

SOX10, a transcription factor regarded as highly specific for Schwann cell and melanocytic origin, was detected in 46% of 13 metaplastic carcinomas, including 5 of 6 matrix-producing metaplastic carcinomas, and 1 of 3 spindle and squamous metaplastic carcinomas (45). SOX10 expression likely constitutes evidence of myoepithelial differentiation (87).

Treatment and Prognosis

Most reported series of metaplastic carcinoma are retrospective, and they include relatively limited numbers of cases or provide only minimal information on tumor morphology. Approximately 20%

of patients in two epidemiological series (2,8) had LN metastases. About 60% of patients presented with stage II disease, and 10% to 14% (8) with stage III. Surgical treatment involved mastectomy in 55% of the cases (2). Radiotherapy was administered to 43% of patients (2), more than 50% received chemotherapy, and only 6% had hormonal therapy (2). Based on SEER data (8), overall survival (OS) at 5 years was 81% for stage I, 59% for stage II, 67% for stage III, and 18% for stage IV. Disease-specific survival (DSS) at 5 years was 93% for patients with stage I disease, 67% for stage II, 71% for stage III, and 20% for stage IV. In a SEER data–based study (14), 38.6% of 1,501 patients with metaplastic carcinoma received radiotherapy. The 10-year OS and DSS for all patients were 53.2% and 68.3%, respectively. Radiotherapy improved OS (64%) and overall DSS (74%).

Most patients with metaplastic carcinoma receive chemotherapy regimens used for usual breast carcinomas, but some patients had received sarcoma-specific chemotherapy. It is unclear as to which chemotherapy regimen is more effective. The use of neoadjuvant chemotherapy has been reported in some series (6,8,9,11,18,88), but the pathologic complete response (pCR) rate was only 10% in one study (8), and in some series the tumors continued to grow during treatment (88,89).

Overall, the prognosis of metaplastic carcinoma is influenced in large part by the stage at diagnosis. Although metaplastic carcinomas have a lower frequency of LN metastases when compared to nonmetaplastic, high-grade carcinomas, their prognosis appears to be significantly worse.

Metaplastic Spindle Cell Carcinomas with Intermediate- to High-grade Morphology

MSpCCs with intermediate- to high-grade morphology have the worst prognosis among all metaplastic carcinomas. About 50% of patients in published series underwent mastectomy (4,17). In one series, (17) 22% had LN macrometastases. Nearly all patients received chemotherapy (4,17). In a series with a median follow-up time of 36 months (4), 47% of the patients developed a local recurrence, including 57% of the patients who did not receive radiotherapy at initial diagnosis, and only 10% of the patients who did. Approximately one-third of the patients died of disease between 4 and 91 months after treatment, two patients were alive with disease at 9 and 87 months, another patient developed a distant recurrence, but her status was unknown. In another series (17), 80% of the patients received chemotherapy, 68%, radiotherapy, and 10%, hormonal therapy. At a median follow-up of 30 months, 28% of the patients developed a locoregional recurrence, 40% developed distant metastases, and 21% had both; 40% of the patients died of disease. Age >50 years and LN macrometastases were associated with significantly decreased disease-free survival (DFS) in stage I to III patients; a metaplastic component representing >95% of the tumor was significantly associated with decreased DFS in stage I to II patients. Patients with MSpCC had decreased DFS when compared to patients with triple-negative breast carcinoma matched by age, stage, tumor grade, chemotherapy, and radiation therapy. The 5-year DFS for patients with stage I to III MSpCC was 44% (vs. 74% in the control group) and 53% for patients with stage I to II MSpCC (vs. 87% in the control group).

Low-grade Fibromatosis-like Metaplastic Spindle Cell Carcinoma

The first series of patients with "fibromatosis-like" MSpCC (46) reported a 44% rate of local recurrence at a median time of 15.5 months after the initial surgery, but no distant metastases or death of disease were reported. Subsequent studies (3,38,47) have documented lung metastases and death due to disease in a few patients. Two patients were alive with disease at 35 and 42 months of follow-up (38). Overall, "low-grade" "fibromatosis-like" MSpCCs appear to have a relatively more indolent behavior than the rapidly aggressive MSpCCs with intermediate- or high-grade morphology.

Metaplastic Carcinoma with Chondroid and/or Osteoid Matrix

About 40% to 60% of patients in the published series underwent mastectomy (21,26,58). LN metastases were detected in 23% to 45% of patients (21,26,58), and they were purely chondroid in 60% of cases (26). In one series (21), 43% of patients received postmastectomy radiation, and most patients received chemotherapy.

Approximately 20% of patients in one study (58) developed a local recurrence or distant metastases within 2 years of initial treatment, and 4 died of disease. The overall 5-year survival rate was 60%. In this study, patients with matrix-producing metaplastic carcinoma had a more favorable prognosis than control patients with invasive ductal carcinoma. In another series (26), the median patient survival was 38.6 months. Sixty-two percent of the patients developed distant metastases, 36% died of disease, two patients (25%) were alive with metastatic disease at 11 and 12 months, and one (12.5%) patient was alive with locally recurrent disease at 35 months. In a recent series of 32 patients with matrix-producing metaplastic carcinomas (21), 22% developed locoregional recurrence and 31% developed distant metastases at a median time of 28 months. Metastatic sites included lung and/or pleural fluid, liver, buttocks, and leptomeninges. At a median follow-up time of 29 months, 25% of patients died due to disease. Factors independently associated with disease recurrence–free survival included LVI and stage IV disease. When compared with a control group of patients with invasive ductal carcinoma not otherwise specified matched by age, stage, and tumor grade, patients with matrix-producing metaplastic carcinoma had significantly lower 9-year actuarial local relapse-free survival (57% vs. 88%; $p = 0.001$) and distant recurrence-free survival (56% vs. 84%; $p = 0.001$). The results of a large retrospective multi-institutional series of matrix-producing carcinomas are limited by the inherent difficulties in integrating clinical, morphologic, and management data from many different centers (90).

LOW-GRADE ADENOSQUAMOUS CARCINOMA

LGASC is an unusual variant of metaplastic mammary carcinoma morphologically similar to cutaneous LGASC.

Clinical Presentation

Incidence and Gender

Only a few more than 100 cases of LGASC have been reported since the first description of this rare tumor (91), but this number likely underestimates the real incidence of LGASC. LGASC occurs in women, usually of peri- or postmenopausal age. LGASCs are also reported in 19- (92) and 20-year-old women (93). Two patients were pregnant at the time of diagnosis (93). Men are not affected.

Predisposing Factors

A patient with LGASC was a *BRCA1* germline mutation carrier (94); two others had a family history of breast carcinoma (93), and another two had personal histories of ipsilateral breast carcinoma (93). A patient had bilateral florid papillomatosis of the nipple (nipple duct adenoma), and another subsequently developed a complex sclerosing lesion (CSL) in the contralateral breast (93).

Presenting Symptoms

Most LGASCs present as a palpable breast mass, and some are detected by mammography. LGASCs may originate in the retroareolar region. Rarely, nipple discharge is the presenting symptom (93).

Imaging Studies

Mammography can detect LGASC, but the findings are nonspecific. Ultrasound examination of a 5-cm tumor was reported as inconclusive (92).

Size

The average size is about 2.0 cm (range 0.5–5.0 cm).

Microscopic Pathology

LGASC is an unusual variant of metaplastic carcinoma with biphasic (epithelial and myoepithelial/squamous) differentiation (91,95). Morphologically, the tumor consists of glandular and squamous epithelium, infiltrating between normal ducts and lobules and surrounded by desmoplastic stroma (**Figs. 13.17–13.19**). The squamous metaplasia ranges from substantial to focal and inconspicuous in predominantly glandular lesions. Syringoma-like foci and microcysts containing keratotic debris are common. The neoplastic squamous epithelium shows low- to intermediate-grade atypia, with scattered apoptosis and rare mitoses. Areas of necrosis are uncommon. The spindle cells around the squamous foci often show a distinctive lamellar arrangement, and in some areas appear to merge with the myoepithelium/epithelium composing the lesion. Transition of LGASC to conventional high-grade spindle cell and squamous sarcomatoid metaplastic carcinoma (96–98) or to MSpCC (93) is exceedingly rare.

DCIS can be present, and sometimes has apocrine features, or exhibits necrosis. The infiltrating glands of LGASC may show peripheral myoepithelial differentiation, and in some cases, it is difficult to distinguish DCIS from infiltrative areas.

LGASC tends to arise in association with sclerosing lesions, such as florid papillomatosis of the nipple (nipple duct adenoma), papilloma, radial sclerosing lesion (RSL), or sclerosing adenosis (SA) (95). The stromal desmoplasia characteristically associated with LGASC is a morphologic feature useful in the differential diagnosis with non-neoplastic sclerosing lesions. An association with adenomyoepithelioma (AME) is also reported (95,99).

Differential Diagnosis at Needle Core Biopsy

The diagnosis of LGASC is especially challenging in NCB samples, as the findings can be very focal and subtle (98).

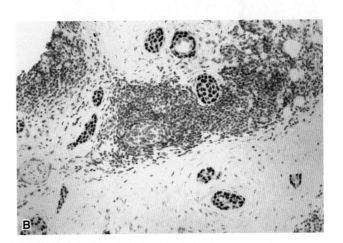

FIGURE 13.17 Metaplastic Carcinoma, Low-grade Adenosquamous Type. A, B: This needle core biopsy sample is from a nonpalpable, mammographically detected stellate tumor. The nests of carcinoma cells with squamous differentiation are accompanied by a lymphocytic infiltrate (**A**). Nuclear reactivity for p63 in areas of squamous differentiation (**B**). **C, D:** The excisional biopsy of the tumor shown in **A, B** revealed cords and clusters of cells with squamoid (**C**) and glandular (**D**) differentiation. The lymphocytic aggregates shown in **A, D** are a characteristic feature of low-grade adenosquamous carcinoma. **E–G:** The needle core biopsy from another tumor showing prominent lymphocytic infiltrates (**E**) and attenuated strands of squamoid epithelial cells (**F**) that were reactive for the cytokeratin 34βE12 (**G**).

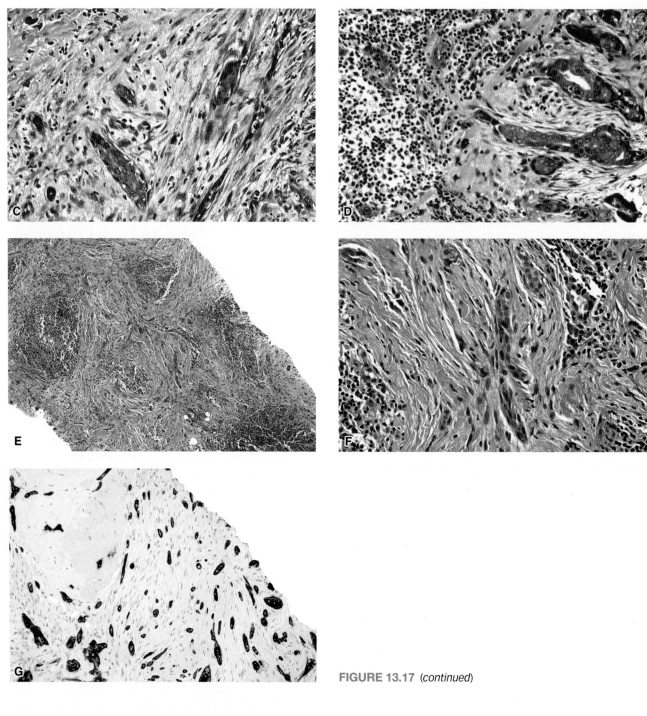

FIGURE 13.17 *(continued)*

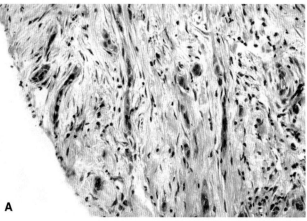

FIGURE 13.18 **Metaplastic Carcinoma, Low-grade Adenosquamous Type.** Images from various tumors are shown.
A: Epithelial strands are shown in mildly cellular stroma in this
needle core biopsy specimen. **B:** Syringoma-like epithelial elements are also present. **C:** In another area of the specimen, a
squamous pearl is surrounded by lymphocytes. **D:** Immunoreactivity for p63. Note myoepithelial cells with p63 reactivity around
a mildly hyperplastic duct in the upper left corner. **E:** Immunoreactivity for cytokeratin MNF116.

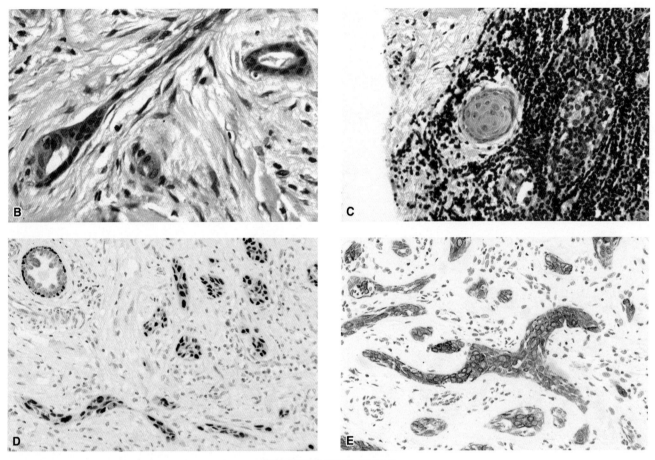

FIGURE 13.18 *(continued)*

Disorganized syringomatous squamous cords and duct-like structures surrounded by spindle cells in a lamellar arrangement should raise the differential diagnosis of LGASC. In some cases, the neoplastic epithelial clusters consist of only few cells with densely eosinophilic and squamoid cytoplasm, admixed with fibrohyalinized or elastotic stroma.

Syringoma closely resembles LGASC morphologically and immunohistochemically, but it does not show cytologic atypia, apoptosis, and dyskeratosis. Syringoma arises primarily in the skin, usually involves the superficial dermis, and rarely extends into the superficial aspect of the breast parenchyma. In contrast, LGASC arises primarily within the breast and may involve the skin secondarily. The differential diagnosis between syringoma and LGASC is particularly challenging when the tumor arises in the nipple **(Fig. 13.19)**.

Sclerosing lesions such as a RSL and a complex sclerosing lesion (CSL) closely mimic LGASC. Furthermore, LGASC tends to arise in association with a sclerosing lesion. It is therefore good practice to entertain the differential diagnosis of LGASC when evaluating a sclerosing lesion that shows unusual features. Compared to benign sclerosing lesions of the breast, LGASC usually shows an infiltrative pattern. The neoplastic glands and squamous nests of LGASC show cytologic atypia, apoptosis, and rare mitoses, which are not common in CSLs. Furthermore, the periductal lamellar fibrosis typically

associated with LGASC is not present in non-neoplastic sclerosing lesions. An inflammatory infiltrate is often present at the periphery and within LGASC.

Immunoreactivity

LGASCs do not show a consistent pattern of immunoreactivity for epithelial and myoepithelial markers. Immunohistochemical studies (93,97) documented staining for AE1:3, CK5/6, CK7, CK14, and CK17 in the epithelial clusters in 50% to 60% of cases, but less-frequent staining for keratin 34βE12 (35%) and CAM5.2 (10%). Some epithelial clusters were CK-negative. The epithelial clusters of LGASC are usually surrounded by myoepithelium, but the latter tends to be incomplete. Complete circumferential staining for p63, SMM-HC, SMA, CD10, and calponin was found only in 11% of the cases in one series (93). The stroma associated with LGASC usually exhibits no reactivity for CKs, although the presence of rare CK7-positive epithelioid stromal cells, and 34βE12- and SMA-positive spindle cells has been reported (93); no p63-positive stromal cells are present. Stromal staining for SMM-HC was identified in 53% of the cases, and for calponin in 57% of the cases (93). Familiarity with the different patterns of immunoreactivity of LGASC is necessary for accurate diagnosis of this rare carcinoma. LGASC is negative for ER, PR, and HER2.

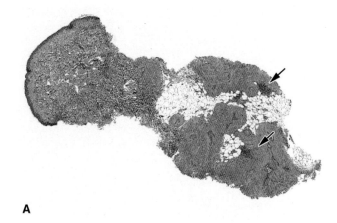

A

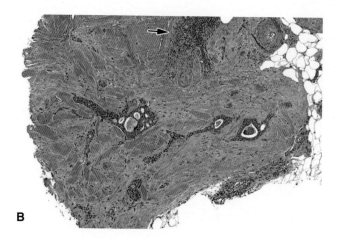

B

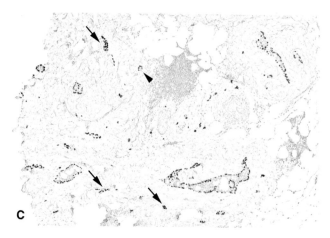

C

FIGURE 13.19 Metaplastic Carcinoma, Low-grade Adeno-squamous Type. The original nipple biopsy material from this patient was erroneously diagnosed as syringoma. The tumor recurred 2 years later in the deep aspect of the nipple. The images in **A–C** illustrate the tumor recurrence. **A:** The lesion in this biopsy material is located in the deep aspect of the nipple, and shows no involvement of the superficial dermis. Aggregates of lymphocytes are associated with the tumor *(arrows)*. **B:** A few neoplastic glands and squamous clusters are present in desmoplastic stroma. An aggregate of lymphocytes is present *(arrow)*. **C:** A p63 stain highlights the myoepithelium around the neoplastic glands. A few small clusters are composed entirely of p63-positive cells *(arrows)*. A neoplastic cluster shows incomplete circumferential staining for p63 *(arrowhead)*.

Prognosis and Treatment

LGASC is characterized by an excellent prognosis. LN involvement by LGASC is extremely rare. The only documented report of systemic disease due to LGASC pertains to a 33-year-old woman with a 8-cm primary breast carcinoma and lung metastases at presentation (91). LGASC, however, may be locally aggressive. A patient with locally recurrent disease developed hemithorax and died due to disease 8.4 years after diagnosis. About 50% of the women treated initially by excisional biopsy developed an ipsilateral recurrence 1 to 3.5 years after the initial treatment, and required mastectomy (91). A LGASC initially diagnosed at NCB as syringomatous adenoma of the nipple recurred after 5 years as a large mass that required mastectomy (93). The surgical management of LGASC is similar to that of other types of invasive breast carcinomas. Radiotherapy can be used in patients treated with breast-conserving surgery. A role for chemotherapy in patients with LGASC has not been determined.

REFERENCES

Metaplastic Carcinomas

1. Kalluri R, Weinberg RA. The basics of epithelial-mesenchymal transition. *J Clin Invest.* 2009;119:1420–1428.
2. Pezzi CM, Patel-Parekh L, Cole K, et al. Characteristics and treatment of metaplastic breast cancer: analysis of 892 cases from the National Cancer Database. *Ann Surg Oncol.* 2007;14:166–173.
3. Kurian KM, Al-Nafussi A. Sarcomatoid/metaplastic carcinoma of the breast: a clinicopathological study of 12 cases. *Histopathology.* 2002;40:58–64.
4. Davis WG, Hennessy B, Babiera G, et al. Metaplastic sarcomatoid carcinoma of the breast with absent or minimal overt invasive carcinomatous component: a misnomer. *Am J Surg Pathol.* 2005;29:1456–1463.
5. Barnes PJ, Boutilier R, Chiasson D, et al. Metaplastic breast carcinoma: clinical-pathologic characteristics and HER2/neu expression. *Breast Cancer Res Treat.* 2005;91:173–178.
6. Beatty JD, Atwood M, Tickman R, et al. Metaplastic breast cancer: clinical significance. *Am J Surg.* 2006;191:657–664.
7. Dave G, Cosmatos H, Do T, et al. Metaplastic carcinoma of the breast: a retrospective review. *Int J Radiat Oncol Biol Phys.* 2006;64:771–775.
8. Hennessy BT, Giordano S, Broglio K, et al. Biphasic metaplastic sarcomatoid carcinoma of the breast. *Ann Oncol.* 2006;17:605–613.
9. Luini A, Aguilar M, Gatti G, et al. Metaplastic carcinoma of the breast, an unusual disease with worse prognosis: the experience of the European Institute of Oncology and review of the literature. *Breast Cancer Res Treat.* 2007;101:349–353.
10. Nassar A, Sookhan N, Santisteban M, et al. Diagnostic utility of Snail in metaplastic breast carcinoma. *Diagn Pathol.* 2010;5:76.
11. Okada N, Hasebe T, Iwasaki M, et al. Metaplastic carcinoma of the breast. *Hum Pathol.* 2010;41:960–970.
12. Park HS, Park S, Kim JH, et al. Clinicopathologic features and outcomes of metaplastic breast carcinoma: comparison with invasive ductal carcinoma of the breast. *Yonsei Med J.* 2010;51:864–869.
13. Gwin K, Buell-Gutbrod R, Tretiakova M, et al. Epithelial-to-mesenchymal transition in metaplastic breast carcinomas with chondroid differentiation: expression of the E-cadherin repressor Snail. *Appl Immunohistochem Mol Morphol.* 2010;18:526–531.
14. Tseng WH, Martinez SR. Metaplastic breast cancer: to radiate or not to radiate? *Ann Surg Oncol.* 2011;18:94–103.

15. Bae SY, Lee SK, Koo MY, et al. The prognoses of metaplastic breast cancer patients compared to those of triple-negative breast cancer patients. *Breast Cancer Res Treat*. 2011;126:471–478.

16. Chen IC, Lin CH, Huang CS, et al. Lack of efficacy to systemic chemotherapy for treatment of metaplastic carcinoma of the breast in the modern era. *Breast Cancer Res Treat*. 2011;130:345–351.

17. Lester TR, Hunt KK, Nayeemuddin KM, et al. Metaplastic sarcomatoid carcinoma of the breast appears more aggressive than other triple receptor-negative breast cancers. *Breast Cancer Res Treat*. 2012;131:41–48.

18. Lee H, Jung SY, Ro JY, et al. Metaplastic breast cancer: clinicopathological features and its prognosis. *J Clin Pathol*. 2012;65:441–446.

19. Choi BB, Shu KS. Metaplastic carcinoma of the breast: multimodality imaging and histopathologic assessment. *Acta Radiol*. 2012;53:5–11.

20. Alvarenga CA, Paravidino PI, Alvarenga M, et al. Reappraisal of immunohistochemical profiling of special histological types of breast carcinomas: a study of 121 cases of eight different subtypes. *J Clin Pathol*. 2012;65:1066–1071.

21. Downs-Kelly E, Nayeemuddin KM, Albarracin C, et al. Matrix-producing carcinoma of the breast: an aggressive subtype of metaplastic carcinoma. *Am J Surg Pathol*. 2009;33:534–541.

22. Yang WT, Hennessy B, Broglio K, et al. Imaging differences in metaplastic and invasive ductal carcinomas of the breast. *AJR Am J Roentgenol*. 2007;189:1288–1293.

23. Rashid MU, Shah MA, Azhar R, et al. A deleterious BRCA1 mutation in a young Pakistani woman with metaplastic breast carcinoma. *Pathol Res Pract*. 2011;207:583–586.

24. Suspitsin EN, Sokolenko AP, Voskresenskiy DA, et al. Mixed epithelial/mesenchymal metaplastic carcinoma (carcinosarcoma) of the breast in BRCA1 carrier. *Breast Cancer*. 2011;18:137–140.

25. Ashida A, Fukutomi T, Tsuda H, et al. Atypical medullary carcinoma of the breast with cartilaginous metaplasia in a patient with a BRCA1 germline mutation. *Jpn J Clin Oncol*. 2000;30:30–32.

26. Gwin K, Wheeler DT, Bossuyt V, et al. Breast carcinoma with chondroid differentiation: a clinicopathologic study of 21 triple negative (ER-, PR-, Her2/neu-) cases. *Int J Surg Pathol*. 2010;18:27–35.

27. Velasco M, Santamaria G, Ganau S, et al. MRI of metaplastic carcinoma of the breast. *AJR Am J Roentgenol*. 2005;184:1274–128.

28. Shin HJ, Kim HH, Kim SM, et al. Imaging features of metaplastic carcinoma with chondroid differentiation of the breast. *AJR Am J Roentgenol*. 2007;188:691–696.

29. Park JM, Han BK, Moon WK, et al. Metaplastic carcinoma of the breast: mammographic and sonographic findings. *J Clin Ultrasound*. 2000;28:179–186.

30. Kaufman MW, Marti JR, Gallager S, et al. Carcinoma of the breast with pseudosarcomatous metaplasia. *Cancer*. 1984;53:1908–1917.

31. Wargotz ES, Norris HJ. Metaplastic carcinomas of the breast. V: Metaplastic carcinoma with osteoclastic giant-cells. *Hum Pathol*. 1990;21:1142–1150.

32. Sugie T, Takeuchi E, Kunishima F, et al. A case of ductal carcinoma with squamous differentiation in malignant phyllodes tumor. *Breast Cancer*. 2007;14:327–332.

33. Ramdass MJ, Dindyal S. Phyllodes breast tumor showing invasive squamous-cell carcinoma with invasive ductal, clear-cell, secretory, and squamous components. *Lancet Oncol*. 2006;7:880.

34. Rostock RA, Bauer TW, Eggleston JC. Primary squamous carcinoma of the breast: a review. 1984;10:27–31.

35. Leiman G. Squamous carcinoma of the breast: diagnosis by aspiration cytology. *Acta Cytol*. 1982;26:201–209.

36. Farrand R, Lavigne R, Lokich J, et al. Epidermoid carcinoma of the breast. *J Surg Oncol*. 1979;12:207–211.

37. DeLair DF, Corben AD, Catalano JP, et al. Non-mammary metastases to the breast and axilla: a study of 85 cases. *Mod Pathol*. 2013;26:343–349.

38. Carter MR, Hornick JL, Lester S, et al. Spindle cell (sarcomatoid) carcinoma of the breast: a clinicopathologic and immunohistochemical analysis of 29 cases. *Am J Surg Pathol*. 2006;30:300–309.

39. Cimino-Mathews A, Subhawong AP, Illei PB, et al. GATA3 expression in breast carcinoma: utility in triple-negative, sarcomatoid, and metastatic carcinomas. *Hum Pathol*. 2013;44:1341–1349.

40. Chia Y, Thike AA, Cheok PY, et al. Stromal keratin expression in phyllodes tumors of the breast: a comparison with other spindle cell breast lesions. *J Clin Pathol*. 2012;65:339–347.

41. Dunne B, Lee AH, Pinder SE, et al. An immunohistochemical study of metaplastic spindle cell carcinoma, phyllodes tumor and fibromatosis of the breast. *Hum Pathol*. 2003;34:1009–1015.

42. Miettinen M, Fetsch JF. Distribution of keratins in normal endothelial cells and a spectrum of vascular tumors: implications in tumor diagnosis. *Hum Pathol*. 2000;31:1062–1067.

43. Kallen ME, Nunes Rosado FG, Gonzalez AL, et al. Occasional staining for p63 in malignant vascular tumors: a potential diagnostic pitfall. *Pathol Oncol Res*. 2012;18:97–100.

44. Jo VY, Fletcher CD. p63 immunohistochemical staining is limited in soft tissue tumors. *Am J Clin Pathol*. 2011;136:762–766.

45. Cimino-Mathews A, Subhawong AP, Elwood H, et al. Neural crest transcription factor Sox10 is preferentially expressed in triple-negative and metaplastic breast carcinomas. *Hum Pathol*. 2013;44:959–965.

46. Gobbi H, Simpson JF, Borowsky A, et al. Metaplastic breast tumors with a dominant fibromatosis-like phenotype have a high risk of local recurrence. *Cancer*. 1999;85:2170–2182.

47. Sneige N, Yaziji H, Mandavilli SR, et al. Low-grade (fibromatosis-like) spindle cell carcinoma of the breast. *Am J Surg Pathol*. 2001;25:1009–1016.

48. Rekhi B, Shet TM, Badwe RA, et al. Fibromatosis-like carcinoma-an unusual phenotype of a metaplastic breast tumor associated with a micropapilloma. *World J Surg Oncol*. 2007;5:24.

49. Gobbi H, Simpson JF, Jensen RA, et al. Metaplastic spindle cell breast tumors arising within papillomas, complex sclerosing lesions, and nipple adenomas. *Mod Pathol*. 2003;16:893–901.

50. Denley H, Pinder SE, Tan PH, et al. Metaplastic carcinoma of the breast arising within complex sclerosing lesion: a report of five cases. *Histopathology*. 2000;36:203–209.

51. Lacroix-Triki M, Geyer FC, Lambros MB, et al. Beta-catenin/Wnt signaling pathway in fibromatosis, metaplastic carcinomas and phyllodes tumors of the breast. *Mod Pathol*. 2010;23:1438–1448.

52. Erickson-Johnson MR, Chou MM, Evers BR, et al. Nodular fasciitis: a novel model of transient neoplasia induced by MYH9-USP6 gene fusion. *Lab Invest*. 2011;91:1427–1433.

53. Lawrence B, Perez-Atayde A, Hibbard MK, et al. TPM3-ALK and TPM4-ALK oncogenes in inflammatory myofibroblastic tumors. *Am J Pathol*. 2000;157:377–384.

54. Wargotz ES, Norris HJ. Metaplastic carcinomas of the breast. I: Matrix-producing carcinoma. *Hum Pathol*. 1989;20:628–635.

55. Tsuda H, Takarabe T, Hasegawa F, et al. Large, central acellular zones indicating myoepithelial tumor differentiation in high-grade invasive ductal carcinomas as markers of predisposition to lung and brain metastases. *Am J Surg Pathol*. 2000;24:197–202.

56. Tsuda H, Takarabe T, Hasegawa T, et al. Myoepithelial differentiation in high-grade invasive ductal carcinomas with large central acellular zones. *Hum Pathol*. 1999;30:1134–1139.

57. Shui R, Bi R, Cheng Y, et al. Matrix-producing carcinoma of the breast in the Chinese population: a clinicopathological study of 13 cases. *Pathol Int*. 2011;61:415–422.

58. Chhieng C, Cranor M, Lesser ME, et al. Metaplastic carcinoma of the breast with osteocartilaginous heterologous elements. *Am J Surg Pathol*. 1998;22:188–194.

59. Rosenblum MK, Purrazzella R, Rosen PP. Is microglandular adenosis a precancerous disease? A study of carcinoma arising therein. *Am J Surg Pathol*. 1986;10:237–245.

60. Geyer FC, Lacroix-Triki M, Colombo PE, et al. Molecular evidence in support of the neoplastic and precursor nature of microglandular adenosis. *Histopathology*. 2012;60:E115–E130.

61. Rakha EA, Aleskandarany MA, Samaka RM, et al. Pleomorphic adenoma-like tumor of the breast. *Histopathology*. 2016;68:405–410.

62. Hayes MM, Lesack D, Girardet C, et al. Carcinoma ex-pleomorphic adenoma of the breast: report of three cases suggesting a relationship to metaplastic carcinoma of matrix-producing type. *Virchows Arch*. 2005;446:142–149.

63. Saigo PE, Rosen PP. Mammary carcinoma with "choriocarcinomatous" features. *Am J Surg Pathol*. 1981;5:773–778.

64. Resetkova E, Sahin A, Ayala AG, et al. Breast carcinoma with choriocarcinomatous features. *Ann Diagn Pathol*. 2004;8:74–79.

65. Canbay E, Bozkurt B, Ergul G, et al. Breast carcinoma with choriocarcinomatous features. *Breast J.* 2010;16:202–203.

66. Siddiqui NH, Cabay RJ, Salem F. Fine-needle aspiration biopsy of a case of breast carcinoma with choriocarcinomatous features. *Diagn Cytopathol.* 2006;34:694–697.

67. Akbulut M, Zekioglu O, Ozdemir N, et al. Fine needle aspiration cytology of mammary carcinoma with choriocarcinomatous features: a report of 2 cases. *Acta Cytol.* 2008;52:99–104.

68. Chell SE, Nayar R, De Frias DV, et al. Metaplastic breast carcinoma metastatic to the lung mimicking a primary chondroid lesion: report of a case with cytohistologic correlation. *Ann Diagn Pathol.* 1998;2:173–180.

69. Adem C, Reynolds C, Adlakha H, et al. Wide spectrum screening keratin as a marker of metaplastic spindle cell carcinoma of the breast: an immunohistochemical study of 24 patients. *Histopathology.* 2002;40:556–562.

70. Reis-Filho JS, Milanezi F, Steele D, et al. Metaplastic breast carcinomas are basal-like tumors. *Histopathology.* 2006;49:10–21.

71. Carpenter PM, Wang-Rodriguez J, Chan OT, et al. Laminin 5 expression in metaplastic breast carcinomas. *Am J Surg Pathol.* 2008;32:345–353.

72. Koker MM, Kleer CG. p63 expression in breast cancer: a highly sensitive and specific marker of metaplastic carcinoma. *Am J Surg Pathol.* 2004;28:1506–1512.

73. Leibl S, Gogg-Kammerer M, Sommersacher A, et al. Metaplastic breast carcinomas: are they of myoepithelial differentiation? Immunohistochemical profile of the sarcomatoid subtype using novel myoepithelial markers. *Am J Surg Pathol.* 2005;29:347–353.

74. Cimino-Mathews A, Sharma R, Illei PB, et al. A subset of malignant phyllodes tumors express p63 and p40: a diagnostic pitfall in breast core needle biopsies. *Am J Surg Pathol.* 2014;38:1689–1696.

75. Kallen ME, Sanders ME, Gonzalez AL, et al. Nuclear p63 expression in osteoblastic tumors. *Tumour Biol.* 2012;33:1639–1644.

76. Popnikolov NK, Ayala AG, Graves K, et al. Benign myoepithelial tumors of the breast have immunophenotypic characteristics similar to metaplastic matrix-producing and spindle cell carcinomas. *Am J Clin Pathol.* 2003;120:161–167.

77. Tse GM, Tsang AK, Putti TC, et al. Stromal CD10 expression in mammary fibroadenomas and phyllodes tumors. *J Clin Pathol.* 2005;58:185–189.

78. Leibl S, Moinfar F. Mammary NOS-type sarcoma with CD10 expression: a rare entity with features of myoepithelial differentiation. *Am J Surg Pathol.* 2006;30:450–456.

79. Weinreb I, Cunningham KS, Perez-Ordonez B, et al. CD10 is expressed in most epithelioid hemangioendotheliomas: a potential diagnostic pitfall. *Arch Pathol Lab Med.* 2009;133:1965–1968.

80. Reis-Filho JS, Milanezi F, Carvalho S, et al. Metaplastic breast carcinomas exhibit EGFR, but not HER2, gene amplification and overexpression: immunohistochemical and chromogenic in situ hybridization analysis. *Breast Cancer Res.* 2005;7:R1028–R1035.

81. Wen YH, Brogi E, Hasanovic A, et al. Immunohistochemical staining with EGFR mutation-specific antibodies: high specificity as a diagnostic marker for lung adenocarcinoma. *Mod Pathol.* 2013;26:1197–1203.

82. Liu H, Shi J, Wilkerson ML, et al. Immunohistochemical evaluation of GATA3 expression in tumors and normal tissues: a useful immunomarker for breast and urothelial carcinomas. *Am J Clin Pathol.* 2012;138:57–64.

83. Miettinen M, McCue PA, Sarlomo-Rikala M, et al. GATA3: a multispecific but potentially useful marker in surgical pathology: a systematic analysis of 2500 epithelial and nonepithelial tumors. *Am J Surg Pathol.* 2014;38:13–22.

84. D'Alfonso TM, Ross DS, Liu YF, et al. Expression of p40 and laminin 332 in metaplastic spindle cell carcinoma of the breast compared with other malignant spindle cell tumors. *J Clin Pathol.* 2015;68:516–521.

85. Sitterding SM, Wiseman WR, Schiller CL, et al. Alpha-B-crystallin: a novel marker of invasive basal-like and metaplastic breast carcinomas. *Ann Diagn Pathol.* 2008;12:33–40.

86. Tsang JY, Lai MW, Wong KH, et al. Alpha-B-crystallin is a useful marker for triple negative and basal breast cancers. *Histopathology.* 2012;61:378–386.

87. Miettinen M, McCue PA, Sarlomo-Rikala M, et al. Sox10—a marker for not only Schwannian and melanocytic neoplasms but also myoepithelial cell tumors of soft tissue: a systematic analysis of 5134 tumors. *Am J Surg Pathol.* 2015;39:826–835.

88. Nagao T, Kinoshita T, Hojo T, et al. The differences in the histological types of breast cancer and the response to neoadjuvant chemotherapy: the relationship between the outcome and the clinicopathological characteristics. *Breast.* 2012;21:289–295.

89. Rayson D, Adjei AA, Suman VJ, et al. Metaplastic breast cancer: prognosis and response to systemic therapy. *Ann Oncol.* 1999;10:413–419.

90. Rakha EA, Tan PH, Shaaban A, et al. Do primary mammary osteosarcoma and chondrosarcoma exist? A review of a large multi-institutional series of malignant matrix-producing breast tumors. *Breast.* 2013;22:13–18.

Low-grade Adenosquamous Carcinoma

91. Rosen PP, Ernsberger D. Low-grade adenosquamous carcinoma: a variant of metaplastic mammary carcinoma. *Am J Surg Pathol.* 1987;11:351–358.

92. Agrawal A, Saha S, Ellis IO, et al. Adenosquamous carcinoma of breast in a 19 years old woman: a case report. *World J Surg Oncol.* 2010;8:44.

93. Kawaguchi K, Shin SJ. Immunohistochemical staining characteristics of low-grade adenosquamous carcinoma of the breast. *Am J Surg Pathol.* 2012;36(7):1009–1020.

94. Noel JC, Buxant F, Engohan-Aloghe C. Low-grade adenosquamous carcinoma of the breast—a case report with a BRCA1 germline mutation. *Pathol Res Pract.* 2010;206:511–513.

95. Van Hoeven KH, Drudis T, Cranor ML, et al. Low-grade adenosquamous carcinoma of the breast: a clinocopathologic study of 32 cases with ultra-structural analysis. *Am J Surg Pathol.* 1993;17:248–258.

96. Suster S, Moran CA, Hurt MA. Syringomatous squamous tumors of the breast. *Cancer.* 1991;67:2350–2355.

97. Geyer FC, Lambros MB, Natrajan R, et al. Genomic and immunohistochemical analysis of adenosquamous carcinoma of the breast. *Mod Pathol.* 2010;23:951–960.

98. Ho BC, Tan HW, Lee VK, et al. Preoperative and intraoperative diagnosis of low-grade adenosquamous carcinoma of the breast: potential diagnostic pitfalls. *Histopathology.* 2006;49:603–611.

99. Foschini MP, Pizzicannella G, Peterse JL, et al. Adenomyoepithelioma of the breast associated with low-grade adenosquamous and sarcomatoid carcinomas. *Virchows Arch.* 1995;427:243–250.

Mucinous Carcinoma

EDI BROGI

Mucinous carcinoma (MC) is composed of neoplastic epithelial clusters admixed with extracellular mucin comprising at least 90% of the tumor. The terms mixed mucinous carcinoma or invasive carcinoma with mucinous features are used for tumors with a mucinous component comprising less than 90% of the lesion. Mention of focal mucinous differentiation should always be included in the diagnostic report of an invasive carcinoma with a lesser mucinous component. MC has a relatively good prognosis. Mixed MC and invasive carcinoma with focal mucinous differentiation are best managed as well-differentiated invasive ductal carcinoma (IFDC) of no special type, as the prognosis is not as good as for MC.

CLINICAL PRESENTATION

Incidence

MC constitutes less than 2% of all breast carcinomas in most series (1–8). A mucinous component of variable extent may be present in up to 2% of other carcinomas.

Age

Women with MC are older than those with nonmucinous carcinoma (1,5,6,8–14). Although MC can occur at any age (range 25–85) (11), the median and the mean age at diagnosis of 11,422 patients with MC in a study based on 1973 to 2002 SEER data (11) were 71 years and 68.3 years, respectively, significantly greater than that for patients with IFDC ($p < 0.01$). More than 80% of patients with MC are postmenopausal (8) and at least 65 years old (11). Most studies (15–17) found no significant difference in the age distribution and median age of women with MC and mixed MC, although in one series (13) the mean age of patients with MC was 75 years (range 59–90) versus 65 years (range 35–89) for patients with mixed MC ($p = 0.02$).

Family History

MC does not appear to be associated with familial breast carcinoma (18) and with *BRCA1* germline mutation carrier status (19). Lacroix-Triki et al. (20) found no evidence of microsatellite instability associated with Lynch syndrome in mammary MC.

Ethnicity

MC is most frequent among Caucasian women (2,11,19,21). In a study based on 1992 to 2007 SEER data (2), 78.5% of women with MC were non-Hispanic whites.

Gender

MC can occur in men. The incidence of MC in males was 0.5% between 1973 and 2002 (11), and 2% between 1985 and 2000 (22). In a series of 759 primary invasive mammary carcinomas in men (23), 21 (2.8%) were MCs and 26 (3.4%) were mixed MCs.

Clinical Findings

MC can present as a palpable, soft mass, or as a nonpalpable mammographic mass or architectural distortion (12,24,25). In one study (26), 44.6% of 56 MCs were self-detected, 37.5% were detected at mammographic screening, and 17.9% were first identified at clinical examination. A palpable mass was the presenting symptom in 87% of cases in another series (27). Primary MC can also arise in ectopic breast tissue, such as in the axilla or vulva.

Radiology

Tumors with a high mucin content tend to be mammographically and sonographically lobulated or circumscribed (25,28–30). The sensitivity of mammograms was only 76.5% for the detection of MC versus 100% for mixed MC (31). Only 37.5% of MC in one series (26) were first detected at mammographic screening. Mammographically detected calcifications in the invasive epithelium and/or in the mucin are found in up to 40% of MCs (12,27,30,32,33). Calcifications can also occur in adjacent ductal carcinoma in situ (DCIS) (14,34) or in a concurrent mucocele-like lesion (35). On ultrasound examination, MC is isoechogenic to the mammary fat (36). The sensitivity of ultrasound was 94.7% for MC versus 100% for mixed MCs in one study (31).

Dhillon et al. (30) reported that 39% of mammographically evident MC ranging in size from 5 to 20 mm (average 11 mm) were not seen on ultrasound. In the same series (30), 38% of MCs were not recognized as abnormal when first encountered in a mammogram or at ultrasound examination. Nonetheless, patients with delayed diagnosis had no lymph node (LN) metastases at the time of surgical excision.

The echographic differential diagnosis of MC includes myxoid fibroadenoma, benign cystic lesions, as well as matrix-producing carcinoma and carcinoma with large central acellular zone (37). MC has a gradually enhancing contrast pattern and very high signal intensity on T2-weighted images at magnetic resonance imaging (MRI) examination (38,39). MC and some types of fibroadenomas are not distinctively different on MRI examination (40,41).

Size

In a study based on 1973 to 2002 SEER data (11), MC had a mean size of 2.2 cm, a median size of 1.6 cm, and 83.2% of tumors measured 3.0 cm or less. More than 50% of MCs in contemporary series measured 2 cm or less (12,16,17,21). MCs larger than 5 cm were observed in only 2.8% (17) and 4.9% (12) of the cases in two studies. The average size of MC without LN metastases was 1.5 cm versus 2.6 cm for MC with LN involvement (21). MCs are smaller than IFDC (11,12) and mixed MCs (15–17).

MICROSCOPIC PATHOLOGY

MC is composed of at least 90% of abundant extracellular mucin admixed with invasive neoplastic epithelial cells **(Fig. 14.1)**. The mucinous component of a mixed MC constitutes less than 90% of the tumor **(Fig. 14.2)**. Extensive sampling of a hypocellular MC composed almost entirely of extracellular mucin may be required to detect the neoplastic epithelium **(Fig. 14.3)**. The carcinoma cells of MC are arranged in a variety of patterns, including strands, alveolar nests, papillary and micropapillary clusters, and large cribriform sheets **(Fig. 14.4)**.

Grade

Most MCs are well to moderately differentiated. In a study based on SEER data (11), 53% of the tumors were well differentiated, 38% were moderately differentiated, and 9% were poorly differentiated or anaplastic. MC with high nuclear grade is rare (16) and has worse prognosis (11).

Calcifications

Calcifications associated with MC tend to be coarse and irregular.

Histological Subtypes of Mucinous Carcinoma

Type A, Type B, and Type AB Mucinous Carcinoma

Capella et al. (42) subclassified MC into three morphologic types: A, B, and AB. They described type A MC as having

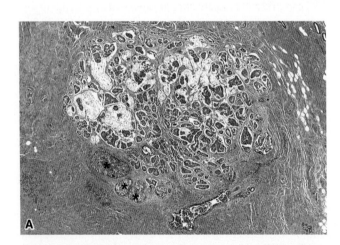

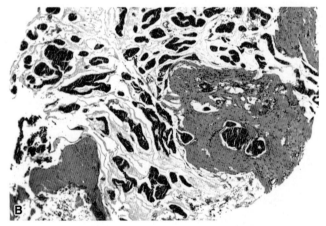

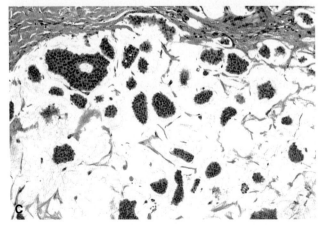

FIGURE 14.1 Mucinous Carcinoma. A: More than 90% of this mucinous carcinoma consists of clusters of carcinoma cells admixed with stromal mucin. Focal solid ductal carcinoma in situ (DCIS) is also present *(asterisks)*. **B, C:** Needle core biopsy specimens showing varying proportions of extracellular mucin and carcinoma cells. The epithelium forms small nests and trabeculae in **B** and nests in **C**.

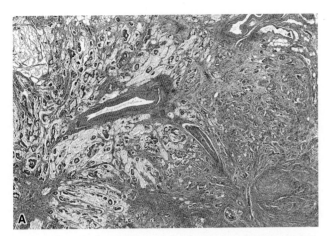
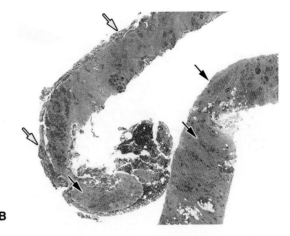

FIGURE 14.2 Mixed Mucinous Carcinoma. A: In this mixed mucinous carcinoma, the mucinous component represents less than 90% of the tumor. **B:** In this needle core biopsy sample of a mixed mucinous carcinoma, the neoplastic clusters are embedded in the stroma in some areas *(dark arrows)*, and admixed with abundant extracellular mucin in others *(white arrows)*.

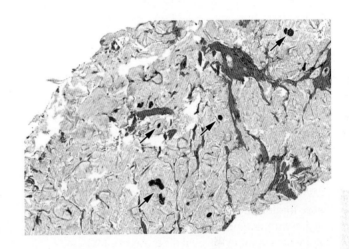

FIGURE 14.3 Mucinous Carcinoma, Hypocellular. Only minute and sparse clusters of carcinoma cells *(arrows)* are present in this core biopsy sample from a hypocellular mucinous carcinoma.

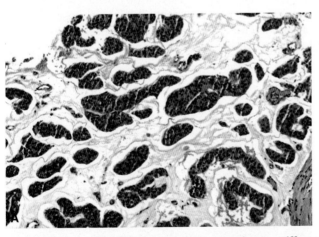
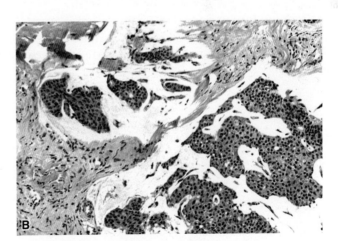

FIGURE 14.4 Mucinous Carcinoma, Different Growth Patterns. Needle core biopsy specimens showing different growth patterns. **A:** Trabecular pattern. **B:** Festoon growth pattern. **C:** Cribriform mucinous carcinoma.

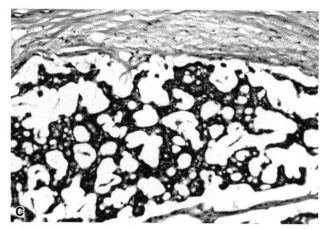

FIGURE 14.4 (*continued*)

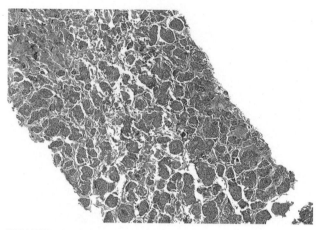

FIGURE 14.6 Mucinous Carcinoma, Type B. The mucinous carcinoma in this needle core biopsy sample is cellular and consists of numerous neoplastic epithelial clusters admixed with relatively limited extracellular mucin.

abundant extracellular mucin and epithelium distributed in "trabeculae and ribbons or festoons" (**Fig. 14.5**). Type B MC had less-abundant extracellular mucin and consisted of "clumps" of cells with intracytoplasmic mucin and often granular cytoplasm (**Fig. 14.6**). Type AB MC had "indeterminate" features and constituted 20% of cases. Patients with type A MC tended to be younger than patients with type B MC. The authors suggested that type B tumors constituted a variant of MC with endocrine differentiation. This classification was not prognostically significant in a subsequent study (5). In a recent series (16), type A MCs were found to be smaller than type B (1.4 cm vs. 1.9 cm, respectively), had lower rates of lymphovascular invasion (LVI) (3% vs. 25%) and LN metastases (8% vs. 25%), and were less often HER2-positive (5.4% vs. 25%). These findings need validation in larger series. At present, the presence of type A, B, or AB morphology is not usually commented upon in the final diagnosis of a MC.

Micropapillary Variant of Mucinous Carcinoma

A micropapillary variant of MC has been described (16,43,44). The micropapillae are arranged in small and tightly cohesive

clusters or in ring-like structures in a space filled with mucin (**Fig. 14.7**). Psammomatous calcifications are common (43) (**Fig. 14.7**). A micropapillary component was recognized in 66.6% (45), 35% (44), and 20% (16) of MC in three separate series, but the percentage of MC with micropapillary morphology required for diagnosis was not defined. In one series (16), MC with and without a micropapillary component had similar average size (1.7 cm and 1.65 cm, respectively), but patients with a micropapillary component were younger (47 years vs. 60 years, respectively). Three of the five (60%) MCs with LN metastases had a micropapillary component, versus only 14% of MCs without LN involvement (16). In another series (46), LVI was present in 9/15 (60%) micropapillary MCs, and LN metastases occurred in 33% of cases. One of 13 patients with follow-up information developed a chest-wall recurrence 9 months after mastectomy. Liu et al. (47) found that 134 patients with MC composed of micropapillary clusters in at least 50% of the tumor were significantly younger (median age 46 years), had more frequent LN involvement (35%), and significantly

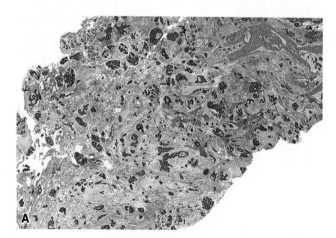

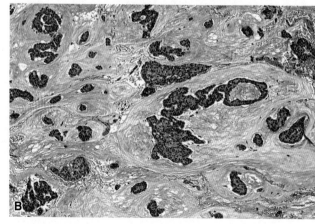

FIGURE 14.5 Mucinous Carcinoma, Type A. A, B: The mucinous carcinoma in this needle core biopsy sample consists of scattered cohesive clusters of neoplastic cells admixed with abundant extracellular mucin.

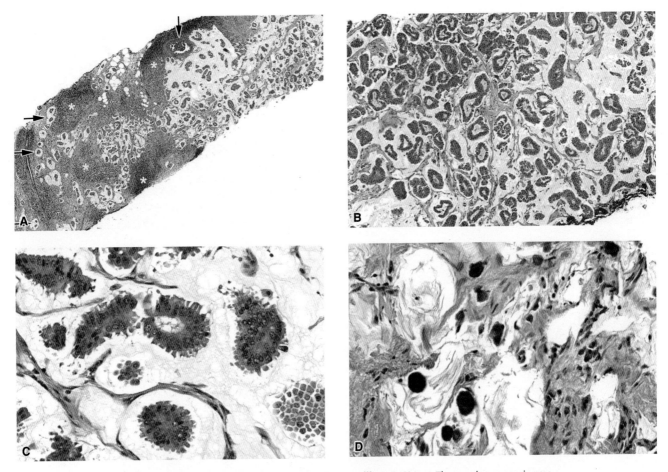

FIGURE 14.7 Mucinous Carcinoma with Micropapillary Pattern. The mucinous carcinoma in this needle core biopsy sample has micropapillary features, best appreciated at high magnification. **A:** Focal micropapillary ductal carcinoma in situ *(vertical arrow)* is associated with the invasive component. Linear arrangement of the neoplastic clusters admixed with mucin at the periphery of the tumor *(horizontal arrows)* suggests lymphovascular invasion, but definitive diagnosis requires confirmation by immunohistochemistry for endothelial antigens. Collections of small lymphocytes, an uncommon finding in this type of carcinoma, are associated with the tumor *(asterisks).* **B:** Some of the neoplastic clusters have a scalloped and irregular outline. **C:** Upon closer examination, the neoplastic clusters are composed of cells with reversed polarity, as typically seen in invasive micropapillary carcinoma. **D:** Psammomatous calcifications are often present.

reduced 10-year overall survival (OS) and relapse-free survival compared to 397 patients with pure MC with absent or less than 50% micropapillary component.

Mucinous Carcinoma with Signet Ring Cells

Carcinomas with extracellular mucin rarely have signet ring cell morphology. Signet ring cells arranged in large solid clusters or as single cells are more common in type B MC with neuroendocrine features (**Fig. 14.8**).

Mucinous Carcinoma Associated with Solid and Papillary Carcinoma

MC can also arise in association with solid–papillary carcinoma. These tumors usually are type B MCs with neuroendocrine morphology, and some may also express neuroendocrine markers.

Ductal Carcinoma In Situ

DCIS is associated with two-thirds (14,15) to 92.5% of MC (34). The nuclear grade of DCIS associated with MC was low

in 29.3% of cases, intermediate in 61%, and high in 9.8% (34). DCIS with necrosis was present in 17% (14) to 30% (34) of the cases. DCIS with high nuclear grade was more common in association with type B MC and mixed MC (14). In one study (34), 86% of DCIS near MC contained intraluminal mucin, and the latter showed neovascularizion in 70% of the cases. Neovascularization of the mucin in the lumen of ducts involved by DCIS does not constitute evidence of stromal invasion (**Fig. 14.9**).

Mucocele-like Lesions

The mucocele-like lesion (MLL), an entity first described by Rosen in 1986 (35), consists of mucin-containing cysts that tend to rupture and discharge the secretion into the adjacent stroma (**Figs. 14.10–14.14**). Some MLLs present as palpable tumors and appear as well-circumscribed and lobulated lesions on mammography. An increasing number of nonpalpable, small MLLs are detected only by mammography as clustered calcifications without a mass, or mass-lesions with associated

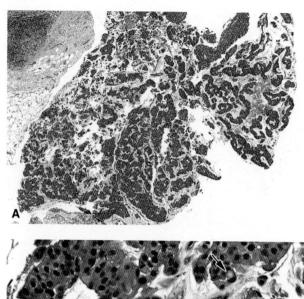

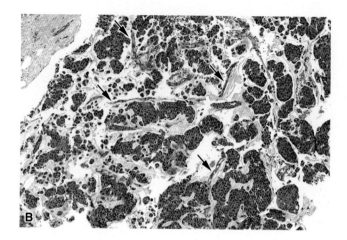

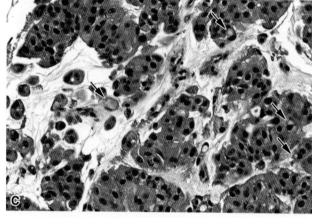

FIGURE 14.8 Mucinous Carcinoma, Type B with Few Signet Ring Cells. **A:** This needle core biopsy from a 40-year-old woman shows fragments of a cellular mucinous carcinoma. **B:** The carcinoma consists of large and somewhat dyshesive clusters admixed with mucin. A few small clusters are composed of two to three cells, and many single cells are present. Capillaries are evident in the mucin *(arrows)*. **C:** Some of the neoplastic cells have the signet ring morphology *(arrows)*.

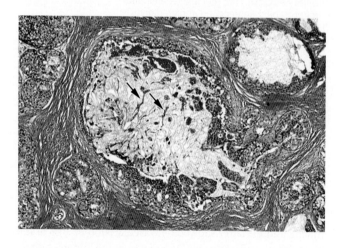

FIGURE 14.9 Ductal Carcinoma In Situ (DCIS) with Mucin Neovascularization. The mucin present within the lumen of a duct involved by DCIS has numerous capillaries *(arrows)*. This finding was present near a focus of mucinous carcinoma (not shown). Neovascularization of the mucin in DCIS does not constitute evidence of invasion.

calcifications (48–54). Ultrasonography shows a hypoechoic, round or lobulated, solid or cystic tumor, sometimes with an ill-defined margin (55–57). In one series (53), the calcifications in eight MLLs with DCIS were all clustered/grouped coarse heterogeneous, whereas those associated with MLLs with atypia were clustered/grouped fine pleomorphic in 67% of the cases, and those in MLLs without atypia were clustered/grouped coarse heterogeneous in 53% of the cases. A sonographic mass was detected in 7/17 (41%) MLLs and complex cysts in 6/17 (36%). In another series (51), calcifications constituted the dominant radiologic abnormality in 84.6%

MLLs, and ultrasound examination was negative in 8 of 13 cases. Predominantly, cystic MLLs tend to be sampled by fine needle aspiration (FNA) biopsy, whereas needle core biopsy (NCB) is often used to sample a more solid component (see also paragraph on MLL in the section dedicated to the differential diagnosis of mucinous lesions at NCB in this chapter).

The biologic behavior of an MLL is likely related to the characteristics of the epithelium composing the lesion, which can be morphologically benign, atypical, or frankly malignant. The epithelium lining the ducts in an MLL without atypia is for most part flat or cuboidal

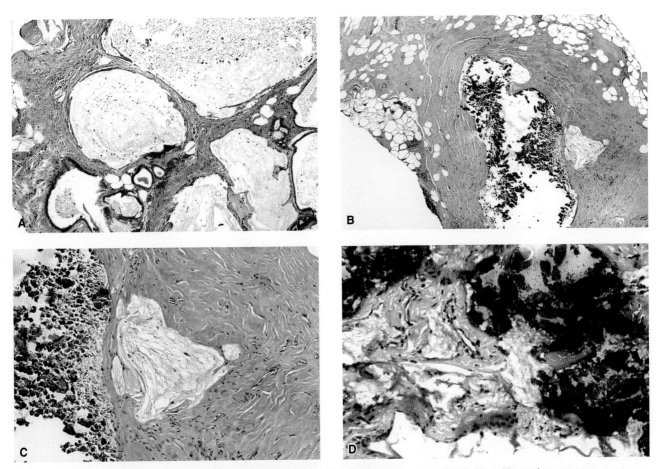

FIGURE 14.10 Mucocele-like Lesion without Atypia. A: A mucocele-like lesion with mucin-filled cysts that also contain finely granular calcifications. **B, C:** Granular calcification near stromal mucin in a needle core biopsy specimen. **D:** Another needle core biopsy sample from a benign mucocele-like lesion consisting of mucin and coarse calcifications.

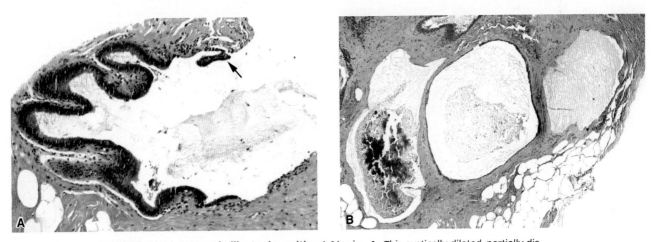

FIGURE 14.11 Mucocele-like Lesion without Atypia. A: This cystically dilated, partially disrupted duct was present in a needle core biopsy specimen taken from a nonpalpable lesion with calcifications. The duct is lined by benign, low columnar epithelium. Note the epithelium curled back toward the duct lumen near the upper border at the site of disruption *(arrow)*. This is a characteristic feature of mucocele-like lesions. **B:** Another specimen with an intact cyst flanked by extruded mucin. Coarse granular calcification is present in the mucin **(left)**. **C:** Slight epithelial hyperplasia in a cyst with calcification in extruded mucin. **D:** This mucin-filled duct in a needle core biopsy specimen from a patient with a nonatypical mucocele-like lesion has strips of detached benign epithelium in mucin. This finding should not be interpreted as mucinous carcinoma.

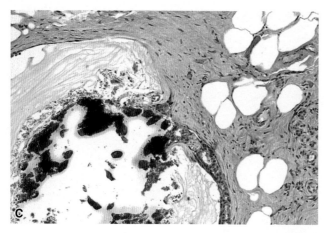

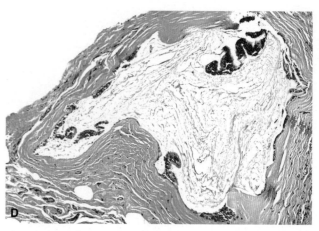

FIGURE 14.11 (*continued*)

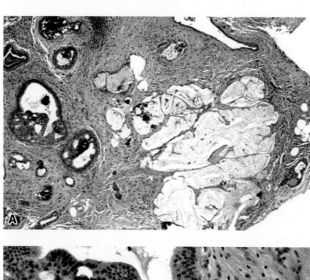

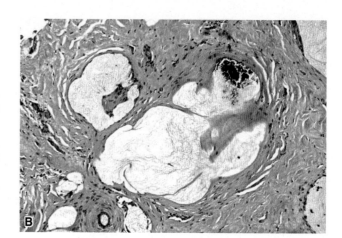

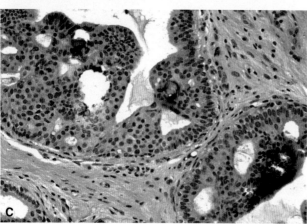

FIGURE 14.12 Mucocele-like Lesion with Atypical Duct Hyperplasia. A: Atypical ductal hyperplasia with calcifications and extruded mucin are evident at low magnification. **B:** Extruded mucin with calcification in the stroma. **C:** Atypical micropapillary and cribriform hyperplasia with calcifications. Note the regular low columnar epithelium focally present at the periphery of the duct in the lower right corner and in the adjacent larger duct.

(**Figs. 14.10 and 14.11**). Epithelial atypia in a MLL ranges from columnar cell change (CCC) with atypia/flat epithelial atypia (FEA) to atypical ductal hyperplasia (ADH) (**Figs. 14.12 and 14.13**) (35,58,59). Clear-cut DCIS can also occur near a MLL (35,58,59) (**Fig. 14.14**). (See also section on NCB of MLLs later in this chapter.)

Verschuur-Maes and Van Diest (60) found acellular stromal mucin in 19/20 (90%) NCB samples targeting mammographic calcifications associated with the mucinous variant of CCC. ADH was present in three of the cases. Abundant powdery and granular calcifications are often present in the mucin of a MLL (**Figs. 14.10–14.13**).

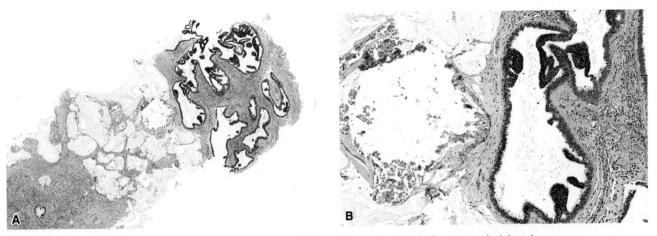

FIGURE 14.13 Mucocele-like Lesion with Atypical Duct Hyperplasia. A: Atypical ductal hyperplasia **(right)** and acellular stromal mucin with calcifications **(center)** are evident at low magnification in this needle core biopsy sample. **B:** Magnified view of **(A)**. Atypical micropapillary ductal hyperplasia partially involves the ducts **(right)**. Stromal mucin devoid of epithelium contains abundant granular calcifications **(left)**. The follow-up surgical excision specimen contained columnar cell change with atypia and pools of acellular stromal mucin (not shown).

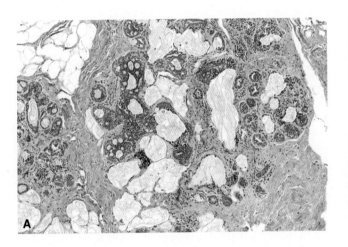

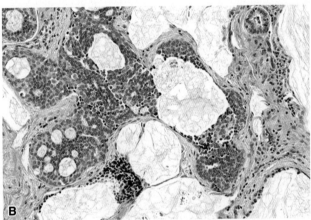

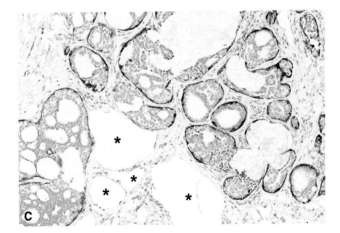

FIGURE 14.14 Mucocele-like Lesion with Intraductal Carcinoma. A, B: Mucin is present in the lumen of cribriform ductal carcinoma in situ involving a few lobules. The acellular mucin pools present in the stroma have irregular outlines. **C:** The calponin stain highlights myoepithelium around the ductal carcinoma in situ. In the immunostained sections, the stromal mucin pools appear as "empty" spaces (*asterisks*) and may be difficult to appreciate.

HISTOCHEMISTRY AND IMMUNOHISTOCHEMISTRY

Mucin

MUC2 is expressed in more than 80% of MC (61,62) but has also been identified in mucinous columnar cell lesions (60). Immunohistochemical detection of *MUC2* has no application in the diagnostic evaluation of MC. Only a small proportion of the cells of a MC contain intracellular mucin that can be demonstrated by histochemical procedures. Intracytoplasmic mucin is only rarely found in the epithelium of a benign MLL.

ER, PR, HER2, and AR

Most MCs are strongly and diffusely positive for estrogen receptor (ER) and progesterone receptor (PR) (10,12,16,63,64). In a review of 1992 to 2007 SEER data (2), 84% of MCs were ER$^+$/PR$^+$, 12.7% ER$^+$/PR$^-$, 0.5% ER$^-$/PR$^+$, and 2.8% ER$^-$/PR$^-$. One study (12) detected ER in 73.4% MCs and PR in 65.4% MCs; the rate of hormone positivity was significantly higher in MC than in control tumors ($p < 0.001$). In another study (16), 95% of MCs were ER-positive, 84% PR-positive, and 9% HER2-positive; 91% of mixed MCs were ER-positive, 87% PR-positive, and 33% HER2-positive. Although the vast majority of MCs are HER2-negative, a small proportion (<5%) overexpress HER2 (10,64). Androgen receptor (AR) was detected in 80.5% of MCs in one study (65). In another series, AR expression was significantly lower in MC than in IFDC of no special type (NST) (21.7% vs. 51.4%, respectively; $p = 0.01$) (66).

Ki67

Ki67 staining was reported as low in 77% (67) and 91.4% of the cases (64); moderate or intermediate in 5.7% (64) and 23% (67), and high (>30%) in only one case (2.9%) (64). The mean and median percentage of Ki67-positive tumor cells was 16.8 and 15, respectively (68).

WT1

Nuclear staining for WT1, an antigen expressed in leukemias and in solid tumors of the urogenital tract, has been detected in 63.7% (64) and 65% (69) of MCs in two series. Staining intensity was weak in 33% of the cases, moderate in 62% of the cases, and strong in only one (5%) case (69). WT1 staining was significantly associated with low tumor grade ($p = 0.01$) and low cellularity ($p = 0.01$). WT1 was also detected in 11/33 (33%) mixed MCs, with similar expression in the mucinous and the nonmucinous components (69).

Neuroendocrine Differentiation

MCs, especially MC type B, often have growth patterns reminiscent of an endocrine tumor. Scopsi et al. (5) detected neuron-specific enolase (NSE), synaptophysin, and chromogranins A and B in most MCs in their series. Neuroendocrine

features and/or differentiation in MC does not appear to have prognostic significance, although a study has documented an association with favorable histologic parameters (70).

DIFFERENTIAL DIAGNOSIS OF MUCINOUS LESIONS AT NEEDLE CORE BIOPSY

Mucinous Carcinoma

A definitive diagnosis of MC requires evaluation of the entire lesion and cannot be rendered based on review of the limited sample obtained by NCB.

The large solid nests of type B MC can sometimes raise the differential diagnosis of DCIS. The finding of mucin-filled clefts around the nests constitutes evidence in favor of stromal invasion (14). In this setting, the use of myoepithelial stains is not always contributory (14).

Ductal Carcinoma In Situ with Mucin

A diagnostic problem can arise when DCIS with intraluminal mucin coexists with stromal mucin devoid of carcinoma. The presence of malignant epithelium within the stromal mucin is required for the diagnosis of MC. Stromal mucin without neoplastic epithelium could represent a focus of hypocellular MC or mucin extruded into the stroma following tissue trauma. In similar cases, additional evaluation is necessary (see the following section on the diagnostic workup of a MLL).

Mucocele-like Lesion

The epithelium associated with an MLL can be benign (**Figs. 14.10 and 14.11**), atypical (**Figs. 14.12 and 14.13**), or frankly malignant (**Fig. 14.14**). If a MLL is associated with ADH or DCIS in an NCB sample, surgical excision is always recommended. NCB sampling of a nonatypical MLL usually yields variable amounts of clean mucin and a few benign cysts lined by inconspicuous flat epithelium (**Figs. 14.10 and 14.11**). Large, granular, and powdery calcifications are usually present in the mucin of a MLL (**Figs. 14.10–14.13**). Histiocytes and inflammatory cells may be present in the extruded mucin, but usually no epithelial elements are identified. Stromal mucin devoid of epithelium is an exceedingly rare finding in a NCB. If this scenario is encountered, it is recommended to evaluate deeper tissue sections to exclude the presence of carcinoma in the mucin pools.

Rarely, sparse, histologically benign epithelial strips displaced by the procedure may be admixed with the mucin (**Fig. 14.11**). Lack of cytologic atypia, epithelium arranged in ribbons and strips of cells with columnar morphology, and no evidence of papillary architecture favor artifactual detachment. The immunohistochemical identification of myoepithelial cells within the benign epithelial ribbons and clusters, and/or along the denuded wall of ducts and acini, also favors artifactual detachment. In this setting, lack of myoepithelium, however, does not constitute evidence of stromal invasion. If malignant cells are identified in the mucin, additional evidence of invasion is usually present, including a smooth, bulbous outline of the stromal mucin pools, papillary arrangement of the epithelial clusters (14), presence of few myofibroblasts and/or capillaries in the mucin pools, and focal inflammatory infiltrate (71,72). These morphologic features support a diagnosis of invasive carcinoma with mucinous features, unless the target lesion was recently sampled by a FNA or a prior NCB. In some instances, it may not be possible to distinguish definitively between artifactual detachment and (micro)invasive MC, particularly if the epithelium shows some atypical features. A pancytokeratin (AE1:AE3) immunostain can be useful to identify epithelial cells in stromal mucin pools apparently devoid of epithelium, as the cells of a MC may have abundant pale cytoplasm and can closely mimic histiocytes. The distinction between MC and MLL can be a challenging clinical, radiologic, and pathologic problem.

Upgrade Rate of Benign MLL at Needle Core Biopsy

NCBs yielding a benign MLL are rare, with only 35 cases (0.38%) identified among 9,286 image-guided NCB specimens obtained between 2006 and 2013 at one institution (54). Few studies evaluated the upgrade rate to carcinoma (invasive carcinoma and/or DCIS) following excision of benign MLLs diagnosed at NCB. Some studies did not report separately the upgrade rate of NCB with or without atypia and/or did not comment on the radiologic–pathologic concordance between the histologic findings in the NCB specimen and the radiologic characteristics of the target lesion. Details of the studies with radiologic–pathologic correlations (48,53,54,73–77) are summarized in **Table 14.1**. It appears that for NCBs with established radiologic–pathologic concordance, surgical excision of a benign MLL yields carcinoma (usually DCIS, rarely invasive carcinoma) in approximately one-third of the cases. The risk of upgrade to carcinoma is approximately 20% following NCB diagnosis of MLL with atypia. Surgical excision following an NCB diagnosis of nonatypical MLL with radiologic–pathologic concordant findings has an upgrade rate to carcinoma ranging from 0% to 1.2%. Surgical excision following an NCB diagnosis of MLL without atypia with radiologic–pathologic concordant findings yields an atypical lesion (ADH, atypical CCC/FEA or atypical lobular hyperplasia) in about 21% of the cases, but no upgrade to carcinoma.

Based on these data, excisional biopsy is recommended following NCB diagnosis of MLL with atypia (ADH or CCC with atypia/FEA) and/or if the radiologic and pathologic findings of the NCB are discordant. Surgical excision of a nonatypical MLL in an NCB can be safely omitted provided that the radiologic and pathologic findings are concordant. Ha et al. (54) suggested that surgical excision following NCB diagnosis

---

TABLE 14.1

Findings at Surgical Excision of MLL with or without Epithelial Atypia at Core Needle Biopsy

Study	Total NCB with EXC	NCB without Atypia[a]			NCB with Atypia		Carcinoma at EXC/ Total NCB	Total Patients with Carcinoma or ADH
		Cases	Atypia at EXC/ cases (%)	Carcinoma at EXC/cases (%)	Cases	Carcinoma at EXC/Cases (%)		
Renshaw 2002 (73)	8	3	1/3 (33%)	0/3	5	0/5	0/8	6/8 (75%)
Carder et al. 2004 (48)	10	6	2/6 (33%)	0/6	4	3/4 (75%)	3/10 (30%)	6/10 (60%)
Wang et al. 2007 (74)	11	7	0/7	0/7	4	0/4	0/11	4/11 (36%)
Begum et al. 2009 (75)	23	10	0/10	1[b]/10 (10%)	13	1/13 (7.6%)	2/23 (8.6%)	2[a]/23 (8.6%)
Carkaci et al. 2011 (53)	12	9	Not specified	0/9	3	1/3 (33%)	1/12 (8.3%)	3/12 (25%)
Sutton et al. 2012 (76)	38	22	Not specified	0/22	16	5/16 (31%)	5/38 (13%)	5/38 (13%)
Edelweiss et al. 2013 (77)	28	10	4/10 (40%)	0/10	18	4/18 (22%)	4/28 (14%)	8/28 (28%)
Ha et al. 2015 (54)	24	12	4/12 (33%) 3 ADH, 1 ALH	0/12	12	1/12 (8.3%)	1/24 (4.1%)	16/24 (66.6%)
TOTAL	**154**	**79**	**11/48 (20.8%)**	**1[a]/79 (1.2%)**	**75**	**15/75 (20%)**	**16/154 (10.3%)**	**50/154 (32.4%)**

ADH, atypical ductal hyperplasia; ALH, atypical lobular hyperplasia; NCB, needle core biopsy; EXC, surgical excision; MLL, mucocele-like lesion.
[a]The radiologic and pathologic findings were concordant in all but one case.
[b]One case with discordant radiologic–pathologic findings

of nonatypical MLL should be considered only if the finding of epithelial atypia in the surgical excision specimen would result in a change in the patient's management; patients with nonatypical MLL at NCB who already carry a diagnosis of atypia and/or carcinoma for another breast lesion could be followed by mammography every 6 months for 2 to 3 years.

Nodular Mucinosis

Rarely, the mammary stroma acquires a myxoid–mucoid quality, referred to as mucinosis. Nodular mucinosis of the breast is an extremely rare entity, usually presenting in young women in the subareolar region. Pathologically, it consists of a myxoid mass of loosely placed benign spindle cells (78).

Nonmucinous Lesions

Cystic Hypersecretory Lesions

Cystic hypersecretory lesions of the breast (see Chapter 17) may bear superficial similarity to MLLs because of the presence of cystically dilated lumina filled with secretion. The latter consists of homogeneous eosinophilic material that resembles thyroid colloid. The dense hypersecretory material tends to fracture along parallel lines, resulting in the characteristic shattering pattern reminiscent of "Venetian blinds." In contrast, mucin has pale, gray to blue color, and is translucent. The cells of a hypersecretory lesion show no reactivity in a mucicarmine stain.

Secretory Carcinoma

Secretory carcinoma (see also Chapter 17) is a rare variant of breast carcinoma and harbors a characteristic chromosomal fusion gene (ETV6-NTRK3). It has amphophilic or pale eosinophilic intraluminal secretion, which is often bubbly in appearance. Intracellular secretion can also occur, but no secretion is present in the stroma. Secretory carcinoma is S-100-positive, and negative for ER and PR. No intracytoplasmic or luminal mucin is detected with a mucicarmine stain. In contrast, MC consists of neoplastic epithelial clusters admixed with stromal mucin. MCs are usually diffusely positive for ER and PR but negative for S-100. Some of the cells of MC are also mucicarmine-positive.

Adenoid Cystic Carcinoma

Adenoid cystic carcinoma (ACC) (see Chapter 16) with delicate myxoid matrix deposits can simulate MC with cribriform growth, but the matrix is devoid of cells and shows at least focal dense eosinophilia. ACC is a biphasic (epithelial and myoepithelial) carcinoma composed of p63-positive myoepithelial cells and CK7-positive epithelial cells (**Fig. 14.15**) and is usually negative for ER and PR.

Mucoepidermoid Carcinoma

Mucoepidermoid carcinoma primary in the breast parenchyma features both mucinous cells and extracellular mucin,

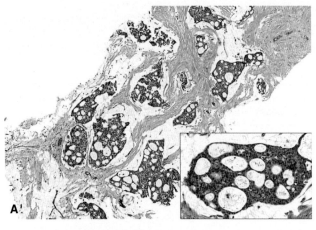

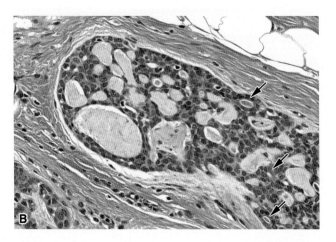

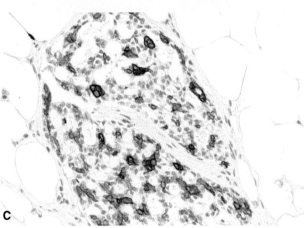

FIGURE 14.15 Mucinous Carcinoma and Adenoid Cystic Carcinoma. A: The mucinous carcinoma with a cribriform growth pattern in this needle core biopsy specimen resembles an adenoid cystic carcinoma. **B:** A cribriform adenoid cystic carcinoma is shown for comparison. A few small glands are visible *(arrows)*. The basophilic material in the duct is basement membrane matrix. **C:** Only the epithelial cells in an adenoid cystic carcinoma are positive for CK7.

resembling its commoner counterpart in the salivary glands. It is negative for ER and PR.

Pleomorphic Adenoma

Pleomorphic adenoma (see Chapter 5) is a rare benign breast tumor that most likely represents a variant of adenomyoepithelioma. It often has areas of myxoid stroma that contain spindly myoepithelial cells. The myxoid stroma is negative for mucicarmine.

Metaplastic Breast Carcinoma with Myxoid Matrix (Matrix-producing Carcinoma)

Most metaplastic carcinomas contain focal or diffuse areas of myxoid change. Although this alteration can raise the differential diagnosis of MC, the malignant cells composing a metaplastic carcinoma tend to have higher nuclear grade, are irregularly distributed, and do not form truly cohesive clusters (see Chapter 13).

Squamous Cell Carcinoma with Prominent Myxoid Stroma

Squamous cell carcinoma with prominent myxoid stroma can also mimic mucinous carcinoma (79).

Metastases from an Extramammary Neoplasm

Metastases from an extramammary neoplasm (see Chapter 22) can have mucinous elements. Metastatic mucinous carcinoma from various extramammary sites has been reported in the breast.

Benign Spindle Cell Lesions with Myxoid Stroma

The myxoid stroma in benign tumors such as myxoid fibroadenoma, myxoma, and neurofibroma with prominent myxoid change can resemble stromal mucin, especially when sampled by NCB or FNA. In all these lesions, the myxoid stroma is admixed with benign-appearing spindle cells of myofibroblastic or neural origin. If displaced epithelial clusters are present, they are also benign-appearing and usually surrounded by myoepithelium and basement membrane. The myxoid stroma is negative for mucicarmine.

Foreign Material

Foreign material can closely resemble extracellular mucin. Clues to the correct diagnosis include a slightly different tinctorial quality, and a foreign body–type giant-cell reaction (72). The latter feature tends to be more evident at the periphery of the foreign material and may be underrepresented in a NCB sample. Injection of hydrophilic polyacrylamide gel for breast augmentation has been used in some countries, especially in Eastern Europe and Asia, but over time it causes breast nodularities and deformity. Polyacrylamide hydrogel resembles mucin in tinctorial quality and translucency (80) (**Fig. 14.16**), and complete and accurate clinical history is of foremost importance in these cases. The gel used during sonographic examination

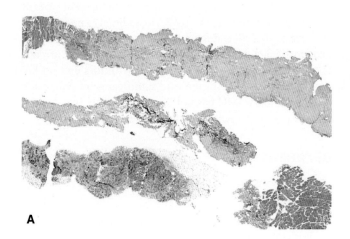

A

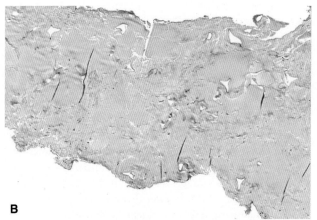

B

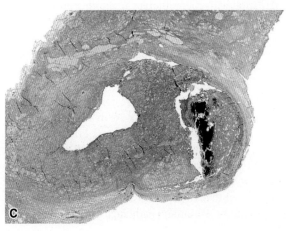

C

FIGURE 14.16 Polyacrylamide Gel Mimics Mucinous Carcinoma. **A:** Polyacrylamide gel injected years earlier for the purpose of breast augmentation is evident in this needle core biopsy specimen obtained from the breast of a 40-year-old woman who complained of breast nodularities. **B:** The polyacrylamide gel closely resembles acellular mucin. **C:** The nipple-sparing mastectomy specimen contained large deposits of polyacrylamide gel with focal coarse calcifications.

is rarely present in the NCB sample, whereas it is commonly present in FNA material. Of note, it is recommended to excise any breast lesion that yields acellular mucin in a FNA sample, even in the absence of epithelial atypia.

TREATMENT AND PROGNOSIS

The relatively favorable prognosis commonly ascribed to MC is supported by numerous studies (1,2,5,11,12,17,21,31,81,82); however, few studies have used a uniform definition for the diagnosis of MC. MC tend to be smaller than tumors with a mixed pattern, and these patients have a lower frequency of axillary lymph node (ALN) metastases (5,13,83). In one study (84), the rate of LN involvement for subcentimeter MC was 2.9%, with no LN metastases in T1a MC and only 3.5% in T1b MC. In another study (21), node-positive patients had a mean tumor size of 2.7 cm compared to 1.5 cm for node-negative patients ($p = 0.0003$), and none of the 31 patients with tumor size <1 cm had LN metastasis. Larger tumor size correlates significantly with LN involvement (11,21).

In contemporary series (12,16,17,21,31,82), patients with LN-negative MC range from 74% to 83% of the cases. Positive nodal status was the most significant predictor of worse prognosis in a large SEER data–based study of 11,422 patients with MC (11). In two studies (10,81), patients with node-positive MC were significantly more likely to develop recurrent disease. In another study (8), the number of involved ALNs was the only significant predictor of patient death ($p = 0.02$). Ranade et al. (16) reported that 18.5% of MCs had sentinel lymph node (SLN) metastases versus 16% of mixed MCs. Non-SLNs were positive in 14% of MC versus 39% of mixed MCs.

In recent series, the surgical treatment of MC consisted of breast-conserving surgery in 15.4% to 81.1% of the cases (12,17,21,31,82). Most patients treated with breast-conserving surgery also received adjuvant radiation therapy (17,21,31,81,82). In a study based on SEER data (11), adjuvant radiotherapy was associated with a small survival advantage on univariate analysis but was not found to be significant on multivariate analysis.

Adjuvant hormonal therapy was administered to patients with MC in 41% to 81.6% of the cases (12,17,31,81,82). Barkly et al. (21) specified that hormonal therapy constituted the only adjuvant treatment in 54% of patients with MC and was used in combination with chemotherapy in another 30%.

Follow-up analysis of MC in one series found that systemic adjuvant chemotherapy is not necessarily indicated for node-negative MC measuring 3 cm or less in diameter (85). Adjuvant chemotherapy for treatment of MC was used in only 3% to 13% of patients in three series from Western countries (21,81,82), but seems more commonly adopted in Asia, where three series reported its use in 40.8% to 63.7% of patients (12,17,31). MCs that overexpress HER2, however, are suitable for HER-targeted treatment in the adjuvant or neoadjuvant setting. In one study (86), the clinical response of 12 MCs treated with neoadjuvant chemotherapy was significantly poorer than that for IFDC, with minimal reduction in the mean tumor size and no pathologic complete response.

When compared with patients who have IFDC or IFDC with a mucinous component, women with MC have had a better RFS 5 and 10 years after mastectomy (5,9,87). In a series of patients treated by lumpectomy (81), with radiotherapy in 90% of the cases, hormonal therapy in 41% of the cases, and chemotherapy in 13% of the cases, local recurrence and locoregional recurrence rates were both 5%, significantly lower than that for IFDC (8% and 10%, respectively). The disease-free survival (DFS) was 91.6% at 5 years and 75.3% at 10 years. The OS rate was 91.8% at 5 years and 74.5% at 10 years.

In a study based on 1973 to 2002 SEER data (11), the 10-, 15-, and 20-year survival for 11,422 patients with MC was 89%, 85%, and 81%, respectively, compared to 72% (10-year), 66% (15-year), and 62% (20 year) for 338,479 patients with IFDC. Scopsi et al. (5) reported no deaths due to disease among 25 patients with node-negative MC. In a series of patients treated between 1997 and 2005 (82), 143 patients with MC had 93% 5-year DFS and 96.3% OS. The DFS of MC and IFDC of similar ER, PR, and HER2 status were not significantly different, but in this study MC had a worse OS when compared to ER$^+$/PR$^+$ and HER2-negative IFDC (hazard ratio = 2.96, 95% confidence interval 1.26–6.95, $p = 0.01$).

MC can develop late metastases (9,85,88,89), even 25 (90) and 30 years (91) after diagnosis. In a series with a mean follow-up of 16 years (9), 42% of the deaths due to disease in patients with MC occurred 12 years or more after diagnosis. Small MCs, however, do not show propensity for late recurrence (92,93) or to cause patient death (6).

Major prognostic factors that are relevant for most types of breast carcinoma also apply to MC. In addition to nodal status, age, tumor size, PR status, and nuclear grade were significant prognostic factors on multivariate analysis (11). Recurrence is least likely for patients with smaller tumors and no LN metastases (21). The prognostic significance of endocrine differentiation in MC has not been sufficiently investigated to be considered a reliable prognostic feature.

REFERENCES

1. Louwman MW, Vriezen M, van Beek MW, et al. Uncommon breast tumors in perspective: incidence, treatment and survival in the Netherlands. *Int J Cancer.* 2007;121:127–135.
2. Li CI. Risk of mortality by histologic type of breast cancer in the United States. *Horm Cancer.* 2010;1:156–165.
3. Albrektsen G, Heuch I, Thoresen SO. Histological type and grade of breast cancer tumors by parity, age at birth, and time since birth: a register-based study in Norway. *BMC Cancer.* 2010;10:226.
4. Rasmussen BB, Rose C, Christensen IB. Prognostic factors in primary mucinous breast carcinoma. *Am J Clin Pathol.* 1987;87:155–160.
5. Scopsi L, Andreola S, Pilotti S, et al. Mucinous carcinoma of the breast: a clinicopathologic, histochemical, and immunocytochemical study with special reference to neuroendocrine differentiation. *Am J Surg Pathol.* 1994;18:702–711.
6. Toikkanen S, Kujari H. Pure and mixed mucinous carcinomas of the breast: a clinicopathologic analysis of 61 cases with long-term follow-up. *Hum Pathol.* 1989;20:758–764.
7. Avisar E, Khan MA, Axelrod D, et al. Pure mucinous carcinoma of the breast: a clinicopathologic correlation study. *Ann Surg Oncol.* 1998;5:447–451.
8. Komenaka IK, El-Tamer MB, Troxel A, et al. Pure mucinous carcinoma of the breast. *Am J Surg.* 2004;187:528–532.

9. Rosen PP, Wang T-Y. Colloid carcinoma of the breast: analysis of 64 patients with long-term follow-up. *Am J Clin Pathol.* 1980;73:30.

10. Diab SG, Clark GM, Osborne CK, et al. Tumor characteristics and clinical outcome of tubular and mucinous breast carcinomas. *J Clin Oncol.* 1999;17:1442–1448.

11. Di Saverio S, Gutierrez J, Avisar E. A retrospective review with long term follow up of 11,400 cases of pure mucinous breast carcinoma. *Breast Cancer Res Treat.* 2008;111:541–547.

12. Cao AY, He M, Liu ZB, et al. Outcome of pure mucinous breast carcinoma compared to infiltrating ductal carcinoma: a population-based study from China. *Ann Surg Oncol.* 2012;19:3019–3027.

13. Paramo JC, Wilson C, Velarde D, et al. Pure mucinous carcinoma of the breast: is axillary staging necessary? *Ann Surg Oncol.* 2002;9:161–164.

14. Kryvenko ON, Chitale DA, Yoon J, et al. Precursor lesions of mucinous carcinoma of the breast: analysis of 130 cases. *Am J Surg Pathol.* 2013;37:1076–1084.

15. Fentiman IS, Millis RR, Smith P, et al. Mucoid breast carcinomas: histology and prognosis. *Br J Cancer.* 1997;75:1061–1065.

16. Ranade A, Batra R, Sandhu G, et al. Clinicopathological evaluation of 100 cases of mucinous carcinoma of breast with emphasis on axillary staging and special reference to a micropapillary pattern. *J Clin Pathol.* 2010;63:1043–1047.

17. Bae SY, Choi MY, Cho DH, et al. Mucinous carcinoma of the breast in comparison with invasive ductal carcinoma: clinicopathologic characteristics and prognosis. *J Breast Cancer.* 2011;14:308–313.

18. Li CI, Daling JR, Malone KE, et al. Relationship between established breast cancer risk factors and risk of seven different histologic types of invasive breast cancer. *Cancer Epidemiol Biomarkers Prev.* 2006;15:946–954.

19. Work ME, Andrulis IL, John EM, et al. Risk factors for uncommon histologic subtypes of breast cancer using centralized pathology review in the Breast Cancer Family Registry. *Breast Cancer Res Treat.* 2012;134:1209–1220.

20. Lacroix-Triki M, Lambros MB, Geyer FC, et al. Absence of microsatellite instability in mucinous carcinomas of the breast. *Int J Clin Exp Pathol.* 2010;4:22–31.

21. Barkley CR, Ligibel JA, Wong JS, et al. Mucinous breast carcinoma: a large contemporary series. *Am J Surg.* 2008;196:549–551.

22. Hodgson NC, Button JH, Franceschi D, et al. Male breast cancer: is the incidence increasing? *Ann Surg Oncol.* 2004;11:751–755.

23. Burga AM, Fadare O, Lininger RA, et al. Invasive carcinomas of the male breast: a morphologic study of the distribution of histologic subtypes and metastatic patterns in 778 cases. *Virchows Arch.* 2006;449:507–512.

24. Cardenosa G, Doudna C, Eklund GW. Mucinous (colloid) breast cancer: clinical and mammographic findings in 10 patients. *AJR Am J Roentgenol.* 1994;162:1077–1079.

25. Lam WW, Chu WC, Tse GM, et al. Sonographic appearance of mucinous carcinoma of the breast. *AJR Am J Roentgenol.* 2004;182:1069–1074.

26. Newcomer LM, Newcomb PA, Trentham-Dietz A, et al. Detection method and breast carcinoma histology. *Cancer.* 2002;95:470–477.

27. Liu H, Tan H, Cheng Y, et al. Imaging findings in mucinous breast carcinoma and correlating factors. *Eur J Radiol.* 2011;80:706–712.

28. Conant EF, Dillon RL, Palazzo J, et al. Imaging findings in mucin-containing carcinomas of the breast: correlation with pathologic features. *AJR Am J Roentgenol.* 1994;163:821–824.

29. Goodman DN, Boutross-Tadross O, Jong RA. Mammographic features of pure mucinous carcinoma of the breast with pathological correlation. *Can Assoc Radiol J.* 1995;46:296–301.

30. Dhillon R, Depree P, Metcalf C, et al. Screen-detected mucinous breast carcinoma: potential for delayed diagnosis. *Clin Radiol.* 2006;61:423–430.

31. Park S, Koo J, Kim JH, et al. Clinicopathological characteristics of mucinous carcinoma of the breast in Korea: comparison with invasive ductal carcinoma-not otherwise specified. *J Korean Med Sci.* 2010;25:361–368.

32. Wilson TE, Helvie MA, Oberman HA, et al. Pure and mixed mucinous carcinoma of the breast: pathologic basis for differences in mammographic appearance. *AJR Am J Roentgenol.* 1995;165:285–289.

33. Ruggieri A, Scola F, Schepps B. Mucinous carcinoma of the breast: mammographic findings. *Breast Dis.* 1995;8:353–361.

34. Gadre SA, Perkins GH, Sahin AA, et al. Neovascularization in mucinous ductal carcinoma in situ suggests an alternative pathway for invasion. *Histopathology.* 2008;53:545–553.

35. Rosen PP. Mucocele-like tumors of the breast. *Am J Surg Pathol.* 1986;10:464–469.

36. Memis A, Ozdemir N, Parildar M, et al. Mucinous (colloid) breast cancer: mammographic and US features with histologic correlation. *Eur J Radiol.* 2000;35:39–43.

37. Yamaguchi R, Tanaka M, Mizushima Y, et al. "High-grade" central acellular carcinoma and matrix-producing carcinoma of the breast: correlation between ultrasonographic findings and pathological features. *Med Mol Morphol.* 2011;44:151–157.

38. Kawashima M, Tamaki Y, Nonaka T, et al. MR imaging of mucinous carcinoma of the breast. *AJR Am J Roentgenol.* 2002;179:179–183.

39. Okafuji T, Yabuuchi H, Sakai S, et al. MR imaging features of pure mucinous carcinoma of the breast. *Eur J Radiol.* 2006;60:405–413.

40. Miller RW, Harms S, Alvarez A. Mucinous carcinoma of the breast: potential false-negative MR imaging interpretation. *AJR Am J Roentgenol.* 1996;167:539–540.

41. Orel SG, Schnall MD, LiVolsi VA, et al. Suspicious breast lesions: MR imaging with radiologic-pathologic correlation. *Radiology.* 1994;190:485–493.

42. Capella C, Eusebi V, Mann B, et al. Endocrine differentiation in mucoid carcinoma of the breast. *Histopathology.* 1980;4:613–630.

43. Ng WK. Fine-needle aspiration cytology findings of an uncommon micropapillary variant of pure mucinous carcinoma of the breast: review of patients over an 8-year period. *Cancer.* 2002;96:280–288.

44. Bal A, Joshi K, Sharma SC, et al. Prognostic significance of micropapillary pattern in pure mucinous carcinoma of the breast. *Int J Surg Pathol.* 2008;16:251–256.

45. Shet T, Chinoy R. Presence of a micropapillary pattern in mucinous carcinomas of the breast and its impact on the clinical behavior. *Breast J.* 2008;14:412–420.

46. Barbashina V, Corben AD, Akram M, et al. Mucinous micropapillary carcinoma of the breast: an aggressive counterpart to conventional pure mucinous tumors. *Hum Pathol.* 2013;44(8):1577–1585.

47. Liu F, Yang M, Li Z, et al. Invasive micropapillary mucinous carcinoma of the breast is associated with poor prognosis. *Breast Cancer Res Treat.* 2015;151:443–451.

48. Carder PJ, Murphy CE, Liston JC. Surgical excision is warranted following a core biopsy diagnosis of mucocoele-like lesion of the breast. *Histopathology.* 2004;45:148–154.

49. Ramsaroop R, Greenberg D, Tracey N, et al. Mucocele-like lesions of the breast: an audit of 2 years at BreastScreen Auckland (New Zealand). *Breast J.* 2005;11:321–325.

50. Kim JY, Han BK, Choe YH, et al. Benign and malignant mucocele-like tumors of the breast: mammographic and sonographic appearances. *AJR Am J Roentgenol.* 2005;185:1310–1316.

51. Farshid G, Pieterse S, King JM, et al. Mucocele-like lesions of the breast: a benign cause for indeterminate or suspicious mammographic microcalcifications. *Breast J.* 2005;11:15–22.

52. Leibman AJ, Staeger CN, Charney DA. Mucocelelike lesions of the breast: mammographic findings with pathologic correlation. *AJR Am J Roentgenol.* 2006;186:1356–1360.

53. Carkaci S, Lane DL, Gilcrease MZ, et al. Do all mucocele-like lesions of the breast require surgery? *Clin Imaging.* 2011;35:94–101.

54. Ha D, Dialani V, Mehta TS, et al. Mucocele-like lesions in the breast diagnosed with percutaneous biopsy: is surgical excision necessary? *AJR Am J Roentgenol.* 2015;204:204–210.

55. Kim Y, Takatsuka Y, Morino H. Mucocele-like tumor of the breast: a case report and assessment of aspirated cytological specimens. *Breast Cancer.* 1998;5:317–320.

56. Yeoh GP, Cheung PS, Chan KW. Fine-needle aspiration cytology of mucocelelike tumors of the breast. *Am J Surg Pathol.* 1999;23:552–559.

57. Park YJ, Kim EK. A pure mucocele-like lesion of the breast diagnosed on ultrasonography-guided core-needle biopsy: is imaging follow-up sufficient? *Ultrasonography.* 2015;34:133–138.

58. Ro JY, Sneige N, Sahin AA, et al. Mucocelelike tumor of the breast associated with atypical ductal hyperplasia or mucinous carcinoma: a clinicopathologic study of seven cases. *Arch Pathol Lab Med.* 1991;115:137–140.

59. Hamele-Bena D, Cranor ML, Rosen PP. Mammary mucocele-like lesions: benign and malignant. *Am J Surg Pathol.* 1996;20:1081–1085.

60. Verschuur-Maes AH, Van Diest PJ. The mucinous variant of columnar cell lesions. *Histopathology*. 2011;58:847–853.

61. Rakha EA, Boyce RW, Abd El-Rehim D, et al. Expression of mucins (MUC1, MUC2, MUC3, MUC4, MUC5AC and MUC6) and their prognostic significance in human breast cancer. *Mod Pathol*. 2005;18:1295–1304.

62. O'Connell JT, Shao ZM, Drori E, et al. Altered mucin expression is a field change that accompanies mucinous (colloid) breast carcinoma histogenesis. *Hum Pathol*. 1998;29:1517–1523.

63. Shousha S, Coady AT, Stamp T, et al. Oestrogen receptors in mucinous carcinoma of the breast: an immunohistological study using paraffin wax sections. *J Clin Pathol*. 1989;42:902–905.

64. Lacroix-Triki M, Suarez PH, MacKay A, et al. Mucinous carcinoma of the breast is genomically distinct from invasive ductal carcinomas of no special type. *J Pathol*. 2010;222:282–298.

65. Collins LC, Cole KS, Marotti JD, et al. Androgen receptor expression in breast cancer in relation to molecular phenotype: results from the Nurses' Health Study. *Mod Pathol*. 2011;24:924–931.

66. Cho LC, Hsu YH. Expression of androgen, estrogen and progesterone receptors in mucinous carcinoma of the breast. *Kaohsiung J Med Sci*. 2008;24:227–232.

67. Kato N, Endo Y, Tamura G, et al. Mucinous carcinoma of the breast: a multifaceted study with special reference to histogenesis and neuroendocrine differentiation. *Pathol Int*. 1999;49:947–955.

68. Alvarenga CA, Paravidino PI, Alvarenga M, et al. Reappraisal of immunohistochemical profiling of special histological types of breast carcinomas: a study of 121 cases of eight different subtypes. *J Clin Pathol*. 2012;65:1066–1071.

69. Domfeh AB, Carley AL, Striebel JM, et al. WT1 immunoreactivity in breast carcinoma: selective expression in pure and mixed mucinous subtypes. *Mod Pathol*. 2008;21:1217–1223.

70. Tse GM, Ma TK, Chu WC, et al. Neuroendocrine differentiation in pure type mammary mucinous carcinoma is associated with favorable histologic and immunohistochemical parameters. *Mod Pathol*. 2004;17:568–572.

71. Molavi D, Argani P. Distinguishing benign dissecting mucin (stromal mucin pools) from invasive mucinous carcinoma. *Adv Anat Pathol*. 2008;15:1–17.

72. Tan PH, Tse GM, Bay BH. Mucinous breast lesions: diagnostic challenges. *J Clin Pathol*. 2008;61:11–19.

73. Renshaw AA. Can mucinous lesions of the breast be reliably diagnosed by core needle biopsy? *Am J Clin Pathol*. 2002;118:82–84.

74. Wang J, Simsir A, Mercado C, et al. Can core biopsy reliably diagnose mucinous lesions of the breast? *Am J Clin Pathol*. 2007;127:124–127.

75. Begum SM, Jara-Lazaro AR, Thike AA, et al. Mucin extravasation in breast core biopsies—clinical significance and outcome correlation. *Histopathology*. 2009;55:609–617.

76. Sutton B, Davion S, Feldman M, et al. Mucocele-like lesions diagnosed on breast core biopsy: assessment of upgrade rate and need for surgical excision. *Am J Clin Pathol*. 2012;138:783–788.

77. Edelweiss M, Corben AD, Liberman L, et al. Focal extravasated mucin in breast core needle biopsies: is surgical excision always necessary? *Breast J*. 2013;19:302–309.

78. Sanati S, Leonard M, Khamapirad T, et al. Nodular mucinosis of the breast: a case report with pathologic, ultrasonographic, and clinical findings and review of the literature. *Arch Pathol Lab Med*. 2005;129:e58–e61.

79. Foschini MP, Fulcheri E, Baracchini P, et al. Squamous cell carcinoma with prominent myxoid stroma. *Hum Pathol*. 1990;21:859–865.

80. Lau PP, Chan AC, Tsui MH. Diagnostic cytological features of polyacrylamide gel injection augmentation mammoplasty. *Pathology*. 2009;41:443–447.

81. Vo T, Xing Y, Meric-Bernstam F, et al. Long-term outcomes in patients with mucinous, medullary, tubular, and invasive ductal carcinomas after lumpectomy. *Am J Surg*. 2007;194:527–531.

82. Colleoni M, Rotmensz N, Maisonneuve P, et al. Outcome of special types of luminal breast cancer. *Ann Oncol*. 2012;23:1428–1436.

83. Komaki K, Sakamoto G, Sugano H, et al. The morphologic feature of mucus leakage appearing in low papillary carcinoma of the breast. *Hum Pathol*. 1991;22:231–236.

84. Maibenco DC, Weiss LK, Pawlish KS, et al. Axillary lymph node metastases associated with small invasive breast carcinomas. *Cancer*. 1999;85:1530–1536.

85. Rosen PP, Groshen S, Kinne DW. Survival and prognostic factors in node-negative breast cancer: results of long-term follow-up studies. *J Natl Cancer Inst Monogr*. 1992;(11):159–162.

86. Nagao T, Kinoshita T, Hojo T, et al. The differences in the histological types of breast cancer and the response to neoadjuvant chemotherapy: the relationship between the outcome and the clinicopathological characteristics. *Breast*. 2012;21:289–295.

87. Andre S, Cunha F, Bernardo M, et al. Mucinous carcinoma of the breast: a pathologic study of 82 cases. *J Surg Oncol*. 1995;58:162–167.

88. Wulsin JH, Schreiber JT. Improved prognosis in certain patterns of carcinoma of the breast: colloid, medullary with lymphoid stroma, and intraductal. *Arch Surg*. 1962;85:791–800.

89. Clayton F. Pure mucinous carcinomas of breast: morphologic features and prognostic correlates. *Hum Pathol*. 1986;17:34–38.

90. Lee YT, Terry R. Surgical treatment of carcinoma of the breast: I: pathological finding and pattern of relapse. *J Surg Oncol*. 1983;23:11–15.

91. Scharnhorst D, Huntrakoon M. Mucinous carcinoma of the breast: recurrence 30 years after mastectomy. *South Med J*. 1988;81:656–657.

92. Komaki K, Sakamoto G, Sugano H, et al. Mucinous carcinoma of the breast in Japan: a prognostic analysis based on morphologic features. *Cancer*. 1988;61:989–996.

93. Rosen PR, Groshen S, Saigo PE, et al. A long-term follow-up study of survival in stage I ($T_1N_0M_0$) and stage II ($T_1N_1M_0$) breast carcinoma. *J Clin Oncol*. 1989;7:355–366.

Apocrine Carcinoma

EDI BROGI

Apocrine cells have abundant, densely eosinophilic cytoplasm and large round nuclei with prominent nucleoli. Apocrine lesions of the breast include apocrine metaplasia, an alteration that is part of FCCs, and atypical and frankly neoplastic apocrine epithelial proliferations. The relationship between the aforementioned lesions remains unclear. Except for apocrine metaplasia, the identification of "apocrine" lesions has somewhat limited reproducibility, and some authors regard "apocrine" morphology as a nonspecific alteration. In this chapter, the designation of "apocrine carcinoma" is used for carcinomas with predominantly apocrine morphology, as well as for carcinomas showing only apocrine features. Cells with apocrine morphology can also be found in some special subtypes of carcinomas.

CLINICAL PRESENTATION

Incidence

The incidence of carcinomas having apocrine cytomorphology in at least 90% of the tumor is unknown. Carcinomas with apocrine features represent 1% (1) to 3% (2) of all breast carcinomas.

Age and Gender

Apocrine carcinomas can occur at any age, but most arise in postmenopausal women (1–6). The mean age of patients with invasive apocrine carcinoma in one series (2) was 58.5 years, significantly higher than the mean age of 54.4 years for women with invasive nonapocrine ductal carcinoma. Apocrine carcinomas are rare in men.

Genetic Predisposition

Breast lesions in patients with Cowden syndrome (germline *PTEN* mutation) often have apocrine morphology (7–9) but not exclusively. Apocrine carcinoma is not specifically linked to Cowden syndrome.

Presenting Symptoms and Imaging Studies

The findings are similar to those in patients with nonapocrine carcinomas. Bilateral apocrine carcinomas are uncommon (10). Apocrine ductal carcinoma in situ (DCIS) can be mass-forming. Apocrine DCIS often involves sclerosing lesions such as radial sclerosing lesion (RSL) and sclerosing adenosis (SA) (11), and can mimic invasive carcinoma clinically, radiologically, and microscopically. Calcifications are common in invasive apocrine carcinomas, in apocrine DCIS, and in atypical apocrine adenosis.

MICROSCOPIC PATHOLOGY

Apocrine Metaplasia

Apocrine metaplasia is a benign epithelial alteration that is part of fibrocystic changes (FCCs). It often involves benign cysts and has a papillary or micropapillary configuration (**Fig. 15.1**). In the absence of a true papilloma/papillary lesion, the qualification of "papillary" should not be used for apocrine metaplasia in the report of a needle core biopsy (NCB) specimen, as it might trigger an unnecessary excision. Calcium oxalate crystals with characteristic "broken glass" appearance are common in apocrine cysts (**Fig. 15.1**). Mammographically, they are detected as "milk of calcium," and might be the target of NCB. Calcium oxalate crystals are almost invariably associated with benign apocrine metaplasia. Rarely, psammomatous calcifications can also occur in apocrine cysts (**Fig. 15.1**).

Atypical Apocrine Proliferations

Atypical apocrine proliferations that are not frankly neoplastic often occur in the context of sclerosing lesions, such as papilloma, RSL, and SA (**Figs. 15.2 and 15.3**), and can raise the differential diagnosis of apocrine DCIS. The atypical cells are cytologically similar to those of low-grade or even intermediate-grade apocrine DCIS, but the proliferation lacks the expansive growth, complex architecture, and/or necrosis and/or mitoses required for the diagnosis of apocrine DCIS (12). The term atypical apocrine adenosis (AAA) has been suggested for these lesions (13).

Size criteria to separate atypical apocrine proliferations from apocrine DCIS have been proposed. Some authors (14) used a 2-mm size cutoff. Another group (15) proposed a combination of cytologic and size criteria (<4 mm, 4–8 mm, and >8 mm). Severely atypical apocrine proliferations spanning at least 4 mm and less atypical lesions measuring at least 8 mm were classified as apocrine DCIS. Apocrine proliferations with modest apocrine atypia and size between 4 mm and 8 mm were referred to as "borderline." Lesions with modest apocrine atypia and size smaller than 4 mm were classified as apocrine adenosis. Given the intrinsic difficulties in the interpretation

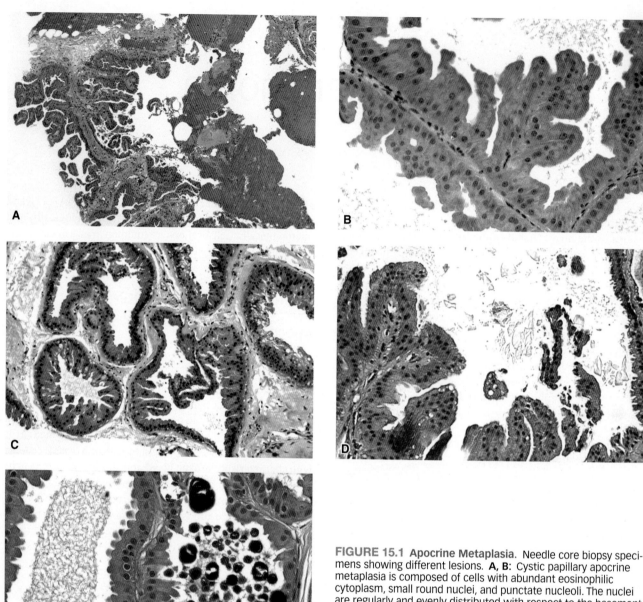

FIGURE 15.1 Apocrine Metaplasia. Needle core biopsy specimens showing different lesions. **A, B:** Cystic papillary apocrine metaplasia is composed of cells with abundant eosinophilic cytoplasm, small round nuclei, and punctate nucleoli. The nuclei are regularly and evenly distributed with respect to the basement membrane. **C:** These glands are lined by a single layer of columnar cells with evenly spaced, basally oriented nuclei. The eosinophilia seen in **A** and **B** and the basophilia in **C** reflect different staining properties in apocrine lesions. **D:** Apocrine metaplasia with oxalate calcifications showing the characteristic "broken glass" appearance. **E:** Cystic apocrine metaplasia with psammomatous calcifications.

of atypical apocrine proliferations, a cautious diagnostic approach is recommended, particularly in the evaluation of NCB material. AAA is also discussed in Chapter 6.

Apocrine DCIS

Apocrine DCIS has the same architectural patterns as nonapocrine DCIS (**Figs. 15.4–15.7**). Involvement of lobules is common. Intermediate- to high-grade neoplastic apocrine cells have enlarged, hyperchromatic, and often pleomorphic nuclei, with prominent, and sometimes multiple and irregular, nucleoli. Binucleation and intranuclear inclusions are common. The nuclear chromatin is coarse and clumped, or deeply basophilic

and smudged. Three-fold or greater variation of the nuclear diameter in adjacent neoplastic cells is common. High-grade apocrine DCIS often shows necrosis. It can have densely eosinophilic cytoplasm and resemble squamous DCIS, but it lacks keratin formation. Apocrine DCIS with intermediate nuclear grade usually shows obvious apocrine cytology. Low-grade apocrine DCIS is less frequent and more difficult to recognize. The nuclei are slightly larger than those of benign apocrine metaplastic cells, and the chromatin is denser; nucleoli are visible, but they are not conspicuous (**Fig. 15.7**). The cytoplasm of neoplastic apocrine cells is usually abundant and shows dense eosinophilia; it can also be granular. Focal cytoplasmic vacuolization or clearing may be present in atypical apocrine lesions,

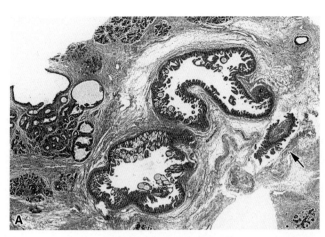 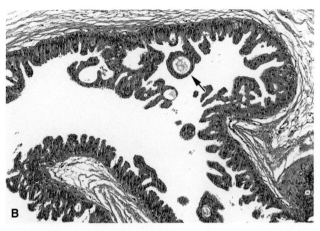

FIGURE 15.2 Apocrine Metaplasia with Atypia. A: Two ducts are involved by an atypical apocrine proliferation. A detached papillary fragment lined by micropapillary apocrine epithelium is also present *(arrow)*. **B:** The apocrine epithelium is arranged in micropapillae and focally shows incipient bridge formation. Focal "button-hole" arrangement is seen *(arrow)*.

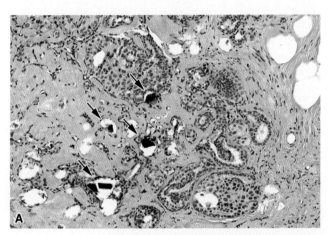 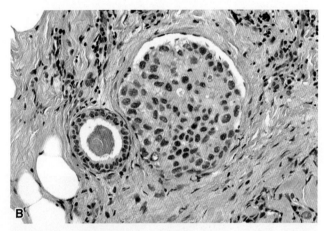

FIGURE 15.3 Apocrine Metaplasia with Atypia in a Radial Scar. A, B: A few sclerosed acini are minimally expanded by atypical apocrine cells. Calcifications are also present in **A** *(arrows)*. The apocrine cytologic atypia is evident **B**, compared to the normal epithelium in an adjacent acinus.

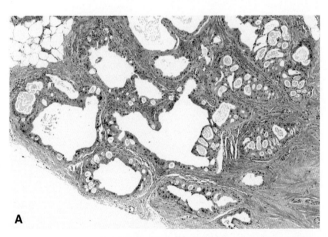 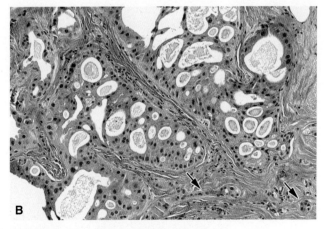

FIGURE 15.4 Apocrine Ductal Carcinoma In Situ (DCIS), Intermediate-Grade, in a Radial Scar. A: This needle core biopsy material shows the periphery of a radial scar with focal DCIS. The elastotic center of the radial scar is on the right. **B:** The glands involved by apocrine DCIS are expanded and show cribriform architecture. Few small nests of carcinoma near the elastotic center of the radial scar simulate stromal invasion *(arrows)*. **C:** The DCIS has intermediate nuclear grade. A mitotic figure is present *(arrow)*. No evidence of invasive carcinoma was present in this case.

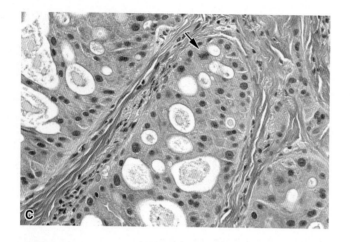

FIGURE 15.4 *(continued)*

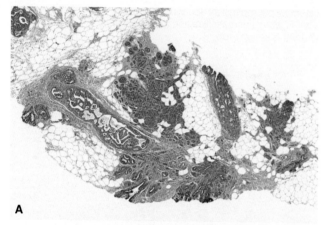

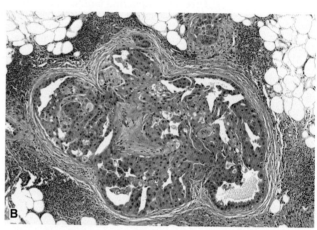

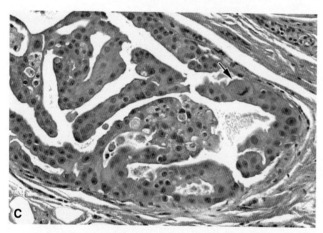

FIGURE 15.5 **Apocrine Ductal Carcinoma In Situ (DCIS), Intermediate-Grade, in a Sclerosing Lesion. A:** This needle core biopsy material shows a sclerosing lesion with apocrine DCIS. **B:** An expanded duct is involved by apocrine DCIS with intermediate nuclear grade. Periductal fibrosis and inflammation are present. **C:** Intermediate-grade apocrine DCIS. A few cells have large nuclei with prominent nucleoli. A mitotic figure is present *(arrow)*.

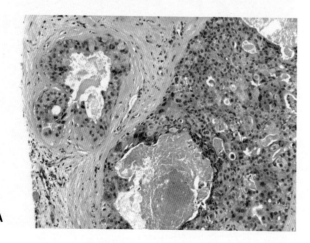

FIGURE 15.6 **Apocrine Ductal Carcinoma In Situ (DCIS), Intermediate- and High-grade. A:** Solid DCIS with necrosis. **B:** Cribriform DCIS with extension into lobular glands **(on the left)**. **C, D:** Micropapillary and papillary foci of apocrine DCIS with pleomorphic, deeply basophilic nuclei. **E:** Flat micropapillary apocrine DCIS with high nuclear grade.

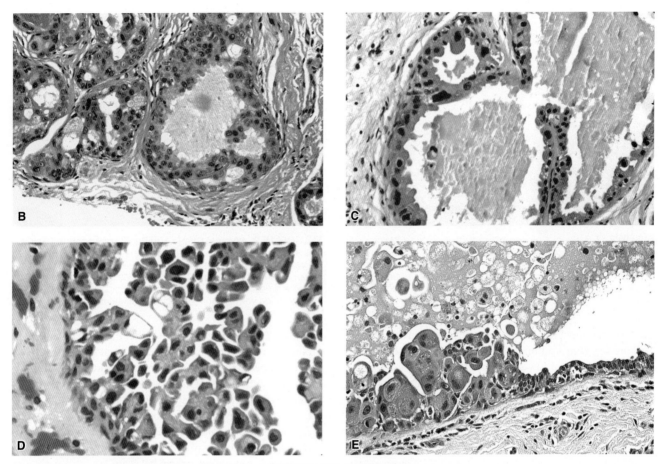

FIGURE 15.6 (*continued*)

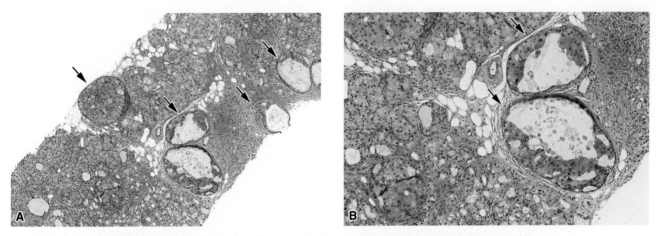

FIGURE 15.7 Invasive and In Situ Apocrine Carcinoma, Low Nuclear Grade. A, B: This needle core biopsy sample from a breast mass in an 80-year-old woman shows invasive apocrine carcinoma with low nuclear grade. Solid and cribriform apocrine ductal carcinoma in situ of low nuclear grade is present in a few scattered ducts *(arrows)*. Minimal stromal inflammation is noted.

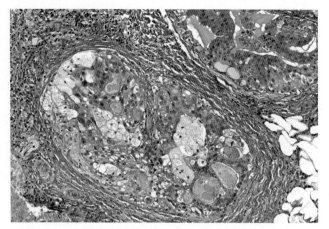

FIGURE 15.8 Foam Cells Admixed with Apocrine Carcinoma. This needle core biopsy sample from a breast mass in a 56-year-old woman shows solid and cribriform ductal carcinoma in situ (DCIS) with low nuclear grade. Stromal inflammation is also present. Foam cells are present in ducts involved by apocrine DCIS.

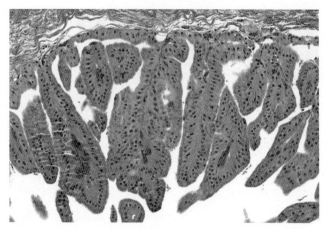

FIGURE 15.9 Atypical Cystic and Papillary Apocrine Lesion. This 3-cm cystic and papillary lesion in the breast of a 47-year-old woman consisted entirely of apocrine cells with no cytologic atypia, arranged in long and filiform papillae. No mitoses or necrosis were present. The entire lesion was devoid of myoepithelium when studied with immunohistochemical stains (not shown).

but it is prominent in high-grade apocrine carcinomas. Foam cells are sometimes admixed with apocrine DCIS (**Fig. 15.8**).

The diagnosis of low-grade apocrine DCIS rests on the identification of expansive growth and/or complex and rigid architectural patterns characteristic of DCIS. The definitive diagnosis of low-grade apocrine DCIS can be very challenging, especially based on review of NCB material. The differential diagnosis includes apocrine atypia and apocrine metaplasia.

Apocrine DCIS often harbors calcifications, which are coarse, heterogenous, and associated with necrosis in high-grade DCIS, and punctate and small in low-grade DCIS. Periductal fibrosis and inflammation are common near ducts and lobules involved by apocrine DCIS or atypical apocrine epithelium. Foamy histiocytes in the stroma adjacent to apocrine DCIS may mimic invasive carcinoma with histiocytoid cells. Foam cells can be present in ducts involved by apocrine DCIS (**Fig. 15.8**).

Apocrine DCIS and AAA often arise within or near sclerosing lesions, such as RSL and SA (11). Papillary lesions often harbor apocrine metaplasia, and apocrine DCIS can be papillary and/or arise in a papillary lesion. When evaluating a papillary apocrine lesion, it is critical to determine whether the apocrine epithelial proliferation has cytologic and architectural atypia, and these parameters need to guide the diagnostic interpretation. The finding of very scant to absent myoepithelium around cytologically benign cystic and papillary apocrine lesions has been described (16–18). In the absence of cytologic and architectural atypia, the absence of myoepithelium does not justify a diagnosis of carcinoma, particularly of invasive carcinoma (**Fig. 15.9**). On the contrary, immunohistochemical stains for cytokeratin and myoepithelial markers are usually very useful for detecting minute invasive foci near apocrine DCIS and for ruling out invasion in cases of apocrine DCIS involving a sclerosing lesion.

Invasive Apocrine Carcinoma

Most invasive apocrine carcinomas are poorly differentiated with high-grade morphology (**Fig. 15.10**) (1,4). Tumor-infiltrating lymphocytes are common (**Fig. 15.11**). Papillary (**Fig. 15.12**) or micropapillary (**Fig. 15.13**) morphology is encountered. The histiocytoid variant consists of large polygonal cells

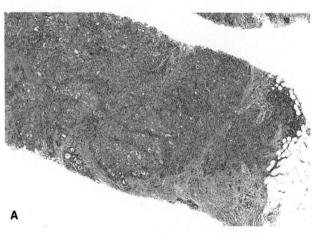

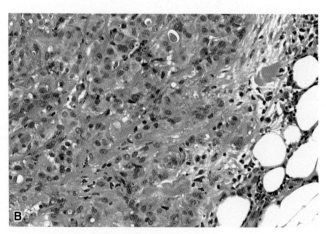

FIGURE 15.10 Invasive Apocrine Carcinoma. A: This needle core biopsy sample from a breast mass shows invasive apocrine carcinoma. **B:** The neoplastic cells infiltrate at the periphery of the tumor.

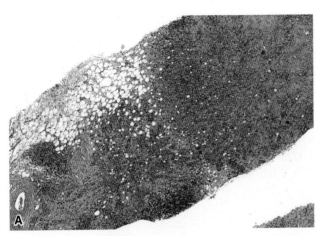
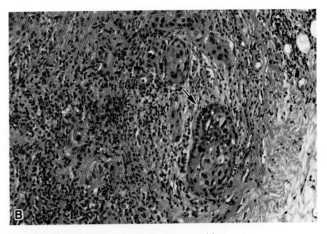

FIGURE 15.11 Invasive Apocrine Carcinoma with Tumor-Infiltrating Lymphocytes. A: This needle core biopsy sample from a breast mass shows invasive apocrine carcinoma with an abundant inflammatory infiltrate. **B:** The inflammatory cells almost mask the invasive carcinoma. A minute focus of solid apocrine ductal carcinoma in situ is also present *(arrow)*.

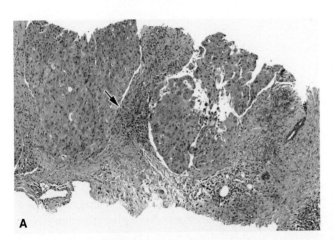
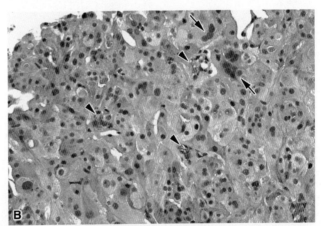

FIGURE 15.12 Invasive Apocrine carcinoma with Solid Papillary Architecture. A: This needle core biopsy sample from a breast mass in a 56-year-old woman shows invasive papillary apocrine carcinoma. Hemosiderin is present in the stroma *(arrow)*, consistent with prior hemorrhage. **B:** The neoplastic cells have a solid growth and low cytologic atypia. A few multinucleated cells are present *(arrows)*. Fibrovascular cores are evident *(arrowheads)*.

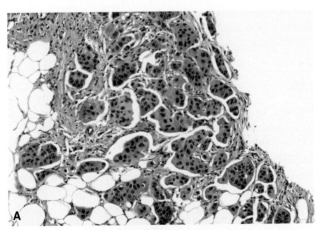
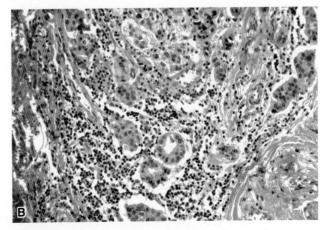

FIGURE 15.13 Invasive Apocrine Carcinoma with Micropapillary Architecture. A: The invasive apocrine carcinoma in this needle core biopsy specimen forms micropapillary clusters. **B:** Another invasive apocrine duct carcinoma forming small glands and micropapillae. A stromal lymphocytic reaction is evident.

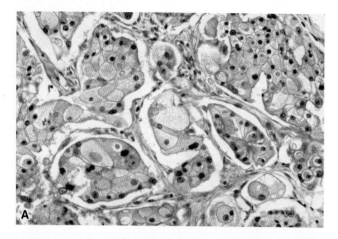

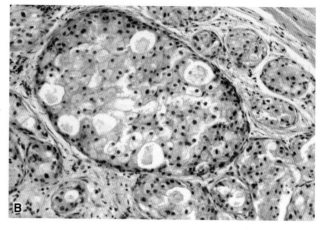

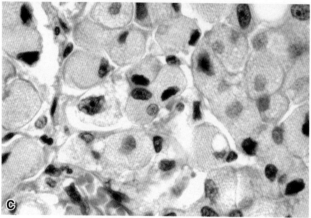

FIGURE 15.14 Apocrine Carcinoma, Clear Cell Type. A: An invasive apocrine carcinoma with marked cytoplasmic clearing. **B:** Cribriform intraductal carcinoma. **C:** Intracytoplasmic mucin is a magenta spot in one cell *(mucicarmine stain).*

with abundant foamy or eosinophilic cytoplasm (19); it closely resembles invasive pleomorphic lobular carcinoma, but shows membranous reactivity for E-cadherin. Lympho-vascular invasion (LVI) is present in 30% to 50% of cases of apocrine carcinoma (1,10,20). In some cases, invasive apocrine carcinoma and invasive lobular carcinoma are very closely associated. Some apocrine carcinomas can have foci of clear-cell morphology. Focal mucicarmine staining may be identified **(Fig. 15.14).** Cells with apocrine morphology can also occur in some mucinous, micropapillary, and invasive lobular carcinomas, especially invasive lobular carcinoma of the pleomorphic type (21). A definitive diagnosis of apocrine carcinoma is not possible based on review of the small tissue sample obtained at NCB.

IMMUNOHISTOCHEMISTRY

ER, PR, AR, and HER2

Apocrine metaplasia is androgen receptor (AR)-positive, but estrogen receptor (ER)- and progesterone (PR)-negative. Most invasive apocrine carcinomas are negative or minimally positive for ER and PR (5,22–25), but some are ER-positive and/or PR-positive, despite apocrine morphology (4,5). AR is detected in most apocrine carcinomas, but it is expressed in other subtypes of breast carcinoma, including ER-positive carcinomas (26). Only about 50% of ER-negative breast

carcinomas are AR-negative (26). Some authors consider as "pure apocrine" only carcinomas having apocrine morphology and ER- and PR-negative, AR-positive immunoprofile, similar to apocrine metaplasia (1,22), and regard those carcinomas with apocrine morphology that are ER-positive and/or AR-positive as "apocrine-like". Nearly 50% of "pure apocrine" carcinomas are HER2-positive (1,4,5,22).

All apocrine DCIS in one study (27) were AR-positive. The low-grade DCIS were also always ER- and PR-negative; about 10% of intermediate- and high-grade apocrine DCIS were ER-positive and/or PR-positive.

Ki67

In one study (4), the mean and median percentage of Ki67-positive cells in apocrine carcinomas were 49% and 42%, respectively; the Ki67-proliferative index was >14% in 82% of the tumors. In a study of apocrine DCIS (27), the Ki67-proliferative index increased significantly between low-, intermediate-, and high-grade apocrine DCIS, but substantial overlap was observed.

GCDFP-15, GATA3, Cytokeratins, and Other Antigens

GCDFP-15 is expressed in most intraductal and invasive apocrine carcinomas (20,28,29), but also in other subtypes of breast carcinoma (29), including some carcinomas with neuroendocrine differentiation (30). In one study (24), most apocrine DCIS and invasive carcinomas were negative for ER, PR, BCL2, and GATA3, akin to apocrine metaplasia, but another group detected GATA3 in most apocrine carcinomas (29).

Apocrine carcinomas tend to be immunoreactive for carcinoembryonic antigen (CEA) and are usually negative to focally positive for S-100 protein. All invasive ductal carcinomas with apocrine features in one study (31) were positive for CK7, CK8, and CK18, and 90% were positive for CK19. Notably, 50% of the carcinomas with apocrine features were CK20-positive, whereas all nonapocrine carcinomas were CK20-negative. None of the carcinomas with apocrine features in this study was positive for CK5/6 and CK14. CK19-positivity was documented in all apocrine carcinomas in one series (32). Reactivity for p53 is detected in 46% (33) to 75% of invasive apocrine carcinomas, and in 40% (27) to 100% (33) of apocrine DCIS, but it is not found in benign apocrine cysts (33). EGFR was detected in 62% apocrine carcinomas, with expression in 76% of "pure apocrine" versus 29% of "apocrine-like" carcinomas (22). EGFR expression in "pure apocrine" carcinoma was inversely correlated with HER2 positivity (22). Apocrine carcinomas are TTF1-negative. One group (34) has reported positivity for napsin in apocrine carcinomas. The cytoplasmic staining for napsin in the published images appears granular. It should be noted that carcinomas with apocrine cytoplasm sometimes show nonspecific granular cytoplasmic immunostaining. Some apocrine carcinoma may contain mucicarmine-positive secretion (**Fig. 15.14C**); intracytoplasmic mucin accumulation resulting in signet ring type cells occurs rarely.

DIFFERENTIAL DIAGNOSIS OF APOCRINE LESIONS AT NEEDLE CORE BIOPSY

Metastasis from an Extramammary Site

Apocrine carcinomas are typically ER- and PR-negative. The carcinoma usually has stellate and infiltrative outline, but in some cases it may be more discretely nodular. The differential diagnosis in a NCB sample with no evidence of DCIS includes metastasis of a carcinoma primary at an extramammary site, such as pulmonary adenocarcinoma (**Fig. 15.15**) or renal cell carcinoma. Metastatic melanoma with epithelioid morphology and large nucleoli can also mimic apocrine carcinoma.

Lymph Node Metastasis of Breast Carcinoma

Tumor-infiltrating lymphocytes associated with apocrine carcinoma may be extensive and raise the differential diagnosis of metastatic carcinoma in a lymph node (LN). In some cases, it is

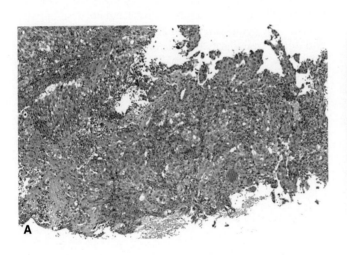

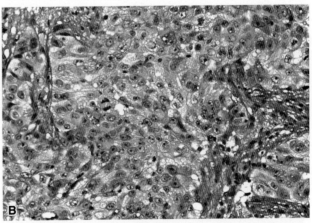

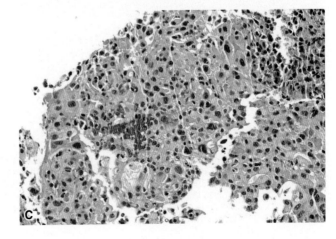

FIGURE 15.15 Metastatic Carcinoma Mimics Triple-negative Apocrine Breast Carcinoma. A: A needle core biopsy specimen from a 2.5-cm superficial mass in the breast of an 80-year-old woman. No breast parenchyma or ductal carcinoma in situ is present. **B:** The carcinoma is poorly differentiated. The neoplastic cells have large and pleomorphic nuclei, with prominent nucleoli. The carcinoma was not reactive for ER, PR, and HER2. **C:** The needle core biopsy specimen of a stellate lung lesion found at imaging workup a few weeks later. The carcinoma in the lung morphologically resembles the carcinoma in **A & B**. Immunohistochemical stains conducted in parallel on the material from the breast and lung lesions showed that both were positive for TTF1 and napsin, while negative for GCDFP-15 and GATA3 (not shown), demonstrating pulmonary origin for the breast lesion.

not possible to determine whether a carcinoma with extensive tumor-infiltrating lymphocytes is in the breast parenchyma or metastatic to a LN. A cautious approach is recommended, as well as clinical and radiologic correlation.

Apocrine DCIS in Sclerosing Lesion Mimics Invasive Carcinoma

Stromal invasion is always best assessed at the periphery of a tumor, and the examination should focus on the interface between the carcinoma and the adjacent breast parenchyma. In the absence of stromal invasion, the stroma around the sclerosing lesion typically lacks reactive desmoplasia and inflammation, and continuous layer of basement membrane is often evident. The identification of focal stromal elastosis in the center of the lesion suggests the possibility of an underlying radial scar. In questionable cases, immunohistochemical stains for myoepithelial markers (calponin and p63) are helpful to document the noninvasive nature of the carcinoma (**Fig. 15.16**).

Apocrine Carcinoma with Pagetoid Spread Mimics Pleomorphic Lobular Carcinoma In Situ

Apocrine DCIS with pagetoid involvement of small ducts and lobules may closely resemble lobular carcinoma in situ (LCIS), particularly pleomorphic LCIS. The neoplastic apocrine cells retain membranous reactivity for E-cadherin and p120, whereas classic and pleomorphic LCIS lack membranous E-cadherin and show diffuse cytoplasmic staining for p120.

Radiation Changes

Irradiated glandular epithelium is characterized by nuclear enlargement, binucleation, intranuclear inclusions, and cytoplasmic vacuolization. Focal necrosis sometimes is present in the lumen of acini in NCB specimens obtained shortly after completion of breast irradiation. All of these changes closely mimic apocrine atypia and raise the differential diagnosis of apocrine DCIS. Cell proliferation is not part of the alterations secondary to radiation treatment, and irradiated epithelium usually consists of a single layer of cells, with no epithelial expansion, and shows no mitotic activity (**Fig. 15.17**). Whenever possible, it is recommended to compare the morphology of the pretreatment carcinoma with that of the posttreatment specimen. In questionable cases, a conservative approach is recommended, which may include surgical excision of the radiologic target for definitive evaluation, as mastectomy is the standard treatment of DCIS recurring after breast-conserving surgery and radiotherapy.

Oncocytic Neoplasms

True oncocytic neoplasms characterized ultrastructurally by abundant mitochondria, strongly immunoreactive with an antimitochondrial antibody, and negative for GCDFP-15 are extremely rare in the breast (35). Definitive diagnosis of an oncocytic neoplasm requires evaluation of the entire tumor.

Granular Cell Tumor

Granular cell tumor (GCT) closely mimics invasive apocrine carcinoma clinically, radiologically, and microscopically. The lesional cells are admixed with sclerotic, but not desmoplastic, stroma. The cytoplasm is abundant and has a characteristic and diffuse granularity because of the presence of abundant lysosomes. The nuclei tend to be small, with no visible nucleoli, and usually lack any atypia (**Fig. 15.18**). Lymphocytes tend to be rare in GCT, but they are common in apocrine carcinoma. GCT is strongly CD68-positive but negative for keratin AE1:3, whereas apocrine carcinoma is keratin AE1:3-positive and CD68-negative. Both tumors are negative for ER and PR. S-100

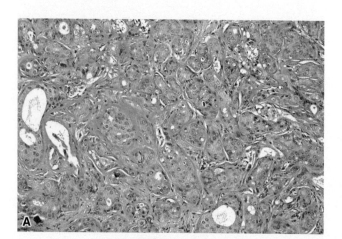
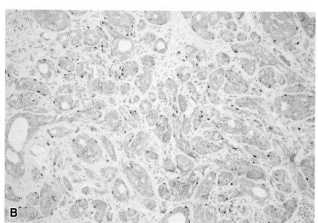

FIGURE 15.16 Ductal Carcinoma In Situ (DCIS) Involving a Sclerosing Lesion Mimics Invasive Carcinoma. A: The carcinoma in this needle core biopsy specimen mimics stromal invasion. The swirling arrangement of the neoplastic epithelium, the presence of basement membranes around the tumor nests, and the absence of stromal desmoplasia suggest the possibility of DCIS involving a sclerosing lesion. **B:** A p63 immunostain highlights the myoepithelial nuclei around the carcinoma, confirming the diagnosis of DCIS.

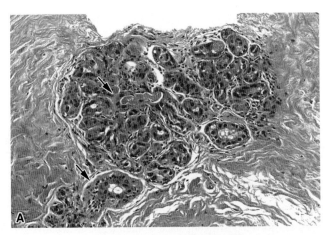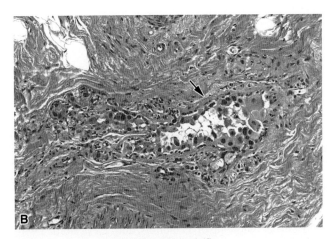

FIGURE 15.17 Radiation Changes. A, B: This needle core biopsy specimen sampled calcification in the breast of a patient who completed radiation therapy 6 months earlier for the treatment of low-grade ductal carcinoma in situ (DCIS). Coarse stromal calcifications were identified (not shown). Two lobules are shown. The epithelium shows nuclear enlargement and hyperchromasia. The differential diagnosis includes lobular involvement of apocrine DCIS. Although the epithelial alterations involve adjacent cells, no proliferation is present. Thickened basement membranes are noted around the acini, consistent with radiation therapy *(arrows)*. Morphologic comparison with the prior low-grade DCIS supported the interpretation of radiation changes in metaplastic apocrine epithelium.

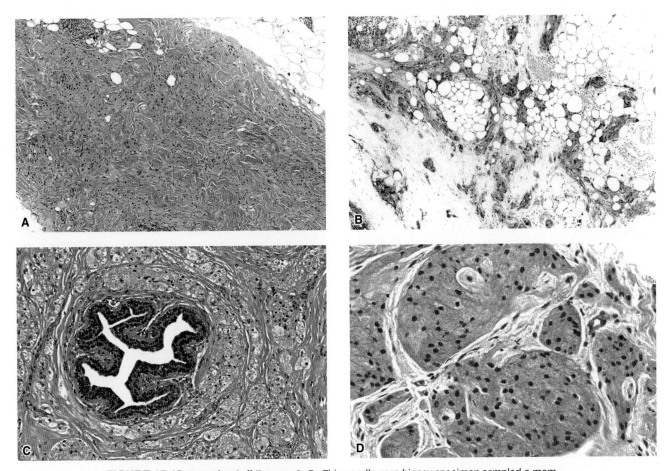

FIGURE 15.18 Granular Cell Tumor. A, B: This needle core biopsy specimen sampled a mammographic area of architectural distortion. The lesion consists of irregularly distributed aggregates of cells with abundant granular cytoplasm admixed with sclerotic stroma. The tumor cells are positive for S-100 **(B)** and negative for cytokeratins (not shown), consistent with the diagnosis. **C:** Another example of granular cell tumor surrounding a benign mammary duct, in a pattern that mimics invasive carcinoma. **D:** The cells of granular cell tumor have abundant amphophilic granular cytoplasm and small nuclei.

is strongly and diffusely positive in GCT, but it can also show some reactivity in apocrine carcinoma, although the staining tends to be focal and less intense.

TREATMENT AND PROGNOSIS

Atypical Apocrine Adenosis

It is unclear whether AAA is a risk factor for the subsequent development of carcinoma (see also discussion in Chapter 6—Adenosis). Carter and Rosen (12) reported no carcinomas in 51 patients with index atypical sclerosing apocrine lesions and a mean follow-up of 35 months, but 11% of women with apocrine adenosis developed carcinoma (3 ipsilateral, 1 contralateral) in another series of 37 patients with a mean follow-up of 8.7 years (13); the reported relapse rate (RR) was 5.5. All patients who developed carcinoma were older than 60 years at diagnosis of AAA, and the RR for developing carcinoma in women 60 years or older with AAA was 14. In a recent study of 37 patients with AAA treated at the Mayo clinic (36) with a median follow-up of 14 years, 8% of the patients developed carcinoma, including two ipsilateral invasive carcinomas and one contralateral DCIS. None of the carcinomas had apocrine morphology. Based on current data, patients with atypical apocrine lesions should be managed clinically with the same follow-up regimen as those with nonapocrine atypical proliferative lesions. The effectiveness of selective ER modulators on atypical apocrine lesions that are typically ER-negative has not been determined.

A lesion yielding AAA at NCB should be surgically excised for its complete and definitive evaluation. A recent study evaluating the upgrade at surgical excision of AAA reported no upgrades to carcinoma (37) (see also detailed discussion of AAA in Chapter 6).

Apocrine DCIS

Apocrine DCIS appears to have the same clinical course as nonapocrine DCIS. Management includes surgical excision and radiation therapy or mastectomy. Hormonal therapy is indicated if at least 1% of apocrine DCIS cells express ER.

Invasive Apocrine Carcinoma

Few studies have found that the prognosis of invasive apocrine mammary carcinoma is similar to that of nonapocrine invasive ductal carcinoma (2). One group (6) studied 29 triple-negative apocrine carcinomas and found LVI in 24% of patients, and LN metastases in 45%. The 5-year overall survival (OS) was 92%, and the disease-free survival (DFS) was 83.7% at 5 years and 67% at 10 years. The outcome of triple-negative apocrine carcinomas in two studies (6,38) was similar to that of triple-negative invasive ductal carcinomas of no special type. Another group (1) reported that pure apocrine carcinomas had worse DFS than nonapocrine carcinomas (HR 1.7; 95%

CI 1.01–2.86), whereas apocrine-like carcinomas and non-apocrine carcinomas had similar DFS and OS.

The prognosis of invasive apocrine carcinoma is determined mainly by conventional prognostic factors such as grade, tumor size, and nodal status. Carcinomas with apocrine differentiation are usually strongly and diffusely AR-positive. Rakha et al. (39) reported that AR-positive triple-negative breast carcinomas had higher nuclear grade, and higher rate of recurrent disease and distant metastases. In a cohort of postmenopausal patients with ER-positive breast carcinoma, AR expression was associated with significantly reduced breast cancer–specific mortality (HR 0.68; 95% CI 0.47–0.99) and overall mortality (HR 0.70; 95% CI 0.53–0.91) by multivariate analysis (40). In the same study, however, postmenopausal women with ER-negative and AR-positive breast carcinoma, such as apocrine carcinomas, had significantly increased breast cancer–specific mortality (HR: 1.59; 95% CI: 0.94–2-68; $p = 0.08$). At present, patients with triple-negative, AR-positive metastatic breast carcinomas can be treated with AR-antagonist drugs in the context of a clinical trial, but also occasionally outside of a trial. A clinical trial evaluating AR-targeted therapy for patients with triple-negative and AR-positive primary breast carcinomas is also planned.

REFERENCES

1. Dellapasqua S, Maisonneuve P, Viale G, et al. Immunohistochemically defined subtypes and outcome of apocrine breast cancer. *Clin Breast Cancer*. 2013;13:95–102.
2. Tanaka K, Imoto S, Wada N, et al. Invasive apocrine carcinoma of the breast: clinicopathologic features of 57 patients. *Breast J*. 2008;14:164–168.
3. Ogiya A, Horii R, Osako T, et al. Apocrine metaplasia of breast cancer: clinicopathological features and predicting response. *Breast Cancer*. 2010;17:290–297.
4. Alvarenga CA, Paravidino PI, Alvarenga M, et al. Reappraisal of immunohistochemical profiling of special histological types of breast carcinomas: a study of 121 cases of eight different subtypes. *J Clin Pathol*. 2012;65:1066–1071.
5. Tsutsumi Y. Apocrine carcinoma as triple-negative breast cancer: novel definition of apocrine-type carcinoma as estrogen/progesterone receptor-negative and androgen receptor-positive invasive ductal carcinoma. *Jpn J Clin Oncol*. 2012;42:375–386.
6. Montagna E, Maisonneuve P, Rotmensz N, et al. Heterogeneity of triple-negative breast cancer: histologic subtyping to inform the outcome. *Clin Breast Cancer*. 2013;13:31–39.
7. Banneau G, Guedj M, MacGrogan G, et al. Molecular apocrine differentiation is a common feature of breast cancer in patients with germline PTEN mutations. *Breast Cancer Res*. 2010;12:R63.
8. Schrager CA, Schneider D, Gruener AC, et al. Similarities of cutaneous and breast pathology in Cowden's Syndrome. *Exp Dermatol*. 1998;7:380–390.
9. Schrager CA, Schneider D, Gruener AC, et al. Clinical and pathological features of breast disease in Cowden's syndrome: an underrecognized syndrome with an increased risk of breast cancer. *Hum Pathol*. 1998;29:47–53.
10. Matsuo K, Fukutomi T, Tsuda H, et al. Apocrine carcinoma of the breast: clinicopathological analysis and histological subclassification of 12 cases. *Breast Cancer*. 1998;5:279–284.
11. Moritani S, Ichihara S, Hasegawa M, et al. Topographical, morphological and immunohistochemical characteristics of carcinoma in situ of the breast involving sclerosing adenosis: two distinct topographical patterns and histological types of carcinoma in situ. *Histopathology*. 2011;58:835–846.
12. Carter DJ, Rosen PP. Atypical apocrine metaplasia in sclerosing lesions of the breast: a study of 51 patients. *Mod Pathol*. 1991;4:1–5.

13. Seidman JD, Ashton M, Lefkowitz M. Atypical apocrine adenosis of the breast: a clinicopathologic study of 37 patients with 8.7-year follow-up. *Cancer*. 1996;77:2529–2537.

14. Tavassoli FA, Norris HJ. Intraductal apocrine carcinoma: a clinicopathologic study of 37 cases. *Mod Pathol*. 1994;7:813–818.

15. O'Malley FP, Page DL, Nelson EH, et al. Ductal carcinoma in situ of the breast with apocrine cytology: definition of a borderline category. *Hum Pathol*. 1994;25:164–168.

16. Cserni G. Benign apocrine papillary lesions of the breast lacking or virtually lacking myoepithelial cells-potential pitfalls in diagnosing malignancy. *APMIS*. 2012;120:249–252.

17. Cserni G. Lack of myoepithelium in apocrine glands of the breast does not necessarily imply malignancy. *Histopathology*. 2008;52:253–255.

18. Tramm T, Kim JY, Tavassoli FA. Diminished number or complete loss of myoepithelial cells associated with metaplastic and neoplastic apocrine lesions of the breast. *Am J Surg Pathol*. 2011;35:202–211.

19. Eusebi V, Foschini MP, Bussolati G, et al. Myoblastomatoid (histiocytoid) carcinoma of the breast: a type of apocrine carcinoma. *Am J Surg Pathol*. 1995;19:553–562.

20. Kasashima S, Kawashima A, Ozaki S, et al. Expression of 5-alpha-reductase in apocrine carcinoma of the breast and its correlation with clinicopathological aggressiveness. *Histopathology*. 2012;60:E51–E57.

21. Eusebi V, Magalhaes F, Azzopardi JG. Pleomorphic lobular carcinoma of the breast: an aggressive tumor showing apocrine differentiation. *Hum Pathol*. 1992;23:655–662.

22. Vranic S, Tawfik O, Palazzo J, et al. EGFR and HER-2/neu expression in invasive apocrine carcinoma of the breast. *Mod Pathol*. 2010;23:644–653.

23. Niemeier LA, Dabbs DJ, Beriwal S, et al. Androgen receptor in breast cancer: expression in estrogen receptor-positive tumors and in estrogen receptor-negative tumors with apocrine differentiation. *Mod Pathol*. 2010;23:205–212.

24. Celis JE, Cabezon T, Moreira JM, et al. Molecular characterization of apocrine carcinoma of the breast: validation of an apocrine protein signature in a well-defined cohort. *Mol Oncol*. 2009;3:220–237.

25. Honma N, Takubo K, Akiyama F, et al. Expression of oestrogen receptor-beta in apocrine carcinomas of the breast. *Histopathology*. 2007;50:425–433.

26. Collins LC, Cole KS, Marotti JD, et al. Androgen receptor expression in breast cancer in relation to molecular phenotype: results from the Nurses' Health Study. *Mod Pathol*. 2011;24:924–931.

27. Leal C, Henrique R, Monteiro P, et al. Apocrine ductal carcinoma in situ of the breast: histologic classification and expression of biologic markers. *Hum Pathol*. 2001;32:487–493.

28. Eusebi V, Betts C, Haagensen DE Jr, et al. Apocrine differentiation in lobular carcinoma of the breast: a morphologic, immunologic, and ultrastructural study. *Hum Pathol*. 1984;15:134–140.

29. Wendroth SM, Mentrikoski MJ, Wick MR. GATA3 expression in morphologic subtypes of breast carcinoma: a comparison with gross cystic disease fluid protein 15 and mammaglobin. *Ann Diagn Pathol*. 2015;19:6–9.

30. Sapino A, Righi L, Cassoni P, et al. Expression of apocrine differentiation markers in neuroendocrine breast carcinomas of aged women. *Mod Pathol*. 2001;14:768–776.

31. Shao MM, Chan SK, Yu AM, et al. Keratin expression in breast cancers. *Virchows Arch*. 2012;461:313–322.

32. Alvarenga CA, Paravidino PI, Alvarenga M, et al. Expression of CK19 in invasive breast carcinomas of special histological types: implications for the use of one-step nucleic acid amplification. *J Clin Pathol*. 2011;64:493–497.

33. Moriya T, Sakamoto K, Sasano H, et al. Immunohistochemical analysis of Ki-67, p53, p21, and p27 in benign and malignant apocrine lesions of the breast: its correlation to histologic findings in 43 cases. *Mod Pathol*. 2000;13:13–18.

34. Vitkovski T, Chaudhary S, Sison C, et al. Aberrant expression of napsin a in breast carcinoma with apocrine features. *Int J Surg Pathol*. 2016;24(5):377–381.

35. Damiani S, Eusebi V, Losi L, et al. Oncocytic carcinoma (malignant oncocytoma) of the breast. *Am J Surg Pathol*. 1998;22:221–230.

36. Fuehrer N, Hartmann L, Degnim A, et al. Atypical apocrine adenosis of the breast: long-term follow-up in 37 patients. *Arch Pathol Lab Med*. 2012;136:179–182.

37. Calhoun BC, Booth CN. Atypical apocrine adenosis diagnosed on breast core biopsy: implications for management. *Hum Pathol*. 2014;45:2130–2135.

38. Dreyer G, Vandorpe T, Smeets A, et al. Triple negative breast cancer: clinical characteristics in the different histological subtypes. *Breast*. 2013;22:761–766.

39. Rakha EA, El-Sayed ME, Green AR, et al. Prognostic markers in triple-negative breast cancer. *Cancer*. 2007;109:25–32.

40. Hu R, Dawood S, Holmes MD, et al. Androgen receptor expression and breast cancer survival in postmenopausal women. *Clin Cancer Res*. 2011;17:1867–1874.

16

Adenoid Cystic Carcinoma

EDI BROGI

Mammary adenoid cystic carcinoma (ACC) is morphologically similar to its counterpart in the salivary glands but has a more indolent behavior. Most ACCs of the breast and salivary glands carry a characteristic *MYB-NFIB* fusion gene, which results from a t(6:9)(q22-23;p23-24) translocation (1–3).

CLINICAL PRESENTATION

Incidence

ACC is one of the least frequent forms of primary mammary carcinoma (4,5), with reported incidence ranging from less than one in a million (6) to about one in a thousand (7). The incidence rate of ACC was relatively constant between 1977 and 2006 (6).

Age and Ethnicity

ACC occurs in women of any age, but the mean and median ages of patients with ACC range from 50 years to 63 years in various studies (4,6–9). Between 70% and 96% of women with ACC in three separate series (6,10,11) were postmenopausal. Most (82%–87%) women with ACC are white (4,7,10). No association with familial syndromes has been described.

Gender

ACC can occur in men, including adolescents. ACC constituted 1% of 759 primary carcinomas of the male breast in one series (12).

Presenting Symptoms

ACC presents as a palpable, discrete, and firm mass in about 80% of cases (10). Pain (10,13,14) and tenderness (14) are rare presenting symptoms and have not been specifically correlated with the histologic finding of perineural invasion. Even though ACC frequently arises in the subareolar region or centrally in the breast (6,15), nipple discharge and Paget disease are rare presenting symptoms.

Site

The most frequent sites of ACC are the upper outer quadrant (6) and the retroareolar region (6,15,16).

Multifocality

ACC is usually unifocal, and only rarely consists of two (10,17) or more distinct foci (10). Bilateral ACC is uncommon.

Risk of Additional Malignancy

The frequency of subsequent carcinoma in either breast or of a solid nonmammary malignant tumor in patients with mammary ACC is not greater than that expected in the general population (6).

Radiology

ACC presents mammographically as a well-defined lobulated mass or an ill-defined lesion (15,18,19); a mammographic spiculated mass can also be observed (14). Only 18% of ACCs in one series (10) were detected by mammography; in another study (19), 12.5% of ACCs were mammographically undetected. Calcifications are rarely associated with ACC.

The sonographic appearance of ACC is that of a heterogenous or hypoechoic mass (14,19). Eight of nine ACCs studied sonographically (19) appeared as irregularly shaped hypoechoic or heterogenous masses, oriented parallel to the skin, with no echogenic halo or posterior shadowing. Doppler sonography detected only minimal flow signal around and within the tumor. One tumor presented as an 8-mm hypoechoic nodule suggestive of an intramammary lymph node (20).

MRI is helpful for defining the extent of the ACC, especially in a dense breast (19). ACC tends to be irregular or lobulated, with rapid and heterogeneous enhancement after injection of gadolinium, and persistent or plateau kinetic (19). T2-weighted images show iso-intensity with the adjacent breast parenchyma or extensive high T2-weighted signal.

Size

Most ACCs measure between 1 and 3 cm. In a recent series of 31 ACCs (21) the mean tumor size was 2.7 cm (range: 0.6–15 cm); the mean size of ACC with conventional histology was 2.9 cm (range: 0.7–12 cm), and that of ACC with basaloid morphology was 2.6 cm (range: 0.6–15 cm). In another series of six cases of solid ACC (22), the mean tumor size was 2 cm.

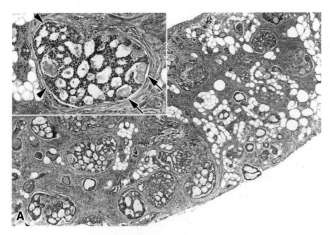

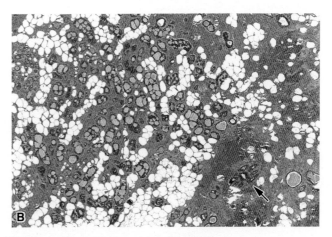

FIGURE 16.1 Adenoid Cystic Carcinoma, Cribriform Growth Pattern. A: A needle core biopsy specimen showing nests of predominantly cribriform adenoid cystic carcinoma. Cribriform growth with basement membrane spherules *(arrows)* and small glandular lumina *(arrowheads)* are shown in the inset. **B:** The surgically excised tumor has similar morphology. Note the diffuse infiltrative growth pattern and lack of stromal desmoplasia. A small duct is also present *(arrow)*.

Microscopic Pathology

ACC is composed of glandular epithelium (adenoid component) and basaloid/myoepithelial cells, which produce abundant basement membrane material **(Figs. 16.1 and 16.2)**. These components are heterogeneously distributed within any given tumor and produce different morphologic appearances.

Cribriform Morphology

Some areas have a predominantly glandular arrangement that closely simulates invasive or in situ cribriform carcinoma **(Fig. 16.1)**. This form of ACC can be mistaken for cribriform carcinoma when the basaloid element and basement membrane material are sparse, especially in the limited material in a needle core biopsy (NCB) sample.

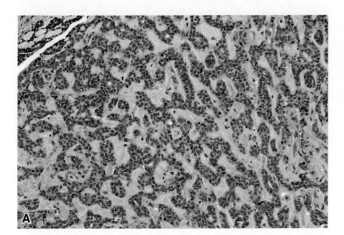

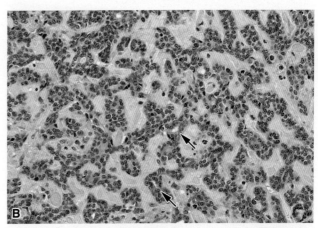

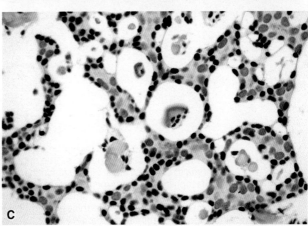

FIGURE 16.2 Adenoid Cystic Carcinoma, Reticular Growth Pattern. A, B: The tumor in this needle core biopsy specimen has a reticular structure. Scattered small glandular spaces are evident *(arrows)* **B**. **C:** Only myoepithelial nuclei are immunoreactive for p63.

Reticular Morphology

The carcinoma consists of trabeculae with a nearly linear arrangement, surrounded by expanded extracellular basement membrane matrix, often with myxoid to mucoid tinctorial quality. Scattered minute glands are visible (**Fig. 16.2**).

Occasionally, different patterns coexist in the same case (**Fig. 16.3**).

Scirrhous Morphology

Abundant basement membrane material can produce a cylindromatous pattern that may be mistaken for dense stromal fibrosis in a scirrhous carcinoma.

Solid and Basaloid Morphology

Solid growth of the basaloid cells yields a pattern referred to as the "solid variant of ACC with basaloid features" (23) (**Fig. 16.4**). The neoplastic cells have scant cytoplasm, relatively large hyperchromatic nuclei, and frequent mitoses. Scattered small glands are usually appreciable, as well as focal minute eosinophilic deposits of basement membrane material.

Ro et al. (24) suggested that ACC be stratified into three grades on the basis of the proportion of solid growth within the lesion: grade I, no solid elements; grade II, less than 30% solid growth; and grade III, solid areas composing more than 30% of the tumor. The authors (24) found that tumors with

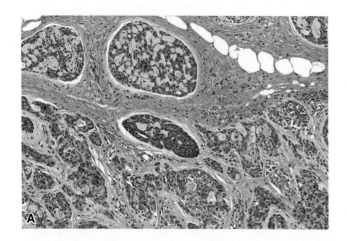
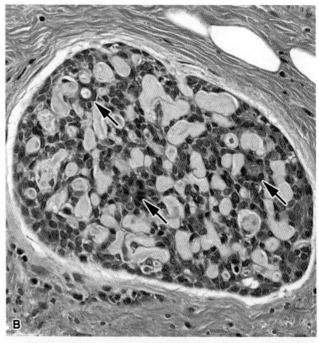
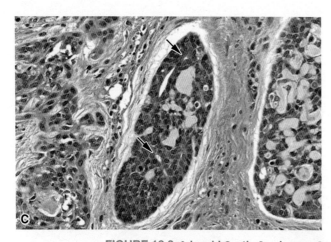
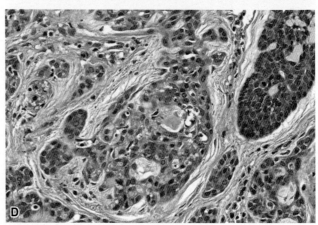

FIGURE 16.3 Adenoid Cystic Carcinoma, Coexisting Patterns. A: Three different growth patterns are present in this tumor. **B:** The cribriform pattern in this nest mimics cribriform ductal carcinoma in situ. Few small glandular lumina are evident *(arrows)*, and there are numerous spherules of basophilic basement membrane material. **C:** A small nest has solid growth with scattered glandular lumina *(arrows)*. Cribriform **(right)** and reticular **(left)** patterns are also represented. **D:** The prevalent growth pattern in this field is reticular. The basaloid solid nest in **C** is partially represented in the right upper corner.

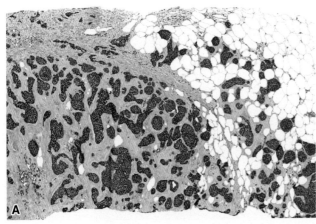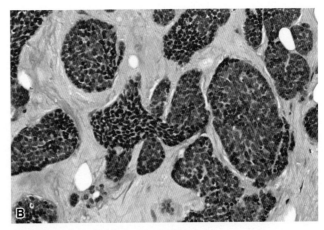

FIGURE 16.4 Adenoid Cystic Carcinoma, Solid and Basaloid Pattern. A: The carcinoma consists of solid nests composed of hyperchromatic cells. The stroma around the neoplastic nests is hypocellular, with a focally pale blue tinctorial quality. **B:** At higher magnification, the neoplastic cells show basaloid morphology. The pale blue staining of the stroma around the invasive nests is a feature commonly associated with high-grade adenoid cystic carcinoma and should not be mistaken for stromal mucin.

a larger proportion of solid component (grades II and III) tended to be larger and were more likely to have recurrences than those without a solid component (grade I). In their series, none of the five patients with a grade I ACC developed distant metastases, whereas two of six patients with grade II ACC had a recurrence distally; the only patient with a grade III ACC also developed distant metastases. The grading scheme proposed by Ro et al. (24) was not prognostically significant in a subsequent study (16).

Metaplastic Alterations

Some ACCs have focal sebaceous metaplasia or squamous differentiation. Adenomyoepitheliomatous (25) and syringomatous areas can be present. Adipocytic differentiation and myofibroblastic hyperplasia can also occur in the stroma of ACC. A high-grade basaloid ACC showed morphologic transition into a metaplastic spindle cell and glandular adenocarcinoma with melanomatous differentiation (26). Another basaloid ACC merged with a "small cell carcinoma" (27). Foschini et al. (22) have suggested that conventional and solid ACCs have a good prognosis, but the latter is more likely to involve lymph nodes (LNs) and recur locally, whereas ACC with areas of overtly malignant transformation has aggressive behavior. This grading scheme needs further validation.

Perineural and Lymphovascular Invasion

Perineural and lymphovascular invasion is uncommon in mammary ACC with conventional morphology, and it is very rarely detected in NCB material. Shrinkage artifact is common, especially in fibrotic portions of ACC, and can mimic lymphovascular invasion (LVI) **(Fig. 16.5)**. Three of six solid ACCs in one series (22) had LVI, including two tumors that also showed perineural invasion.

Adenoid Cystic Carcinoma In Situ

It is difficult to distinguish invasive from in situ ACC. ACC in situ lacks the periductal cuff of cellular myxoid stroma that

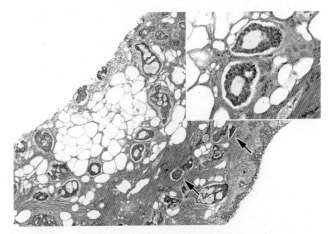

FIGURE 16.5 Shrinkage Artifact Can Mimic Lymphovascular Invasion. Shrinkage artifact around nests of adenoid cystic carcinoma is common and can simulate lymphovascular invasion *(arrows)*. On high-power examination **(inset)**, the space around the nests of adenoid cystic carcinoma is devoid of endothelium.

typically surrounds the nests of invasive ACC, but this finding can be very subtle. Calponin decorates the native myoepithelium of the ducts and acini harboring in situ ACC, but it is absent within and around the nests of invasive ACC. Lobules and ducts adjacent to invasive ACC can display adenoid cystic traits, with small cylindromatous areas, which represent in situ carcinoma.

Other Associated Carcinomas

Patients with ACC can also develop other types of breast carcinoma in the same or opposite breast coincidentally or asynchronously. Merging of ACC with well-differentiated ER-positive invasive ductal carcinoma has been observed **(Fig. 16.6)**.

Immonohistochemistry

The glandular (luminal) and basaloid/myoepithelial components of ACC have different immunoprofiles.

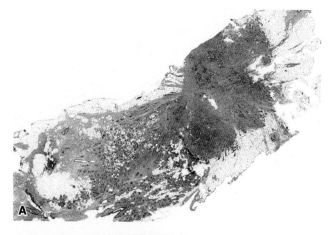

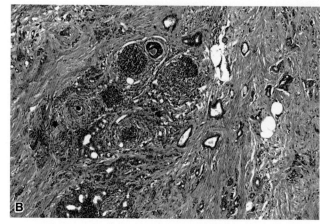

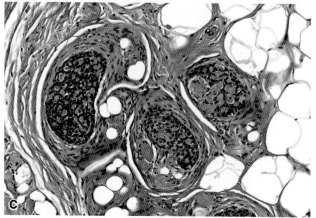

FIGURE 16.6 Adenoid Cystic Carcinoma and Well-differentiated Ductal Carcinoma. A: This core biopsy sampled an invasive carcinoma with dual morphology. One half **(right)** consists of a well-differentiated invasive ductal carcinoma, and the other half **(left)** is adenoid cystic carcinoma. **B:** The two morphologic components merge in the center of the tumor. **C:** A close-up view of the adenoid cystic component with cylindromatous features.

Glandular Component

The glandular cells of ACC are positive for CK7 **(Fig. 16.7)**, CEA, EMA, CK5/6, CK8/18, and CD117/C-KIT **(Fig. 16.7)** (28). The glandular component is present focally in solid ACC. In most basaloid ACCs, CK7 highlights scattered and glandular lumina (21), but some cases show diffuse staining for CK7 (22).

Myoepithelial/Basaloid Cells

The basaloid cells of ACC express the myoepithelial markers p63 **(Figs. 16.2 and 16.7)** (28,29), smooth muscle actin (SMA) (29,30) **(Fig. 16.7)**, and maspin (31), but show no reactivity for calponin (29), smooth muscle myosin heavy chain (23,29), and CD10 (32). The basaloid cells are also positive for basal keratins CK5/6, CK14, and CK17 (2). Glandular and myoepithelial cells stain with keratin 34βE12, albeit not uniformly **(Fig. 16.7)**. Most basaloid ACCs are diffusely positive for p63, but some cases are p63-negative or only focally positive (22), including cases with documented *MYB* rearrangement by FISH (21).

ER, PR, AR, and HER2

Most ACCs are negative for ER (2,28,33), PR, and AR (34). Very limited positivity for ER has been detected in some ACCs (10,19,23,35). HER2 is also negative (28). Based on its triple-negative profile and reactivity for basal cytokeratins, ACC qualifies as a "basal-like" triple-negative breast carcinoma, but it differs from other "basal-like" mammary carcinomas because it harbors a characteristic genetic alteration and has a relatively good prognosis.

Ki67

Ki67 staining in ACC ranges from 4% to 70%, depending on the tumor grade, with a trend to a higher positivity in higher-grade tumors (35). In one study (36), three ACCs with a low Ki67 index and no expression of p53 protein had no LN involvement, whereas a fourth tumor with a high Ki67 index and p53 expression presented with LN metastases. Other investigators found that the Ki67 index is not significantly related to prognosis (16).

CD117/KIT

KIT, a transmembrane tyrosine kinase receptor encoded by the protooncogene *CKIT* located on chromosome 4(q11–12), is involved in the regulation of cell growth, and is expressed in normal mammary glandular epithelium. Mammary ACC is typically CD117/KIT-positive (2,28,29,35,37) **(Fig. 16.7)**. CD117/KIT staining in cribriform ACC is reported to be limited to the epithelial component (28,37), with positivity in 50% or more of the cells; however, diffuse positivity in all (epithelial and myoepithelial/basaloid) cells of ACC was detected in some laboratories, and may be antibody- and/or protocol-dependent. CD117/KIT decorates nearly all cells in ACC with solid and basaloid morphology (28,37). CD117/KIT does not decorate ductal carcinoma in situ (DCIS) or invasive cribriform ductal carcinoma. CD117/KIT is also reportedly negative in the benign epithelium associated with collagenous spherulosis (29).

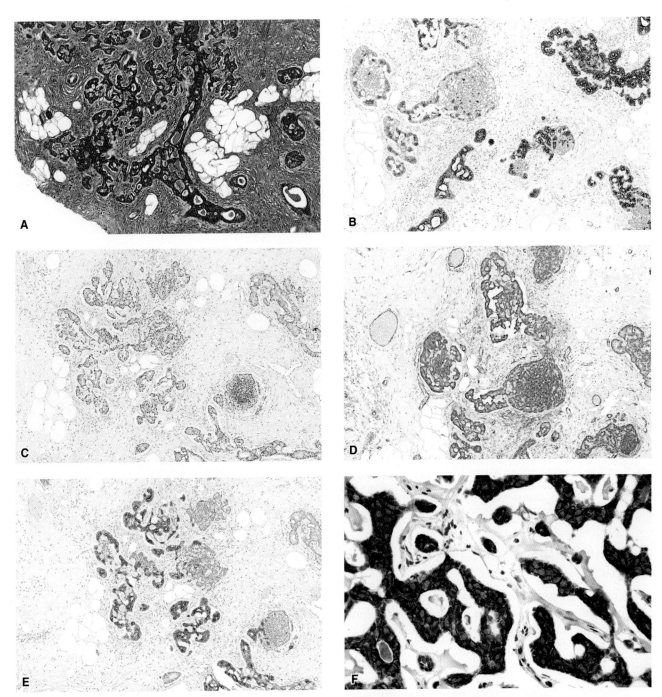

FIGURE 16.7 Adenoid Cystic Carcinoma, Immunohistochemistry. The adenoid cystic carcinoma **(A)** shows positive reactivity for CK7 in the epithelial component **(B)**, and for p63 **(C)** and SMA **(D)** in the myoepithelial/basaloid cells. A calponin stain was negative in all cells (not shown). **E:** A 34βE12 cytokeratin immunostain highlights a mixed population of basaloid and epithelial cells in the same tumor. **F:** CD117/KIT staining in another ACC.

Neuroendocrine Markers

Neuroendocrine markers, such as chromogranin and synaptophysin, are negative in ACC.

MYB

Most ACCs harbor a t(6:9)(q22-23;p23-24) translocation (1–3) that produces a *MYB-NFIB* fusion gene, leading to overexpression of the *MYB* oncogene. Immunohistochemical evidence of nuclear MYB expression **(Fig. 16.8)** is detected in both *MYB-NFIB* fusion-positive and fusion-negative tumors, suggesting that mechanisms other than *MYB-NFIB* gene fusion can also be involved. In the absence of the appropriate tumor morphology, MYB immunoreactivity is not diagnostic of ACC, as it can also be expressed in some high-grade breast carcinomas.

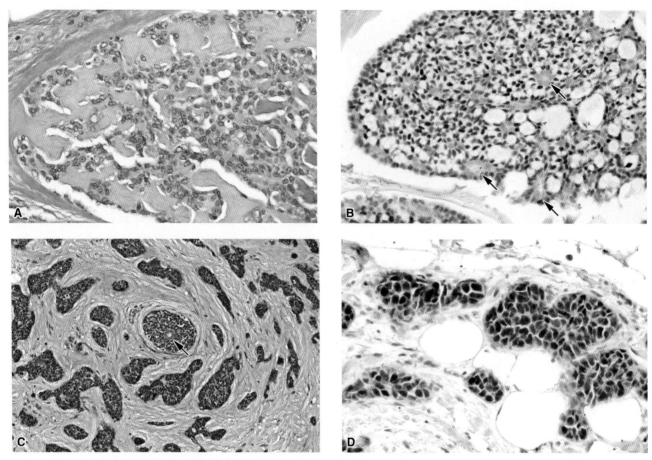

FIGURE 16.8 MYB Reactivity in Adenoid Cystic Carcinoma. The basaloid cells of this adenoid cystic carcinoma **(A)** with cribriform pattern express MYB protein. **B:** The glandular cells appear negative *(arrows)*. **C:** The basaloid cells in this solid adenoid cystic carcinoma express strong nuclear reactivity for the MYB protein **(D)**. A small glandular lumen is identified in **C** *(arrow)*.

Differential Diagnosis in Needle Core Biopsy Material

Invasive Cribriform Carcinoma

Invasive cribriform carcinoma is a monophasic ER-positive adenocarcinoma and has no myoepithelial component or intrinsic matrix deposition.

Cribriform DCIS

Cribriform DCIS shows no internal reactivity for myoepithelial markers, but it is usually surrounded by myoepithelium and basement membrane that are normal components of the duct wall.

Carcinoma with Neuroendocrine Features

Solid ACC can mimic invasive or in situ solid-papillary carcinoma. The presence of scattered CK-positive small glands and focal basement membrane deposits admixed with the solid basaloid proliferation supports the diagnosis of ACC. The differential diagnosis of solid ACC should be considered whenever an invasive carcinoma with apparent neuroendocrine morphology is negative for ER and PR. The stroma associated with solid ACC can have a pale blue tinctorial quality that mimics stromal mucin.

Small Cell Carcinoma

Solid ACC with necrosis can closely resemble a high-grade neuroendocrine carcinoma (small cell carcinoma) primary in the breast or metastatic from another site. In contrast to small cell carcinoma, solid ACC is TTF1-negative. In addition, ACC has no detectable neuroendocrine differentiation with immunohistochemical stains. In a study of basaloid, small cell, and ACCs of the oropharynx (38), staining for high-molecular-weight keratin 34βE12 was present in basaloid carcinomas and ACCs but absent in small cell carcinomas. The diagnostic utility of 34βE12 staining in the differential diagnosis of ACC and small cell carcinoma in breast NCB material has not been evaluated. A case of ACC merging with small cell carcinoma has been reported (27). The nests of solid ACC are usually surrounded by pale blue stroma **(Fig. 16.9)**.

High-grade Carcinoma Arising in Microglandular Adenosis

High-grade carcinoma arising in microglandular adenosis (MGA) can resemble the solid, basaloid variant of ACC. MGA and MGA-associated carcinomas are characteristically negative for all myoepithelial markers, whereas solid ACC is typically positive for p63 and SMA.

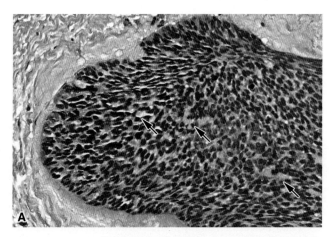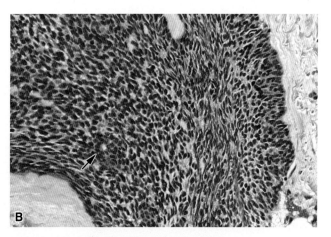

FIGURE 16.9 Solid Adenoid Cystic Carcinoma. A, B: The basaloid cells of this adenoid cystic carcinoma are surrounded by a pale blue rim of basement membrane–like material that superficially resembles stromal mucin. Note that the same pale blue material is also present within the carcinoma *(arrows)*. A small glandular lumen is identified in **B** *(arrowhead)*.

Cylindroma and Syringomatous Adenoma

ACC arising in the nipple can resemble a syringomatous adenoma, a benign lesion that does not produce Paget disease. A cylindroma of the skin overlying the breast can also simulate a mammary ACC if one overlooks its superficial location and cutaneous origin. In contrast to ACC, syringomatous adenoma and cylindroma show no cytologic atypia.

Adenomyoepithelioma

ACC can arise in association with an adenomyoepithelioma (AME). Both lesions are biphasic (epithelial and myoepithelial), and sometimes they can be difficult to differentiate. The myoepithelial cells of AME are calponin-positive, whereas the basaloid/myoepithelial cells of ACC are typically calponin-negative (see Chapter 5).

Solid Usual Duct Hyperplasia

Solid usual duct hyperplasia (UDH) involving a papilloma can occasionally resemble a solid ACC but lacks nuclear atypia.

Collagenous Spherulosis

Collagenous spherulosis (CS) (see Chapter 4) is a lobular alteration in which benign acini are admixed with globoid deposits of eosinophilic and/or myxoid basement membrane material produced by the myoepithelium. Atypical lobular hyperplasia (ALH) and classic lobular carcinoma in situ (LCIS) frequently involve CS. CS may constitute an incidental focal finding in aNCB sample targeting another lesion, such as a papilloma or mass-forming FCC. Occasionally, CS is detected mammographically as clustered calcifications in the basement membrane deposits (39). The combination of glands and spherules of basement membrane material surrounded by myoepithelium found in CS may simulate a cribriform ACC, especially in limited NCB material. The myoepithelium surrounding the spherules of CS reacts with p63, SMA, calponin, and smooth muscle myosin heavy chain, but the latter two antigens are not expressed in the basaloid/myoepithelial cells of ACC (29). CD117/KIT decorates ACC, but it does not stain the glandular epithelium of CS (28,29,35–37) (**Table 16.1**).

TABLE 16.1

Differential Staining in ACC and Collagenous Spherulosis

	ACC	CS
p63	MECs positive	MECs positive
SMA	MECs positive	MECs positive
Calponin	MECs negative	MECs positive
SMM-HC	MECs negative	MECs positive
CD10	MECs negative	MECs positive
ER and PR	All cells negative	Scattered glandular cells positive *and* MECs negative
CD117/c-kit	Glandular cells positive *and* MECs negative *OR* all cells positive	All cells negative

ACC, adenoid cystic carcinoma; CS, collagenous spherulosis; MEC, myoepithelial cells.

ACC often shows intratumoral heterogeneity and sometimes can be difficult to recognize in the limited material obtained by NCB. ACC with conspicuous cylindromatous material compressing the glandular elements can simulate invasive lobular carcinoma or a scirrhus carcinoma.

Prognosis and Treatment

Breast-conserving surgery is the preferred primary therapy for mammary ACC (10,11,28,40,41), with the exception of large tumors that require a mastectomy to achieve a negative margin (10). ACC tends to show peripheral infiltration beyond the obvious tumor mass, and wide excision margins are usually recommended (13,16).

Adjuvant radiotherapy is recommended in patients treated with breast-conserving surgery. In a study (41) of 376 women with mammary ACC recorded in the SEER database for the years 1988 to 2005, 53% of 227 patients treated surgically with lumpectomy received adjuvant radiotherapy and showed a survival benefit of 12.4% at 5 years and 19.7% at 10 years compared to patients who were not treated with radiotherapy. Radiotherapy was administered to 66% of 61 patients in one series (10), including 35 patients who received whole-breast irradiation after breast-conserving surgery. After a median follow-up of 79 months, local recurrence developed in 5.7% of the patients who received radiotherapy and in 33% of the patients who did not receive radiotherapy.

ACC metastasizes rarely to LNs. In one study (10), none of the 51 patients with ACC who underwent axillary lymph node dissection (ALND) or sentinel lymph node biopsy had LN involvement. Only 4.9% of 244 women with mammary ACC treated between 1988 and 2006 and recorded in the California Cancer Registry (4) had ALN metastases. The mean tumor size of ACC with LN metastases was 3.7 cm (range: 1.4–7.7 cm) versus 2.2 cm (range: 0.1–8 cm) for ACC without LN metastases, but the difference was not statistically significant. LN metastases were identified in 5.1% of 703 patients with ACC in the National Cancer Database between 1998 and 2008 (6). ALN involvement appears to be relatively more frequent in patients with basaloid ACC, but data are limited. Shin and Rosen (23) documented LN metastases in two of seven patients with basaloid ACC. D'Alfonso et al. (21) reported that 2 of 10 patients with basaloid ACC had LN involvement; an 83-year-old woman with LN metastases was included in both series. Two of six patients with solid ACC in another series (22) also had LN metastases at presentation.

Axillary LN involvement usually carries a negative prognosis, even though distant metastases can occur independent of LN involvement. Two patients with LN metastases at the time of mastectomy (24,42) developed pulmonary metastases and died of disease. Clinical follow-up information was available for 11 patients with solid ACC in one series (21). One patient developed pulmonary metastases 7 months after initial mastectomy; she underwent lung wedge resection and had no evidence of disease at 4 years of follow-up. Another patient developed local recurrence 5 years following initial treatment with surgical excision without radiotherapy; she underwent mastectomy and had no evidence of disease 11 years later. Two patients in another series developed local recurrence 13 and 16 months after initial diagnosis; a third patient died of another tumor (pulmonary small cell carcinoma); the remaining three patients had no evidence of disease with a mean follow-up of 42 months.

Adjuvant chemotherapy is rarely administered to patients with ACC. Only 11.3% of 933 patients with ACC in the 1998 to 2008 National Cancer Database received chemotherapy versus 45.4% of all patients with breast carcinoma treated in the same period ($p < 0.0001$) (7). In one series (10), only 24.5% of 61 women with ACC received adjuvant chemotherapy, and none of the 18 patients in another series did (28).

In a study of 23 patients (11), 70% had no adjuvant therapy, 26% had hormonal therapy, and only one patient received chemotherapy.

Hormonal therapy usually is not prescribed for ACC, as most are hormone receptor–negative.

The overall survival of 61 patients with ACC in the Rare Cancer Network (10) was 94% and 86% at 5 and 10 years, respectively, and the corresponding disease-free survival was 82% and 74%. In one study (4), women with ACC had a relative cumulative survival advantage of approximately 20% after 10 years of follow-up when compared to women with breast carcinoma in general.

In another study (7), a patient with ACC treated only by radiotherapy died of disease 2 years after diagnosis. Two patients initially treated with breast-conserving surgery developed local recurrence after 11 and 13 years and were treated surgically; both patients were alive 16 and 19 years after treatment. All patients with distant metastases have had pulmonary involvement, which usually occurred 6 to 12 years after initial diagnosis (7,43–45), although some patients developed metastases earlier (21). Other sites of distant metastases include bone (24), liver (24), brain (45,46), and kidneys (43).

At present, the prognosis of ACC with basaloid morphology does not appear to be substantially different, although the available data are limited (21,22).

Overall, patients with mammary ACC have a very good prognosis with a low risk of systemic metastases and death due to ACC.

REFERENCES

1. Persson M, Andren Y, Mark J, et al. Recurrent fusion of MYB and NFIB transcription factor genes in carcinomas of the breast and head and neck. *Proc Natl Acad Sci U S A*. 2009;106:18740–18744.
2. Wetterskog D, Lopez-Garcia MA, Lambros MB, et al. Adenoid cystic carcinomas constitute a genomically distinct subgroup of triple-negative and basal-like breast cancers. *J Pathol*. 2012;226:84–96.
3. Brill LB II, Kanner WA, Fehr A, et al. Analysis of MYB expression and MYB-NFIB gene fusions in adenoid cystic carcinoma and other salivary neoplasms. *Mod Pathol*. 2011;24:1169–1176.
4. Thompson K, Grabowski J, Saltzstein SL, et al. Adenoid cystic breast carcinoma: is axillary staging necessary in all cases? Results from the California Cancer Registry. *Breast J*. 2011;17:485–489.
5. McClenathan JH, de la Roza G. Adenoid cystic breast cancer. *Am J Surg*. 2002;183:646–649.
6. Ghabach B, Anderson WF, Curtis RE, et al. Adenoid cystic carcinoma of the breast in the United States (1977 to 2006): a population-based cohort study. *Breast Cancer Res*. 2010;12:R54.

7. Kulkarni N, Pezzi CM, Greif JM, et al. Rare breast cancer: 933 adenoid cystic carcinomas from the National Cancer Data Base. *Ann Surg Oncol.* 2013;20(7):2236–2241.

8. Rosen PP. Adenoid cystic carcinoma of the breast: a morphologically heterogeneous neoplasm. *Pathol Annu.* 1989;24(pt 2):237–254.

9. Delanote S, Van den Broecke R, Schelfhout VR, et al. Adenoid cystic carcinoma of the breast in a 19-year-old girl. *Breast.* 2003;12:75–77.

10. Khanfir K, Kallel A, Villette S, et al. Management of adenoid cystic carcinoma of the breast: a Rare Cancer Network study. *Int J Radiat Oncol Biol Phys.* 2012;82:2118–2124.

11. Arpino G, Clark GM, Mohsin S, et al. Adenoid cystic carcinoma of the breast: molecular markers, treatment, and clinical outcome. *Cancer.* 2002;94:2119–2127.

12. Burga AM, Fadare O, Lininger RA, et al. Invasive carcinomas of the male breast: a morphologic study of the distribution of histologic subtypes and metastatic patterns in 778 cases. *Virchows Arch.* 2006;449:507–512.

13. Hodgson NC, Lytwyn A, Bacopulos S, et al. Adenoid cystic breast carcinoma: high rates of margin positivity after breast conserving surgery. *Am J Clin Oncol.* 2010;33:28–31.

14. Sarnaik AA, Meade T, King J, et al. Adenoid cystic carcinoma of the breast: a review of a single institution's experience. *Breast J.* 2010;16:208–210.

15. Santamaria G, Velasco M, Zanon G, et al. Adenoid cystic carcinoma of the breast: mammographic appearance and pathologic correlation. *AJR Am J Roentgenol.* 1998;171:1679–1683.

16. Kleer CG, Oberman HA. Adenoid cystic carcinoma of the breast: value of histologic grading and proliferative activity. *Am J Surg Pathol.* 1998;22:569–575.

17. Montagna E, Maisonneuve P, Rotmensz N, et al. Heterogeneity of triple-negative breast cancer: histologic subtyping to inform the outcome. *Clin Breast Cancer.* 2013;13:31–39.

18. Bourke AG, Metcalf C, Wylie EJ. Mammographic features of adenoid cystic carcinoma. *Australas Radiol.* 1994;38:324–325.

19. Glazebrook KN, Reynolds C, Smith RL, et al. Adenoid cystic carcinoma of the breast. *AJR Am J Roentgenol.* 2010;194:1391–1396.

20. Saqi A, Mercado CL, Hamele-Bena D. Adenoid cystic carcinoma of the breast diagnosed by fine-needle aspiration. *Diagn Cytopathol.* 2004;30:271–274.

21. D'Alfonso TM, Mosquera JM, MacDonald TY, et al. MYB-NFIB gene fusion in adenoid cystic carcinoma of the breast with special focus paid to the solid variant with basaloid features. *Hum Pathol.* 2014;45(11):2270–2280.

22. Foschini MP, Rizzo A, De Leo A, et al. Solid variant of adenoid cystic carcinoma of the breast: a case series with proposal of a new grading system. *Int J Surg Pathol.* 2016;24:97–102.

23. Shin SJ, Rosen PP. Solid variant of mammary adenoid cystic carcinoma with basaloid features: a study of nine cases. *Am J Surg Pathol.* 2002;26:413–420.

24. Ro JY, Silva EG, Gallager HS. Adenoid cystic carcinoma of the breast. *Hum Pathol.* 1987;18:1276–1281.

25. Van Dorpe J, De Pauw A, Moerman P. Adenoid cystic carcinoma arising in an adenomyoepithelioma of the breast. *Virchows Arch.* 1998;432:119–122.

26. Noske A, Schwabe M, Pahl S, et al. Report of a metaplastic carcinoma of the breast with multi-directional differentiation: an adenoid cystic carcinoma, a spindle cell carcinoma and melanoma. *Virchows Arch.* 2008;452:575–579.

27. Cabibi D, Cipolla C, Maria Florena A, et al. Solid variant of mammary "adenoid cystic carcinoma with basaloid features" merging with "small cell carcinoma". *Pathol Res Pract.* 2005;201:705–711.

28. Azoulay S, Lae M, Freneaux P, et al. KIT is highly expressed in adenoid cystic carcinoma of the breast, a basal-like carcinoma associated with a favorable outcome. *Mod Pathol.* 2005;18:1623–1631.

29. Rabban JT, Swain RS, Zaloudek CJ, et al. Immunophenotypic overlap between adenoid cystic carcinoma and collagenous spherulosis of the breast: potential diagnostic pitfalls using myoepithelial markers. *Mod Pathol.* 2006;19:1351–1357.

30. Kasami M, Olson SJ, Simpson JF, et al. Maintenance of polarity and a dual cell population in adenoid cystic carcinoma of the breast: an immunohistochemical study. *Histopathology.* 1998;32:232–238.

31. Reis-Filho JS, Milanezi F, Silva P, et al. Maspin expression in myoepithelial tumors of the breast. *Pathol Res Pract.* 2001;197:817–821.

32. Cabibi D, Giannone AG, Belmonte B, et al. CD10 and HHF35 actin in the differential diagnosis between collagenous spherulosis and adenoid-cystic carcinoma of the breast. *Pathol Res Pract.* 2012;208:405–409.

33. Marchio C, Weigelt B, Reis-Filho JS. Adenoid cystic carcinomas of the breast and salivary glands (or 'The strange case of Dr Jekyll and Mr Hyde' of exocrine gland carcinomas). *J Clin Pathol.* 2010;63:220–228.

34. Vranic S, Gatalica Z, Deng H, et al. ER-alpha36, a novel isoform of ER-alpha66, is commonly over-expressed in apocrine and adenoid cystic carcinomas of the breast. *J Clin Pathol.* 2011;64:54–57.

35. Mastropasqua MG, Maiorano E, Pruneri G, et al. Immunoreactivity for c-Kit and p63 as an adjunct in the diagnosis of adenoid cystic carcinoma of the breast. *Mod Pathol.* 2005;18:1277–1282.

36. Pastolero G, Hanna W, Zbieranowski I, et al. Proliferative activity and p53 expression in adenoid cystic carcinoma of the breast. *Mod Pathol.* 1996;9:215–219.

37. Crisi GM, Marconi SA, Makari-Judson G, et al. Expression of c-Kit in adenoid cystic carcinoma of the breast. *Am J Clin Pathol.* 2005;124:733–739.

38. Morice WG, Ferreiro JA. Distinction of basaloid squamous cell carcinoma from adenoid cystic and small cell undifferentiated carcinoma by immunohistochemistry. *Hum Pathol.* 1998;29:609–612.

39. Resetkova E, Albarracin C, Sneige N. Collagenous spherulosis of breast: morphologic study of 59 cases and review of the literature. *Am J Surg Pathol.* 2006;30:20–27.

40. Millar BA, Kerba M, Youngson B, et al. The potential role of breast conservation surgery and adjuvant breast radiation for adenoid cystic carcinoma of the breast. *Breast Cancer Res Treat.* 2004;87:225–232.

41. Coates JM, Martinez SR, Bold RJ, et al. Adjuvant radiation therapy is associated with improved survival for adenoid cystic carcinoma of the breast. *J Surg Oncol.* 2010;102:342–347.

42. Wells CA, Nicoll S, Ferguson DJ. Adenoid cystic carcinoma of the breast: a case with axillary lymph node metastasis. *Histopathology.* 1986;10:415–424.

43. Herzberg AJ, Bossen EH, Walther PJ. Adenoid cystic carcinoma of the breast metastatic to the kidney: a clinically symptomatic lesion requiring surgical management. *Cancer.* 1991;68:1015–1020.

44. Peters GN, Wolff M. Adenoid cystic carcinoma of the breast: report of 11 new cases: review of the literature and discussion of biological behavior. *Cancer.* 1983;52:680–686.

45. Koller M, Ram Z, Findler G, et al. Brain metastasis: a rare manifestation of adenoid cystic carcinoma of the breast. *Surg Neurol.* 1986;26:470–472.

46. Silva I, Tome V, Oliveira J. Adenoid cystic carcinoma of the breast with cerebral metastasis: a clinical novelty. *BMJ Case Rep.* 2011;2011.

17

Other Special Types of Invasive Ductal Carcinoma

FREDERICK C. KOERNER

INVASIVE MICROPAPILLARY CARCINOMA

Invasive micropapillary carcinoma is a distinctive form of ductal carcinoma in which the tumor cells grow in morule-like clusters creating an "exfoliative appearance" (1). This growth pattern may be found throughout the lesion (*pure invasive micropapillary carcinoma*) or as part of an otherwise conventional invasive ductal carcinoma (*mixed invasive micropapillary carcinoma*). Pure invasive micropapillary carcinomas account for 1% to 2% of the cases in two study groups, each consisting of approximately 1,000 breast carcinomas (2,3). Mixed invasive micropapillary carcinoma occurs more commonly. For example, Pettinato et al. (4) observed a micropapillary pattern in 3.8% of 1,635 breast carcinomas, and Luna-Moré et al. (5) detected micropapillary differentiation in 27 of 986 (2.7%) consecutive breast carcinomas. For practical purposes, one should reserve the category of pure invasive micropapillary carcinoma for those tumors in which at least 75% of the entire excised carcinoma demonstrates the characteristic micropapillary growth pattern. Needle core biopsy (NCB) specimens do not allow one to evaluate this criterion; so one can only suggest the diagnosis of invasive micropapillary carcinoma based on examination of such a specimen.

Clinical Presentation

The reported age at diagnosis ranges from 25 to 92 years, and the mean ages in several series fall in the sixth decade. Patients with lesions composed of more than 50% invasive micropapillary carcinoma tend to be older than patients with less extensive micropapillary growth (5). The literature contains only a few well-documented reports of pure invasive micropapillary carcinoma in men (6–8).

The majority of patients present with a palpable mass. Less frequently, screening mammography or other imaging reveals a suspicious density, an irregular mass, a region of calcifications, or another suspicious finding (9–11).

The reported carcinomas span from 0.1 to 11 cm. Tumors with more than 50% micropapillary growth tend to be larger (mean size 6 cm) than those with a lesser amount of this pattern (mean size 3.5 cm) (5). The presence of several nodules has been noted (4).

Microscopic Pathology

The invasive carcinoma cells are cuboidal to columnar and they contain finely granular or dense, eosinophilic cytoplasm. The nuclei usually display intermediate- to high-grade atypia. The tumor cells grow in small clusters, which have serrated peripheral borders and sometimes surround central lumina **(Fig. 17.1)**. The clusters lack fibrovascular cores and they exhibit an "inside-out" arrangement with the luminal aspect of the cell facing the outer surface of the cluster (12). A central clear space is often present, but solid groups may also occur. Uncommon variants feature microcystic dilatation of lumina within cell clusters and apocrine change. Mucin may be present in the tumor cells rarely. Necrosis and lymphocytic infiltration are not typical features; however, large tumors may undergo necrosis, and a lymphoid infiltrate may come to permeate the stroma. Microcalcifications, sometimes with psammomatous features, are variably present.

A clear space outlined by stroma surrounds each tumor cell cluster. Endothelial cells do not line these spaces, and they are usually attributed to shrinkage of the clusters during tissue fixation. The spaces generally appear empty, but in some instances mucinous material has been demonstrated using special stains (5). The stroma consists of dense collagenous tissue or a network of delicate collagen bundles. Myxoid stroma has been noted in a minority of cases (10). The sponge-like pattern of spaces filled by tumor cell clusters is duplicated in metastatic foci.

The proclivity of the carcinoma to grow in a sponge-like pattern makes it difficult to identify lymphatic tumor emboli in the vicinity of the primary tumor. By using antibodies to factor VIII and CD31 to mark vascular endothelium, Pettinato et al. (4) demonstrated vascular invasion in 63% of tumors. Intravascular carcinoma cells form papillary clusters identical to the invasive groups present in the mammary parenchyma.

Mixed invasive micropapillary carcinomas usually show a sharp demarcation between the micropapillary and conventional components. The latter usually has the conventional not otherwise specified (NOS) pattern, but invasive mucinous, lobular, cribriform, metaplastic, and tubular types have been reported (11,13–16).

Ductal carcinoma in situ (DCIS) coexists with the invasive carcinoma in most cases. In pure invasive micropapillary

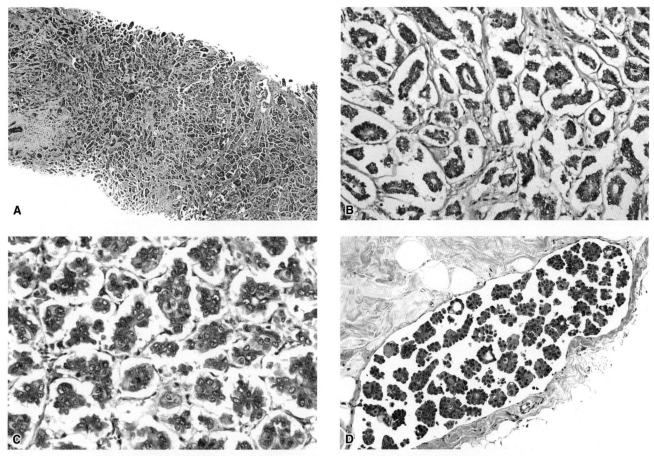

FIGURE 17.1 Invasive Micropapillary Carcinoma. A: This needle core biopsy specimen shows small nests of carcinoma cells outlined by clear spaces. **B, C:** The "inside-out" pattern consists of morule-like solid clusters of tumor cells with serrated outer borders. The spaces between the carcinoma cells and the stroma are devoid of secretion. **D:** Clusters of invasive micropapillary carcinoma occupy the lumen of a lymphatic vessel.

carcinoma, the DCIS usually has a micropapillary or cribriform architecture, but solid DCIS sometimes occurs. The noninvasive cells usually possess intermediate-grade, hyperchromatic nuclei unlike the bland nuclei characteristic of conventional micropapillary/cribriform DCIS. Prominent necrosis tends to occur in tumors with only a focal invasive micropapillary pattern, and the carcinoma cells in these cases usually have high-grade hyperchromatic nuclei. Calcifications are sometimes found in the noninvasive component.

Ultrastructure and Immunohistochemistry

Ultrastructural study has revealed microvilli on the cell surfaces that border the clear spaces. This finding suggests that the cells are oriented as though the spaces around the tumor cell clusters were glandular lumina (5). The distribution of MUC-1 glycoprotein and epithelial membrane antigen (EMA) supports this interpretation. MUC-1 localizes to the apical cell membrane in conventional, gland-forming breast carcinomas, where the glycoprotein contributes to the formation of lumina. In invasive micropapillary carcinoma, MUC-1 localizes on the external surfaces of papillary tumor clusters, adjacent to the surrounding stroma (17). The expression of EMA displays the same pattern

(5). This reversal of cell polarity has also been observed as a feature of intralymphatic clusters of carcinoma cells (18,19).

Most cases of invasive micropapillary carcinoma stain for E-cadherin, although Pettinato et al. (4) noted that reactivity was limited to cell membranes between carcinoma cells and that the cell membranes abutting the stroma did not stain. In one series (20), all 12 examples of invasive micropapillary carcinoma stained for GATA3. The tumors typically do not stain for CK5/6, CK14, CK20, EGFR, or c-kit. The majority of invasive micropapillary carcinomas stain for estrogen receptor (ER) and progesterone receptor (PR), and evidence of HER2 overexpression or gene amplification occurs in 10% to 50% of the cases (7,11,21).

Differential Diagnosis

The differential diagnosis of invasive micropapillary carcinoma includes conventional invasive breast carcinoma with prominent retraction of the malignant cells from the stroma and metastatic micropapillary carcinoma. The carcinoma cells in commonplace invasive carcinoma with prominent retraction artifact do not display the complete reversal of cell polarity characteristic of invasive micropapillary carcinoma, nor do conventional carcinoma cells with retraction artifact exhibit strong peripheral linear membrane staining for EMA. One can detect focal (less than 5% of the tumor area) peripheral linear membrane EMA staining in as many as 50% of conventional invasive carcinomas (22) and robust linear membrane staining in clusters of conventional carcinoma cells within lymphatic vessels (18,19). These observations make clear that one must interpret the results of staining for EMA carefully when evaluating a carcinoma whose appearance suggests the diagnosis of invasive micropapillary carcinoma.

The ovary represents the most common origin of metastatic micropapillary carcinoma in the breast. Other possible sites include the lung, urinary bladder, and colon. The presence of an intraductal component serves as strong evidence to exclude metastatic carcinoma. In the absence of an in situ component, immunohistochemical staining for CA125 and WT1 may help to distinguish metastatic ovarian serous carcinoma from a mammary carcinoma. Lee et al. (23) observed membranous staining for CA125 in 18% of invasive micropapillary breast carcinomas and cytoplasmic staining for the protein in 3% of the same group. This marker was identified in more than 90% of serous papillary ovarian carcinomas, usually in 80% to 100% of the cells. WT1 nuclear staining was found in 26% of invasive micropapillary carcinomas, typically in fewer than 10% of cells, and weak cytoplasmic staining, which usually required high magnification to detect, was seen in 59% of the tumors. Only 1 of 34 invasive micropapillary breast carcinomas displayed both nuclear reactivity for WT1 and cytoplasmic reactivity for CA125. The presence of diffuse nuclear expression of WT1 and strong staining for CA125 of a papillary carcinoma in the breast strongly favors the diagnosis of metastatic serous papillary carcinoma over the diagnosis of invasive micropapillary carcinoma. Detection of proteins suggestive of müllerian origin such as PAX8 and PAX2 or those typical of mammary origin such as mammaglobin and GATA3 (24,25) may also help to evaluate the possibility of metastatic serous carcinoma. The results of immunohistochemical staining for other markers and clinical investigations will usually exclude the diagnosis of metastatic carcinoma originating from the lung, urinary bladder, and other sites (25).

Uncommon examples of invasive micropapillary carcinoma feature the presence of abundant extracellular mucin. Pathologists may find it difficult to distinguish such tumors, termed *invasive micropapillary mucinous carcinoma*, from conventional mucinous carcinomas. The tumor cell clusters in conventional mucinous carcinoma usually exhibit a smooth outer contour rather than the serrated shape seen in invasive micropapillary carcinoma; furthermore, the cell clusters in the former do not display the "inside-out" micropapillary arrangement characteristic of the latter. To render the diagnosis of invasive micropapillary mucinous carcinoma, one should observe the typical features of invasive micropapillary carcinoma in at least 50% of the neoplastic cells in conjunction with the presence of a large amount of extracellular mucin.

Prognosis and Treatment

One has difficulty determining the prognosis of patients with invasive micropapillary carcinoma, because most studies have not separately analyzed data from pure and mixed forms, nor have the investigations taken into account many of the well-established prognostic parameters when comparing findings of invasive micropapillary carcinomas with those of conventional ductal carcinomas. Nonetheless, the accumulated experience indicates that invasive micropapillary carcinomas tend to be larger, that they more often have an intermediate or high histologic grade, and that they have a higher likelihood of metastasis to local lymph nodes than do conventional breast carcinomas (26). Despite these ominous features, the 5-year disease-specific survival and overall survival of patients with invasive micropapillary carcinoma did not differ from those of patients with conventional breast carcinoma in a large study using the SEER database (26). In one study (16), patients with stage I invasive micropapillary mucinous carcinoma experienced the same overall survival and recurrence-free survival as patients with pure conventional mucinous carcinoma. Patients with higher-stage (II and III) invasive micropapillary mucinous carcinoma had survival rates between those of patients with pure mucinous carcinoma and conventional invasive micropapillary carcinoma.

Because of the propensity of micropapillary carcinoma to spread to axillary lymph nodes, careful staging of the axilla is recommended. Recommendations for treatment would usually follow those for conventional invasive ductal carcinomas.

CRIBRIFORM CARCINOMA

Invasive cribriform carcinoma consists of well-differentiated ductal carcinoma cells growing in cribriform and tubular patterns. Published information does not allow one to determine whether invasive cribriform carcinoma represents a low-grade variant of invasive ductal carcinoma or a specific subtype of carcinoma. One should distinguish two subtypes of invasive cribriform carcinoma: *classic invasive cribriform carcinoma*, in which the invasive carcinoma exhibits a cribriform pattern with or without tubular elements, and *mixed invasive cribriform carcinoma*, in which less than 50% of the mass has an invasive cribriform pattern and the majority displays neither cribriform nor tubular patterns. Fewer than 6% of invasive mammary carcinomas are invasive cribriform carcinomas, and classic and mixed forms account for approximately equal proportions (27–30).

Clinical Presentation

The ages of the female patients range from 7 to 91 years. Two reported patients were men (28,31). Choi et al. (32) described a 6-cm invasive cribriform carcinoma occupying a 10-cm malignant phyllodes tumor in a 62-year-old woman.

In a study of eight cases, mammograms revealed spiculated masses spanning 20 to 35 mm in four patients (33). Two of these carcinomas contained calcifications, and so did the carcinoma described by Nishimura et al. (31). Invasive cribriform carcinomas do not have consistent sonographic findings (31,33,34). Magnetic resonance imaging (MRI) performed on one tumor

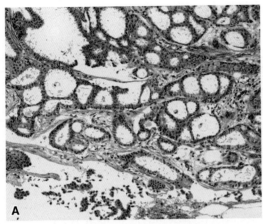
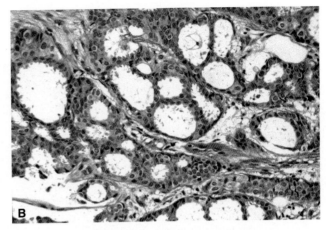

FIGURE 17.2 **Invasive Cribriform Carcinoma. A, B:** The invasive carcinoma in this needle core biopsy specimen has a cribriform structure composed of round or oval glandular spaces formed by thin, rigid bands of tumor cells with low-grade nuclei.

displayed findings compatible with a carcinoma (34). Data from three studies suggest that a small number of invasive cribriform carcinomas occur as multifocal masses (27,29,30).

Microscopic Pathology

Invasive cribriform carcinoma exhibits the same sieve-like growth pattern that characterizes conventional cribriform DCIS. The rounded and angular masses of uniform, well-differentiated tumor cells are embedded in variable amounts of collagenous stroma. Sharply outlined, round, or oval glandular spaces are distributed throughout these tumor aggregates, creating a fenestrated appearance **(Fig. 17.2)**. Variable amounts of mucin-positive secretion occupies the lumina (35), which may also contain calcifications (36). The in situ component has a cribriform pattern in most, but not all, classic invasive cribriform carcinomas.

Besides displaying a cribriform pattern, invasive cribriform carcinomas can show areas of tubular growth **(Fig. 17.3)**, and such foci can comprise a substantial proportion of the lesion (28–30). The presence of regions showing a tubular pattern does not itself justify the use of the diagnosis of tubular carcinoma. Tumors composed of both cribriform and tubular areas in which the cribriform pattern accounts for more than 25% of the mass should be classified as invasive cribriform carcinomas rather than tubular carcinomas. When the tubular pattern represents more than 75% of the mass, one could consider the diagnosis of tubular carcinoma if the cytologic and architectural features of the tubules seem appropriate. Most NCB specimens do not provide sufficient material to allow one to evaluate the proportions of these two patterns.

Immunohistochemistry

Venable et al. (28) reported that 16 of 16 classic and mixed invasive cribriform carcinomas were ER-positive and that 11 of the tumors (69%) were PR-positive. The classic and mixed cribriform carcinomas did not differ appreciably in their degrees of PR positivity. Other case reports describe positive staining for ER, variable staining for PR, and lack of staining for HER2 (31,37,38), although Zhang et al. (29) noted staining of one carcinoma for HER2.

Differential Diagnosis

Invasive cribriform carcinoma should be distinguished from adenoid cystic carcinoma. Cribriform growth of an invasive cribriform carcinoma produces a fenestrated structural pattern that lacks the cylindromatous components composed of basal lamina material characteristic of adenoid cystic carcinoma. Although adenoid cystic carcinomas can contain regions showing prominent cribriform gland formation, (39) one should not interpret the presence of such regions in an adenoid cystic carcinoma as evidence of a component of invasive cribriform carcinoma. Carcinomas with osteoclast-like giant cells often demonstrate regions showing a cribriform growth pattern (37). One should classify such tumors as carcinomas with osteoclast-like giant cells.

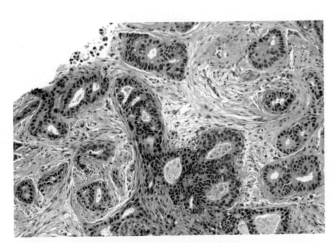

FIGURE 17.3 **Invasive Cribriform Carcinoma.** In the region shown, the cribriform carcinoma in this needle core biopsy specimen has tubular features.

Prognosis and Treatment

The majority of patients described in published reports were treated by mastectomy and axillary dissection. The authors of three studies concluded that patients with classic invasive cribriform carcinoma were less likely to develop axillary lymph node metastases than women with mixed invasive cribriform carcinoma (29,30) or ordinary invasive ductal carcinoma (28,29). One case report (38) documents spread to an internal mammary lymph node without involvement of the axillary sentinel lymph node. Nodal metastases from classic tumors usually also have a cribriform structure, whereas metastases derived from mixed tumors are more likely to lack a cribriform pattern (28,30).

Deaths attributable to classic invasive cribriform carcinoma did not occur among 34 patients studied by Page et al. (30) with follow-up intervals of 10 to 21 years. One patient was alive with recurrent classic invasive cribriform carcinoma, and another died of metastases from a contralateral carcinoma. Venable et al. (28) reported a disease-free survival of 100% among 45 patients with classic invasive cribriform carcinoma followed up for 1 to 5 years. In the study of Cong et al. (40), one of eight patients with classic invasive cribriform carcinoma developed a local recurrence, but the other seven remained free of carcinoma with a median follow-up time of 38 months.

Using the SEER database, Liu et al. (41) compared clinical and pathologic findings of more than 600 invasive cribriform carcinomas with those of conventional invasive ductal carcinomas. The investigators found that invasive cribriform carcinomas were smaller, more often grade 1, less likely to involve lymph nodes, more often positive for ER and PR, and less often positive for HER2 than were conventional invasive carcinomas. Approximately 60% of patients in this study were treated with breast-conservation therapy. Patients with invasive cribriform carcinoma experienced greater disease-specific survival and overall survival than those with conventional carcinomas. The improvement in survival appears to depend on the more favorable staging and receptor profile associated with invasive cribriform carcinoma. When corrected for these confounding features, patients with invasive cribriform carcinoma did not show more favorable survival than those with conventional carcinomas.

The foregoing data suggest that breast-conservation therapy is feasible if an adequate excision can be performed, but the possibility of encountering multifocal lesions should be borne in mind. Axillary staging by sentinel lymph node mapping is appropriate.

SECRETORY CARCINOMA

Secretory carcinoma features the presence of abundant, pale pink or amphophilic secretory material within the cytoplasm of the carcinoma cells and the lumina of the spaces formed by the carcinoma cells. Although secretory carcinoma occurs in children, the majority of cases occur in adults. Consequently, the term "secretory" is preferable to the original designation, "juvenile." The cellular characteristics of the lesion are identical in patients of all ages.

Clinical Presentation

Secretory carcinoma affects individuals throughout life; only the very young escape the disease. The reported ages of females with secretory carcinoma range from 3 to 91 years (42–44). Male patients exhibit a similar age range (3–79 years) (45–47). There is a dearth of cases of secretory carcinoma in girls 10 to 15 years of age, and cases in males cluster in the pediatric and adolescent age groups.

Most patients describe a painless, circumscribed mass that may have been present for one or more years. A subareolar tumor is most common in prepubertal girls and males of all ages because their breast tissue is localized in this region; however, even among women, the central region of the breast stands out as a favored location. Secretory carcinoma usually grows as a single mass, but rare cases present with two or more nodules (48–50). Secretory carcinomas have arisen in axillary breast tissue (51,52) and from adnexal glands of the axillary skin (53).

Pregnancy has not been implicated in the development of secretory carcinoma, nor has clinical evidence of a hormonal abnormality that would explain the secretory properties of the carcinoma been described. Secretory carcinoma developed in the breast of a male-to-female transgender individual, who had undergone "long-term cross-sex hormone treatment" of an unspecified nature (54).

Associated breast conditions have been described in a few cases. Gynecomastia accompanied a minority of the secretory carcinomas in male patients. The coexistence of juvenile papillomatosis and secretory carcinoma has been reported (55), but the evidence presented to substantiate the diagnosis of juvenile papillomatosis is not convincing in several other reports.

Mammography typically reveals a discrete tumor with smooth or irregular borders (48,56,57), which one could mistake for a fibroadenoma or papilloma. Sonography discloses a solid, hypoechoic to isoechoic mass, which may have a microlobulated border (48,58).

Secretory carcinoma usually forms a circumscribed, firm mass, which may be lobulated; rarely, the tumor has infiltrative margin. The tumors tend to be 3 cm or fewer in diameter (59), although carcinomas spanning 10 cm were reported in two women (60,61) and another spanning 12.5 cm tumor was reported in a man (62).

Microscopic Pathology

Like other forms of ductal carcinoma, secretory carcinoma may exhibit an intraductal component. Kameyama et al. (57) described a purely noninvasive form of secretory carcinoma. Most commonly, the DCIS has a papillary or cribriform (57) pattern of growth, but solid foci and, rarely, comedonecrosis may also be found. The invasive component tends to form a compact mass subdivided by fibrous septa. The borders of the carcinoma usually appear circumscribed, but overtly infiltrative

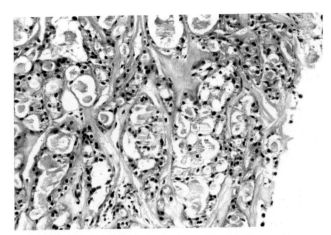

FIGURE 17.4 Secretory Carcinoma. This needle core biopsy specimen comes from a circumscribed 2-cm tumor in a 68-year-old woman. The carcinoma has the characteristic microcystic architecture. The tumor cells in this example have small, low-grade nuclei.

growth is sometimes present. The neoplastic cells grow in papillary, microcystic, and glandular formations.

The tumor cells vary from secretory to apocrine in their appearance. Cells of a secretory nature possess pale to clear, pink or amphophilic cytoplasm that contains abundant secretion. The low-grade nuclei vary from small to modest in size, and their chromatin from dark and finely dispersed to pale and granular (**Fig. 17.4**). Nuclei with pale chromatin usually contain small, uniform nucleoli. Cells with apocrine features contain granular, eosinophilic cytoplasm and nuclei with features similar to those of conventional apocrine cells (**Fig. 17.5**). One usually finds both types of cells in a carcinoma, although one type or the other can predominate. On occasion, cells with apocrine features growing in a solid pattern comprise most of the tumor and thereby obscure the secretory nature of the carcinoma. The cells do not display noticeable mitotic activity or necrosis. One does not usually find microcalcifications in the neoplastic glands or the stroma.

Secretion accumulates in the tumor cells, in the glands formed by the tumor cells, and in the microcystic spaces associated with the tumor cells. The secretory material appears pale pink or amphophilic with H&E staining, and it often contains lacunae, which create a "bubbly" appearance. The secretion stains with the periodic acid–Schiff (PAS) and Alcian blue methods, and PAS staining persists after diastase digestion. The secretory material reacts variably for mucin. The secretion in microcystic areas resembles thyroid colloid

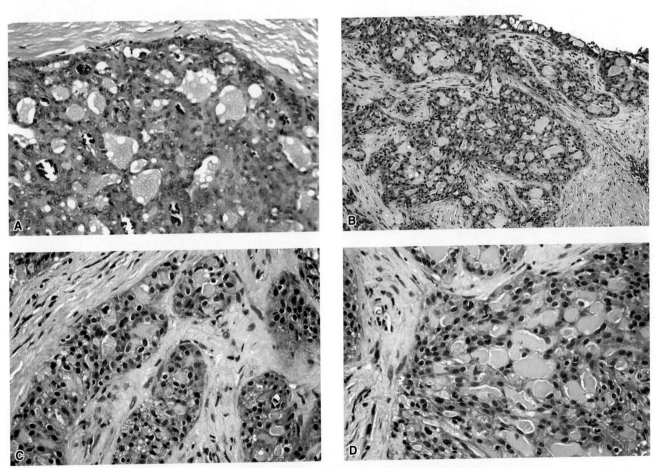

FIGURE 17.5 Secretory Carcinoma with Apocrine Cytology. A: The lesion has a well-circumscribed border and a microcystic growth pattern. The nuclei have prominent nucleoli typically associated with apocrine differentiation. **B–D:** Secretory carcinoma in needle core biopsy samples from a 41-year-old woman. Note the apocrine cytologic features, the irregular shapes of the microcystic spaces, and the dense secretions.

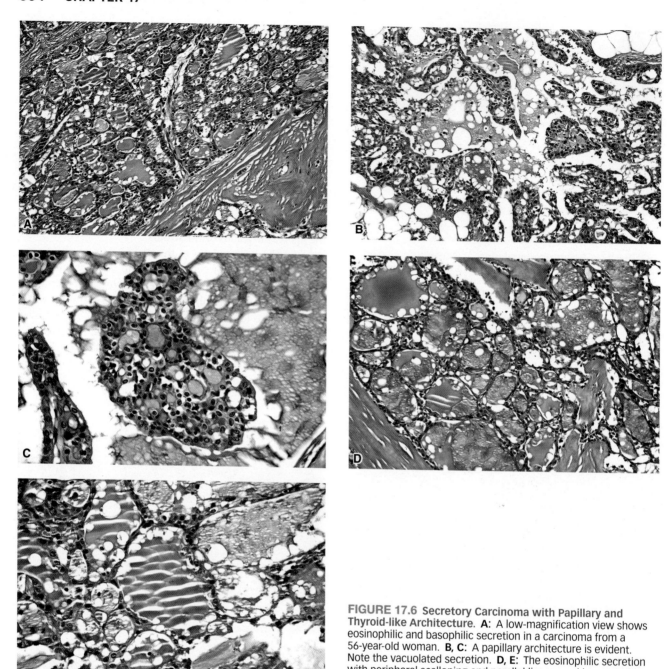

FIGURE 17.6 Secretory Carcinoma with Papillary and Thyroid-like Architecture. A: A low-magnification view shows eosinophilic and basophilic secretion in a carcinoma from a 56-year-old woman. **B, C:** A papillary architecture is evident. Note the vacuolated secretion. **D, E:** The eosinophilic secretion with peripheral scalloping and parallel linear cracking resembles thyroid colloid and the secretion in cystic hypersecretory lesions of the breast.

and the secretion that accumulates in cystic hypersecretory lesions of the breast **(Fig. 17.6)**.

Differential Diagnosis

Pathologists should not have difficulty recognizing secretory carcinoma when they have sufficient material to study. It may require an excision of the mass to provide an adequate sample, but the diagnosis can be suspected in a needle aspiration or NCB specimen (48). Other lesions to consider include acinic cell carcinoma, cystic hypersecretory carcinoma (CHC), apocrine carcinoma, and microglandular adenosis.

Mammary acinic cell carcinoma (63) is composed of cells with abundant granular cytoplasm in solid, microglandular, and microcystic formations. The cells stain for salivary-type amylase, a protein not characteristic of secretory carcinomas, but acinic cell carcinomas fail to demonstrate the vacuolar and punctate staining for acidophilin seen in secretory carcinomas (64). In most CHCs, DCIS constitutes either the exclusive or the dominant component. It gives rise to dilated ducts and acini lined by cells that possess intermediate- to high-grade nuclei and lack prominent cytoplasmic vacuolization. Apocrine carcinomas do not demonstrate the evidence of secretory activity seen in secretory carcinomas. Microglandular adenosis consists of an orderly proliferation of uniform small, round glands displaying open lumina, lined by small uniform cells with bland nuclei, and encircled by basement membrane.

Immunohistochemistry and Molecular Studies

To the extent that it can be determined from the reported data, the results of staining for cellular markers do not differ among secretory carcinomas from females and males nor among tumors from children and adults. Strong staining for α-lactalbumin has been reported (65). The carcinoma cells stain for cytokeratin, EMA, E-cadherin, mammaglobin and, with rare exceptions (61,66), S-100 protein. One report (67) documents nuclear staining for p63 in three of seven cases and staining of the cytoplasm and secretory material for p63 in the remaining four cases. The latter observation may reflect the secretory nature of the carcinoma cells. Variable reactivity for carcinoembryonic antigen (CEA) and GCDFP-15 has been observed, and stains for proteins indicative of endocrine, muscle, and melanocytic differentiation have been negative.

Most secretory carcinomas lack ER and PR. Three carcinomas did not express the androgen receptor (45,54,68). Strong expression of HER2 protein has been detected in one secretory carcinoma (50).

Tognon et al. (69) and Euhus et al. (70) described the presence of the *ETV6-NTRK3* fusion gene, a gene previously detected in congenital fibrosarcoma and congenital cellular mesoblastic nephroma, in secretory carcinomas (see Chapter 26). Using fluorescence in situ hybridization, sequencing of reverse transcription polymerase chain reaction (RT-PCR) products, and immunoprecipitation, evidence of this oncoprotein was found in 12 of 13 (92%) secretory carcinomas and in only 1 of 50 (2%) of invasive ductal carcinomas (69). The single conventional invasive carcinoma that demonstrated fusion transcripts contained regions with features suggestive of secretory carcinoma. Testing of other cases of secretory carcinoma and of commonplace breast carcinomas has confirmed the presence of this fusion gene in most secretory carcinomas and the absence of the gene in conventional breast carcinomas (71) and several other lesions with features similar to those of secretory carcinoma (64).

STAT5a, a mammary growth factor, is one of several molecules involved in the transcription of differentiation proteins. Activation of STAT5a in the breast occurs largely as a result of the binding of prolactin to its receptor (72). STAT5a expression is present in the majority of normal mammary gland cells and largely absent in atypical ductal hyperplasia and carcinoma (73). Overexpression of STAT5a occurs in physiologic secretory and lactating mammary epithelium as well as in secretory mammary carcinoma (74).

Prognosis and Treatment

Axillary lymph node metastases have been observed in approximately one-third of all patients (59), but the risk in males is approximately 50% (47). The risk of nodal involvement in children is at least as great as it is in adults (46,75). The metastatic deposits rarely involve more than three lymph nodes. Metastatic foci display the characteristics features of secretory carcinoma. Sentinel lymph node mapping can be an effective method for studying the axilla.

In the majority of patients, secretory carcinoma has an indolent clinical course resulting in an exceptionally favorable prognosis. A study using the SEER database revealed a 10-year cause-specific survival of 91.4% (59). The treatment of secretory carcinoma is surgical, but the extent of surgery and the use of adjuvant therapies remain undetermined. In earlier times, most adult patients were treated with mastectomy, whereas excision was the preferred initial treatment in children (75). Local recurrence in residual breast tissue after a mastectomy has been reported (76). Currently, in postmenarchal girls and women, wide local excision will suffice for small lesions, but quadrantectomy may be necessary to obtain negative margins around larger tumors. Because of the small size of the male breast, surgical excision usually constitutes a mastectomy. The value of postoperative irradiation and adjuvant systemic therapy, radiotherapy, and chemotherapy in the treatment of recurrent or metastatic secretory carcinoma not has been determined.

CYSTIC HYPERSECRETORY CARCINOMA

First described by Rosen and Scott (77), cystic hypersecretory carcinoma (CHC) displays cysts containing eosinophilic secretory material bearing a striking resemblance to thyroid colloid. The majority of cases have been DCIS.

Clinical Presentation

The age distribution of CHC ranges from 34 to 79 years. The mean age falls in the sixth or seventh decade (78,79). All patients, including one African-American, (80) have been women. The presenting symptom is usually a mass or other palpable abnormality. Nipple discharge occurs rarely and can appear bloody (81). Paget disease of the nipple was present in one case (82).

Radiologic imaging has not revealed distinctive findings. Mammograms of cases with invasive components have shown a region of increased density with trabecular thickening (80), a prominent ductal pattern and an irregular density (83), and spiculated masses with calcifications (84). Sonography in one case revealed "...multiple small aggregated anechoic cysts with good through transmission" (85).

To the unaided eye, CHC displays cysts measuring as much as 1.5 cm. Prosectors have described the secretion within cysts as sticky, mucinous, gelatinous, and resembling thyroid colloid. An invasive component associated with CHC produces a distinct solid mass.

Microscopic Pathology

The microscopic hallmark of all types of cystic hypersecretory lesions is the presence of cysts that contain eosinophilic

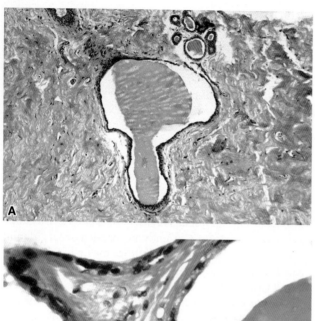

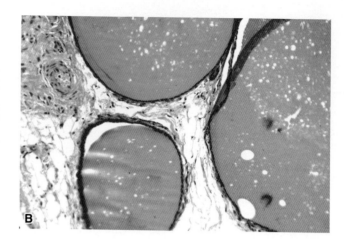

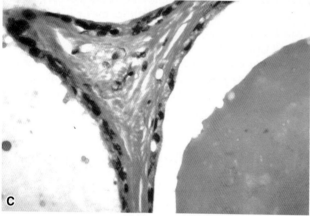

FIGURE 17.7 Cystic Hypersecretory Hyperplasia. A, B: The dilated ducts in two needle core biopsy specimens contain dense, eosinophilic secretion, which retracts from the inconspicuous epithelium. The secretion has developed cracks and small punctate holes. **C:** The cystic spaces are lined by single layers of flat cells.

secretion similar in appearance to thyroid colloid (**Fig. 17.7**). The homogeneous and virtually acellular secretion often retracts from the surrounding epithelium, resulting in a smooth or scalloped margin duplicating the contour of the epithelial proliferation. Folds, linear cracks, or small punched out holes occur in the secretion. Positive reactions of the cyst contents for CEA, α-lactalbumin, and mucin have been observed.

The secretion stains with the PAS method but does not stain for thyroglobulin. Disruption of cysts results in discharge of their contents into the stroma, eliciting an intense inflammatory reaction consisting of lymphocytes, histiocytes, and sometimes giant cells.

In CHC, the epithelium of involved cysts and ducts grows as micropapillary DCIS (**Fig. 17.8**). One often observes a

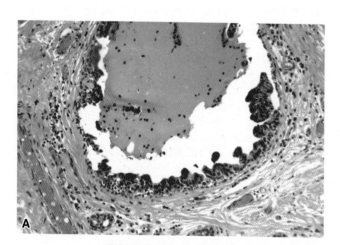

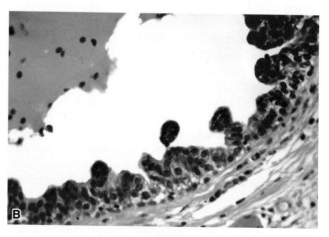

FIGURE 17.8 Cystic Hypersecretory Ductal Carcinoma In Situ. A, B: Low micropapillary fronds line the wall of this dilated duct. The retracted eosinophilic secretion has a scalloped border. **C:** In this micropapillary DCIS, an area of flat growth merges with a region composed of elongated micropapillary fronds. As depicted in this example, the almost complete absence of secretion can be encountered in foci of florid cystic hypersecretory DCIS.

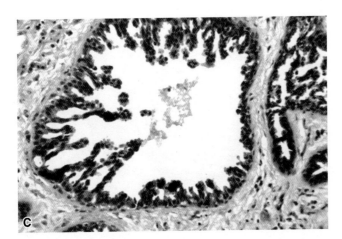

FIGURE 17.8 *(continued)*

spectrum of architectural patterns of the noninvasive component within a single case. The formations range from short, knobby epithelial tufts to complex branching fronds, which may traverse the duct lumen. The so-called Roman arch, or bridging pattern, commonly seen in other forms of micropapillary DCIS is uncommon in hypersecretory lesions, but the solid pattern can occur. One observes fibrovascular stroma within the micropapillary fronds only rarely. Ducts with DCIS may not contain the characteristic colloid-like secretion.

The cells in the fronds of micropapillary DCIS have crowded, hyperchromatic nuclei with sparse cytoplasm. The nuclei display an intermediate or high grade, they usually have irregular contours and easily seen nucleoli, and they may contain intranuclear inclusions. One does not see secretory material within the cytoplasm of the tumor cells, but the presence of frayed, apical cell borders and cytoplasmic blebs suggests a degree of secretory activity. Calcifications form within ducts in many cases.

Invasive CHC consists of intraductal CHC accompanied by an invasive component. Most invasive carcinomas encountered in this setting have been poorly differentiated ductal carcinomas with a solid growth pattern. The nuclei in the invasive

carcinoma cells usually have a clear vacuolated appearance similar to that of the cells in papillary thyroid carcinoma. Scattered lymphocytes often mingle with the invasive carcinoma (81). The carcinoma cells do not display noticeable evidence of secretory activity. The metastases in the axillary lymph nodes of two patients displayed cystic elements that contained eosinophilic secretions (78).

Cystic hypersecretory carcinoma usually coexists with other cystic hypersecretory lesions, most commonly *cystic hypersecretory hyperplasia* (CHH) (78,79). In this lesion, orderly columnar epithelial cells with round to oval vesicular nuclei and eosinophilic cytoplasm, often with apical blebs, line the cysts **(Fig. 17.9)**. When the lining cells display cytologic atypia, the lesion is termed *cystic hypersecretory hyperplasia with atypia*. Atypical features in this setting are epithelial crowding sometimes resulting in micropapillary hyperplasia, hyperchromasia, and enlargement of nuclei, which may contain nucleoli **(Fig. 17.10)**. One occasionally observes cysts lined by a single layer of inconspicuous, flat, cuboidal, or low columnar cells with bland nuclei and scant cytoplasm. This form of cystic hypersecretory lesion, referred to as *cystic hypersecretory change*, does not commonly coexist with CHC.

The finding of areas with the typical features of CHH, sometimes with atypia, associated with CHC suggests that these processes are related, but convincing evidence of progression through these stages has not been observed, yet. Review of prior biopsies from women with CHC has disclosed various lesions, including seemingly unrelated common proliferative changes as well as CHH and CHC. Follow-up of eight patients with CHH revealed subsequent breast carcinoma in two cases. One woman developed a fatal contralateral invasive ductal carcinoma that lacked cystic hypersecretory features. The other patient had DCIS separate from CHH in a biopsy specimen and residual CHH in the mastectomy specimen. Bogomoletz (86) described a 55-year-old woman who was well without recurrence 6 years after excision of a 7-cm focus of CHH.

The mammary lobules adjacent to cystic hypersecretory lesions often exhibit hypersecretory changes that include the accumulation of secretion in lobular gland lumina. This

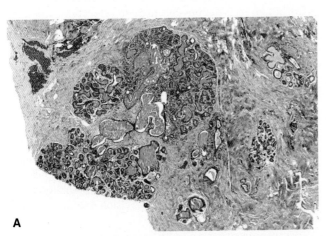

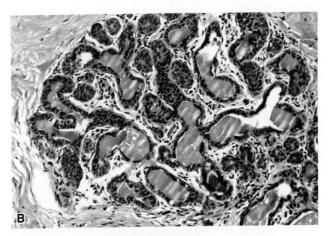

FIGURE 17.9 **Cystic Hypersecretory Hyperplasia in Lobules. A, B:** The characteristic eosinophilic secretion is present in the terminal ducts and lobular glands in this needle core biopsy specimen.

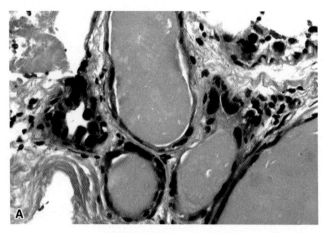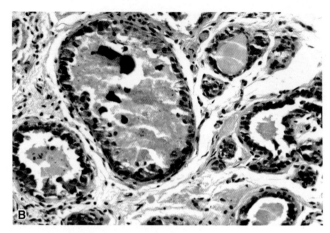

FIGURE 17.10 Cystic Hypersecretory Hyperplasia with Atypia. A: The cells in this cystic hypersecretory lesion have hyperchromatic, pleomorphic nuclei. **B:** Cells with hyperchromatic, enlarged nuclei are present in this atypical cystic hypersecretory lesion. Calcifications like those in one cyst are not present in this condition often.

lobular abnormality may occur as an isolated finding in the absence of a fully developed cystic hypersecretory lesion, an observation that suggests that hypersecretory lesions may originate in such foci.

A few examples of intraductal CHC have been encountered in which there is pronounced vacuolization of the cytoplasm of the carcinoma cells and secretion, a pattern reminiscent of pregnancy-like hyperplasia (PLH). Secretion of the type found in a cystic hypersecretory lesion may be found in glands lined by epithelium showing the appearance of pregnancy-like hyperplasia. Moreover, one occasionally encounters cases wherein CHH or CHC and PLH coexist, and aspects of the two conditions seem to overlap when this occurs (87,88). This convergence is usually marked by cytologic and structural atypia that may be severe. Rarely, the proliferative and cytologic abnormalities warrant a diagnosis of CHC that has features of PLH (87). The relationship between cystic hypersecretory lesions and PLH has not been elucidated.

Immunohistochemistry

In the small number of cases of CHC studied, the carcinoma cells have not stained for CK5 or CK14 (79). Many of the tumors stained for ER, and a lesser number stained for PR (79,81). Three of ten cases in one report (81) stained for androgen receptor. Two of the associated invasive carcinomas showed overexpression of HER2 (81). Staining for p63, smooth muscle myosin heavy chain, and CK5 failed to detect myoepithelial cells around the cysts in one case of CHC and another of CHH (79).

Differential Diagnosis

The differential diagnosis of CHC includes fibrocystic changes (FCCs), conventional micropapillary DCIS, juvenile papillomatosis (JP), and secretory carcinoma. The eosinophilic secretions that fill cysts of FCC do not stain as densely as the contents of the cysts in cystic hypersecretory lesions; furthermore, the former lack the scalloping and linear cracking characteristic

of the latter. Lipid-laden histiocytes usually sit in the cysts of FCC, but they do not do so in hypersecretory cysts. Cells lining the cysts of FCC do not display the atypia demonstrated by the cells of CHC. The usual examples of micropapillary DCIS do not contain secretions like those seen in CHC, and the carcinoma cells display a low nuclei grade, in contrast to the intermediate or high grade of the nuclei seen in CHC. The intraductal component of CHC grows in a predominantly micropapillary architecture and does not blend with areas showing a cribriform pattern as conventional micropapillary DCIS does. The large cysts seen in JP contain secretory material like that seen in FCC. The benign apocrine cells and bland ductal cells lining the cysts of JP do not resemble the atypical cells seen in CHC. Secretory carcinoma is a low-grade carcinoma in which eosinophilic secretions accumulate within cells and in microcystic spaces created by the carcinoma cells. The tumor cells contain the characteristic *ETV6-NTRK3* fusion gene.

Prognosis and Treatment

Excision of the abnormality is required if CHH is present in a NCB, because it is not possible to exclude focal carcinoma on the basis of such a sample. Some lesions have been misclassified as cystic disease, and the true nature of the process became apparent only after the lesion recurred (77,83).

The clinical course of intraductal CHC does not differ from that of other forms of DCIS thus far. All patients had negative lymph nodes. Therapeutic options for women with noninvasive CHC are similar to those available for women with other forms of DCIS. There have been only rare recurrences in women treated by mastectomy alone after a mean follow-up of 8 years and extending in one case to 23 years (78,81). Breast recurrence has also been reported after excision alone. Too few patients have been treated by excision and radiotherapy to assess this form of treatment.

Because several women with invasive CHC had metastases in axillary lymph nodes (78,81), sentinel node mapping is indicated when invasive carcinoma is present. A patient who presented with locally advanced or inflammatory carcinoma and died of her carcinoma 9 months later stands as the single reported death from CHC (78) to date. In view of the poorly differentiated character of these tumors, adjuvant chemotherapy would be prudent when invasive carcinoma is present.

MAMMARY CARCINOMA WITH OSTEOCLAST-LIKE GIANT CELLS

One can detect benign, osteoclast-like giant cells as a component of several otherwise conventional types of mammary carcinoma. The presence of these cells defines such a carcinoma as *mammary carcinoma with osteoclast-like giant cells*. Since the first series was published in 1979, (89) more than 200 examples of this type of mammary carcinoma have been reported.

Clinical Presentation

The clinical features are similar to those of breast carcinoma generally. Patients' ages range from 28 to 88 years, and the average age at diagnosis in the largest series is 43.8 years (90). One reported case affected a man (90). Multifocal lesions were clinically described in three cases (91,92). Bilateral primary carcinomas with osteoclast-like giant cells are exceedingly rare (90,93).

On mammography and ultrasonography, the well-circumscribed margin of most tumors may bring to mind a benign lesion such as a cyst or a fibroadenoma (92,94,95). MRI of one carcinoma exhibited "rich vascularity, especially in the periphery" (96).

Reported diameters range from 0.5 to 10 cm. The mean size in one series is 1.7 cm (90). The dark brown or red-brown color of most examples presents a striking macroscopic appearance (97). Tumors with relatively few osteoclast-like giant cells or with little hemorrhage may appear tan or white.

Microscopic Pathology

Most of these lesions are invasive ductal carcinomas of no special type (**Fig. 17.11**). The publication of Zhou et al. (90) tabulates the types of carcinomas showing osteoclast-like giant cells in 112 published cases. A cribriform growth pattern

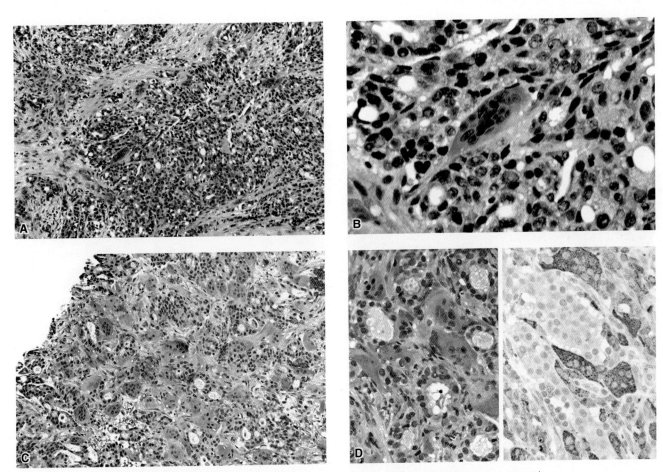

FIGURE 17.11 Carcinoma with Osteoclast-like Giant Cells. A, B: One can see scattered multinucleate osteoclast-like giant cells in this invasive, poorly differentiated ductal carcinoma. The tumor shown in this needle core biopsy specimen is unusual because it lacks the typical stromal elements, which include erythrocytes, hemosiderin, and lymphocytes. **C:** The invasive ductal carcinoma in another needle core biopsy specimen contains many osteoclast-like giant cells nestled among the neoplastic glands. Extravasated erythrocytes populate the stroma. **D:** The nuclei of the osteoclast-like giant cells differ from those of the neoplastic cells (**left panel**). The osteoclast-like giant cells stain for KP1 (**right panel**).

occurs relatively more often than among ductal carcinomas generally, and metaplastic carcinomas constitute another frequently seen type (90,98–101). Uncommon patterns include well-differentiated (**Fig. 17.12**) or tubular (99,102), lobular (89,93,95), squamous, papillary (89), apocrine, mucinous (103), neuroendocrine (104,105), and pure invasive micropapillary (106) carcinomas. Rarely, the carcinoma has a glandular pattern reminiscent of that of infiltrating colonic carcinoma. When present, the DCIS has the appearance of one of the conventional variants, usually cribriform, solid, or papillary. Osteoclast-like giant cells are not always present in the associated DCIS. It is very uncommon to find osteoclast-like giant cells in DCIS in the absence of an invasive lesion (107).

The osteoclast-like giant cells range from 20 to 180 μ in diameter, and they number from fewer than 1 to more than 10 per high-power field. The giant cells contain abundant cytoplasm and many evenly distributed and usually centrally located oval nuclei, some of which contain small nucleoli. The giant cells tend to cluster close to the edges of carcinomatous glands or in the intervening stroma, and they may be found in the glandular lumina. The stroma typically contains mononuclear histiocytes whose cytologic features resemble those of the multinuclear cells. The extravasated erythrocytes and hemosiderin, which one finds in the vascular stroma in most cases, reflect repeated episodes of hemorrhage. Erythrophagocytosis by the giant cells is uncommon, and they contain little hemosiderin detectable by light microscopy. Fibroblastic reaction, collagenization, angiogenesis, and lymphocytic infiltration are variably present.

Immunohistochemistry

The immunohistochemical profile of the carcinoma cells depends on the type of the carcinoma. The malignant cells typically stain for keratin, and they often stain for EMA. Staining for CEA, ER, PR, GCDFP-15, and HER2 has yielded variable results. The carcinoma cells in several tumors demonstrated high levels of PR (92,94,99). In one group of tumors in which the carcinoma was of no special type (90), all of the 36 cases demonstrate a luminal phenotype (ER$^+$ and/or PR$^+$).

The giant cells stain for proteins characteristic of macrophages such as α_1-antitrypsin and CD68 and for proteins found in osteoclasts such as acid phosphatase and, especially, tartrate-resistant acid phosphatase. These results suggest that the giant cells represent a specific type of histiocyte with osteoclastic features.

Differential Diagnosis

The differential diagnosis includes several noncarcinomatous lesions. Megakaryocytes in myeloid metaplasia in the breast might be mistaken for osteoclast-like giant cells, but these lesions have abundant myeloid elements in various stages of maturation, a feature not found in carcinomas with osteoclast-like

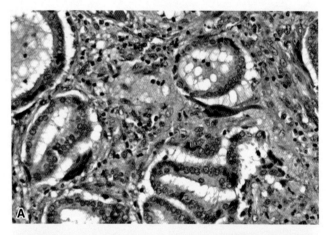

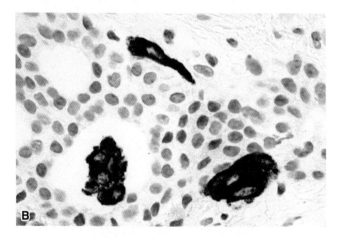

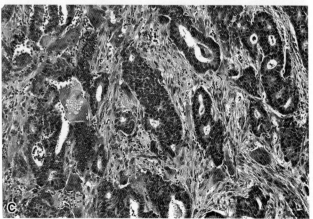

FIGURE 17.12 Carcinomas with Osteoclast-like Giant Cells. A: This infiltrating ductal carcinoma with osteoclast-like giant cells has a well-differentiated glandular pattern and the characteristic stroma. The giant cells are attenuated and apposed to the outer surfaces of the glands. **B:** Osteoclast-like giant cells in and around the carcinoma glands are KP1-positive. **C:** The stroma of this low-grade invasive ductal carcinoma with a cribriform structure contains osteoclast-like giant cells and many red blood cells.

giant cells. Granulomatous foci in inflammatory conditions such as sarcoidosis or coexistent with carcinoma also contain giant cells. Because the giant cells in these situations do not resemble osteoclasts and the lesions have a granulomatous pattern, one can distinguish mammary carcinoma with osteoclast-like giant cells from sarcoid or tuberculoid reactions without difficulty in histologic sections. The multinucleated giant cells in the nonspecialized stroma, which occasionally occur as an incidental finding, lack the relatively abundant cytoplasm seen in the osteoclast-like giant cells associated with mammary carcinomas.

Osteoclast-like giant cells are found in some but not all metastases. The presence of osteoclast-like giant cells within intralymphatic carcinomatous emboli (94) suggests that these stromal cells can be transported to regional lymph nodes and to distant metastases.

Prognosis and Treatment

Primary treatment in many retrospective reports was mastectomy with axillary dissection, but breast conservation with radiotherapy has been used more recently (90). Axillary lymph node metastases have been reported in a small proportion of cases, and metastases in the lungs and other sites have also been reported (89,90). Nearly two-thirds of reported patients have remained alive and well, but most follow-up does not extend beyond 5 years (90,92,99,102).

SMALL CELL CARCINOMA

Carcinoma resembling small cell carcinoma of the lung is an especially uncommon variant of breast carcinoma. The diagnosis of primary small cell mammary carcinoma can be made only if a nonmammary site is excluded as a source of metastasis to the breast or an in situ component is demonstrated histologically. Several reports fail to meet these criteria, and a few others do not provide sufficient details to substantiate the diagnosis of mammary small cell carcinoma. Moreover, one should reserve the diagnosis of small cell carcinoma for carcinomas displaying both the characteristic morphologic features and the immunohistochemical evidence of neuroendocrine differentiation. Mammary carcinomas that stain for neuroendocrine proteins while showing conventional morphologic features and carcinomas composed of small malignant cells that do not display evidence of neuroendocrine differentiation should not be classified as small cell carcinomas.

Clinical Presentation

The ages of patients with mammary small cell carcinoma range from 25 (108) to 81 years (109). The mean is 53 years. With the exception of two cases (110,111), all patients have been women. Small cell carcinoma typically forms a single mass, but multiple nodules have been described (109,112).

Mammograms of patients with small cell carcinomas reveal well-defined or irregular masses with borders often described as microlobulated. Using sonography, the masses appear solid, and MRI displays early enhancement (113–117). The pattern of enhancement on computed tomography and MRI scans may be indicative of extensive DCIS (118).

Microscopic Pathology

The histologic characteristics of mammary small cell carcinomas resemble those of small cell carcinomas arising in other organs. The noninvasive component usually consists of small cells with scant cytoplasm and hyperchromatic nuclei. These cells may constitute the entire noninvasive neoplastic population as they did in the four cases described by Papotti et al. (119) and five of the nine cases reported by Shin et al. (120), or the small cells may represent one component of an in situ carcinoma with mixed features. Other patterns of coexisting DCIS include cribriform, solid, comedo, and micropapillary (120,121). The two types of neoplastic cells sometimes mingle in such a way that the non-small cell component surrounds the small cell carcinoma cells. Squamous metaplasia may occur in small cell carcinomas.

The invasive component typically consists of patternless sheets and clusters of cells that often contain zones of coagulative necrosis and foci of hemorrhage (**Fig. 17.13**). Regions sometimes display architectural patterns of a neuroendocrine nature: organoid groups, trabeculae, or rosette-like structures surrounded by delicate blood vessels and stroma. The neoplastic cells appear small and round, polygonal, or spindly. They contain round to oval nuclei, homogeneous dark chromatin, inconspicuous nucleoli, and scant eosinophilic cytoplasm. The nuclear-cytoplasmic ratio is high. Nuclear molding can be seen, but it usually does not appear as prominent in tissue sections as it does in cytologic specimens (120). Mitotic figures abound in most examples, and mitotic counts as high as 10 per high-power field, have been recorded (114). Disruption of nuclei occasionally leads to deposition of the nuclear material around blood vessels (the "Azzopardi effect"). Vascular invasion often appears prominent.

Certain invasive small cell carcinomas, termed *dimorphic small cell carcinomas*, display an abrupt juxtaposition of carcinoma cells of the small cell type with carcinoma cells displaying different characteristics without transitional forms. The second population can have lobular or tubulolobular, squamous, or glandular features (119,120,122–126). For example, four of the nine carcinomas in one study (120) displayed dimorphic histologic patterns: two carcinomas had glandular elements, one showed foci of squamous differentiation, and the fourth consisted of a mixture of small cell carcinoma and invasive lobular carcinoma. In tumors like the latter case, the small cell carcinoma will stain for E-cadherin and lack hormone receptors, whereas the lobular component will not stain for E-cadherin or neuroendocrine markers but will usually express hormone receptors.

The malignant cells of small cell carcinoma can involve the epidermis in a pagetoid pattern (120,127), but the clinical manifestations of Paget disease of the nipple have not been reported.

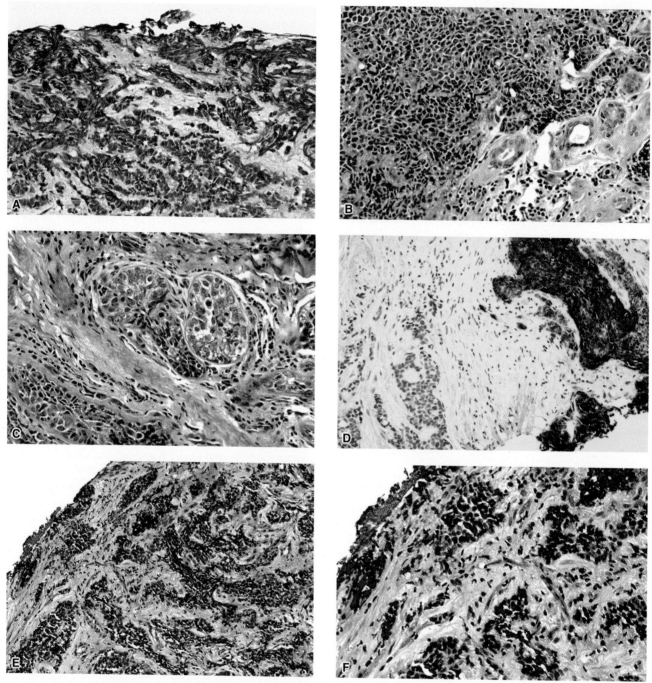

FIGURE 17.13 Small Cell Carcinoma. A: This needle core biopsy specimen shows small carcinoma cells growing in ill-defined bands. Characteristic crush artifact is evident at the edge of the tumor. **B, C:** The excision specimen from the tumor shown in **A** shows small cell carcinoma infiltrating the mammary parenchyma and in situ carcinoma in a terminal duct-lobular unit **(C).** **D:** The small cell carcinoma in situ is immunoreactive for CD56 **(right).** The invasive carcinoma **(left)** is CD56-negative. **E, F:** Invasive small cell carcinoma with a trabecular growth pattern is present in this needle core biopsy sample.

Immunohistochemistry

Investigators have not reported consistent patterns of immunoreactivity in mammary small cell carcinomas. With rare exceptions (114,121,128), almost all cases have stained for AE1/AE3, CK7, and CAM 5.2. Most failed to stain for CK20, and the results of staining for CK5/6 and 34βE12 have been variable or negative. Staining for EMA usually yields a positive reaction, whereas testing for GCDFP-15 usually does not. Except for two examples (129,130), small cell carcinomas have expressed E-cadherin. The later observation suggests that the majority of mammary small cell carcinomas are ductal in their nature, but that they rarely may have a lobular immunophenotype.

Among proteins suggestive of neuroendocrine differentiation, expression of neuron-specific enolase (NSE) represents the most consistent finding. Staining for chromogranins (A, B, and C), synaptophysin, gastrin-releasing peptide (bombesin), serotonin, PGP9.5, CD56, and leu 7 has produced variable results, but almost all mammary small cell carcinomas have expressed at least one of these molecules (119,120,123,128,130,131).

A few investigators reported the staining results of both the noninvasive and invasive components of small cell carcinomas. The two components displayed identical staining properties in two tumors (127,131), but in two instances, the noninvasive and invasive cells exhibited different staining reactions (125,132).

Small cell carcinomas demonstrate variable immunoreactivity for ER and PR. About 25% of cases have expressed ER, and slightly more have stained for PR. Androgen receptor reactivity was absent in one case (108). Except for four tumors (111,130,133,134), the carcinomas have not overexpressed HER2.

Because a small cell carcinoma in the breast sometimes represents a metastasis rather than a primary carcinoma, investigators have studied the expression of TTF-1 and CD117 in *bona fide* mammary small cell carcinomas. Eight of nineteen reported mammary small cell carcinomas stained for TTF-1 (114–116,118,125,127,130,132,134,135), and researchers detected CD117 in three out of four tumors (113,117,129,136). These findings make clear that one cannot rely on the presence of either TTF-1 or CD117 to distinguish a mammary small cell carcinoma from a metastasis from a small cell carcinoma arising in the lung or another site.

Differential Diagnosis

The differential diagnosis of mammary small cell carcinoma includes lymphomas and related neoplasms, certain sarcomas, and metastatic carcinomas. Evaluation of the growth pattern and cytologic features of the malignant cells, the presence of noninvasive carcinoma, and the results of commonly employed immunohistochemical stains for epithelial and lymphoid proteins should allow one to exclude the diagnosis of a lymphoproliferative malignancy. Sarcomas such as Ewing sarcoma, osteosarcoma, mesenchymal chondrosarcoma, and synovial sarcoma would belong in the differential diagnosis in certain cases. Evaluation of problematic tumors with immunohistochemical staining and genetic studies allows one to exclude these possibilities. Pathologists must keep in mind that mammary small cell carcinomas can stain for CD99 (121,129), a protein usually present in the aforementioned mesenchymal tumors. To exclude the possibility of a metastatic lesion of any type, pathologists should sample the specimen extensively to detect an in situ component. When the primary site is in doubt, clinicians should undertake a careful search for evidence of a primary carcinoma in another organ.

Small cell carcinoma of the lung stands out as the most likely primary source for metastatic neuroendocrine carcinoma in the breast, and the mammary metastasis may be the first manifestation of an occult pulmonary small cell carcinoma.

Spread from a Merkel cell carcinoma of the skin represents another possibility, which one can exclude using the results of staining for CK20 and neurofilaments (131,137). In most reported examples of metastatic nonmammary small cell carcinoma in the breast (125), the existence of an extramammary primary was known.

Prognosis and Treatment

The small number of cases, the variation in their treatment, and the short duration of their follow-up prevent one from drawing secure conclusions regarding either the prognosis or the optimum treatment of patients with mammary small cell carcinoma. Among the patients in published reports, approximately 20% succumbed to the carcinoma during intervals from 3 months (127) to approximately 2 years (113), and approximately 20% developed recurrences during the same interval yet remained alive with disease. Finally, about one-half of the patients followed up for 3 months (120) to 49 months (123) remained free of carcinoma. Prognosis is substantially dependent on tumor size and stage at clinical diagnosis. Patients with relatively small tumors described in certain recent studies have experienced a much more favorable prognosis than those with advanced disease described in retrospective reports (120). Surgery followed by chemotherapy may cure patients with early-stage disease (120), but the use of radiation therapy does not seem to improve survival (138). Neoadjuvant administration of chemotherapeutic agents may benefit patients with locally advanced carcinomas (108).

GLYCOGEN-RICH CARCINOMA

Malignant cells containing abundant glycogen compose this variety of mammary carcinoma. Extraction of the glycogen during tissue processing leaves the cytoplasm of these carcinomas vacuolated or completely clear in routine sections. In one series, 3% of 1,555 breast carcinomas were classified as clear cell, glycogen-rich carcinomas (139). Others (140) reported that glycogen-rich clear cell carcinoma account for less than 1% of mammary ductal carcinomas.

Clinical Presentation

The age of reported patients with glycogen-rich carcinoma ranges from 31 to 81 years (141,142). The patients presented with a mass accompanied by skin dimpling, nipple retraction, or pain in some cases.

Both in situ and invasive lesions may be detected by mammography (140,143,144) and sonography (140). The images often reveal an ill-defined mass (142,143), which may contain calcifications (142,145).

Most tumors measure between 2 and 5 cm; the largest spanned "about 15 cm" (145). The mean sizes in two series are 3 cm (141) and 3.2 cm (142). The carcinoma can form multifocal or multicentric masses (146).

Microscopic Pathology

Glycogen-rich carcinomas grow in both noninvasive and invasive forms. The noninvasive component can create papillary, solid, cribriform, micropapillary, and intracystic patterns. Cytoplasmic clearing appears most evident in solid areas, in which the cells exhibit moderate nuclear atypia. Those in cribriform and micropapillary regions usually have low-grade atypia and less often appear water-clear. The neoplastic cells can undergo focal necrosis, but abundant, comedo-like necrosis associated with high-grade nuclear atypia does not occur commonly. In most cases, one can detect small regions in which the cells contain eosinophilic and granular cytoplasm or exhibit other clear-cut apocrine features.

The invasive component usually exhibits the histologic growth pattern of a conventional invasive ductal carcinoma. The tumor cells form cords, solid nests, or papillary structures, but the formation of ductular or tubular structure occurs only rarely. A linear pattern consisting of strands of cells resembling invasive lobular carcinoma may be seen, and glycogen-rich variants of tubular, medullary, micropapillary, and endocrine carcinomas have been described (139,141,147,148). The cells exhibit sharply defined borders and polygonal rather than rounded contours. The cytoplasm is clear or, less often, finely granular or foamy. Like the noninvasive component, the invasive carcinoma sometimes contains foci in which the cells have eosinophilic and granular cytoplasm that suggests an apocrine nature, and these cells often form a continuum with the clear cells. Observers have noted PAS-positive, diastase-resistant, intracytoplasmic hyalin droplets in rare cases (144). The nuclei appear hyperchromatic and sometimes contain clumped chromatin and nucleoli (**Fig. 17.14**). Mitotic figures are easily identified in most cases. One report (149) recorded the presence of 65 mitotic figures in 10 high-power fields. Large tumors often show foci of necrosis. The carcinoma cells can invade lymphatic vessels and nerves. The histologic appearance of the primary tumor is duplicated in the metastases, which also contain abundant glycogen (150).

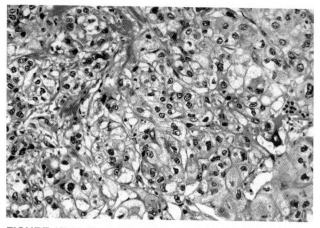

FIGURE 17.14 Glycogen-rich Carcinoma. The neoplastic cells have pale eosinophilic or clear cytoplasm.

Immunohistochemistry

The cytoplasm of glycogen-rich clear cell carcinomas gives a positive, diastase-labile reaction with the PAS stain. The tumor cells are reactive for CK7, AE1/AE3, CK8/18, CAM 5.2, and E-cadherin and variably or weakly reactive for CK19, CK34βE12, and EMA. Glycogen-rich carcinomas do not display a consistent pattern of staining for hormone receptors. The reported frequency of ER and PR expression varies from 35% to 62%, and 12% to 43% of cases have stained for HER2 (141,142,151).

Differential Diagnosis

The differential diagnosis of glycogen-rich carcinoma includes both benign and malignant mammary and extramammary neoplasms. The clear-cell type of hidradenoma (eccrine acrospiroma) shares the presence of many glycogen-laden clear cells with glycogen-rich carcinoma; however, hidradenomas are centered in the dermis, they have well-defined, smooth contours, and they consist of uniform bland cells. Atypical and malignant hidradenomas pose greater challenges in differential diagnosis. Myoepithelial cells with clear cytoplasm can dominate in uncommon examples of mammary adenomyoepithelioma. Detection of a second population consisting of glandular cells and immunohistochemical demonstration of proteins characteristic of myoepithelial cells will distinguish such a tumor from glycogen-rich carcinoma.

Among the types of primary mammary carcinomas, lipid-rich, secretory, histiocytoid lobular, and apocrine carcinomas exhibit certain features that may bring to mind the appearance of glycogen-rich carcinoma, but one can usually distinguish these tumors without difficulty. Lipid-rich carcinomas contain lipid rather than glycogen. Secretory carcinomas feature microcystic spaces containing mucin and eosinophilic secretions. Invasive lobular carcinomas of the histiocytoid type possess intracytoplasmic mucin rather than glycogen. Apocrine carcinomas can contain clear cells, and focal apocrine features are identified in the majority of glycogen-rich carcinomas. This association suggests that that glycogen-rich carcinoma might constitute a variant of apocrine carcinoma (144). These overlapping findings and the possibility of an etiological relationship notwithstanding, the usual apocrine carcinoma contains intracytoplasmic, diastase-resistant eosinophilic granules or droplets, a finding that does not characterize glycogen-rich carcinomas.

Metastatic clear cell carcinomas can mimic the appearance of glycogen-rich carcinoma. Carcinoma of the kidney is the most notable culprit in this regard.

Finally, the mere presence of glycogen in a mammary carcinoma does not establish the diagnosis of glycogen-rich carcinoma, because Fisher et al. (139) found that 58% of breast carcinomas lacking clear cells contained intracytoplasmic glycogen. To substantiate the diagnosis of glycogen-rich carcinoma, one must both observe the characteristic morphologic findings and establish the presence of abundant glycogen by means of histochemical staining.

Prognosis and Treatment

In one series (142), 46% of patients had metastatic carcinoma in their axillary lymph nodes. The limited follow-up data suggest that the prognosis of patients with glycogen-rich mammary carcinoma is not particularly favorable and that it may be similar to that of ordinary invasive duct carcinoma when analyzed on a stage- and grade-matched basis (139,142,144). Treatment recommendations should probably follow those proposed for conventional breast carcinomas.

LIPID-RICH CARCINOMA

This rare variant of infiltrating ductal carcinoma features large cells with abundant cytoplasmic lipid, which imparts a vacuolated or foamy appearance to the cytoplasm. The tumor was first described in a case report by Aboumrad et al. (152) as *lipid-secreting carcinoma*; later, Ramos and Taylor (153) proposed the less committal term, *lipid-rich carcinoma*.

Clinical Presentation

With one exception (154), all adult patients have been women between the ages of 22 and 81 years. One patient was a 10-year-old girl (155). Most patients presented with a palpable mass. Attachment to the skin with dimpling, retraction, ulceration, and *peau d'orange* has been reported.

Imaging studies revealed spiculated masses in three patients, and ultrasonography and MRI in one patient demonstrated findings suspicious for malignancy (156).

Microscopic Pathology

In most cases, tissue sections demonstrate a predominantly invasive carcinoma composed of sheets, nests, and cords of large, polygonal cells, which may have poorly defined borders. Two examples seem to represent entirely noninvasive form of lipid-rich carcinoma (156,157). van Bogaert and Maldague (158) described three histopathologic patterns created by the malignant cells. The histiocytoid pattern, which represents the most common variety, consists of large cells with pale foamy cytoplasm and small dark nuclei that lack pleomorphism **(Fig. 17.15)**. Cells with large, irregular, and bubbly vacuoles, pleomorphic nuclei, and prominent nucleoli characterize the sebaceous pattern of lipid-rich carcinoma. The third pattern consists of cells with apocrine qualities. They possess abundant, finely granular, eosinophilic cytoplasm and nuclei with coarse chromatin and prominent nucleoli. Cells with these different appearances sometimes mingle in a single carcinoma. One can usually detect mitotic figures without difficulty, and the carcinomas usually fall in the category of histologic grade 2 or 3. Scalloping of the nuclei by the cytoplasmic vacuoles can bring to mind the appearance of sebaceous cells or brown fat. Unusual histologic findings include focal chrondroid metaplasia (159) and cytologic findings similar to those seen in pregnancy-like change (160,161).

The cytoplasmic vacuolization arises because histologic processing extracts the cytoplasmic lipid. To document the presence of lipid, one can employ oil red O or Sudan III stains using frozen sections of fresh tissue or tissue processed in a fashion that preserves cytoplasmic lipids, or one can carry out ultrastructural studies.

Immunohistochemistry

Lipid-rich carcinomas do not stain with PAS, Alcian blue, or mucicarmine stains, nor do they stain for CK5/6, CK14, S-100 protein, SMA, or p63. Staining for E-cadherin, CK7, mammaglobin, and CEA was observed in one case (162). The results of studies of ER and PR expression vary. Most investigators report little or no detection of ER but modest expression of PR. Many cases showed strong membrane staining for HER2 and amplification of the *HER2* gene (161–163).

Differential Diagnosis

The diagnosis of lipid-rich carcinoma requires the presence of two types of evidence: the characteristic cellular features, which include clear, pale, or vacuolated cytoplasm, and intracytoplasmic

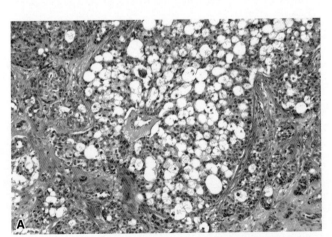
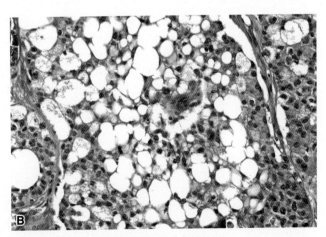

FIGURE 17.15 Lipid-rich Carcinoma. A, B: The carcinoma cells contain prominent cytoplasmic vacuoles resulting from extraction of lipid during tissue processing. (Courtesy of Dr. Frank Brazza.)

lipid demonstrated by special studies. Neither type of evidence alone can establish the diagnosis of lipid-rich carcinoma. The most commonly encountered carcinomas that superficially resemble lipid-rich carcinoma include glycogen-rich carcinoma, apocrine carcinoma, and secretory carcinoma; rare malignancies such as myoepithelial carcinoma and liposarcoma might also enter into consideration. The cytoplasm of glycogen-rich carcinomas appears clear rather than foamy and it contains diastase-sensitive, PAS-positive glycogen rather than lipid. Apocrine carcinomas typically stain for GCDFP-15 strongly, whereas lipid-rich carcinomas show only focal staining for this molecule. PAS-positive, Alcian blue-positive acid mucopolysaccharides form cytoplasmic vacuoles in secretory carcinomas, and genetic studies demonstrate the characteristic fusion gene. Myoepithelial carcinomas express characteristic proteins not seen in lipid-rich carcinomas, and the cells of liposarcoma do not commonly express keratin.

The accumulated information notwithstanding, the nature of lipid-rich carcinoma remains undefined. Lipids accumulate in carcinomas classified as ductal, lobular, and apocrine among others, and carcinomas classified as lipid-rich might simply represent conventional types of carcinoma with especially abundant lipid accumulation. Additional studies of more patients will be required to determine whether lipid-rich tumors constitute a morphologically and clinically distinctive type of carcinoma.

Treatment and Prognosis

Axillary nodal metastases have been found mostly associated with tumors measuring more than 3 cm. Patients with nodal metastases at the time of diagnosis have a poor prognosis, but those with negative lymph nodes have survived as long as 20 years (161). Treatment of patients with lipid-rich carcinoma reported in the literature has been by mastectomy and axillary dissection in most cases, but breast-conserving surgery could be an alternative in appropriate situations.

OTHER RARE TYPES OF CARCINOMA

Other rare types of mammary carcinoma include acinic cell carcinoma (164), mucoepidermoid carcinoma (165), oncocytic carcinoma (166), polymorphous adenocarcinoma (167), and sebaceous carcinoma (168). Although one might suspect one of these diagnoses when examining a NCB specimen, it would probably require thorough evaluation of the excised specimen to make a secure diagnosis of such rare types of mammary carcinoma.

REFERENCES

Invasive Micropapillary Carcinoma

1. Fisher ER, Palekar AS, Redmond C, et al. Pathologic findings from the National Surgical Adjuvant Breast Project (Protocol No. 4): VI: Invasive papillary cancer. *Am J Clin Pathol*. 1980;73:313–322.

2. Guo X, Chen L, Lang R, et al. Invasive micropapillary carcinoma of the breast: association of pathologic features with lymph node metastasis. *Am J Clin Pathol*. 2006;126:740–746.

3. Paterakos M, Watkin WG, Edgerton SM, et al. Invasive micropapillary carcinoma of the breast: a prognostic study. *Hum Pathol*. 1999;30:1459–1463.

4. Pettinato G, Manivel CJ, Panico L, et al. Invasive micropapillary carcinoma of the breast: clinicopathologic study of 62 cases of a poorly recognized variant with highly aggressive behavior. *Am J Clin Pathol*. 2004;121:857–866.

5. Luna-Moré S, Gonzalez B, Acedo C, et al. Invasive micropapillary carcinoma of the breast: a new special type of invasive mammary carcinoma. *Pathol Res Pract*. 1994;190:668–674.

6. Erhan Y, Zekioglu O. Pure invasive micropapillary carcinoma of the male breast: report of a rare case. *Can J Surg*. 2005;48:156–157.

7. Marchio C, Iravani M, Natrajan R, et al. Genomic and immunophenotypical characterization of pure micropapillary carcinomas of the breast. *J Pathol*. 2008;215:398–410.

8. Trepant AL, Hoorens A, Noel JC. Pure invasive micropapillary carcinoma of the male breast: report of a rare case with C-MYC amplification. *Pathol Res Pract*. 2014;210(12):1164–1166.

9. Alsharif S, Daghistani R, Kamberoglu EA, et al. Mammographic, sonographic and MR imaging features of invasive micropapillary breast cancer. *Eur J Radiol*. 2014;83:1375–1380.

10. Siriaunkgul S, Tavassoli FA. Invasive micropapillary carcinoma of the breast. *Mod Pathol*. 1993;6:660–662.

11. Yun SU, Choi BB, Shu KS, et al. Imaging findings of invasive micropapillary carcinoma of the breast. *J Breast Cancer*. 2012;15:57–64.

12. Petersen J. Breast carcinoma with an unexpected inside out growth pattern, rotation of polarisation associated with angioinvasion. *Path Res Pract*. 1993;189:780.

13. Aggarwal G, Reid MD, Sharma S. Metaplastic variant of invasive micropapillary breast carcinoma: a unique triple negative phenotype. *Int J Surg Pathol*. 2012;20:488–493.

14. Chen L, Fan Y, Lang RG, et al. Breast carcinoma with micropapillary features: clinicopathologic study and long-term follow-up of 100 cases. *Int J Surg Pathol*. 2008;16:155–163.

15. Barbashina V, Corben AD, Akram M, et al. Mucinous micropapillary carcinoma of the breast: an aggressive counterpart to conventional pure mucinous tumors. *Hum Pathol*. 2013;44:1577–1585.

16. Liu F, Yang M, Li Z, et al. Invasive micropapillary mucinous carcinoma of the breast is associated with poor prognosis. *Breast Cancer Res Treat*. 2015;151:443–451.

17. Nassar H, Pansare V, Zhang H, et al. Pathogenesis of invasive micropapillary carcinoma: role of MUC1 glycoprotein. *Mod Pathol*. 2004;17:1045–1050.

18. Acs G, Esposito NN, Rakosy Z, et al. Invasive ductal carcinomas of the breast showing partial reversed cell polarity are associated with lymphatic tumor spread and may represent part of a spectrum of invasive micropapillary carcinoma. *Am J Surg Pathol*. 2010;34:1637–1646.

19. Adams SA, Smith ME, Cowley GP, et al. Reversal of glandular polarity in the lymphovascular compartment of breast cancer. *J Clin Pathol*. 2004;57:1114–1117.

20. Wendroth SM, Mentrikoski MJ, Wick MR. GATA3 expression in morphologic subtypes of breast carcinoma: a comparison with gross cystic disease fluid protein 15 and mammaglobin. *Ann Diagn Pathol*. 2015;19:6–9.

21. Yamaguchi R, Tanaka M, Kondo K, et al. Characteristic morphology of invasive micropapillary carcinoma of the breast: an immunohistochemical analysis. *Jpn J Clin Oncol*. 2010;40:781–787.

22. Kuba S, Ohtani H, Yamaguchi J, et al. Incomplete inside-out growth pattern in invasive breast carcinoma: association with lymph vessel invasion and recurrence-free survival. *Virchows Arch*. 2011;458:159–169.

23. Lee AH, Paish EC, Marchio C, et al. The expression of Wilms' tumour-1 and Ca125 in invasive micropapillary carcinoma of the breast. *Histopathology*. 2007;51:824–828.

24. Chivukula M, Dabbs DJ, O'Connor S, et al. PAX 2: a novel Mullerian marker for serous papillary carcinomas to differentiate from micropapillary breast carcinoma. *Int J Gynecol Pathol*. 2009;28:570–578.

25. Lotan TL, Ye H, Melamed J, et al. Immunohistochemical panel to identify the primary site of invasive micropapillary carcinoma. *Am J Surg Pathol*. 2009;33:1037–1041.

26. Chen AC, Paulino AC, Schwartz MR, et al. Population-based comparison of prognostic factors in invasive micropapillary and invasive ductal carcinoma of the breast. *Br J Cancer.* 2014;111:619–622.

Cribriform Carcinoma

27. Marzullo F, Zito FA, Marzullo A, et al. Infiltrating cribriform carcinoma of the breast: a clinico-pathologic and immunohistochemical study of 5 cases. *Eur J Gynaecol Oncol.* 1996;17:228–231.

28. Venable JG, Schwartz AM, Silverberg SG. Infiltrating cribriform carcinoma of the breast: a distinctive clinicopathologic entity. *Hum Pathol.* 1990;21:333–338.

29. Zhang W, Zhang T, Lin Z, et al. Invasive cribriform carcinoma in a Chinese population: comparison with low-grade invasive ductal carcinoma-not otherwise specified. *Int J Clin Exp Pathol.* 2013;6:445–457.

30. Page DL, Dixon JM, Anderson TJ, et al. Invasive cribriform carcinoma of the breast. *Histopathology.* 1983;7:525–536.

31. Nishimura R, Ohsumi S, Teramoto N, et al. Invasive cribriform carcinoma with extensive microcalcifications in the male breast. *Breast Cancer.* 2005;12:145–148.

32. Choi Y, Lee KY, Jang MH, et al. Invasive cribriform carcinoma arising in malignant phyllodes tumor of breast: a case report. *Korean J Pathol.* 2012;46:205–209.

33. Stutz JA, Evans AJ, Pinder S, et al; Nottingham Breast Team. The radiological appearances of invasive cribriform carcinoma of the breast. *Clin Radiol.* 1994;49:693–695.

34. Lim HS, Jeong SJ, Lee JS, et al. Sonographic findings of invasive cribriform carcinoma of the breast. *J Ultrasound Med.* 2011;30:701–705.

35. Wells CA, Ferguson DJ. Ultrastructural and immunocytochemical study of a case of invasive cribriform breast carcinoma. *J Clin Pathol.* 1988;41:17–20.

36. Shousha S, Schoenfeld A, Moss J, et al. Light and electron microscopic study of an invasive cribriform carcinoma with extensive microcalcification developing in a breast with silicone augmentation. *Ultrastruct Pathol.* 1994;18:519–523.

37. Gjerdrum LM, Lauridsen MC, Sorensen FB. Breast carcinoma with osteoclast-like giant cells: morphological and ultrastructural studies of a case with review of the literature. *Breast.* 2001;10:231–236.

38. Gatti G, Pruneri G, Gilardi D, et al. Report on a case of pure cribriform carcinoma of the breast with internal mammary node metastasis: description of the case and review of the literature. *Tumori.* 2006;92:241–243.

39. Rosen PP. Adenoid cystic carcinoma of the breast: a morphologically heterogeneous neoplasm. *Pathol Annu.* 1989;24(pt 2):237–254.

40. Cong Y, Qiao Q, Zou H, et al. Invasive cribriform carcinoma of the breast: a report of nine cases and a review of the literature. *Oncol Lett.* 2015;9:1753–1758.

41. Liu XY, Jiang YZ, Liu YR, et al. Clinicopathological characteristics and survival outcomes of invasive cribriforma carcinoma of breast: a SEER population-based study. *Medicine (Baltimore).* 2015;94:e1309.

Secretory Carcinoma

42. Gupta K, Lallu SD, Fauck R, et al. Needle aspiration cytology, immunocytochemistry, and electron microscopy in a rare case of secretory carcinoma of the breast in an elderly woman. *Diagn Cytopathol.* 1992;8:388–391.

43. McDivitt RW, Stewart FW. Breast carcinoma in children. *JAMA.* 1966;195:388–390.

44. Noh WC, Paik NS, Cho KJ, et al. Breast mass in a 3-year-old girl: differentiation of secretory carcinoma versus abnormal thelarche by fine needle aspiration biopsy. *Surgery.* 2005;137:109–110.

45. Alenda C, Aranda FI, Segui FJ, et al. Secretory carcinoma of the male breast: correlation of aspiration cytology and pathology. *Diagn Cytopathol.* 2005;32:47–50.

46. Karl SR, Ballantine TV, Zaino R. Juvenile secretory carcinoma of the breast. *J Pediatr Surg.* 1985;20:368–371.

47. Ding J, Jiang L, Gan Y, et al. A rare case of secretory breast carcinoma in a male adult with axillary lymph node metastasis. *Int J Clin Exp Pathol.* 2015;8:3322–3327.

48. Beatty SM, Orel SG, Kim P, et al. Multicentric secretory carcinoma of the breast in a 35-year-old woman: mammographic appearance and the use of core biopsy in preoperative management. *Breast J.* 1998;4:200–203.

49. Ben Romdhane K, Ben Ayed M, Labbane N, et al. Carcinome secretant juvenile du sein: a propos d'une observation chez une fille de 4 ans. *Ann Pathol.* 1987;7:227–230.

50. Diallo R, Schaefer KL, Bankfalvi A, et al. Secretory carcinoma of the breast: a distinct variant of invasive ductal carcinoma assessed by comparative genomic hybridization and immunohistochemistry. *Hum Pathol.* 2003;34:1299–1305.

51. Shin SJ, Sheikh FS, Allenby PA, et al. Invasive secretory (juvenile) carcinoma arising in ectopic breast tissue of the axilla. *Arch Pathol Lab Med.* 2001;125:1372–1374.

52. Li D, Xiao X, Yang W, et al. Secretory breast carcinoma: a clinicopathological and immunophenotypic study of 15 cases with a review of the literature. *Mod Pathol.* 2012;25:567–575.

53. Brandt SM, Swistel AJ, Rosen PP. Secretory carcinoma in the axilla: probable origin from axillary skin appendage glands in a young girl. *Am J Surg Pathol.* 2009;33:950–953.

54. Grabellus F, Worm K, Willruth A, et al. ETV6-NTRK3 gene fusion in a secretory carcinoma of the breast of a male-to-female transsexual. *Breast.* 2005;14:71–74.

55. Rosen PP, Holmes G, Lesser ML, et al. Juvenile papillomatosis and breast carcinoma. *Cancer.* 1985;55:1345–1352.

56. de Bree E, Askoxylakis J, Giannikaki E, et al. Secretory carcinoma of the male breast. *Ann Surg Oncol.* 2002;9:663–667.

57. Kameyama K, Mukai M, Iri H, et al. Secretory carcinoma of the breast in a 51-year-old male. *Pathol Int.* 1998;48:994–997.

58. Paeng MH, Choi HY, Sung SH, et al. Secretory carcinoma of the breast. *J Clin Ultrasound.* 2003;31:425–429.

59. Horowitz DP, Sharma CS, Connolly E, et al. Secretory carcinoma of the breast: results from the survival, epidemiology and end results database. *Breast.* 2012;21:350–353.

60. Din NU, Idrees R, Fatima S, et al. Secretory carcinoma of breast: clinicopathologic study of 8 cases. *Ann Diagn Pathol.* 2013;17:54–57.

61. Yildirim E, Turhan N, Pak I, et al. Secretory breast carcinoma in a boy. *Eur J Surg Oncol.* 1999;25:98–99.

62. Woto-Gaye G, Kasse AA, Dieye Y, et al. Carcinome secretoire du sein chez l' hommme: a propos d'un cas d'evolution rapide. *Ann Pathol.* 2004;24:432–435; quiz 393.

63. Roncaroli F, Lamovec J, Zidar A, et al. Acinic cell-like carcinoma of the breast. *Virchows Arch.* 1996;429:69–74.

64. Osako T, Takeuchi K, Horii R, et al. Secretory carcinoma of the breast and its histopathological mimics: value of markers for differential diagnosis. *Histopathology.* 2013;63:509–519.

65. Lamovec J, Bracko M. Secretory carcinoma of the breast: light microscopical, immunohistochemical and flow cytometric study. *Mod Pathol.* 1994;7:475–479.

66. Lae M, Freneaux P, Sastre-Garau X, et al. Secretory breast carcinomas with ETV6-NTRK3 fusion gene belong to the basal-like carcinoma spectrum. *Mod Pathol.* 2009;22:291–298.

67. Choi J, Kim D, Koo JS. Secretory carcinoma of breast demonstrates nuclear or cytoplasmic expression in p63 immunohistochemistry. *Int J Surg Pathol.* 2012;20:367–372.

68. Lambros MB, Tan DS, Jones RL, et al. Genomic profile of a secretory breast cancer with an ETV6-NTRK3 duplication. *J Clin Pathol.* 2009;62:604–612.

69. Tognon C, Knezevich SR, Huntsman D, et al. Expression of the ETV6-NTRK3 gene fusion as a primary event in human secretory breast carcinoma. *Cancer Cell.* 2002;2:367–376.

70. Euhus DM, Timmons CF, Tomlinson GE. ETV6-NTRK3—Trk-ing the primary event in human secretory breast cancer. *Cancer Cell.* 2002;2:347–348.

71. Makretsov N, He M, Hayes M, et al. A fluorescence in situ hybridization study of ETV6-NTRK3 fusion gene in secretory breast carcinoma. *Genes Chromosomes Cancer.* 2004;40:152–157.

72. Nevalainen MT, Xie J, Bubendorf L, et al. Basal activation of transcription factor signal transducer and activator of transcription (Stat5) in nonpregnant mouse and human breast epithelium. *Mol Endocrinol.* 2002;16:1108–1124.

73. Bratthauer GL, Strauss BL, Tavassoli FA. STAT 5a expression in various lesions of the breast. *Virchows Arch.* 2006;448:165–171.

74. Strauss BL, Bratthauer GL, Tavassoli FA. STAT 5a expression in the breast is maintained in secretory carcinoma, in contrast to other histologic types. *Hum Pathol.* 2006;37:586–592.

75. Rosen PP, Cranor ML. Secretory carcinoma of the breast. *Arch Pathol Lab Med.* 1991;115:141–144.

76. Mies C. Recurrent secretory carcinoma in residual mammary tissue after mastectomy. *Am J Surg Pathol.* 1993;17:715–721.

Cystic Hypersecretory Carcinoma

77. Rosen PP, Scott M. Cystic hypersecretory duct carcinoma of the breast. *Am J Surg Pathol.* 1984;8:31–41.

78. Guerry P, Erlandson RA, Rosen PP. Cystic hypersecretory hyperplasia and cystic hypersecretory duct carcinoma of the breast: pathology, therapy, and follow-up of 39 patients. *Cancer.* 1988;61:1611–1620.

79. D'Alfonso TM, Ginter PS, Liu YF, et al. Cystic hypersecretory (in situ) carcinoma of the breast: a clinicopathologic and immunohistochemical characterization of 10 cases with clinical follow-up. *Am J Surg Pathol.* 2014;38:45–53.

80. Resetkova E, Padula A, Albarraccin CT, et al. Pathologic quiz case: a large, ill-defined cystic breast mass: invasive cystic hypersecretory duct carcinoma. *Arch Pathol Lab Med.* 2005;129:e79–e80.

81. Skalova A, Ryska A, Kajo K, et al. Cystic hypersecretory carcinoma: rare and poorly recognized variant of intraductal carcinoma of the breast: report of five cases. *Histopathology.* 2005;46:43–49.

82. Sahoo S, Gopal P, Roland L, et al. Cystic hypersecretory carcinoma of the breast with Paget disease of the nipple: a diagnostic challenge. *Int J Surg Pathol.* 2008;16:208–212.

83. Colandrea JM, Shmookler BM, O'Dowd GJ, et al. Cystic hypersecretory duct carcinoma of the breast: report of a case with fine-needle aspiration. *Arch Pathol Lab Med.* 1988;112:560–563.

84. Park JM, Seo MR. Cystic hypersecretory duct carcinoma of the breast: report of two cases. *Clin Radiol.* 2002;57:312–315.

85. Park C, Jung JI, Lee AW, et al. Sonographic findings in a patient with cystic hypersecretory duct carcinoma of the breast. *J Clin Ultrasound.* 2004;32:29–32.

86. Bogomoletz WV. Cystic hypersecretory hyperplasia of the breast: a rare diagnosis in breast pathology. *Ann Pathol.* 1994;14:131–132.

87. Shin SJ, Rosen PP. Carcinoma arising from preexisting pregnancy-like and cystic hypersecretory hyperplasia lesions of the breast: a clinicopathologic study of 9 patients. *Am J Surg Pathol.* 2004;28:789–793.

88. Shin SJ, Rosen PP. Pregnancy-like (pseudolactational) hyperplasia: a primary diagnosis in mammographically detected lesions of the breast and its relationship to cystic hypersecretory hyperplasia. *Am J Surg Pathol.* 2000;24:1670–1674.

Mammary Carcinoma with Osteoclast-Like Giant Cells

89. Agnantis NT, Rosen PP. Mammary carcinoma with osteoclast-like giant cells: a study of eight cases with follow-up data. *Am J Clin Pathol.* 1979;72:383–389.

90. Zhou S, Yu L, Zhou R, et al. Invasive breast carcinomas of no special type with osteoclast-like giant cells frequently have a luminal phenotype. *Virchows Arch.* 2014;464:681–688.

91. Richter G, Uleer C, Noesselt T. Multifocal invasive ductal breast cancer with osteoclast-like giant cells: a case report. *J Med Case Rep.* 2011;5:85.

92. Saimura M, Fukutomi T, Tsuda H, et al. Breast carcinoma with osteoclast-like giant cells: a case report and review of the Japanese literature. *Breast Cancer.* 1999;6:121–126.

93. Iacocca MV, Maia DM. Bilateral infiltrating lobular carcinoma of the breast with osteoclast-like giant cells. *Breast J.* 2001;7:60–65.

94. Holland R, van Haelst UJ. Mammary carcinoma with osteoclast-like giant cells: additional observations on six cases. *Cancer.* 1984;53:1963–1973.

95. Takahashi T, Moriki T, Hiroi M, et al. Invasive lobular carcinoma of the breast with osteoclastlike giant cells: a case report. *Acta Cytol.* 1998;42:734–741.

96. Shishido-Hara Y, Kurata A, Fujiwara M, et al. Two cases of breast carcinoma with osteoclastic giant cells: Are the osteoclastic giant cells pro-tumoural differentiation of macrophages? *Diagn Pathol.* 2010;5:55.

97. Ginter PS, Petrova K, Hoda SA. The grossly "rusty" tumor of breast: invasive ductal carcinoma with osteoclast-like giant cells. *Int J Surg Pathol.* 2015;23:32–33.

98. Boccato P, Briani G, d'Atri C, et al. Spindle cell and cartilaginous metaplasia in a breast carcinoma with osteoclastlike stromal cells: a difficult fine needle aspiration diagnosis. *Acta Cytol.* 1988;32:75–78.

99. Tavassoli FA, Norris HJ. Breast carcinoma with osteoclastlike giant cells. *Arch Pathol Lab Med.* 1986;110:636–639.

100. Wargotz ES, Norris HJ. Metaplastic carcinomas of the breast. V: Metaplastic carcinoma with osteoclastic giant cells. *Hum Pathol.* 1990;21:1142–1150.

101. Lee JS, Kim YB, Min KW. Metaplastic mammary carcinoma with osteoclast-like giant cells: identical point mutation of p53 gene only identified in both the intraductal and sarcomatous components. *Virchows Arch.* 2004;444:194–197.

102. Ichijima K, Kobashi Y, Ueda Y, et al. Breast cancer with reactive multinucleated giant cells: report of three cases. *Acta Pathol Jpn.* 1986;36:449–457.

103. Nielsen BB, Kiaer HW. Carcinoma of the breast with stromal multinucleated giant cells. *Histopathology.* 1985;9:183–193.

104. Fadare O, Gill SA. Solid neuroendocrine carcinoma of the breast with osteoclast-like giant cells. *Breast J.* 2009;15:205–206.

105. Cozzolino I, Ciancia G, Limite G, et al. Neuroendocrine differentiation in breast carcinoma with osteoclast-like giant cells: report of a case and review of the literature. *Int J Surg.* 2014;12(Suppl 2):S8–S11.

106. Marchio C, Pietribiasi F, Castiglione R, et al. "Giants in a microcosm": multinucleated giant cells populating an invasive micropapillary carcinoma of the breast. *Int J Surg Pathol.* 2015;23:654–655.

107. Krishnan C, Longacre TA. Ductal carcinoma in situ of the breast with osteoclast-like giant cells. *Hum Pathol.* 2006;37:369–372.

Small Cell Carcinoma

108. Ochoa R, Sudhindra A, Garcia-Buitrago M, et al. Small-cell cancer of the breast: what is the optimal treatment? A report and review of outcomes. *Clin Breast Cancer.* 2012;12:287–292.

109. Rineer J, Choi K, Sanmugarajah J. Small cell carcinoma of the breast. *J Natl Med Assoc.* 2009;101:1061–1064.

110. Jundt G, Schulz A, Heitz PU, et al. Small cell neuroendocrine (oat cell) carcinoma of the male breast: immunocytochemical and ultrastructural investigations. *Virchows Arch A Pathol Anat Histopathol.* 1984;404:213–221.

111. Jiang J, Wang G, Lv L, et al. Primary small-cell neuroendocrine carcinoma of the male breast: a rare case report with review of the literature. *Onco Targets Ther.* 2014;7:663–666.

112. Jochems L, Tjalma WA. Primary small cell neuroendocrine tumour of the breast. *Eur J Obstet Gynecol Reprod Biol.* 2004;115:231–233.

113. Hojo T, Kinoshita T, Shien T, et al. Primary small cell carcinoma of the breast. *Breast Cancer.* 2009;16:68–71.

114. Kitakata H, Yasumoto K, Sudo Y, et al. A case of primary small cell carcinoma of the breast. *Breast Cancer.* 2007;14:414–419.

115. Latif N, Rosa M, Samian L, et al. An unusual case of primary small cell neuroendocrine carcinoma of the breast. *Breast J.* 2010;16:647–651.

116. Mariscal A, Balliu E, Diaz R, et al. Primary oat cell carcinoma of the breast: imaging features. *AJR Am J Roentgenol.* 2004;183:1169–1171.

117. Yamaguchi R, Tanaka M, Otsuka H, et al. Neuroendocrine small cell carcinoma of the breast: report of a case. *Med Mol Morphol.* 2009;42:58–61.

118. Amano M, Ogura K, Ozaki Y, et al. Two cases of primary small cell carcinoma of the breast showing non-mass-like pattern on diagnostic imaging and histopathology. *Breast Cancer.* 2015;22:437–441.

119. Papotti M, Gherardi G, Eusebi V, et al. Primary oat cell (neuroendocrine) carcinoma of the breast: report of four cases. *Virchows Arch A Pathol Anat Histopathol.* 1992;420:103–108.

120. Shin SJ, DeLellis RA, Ying L, et al. Small cell carcinoma of the breast: a clinicopathologic and immunohistochemical study of nine patients. *Am J Surg Pathol.* 2000;24:1231–1238.

121. Hoang MP, Maitra A, Gazdar AF, et al. Primary mammary small-cell carcinoma: a molecular analysis of 2 cases. *Hum Pathol.* 2001;32:753–757.

122. Fukunaga M, Ushigome S. Small cell (oat cell) carcinoma of the breast. *Pathol Int.* 1998;48:744–748.

123. Kawasaki T, Bussolati G, Castellano I, et al. Small-cell carcinoma of the breast with squamous differentiation. *Histopathology.* 2013;63:739–741.

124. Kinoshita S, Hirano A, Komine K, et al. Primary small-cell neuroendocrine carcinoma of the breast: report of a case. *Surg Today*. 2008;38:734–738.

125. Salman WD, Harrison JA, Howat AJ. Small-cell neuroendocrine carcinoma of the breast. *J Clin Pathol*. 2006;59:888.

126. Sridhar P, Matey P, Aluwihare N. Primary carcinoma of breast with small-cell differentiation. *Breast*. 2004;13:149–151.

127. Christie M, Chin-Lenn L, Watts MM, et al. Primary small cell carcinoma of the breast with TTF-1 and neuroendocrine marker expressing carcinoma in situ. *Int J Clin Exp Pathol*. 2010;3:629–633.

128. Salmo EN, Connolly CE. Primary small cell carcinoma of the breast: report of a case and review of the literature. *Histopathology*. 2001;38:277–278.

129. Bergman S, Hoda SA, Geisinger KR, et al. E-cadherin-negative primary small cell carcinoma of the breast: report of a case and review of the literature. *Am J Clin Pathol*. 2004;121:117–121.

130. Yamamoto J, Ohshima K, Nabeshima K, et al. Comparative study of primary mammary small cell carcinoma, carcinoma with endocrine features and invasive ductal carcinoma. *Oncol Rep*. 2004;11:825–831.

131. Adegbola T, Connolly CE, Mortimer G. Small cell neuroendocrine carcinoma of the breast: a report of three cases and review of the literature. *J Clin Pathol*. 2005;58:775–778.

132. Ersahin C, Bandyopadhyay S, Bhargava R. Thyroid transcription factor-1 and "basal marker"—expressing small cell carcinoma of the breast. *Int J Surg Pathol*. 2009;17:368–372.

133. An JK, Woo JJ, Kang JH, et al. Small-cell neuroendocrine carcinoma of the breast. *J Korean Surg Soc*. 2012;82:116–119.

134. Ge QD, Lv N, Cao Y, et al. A case report of primary small cell carcinoma of the breast and review of the literature. *Chin J Cancer*. 2012;31:354–358.

135. Shin SJ, DeLellis RA, Rosen PP. Small cell carcinoma of the breast—additional immunohistochemical studies. *Am J Surg Pathol*. 2001;25:831–832.

136. Yamasaki T, Shimazaki H, Aida S, et al. Primary small cell (oat cell) carcinoma of the breast: report of a case and review of the literature. *Pathol Int*. 2000;50:914–918.

137. Bobos M, Hytiroglou P, Kostopoulos I, et al. Immunohistochemical distinction between Merkel cell carcinoma and small cell carcinoma of the lung. *Am J Dermatopathol*. 2006;28:99–104.

138. Hare F, Giri S, Patel JK, et al. A population-based analysis of outcomes for small cell carcinoma of the breast by tumor stage and the use of radiation therapy. *Springerplus*. 2015;4:138.

Glycogen-Rich Carcinoma

139. Fisher ER, Tavares J, Bulatao IS, et al. Glycogen-rich, clear cell breast cancer: with comments concerning other clear cell variants. *Hum Pathol*. 1985;16:1085–1090.

140. Hull MT, Priest JB, Broadie TA, et al. Glycogen-rich clear cell carcinoma of the breast: a light and electron microscopic study. *Cancer*. 1981;48:2003–2009.

141. Akbulut M, Zekioglu O, Kapkac M, et al. Fine needle aspiration cytology of glycogen-rich clear cell carcinoma of the breast: review of 37 cases with histologic correlation. *Acta Cytol*. 2008;52:65–71.

142. Ma X, Han Y, Fan Y, et al. Clinicopathologic characteristics and prognosis of glycogen-rich clear cell carcinoma of the breast. *Breast J*. 2014;20:166–173.

143. Sorensen FB, Paulsen SM. Glycogen-rich clear cell carcinoma of the breast: a solid variant with mucus: a light microscopic, immunohistochemical and ultrastructural study of a case. *Histopathology*. 1987;11:857–869.

144. Hayes MM, Seidman JD, Ashton MA. Glycogen-rich clear cell carcinoma of the breast: a clinicopathologic study of 21 cases. *Am J Surg Pathol*. 1995;19:904–911.

145. Martin-Martin B, Berna-Serna JD, Sanchez-Henarejos P, et al. An unusual case of locally advanced glycogen-rich clear cell carcinoma of the breast. *Case Rep Oncol*. 2011;4:452–457.

146. Salemis NS. Intraductal glycogen-rich clear cell carcinoma of the breast: a rare presentation and review of the literature. *Breast Care (Basel)*. 2012;7:319–321.

147. Gurbuz Y, Ozkara SK. Clear cell carcinoma of the breast with solid papillary pattern: a case report with immunohistochemical profile. *J Clin Pathol*. 2003;56:552–554.

148. Di Tommaso L, Pasquinelli G, Portincasa G, et al. Glycogen-rich clear-cell breast carcinoma with neuroendocrine differentiation features. *Pathologica*. 2001;93:676–680.

149. Sato A, Kawasaki T, Kashiwaba M, et al. Glycogen-rich clear cell carcinoma of the breast showing carcinomatous lymphangiosis and extremely aggressive clinical behavior. *Pathol Int*. 2015;65:674–676.

150. Hull MT, Warfel KA. Glycogen-rich clear cell carcinomas of the breast: a clinicopathologic and ultrastructural study. *Am J Surg Pathol*. 1986;10:553–559.

151. Kuroda H, Sakamoto G, Ohnisi K, et al. Clinical and pathological features of glycogen-rich clear cell carcinoma of the breast. *Breast Cancer*. 2005;12:189–195.

Lipid-Rich Carcinoma

152. Aboumrad MH, Horn RC Jr, Fine G. Lipid-secreting mammary carcinoma: report of a case associated with Paget's disease of the nipple. *Cancer*. 1963;16:521–525.

153. Ramos CV, Taylor HB. Lipid-rich carcinoma of the breast: a clinico-pathologic analysis of 13 examples. *Cancer*. 1974;33:812–819.

154. Mazzella FM, Sieber SC, Braza F. Ductal carcinoma of male breast with prominent lipid-rich component. *Pathology*. 1995;27:280–283.

155. Balik E, Taneli C, Cetinkursun S, et al. Lipid secreting breast carcinoma in childhood: a case report. *Eur J Pediatr Surg*. 1993;3:48–49.

156. Nagata Y, Hanagiri T, Ono K, et al. A non-invasive form of lipid-secreting carcinoma of the breast. *Breast Cancer*. 2012;19:83–87.

157. Kurisu Y, Tsuji M, Shibayama Y, et al. Intraductal lipid-rich carcinoma of the breast with a component of glycogen-rich carcinoma. *J Breast Cancer*. 2012;15:135–138.

158. van Bogaert LJ, Maldague P. Histologic variants of lipid-secreting carcinoma of the breast. *Virchows Arch A Pathol Anat Histol*. 1977;375:345–353.

159. Varga Z, Robl C, Spycher M, et al. Metaplastic lipid-rich carcinoma of the breast. *Pathol Int*. 1998;48:912–916.

160. Tsubura A, Hatano T, Murata A, et al. Breast carcinoma in patients receiving neuroleptic therapy: morphologic and clinicopathologic features of thirteen cases. *Acta Pathol Jpn*. 1992;42:494–499.

161. Kimura A, Miki H, Yuri T, et al. A case report of lipid-rich carcinoma of the breast including histological characteristics and intrinsic subtype profile. *Case Rep Oncol*. 2011;4:275–280.

162. Machalekova K, Kajo K, Bencat M. Unusual occurrence of rare lipid-rich carcinoma and conventional invasive ductal carcinoma in the one breast: case report. *Case Rep Pathol*. 2012;2012:387045.

163. Guan B, Wang H, Cao S, et al. Lipid-rich carcinoma of the breast clinicopathologic analysis of 17 cases. *Ann Diagn Pathol*. 2011;15:225–232.

Other Rare Tpes of Mammary Carcinoma

164. Limite G, Di Micco R, Esposito E, et al. Acinic cell carcinoma of the breast: review of the literature. *Int J Surg*. 2014;12(Suppl 1):S35–S39.

165. Basbug M, Akbulut S, Arikanoglu Z, et al. Mucoepidermoid carcinoma in a breast affected by burn scars: comprehensive literature review and case report. *Breast Care (Basel)*. 2011;6:293–297.

166. Ragazzi M, de Biase D, Betts CM, et al. Oncocytic carcinoma of the breast: frequency, morphology and follow-up. *Hum Pathol*. 2011;42:166–175.

167. Asioli S, Marucci G, Ficarra G, et al. Polymorphous adenocarcinoma of the breast: report of three cases. *Virchows Arch*. 2006;448:29–34.

168. Hisaoka M, Takamatsu Y, Hirano Y, et al. Sebaceous carcinoma of the breast: case report and review of the literature. *Virchows Arch*. 2006;449:484–488.

18

Lobular Carcinoma In Situ and Atypical Lobular Hyperplasia

SYED A. HODA

TERMINOLOGY OF "LOBULAR" LESIONS

Foote and Stewart (1) had coined the term "lobular carcinoma in situ" (LCIS) for a group of in situ carcinomas of the breast that occurred in the terminal ducts and lobules and were characterized by loss of cellular cohesion, presence of cytoplasmic vacuoles, pagetoid extension, and multifocality.

Classic LCIS (C-LCIS) refers to an architectural pattern of LCIS in which the affected acini are minimally distended, and the affected lobules are generally scattered amid breast tissue (**Figs. 18.1–18.3**). In objective terms, distention is defined as "the presence of 8 or more cells in the cross-sectional diameter of an acinus" (2). C-LCIS may be populated by cells of type "A" or type "B."

LCIS with type "A" cytology is characterized by smaller cells (<1.5X size of lymphocyte) with minimal cytoplasm, low-grade nuclei, inconspicuous nucleoli, and extremely rare mitoses. LCIS with type "B' cytology is typified by larger cells (2X size of lymphocyte) with relatively more cytoplasm, intermediate-grade nuclei, presence of micronucleoli, and rare mitoses (**Fig. 18.4**).

The classification of C-LCIS into types "A" and "B" is of no known clinical significance; however, such categorization serves as a reminder that "some cytologic variation can be observed in *bona fide* cases of C-LCIS, and these features should not be over-interpreted as representing the pleomorphic variant of LCIS" (2). Nevertheless, in recent years, the cytologic classification of LCIS as "type A" and "type B" has been largely abandoned, in favor of grouping into classic, florid, and pleomorphic variants.

LCIS can be architecturally as well as cytologically (if not molecularly) heterogeneous. Minimal distention of acini is the hallmark of C-LCIS, whereas confluent lobular involvement with marked distention of acini is observed in *florid LCIS* (F-LCIS). The *pleomorphic variant of LCIS* (P-LCIS) is typically characterized by high-grade nuclei populating LCIS with florid-type features.

F-LCIS may be populated by cells of types "A" or "B" and can show central necrosis (**Fig. 18.5**). F-LCIS with signet ring cells has also been described (3). F-LCIS shares several features with C-LCIS including some cytologic characteristics, loss of E-cadherin, gain of 1q, and loss of 16q; however, F-LCIS has been shown to demonstrate more genomic alterations than C-LCIS (4).

P-LCIS refers to an architectural as well as cytologic pattern of LCIS in which there is diffusely confluent involvement of several contiguous lobules, and the individual acini are considerably distended (**Fig. 18.6**). P-LCIS is populated by cells with variable size and shape (hence, the designation: pleomorphic). P-LCIS cells are much larger (4X size of lymphocyte) and bear high-grade nuclei, irregular nuclear membrane, prominent nucleoli, and frequent mitoses. Central necrosis of the so-called "comedo" type usually accompanies P-LCIS. LCIS that is *cytologically* pleomorphic can be rarely found with classic *architectural* morphology in the vicinity of typical examples of P-LCIS. Some cases of P-LCIS possess abundant eosinophilic (apocrine-type) cytoplasm.

The issue of how much lobular involvement is necessary for the diagnosis of LCIS is of questionable relevance in the diagnosis of needle core biopsies (NCBs) that provide limited samples. Because the number of affected lobules in a biopsy has not proven to be related to the risk for subsequent carcinoma among patients not treated by mastectomy (5,6), there is presently no reason for drawing a distinction between one and two or more involved lobules as a basis for the diagnosis of LCIS (5). In some instances, the only evidence of a neoplastic lobular proliferation is one lobule in which some, but not all, acini are involved. It has been suggested, rather arbitrarily, that at least 50% (7) or 75% (8) of one lobule should be involved to establish a diagnosis of LCIS. Specimens with lesser lesions should be included in the category of *atypical lobular hyperplasia* (ALH).

The umbrella diagnostic term *lobular neoplasia* (LN), encompassing ALH and LCIS, was introduced by Haagensen et al. (9) in an era when breast conservation therapy was uncommon mainly for the purpose of avoiding overtreatment of the disease by removing the word "carcinoma" (**Fig. 18.7**). This rationale is no longer valid in the era of breast conservation. Furthermore, the spectrum of lesions encompassed by LN, from ALH to P-LCIS, is so broad as to render it a useless term. The use of this misleading term demonstrates a lack of regard for criteria-based diagnosis.

Gomes et al. (10) have reported good interobserver agreement between general pathologists and specialized breast pathologists in the diagnosis of ALH (Kappa = 0.62) and LCIS (Kappa = 0.66); however, poor agreement was observed for P-LCIS (Kappa = 0.22). It is likely that the presence of overt central necrosis in P-LCIS is the most likely reason for it to be mistaken for high-grade DCIS.

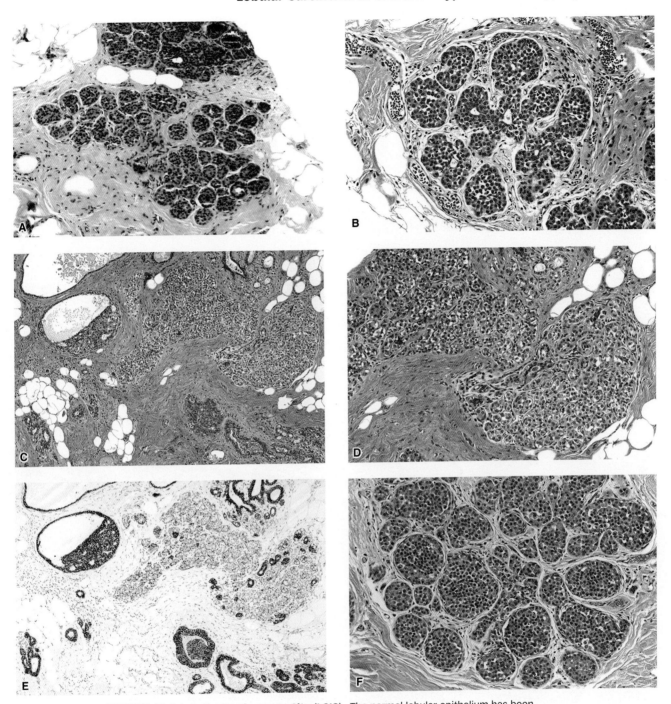

FIGURE 18.1 Lobular Carcinoma In Situ (LCIS). The normal lobular epithelium has been replaced by neoplastic cells that fill the acinar lumina in these needle core biopsy specimens. **A:** Two contiguous lobules are affected. The biopsy was performed for mammographically detected calcifications that were present in lobular glands not involved by in situ carcinoma. **B:** Magnified view of classic LCIS in a lobule is shown. **C, D:** Classic form of LCIS. **E:** The neoplastic cells are negative for E-cadherin. **F, G:** Two additional cases of classic LCIS. The "cloverleaf" pattern of lobular involvement is seen in **(G)**.

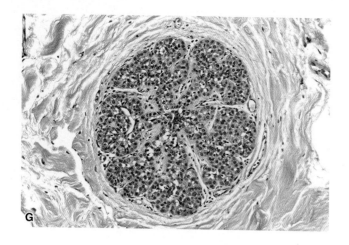

G

FIGURE 18.1 (*continued*)

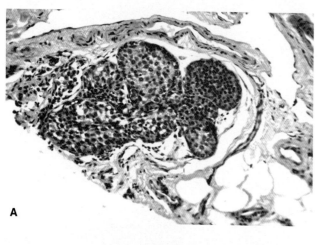

A

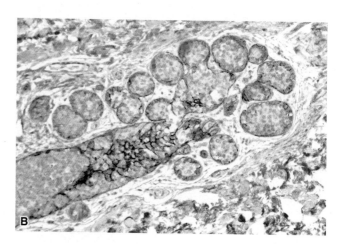

B

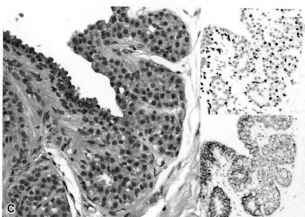

C

FIGURE 18.2 Lobular Carcinoma In Situ (LCIS). A: A needle core biopsy specimen with a completely involved lobule. **B:** E-cadherin reactivity is present in residual ductal epithelium and in lobular myoepithelial cells in this example of LCIS in a terminal duct–lobular unit. The neoplastic cells are not reactive. **C:** Another example of LCIS involving a terminal duct lobular unit. Top inset shows abundant presence of myoepithelial cells (p63-positive) around the LCIS. Bottom inset shows E-cadherin reactivity in myoepithelial cells and the absence of E-cadherin in the neoplastic cells. Such a lesion can be mistaken for myoepithelial hyperplasia.

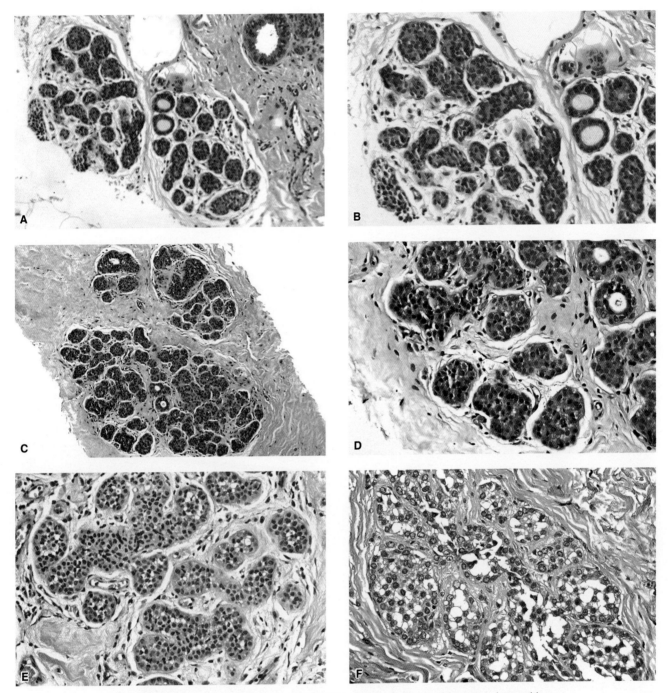

FIGURE 18.3 Lobular Carcinoma In Situ (LCIS). A, B: A needle core biopsy specimen with minimal diagnostic evidence. Approximately 85% of the lobular glands are involved. **C, D:** Another example of minimal evidence for LCIS in a needle core biopsy sample. Note the distinct lobular glands. **E:** Loss of cohesion and focal cellular degeneration have resulted in the formation of spaces in some lobular glands. These are not true acinar lumina. Extreme loss of cohesion in LCIS **(F)**.

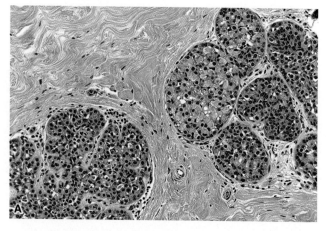

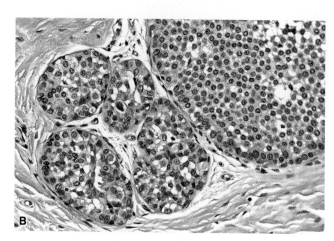

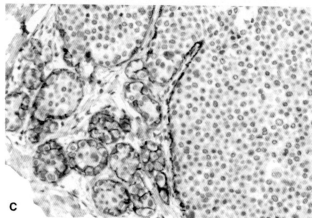

FIGURE 18.4 Lobular Carcinoma In Situ (LCIS): Types A and B. A, B: LCIS with type "A" cytology is characterized by smaller cells with minimal cytoplasm and low-grade nuclei. LCIS with type "B" cytology is typified by larger cells with relatively more cytoplasm, intermediate-grade nuclei. Type "A" LCIS is on the top right and type "B" LCIS is on the lower left in **(B)**. **C:** The E-cadherin immunostain is negative in both types of LCIS (same case as shown in **B**).

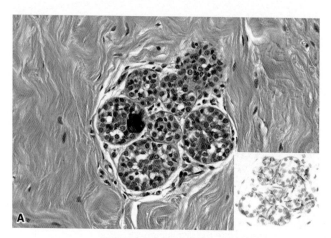

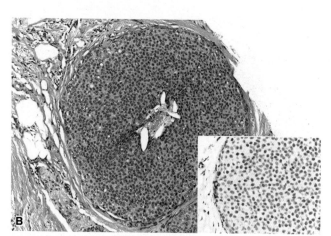

FIGURE 18.5 Lobular Carcinoma In Situ (LCIS), Classic and Florid Patterns. A: Low-grade neoplastic cells fill acini in this example of classic LCIS. This particular lesion has a calcification. **B:** A markedly enlarged duct is filled with a solid growth of florid LCIS with punctate central necrosis (insets show negativity for E-cadherin in each case). **C, D:** Two examples of florid LCIS with "macroacini," intermediate-grade nuclei, necrosis, and calcifications are shown. Insets show negativity for E-cadherin in each case.

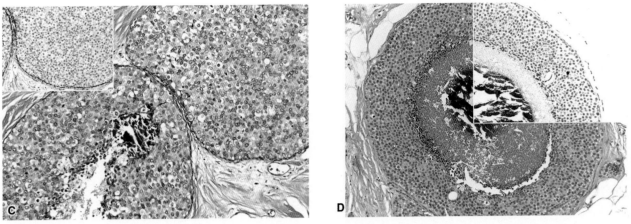

FIGURE 18.5 (*continued*)

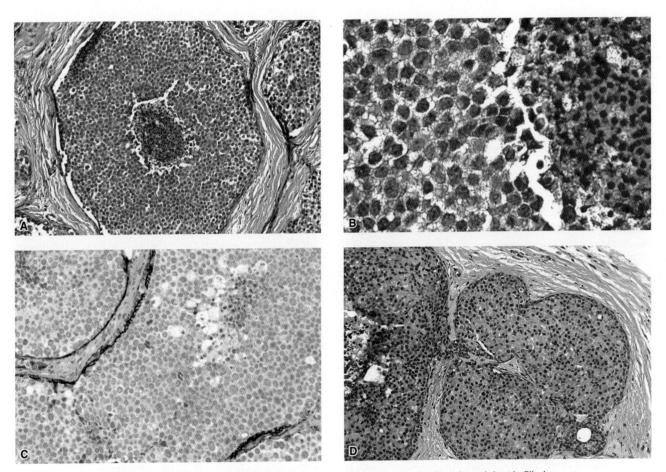

FIGURE 18.6 **Florid Lobular Carcinoma In Situ (LCIS).** **A:** A markedly enlarged duct is filled with a solid growth of pleomorphic LCIS. Central "comedo-type" necrosis is evident. **B:** This magnified view of the carcinoma shows necrosis and loss of cohesion between tumor cells. **C:** The LCIS is E-cadherin-negative. Reactivity is demonstrated in persisting myoepithelium. **D–F:** Another example of florid LCIS composed of cells with cytoplasmic mucin. The LCIS is E-cadherin-negative **(F).**

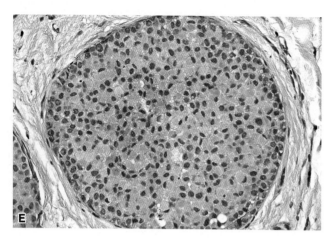 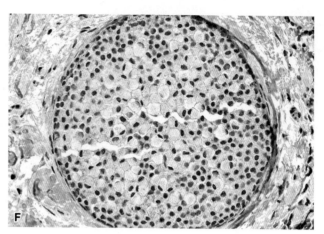

FIGURE 18.6 (*continued*)

CLINICAL PRESENTATION

The classic form of lobular carcinoma in situ (C-LCIS) is a lesion that is evident only on microscopic examination; it almost never forms a palpable tumor (11). C-LCIS is rarely detectable with various imaging modalities. Typically, C-LCIS is discovered incidentally in breast tissue biopsied for lesions that produce masses or cause abnormalities on imaging studies. Calcifications are infrequently formed in C-LCIS (12), and when present are usually associated with an underlying lesion. No radiologic technique has proven to be an effective method for detecting C-LCIS, and thus imaging studies cannot be depended upon to assess the presence of the disease (5,13).

Exceptional situations exist in the relatively infrequent instances of F-LCIS and P-LCIS, the two variant forms of LCIS. These forms of LCIS show marked expansion of acini within lobules. F-LCIS and P-LCIS may involve the breast extensively, and can sometimes involve foci of sclerosing adenosis. As stated earlier, F-LCIS can be populated by cells with either low-grade (type "A"), intermediate-grade (type "B"), or high-grade ("pleomorphic") nuclei. Necrosis and calcification can be associated with F-LCIS inhabited by neoplastic cells that possess either intermediate- or high-grade nuclei, and with nearly every case of P-LCIS. Such lesions display a pattern and distribution more commonly encountered with ductal carcinoma in situ (DCIS) rather than LCIS (14). Thus, the resultant appearance on mammography is likely to suggest DCIS. The most compelling evidence supporting classification of such cases as LCIS is the lack of E-cadherin immunoreactivity as well as the finding of associated C-LCIS and/or invasive lobular carcinoma in some cases.

INCIDENCE

In a retrospective cohort analysis of SEER (Surveillance, Epidemiology and End Results) database, including 14,048 patients diagnosed with LCIS, a 38% increase in the incidence of LCIS (15) was reported, from 2.0/100,000 to 2.75/100,000,

from 2000 to 2009. Ten percent of the LCIS patients reportedly underwent biopsy alone, seventy-four percent underwent excision, and sixteen percent had mastectomy.

In retrospective reviews, published in previous decades, each involving several thousand breast specimens, the frequency of LCIS was 0.5% to 1.5% (16–18). Analysis of population-based data from 1978 to 1998 in the United States revealed an increase in the incidence rate of LCIS from 0.90 per 100,000 person years to 3.19 per 100,000 person years (19). Incidence rates increased continuously throughout the two decades–long study period among postmenopausal women with the highest incidence rate among women 50 to 59 years of age in 1996 to 1998 (11.47/100,000 person years). The absence of consistent pathology review creates uncertainty about the reliability of the data, but if it is correct, the increasing use of breast imaging leading to more frequent biopsies is probably the most important factor responsible for this change. In particular, columnar cell alterations, which are predisposed to develop calcifications, often coexist with LCIS (20,21).

Parenthetically, *The Rosen Triad* comprises LCIS, columnar cell changes, and tubular carcinoma (**Fig. 18.8**) (22). The latter two lesions are often responsible for mammographically detected calcifications in the absence of a palpable lesion. ALH and LCIS are commonly associated with various types of columnar change (**Fig. 18.9**). An instance of the Rosen Triad with LCIS of the signet ring cell type has been reported (23).

Up to 25% of LCIS patients are postmenopausal at the time of first diagnosis (24). LCIS occurs infrequently in women younger than 35 years. In a consecutive series of more than 1,000 patients treated for breast carcinoma, the mean age of women with LCIS (53 years) was not significantly different from the mean age of patients who had invasive ductal carcinoma (57 years) (25).

Some conclusions based on the earliest studies of LCIS are still valid and provide invaluable insight into its behavior. These conclusions include the relatively high frequency of ipsilateral multicentric carcinoma, including occult invasive carcinoma in 5% to 6% of women who undergo mastectomy (26,27). Urban (28) had reported finding LCIS in the contralateral breast in

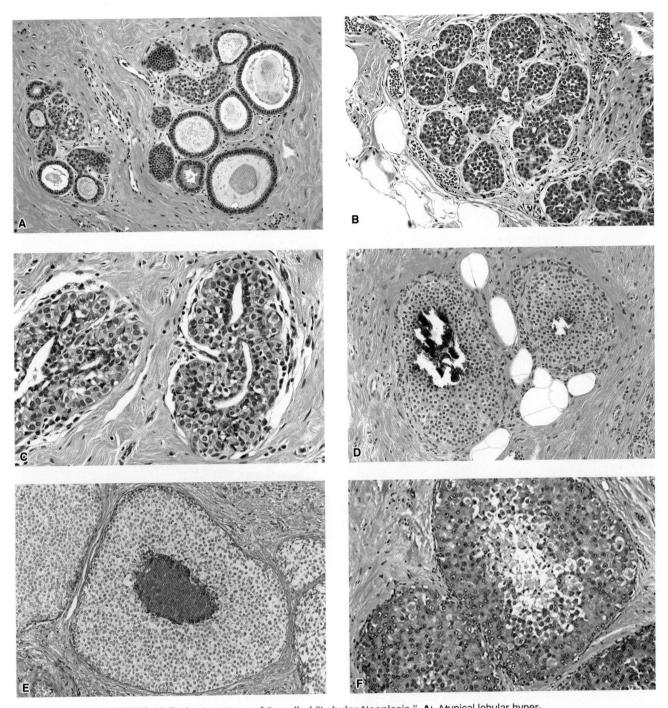

FIGURE 18.7 The Spectrum of So-called "Lobular Neoplasia." A: Atypical lobular hyperplasia. **B:** Classic lobular carcinoma in situ (LCIS), type "A." **C:** LCIS, type "B." **D:** Florid LCIS with calcifications. **E:** Florid LCIS with markedly distended acini, intermediate-grade nuclei, and central necrosis. **F:** Pleomorphic LCIS with markedly distended acini, high-grade nuclei, slightly apocrine cytoplasmic traits, and central necrosis.

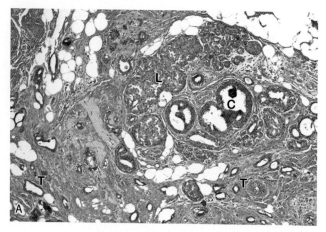
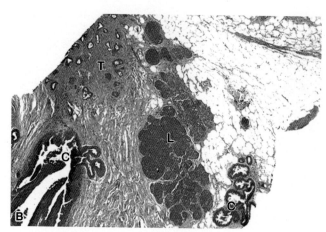

FIGURE 18.8 The Rosen Triad. A, B: Two examples of "The Rosen Triad" comprising lobular carcinoma in situ (labeled *L*), columnar cell changes (labeled *C*), and tubular carcinoma (labeled *T*) are shown. The entire triad is seen in a needle core biopsy sampling in **(A)**.

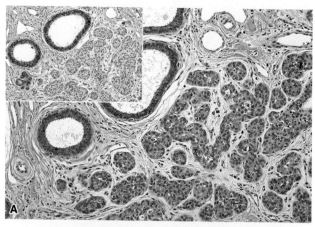
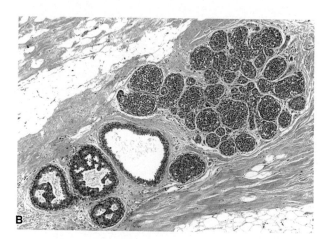
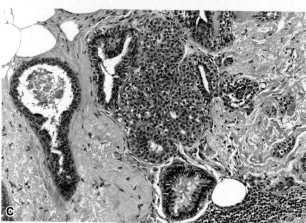

FIGURE 18.9 Lobular Carcinoma In Situ (LCIS)/Atypical Lobular Hyperplasia (ALH) and Columnar Cell Changes. A: LCIS associated with columnar cell change (inset shows E-cadherin negativity in LCIS and E-cadherin positivity in columnar cell change). **B:** LCIS associated with atypical columnar cell hyperplasia. **C:** ALH associated with columnar cell change.

40% of the cases when a random biopsy was performed even in the absence of any clinical abnormality. This procedure is rarely done today.

HISTOPATHOLOGY OF LCIS

The anatomic distribution of LCIS in lobules and terminal ducts (and occasionally in ducts) as well as morphologic alterations in these structures influence the histopathologic appearance of LCIS in any given case. In the typical lobular form, a population of neoplastic cells replaces the normal epithelium of acini within lobules. Intralobular ductules are also characteristically involved **(Fig. 18.10)**. The LCIS cells must be sufficiently numerous to cause expansion of these structures. There may be enlargement of the entire lobule in comparison with uninvolved lobules in the adjacent breast tissues; however, the lobular enlargement is not an absolute diagnostic criterion

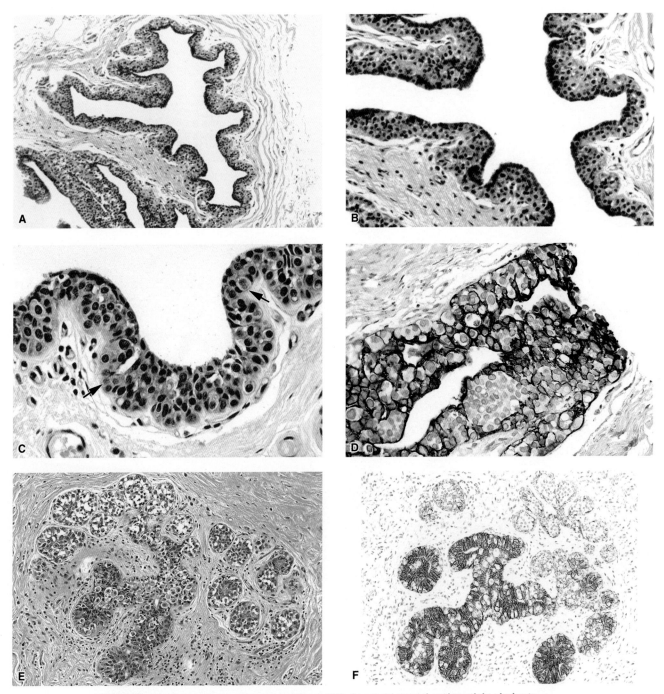

FIGURE 18.10 Lobular Carcinoma In Situ (LCIS), Pagetoid Ductal and Partial Lobular Involvement. A, B: These dilated ducts involved by pagetoid spread of LCIS were found in a needle core biopsy specimen. **C:** Intracytoplasmic mucin is demonstrated with the mucicarmine stain in carcinoma cells *(arrows)* but not in the overlying residual benign ductal epithelium. **D:** Pagetoid LCIS in this duct is highlighted by absence of E-cadherin reactivity. The hyperplastic ductal epithelium is E-cadherin-positive. **E, F:** LCIS with partial (>50%) involvement of a lobule. E-cadherin immunostain (in **F**) shows reactivity limited to residual ductal cells.

(Fig. 18.11). The drift to lobular atrophy in postmenopausal women makes expansion of lobules an unreliable diagnostic feature in that patient group. If the diagnosis of LCIS is to be meaningful because it identifies a lesion associated with a substantial risk of later carcinoma, then the *architectural or quantitative finding of lobular enlargement* cannot be regarded as the paramount diagnostic criterion in lesions that have reached an acceptable *qualitative level of cytologic abnormality*.

Loss of intercellular cohesion is a characteristic of LCIS, although this is not always readily apparent in acini filled and expanded by the process. When loss of cohesion is prominent, the resultant spaces may be mistaken for glandular lumina.

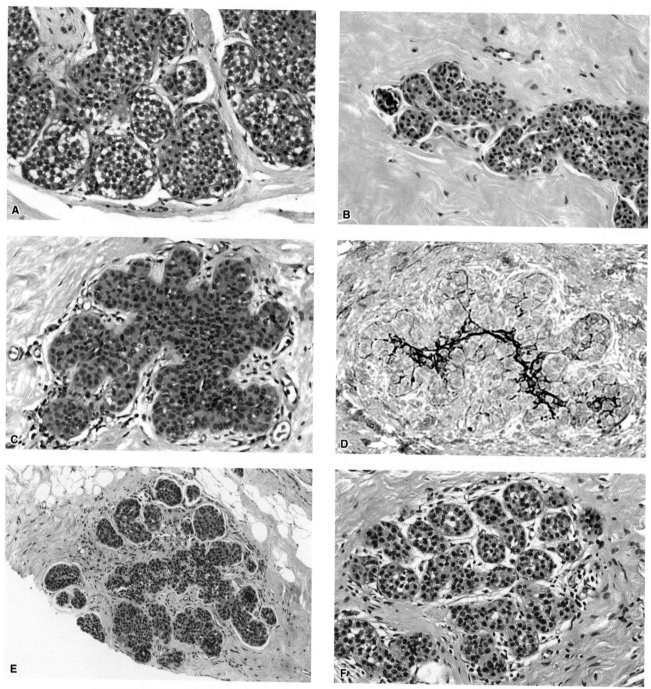

FIGURE 18.11 Lobular Carcinoma In Situ (LCIS). **A:** LCIS as it appeared when the patient was premenopausal. The lobular glands are fully expanded. **B, C:** LCIS as it appeared in a biopsy specimen taken from the same breast after the menopause. The lobules are markedly shrunken. One lobular gland contains a calcification **(B)**. **D:** The lobule shown in **(C)** stained for E-cadherin showing strong reactivity in residual non-neoplastic epithelium and weak, fragmented reactivity in the LCIS. Reactivity is present in residual ductal epithelial cells in the center of the ductule. The LCIS cells are E-cadherin-negative. **E:** The only histopathologic lesion in this needle core biopsy specimen was this lobule with LCIS. **F:** This is one of several foci of LCIS found in the subsequent excisional biopsy specimen.

Degenerative changes may also disrupt the cellular composition of LCIS. In these situations, the neoplastic cells are not arranged in the polarized fashion. The latter is a trait of non-neoplastic cells persisting around true glandular lumina. Loss of cohesion in lobular neoplastic lesions is attributable to

genetic alterations in the *E-cadherin* gene that are manifested by greatly reduced, fragmented, or absent membrane E-cadherin immunoreactivity (29,30).

Intracytoplasmic vacuoles that contain mucin are present in some LCIS cells **(Fig. 18.12)**. The presence of mucin can

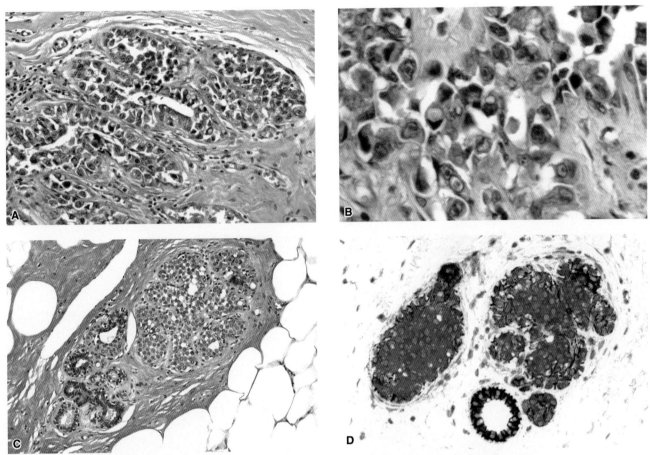

FIGURE 18.12 Lobular Carcinoma In Situ (LCIS), Postmenopausal. A, B: The lesion is characterized by loss of cohesion and shrinkage of the tumor cells in lobular glands. Intracytoplasmic mucin is demonstrated with the mucicarmine stain **(B)**. **C, D:** In this example of LCIS in the elderly, the entire lobule is small. The lesional cells are p120-positive (depicted by red cytoplasmic staining). Benign epithelial cells are strongly positive for E-cadherin (depicted by brown staining), and myoepithelial cells show weaker staining with E-cadherin (double immunostain with p120 and E-cadherin). The LCIS cells are not reactive for E-cadherin.

be an inconspicuous feature that can be highlighted with mucicarmine, Alcian blue, or periodic acid–Schiff (PAS) stains (31,32). An extreme manifestation of this phenomenon is the formation of signet ring cells having a distended cytoplasmic vacuole that causes the nucleus to appear eccentric, crescentic, or indented. Signet ring cells can have low-, intermediate-, or high-grade nuclei. Intracytoplasmic mucin vacuoles are uncommon in ductal carcinoma cells and are also uncommon in hyperplastic lesions of ductal or lobular epithelium. Thus, the presence of intracellular mucin is an important but not a necessary criterion for the diagnosis of LCIS. Intracytoplasmic mucin is also present in LCIS with clear cell change.

Several uncommon cytologic features can be found in LCIS. Cytoplasmic pallor or cytoplasmic clearing occurs rarely in LCIS. These cells may have intracytoplasmic mucin that is not restricted to vacuoles, an occurrence manifested by diffuse cytoplasmic staining with the mucicarmine or Alcian blue stain. Apocrine change has been described in LCIS (33). Mucin in the cytoplasm of cells in apocrine LCIS is usually evident in H&E-stained sections as cytoplasmic amphophilia or basophilia. Apocrine LCIS often has pleomorphic cytology and tends to grow in a pagetoid manner into ducts where it

can be difficult to distinguish from apocrine DCIS. However, apocrine LCIS is E-cadherin-negative, and it is often estrogen receptor (ER)-positive, whereas apocrine DCIS is E-cadherin-positive and almost always ER-negative. LCIS in atrophic lobules and terminal ducts of postmenopausal women sometimes features cells with dark, eosinophilic-to-basophilic cytoplasm and deeply basophilic, eccentric nuclei. This appearance is probably the result of cytoplasmic condensation associated with loss of cohesion and shrinkage of cells. These cells frequently contain intracytoplasmic mucin. In another variant, the cells of LCIS have a *mosaic* appearance that results from the presence of distinct cell borders between cells and prominent, round, centrally placed nuclei surrounded by pale cytoplasm **(Fig. 18.13)**. Intracytoplasmic mucin vacuoles can usually be found in this type of LCIS.

LCIS typically involves intralobular and extralobular or terminal ductules as well as acinar units within the lobule **(Fig. 18.14)**. In postmenopausal patients with atrophic lobules, ductal involvement may be the only manifestation of LCIS (34). The irregular configuration of ductules affected by LCIS has been described as "saw-toothed" or as resembling a cloverleaf. Pagetoid LCIS cells growing beneath the non-neoplastic ductal

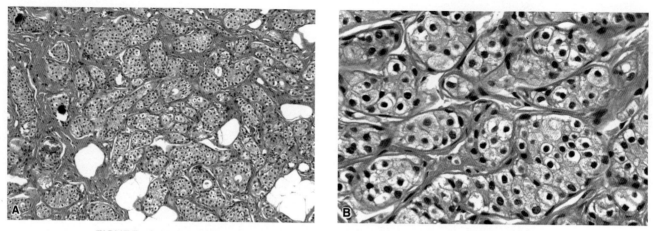

FIGURE 18.13 Lobular Carcinoma In Situ (LCIS), Mosaic Pattern. A, B: The lesion involves sclerosing adenosis. Calcifications are shown in **(A).** The cells have distinct cytoplasmic borders, abundant pale cytoplasm, and punctate centrally placed nuclei.

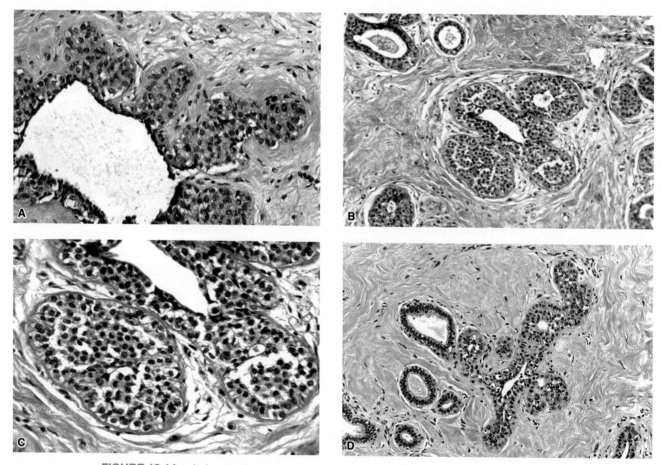

FIGURE 18.14 Lobular Carcinoma In Situ (LCIS), Ductal Involvement. A: The cloverleaf pattern of ductal involvement is shown. The presence of lobule-like structures around the perimeter of the duct suggests that the neoplasm arose de novo at this site. **B, C:** This small duct exhibits florid LCIS and pagetoid spread in adjacent ductules. **D:** Another example of LCIS with pagetoid spread into a terminal duct.

epithelium may be distributed continuously or discontinuously along the ductal system, undermining, and ultimately displacing the normal ductal epithelium. The cloverleaf pattern of LCIS sometimes involves the terminal ducts, seemingly without lobular involvement. The myoepithelial layer is preserved to a variable extent, and it may require p63 and actin immunostains to confirm that it is present. LCIS can be found in lesions with intra-acinar myoepithelial cell hyperplasia (35).

Pagetoid spread of LCIS may also be encountered in papillomas or radial scar lesions. F-LCIS may proliferate to form a solid mass of tumor cells that fill and expand the ductal lumen, and develop central necrosis and calcifications that are detectable in mammograms. A negative, weak, or fragmented E-cadherin immunostain distinguishes this pattern of F-LCIS from E-cadherin-positive solid type of high-grade DCIS (36).

LCIS WITH COLLAGENOUS SPHERULOSIS

An unusual pattern of ductal involvement occurs when LCIS develops in ducts altered by collagenous spherulosis (37,38).

This configuration mimics cribriform DCIS (**Fig. 18.15**). However, myoepithelial cells outline the spherule material. The latter should be distinguished from true microlumina of cribiform carcinoma. The neoplastic cells in such foci display loss of cohesion and intracytoplasmic vacuoles characteristic of lobular carcinoma. When LCIS involves collagenous spherulosis, myoepithelium can be highlighted with immunostains such as p63 and myosin. LCIS cells will be E-cadherin-negative. LCIS in collagenous spherulosis only rarely occurs as an isolated finding even in NCB samplings. In the series reported by Eisenberg and Hoda (38), LCIS was identified beyond the index lesion in 4 of 38 cases (14%). In this series, 22 of the 38 specimens were NCB samplings.

MOLECULAR ALTERATIONS

Losses in chromosome 16q22.1, the site of the *CDH1* gene, are the most common cytogenetic abnormality found in LCIS (39). E-cadherin is the protein product of the *CDH1* gene. Despite the high frequency of somatic E-cadherin mutations

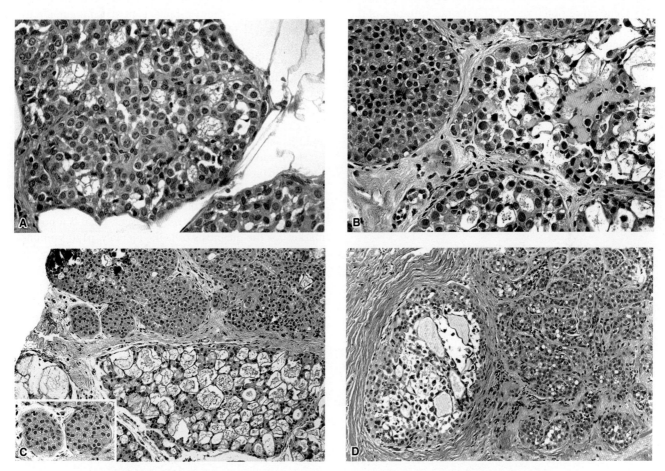

FIGURE 18.15 Lobular Carcinoma In Situ (LCIS) in Collagenous Spherulosis. A: LCIS is shown involving collagenous spherulosis above. Indistinct fibrillary material in the spherules contributes to the cribriform-like appearance. **B:** Pleomorphic LCIS in collagenous spherulosis. **C:** LCIS with apocrine traits and calcifications in degenerative collagenous spherulosis. LCIS is shown in the inset. **D:** LCIS in collagenous spherulosis with "mucoid" features. **E:** LCIS with collagenous spherulosis mimicking cribriform type of ductal carcinoma in situ (DCIS). **F:** LCIS in collagenous spherulosis that resembles cribriform/solid DCIS with calcifications. Inset shows absence of E-cadherin immunoreactivity.

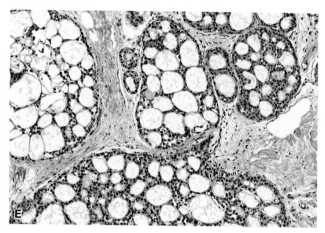
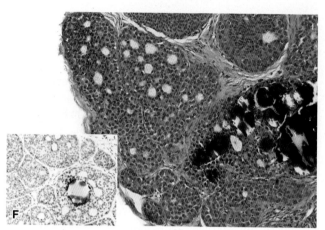

FIGURE 18.15 (*continued*)

in LCIS, germline E-cadherin mutations are rarely detected in these patients (39,40).

The heterogeneity of LCIS has been demonstrated at the transcriptomic level, and several candidate precursor genes that may play a role in disease progression have been identified (41). Gene expression profiling and the identification of the molecular drivers of LCIS may further our understanding of this enigmatic disease (42).

The data most closely linking LCIS to invasive lobular carcinoma come from molecular studies of the two lesions when they coexist. For example, Vos et al. (29) demonstrated that LCIS and invasive lobular carcinomas had losses of the same alleles in 16q22.1 and the same E-cadherin mutations. Similar results were obtained by Sarrió et al. (43) who found that coincidental LCIS and invasive lobular carcinomas shared the same E-cadherin mutations and the same distribution of loss of heterozygosity. Additional supporting studies were published by Nayar et al. (44) and Hwang et al. (45).

IMMUNOHISTOCHEMISTRY

The distinction between LCIS and DCIS on NCB sampling is of clinical significance because a subsequent excisional biopsy may not, on occasions, be performed for LCIS. Furthermore, there may be long-term implications for nonsurgical risk reducing management. Immunohistochemical features of LCIS are listed in **Table 18.1**.

C-LCIS is strongly and diffusely positive for ER and for progesterone receptors (PRs), and only rarely express HER2 or p53 protein. F-LCIS shows a similar pattern of immunoreactivity. Khoury et al. (46) reported the results of ancillary studies on P-LCIS. Seven of the twenty-five (28%) cases were negative for ER, nine (36%) were negative for PR, and five (20%) were negative for both ER and PR. Seven of the seventeen cases (41%) were HER2-positive, and eight (47%) were equivocal for HER2. There were two triple-negative cases. P-LCIS with apocrine features are even more likely to be negative for ER and PR, and show HER2 expression (47).

The E-cadherin complex is composed of transmembrane E-cadherin protein and various catenins (including alpha- and beta-catenin as well as p120 catenin). The catenins serve to anchor the E-cadherin protein to cytoplasmic actin filaments. When E-cadherin is defective or absent, p120 is a positive marker for the diagnosis of LCIS. Notably, p120 immunoreactivity is evident in cytosol of ALH, LCIS, and invasive lobular carcinoma cells. Beta-catenin as well as alpha-catenin are absent in ALH and LCIS (48,49). LCIS is negative for E-cadherin in at least 90% of all LCIS cases. It is important to ensure that there is cytoplasmic membrane positivity of

TABLE 18.1

Immunohistochemical Stains in the Differential Diagnosis of Three Forms of LCIS

	C-LCIS	**F-LCIS**	**P-LCIS**
ER	(+)	(+)	(−/+)
PR	(+)	(+)	(−/+)
HER2	(−)	(−)	(−/+)
E-cadherin	(−)	(−)	(−)
p120	Cytoplasmic+	Cytoplasmic+	Cytoplasmic+
Ki67	Low	Intermediate	High

C-LCIS, classic lobular carcinoma in situ; F-LCIS, florid lobular carcinoma in situ; P-LCIS, pleomorphic lobular carcinoma in situ.

E-cadherin in normal breast epithelium before interpreting the lack of lesional staining as negative.

Rarely, the cells of ALH or LCIS display weak, fragmented, and discontinuous E-cadherin reactivity that is substantially weaker than reactivity in ductal epithelium, so-called "aberrant reactivity" (36,50–53). Approximately 10% of LCIS cases express E-cadherin, that is, they show aberrant (that is, either patchy, or weak, or "dot-like") immunoreactivity for E-cadherin (54,55). Cases of LCIS that have aberrant E-cadherin reactivity may also be positive for beta-catenin and p120—a finding that is consistent with loss of function of the E-cadherin and catenin complex in such cases (56). Aberrant reactivity for E-cadherin should not preclude the diagnosis of LCIS if the cytologic and histologic characteristics are indicative of lobular rather than ductal differentiation. It is notable that true E-cadherin negativity in carcinomas of ductal phenotype (except those of the metaplastic type) is extremely rare (<1%) (57).

Some cases of LCIS show concomitant classic and pleomorphic cell types, both of which are E-cadherin-negative (29). Variable E-cadherin reactivity has been reported when different antibodies were used (52).

In some cases, apparent positivity of LCIS cells for E-cadherin may be due to admixture of reactive myoepithelial cells or residual ductal epithelial cells. The presence of residual, non-neoplastic ductal or lobular epithelial cells or myoepithelial cells is most commonly responsible for traces of reactivity that can be found in some cases of LCIS. Indeed, there may be marked intra-acinar myoepithelial proliferation in certain LCIS lesions (58). In such cases, E-cadherin shows negativity in LCIS, and diffuse, albeit weak, positivity in myoepithelial cells. There is a potential for such biphasic staining to be misinterpreted, and for the lesion to be diagnosed as mixed LCIS and DCIS.

DIFFERENTIAL DIAGNOSIS

DCIS is the most frequent entity that is mistaken for LCIS, and vice versa. Low-grade solid DCIS can be mistaken for C-LCIS and F-LCIS (**Table 18.2**), and P-LCIS may be difficult to distinguish from high-grade DCIS. The E-cadherin immunostain is the most effective method to differentiate between LCIS and DCIS.

Intraepithelial histiocytes can be confused with pagetoid LCIS. Histiocytes possess foamy cytoplasm, sometimes with lipofuscin or hemosiderin pigment, and small dark nuclei. Intracytoplasmic mucin is typically absent from histiocytes, and the cells are not immunoreactive for cytokeratin. The overlying non-neoplastic epithelium is attenuated and flattened over intraepithelial histiocytes as well as over pagetoid spread of LCIS. Intraepithelial histiocytes may be relatively sparse, or they may form a continuous layer, which may be one or more cells thick. The CD68 immunostain highlights histiocytes.

Epithelioid myoepithelial hyperplasia is more likely to be mistaken for pagetoid spread of LCIS than the presence of intraepithelial histiocytes. Epithelioid myoepithelial cells have abundant clear vesicular cytoplasm. Except in papillomas, hyperplastic myoepithelial cells tend to be distributed in a single layer causing less attenuation of the overlying epithelium than pagetoid LCIS. Some "myoid" immunohistochemical properties are usually retained in epithelioid myoepithelial hyperplasia. p63 immunostain is reliable in this circumstance because nuclear reactivity is retained in epithelioid myoepithelial cells, whereas LCIS cells are p63-negative.

Coexistence of LCIS and DCIS in a single duct is an extremely unusual phenomenon (**Figs. 18.16 and 18.17**). When this occurs, LCIS often grows in a cloverleaf pattern around the perimeter of a ductal lumen that contains cytologically and histologically different DCIS. Immunostaining is helpful in confirming the diagnosis of coexistent LCIS and DCIS in a single ductal–lobular unit: LCIS is E-cadherin-negative, and the DCIS is E-cadherin-positive (36).

Lobules structurally altered by various benign proliferative processes can harbor LCIS (37,38). As a consequence, LCIS has been encountered in sclerosing adenosis, radial scars, collagenous spherulosis, fibroadenoma, phyllodes tumor, papilloma, and papillary carcinoma (**Fig. 18.18**). The diagnosis of LCIS under these circumstances rests largely on the identification of the appropriate cytologic features and absence of E-cadherin reactivity. The demonstration of intracytoplasmic mucin

---

TABLE 18.2

Staining Patterns of Classic LCIS and Low-grade Solid DCIS

	Classic LCIS	Low-grade Solid DCIS
Mucin stains[a]	(+)	(−)
E-cadherin	(−)	(+)
Beta-catenin	(−)	(+)
Alpha-catenin	(−)	(+)
p120 localization	(+) cytoplasmic	(+) cytoplasmic membrane
cytokeratin 34βE12	(+)	(−), or weakly (+)

[a]Either mucicarmine, Alcian blue, or periodic acid–Schiff histochemical stains can be utilized.
LCIS, lobular carcinoma in situ; DCIS, ductal carcinoma in situ.

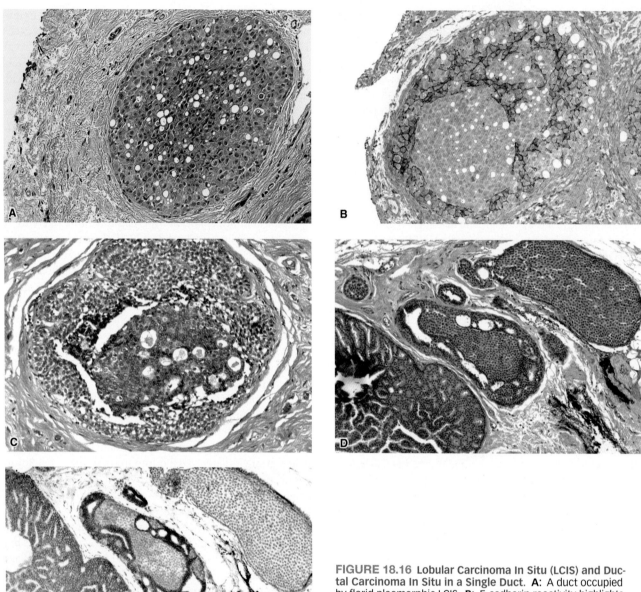

FIGURE 18.16 Lobular Carcinoma In Situ (LCIS) and Ductal Carcinoma In Situ in a Single Duct. **A:** A duct occupied by florid pleomorphic LCIS. **B:** E-cadherin reactivity highlights residual ductal epithelial cells. The LCIS cells are E-cadherin-negative. **C:** The lumen of the duct contains cribriform intraductal carcinoma. LCIS has a cloverleaf pattern around the perimeter of the duct. **D:** Another case in which LCIS merges with cribriform intraductal carcinoma. **E:** E-cadherin reactivity is present only in the ductal carcinoma. (Images **D** and **E** courtesy of Dr. Malini Harigopal.)

droplets is helpful for distinguishing LCIS from florid adenosis because intracellular mucin may be present in the former but not in the latter. LCIS in tubular adenosis, and in sclerosing adenosis, has a striking histologic appearance (**Fig. 18.19**). In all of the foregoing situations, the most reliable method for confirming the presence of LCIS is the demonstration of weak, fragmented, or absent E-cadherin immunoreactivity.

Normal lobular architecture is radically distorted in sclerosing lesions, and as a result it is difficult to exclude invasion when LCIS occurs in such foci (59). Careful inspection usually

reveals the underlying adenosis pattern in which glandular units are surrounded by myoepithelial cells and basement membrane. The latter structure can be highlighted with reticulin stain and by laminin or type IV collagen immunostain. p63, CD10, calponin, and actin immunostains highlight the myoepithelial layer. The spindle-shaped myoepithelial cells persist in sclerosing adenosis, albeit in an extremely slender form, even when the lesion is colonized by LCIS (60). Invasive carcinoma cannot be diagnosed as long as the neoplastic cells remain confined to the configuration of sclerosing adenosis.

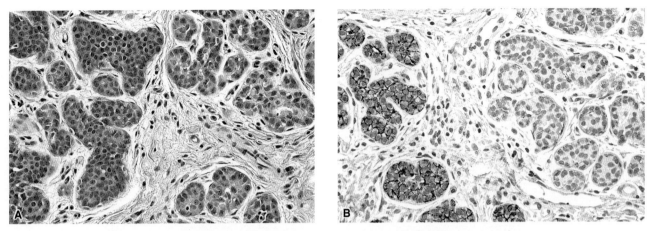

FIGURE 18.17 Lobular Carcinoma In Situ (LCIS) in the Vicinity of Ductal Carcinoma In Situ (DCIS). **A, B:** In this example, LCIS **(right)** and DCIS **(left)** of the solid type lie in juxtaposition. LCIS cells appear discohesive. E-cadherin differentiates LCIS (negative stain) from DCIS (positive staining).

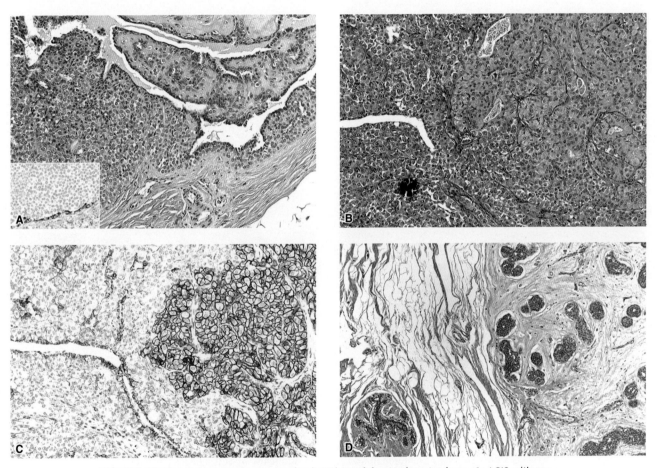

FIGURE 18.18 Lobular Carcinoma In Situ (LCIS) Involving Various Lesions. **A:** LCIS with partial involvement of an intraductal papilloma (inset shows negative E-cadherin staining in LCIS). **B, C:** LCIS with partial involvement of a solid-papillary carcinoma. LCIS cells are negative for E-cadherin **(C). D:** LCIS in a myxoid fibroadenoma. **E, F:** LCIS in a benign phyllodes tumor. There is moderate epithelial hyperplasia in the elongated ducts on the left. LCIS cells are negative for E-cadherin **(F).**

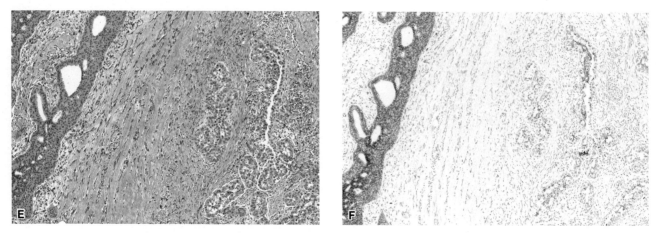

FIGURE 18.18 (*continued*)

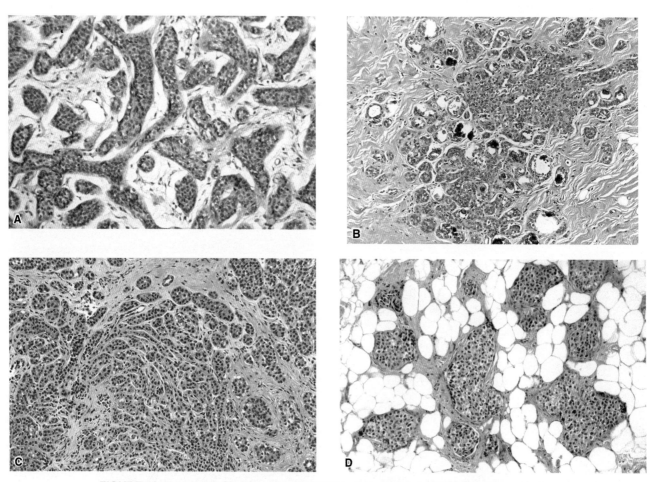

FIGURE 18.19 **Lobular Carcinoma In Situ (LCIS) in Adenosis.** **A:** LCIS inhabits a network of elongated adenosis tubules (tubular adenosis). **B, C:** LCIS populates sclerosing adenosis—with calcifications **(B)** and without calcifications **(C)**. **D, E:** Glandular structures occupied by LCIS are shown in fat. This pattern suggests invasive carcinoma. Each glandular structure is outlined by an actin-positive border indicative of a myoepithelial cell layer **(E)**. This confirms the in situ nature of the lesion.

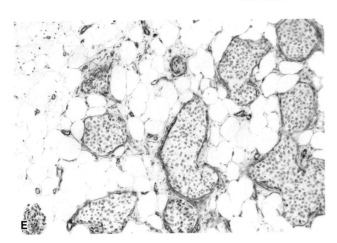

FIGURE 18.19 (*continued*)

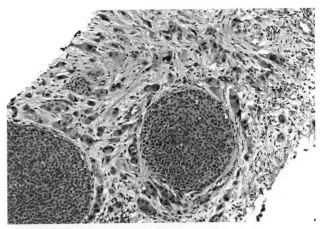

FIGURE 18.21 Pleomorphic Type of Invasive Lobular Carcinoma Associated with Lobular Carcinoma In Situ of the Classic Type. The invasive lobular carcinoma cells contain high-grade nuclei. Both, invasive and in situ, carcinoma cells were negative for E-cadherin (not shown).

MICROINVASIVE LOBULAR CARCINOMA

The diagnosis of invasive lobular carcinoma can be rendered by finding carcinoma cells in the stroma outside the confines of the periglandular myoepithelial cells and basement membrane (**Figs. 18.20 and 18.21**). Foci of microinvasive (<0.1 cm) carcinoma are more easily detected and can be highlighted with double immunostaining, typically myoepithelial (myosin) and epithelial (cytokeratin).

Most lobules in premenopausal women are surrounded by fibrous stroma, but infrequently lobules are distributed amid adipose tissue. Lobules in fat are subject to the same histopathological alterations that occur in parenchymal lobules, including the development of sclerosing adenosis and LCIS. These conditions may resemble invasive carcinoma. Important distinguishing features of LCIS in fat are the presence of well-circumscribed glands containing LCIS often encircled by myoepithelial cells and the linear pattern of most invasive lesions. However, the distinction between LCIS and the alveolar-type of invasive lobular carcinoma in fat can be difficult.

Ross and Hoda (61) published the clinicopathological profile of 16 cases of microinvasive (invasion: <1 mm) lobular carcinoma. The mean age of patients with this rare disease was 52 (range: 41–65) years. Most (13/16) patients had presented with a radiographic abnormality. All cases of microinvasive lobular carcinoma were unilateral and were associated with LCIS. LCIS was of the classic type in 11 cases, florid type in 4, and pleomorphic type in 1. Mean number of microinvasive foci was 1.5 (range: 1–5). Axillary lymph node biopsies were negative in 13 of 13 cases. In a mean follow-up of 24 months, there was no evidence of recurrence or metastases. It is noteworthy that a "slight enhancement of stromal cellularity was the only histologic hint of microinvasive disease at low-power microscopy." This finding emphasizes the need for careful scrutiny of all cases of LCIS—especially in the limited samplings obtained on NCBs wherein such a subtle finding is evident only on high-power microscopic evaluation.

PROGNOSIS OF LCIS

Until recently, follow-up studies of LCIS have consisted of patients who were biopsied for palpable clinical abnormalities in which LCIS was an incidental, sometimes unrecognized, abnormality. The risk associated with not treating LCIS by mastectomy has been estimated in several retrospective studies. The frequency of subsequent carcinoma other than LCIS varied from 12% to 36.4% (5,12,13,34,62,63,64). Studies with longer follow-up tend to report a higher frequency of subsequent carcinoma. When compared with control populations, the relative risk to LCIS patients for the development of carcinoma other than LCIS has been 4.0 to 12.0. In most studies, the risk of subsequent carcinoma was slightly higher in the ipsilateral than in the contralateral breast, although the difference has not been significant.

Several studies prospectively assessed the follow-up of patients with LCIS following a surgical biopsy alone. After approximately 5 years, in three studies, subsequent ipsilateral carcinoma other than LCIS developed in 7% to 17% of patients

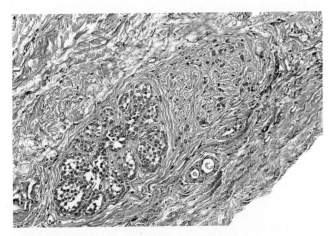

FIGURE 18.20 Microinvasive (<0.1 cm) Lobular Carcinoma Associated with Lobular Carcinoma In Situ of the Classic Type. Microinvasive lobular carcinoma cells have low-grade nuclei (**right**).

managed by follow-up only (6,65). Ottesen et al. (65) evaluated 100 women with a median prospective follow-up of 120 months. Subsequent carcinoma was detected in 18 (18%), consisting of invasive carcinoma in 13 and DCIS in 5. Sixteen carcinomas occurred in the ipsilateral and two in the contralateral breast. The risk of subsequent carcinoma was significantly greater when the initial LCIS had "large" nuclear size when compared with those with "small" nuclear size. The terms C-LCIS and P-LCIS were not used by these authors, but they are probably equivalent. In this prospective study, the risk for developing subsequent carcinoma other than LCIS was not significantly related to the number of lobules with LCIS in the initial biopsy.

Zurrida et al. (66) reported the prospective follow-up of 157 patients in whom LCIS was detected in a biopsy performed for a mammographic or palpable lesion. The ipsilateral breast was conserved in 135 cases. After a mean follow-up of 5 years, eight patients (5%) had developed invasive carcinoma. The observed rate of carcinoma in the ipsilateral breast with LCIS (4 carcinomas per 639 person years at risk = 0.00625) was significantly greater ($p < 0.05$) than the expected rate (0.98 carcinomas per 639 person years at risk = 0.00152), resulting in a relative risk of 4.1 (CI: 1.1–10.5). The person years at risk for carcinoma in either breast was 865, with an expected rate of 0.0015, an observed rate of 0.00925 (8/865), and a relative risk of 5.93 (CI: 2.6–11.7).

Reliable pathologic predictors of increased risk for the subsequent development of carcinoma after LCIS has been diagnosed by needle core or surgical biopsy have not been found. Three studies reported a greater risk in patients with LCIS that were of classic and pleomorphic types in comparison with patients who had LCIS of either type alone (5,6,9,34). Increased risk has also been associated with marked lobular distention (6). Lesions with marked ductal distention, necrosis, and calcification are special concern because the authors have found an unexpectedly high frequency of microinvasive carcinoma in such cases. Specimens with these features should be examined carefully with cytokeratin and E-cadherin immunostains accompanied by contemporaneous H&E-stained recuts.

Goldstein et al. (53) conducted a retrospective study of 82 patients with LCIS who did not undergo mastectomy. The actuarial rates for subsequent carcinoma were 7.8% after 10 years of follow-up and 15.4% after 20 years. Six of the subsequent twenty-one carcinomas (29%) developed 20 or more years after diagnosis. No E-cadherin immunoreactivity was present in 73 LCIS lesions (89%), and 9 had focal weak and discontinuous reactivity. When compared with patients with E-cadherin-negative LCIS, the presence of focal E-cadherin reactivity was associated with a higher risk for developing subsequent carcinoma, earlier onset of carcinoma, and more frequent ductal carcinoma. This observation based on a small number of cases with focal E-cadherin reactivity remains to be confirmed by other investigators.

In a prospective study of 1,004 women who chose surveillance instead of mastectomy after a diagnosis of LCIS, King et al. (67) reported that the incidence of subsequent carcinoma other than LCIS was significantly reduced among those entered into a chemoprevention program. The assignment of patients

was not randomized, with 173 choosing chemoprevention and 831 opting for surveillance alone. Overall, the annual incidence of carcinoma during surveillance follow-up with or without chemoprevention was 2%. The 10-year cumulative risk for subsequent carcinoma among those in the chemoprevention group was 7% compared to 21% in the surveillance-alone group. The investigators did not distinguish between subgroups of patients with classic LCIS, F-LCIS, and P-LCIS, but it is likely that the majority of patients had classic LCIS. These data strongly support the use of chemoprevention in women with LCIS who choose follow-up surveillance.

Various aspects of the clinical management of P-LCIS were summarized by Murray et al. (68) and Massant et al. (69).

ATYPICAL LOBULAR HYPERPLASIA

There are no specific clinical features associated with the diagnosis of ALH. The clinical indications for biopsy are the same as those that lead to the detection of LCIS: a palpable lesion or an imaging abnormality. ALH is usually an incidental finding not specifically associated with the abnormality that prompted the biopsy.

The glandular proliferation in ALH has some features of LCIS, but they are not sufficiently developed to qualify for the latter diagnosis (**Figs. 18.22–18.26**). There are no universally accepted criteria for the precise distinction between ALH and LCIS. Qualitative and quantitative factors must be considered. The cells that form ALH are E-cadherin-negative.

Quantitative criteria for the diagnosis of LCIS influence the distribution of cases classified as ALH. The diagnosis of ALH is made if less than 50% (7) or 75% (8) of the only-affected lobule shows the features of LCIS. ALH is characterized by the presence, within one or more lobules, of abnormal cells similar to those found in LCIS. In the least conspicuous configuration, these cells replace a portion of the normal lobular glandular epithelium, effacing some lumina. The acini are not enlarged at this level of proliferation. As the process evolves, the accumulation of a greater number of cells causes progressive acinar expansion, but the borders of individual acini and intralobular ductules remain indistinct in ALH. Clear delineation of intralobular acinar units filled by the abnormal cell population is an important feature that characterizes LCIS and reflects the accumulation of enough neoplastic cells to cause the individual glands to have a distinct configuration.

Similar criteria apply to the diagnosis of lobular proliferations in terminal ductal structures. These alterations tend to create a cloverleaf pattern similar to LCIS. The peripheral lobule-like bulges are sometimes inhabited by a mixture of normal and neoplastic cells. ALH of terminal ducts may also occur in a solid form that develops when the neoplastic growth is distributed in a continuous layer around the ductal lumen. ALH is E-cadherin-negative, a property it shares with LCIS (70).

Estimates of the risk for subsequent carcinoma in women with ALH are clouded by the absence of a clear definition for this lesion. Some investigators who did not distinguish

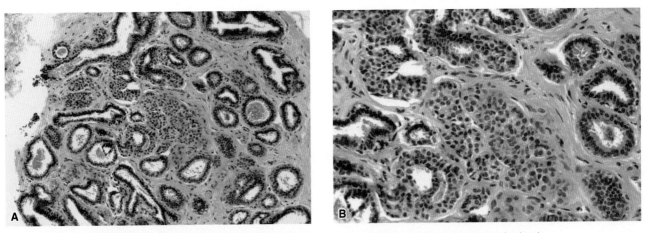

FIGURE 18.22 Atypical Lobular Hyperplasia. A, B: A needle core biopsy specimen obtained for calcifications revealed tubular carcinoma. One of the additional tissue samples had this focus of atypical lobular hyperplasia in adenosis.

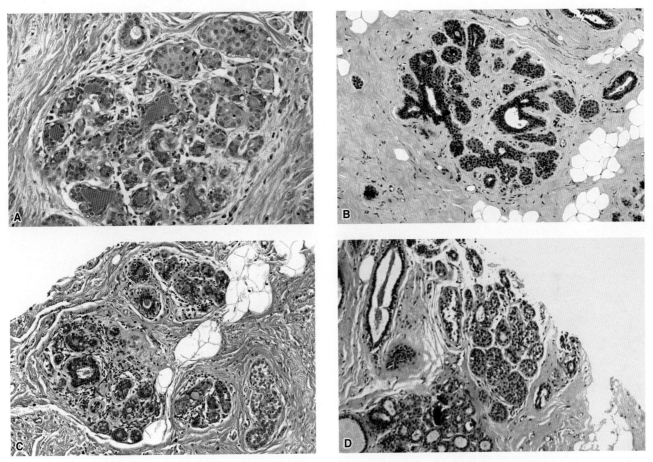

FIGURE 18.23 Atypical Lobular Hyperplasia (ALH). A, B: Examples of partially involved lobules that qualify as ALH found in needle core biopsy specimens. **C:** ALH **(lower right)** next to normal lobules in a needle core biopsy sample. **D, E:** One partially involved lobule is present at the edge of this needle core biopsy specimen. The procedure was performed for calcifications that were present in sclerosing adenosis next to the ALH in a premenopausal patient.

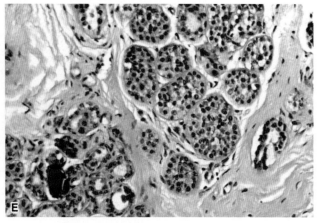

FIGURE 18.23 (*continued*)

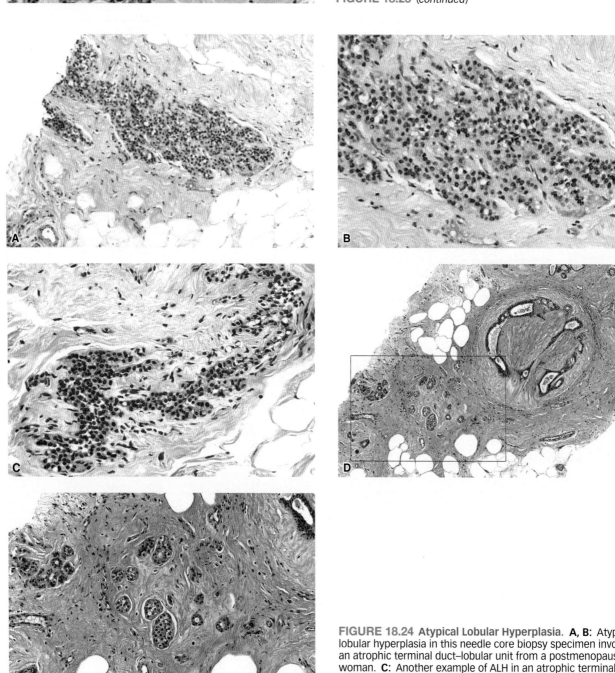

FIGURE 18.24 Atypical Lobular Hyperplasia. A, B: Atypical lobular hyperplasia in this needle core biopsy specimen involves an atrophic terminal duct–lobular unit from a postmenopausal woman. **C:** Another example of ALH in an atrophic terminal duct–lobular unit. **D, E:** An example of ALH next to a minute fibroadenoma in a needle core biopsy sample. (**E** shows area highlighted in the box in **D**).

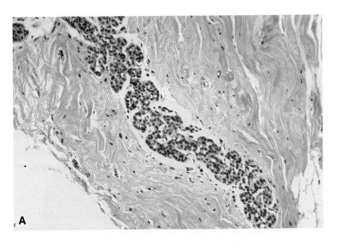

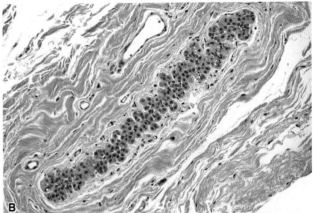

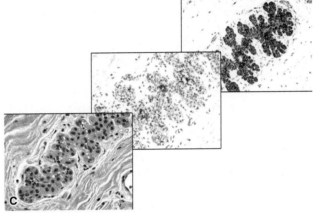

FIGURE 18.25 Atypical Lobular Hyperplasia, Ductal Involvement. A: Atypical lobular hyperplasia in a duct from a postmenopausal patient cut in a longitudinal plane. **B, C:** Another example of lobular carcinoma in situ with ductal involvement in an elderly woman. The lesional cells are negative for E-cadherin **(center figure)** and show cytoplasmic positivity for p120 **(upper right)** in **C**.

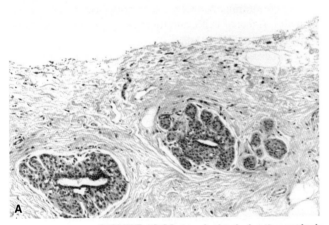

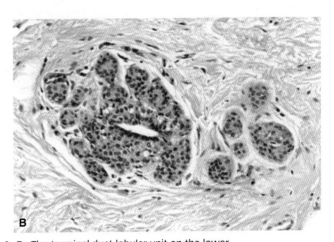

FIGURE 18.26 Atypical Lobular Hyperplasia. A, B: The terminal duct lobular unit on the lower left in **(A)** shows atypical hyperplasia with a cloverleaf pattern. The unit on the right has a more distinct lobular pattern, which approaches lobular carcinoma in situ.

between ALH and LCIS have reported relative risk estimates for both lesions under the heading of lobular neoplasia (9,62). The relative risk for developing carcinoma after the finding of ALH is three to four times the expected frequency when compared to age-matched controls (63,64). The risk is higher in women with a family history of breast carcinoma, when there is ductal involvement by the ALH (71), and when there is coexistent atypical ductal hyperplasia (64).

IS EXCISIONAL BIOPSY ALWAYS INDICATED AFTER THE NEEDLE CORE BIOPSY DIAGNOSIS OF LCIS?

The management of a patient with LCIS in a mammographically directed NCB specimen is a relatively recent concern. Liberman et al. (72) found LCIS as the only neoplastic lesion in 16 (1.2%) of 1,315 consecutive NCB specimens at Memorial

Hospital in New York City. Other significant proliferative lesions in the core biopsy specimens with LCIS included "radial scar" in three and atypical ductal hyperplasia in two cases. Subsequent excision revealed DCIS in the region of the LCIS in two cases and invasive carcinoma in a third. F-LCIS involving markedly expanded ducts was present in two core biopsy specimens after which surgery revealed DCIS in one case and invasive carcinoma in the other. ADH accompanied LCIS in another core biopsy specimen that was followed by DCIS at surgery. The authors concluded that surgical biopsy should be performed when a core biopsy specimen contains LCIS accompanied by a "high-risk" proliferative lesion, when F-LCIS resembling DCIS is present or if there is discordance between histopathologic and imaging findings. These conclusions were supported by a subsequent study (73).

A larger series of patients with LCIS and ALH diagnosed in NCBs performed for mammographic indications was reported by Lechner et al. (74). This multi-institutional study of 32,424 biopsies revealed 89 (0.3%) examples of LCIS. Surgical biopsies were performed on 58 (65%) of the LCIS lesions yielding invasive lobular carcinoma in 8 (14%), invasive ductal carcinoma in 2 (3%), tubular carcinoma in 8 (14%), and DCIS in 2 (3%). Thus, 20 of the 89 (22%) patients with LCIS in a core biopsy specimen had intraductal or invasive carcinoma in a subsequent surgical biopsy. Foster et al. (75) described 12 patients with LCIS in a core biopsy specimen who had a surgical excision performed. Four patients (25%) were found to have invasive carcinoma or DCIS. Crisi et al. (76) found invasive carcinoma in two of nine (22%) surgical specimens after a NCB specimen showed LCIS.

A summary of the foregoing reports and other studies including a total of 140 patients with LCIS diagnosed in a NCB specimen who later underwent surgical biopsy was compiled by Arpino et al. (77). Carcinoma, either intraductal or invasive, was found in 40 cases (26%). These data support a recommendation to perform a surgical biopsy in most patients after LCIS is detected in a NCB specimen (78). The final decision for the management of individual patients may be influenced by clinical and imaging factors. Londero et al. (79) and Brem et al. (80) reported that the likelihood of finding intraductal or invasive carcinoma in a surgical biopsy was greater if the mammogram was classified as BIRADS 4 or 5 than if it was BIRADS 3.

Reports of follow-up studies of LCIS diagnosed by NCB have not always identified the LCIS as classic, florid, or pleomorphic type, and in some instances they have not clearly distinguished between LCIS and ALH. Chivukula et al. (81) described a substantial series of patients with pleomorphic LCIS diagnosed by NCB. In this series of 12 cases, 11 (92%) were ER-positive, 6 (50%) were PR-positive, 3 (25%) were HER2-positive, and all were E-cadherin-negative. Subsequent surgical excisions revealed residual pleomorphic LCIS in 10 (83%) and invasive lobular carcinoma in 3 of the cases (25%). One invasive carcinoma was classified as classic, one as pleomorphic, and one as classic/pleomorphic.

The current National Comprehensive Cancer Network (NCCN) guidelines recommend consideration of an excisional biopsy after a core biopsy diagnosis of LCIS or ALH is rendered to rule out a more significant lesion in the vicinity of the biopsied area (82). There is ample published evidence to support this recommendation. Multiple reports published earlier, that is, in the years that followed relatively soon after the widespread adoption of NCB, had reported an "upgrade rate" of up to 50% in excisional biopsies after NCB diagnosis of LCIS or ALH. Hussain et al., upon compilation of multiple series, computed that 32% (77/241) of LCIS cases diagnosed on NCBs contained malignancy (either DCIS or invasive carcinoma) on subsequent excision (83).

More recent series have generally reported a lower upgrade rate of <10% on excisional biopsy of consecutive cases of LCIS. The lower upgrade rate most likely reflects increasing adoption of a multidisciplinary approach to disease management with enhanced assessment of radiologic–pathologic concordance as well as careful exclusion of other high-risk lesions. It is increasingly becoming evident that not all patients with a NCB diagnosis of LCIS or ALH require excisional biopsy and that a more nuanced approach to this issue is required.

Because most cases of LCIS that are currently diagnosed on NCBs are performed for an abnormality found on imaging studies, radiologic–pathologic correlation is an important element in the decision to perform an excisional biopsy thereafter. This entails determination of whether or not there is concordance between the intended target lesion and findings in the NCB.

A *concordant biopsy* is one wherein the histopathologic findings provide adequate explanation for the target on imaging, typically microcalcifications in LCIS (or in benign tissue) or fibroadenomas (with incidental LCIS within or beyond the benign tumor). Notably, calcifications can be associated with all variants of LCIS, and therefore the findings could be concordant on NCB (84).

A *discordant biopsy* is one wherein the histopathologic findings do not provide adequate explanation for the imaging abnormality (typically: insufficient explanation for a mass, inadequate sampling, no microcalcifications in NCB).

In a carefully conducted study at Memorial Sloan Kettering Cancer Center, Murray et al. (73) found that excisional biopsy identified carcinoma in 3% (2 of 72) of concordant cases, and excisions in discordant cases yielded carcinoma in 38% (3/8) of the cases. The two carcinomas found in concordant cases included one low-grade DCIS and one grade 1 invasive carcinoma, each of which spanned 2 mm. Rendi et al. (85) reported an upgrade rate of 4.4% (3/68) after excision following the diagnosis of LCIS.

The upgrade rate for P-LCIS is much higher. The combined results of four studies show that the incidence of invasive carcinoma on excision after pleomorphic LCIS diagnosed on NCB in 22 patients was 41% (9/22) (83,84,86–88). In Flanagan et al.'s study of P-LCIS diagnosed on NCB, the overall upgrade rate to either invasive carcinoma or DCIS was 48% (11/23) (89). All three patients with P-LCIS on NCB in Niell's series were found to have invasive carcinoma upon excision (that is, the upgrade rate was 100%) (90). These data support the performance of an excisional biopsy after the diagnosis of P-LCIS on NCB sampling. Until the clinicopathologic and biologic significance of F-LCIS are fully characterized, an excisional biopsy should follow upon its diagnosis on NCB samplings.

Some of the many reports evaluating the management of LCIS and ALH after diagnosis by a NCB were summarized by Rendi et al. (85). This review of 18 studies (including one cited above by these authors) found that the excision rate varied from 41% to 89%, with no data for this factor in three reports and excisions in less than 50% of cases in six other reports. Eight of the eighteen studies included instances of P-LCIS or "mixed CIS." Some investigators lumped ALH and LCIS under the term "lobular neoplasia." The limitations inherent in these reports are representative of most of the numerous other studies that have been undertaken to determine how often and under which conditions excisional biopsy is beneficial because it reveals DCIS, invasive carcinoma, or another significant lesion that would be detrimental to the patient if left undetected after core biopsy sample reveals LCIS.

In the face of these very heterogeneous data, definitive conclusions are somewhat tenuous, but some indications seem to be reasonably well substantiated with respect to performing an excisional biopsy in certain circumstances after a NCB diagnosis of LCIS. These are as follows:

a. When the imaging and biopsy findings are discordant (e.g., calcifications seen on mammogram are not present in the core biopsy specimen);
b. Patients at significantly increased risk for breast carcinoma such as those with concurrent or prior atypical ductal hyperplasia (ADH), a family history of breast carcinoma, positive BRCA status, or contralateral breast carcinoma;
c. The presence of P-LCIS even when calcifications in the P-LCIS correspond to those seen in a mammogram; and
d. The presence of F-LCIS even if the core biopsy findings are concordant with the mammogram.

IS EXCISIONAL BIOPSY INDICATED AFTER A NEEDLE CORE BIOPSY DIAGNOSIS OF ALH?

Many of the foregoing limitations in the data about LCIS also hinder our understanding of the optimal management of ALH diagnosed in a NCB sample. This is illustrated in some of the following reports.

Lechner et al. (74) reported the results of a multi-institutional study that included 154 (0.5%) instances of ALH in 32,424 NCB specimens. Surgical biopsies performed in only 84 of the 154 cases of ALH (55%) revealed invasive lobular carcinoma in 3 (4%) and DCIS in 4 (5%) for a total yield of 9 (11%) carcinomas. A review of 6,081 consecutive breast NCB procedures performed at two institutions uncovered 20 (0.3%) cases of ALH (75). Surgical biopsies performed in 14 of the 20 cases revealed DCIS in 2. The six patients who did not have a surgical biopsy had not developed clinical evidence of carcinoma after a mean follow-up of 36 months, an exceedingly short time in the context of ALH.

Perhaps the most disconcerting report comes from Subhawong et al. (91) who reported that none of the 56 cases of ALH diagnosed on NCB at a single institution was upgraded on excision. However, the illustrations provided in their Figure 1 for ALH are diagnostic of LCIS. A lesion described by these authors as "mild atypical ductal hyperplasia" in their Figure 2A appears to be micropapillary DCIS. Furthermore, Figure 2B in this report described as "lobular carcinoma in situ" appears to be an example of extreme F-LCIS, possibly with microinvasive lobular carcinoma in the upper left corner of the image.

Arpino et al. (77) reviewed 16 studies of patients with ALH diagnosed by NCB, included the foregoing reports. A total of 184 women had subsequent surgical excisions that revealed either intraductal or invasive carcinoma in 30 (16%). The frequency of carcinoma detected in these excisions was somewhat lower than that for LCIS, but not inconsequential.

Close clinical and radiologic follow-up ought to be ensured in all cases of ALH or LCIS diagnosed on NCB that are not subjected to excisional biopsy. Larger tissue sampling (s/p NCB with LCIS or ALH) via use of vacuum-assisted biopsy has been proposed as an alternative to excisional biopsy in selected cases (92). The optimal management of ALH and LCIS diagnosed on NCB remains an area of active research (93–97).

LCIS: PRECUSOR LESION OR MARKER OF INVASIVE CARCINOMA?

LCIS is a morphologically and clinically heterogeneous disease. The concept that LCIS is simply a "marker" lesion has been widely promulgated. The impression created by this idea is that LCIS is a proliferative abnormality associated with an increased risk for the development of breast carcinoma, but it implies that, in contrast to DCIS, LCIS does not itself progress to invasive carcinoma. This misperception is incorrect and can have unfortunate consequences. There is sufficient cumulative evidence to support the conclusion that LCIS is a direct precursor to invasive lobular carcinoma, and possibly in a minority of instances to invasive ductal carcinoma (e.g., ductal–lobular and tubulolobular), but that this progression is not observed in the lifetime of every patient with LCIS.

It appears that progression of LCIS to the invasive phenotype is less frequent and takes longer than in DCIS. Because LCIS and DCIS coexist in a number of patients, it is not surprising that some of them might develop invasive ductal carcinoma sooner and therefore more frequently than invasive lobular carcinoma. This phenomenon most likely reflects differences in the rates of progression of the two diseases so that the earlier appearance of invasive ductal carcinoma results in treatment before the LCIS has had an opportunity to evolve into invasive lobular carcinoma.

LCIS is a heterogeneous disease in both cytologic and architectural terms. The relationships of these differences to prognosis or to the risk of progression have not been well characterized. Perhaps the greatest challenge to regarding LCIS as a "marker" lesion has come from the recent recognition of the florid and pleomorphic variants of LCIS characterized by marked glandular expansion with a tendency to necrosis and calcification.

Contrary to the widely held perception that LCIS is not detected by mammography except as an incidental lesion, F-LCIS and P-LCIS are likely to present with calcifications and a mammographic pattern that resembles DCIS. The paradigm of LCIS as an incidental "marker" lesion does not fit well with this clinical presentation and the histopathological findings. On the basis of limited published and, admittedly anecdotal personal observations, including a number of instances of microinvasive lobular carcinoma that arose in F-LCIS and P-LCIS, the authors are of the opinion that these variant forms of LCIS might in some cases be treated as if they were DCIS, at least with respect to local surgical control in the conserved breast. The effectiveness of radiotherapy for treating any of these forms of LCIS has, thus far, not been determined.

REFERENCES

1. Foote FW, Stewart FW. Lobular carcinoma in situ: a rare form of mammary cancer. *Am J Pathol*. 1941;17:491–496.
2. King TA, Reis-Filho JS. Lobular neoplasia. *Surg Oncol Clin N Am*. 2014;23:487–503.
3. Alvarado-Cabrero I, Coronel GP, Cedillo RV, et al. Florid lobular intraepithelial neoplasia with signet ring cells, central necrosis and calcifications: a clinicopathological and immunohistochemical analysis of ten cases associated with invasive lobular carcinoma. *Arch Med Res*. 2010;41:436–441.
4. Shin SJ, Lal A, De Vries S, et al. Florid lobular carcinoma in situ: molecular profiling and comparison to classic lobular carcinoma in situ and pleomorphic lobular carcinoma in situ. *Hum Pathol*. 2013;44:1998–2009.
5. Mackaren G, Yacoub LK, Lee AKC, et al. Effects of screening on detection of lobular carcinoma in situ of the breast: nonspecificity of mammography and physical examination. *Breast Dis*. 1994;7:339–345.
6. Fisher ER, Costantino J, Fisher B, et al; for the National Surgical Adjuvant Breast and Bowel Project Collaborating Investigators. Pathologic findings from the National Surgical Adjuvant Breast Project (NSABP) Protocol B-17: five-year observations concerning lobular carcinoma in situ. *Cancer*. 1996;78:1403–1416.
7. Page DL, Andersen TJ. *Diagnostic Histopathology of the Breast*. New York, NY: Churchill Livingstone; 1987.
8. Rosen PP. Lobular carcinoma in situ and intraductal carcinoma of the breast. In: McDivitt RW, Oberman HA, Ozello L, et al, eds. *The Breast*. Baltimore, MD: Williams & Wilkins; 1984:59–105.
9. Haagensen CD, Lane N, Lattes R, et al. Lobular neoplasia (so-called lobular carcinoma in situ) of the breast. *Cancer*. 1978;42:737–769.
10. Gomes DS, Porto SS, Balabram D, et al. Inter-observer variability between general pathologists and a specialist in breast pathology in the diagnosis of lobular neoplasia, columnar cell lesions, atypical ductal hyperplasia and ductal carcinoma in situ of the breast. *Diagn Pathol*. 2014;9:121.
11. Christiano JG, Duncan LD, Bell JL. Lobular carcinoma in situ of the breast presenting as a discrete mass. *Am Surg*. 2012;78:e38–e40.
12. Hutter RVP, Snyder RE, Lucas J, et al. Clinical and pathologic correlation with mammographic findings in lobular carcinoma in situ. *Cancer*. 1969;23:826–839.
13. Morris DM, Walker AP, Cocker DC. Lack of efficacy of xeromammography in preoperatively detecting lobular carcinoma in situ of the breast. *Breast Cancer Res Treat*. 1982;1:365–368.
14. Fadare O, Dadmanesh F, Alvarado-Cabrero I, et al. Lobular intraepithelial neoplasia (lobular carcinoma in situ) with comedo-type necrosis: a clinicopathologic study of 18 cases. *Am J Surg Pathol*. 2006;30:1445–1453.
15. Portschy PR, Marmor S, Nzara R, et al. Trends in incidence and management of lobular carcinoma in situ: a population-based analysis. *Ann Surg Oncol*. 2013;20:3240–3246.
16. Andersen J. Lobular carcinoma in situ: a long-term follow-up in 52 cases. *Acta Pathol Microbiol Scand Sect A*. 1974;82:519–533.
17. Rosen PP, Lieberman PH, Braun DW Jr, et al. Lobular carcinoma in situ of the breast: detailed analysis of 99 patients with average follow-up of 24 years. *Am J Surg Pathol*. 1978;2:225–251.
18. Page DL, Kidd TE Jr, Dupont WD, et al. Lobular neoplasia of the breast: higher risk for subsequent invasive cancer predicted by more extensive disease. *Hum Pathol*. 1991;22:1232–1239.
19. Li CI, Anderson BO, Daling JR, et al. Changing incidence of lobular carcinoma in situ of the breast. *Breast Cancer Res Treat*. 2002;75:259–268.
20. Rosen PP. Columnar cell hyperplasia is associated with lobular carcinoma in situ and tubular carcinoma. *Am J Surg Pathol*. 1999;23:1561.
21. Carley AM, Chivukula M, Carter GJ, et al. Frequency and clinical significance of simultaneous association of lobular neoplasia and columnar cell alterations in breast tissue specimens. *Am J Clin Pathol*. 2008;130:254–258.
22. Brandt SM, Young GQ, Hoda SA. The "Rosen Triad": tubular carcinoma, lobular carcinoma in situ, and columnar cell lesions. *Adv Anat Pathol*. 2008;15:140–146.
23. Bezic J, Gugic D. Signet ring lobular carcinoma in situ as a part of the "Rosen Triad" (tubular carcinoma, columnar cell hyperplasia, and lobular carcinoma in situ). *Turk Patoloji Derg*. 2013;29:134–137.
24. Rosen PP, Senie R, Ashikari R, et al. Age, menstrual status, and exogenous hormone usage in patients with lobular carcinoma in situ (LCIS). *Surgery*. 1979;85:219–224.
25. Rosen PP, Lesser ML, Senie RT, et al. Epidemiology of breast carcinoma IV: age and histologic tumor type. *J Surg Oncol*. 1982;19:44–47.
26. Shah JP, Rosen PP, Robbins GF. Pitfalls of local excision in the treatment of carcinoma of the breast. *Surg Gynecol Obstet*. 1973;136:721–725.
27. Carter D, Smith AL. Carcinoma in situ of the breast. *Cancer*. 1977;40:1189–1193.
28. Urban JA. Biopsy of the 'normal' breast in treating breast cancer. *Surg Clin North Am*. 1969;49:291–301.
29. Vos CB, Cleton-Jones AM, Berx G, et al. E-cadherin inactivation in lobular carcinoma in situ of the breast: an early event in tumor genesis. *Br J Cancer*. 1997;76:1131–1133.
30. Moll R, Mitze M, Frixen UH, et al. Differential loss of E-cadherin expression in infiltrating ductal and lobular carcinomas. *Am J Pathol*. 1993;143:1737–1742.
31. Andersen JA, Vendelhoe ML. Cytoplasmic mucous globules in lobular carcinoma in situ: diagnosis and prognosis. *Am J Surg Pathol*. 1981;5:251–255.
32. Gad A, Azzopardi JG. Lobular carcinoma of the breast: a special variant of mucin secreting carcinoma. *J Clin Pathol*. 1975;28:711–716.
33. Chen YY, Hwang ES, Roy R, et al. Genetic and phenotypic characteristics of pleomorphic lobular carcinoma in situ of the breast. *Am J Surg Pathol*. 2009;33:1683–1694.
34. Haagensen CD, Lane N, Lattes R. Neoplastic proliferation of the epithelium of the mammary lobules: adenosis, lobular neoplasia and small cell carcinoma. *Surg Clin North Am*. 1972;52:497–524.
35. Shousha S. In situ lobular neoplasia of the breast with marked myoepithelial proliferation. *Histopathology*. 2011;58:1081–1085.
36. Acs G, Lawton TJ, Rebbeck TR, et al. Differential expression of E-cadherin in lobular and ductal neoplasms of the breast and its biological and diagnostic implications. *Am J Clin Pathol*. 2001;115:85–89.
37. Sgroi D, Koerner FC. Involvement of collagenous spherulosis by lobular carcinoma in situ: potential confusion with cribriform ductal carcinoma in situ. *Am J Surg Pathol*. 1995;19:1366–1370.
38. Eisenberg RE, Hoda SA. Lobular carcinoma in situ with collagenous spherulosis: clinicopathologic characteristics of 38 cases. *Breast J*. 2014;20:440–441.
39. Etzell JE, Devries S, Chew K, et al. Loss of chromosome 16q in lobular carcinoma in situ. *Hum Pathol*. 2001;32:292–296.
40. Rahman N, Stone JG, Coleman G, et al. Lobular carcinoma in situ of the breast is not caused by constitutional mutations in the E-cadherin gene. *Br J Cancer*. 2000;82:568–570.
41. Andrade VP, Morrogh M, Qin LX, et al. Gene expression profiling of lobular carcinoma in situ reveals candidate precursor genes for invasion. *Mol Oncol*. 2015;9:772–782.
42. Logan GJ, Dabbs DJ, Lucas PC, et al. Molecular drivers of lobular carcinoma in situ. *Breast Cancer Res*. 2015;17:76.
43. Sarrió D, Moreno-Bueno G, Hardisson E, et al. Epigenetic and genetic alterations of APC and CDH1 genes in lobular breast cancer: relationships

with abnormal E-cadherin and catenin expression and microsatellite instability. *Int J Cancer.* 2003;106:208–215.

44. Nayar R, Zhuang Z, Merino MJ, et al. Loss of heterozygosity on chromosome 11q13 in lobular lesions of the breast using microdissection and polymerase chain reaction. *Hum Pathol.* 1996;28:277–282.

45. Hwang ES, Nyante SJ, Chen YY, et al. Clonality of lobular carcinoma in situ and synchronous invasive lobular carcinoma. *Cancer.* 2004;100:2562–2572.

46. Khoury T, Karabakhtsian RG, Mattson D, et al. Pleomorphic lobular carcinoma in situ of the breast: clinicopathological review of 47 cases. *Histopathology.* 2014;64:981–993.

47. Lien HC, Chen YL, Juang YL, et al. Frequent alterations of HER2 through mutation, amplification, or overexpression in pleomorphic lobular carcinoma of the breast. *Breast Cancer Res Treat.* 2015;150:447–455.

48. Gomes DS, Porto SS, Rocha RM, et al. Usefulness and limitations of E-cadherin and β-catenin in the classification of breast carcinomas in situ with mixed pattern. *Diagn Pathol.* 2013;8:114.

49. Morrogh M, Andrade VP, Giri D, et al. Cadherin-catenin complex dissociation in lobular neoplasia of the breast. *Breast Cancer Res Treat.* 2012;132:641–652.

50. Goldstein NS, Bassi D, Watts JC, et al. E-cadherin reactivity of 95 noninvasive ductal and lobular lesions of the breast: implications for the interpretation of problematic lesions. *Am J Clin Pathol.* 2001;115:534–542.

51. Jacobs TW, Pliss N, Kouria G, et al. Carcinomas in situ of the breast with indeterminate features: role of E-cadherin staining in categorization. *Am J Surg Pathol.* 2001;25:229–236.

52. Choi YJ, Pinto MM, Hao L, et al. Interobserver variability and aberrant E-cadherin immunostaining of lobular neoplasia and infiltrating lobular carcinoma. *Mod Pathol.* 2008;21:1224–1237.

53. Goldstein NS, Kestin LL, Vicini FA. Clinicopathologic implications of E-cadherin reactivity in patients with lobular carcinoma in situ of the breast. *Cancer.* 2001;92:738–747.

54. Harigopal M, Shin SJ, Murray MP, et al. Aberrant E-cadherin staining patterns in invasive mammary carcinoma. *World J Surg Oncol.* 2005;3:73.

55. Lee AH. Use of immunohistochemistry in the diagnosis of problematic breast lesions. *J Clin Pathol.* 2013;66:471–477.

56. Dabbs DJ, Schnitt SJ, Geyer FC, et al. Lobular neoplasia of the breast revisited with emphasis on the role of E-cadherin immunohistochemistry. *Am J Surg Pathol.* 2013;37:e1–e11.

57. de Deus Moura R, Wludarski SC, Carvalho FM, et al. Immunohistochemistry applied to the differential diagnosis between ductal and lobular carcinoma of the breast. *Appl Immunohistochem Mol Morphol.* 2013;21:1–12.

58. Shousha S. In situ lobular neoplasia of the breast with marked myoepithelial proliferation. *Histopathology.* 2011;58:1081–1085.

59. Fechner RE. Lobular carcinoma in situ in sclerosing adenosis: a potential source of confusion with invasive carcinoma. *Am J Surg Pathol.* 1981;5:233–239.

60. Oberman HA, Markey BA. Noninvasive carcinoma of the breast presenting in adenosis. *Mod Pathol.* 1991;4:31–35.

61. Ross DS, Hoda SA. Microinvasive (T1mic) lobular carcinoma of the breast: clinicopathologic profile of 16 cases. *Am J Surg Pathol.* 2011;35:750–756.

62. Bodian CA, Perzin KH, Lattes R. Lobular neoplasia: long term risk of breast cancer and relation to other factors. *Cancer.* 1996;78:1024–1034.

63. Page DL, Dupont WD, Rogers LW, et al. Atypical hyperplastic lesions of the female breast: a long-term follow-up study. *Cancer.* 1985;55:2698–2708.

64. Page DL, Schuyler PA, Dupont WD, et al. Atypical lobular hyperplasia as a unilateral predictor of breast cancer risk: a retrospective cohort study. *Lancet.* 2003;361:125–129.

65. Ottesen GL, Graversen HP, Blichert-Toft M, et al. Lobular carcinoma in situ of the female breast: short-term results of a prospective nationwide study. *Am J Surg Pathol.* 1993;17:14–21.

66. Zurrida S, Bartoli C, Galimberti V, et al. Interpretation of the risk associated with the unexpected finding of lobular carcinoma in situ. *Ann Surg Oncol.* 1996;3:57–61.

67. King TA, Pilewskie M, Muhsen S, et al. Lobular carcinoma in situ: a 29-year longitudinal experience evaluating clinicopathologic features and breast cancer risk. *J Clin Oncol.* 2015;33:3945–3952.

68. Murray L, Reintgen M, Akman K, et al. Pleomorphic lobular carcinoma in situ: treatment options for a new pathologic entity. *Clin Breast Cancer.* 2012;12:76–79.

69. Masannat YA, Bains SK, Pinder SE, et al. Challenges in the management of pleomorphic lobular carcinoma in situ of the breast. *Breast.* 2013;22:194–196.

70. Mastracci TL, Tjan S, Ban AL, et al. E-cadherin alterations in atypical lobular hyperplasia and lobular carcinoma in situ of the breast. *Mod Pathol.* 2005;18:741–751.

71. Page DL, Dupont WD, Rogers LW. Ductal involvement by cells of atypical lobular hyperplasia in the breast: a long-term follow-up study of cancer risk. *Hum Pathol.* 1988;19:201–207.

72. Liberman L, Sama M, Susnik B, et al. Lobular carcinoma in situ at percutaneous breast biopsy: surgical biopsy findings. *AJR Am J Roentgenol.* 1999;173:291–299.

73. Murray MP, Luedtke C, Liberman L, et al. Classic lobular carcinoma in situ and atypical lobular hyperplasia at percutaneous breast core biopsy: outcomes of prospective excision. *Cancer.* 2013;119:1073–1079.

74. Lechner MD, Park SL, Jackman RJ, et al. Lobular carcinoma in situ and atypical lobular hyperplasia at percutaneous biopsy with surgical correlation: multi-institutional study. *Radiology.* 1999;213:106.

75. Foster MC, Helvie MA, Gregory NE, et al. Lobular carcinoma in situ or atypical lobular hyperplasia at core-needle biopsy: is excisional biopsy necessary? *Radiology.* 2004;231:813–819.

76. Crisi GM, Mandavilli S, Cronin E, et al. Invasive mammary carcinoma after immediate and short-term follow-up for lobular neoplasia on core biopsy. *Am J Surg Pathol.* 2003;27:325–333.

77. Arpino G, Allred DC, Mohsin SK, et al. Lobular neoplasia on core-needle biopsy-clinical significance. *Cancer.* 2004;101:242–250.

78. Cohen MA. Cancer upgrades at excisional biopsy after diagnosis of atypical lobular hyperplasia or lobular carcinoma in situ at core-needle core biopsy: some reasons why. *Radiology.* 2004;231:671–621.

79. Londero V, Zuiani C, Linda A, et al. Lobular neoplasia: core needle breast biopsy underestimation of malignancy in relation to radiologic and pathologic features. *The Breast.* 2008;17:623–630.

80. Brem RF, Lechner MC, Jackman RJ, et al. Lobular neoplasia at percutaneous breast biopsy: variables associated with carcinoma at surgical excision. *AJR Am J Roentgenol.* 2008;190:637–641.

81. Chivukula M, Haynik DM, Brufsky A, et al. Pleomorphic lobular carcinoma in situ (PLCIS) on breast core needle biopsies: clinical significance and immunoprofile. *Am J Surg Pathol.* 2008;32:1721–1726.

82. National Comprehensive Cancer Network. http://www.nccn.org.

83. Hussain M, Cunnick GH. Management of lobular carcinoma in situ and atypical lobular hyperplasia of the breast—a review. *Eur J Surg Oncol.* 2011;37:279–289.

84. Georgian-Smith D, Lawton TJ. Calcifications of lobular carcinoma in situ of the breast: radiologic-pathologic correlation. *AJR Am J Roentgenol.* 2001;176:1255–1259.

85. Rendi MH, Dintzis SM, Lehman CD, et al. Lobular in situ neoplasia on breast core needle biopsy: imaging indication and pathologic extent can identify which patients require excisional biopsy. *Ann Surg Oncol.* 2012;19:914–921.

86. Pacelli A, Rhodes DJ, Amrami KK, et al. Outcome of atypical lobular hyperplasia and lobular carcinoma in situ diagnosed by core needle biopsy: clinical and surgical follow-up of 30 cases. *Am J Clin Pathol.* 2001;116:591–592.

87. Mahoney MC, Robinson-Smith TM, Shaughnessy EA. Lobular neoplasia at 11-gauge vacuum-assisted stereotactic biopsy: correlation with surgical excisional biopsy and mammographic follow-up. *AJR Am J Roentgenol.* 2006;187:949–954.

88. Lavoue V, Graesslin O, Classe JM, et al. Management of lobular neoplasia diagnosed by core needle biopsy: study of 52 biopsies with follow-up surgical excision. *Breast.* 2007;16:533–539.

89. Flanagan MR, Rendi MH, Calhoun KE, et al. Pleomorphic lobular carcinoma in situ: radiologic-pathologic features and clinical management. *Ann Surg Oncol.* 2015;22(13):4263–4269.

90. Niell B, Specht M, Gerade B, et al. Is excisional biopsy required after a breast core biopsy yields lobular neoplasia? *AJR Am J Roentgenol.* 2012;199:929–935.

91. Subhawong AP, Subhawong TK, Khouri N, et al. Incidental minimal atypical lobular hyperplasia on core needle biopsy: correlation with findings on follow-up excision. *Am J Surg Pathol.* 2010;34:822–828.

92. Parkin CK, Garewal S, Waugh P, et al. Outcomes of patients with lobular in situ neoplasia of the breast: the role of vacuum-assisted biopsy. *Breast.* 2014;23:651–655.

93. Shah-Khan MG, Geiger XJ, Reynolds C, et al. Long-term follow-up of lobular neoplasia (atypical lobular hyperplasia/lobular carcinoma in situ) diagnosed on core needle biopsy. *Ann Surg Oncol.* 2012;19:3131–3138.

94. Atkins KA, Cohen MA, Nicholson B, et al. Atypical lobular hyperplasia and lobular carcinoma in situ at core breast biopsy: use of careful radiologic-pathologic correlation to recommend excision or observation. *Radiology.* 2013;269:340–347.

95. Middleton LP, Sneige N, Coyne R, et al. Most lobular carcinoma in situ and atypical lobular hyperplasia diagnosed on core needle biopsy can be managed clinically with radiologic follow-up in a multidisciplinary setting. *Cancer Med.* 2014;3:492–499.

96. Chaudhary S, Lawrence L, McGinty G, et al. Classic lobular neoplasia on core biopsy: a clinical and radio-pathologic correlation study with follow-up excision biopsy. *Mod Pathol.* 2013;26:762–771.

97. D'Alfonso TM, Wang K, Chiu YL, et al. Pathologic upgrade rates on subsequent excision when lobular carcinoma in situ is the primary diagnosis in the needle core biopsy with special attention to the radiographic target. *Arch Pathol Lab Med.* 2013;137:927–935.

19

Invasive Lobular Carcinoma

SYED A. HODA

The classic type of invasive lobular carcinoma (ILC) either infiltrates mammary stroma in linear cords or in a concentric pattern around uninvolved native glands. The noncohesive individual invasive carcinoma cells are small with round-to-ovoid nuclei and minimal occasionally vacuolated cytoplasm. "Skip areas," that is, poorly delimited foci of invasive carcinoma separated by unremarkable mammary glandular and stromal tissue without desmoplastic reaction, impart the impression of multifocality. There is minimal disruption of the native mammary glandular architecture.

CLINICAL PRESENTATION

When the diagnosis is restricted to the histologic and cytologic features of an invasive carcinoma, as described in the preceding paragraph, less than 5% of carcinomas qualify for the diagnosis of the classic type of ILC (1–3). If the classification is broadened to include variant forms, the frequency of ILC has reportedly been as high as 10% to 14% of all invasive carcinomas (4–6). ILC occurs almost throughout the entire age range of breast carcinoma in adult women (28–86 years). Most studies have placed the median age at diagnosis between 45 and 56 years (2,3,5–7). ILC is relatively more common among women older than 75 years (11%) than in women 35 years or younger. A population-based study of women with invasive breast carcinoma diagnosed from 1987 to 1999 revealed that the incidence rate of lobular carcinoma increased during this period (8). The increased incidence rate of ILC was greatest in women 50 years of age or older. On the other hand, the incidence rate for invasive ductal carcinoma (IDC) was relatively constant. In the absence of a systematic histopathologic review, these data have marginal reliability. ILC of classic as well as pleomorphic types occurs, albeit rarely, in the male breast (9–12).

The presenting symptom of ILC in almost all cases is either a mass or a radiologically evident lesion. In a minority of cases, the only physical evidence of the neoplasm is vague thickening or diffuse nodularity of the breast.

IMAGING

On *mammography*, ILC usually manifests as a spiculated mass or architectural distortion, and it is not prone to exhibit calcifications. Calcifications may be present coincidentally in benign proliferative lesions such as sclerosing adenosis associated with ILC (13). A lower frequency of calcifications detected by mammography has been reported in ILC than in ductal carcinomas (14–16). Exceptions are ILC arising in florid lobular carcinoma in situ (F-LCIS) or pleomorphic lobular carcinoma in situ (P-LCIS), both of which show central necrosis and calcifications within glands (see Chapter 18). In the screening setting, ILC is found more often clinically during intervals between examinations than by mammography (so-called "*interval carcinomas*") (17). The mammographic size of ILC tends to be lesser when determined mammographically than grossly (18), although the latter methodology has its own disadvantages (19).

The most common mammographic manifestation of ILC is an asymmetric, ill-defined or irregular, spiculated mass (13,14,16,20). In one study, 46% of mammograms from patients who ultimately proved to have ILC were initially reported to be negative (15). The absence of well-defined margins and a tendency to form multiple subtle nodules of variable extent throughout the breast in some cases are features that hinder the radiologic detection of ILC and lead to a false-negative interpretation of mammograms. Patients with a spiculated ILC are less likely to have residual carcinoma when re-excision is performed than are those with ill-defined or asymmetric lesions (21). A minority of ILC present with mammographically round or ovoid tumors (22). In a radiologic study of 27 ILCs and 85 IDCs, "normal" findings and mass lesions on mammography and posterior acoustic shadowing on ultrasound evaluation were more frequently associated with ILC than with IDC (23).

Ultrasonography has been useful for detecting multifocal and multicentric ILC (24), and it may be more accurate than mammography for predicting tumor size (25). Selinko et al. (26) reported that the sensitivity of sonography for detecting ILC (98%) was substantially higher than the sensitivity of mammography (65%).

Rodenko et al. (27) found that *magnetic resonance imaging* (MRI) was more effective than mammography in a significant proportion of cases for determining the extent of a primary ILC, but the presence of metastatic carcinoma in axillary lymph nodes was not detected in four cases examined. Yeh et al. (28) reported that tumor morphology as seen on MRI combined with quantitative measurement of gadolinium uptake was effective for detecting ILC in most cases. However, in the absence of an enhancing mass, ILC may not be detectable by MRI. ILC enhances slower than IDC on MRI, but peak enhancement is not significantly less (29). In the context of ILC, the effectiveness of MRI is somewhat diminished by the high rate of false-positives and overestimation of extent of disease limit.

Breast-specific gamma imaging (BSGI) has potential to be the most effective radiologic tool for the detection of ILC. In a study by Brem et al. (30), 26 women with a total of 28 biopsy-proven ILC, BSGI was shown to have the highest sensitivity for the detection of ILC with a sensitivity of 93%, whereas mammography, sonography, and MRI showed sensitivities of 79%, 68%, and 83%, respectively.

BILATERALITY

Patients with ILC are reported to have a relatively high frequency of *bilateral* carcinoma when compared with women who have other types of carcinoma (31–33). The reported relative risk for contralateral carcinoma in women with ILC when compared with those with ductal carcinoma ranged from 1.6 to 2 (34,35). Synchronous and metachronous contralateral carcinomas have been described in 6% to 28% of ILC cases (5,7,36). The reported incidence of subsequent contralateral carcinoma ranges from 1.0 (36,37) to 2.38 (38) per 100 women per year. There is some evidence that the frequency of bilaterality is higher in patients with classic ILC than in patients with the variant subtypes (38). A lobular

component has been found in the majority of synchronous or metachronous contralateral carcinomas, and at least 50% of these have been invasive (7,36,37). In one series, random concurrent contralateral biopsies in 108 patients revealed intraductal carcinoma in 6% and invasive carcinoma in 10% of patients (39). Biopsies performed for clinical indications in an additional 22 cases yielded intraductal carcinoma in 5% and invasive carcinoma in 32%. The probability of detecting contralateral invasive carcinoma was significantly greater in women who had multicentric ILC in the ipsilateral breast or who had ipsilateral lymph node metastases.

MICROSCOPIC PATHOLOGY

Several *growth patterns* may be encountered in lesions classified as classic ILC. The common denominator is the virtual absence of solid, alveolar, papillary, and gland-forming aggregates of cells. In the two-dimensional plane of a histologic section, the slender strands of cells are arranged in a linear fashion, with one or two cells across **(Fig. 19.1)**. If the tumor cells are arranged around ducts and lobules in a concentric fashion, the distribution is described as having a "targetoid" (or "bull's eye") appearance **(Fig. 19.2)**. In a minority of cases, the linear strand-forming pattern is not conspicuous, and the tumor cells tend to grow mainly in dispersed, disorderly foci

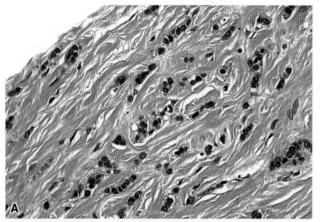

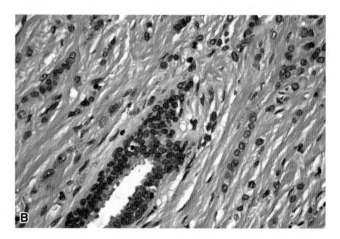

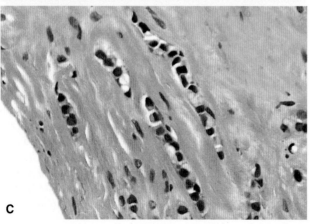

FIGURE 19.1 Histology and Cytology of Invasive Lobular Carcinoma, Classic Type. A–C: The "small" malignant cells with scant cytoplasm and dark, homogeneous nuclei are arranged in a linear pattern in these three different needle core biopsy specimens. **D:** Invasive lobular carcinoma cells of the classic type are seen in a linear array in this Papanicolaou-stained smear preparation from a fine needle aspiration procedure. **E:** A characteristic linear array of invasive lobular carcinoma cells was found in the corresponding monolayer ThinPrep preparation.

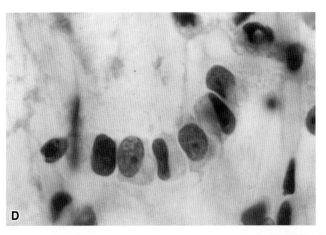

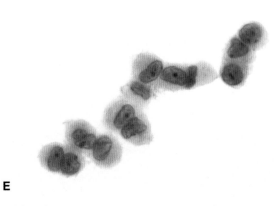

FIGURE 19.1 (*continued*)

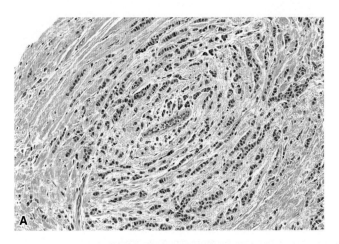

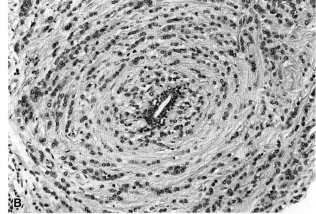

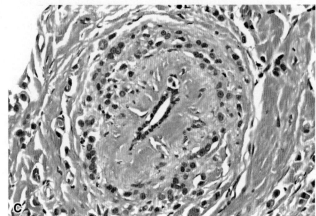

FIGURE 19.2 Invasive Lobular Carcinoma, Classic Type with "Targetoid" Growth. A–C: The linear infiltrates of carcinoma cells are distributed circumferentially around ducts. The "targetoid" ("bull's eye" or "satellitosis") appearance can occasionally be quite subtle, as seen in **C**.

(Fig. 19.3). The tumor cells in such foci may be small enough to be mistaken for lymphocytes or plasma cells, especially in areas of fibrosis or amid adipose tissue when sections are examined at lower magnification in a frozen section or in a needle core biopsy (NCB) specimen **(Figs. 19.4 and 19.5)**. ILC is only rarely accompanied by a notable lymphocytic reaction **(Fig. 19.6)**, although the term "lymphoepithelioma-like carcinoma" has been applied to an ILC with prominent lymphocytic reaction (40). One such tumor proved to be negative for Epstein–Barr virus.

Occasionally, the sample obtained in a NCB procedure contains minimal, histologically inconspicuous, evidence of ILC that can easily be overlooked after being mistaken for a lymphocytic infiltrate (41) **(Figs. 19.7 and 19.8)**. When LCIS is identified in a NCB specimen, all sections should be vigilantly inspected for foci of occult invasion. A cytokeratin immunostain can be helpful in detecting inconspicuous ILC **(Fig. 19.9)**.

All of the *cytologic appearances* found in LCIS may also be present in ILC. Classic ILC consists of small, uniform cells with

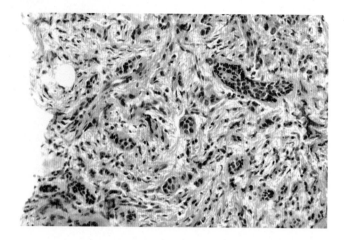

FIGURE 19.3 Invasive Lobular Carcinoma, Classic Type. The linear growth pattern is obscured by stromal reaction around a terminal duct and lobular glands in this needle core biopsy specimen.

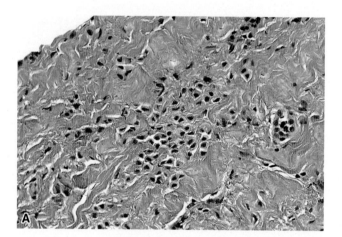

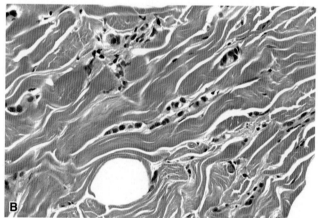

FIGURE 19.4 Invasive Lobular Carcinoma, Classic Type, Obscured by Fibrosis. A, B: The invasive carcinoma cells in these two needle core biopsy specimens are obscured by dense fibrosis and subtle forms of pseudoangiomatous stromal hyperplasia.

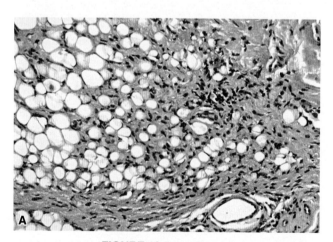

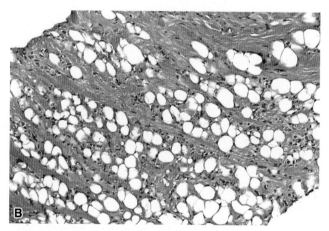

FIGURE 19.5 Invasive Lobular Carcinoma, Classic Type, Obscured by Fat. A–D: Carcinoma cells infiltrating fat in these four needle core biopsy specimens create an appearance that superficially resembles fat necrosis.

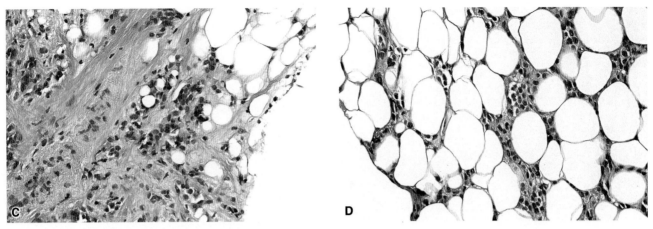

FIGURE 19.5 (*continued*)

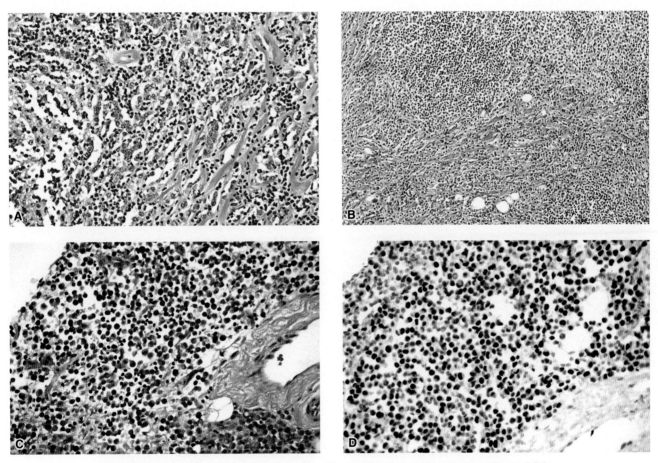

FIGURE 19.6 Invasive Lobular Carcinoma with Prominent Lymphocytic Reaction and "Plasmacytoid" Type of Invasive Lobular Carcinoma. A, B: The invasive lobular carcinoma cells have a linear growth pattern that is difficult to appreciate in the midst of the lymphocytic reaction. **C:** In this needle core biopsy specimen, the invasive lobular carcinoma cells display plasma cell-like cytology. **D:** The neoplastic cells of the case shown in **C** are strongly and diffusely immunoreactive for estrogen receptors.

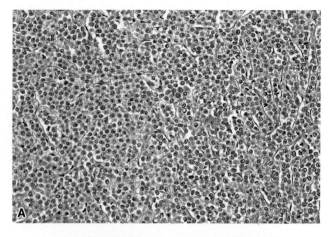

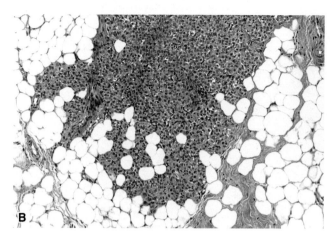

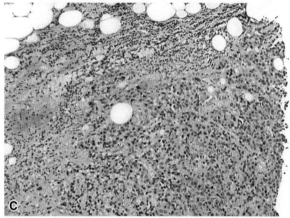

FIGURE 19.7 Invasive Lobular Carcinoma, Solid Variant.
A: Solid growth pattern, albeit with loss of cohesion (a feature commonly present in invasive lobular carcinoma), is illustrated in this area. Slender strands of stroma are present. **B:** The tumor cells form a solid mass with uneven borders infiltrating fat (hematoxylin–phloxine–saffranin). **C:** A needle core biopsy specimen in which the border of solid invasive lobular carcinoma is defined by a lymphocytic reaction.

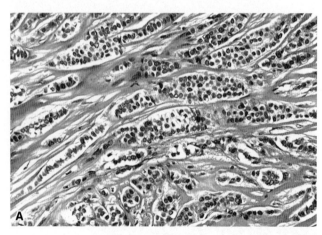

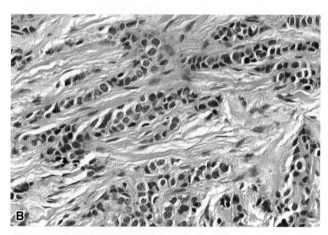

FIGURE 19.8 Invasive Lobular Carcinoma, Trabecular Variant. A, B: Both tumors shown here display a trabecular growth pattern formed by bands of cells. The latter are arrayed two to four cell across.

round nuclei and inconspicuous nucleoli. A variable proportion of cells have intracytoplasmic lumina (**Fig. 19.10**). Mucin is demonstrable in these vacuoles with the mucicarmine and Alcian blue stains (42,43). When the secretion is prominent, the cells assume a signet ring configuration. The majority of so-called signet ring cell carcinomas, but not all, are forms of ILC (5,42–44).

Classic type of ILC exhibits negligible duct (gland) formation, cytologic blandness as well as monotony, and negligible

mitotic activity. As such, when classic ILCs are graded according to the Nottingham scheme, most are accorded grade 2 (usually 3+2+1).

Some *variants of ILC* (solid, alveolar, or trabecular) are based on architectural variance from the classic type. Other variants (signet ring cell, pleomorphic) differ in cytologic appearance (**Table 19.1**). The typical pattern of linear and concentric infiltration of noncohesive neoplastic cells are common features in some of these variants (2,5,6). One or more variants of ILC

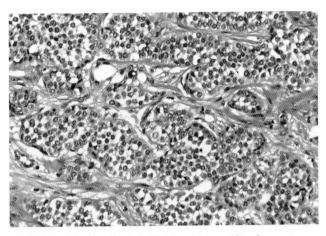

FIGURE 19.9 Invasive Lobular Carcinoma, Alveolar Type. The tumor cells form rounded masses that duplicate the appearance of lobular carcinoma in situ (LCIS). Immunostains for myoepithelial cells (not shown here) are useful to distinguish alveolar type of invasive lobular carcinoma and LCIS.

TABLE 19.1
Variants of Invasive Lobular Carcinoma
Architectural Variants
Solid Alveolar Trabecular Mixed group
Cytological Variants
Signet ring cell Pleomorphic (including those described as histiocytoid and apocrine) Mixed group

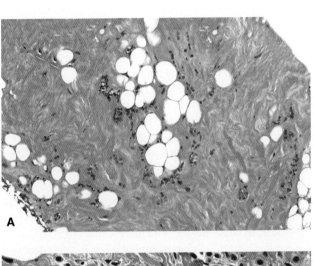

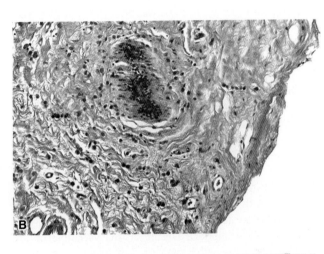

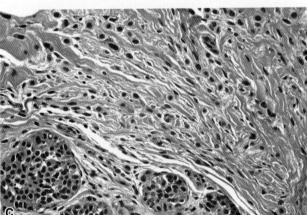

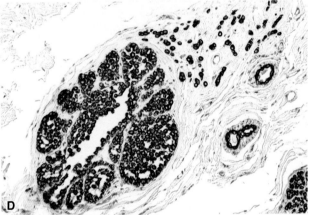

FIGURE 19.10 Invasive Lobular Carcinoma, Classic Type, Subtle Lesions. A–D: The only evidence of invasive carcinoma in these four needle core biopsies were subtle and inconspicuous foci, each of which spanned less than 1 mm. Microinvasive lobular carcinoma, next to lobular carcinoma in situ, is highlighted by the cytokeratin (CK7) immunostain in **D**.

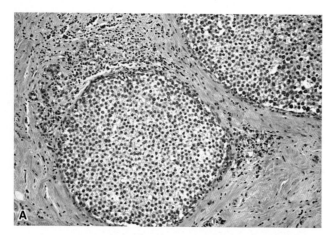
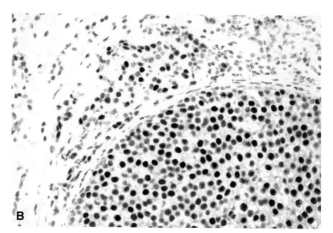

FIGURE 19.11 Microinvasive Lobular Carcinoma. A, B: Lobular carcinoma in situ of the florid type associated with a solitary focus of microinvasive lobular carcinoma. The latter is highlighted by the estrogen receptor immunostain (shown in **B**).

may coexist with classic ILC in cases that should be regarded as a *mixed group*. Areas of classic ILC with a linear pattern are found (at least focally) in most variant forms, but they may not be necessarily represented in a NCB sampling.

The *solid* type of ILC consists of compact nests or sheets of tumor cells **(Fig. 19.11)**. *Trabecular* ILC refers to tumors with prominent bands more than two cells broad **(Fig. 19.12)**. Usually, the trabecular pattern is found in association with other variants, and the tumors are classified as mixed. The *alveolar* pattern of ILC is defined by rounded ("globular") aggregates of cells that may simulate LCIS, particularly in NCB sampling (45) **(Fig. 19.13)**. LCIS coexists with about 85% of variant tumors. The observation that many examples of classic ILC have minor components of alveolar, tubular, trabecular, or solid growth is further evidence for classifying neoplasms that express these features prominently as variants of ILC. This conclusion is also supported by the fact that variant forms are not immunoreactive with E-cadherin. Tubulolobular carcinoma is immunoreactive for E-cadherin and should be regarded as a variant of tubular carcinoma, rather than of lobular carcinoma (see Chapter 10).

Perineural invasion is uncommon in ILC but may occur when the lesion is either diffusely extensive or is of the solid type. Lymphovascular involvement is rarely identified in ILC, and in some situations shrinkage artifacts may simulate carcinoma in lymphovascular spaces. When lymphovascular tumor emboli are present, the tumor cells tend to form cohesive aggregates rather than being singly dispersed.

Some ILC consist entirely, or in part, of cells with relatively abundant cytoplasm and enlarged hyperchromatic nuclei **(Fig. 19.14)**. These distinctive cells have been referred to as *pleomorphic* (from Greek, *pleo*: more than one, *morphe*: form) lobular carcinoma (35–38,46–49). The cytoplasm of the cells in pleomorphic ILC may display apocrine or histiocytoid traits (47,50) **(Fig. 19.15)** and is usually associated with LCIS that is composed of cytologically similar pleomorphic cells (that is, pleomorphic variant of LCIS). Most forms of ILC described previously as either histiocytoid or apocrine ought to qualify for the designation of pleomorphic ILC. A low frequency of reactivity for estrogen receptor (ER) and progesterone receptor (PR) is found in pleomorphic ILC (51), and apocrine carcinomas are also typically not reactive for these receptors. Androgen

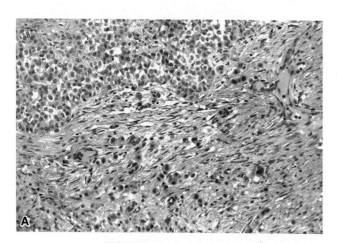
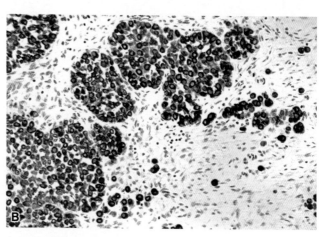

FIGURE 19.12 In Situ and Invasive Lobular Carcinoma, Classic Type, in a Benign Phyllodes Tumor. A: In situ lobular carcinoma is shown in enlarged lobules (top). The stroma contains "small" round cells suggestive of invasive lobular carcinoma. **B:** Scattered invasive carcinoma cells are highlighted with a cytokeratin (CK7) immunostain.

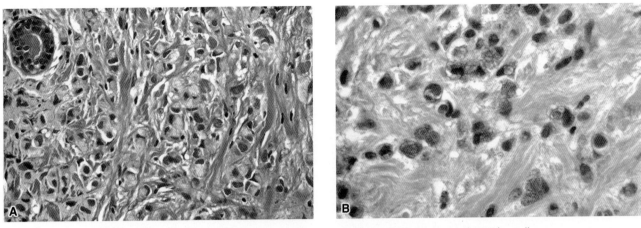

FIGURE 19.13 Invasive Lobular Carcinoma with Signet Ring Cells. A, B: Signet ring cells are shown in *this* invasive lobular carcinoma found in a needle core biopsy specimen. The intracytoplasmic mucin in the signet ring cells is highlighted by a mucicarmine stain in **B**.

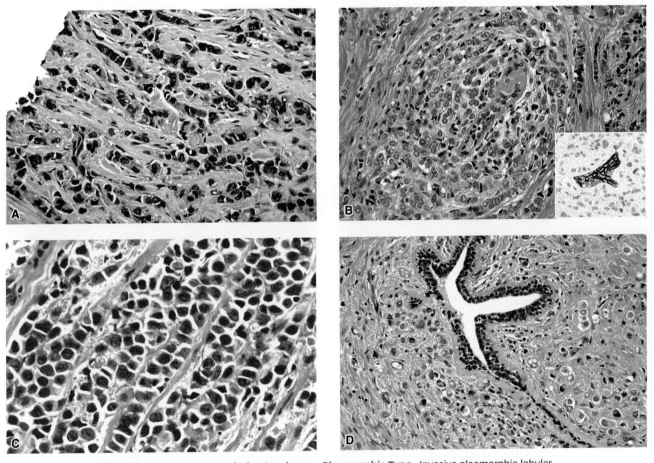

FIGURE 19.14 Invasive Lobular Carcinoma, Pleomorphic Type. Invasive pleomorphic lobular carcinoma with marked variation in nuclear morphology is shown in these biopsies. **A, B:** The invasive carcinoma cells are arranged in linear strands in **A**, and in a "targetoid" manner in **B**. Inset shows E-cadherin negativity in invasive pleomorphic lobular carcinoma cells, and E-cadherin positivity in the benign ductal cells **(center)**. **C, D:** The pleomorphic cells show a trabecular arrangement in **C** and show apocrine (pink cytoplasmic) features in **D**. **E:** A prominent lymphocytic reaction around rare dispersed pleomorphic carcinoma cells is shown. **F:** A touch-imprint cytology preparation of a sentinel lymph node with metastatic pleomorphic lobular carcinoma and many lymphocytes. Note marked anisonucleosis of the malignant cells. **G:** The histopathologic appearance of the corresponding "positive" sentinel lymph node is shown.

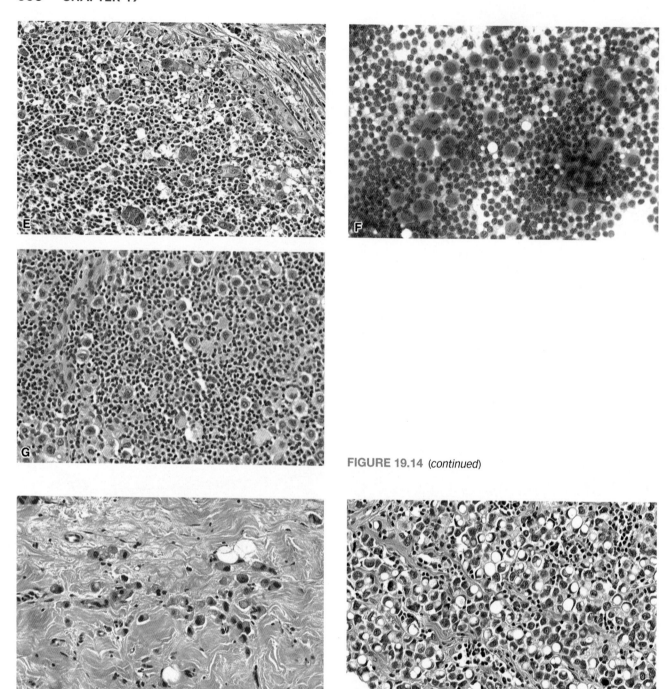

FIGURE 19.14 (continued)

FIGURE 19.15 Invasive Lobular Carcinoma, Pleomorphic Type with Variable Cytologic and Histologic Appearances. **A:** These invasive pleomorphic lobular carcinoma cells show "histiocytoid" cytoplasm and pleomorphic hyperchromatic nuclei. **B:** This invasive pleomorphic lobular carcinoma has almost exclusively signet ring cell features. **C:** Another example of invasive pleomorphic lobular carcinoma showing neoplastic cells in minute aggregates amid lymphocytes. **D:** This invasive pleomorphic lobular carcinoma, associated with dense calcification, is infiltrative in linear arrays in a manner reminiscent of classic type of invasive lobular carcinoma.

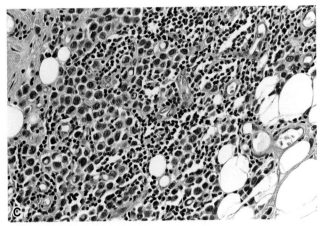

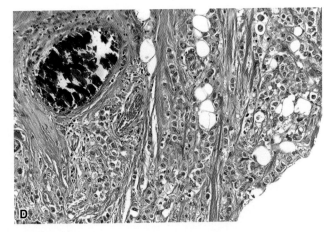

FIGURE 19.15 (*continued*)

receptors have been detected in pleomorphic lobular carcinomas (52), and are also typically present in apocrine carcinomas. Pleomorphic ILC exhibits a relatively high nuclear grade and brisk mitotic rate; as such, per the Nottingham system, these carcinomas are accorded grade 3 (usually 3+3+2).

GENETIC ALTERATIONS AND IMMUNOHISTOCHEMISTRY

Molecular alterations in pleomorphic ILC are more typical of high-grade IDC than classic ILC, that is, p53(+) and HER2(+),

8q(+), 17q24-q25(+), 13q(−) and amplification of 8q24, 12q14, 17q12, and 20q13 purportedly propel the relatively more assertive pathobiology of pleomorphic ILC (53).

E-cadherin is an epithelium-associated molecule involved in cell-to-cell adhesion that acts as a tumor invasion–suppressor gene. When compared with IDC, E-cadherin immunoreactivity is either markedly diminished or absent in the majority of ILCs (54–57) (**Fig. 19.16**). Loss of immunoreactivity for α-, β-, and λ-catenins also occurs in ILC (55). Mutations have been reported in the E-cadherin gene in classic (58–60) and in pleomorphic (61) ILCs. Loss of E-cadherin immunoreactivity is consistently observed in LCIS of classic, florid, and

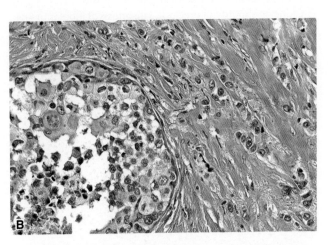

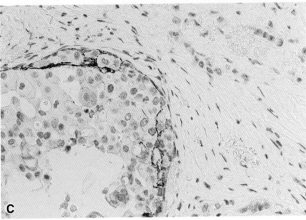

FIGURE 19.16 Invasive and In Situ Carcinoma, Immunostaining. A: Smooth muscle myosin immunoreactivity is observed only in the myoepithelial cells around the in situ component of this classic type of invasive and in situ lobular carcinoma.
B, C: This case of invasive and in situ pleomorphic lobular carcinoma shows E-cadherin negativity in the malignant cells **(C)**. Attenuated and interrupted immunoreactivity of the myoepithelial cells (or possibly of some rare residual epithelial cells) in the in situ lobular carcinoma can occasionally be misinterpreted **(C)**.

TABLE 19.2		
Immunohistochemical Results for Invasive Ductal and Invasive Lobular Carcinoma		
	Invasive Lobular Carcinoma	**Invasive Ductal Carcinoma**
E-cadherin	Negative	Positive
p120	Positive (cytoplasmic membrane)	Positive (cytoplasmic)
β-catenin	Negative	Positive
HMW-CK (K903/34β12)	Positive (perinuclear)	Negative

HMW-CK, high-molecular-weight cytokeratin.

pleomorphic types in the presence or absence of concomitant ILC (60–62). In one study of paired LCIS and ILC samples from 24 patients, loss of the entire 16q arm was detected in all tumors, and it was concluded that "the striking similarity in genomic changes between the in situ and invasive components of these lesions clearly demonstrated the common clonality of the two lesions" (63).

Because the E-cadherin staining pattern is so highly associated with histologic tumor type, lesions that depart from expected E-cadherin reactivity are described as having *aberrant E-cadherin staining* (64). Da Silva et al. (65) reported that the cadherin–catenin complex may not be functional in lobular carcinomas with aberrant E-cadherin expression. These authors concluded that when the H&E histologic appearance is characteristic for lobular carcinoma, "positive staining for E-cadherin should not preclude a diagnosis of lobular in favor of ductal carcinoma."

Several additional *immunohistochemical markers*, including p120, β-catenin, and low-molecular-weight and high-molecular-weight cytokeratins, have been reported to help distinguish between lobular and ductal carcinoma (**Table 19.2**) (66). The vast majority of ILCs exhibit nuclear immunoreactivity for ER and PR (**Fig. 19.17**). Pleomorphic ILCs are typically positive for gross cystic disease fluid protein-15 (GCDFP-15, BRST2) (67). HER2 is only rarely positive (that is, 3+, on a scale of 0 to 3+) in classic types of ILC (and LCIS) (35). ILC is typically negative for p53 protein, p63, and vimentin (68). About 20% of ILCs are positive for CK 5/6 (69). The CK5/6-positive carcinomas tend to be negative for ER and may represent a "basal-like" subset of ILCs.

Inactivation of E-cadherin is the most commonly identified genetic alteration in ILC. Classic ILCs typically show loss of chromosomal arm 16q and gain of material on 1q and 16p. Pleomorphic ILCs exhibit similar alterations and also display amplification of 8q24, 1q12, and 20q13. These amplifications are also found in high-grade ductal carcinomas (70).

METASTATIC LOBULAR CARCINOMA

Metastatic deposits of ILC tend to duplicate the cytologic (and sometimes the architectural) features of the primary tumor

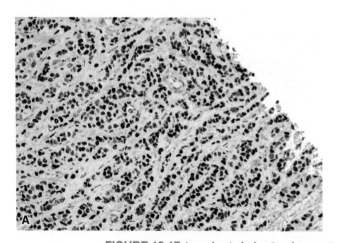
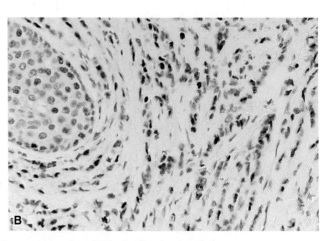

FIGURE 19.17 Invasive Lobular Carcinoma, Estrogen Receptors (ER). A: The characteristic strong and diffuse nuclear immunoreactivity for ER is evident in this classic type of invasive lobular carcinoma. This is the most common pattern of ER immunoreactivity in invasive classic lobular carcinoma. **B:** This immunostained section of another needle core biopsy specimen displays intermediate-to-strong nuclear immunoreactivity for ER in the majority of the invasive lobular carcinoma cells of the classic type. This is the second most common pattern of ER-positivity in invasive lobular carcinoma of the classic type.

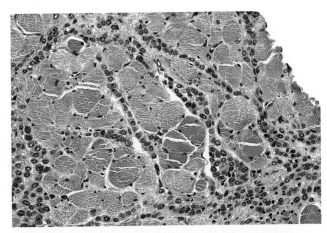

FIGURE 19.18 Metastatic Lobular Carcinoma. Lobular carcinoma with a linear growth pattern is shown infiltrating around fibers of skeletal muscle.

(**Fig. 19.18**). Axillary lymph node metastases derived from ILC of the classic type may be distributed largely in sinusoids, sparing lymphoid areas. If lymph node involvement is sparse, the distinction between tumor cells and histiocytes may be difficult to appreciate in H&E-stained NCB samples.

When compared with ductal carcinoma, there is a statistically significant greater frequency of metastases of lobular carcinoma to the peritoneum, meninges, gastrointestinal tract, and gynecological organs, and a lower frequency of pulmonary metastases (71). Metastatic ILC cells can be rather difficult to identify in cytologic examination of pleural, ascetic, or cerebrospinal fluid. In the uterus, metastatic lobular carcinoma cells blend with normal endometrial stromal cells and may be overlooked in endometrial curettings (72). Metastatic lobular carcinoma has been described in endometrial polyps associated with tamoxifen therapy (73). Metastases involving the stomach can produce clinical and pathologic findings indistinguishable from those of a primary gastric carcinoma (74). ER immunoreactivity has been reported in primary gastric adenocarcinomas; however, in the appropriate clinical setting, diffusely strong immunoreactivity of carcinoma cells in gastric mucosa favors metastatic lobular carcinoma (75,76). Isolated metastatic lobular carcinoma cells in the bone marrow may resemble normal hematopoietic elements (77). No significant differences have been found in the distribution of metastases between patients with the classic and variant patterns of ILC (5).

PROGNOSIS

Data from several studies suggest that the pleomorphic variant of ILC may have a less-favorable prognosis than classic variants (47–49). The prognosis of pleomorphic ILC has been related specifically to mitotic activity rather than nuclear pleomorphism (78). Monhollen et al. (79) reported on 40 cases of pleomorphic ILC, which included five triple-negative cases and 14 HER2-positive cases. Older patients and negative hormonal receptor status correlated significantly with worse clinical outcome ($P < 0.03$). The 5-year recurrence-free and

overall survival rates were 54.9% and 76.2%, respectively. Based on these data, the authors concluded that pleomorphic ILC has "hybrid clinicopathological characteristics" between ILC and IDC.

Several studies of prognosis in patients with nonpleomorphic ILC have not shown a consistent difference from patients with IDC treated by mastectomy when stage at diagnosis is taken into consideration (2,5,38,80,81). Patients with classic ILC have a slightly better prognosis than those with variant forms as a group, but the differences have not been statistically significant. No reproducible differences in prognosis have been demonstrated among patients with different nonpleomorphic variant carcinomas, and it is evident that large numbers of cases would be needed to document significant differences if they exist. Consequently, no distinction should be made between classic and nonpleomorphic variant forms of ILC with regard to therapy. At this time, size of ILC and nodal status remain the most important determinants of treatment and prognosis.

TREATMENT

Many reports of successful treatment by breast conservation with radiotherapy have appeared (20,82–89). These studies indicate that survival for patients with ILC treated by breast conservation is similar to the result obtained for ductal carcinoma. Patients with multifocal ILC had a greater frequency of breast recurrence than those with unifocal tumors (87).

Biglia et al. (90) undertook a retrospective analysis of 1,407 patients with IDC and 243 with ILC to compare histopathologic and immunohistochemical characteristics, surgical treatment, and clinical outcome in the two groups. ILC, when treated with conservative surgery, required re-excision or mastectomy more frequently owing to margin-positivity. No difference was observed in terms of 5-year disease-free survival and local relapse-free survival between the two groups in the whole series, and in the subgroup of patients treated with breast conservation. The study concluded that ILC can be successfully treated with conservative surgery, although accurate preoperative estimation of extent and multifocality of ILC may facilitate the goal.

Limited information is available about the treatment of invasive pleomorphic lobular carcinoma by conservation therapy. If the latter option is exercised, pleomorphic lobular carcinoma in situ (P-LCIS) ought to be viewed as being similar to intraductal carcinoma with respect to assessing margins.

ILC responds poorly to neoadjuvant chemotherapy when compared to IDC (91,92). Thus, determination of differentiation (ductal vs. lobular) of invasive carcinoma in NCB samples can be of extreme significance *vis a vis* initiation of appropriate treatment.

REFERENCES

1. Henson D, Tarone R. A study of lobular carcinoma of the breast based on the Third National Cancer Survey in the United States of America. *Tumori.* 1979;65:133–142.

2. Dixon JM, Anderson TJ, Page DL, et al. Infiltrating lobular carcinoma of the breast. *Histopathology.* 1982;6:149–161.

3. Ashikari R, Huvos AG, Urban JA, et al. Infiltrating lobular carcinoma of the breast. *Cancer.* 1973;31:110–116.

4. Martinez V, Azzopardi JG. Invasive lobular carcinoma of the breast: incidence and variants. *Histopathology.* 1979;3:467–488.

5. DiCostanzo D, Rosen PP, Gareen I, et al. Prognosis in infiltrating lobular carcinoma: an analysis of 'classical' and variant tumors. *Am J Surg Pathol.* 1990;14:12–23.

6. Fechner RE. Histologic variants of infiltrating lobular carcinoma of the breast. *Hum Pathol.* 1975;6:373–378.

7. Fechner RE. Infiltrating lobular carcinoma without lobular carcinoma in situ. *Cancer.* 1972;29:1539–1545.

8. Li CL, Anderson BO, Daling JR, et al. Trends in incidence rates of invasive lobular and ductal breast carcinoma. *JAMA.* 2003;289:1421–1424.

9. Spencer JT, Shutter J. Synchronous bilateral invasive lobular breast cancer presenting as carcinomatosis in a male. *Am J Surg Pathol.* 2009;33:470–474.

10. Moten A, Obirieze A, Wilson LL. Characterizing lobular carcinoma of the male breast using the SEER database. *J Surg Res.* 2013;185:e71–e76.

11. Ishida M, Mori T, Umeda T, et al. Pleomorphic lobular carcinoma in a male breast: case report with review of the literature. *Int J Clin Exp Pathol.* 2013;6:1441–1444.

12. Zahir MN, Minhas K, Shabbir-Moosajee M. Pleomorphic lobular carcinoma of the male breast with axillary lymph node involvement: a case report and review of literature. *BMC Clin Pathol.* 2014;14:16. doi: 10.1186/1472-6890-14-16.24795533

13. Mendelson EB, Harris KM, Doshi N, et al. Infiltrating lobular carcinoma: mammographic patterns with pathologic correlation. *Am J Radiol.* 1989;153:265–271.

14. Helvie MA, Paramagul C, Oberman HA, et al. Invasive lobular carcinoma: imaging features and clinical detection. *Invest Radiol.* 1993;28:202–207.

15. Krecke KN, Gisvold JJ. Invasive lobular carcinoma of the breast: mammographic findings and extent of disease at diagnosis in 184 patients. *AJR Am J Roentgenol.* 1993;161:957–960.

16. Le Gal M, Ollivier L, Asselain B, et al. Mammographic features of 455 invasive lobular carcinomas. *Radiology.* 1992;185:705–708.

17. Porter PL, El-Bastawissi AY, Mendelson MT, et al. Breast tumor characteristics as predictors of mammographic detection: comparison of interval-and screen-detected cancers. *J Natl Cancer Inst.* 1999;91:2020–2028.

18. Yeatman TJ, Cantor AB, Smith TJ, et al. Tumor biology of infiltrating lobular carcinoma: implications for management. *Ann Surg.* 1995;222:549–561.

19. Varma S, Ozerdem U, Hoda SA. Complexities and challenges in the pathologic assessment of size (T) of invasive breast carcinoma. *Adv Anat Pathol.* 2014;21:420–432.

20. White JR, Gustafson GS, Wimbish K, et al. Conservative surgery and radiation therapy for infiltrating lobular carcinoma of the breast: the role of preoperative mammograms in guiding treatment. *Cancer.* 1994;74:640–647.

21. Porter AJ, Evans EB, Foxcroft LM, et al. Mammographic and ultrasound features of invasive lobular carcinoma of the breast. *J Med Imaging Radiat Oncol.* 2014;58:1–10.

22. Evans WP, Burhenne LJW, Laurie L, et al. Invasive lobular carcinoma of the breast: mammographic characteristics and computer-aided detection. *Radiology.* 2002;225:182–189.

23. Kim SH, Cha ES, Park CS, et al. Imaging features of invasive lobular carcinoma: comparison with invasive ductal carcinoma. *Jpn J Radiol.* 2011;29:475–482.

24. Berg WA, Gilbreath PL. Multicentric and multi-focal cancer: whole breast US in preoperative evaluation. *Radiology.* 2000;214:59–66.

25. Skaane P, Skjorken G. Ultrasonographic evaluation of invasive lobular carcinoma. *Acta Radiol.* 1999;40:369–375.

26. Selinko VL, Middleton LP, Dempsey PJ. Role of sonography in diagnosing and staging invasive lobular carcinoma. *J Clin Ultrasound.* 2004;32:323–332.

27. Rodenko GN, Harms SE, Pruneda JM, et al. MR imaging in the management before surgery of lobular carcinoma of the breast: correlation with pathology. *AJR Am J Roentgenol.* 1996;167:1415–1419.

28. Yeh ED, Slanetz PJ, Edmister WB, et al. Invasive lobular carcinoma: spectrum of enhancement and morphology on magnetic resonance imaging. *Breast J.* 2003;9:13–18.

29. Mann RM, Veltman J, Huisman H, et al. Comparison of enhancement characteristics between invasive lobular carcinoma and invasive ductal carcinoma. *J Magn Reson Imaging.* 2011;34:293–300.

30. Brem RF, Ioffe M, Rapelyea JA, et al. Invasive lobular carcinoma: detection with mammography, sonography, MRI, and breast-specific gamma imaging. *AJR Am J Roentgenol.* 2009;192:379–383.

31. Broët P, de la Rochefordière A, Scholl SM, et al. Contralateral breast cancer: annual incidence and risk parameters. *J Clin Oncol.* 1995;13:1578–1583.

32. Bernstein JL, Thompson WD, Risch N, et al. Risk factors predicting the incidence of second primary breast cancer among women diagnosed with a first primary breast cancer. *Am J Epidemiol.* 1992;136:925–936.

33. Lesser ML, Rosen PP, Kinne DW. Multicentricity and bilaterality in invasive breast carcinoma. *Surgery.* 1982;1:234–240.

34. Horn PL, Thompson WD. Risk of contralateral breast cancer: associations with factors related to initial breast cancer. *Am J Epidemiol.* 1988;128:309–323.

35. Kollias J, Ellis IO, Elston CW, et al. Clinical and histologic predictors of contralateral breast cancer. *Eur J Surg Oncol.* 1999;25:584–589.

36. Dixon JM, Anderson TJ, Page DL, et al. Infiltrating lobular carcinoma of the breast: an evaluation of the incidence and consequence of bilateral disease. *Br J Surg.* 1983;70:513–516.

37. Hislop TG, Ng V, McBride ML, et al. Incidence and risk factors for second breast primaries in women with lobular breast carcinoma. *Breast Dis.* 1990;3:95–105.

38. du Toit RS, Locker AP, Ellis IO, et al. Invasive lobular carcinomas of the breast—the prognosis of histopathological subtypes. *Br J Cancer.* 1989;60:605–609.

39. Simkovich AH, Sclafani LM, Masri M, et al. Role of contralateral breast biopsy in infiltrating lobular cancer. *Surgery.* 1993;114:555–557.

40. Cristina S, Boldorini R, Brustia F, et al. Lymphoepithelioma-like carcinoma of the breast: an unusual pattern of infiltrating lobular carcinoma. *Virchows Arch.* 2000;437:198–202.

41. Ross DS, Hoda SA. Microinvasive (T1mic) lobular carcinoma of the breast: clinicopathologic profile of 16 cases. *Am J Surg Pathol.* 2011;35:750–756.

42. Breslow A, Brancaccio ME. Intracellular mucin production by lobular breast carcinoma cells. *Arch Pathol Lab Med.* 1976;100:620–621.

43. Gad A, Azzopardi JG. Lobular carcinoma of the breast: a special variant of mucin secreting carcinoma. *J Clin Pathol.* 1975;28:711–716.

44. Steinbrecher JS, Silverberg SG. Signet ring cell carcinoma of the breast: the mucinous variant of infiltrating lobular carcinoma. *Cancer.* 1976;37:828–840.

45. Butler R, Pinsky R, Jorns JM. Alveolar variant of invasive lobular carcinoma in a fibroadenoma. *Breast J.* 2012;18:613–614.

46. Allenby PL, Chowdhury LN. Histiocytic appearance of metastatic lobular breast carcinoma. *Arch Pathol Lab Med.* 1986;110:759–760.

47. Eusebi V, Magalhaes F, Azzopardi JG. Pleomorphic lobular carcinoma of the breast: an aggressive tumor showing apocrine differentiation. *Hum Pathol.* 1992;23:655–662.

48. Weidner N, Semple JP. Pleomorphic variant of invasive lobular carcinoma of the breast. *Hum Pathol.* 1992;23:1167–1171.

49. Bentz JS, Yassa N, Clayton F. Pleomorphic lobular carcinoma of the breast: clinicopathologic features of 12 cases. *Mod Pathol.* 1998;11:814–822.

50. Walford N, Ten Velden J. Histiocytoid breast carcinoma: an apocrine variant of lobular carcinoma. *Histopathology.* 1989;14:515–522.

51. Shimzu S, Kitamura H, Ito T, et al. Histiocytoid breast carcinoma: histological, immunohistochemical, ultrastructural, cytological and clincopathological studies. *Pathol Int.* 1998;48:849–856.

52. Augros M, Buenerd A, Decouassoux-Shisheboran M, et al. Infiltrating lobular carcinoma of the breast with histiocytoid features. *Ann Pathol.* 2004;24:259–263.

53. Simpson PT, Reis-Filho JS, Lambros MB, et al. Molecular profiling pleomorphic lobular carcinomas of the breast: evidence for a common molecular genetic pathway with classic lobular carcinomas. *J Pathol.* 2008;215:231–244.

54. Moll R, Mitze M, Frixen UH, et al. Differential loss of E-cadherin expression in infiltrating ductal and lobular breast carcinomas. *Am J Pathol.* 1993;143:1731–1742.

55. DeLeeuw WJ, Berx G, Vos CB, et al. Simultaneous loss of E-cadherin and catenins in invasive lobular breast cancer and lobular carcinoma in situ. *J Pathol.* 1997;183:404–411.

56. Lehr HA, Folpe A, Yaziji H, et al. Cytokeratin 8 immunostaining pattern and E-cadherin expression distinguish lobular from ductal breast carcinoma. *Am J Clin Pathol*. 2000;114:190–196.

57. Morrogh M, Andrade VP, Giri D, et al. Cadherin-catenin complex dissociation in lobular neoplasia of the breast. *Breast Cancer Res Treat*. 2012;132:641–652.

58. Kanai Y, Oda T, Tsuda H, et al. Point mutation of the E-cadherin gene in invasive lobular carcinoma of the breast. *Jpn J Cancer Res*. 1994;85:1035–1039.

59. Berx G, Cleton-Jansen AM, Strumane K, et al. E-cadherin is inactivated in a majority of invasive human lobular breast cancers by truncation mutations throughout its extracellular domain. *Oncogene*. 1996;13:1919–1925.

60. Huiping C, Sigurgeirdottir JR, Jonasson JG, et al. Chromosome alterations and E-cadherin gene mutations in human lobular breast cancer. *Br J Cancer*. 1999;81:1103–1110.

61. Palacios J, Sarrio D, Garcia-Macias MC, et al. Frequent E-cadherin gene inactivation by loss of heterozygosity in pleomorphic lobular carcinoma of the breast. *Mod Pathol*. 2003;16:674–678.

62. Wahed A, Connelly J, Reese T. E-cadherin expression in pleomorphic lobular carcinoma: an aid to differentiation from ductal carcinoma. *Ann Diagn Pathol*. 2002;6:349–351.

63. Hwang ES, Nyante SJ, Chen YY, et al. Clonality of lobular carcinoma in situ and synchronous invasive lobular carcinoma. *Cancer*. 2004;100:2562–2572.

64. Harigopal M, Shin SJ, Murray M, et al. Aberrant E-cadherin staining patterns in invasive mammary carcinoma. *World J Surg Oncol*. 2005;3:73–83.

65. Da Silva L, Parry S, Reid L, et al. Aberrant expression of E-cadherin in lobular carcinomas of the breast. *Am J Surg Pathol*. 2008;32:773–783.

66. de Deus Moura R, Wludarski SC, Carvalho FM, et al. Immunohistochemistry applied to the differential diagnosis between ductal and lobular carcinoma of the breast. *Appl Immunohistochem Mol Morphol*. 2013;21:1–12.

67. Porter PL, Garcia R, Moe R, et al. C-erbB-2 oncogene protein in in situ and invasive lobular breast neoplasia. *Cancer*. 1991;68:331–334.

68. Domagala W, Markiewski M, Kubiak R, et al. Immunohistochemical profile of invasive lobular carcinoma of the breast: predominantly vimentin and p53 protein negative cathepsin D and oestrogen receptor positive. *Virchows Arch (A)*. 1993;423:497–502.

69. Fadare O, Wang SA, Hileeto D. The expression of cytokeratin 5/6 in invasive lobular carcinoma of the breast: evidence of a basal-like subset? *Hum Pathol*. 2008;39:331–336.

70. Vargas AC, Lakhani SR, Simpson PT. Pleomorphic lobular carcinoma of the breast: molecular pathology and clinical impact. *Future Oncol*. 2009;5:233–243.

71. Harris M, Howell A, Chrissohou M, et al. A comparison of the metastatic pattern of infiltrating lobular carcinoma and infiltrating duct carcinoma of the breast. *Br J Cancer*. 1984;50:23–30.

72. Kumar NB, Hart WR. Metastases to the uterine corpus from extragenital cancers: a clinicopathologic study of 63 cases. *Cancer*. 1982;50:2163–2169.

73. Houghton JP, Ioffe OB, Silverberg SG, et al. Metastatic breast lobular carcinoma involving tamoxifen-associated endometrial polyps: report of two cases and review of tamoxifen-associated polypoid uterine lesions. *Mod Pathol*. 2003;16:395–398.

74. Cormier WJ, Gaffey TA, Welch JM, et al. Linitis plastica caused by metastatic carcinoma of the breast. *Mayo Clin Proc*. 1980;55:747–753.

75. Harrison JD, Morris DL, Ellis IO, et al. The effect of tamoxifen and estrogen receptor status on survival in gastric carcinoma. *Cancer*. 1989;64:1007–1010.

76. Yokozaki H, Takemura N, Takanashi A, et al. Estrogen receptors in gastric adenocarcinoma: a retrospective immunohistochemical analysis. *Virchows Arch (A)*. 1988;413:297–302.

77. Bitter MA, Fiorito D, Corkell ME, et al. Bone marrow involvement by lobular carcinoma of the breast cannot be identified reliably by routine histological examination alone. *Hum Pathol*. 1994;25:781–788.

78. Rakha EA, van Deurzen CH, Paish EC, et al. Pleomorphic lobular carcinoma of the breast: is it a prognostically significant pathological subtype independent of histological grade? *Mod Pathol*. 2013;26:496–501.

79. Monhollen L, Morrison C, Ademuyiwa FO, et al. Pleomorphic lobular carcinoma: a distinctive clinical and molecular breast cancer type. *Histopathology*. 2012;61:365–377.

80. Frost AR, Terahata S, Siegel RS, et al. An analysis of prognostic features in infiltrating lobular carcinoma of the breast. *Mod Pathol*. 1995;8:830–836.

81. Jayasinghe VW, Bilous AM, Boyages J. Is survival from infiltrating lobular carcinoma different from that of infiltrating ductal carcinoma? *Breast J*. 2007;13:479–485.

82. Cha I, Weidner N. Correlation of prognostic factors and survival with classical and the pleomorphic variants of invasive lobular carcinoma. *Breast J*. 1996;2:385–393.

83. Kurtz JM, Jacquemier J, Torhorst J, et al. Conservation therapy for breast cancers other than infiltrating ductal carcinoma. *Cancer*. 1989;63:1630–1635.

84. Poen JC, Tran L, Juillard G, et al. Conservation therapy for invasive lobular carcinoma of the breast. *Cancer*. 1992;69:2789–2795.

85. Sastre-Garau X, Jouve M, Asselain B, et al. Infiltrating lobular carcinoma of the breast: clinicopathologic analysis of 975 cases with reference to data on conservative therapy and metastatic patterns. *Cancer*. 1996;77:113–120.

86. Warneke J, Berger R, Johnson C, et al. Lumpectomy and radiation treatment for invasive lobular carcinoma of the breast. *Am J Surg*. 1996;172:496–500.

87. Schnitt SJ, Connolly JL, Recht A, et al. Influence of lobular histology on local tumor control in breast cancer patients treated with conservative surgery and radiotherapy. *Cancer*. 1989;64:448–454.

88. Morrow M, Keeney K, Scholtens D, et al. Selecting patients for breast conserving therapy: the importance of lobular histology. *Cancer*. 2006;106:2563–2568.

89. Santiago RJ, Harris EER, Quin L, et al. Similar long-term results of breast conservation treatment for stage I and II invasive lobular carcinoma compared with invasive duct carcinoma of the breast: the University of Pennsylvania experience. *Cancer*. 2006;103:2447–2454.

90. Biglia N, Maggiorotto F, Liberale V, et al. Clinical-pathologic features, long term-outcome and surgical treatment in a large series of patients with invasive lobular carcinoma and invasive ductal carcinoma. *Eur J Surg Oncol*. 2013;39:455–460.

91. Sullivan PS, Apple SK. Should histological type be taken into account when considering neoadjuvant chemotherapy in breast carcinoma? *Breast J*. 2009;15:146–154.

92. Nagao T, Kinoshita T, Hojo T, et al. The differences in the histological types of breast cancer and the response to neoadjuvant chemotherapy: the relationship between the outcome and the clinicopathological characteristics. *Breast*. 2012;21:289–295.

20

Mesenchymal Lesions

FREDERICK C. KOERNER

The diagnosis of mesenchymal mammary lesions using core biopsy specimens often challenges the pathologist. The limitations posed by the small size of the tissue samples and the overlapping features of many mesenchymal tumors impede the pathologist's ability to provide a specific diagnosis. Ever-present difficulties include recognizing phyllodes tumors and metaplastic carcinomas, and distinguishing low-grade sarcomas from their benign counterparts. Making such distinctions usually requires evaluation of the excised mass to search for the presence of benign glandular tissue, which would suggest the diagnosis of phyllodes tumor, and for immunohistochemical evidence of epithelial differentiation, which would point to the diagnosis of metaplastic carcinoma.

Despite these limitations, the study of specimens obtained by core biopsy can establish definite diagnoses in certain cases and can narrow the range of possible diagnoses in most others. By integrating conventional morphologic findings with the results of immunohistochemical staining or genetic analysis, one can usually establish secure diagnoses of granular cell tumor, fibromatosis, myofibroblastoma, schwannoma, hemangiopericytoma (solitary fibrous tumor), rhabdomyosarcoma, primitive neuroectodermal tumor, liposarcoma, and synovial sarcoma, among others. Even if one cannot make an exact diagnosis, one can often provide valuable clinical information. One can establish the vascular or leiomyomatous nature of a mass, for instance, and one can often suggest the diagnosis of hamartoma.

BENIGN LESIONS

Fibromatosis

Fibromatosis is an infiltrating, histologically low-grade, spindle cell proliferation composed of fibroblastic cells and variable amounts of collagen. Other terms applied to this lesion include extra-abdominal desmoid, low-grade fibrosarcoma, and aggressive fibromatosis, but most authors prefer the designation of fibromatosis.

Patients with mammary fibromatosis range from 14 to 83 years at diagnosis. Three series (1–3) report average ages from 37 to 49 years. Females are more commonly affected than males. Patients with mammary fibromatosis almost always present with a palpable, firm or hard tumor, which may suggest carcinoma on clinical examination. Dimpling or retraction of

the skin may reinforce this clinical impression. Fibromatosis affects the left and right breasts approximately equally. It rarely involves the subareolar region. The masses are usually painless, but pain and tenderness have been described. Several cases of bilateral mammary fibromatosis have been reported; in most of the cases, the bilateral tumors presented simultaneously (4). Fibromatosis has arisen in axillary breast tissue (5).

Antecedent injury from trauma or surgery was noted in a few cases, and several examples developed following breast augmentation (1,6–8). The tumors came to attention after a mean interval of 3 years from the time of implant placement. They are typically unilateral and arise in or around the implant capsule. Current evidence does not suggest that the biomaterials by themselves cause fibromatosis. Rare examples of mammary fibromatosis have been associated with familial adenomatous polyposis, a condition in which somatic fibromatosis (desmoid tumor) frequently occurs (4). Other potential predisposing genetic conditions are not known. The positive family history of breast carcinoma mentioned in a few case reports is probably coincidental. Rarely, patients had invasive ductal carcinoma of the contralateral breast. A 22-year-old woman developed unilateral mammary fibromatosis 5 years after treatment of Hodgkin's disease by chemotherapy alone (1). Despite the frequent association of abdominal desmoid tumors with pregnancy, only a few cases of mammary fibromatosis have been pregnancy-related. It seems likely that the two conditions occasionally coexist because of the broad age range of women with fibromatosis, many of whom are younger than 40 years.

Mammography reveals a stellate tumor that may be indistinguishable from carcinoma. Calcifications are rarely formed in mammary fibromatosis, but they may be present in a benign lesion such as sclerosing adenosis, which has been engulfed by the tumor.

The sizes of reported tumors vary from less than 1 to 17 cm and average 2.5 to 3.0 cm (1,2,9–11). Some examples of fibromatosis have a distinct stellate configuration; others are described as circumscribed or well-demarcated nodules. The masses consist of firm, white, tan, or gray fibrous tissue. Occasionally, the cut surface is said to have a whorled or trabecular appearance.

The histologic features of mammary fibromatosis are identical to those of the lesion when it develops in extramammary sites. Although the mass often exhibits varied growth patterns, spindle cells and collagen constitute consistent components. The spindle cells are usually distributed in broad sheets,

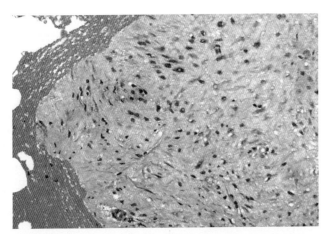

FIGURE 20.1 Fibromatosis. A needle core biopsy specimen shows average cellularity and slight stromal edema. The tumor cells have uniform round-to-oval nuclei.

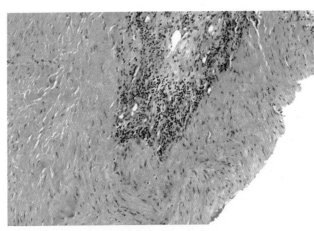

FIGURE 20.3 Fibromatosis. One can see a perivascular lymphocytic infiltrate in this needle core biopsy specimen.

sometimes in a storiform configuration, or in interlacing bundles with a herringbone pattern. The cells usually have small, pale, oval or spindly, uniform nuclei **(Fig. 20.1)**. Nuclear atypia and pleomorphism are uncommon. Mitotic figures are inconspicuous or undetectable in most cases, although a rate of 3 mitotic figures per 10 HPF has been reported (1). Areas in which the collagenous element overshadows the spindle cells have a keloidal appearance **(Fig. 20.2)**. In certain tumors, the center appears more fibrous than the periphery, whereas others exhibit more pronounced collagenization in the outer regions. Myxoid areas sometimes occur. Focal lymphocytic infiltrates, some with germinal centers, are found in nearly half of the tumors **(Fig. 20.3)** and usually appear more prominent at the periphery. Small blood vessels are evenly distributed throughout the tumor. Stromal calcification is seen rarely.

Cytoplasmic inclusion bodies identical to those seen in infantile digital fibromatosis have been described in two mammary tumors that appear to be fibromatosis (12). Round eosinophilic cytoplasmic inclusions measuring 3 to 10 μm were observed in the cytoplasm of tumor cells, often in a juxtanuclear location. The inclusions stained red with Masson's trichrome but did not stain with the periodic acid–Schiff method, nor did they stain for cytokeratin, desmin, or S-100. A ring of immunoreactivity for muscle-specific actin was apparent around the inclusion bodies. Similar inclusions in mammary fibroepithelial neoplasms consist of tightly packed actin filaments. These findings suggest that myofibroblasts play a role in this form of mammary fibromatosis.

No matter how well demarcated the masses appear grossly, all have invasive stellate extensions into the surrounding mammary parenchyma. It is generally possible to identify mammary ducts and lobules engulfed by these peripheral extensions **(Fig. 20.4)**. The appearance created in these infiltrative areas may mimic the growth pattern of a phyllodes tumor. Glandular parenchymal elements are less conspicuous or absent toward the center of the mass. Rare cases of fibromatosis are entirely or almost entirely limited to the mammary subcutaneous fat with little or no parenchymal involvement.

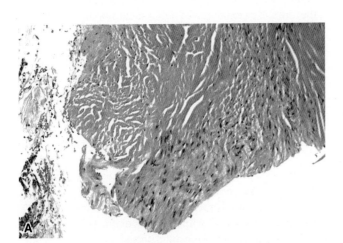
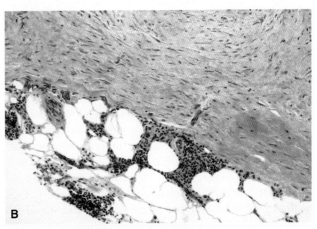

FIGURE 20.2 Fibromatosis, Keloidal. A: This needle core biopsy specimen displays an area of dense collagenous tissue adjacent to a more cellular component of the mass. The slit-shaped spaces in the keloidal tissue resemble pseudoangiomatous hyperplasia of mammary stroma. **B:** Fibromatosis with a peripheral lymphoid aggregate is shown.

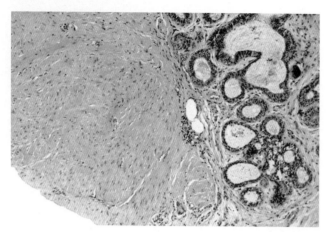

FIGURE 20.4 Fibromatosis. The tumor abuts a lobule in this part of a needle core biopsy specimen.

The surrounding breast parenchyma usually appears inactive. Mild epithelial hyperplasia is sometimes present in ducts trapped by the infiltrating extensions of the tumor.

Nuclear localization of β-catenin, commonly seen in somatic fibromatosis, is also seen in mammary fibromatosis. Among 53 examples of mammary fibromatosis pooled from three series (9,11,13), 83% demonstrated nuclear β-catenin reactivity. The majority showed diffuse and intense nuclear staining, although occasional tumors demonstrated only focal reactivity. Nuclear staining for β-catenin is not limited to fibromatosis. One can observe it in spindle cell carcinomas, phyllodes tumors, and fibroadenomas. The intensity of the staining in the latter lesions varies, but it can appear moderate to strong, particularly in fibroepithelial tumors. The absence of β-catenin reactivity does not exclude the diagnosis of fibromatosis.

The spindle cells of fibromatosis virtually never react for CD34, but they demonstrate variable reactivity for actin and desmin. Anecdotal observations suggest that actin and desmin reactivity may be more common in subcutaneous than in parenchymal fibromatosis. The tumor cells are negative for cytokeratin. Mammary fibromatosis usually does not stain for estrogen receptor (ER)-α or progesterone receptor (PR).

It seems that pathologists do not commonly consider the diagnosis of fibromatosis when examining a needle core biopsy (NCB) specimen composed of bland spindle cells. In one group of 12 cases (11), the diagnosis of fibromatosis was either suggested or proposed in just three. Diagnoses such as fibroadenoma and stromal fibrosis were proffered for the remaining nine specimens.

The differential diagnosis of mammary fibromatosis includes neoplasms such as fibrous histiocytoma, spindle cell carcinoma, and sarcoma. Mammary fibromatosis may have storiform areas, but rarely does this pattern dominate, as it does in fibrous histiocytomas; furthermore, the epithelioid, histiocytic, and multinucleated cells often found in fibrous histiocytoma are not features of fibromatosis. One would not confuse spindle cell carcinomas showing obvious squamous or glandular elements with mammary fibromatosis, but certain spindle cell carcinomas are virtually devoid of such epithelial elements. One feature favoring metaplastic carcinoma or

sarcoma is a highly cellular and pleomorphic spindle cell component with mitoses. Although a mitotic rate of 3 per 10 HPF has been described in fibromatosis, this value is exceptional, and such a lesion is more likely to be a low-grade malignant tumor. The typical mitotic rate in fibromatosis does not exceed 1 per 10 HPF, and usually one cannot find mitotic figures. Nuclear reactivity for Ki67 is very much lower in fibromatosis than in spindle cell carcinoma or sarcoma. An inflammatory reaction, which may be predominantly lymphocytic, occurs more diffusely in and around most metaplastic carcinomas than it does in fibromatosis. Immunoreactivity for proteins such as cytokeratin, p63, and CD10 characterizes metaplastic carcinoma, whereas nuclear reactivity for β-catenin commonly occurs in fibromatosis.

One can also confuse mammary fibromatosis with reparative and reactive processes. Scars from healed fat necrosis, remote trauma, and surgery must be distinguished from fibromatosis. Calcifications are more likely to be associated with fat necrosis, but they can occur in fibromatosis rarely. Foreign body granulomas, sometimes with partly absorbed suture material, indicate prior surgery. If the patient has recurrent fibromatosis, reparative changes caused by an earlier operation may mingle with recurrent tumor, further complicating the diagnosis. The presence of lymphoid infiltrates, which commonly occur in fibromatosis, should not lead to the erroneous diagnosis of an inflammatory condition such as nodular fasciitis. The inflammatory component of fibromatosis is typically limited to isolated separate lymphoid aggregates at the periphery of the lesion. In fasciitis, inflammatory cells are dispersed more diffusely at the periphery as well as within the lesion, although localized areas of inflammation also occur. Myoid and multinucleated cells characteristically found in nodular fasciitis are not a feature of fibromatosis.

Recommended treatment is wide local excision. When a tumor is adherent to fascia, muscle, or skin, the excision should be extended to include the involved tissue, and it may be necessary to perform a mastectomy to achieve adequate margins of resection around a bulky tumor.

Immediate re-excision of the biopsy site should be considered if the initial excision removed only a small amount of tissue, or the margins are positive. Re-excision seems especially important for lesions located deep in the breast or near the chest wall, because recurrences at these sites may be difficult to control. On the other hand, follow-up is preferable to re-excision for relatively superficial lesions or subareolar nodules, which might require excision of the nipple.

The frequency of local recurrence ranges from 23% to 29% (1–3,10). Although the risk of recurrence is higher in patients with positive margins, recurrences have been observed in cases with apparently negative margins. Patients with positive margins do not always develop recurrences, and locally advanced lesions have stabilized or regressed after incomplete excision (3). Most recurrences occur within 3 years of diagnosis; however, in a few instances, they were not detected for nearly a decade. Multiple recurrences have been documented (10). Evaluation of histologic features such as cellularity, mitotic activity, and cellular pleomorphism does not help to predict recurrence.

Oncologists have used irradiation, hormonal therapy, and chemotherapy to treat cases of fibromatosis arising outside the breast, but none of these approaches represents an established modality for the treatment of mammary fibromatosis.

Nodular Fasciitis

Nodular fasciitis is a benign reactive fibroblastic and myofibroblastic proliferation. Although it is a common tumor-like lesion of the soft tissues, it affects the mammary gland only rarely. Most reports illustrate superficial, palpable nodules, but masses abutting the deep fascia have been described as well (14,15). A few descriptions (16,17) mention the presence of mammary glands at the edges of the masses, but none of the publications provides clear evidence that the nodules arose within the mammary parenchyma. Nevertheless, clinicians usually regard such nodules as breast masses, and pathologists must distinguish these tumors from spindle cell carcinoma with a fasciitis-like appearance and from fibromatosis. Because the latter two lesions involve the mammary glandular tissue, attention to the location of a mass as well as its morphologic characteristics provides important diagnostic information.

Nodular fasciitis of the mammary region occurs in both females and males. The ages of the patients range from 15 to 84 years. Most patients present with a recently discovered, palpable firm mass and they often describe rapid enlargement of the mass. Prior trauma is not usually mentioned.

The radiographic findings are often suspicious for carcinoma. Mammography demonstrates a high-density mass with spiculated or irregular margins, and ultrasonography reveals a hypoechoic mass with irregular borders (14,15,18). Magnetic resonance imaging (MRI) may also suggest the presence of a malignancy (19).

In a literature review by Squillaci et al. (18), reported examples ranged from 1 to 7 cm with an average size of 2.4 cm. The typical example is a firm, white-gray mass, which may display gelatinous areas.

The proliferative spindle cells form short bundles and fascicles randomly dispersed in a loose myxoid stroma (**Fig. 20.5**). The appearance is often described as having a feathery or tissue culture-like quality. Older lesions show greater collagenization. The spindle cells have bipolar to oval nuclei with delicate chromatin and small nucleoli. Atypia is lacking. Cellularity is high in early lesions, and mitotic activity may be brisk. Inflammatory cells, extravasated red blood cells, and prominent thin-walled vessels are present within the nodule. The borders of the mass are irregular. Benign ducts and lobules can become entrapped in the proliferation, but they usually do not do so.

The spindle cells in nodular fasciitis are positive for smooth muscle actin (SMA) and muscle-specific actin. The proliferative cells do not stain for CD34, nor do their nuclei stain for β-catenin. The cells are typically negative for keratin, but rare spindle cells may stain using the keratin AE1/AE3 mixture.

The differential diagnosis includes spindle cell carcinoma, fibromatosis, myofibroblastoma, and sarcoma. Spindle cell carcinoma can closely mimic the appearance of nodular fasciitis. The presence of nuclear atypia, clustered cell aggregates, or in situ carcinoma favors a diagnosis of spindle cell carcinoma. Some spindle cell carcinomas consist of bland cells that lack overt epithelial differentiation. Immunohistochemistry can be helpful to clarify the diagnosis in such cases, because spindle cell carcinoma usually demonstrates at least some reactivity for one or more cytokeratins and for p63. Fibromatosis is characterized by longer, sweeping fascicles and greater infiltration of the surrounding parenchyma, and most cases display nuclear reactivity for β-catenin cases. Myofibroblastoma demonstrates more clearly defined fascicles intermixed with conspicuous bands of bright, eosinophilic collagen. The usual example appears sharply circumscribed and stains for CD34. The absence of nuclear atypia and pleomorphism helps to distinguish nodular fasciitis from sarcoma.

Nodular fasciitis is a benign, self-limited process. Several reports document spontaneous resolution of mammary lesions within 3 to 6 months from the time of diagnosis (14,15,20). A conservative approach that includes careful and close monitoring for several months may provide adequate treatment for certain patients. Nevertheless, it may be difficult to exclude the diagnosis of other lesions such as spindle cell carcinoma based on the findings in a NCB sample, and excision of the mass should be considered in most circumstances. Recurrence after surgical excision is rare.

Fibrous Tumor

Fibrous tumor (focal fibrous disease) presents as a discrete breast mass composed of collagenized mammary stroma. It was first characterized by Haagensen as fibrous disease. Other names given to this entity include fibrous mastopathy, fibrosis of the breast, and focal fibrous disease. Because of the clinical presentation as a distinct mass, the term *fibrous tumor* is preferable to distinguish it from more frequent, nonspecific, and involutional stromal changes (21). A few tumors illustrated and described as focal fibrous disease and fibrous tumor appear to be examples of pseudoangiomatous hyperplasia of mammary stroma. On the other hand, certain cases sampled by NCB and classified as focal fibrosis probably represent examples of fibrous tumor (22).

Fibrous tumor is a disease of premenopausal women. Harvey et al. (23) studied 14 patients with "fibrous nodules," which appear to correspond histologically to fibrous tumors. Ten patients (71%) were premenopausal, and three of the four postmenopausal women were receiving hormone replacement therapy. On palpation, fibrous tumor is a firm to hard, distinct tumor measuring 2 to 5 cm. Skin retraction and dimpling are not evident. Many examples are not palpable and are detected only by radiologic imaging.

Mammography often reveals a mass, asymmetric density, or architectural distortion, but imaging sometimes fails to disclose the lesion. When demonstrated, the abnormality may display a round, oval, irregular, or spiculated shape with either well-defined or indistinct margins (23). Calcifications are usually not a feature of fibrous tumor, but they have been reported in one example (24).

Fibrous tumor forms a firm to hard mass spanning a few centimeters. The excised specimen typically has the appearance

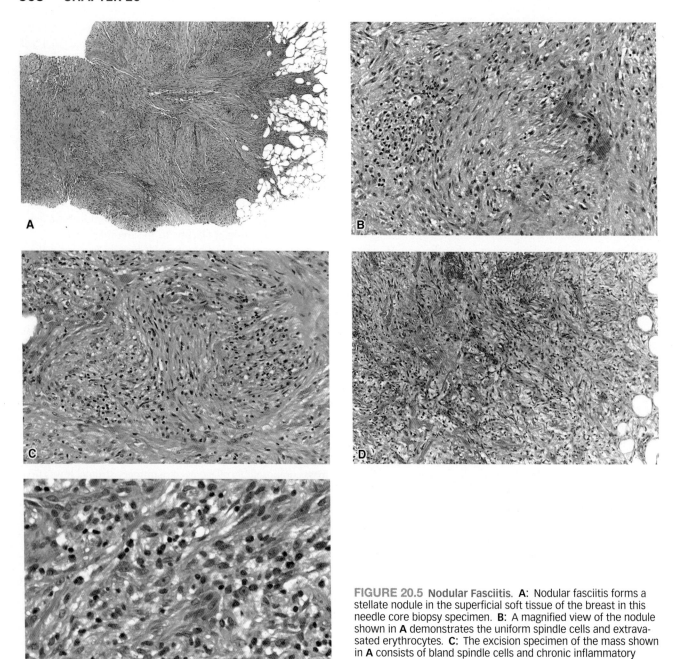

FIGURE 20.5 Nodular Fasciitis. A: Nodular fasciitis forms a stellate nodule in the superficial soft tissue of the breast in this needle core biopsy specimen. **B:** A magnified view of the nodule shown in **A** demonstrates the uniform spindle cells and extravasated erythrocytes. **C:** The excision specimen of the mass shown in **A** consists of bland spindle cells and chronic inflammatory cells. **D, E:** A needle core biopsy specimen from another example of nodular fasciitis demonstrates the "feathery" growth pattern of the spindle cells (**D**) and the mixed inflammatory infiltrate (**E**).

of a discrete tumor composed of white, homogeneous rubbery tissue.

Fibrous tumor consists of collagenous stroma that contains markedly decreased or absent ductal and lobular elements, which are atrophic. The findings in a NCB specimen are not specific and are usually reported as fibrosis (**Fig. 20.6**). Capillaries, other vascular structures, and nerves are very sparse; perivascular and perilobular inflammatory infiltrates are absent. Cysts, apocrine metaplasia, sclerosing adenosis, and duct hyperplasia are not features of fibrous tumor. One could suggest the diagnosis of fibrous tumor when a NCB sample from a nonpalpable, relatively discrete mammographically

detected lesion consists of hypocellular collagenous tissue devoid of glandular structures.

Fibrous tumor is a benign, self-limited stromal proliferation adequately treated by local excision.

Pseudoangiomatous Hyperplasia of Mammary Stroma

Pseudoangiomatous hyperplasia of mammary stroma (PASH) is a benign stromal proliferation characterized by the formation of slit-like spaces within dense collagenous stroma. The term "pseudoangiomatous" was introduced by Vuitch et al. (25) to

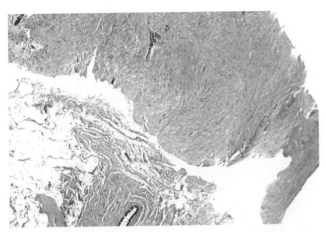

FIGURE 20.6 Fibrous Tumor. The upper sample in this needle core biopsy specimen shows a broad expanse of collagenous tissue representing the tumor. In the lower sample, normal fibrofatty tissue surrounds a duct.

acknowledge the vascular-like appearance of the stromal proliferation. It has been suggested that the spaces in PASH are part of a prelymphatic pathway (26). The presence of myoid differentiation in examples of PASH has led some authors to classify certain examples as hamartomas; however, PASH is a myofibroblastic proliferation with entrapment of preexisting glandular elements rather than a malformation of mammary tissues.

Pseudoangiomatous stromal hyperplasia appears to be an exaggerated and localized form of physiologic proliferation of stromal cells. Ibrahim et al. (27) found microscopic foci of PASH in 23% of 200 consecutive breast specimens, and Degnim et al. (28) found evidence of PASH in 6% of 9,065 consecutive excision specimens showing only benign lesions. The nonlocalized form of PASH often accounts for the clinical impression of a mass in specimens in which the histologic findings are described as fibrocystic changes. In its localized form, the lesion can give rise to a palpable or radiographically detected mass.

With rare exceptions, reported patients with tumor-forming PASH have been females. The age at diagnosis ranges from 3 to 86 years, and the mean age in several series (25,29–34) ranges from 37 to 51 years. The vast majority of women are premenopausal, and postmenopausal women with PASH often have a history of hormone replacement therapy. Rare examples of mass-forming PASH have been described in children and adolescents. One of the youngest patients was a 3-year-old boy, who had a 5.5-cm tumor in the right breast (33). Singh et al. (35) described a menarchal 12-year-old girl with marked bilateral breast enlargement due to PASH. When it occurs in males, PASH usually represents an incidental component of gynecomastia. Investigators have observed nontumorous PASH in 24% to 54% of cases of gynecomastia (36,37), and 98% of samples showing PASH in men also harbored gynecomastia (38). Unusual examples include an 11-cm mass associated with gynecomastia in a 50-year-old man (39), 10-cm masses in both axillae of a 44-year-old man (40), and PASH associated with rapidly growing gynecomastia-like changes in the axilla of an immunosuppressed 39-year-old man (41). Immune system suppression was described in two other cases (42,43).

Patients typically describe a palpable, painless, unilateral mass, which feels rubbery or firm. Although the lesion tends to arise in the upper outer quadrant, any part of the breast, including the subareolar region, can be affected (44). Rare examples are located in the axillary tail (32) or vulva (45). Occasional patients have had asynchronous or concurrent, bilateral PASH. Diffuse breast enlargement is seen rarely, and rapid growth of the lesion may occur (46). One patient presented with unilateral, mildly painful breast enlargement with *peau d'orange* change suggesting inflammatory carcinoma (27), and *peau d'orange* change and skin necrosis have been observed during pregnancy in patients who have massive breast enlargement caused by diffuse PASH.

PASH is occasionally an incidental finding in breast specimens containing invasive or in situ carcinoma. The carcinomas and PASH are generally anatomically separate. In one unusual case, a 0.9-cm invasive ductal carcinoma was present within a 4-cm PASH tumor (32).

PASH has been detected by mammography in asymptomatic patients. Mammograms usually demonstrate a mass without calcification or, less frequently, a focal asymmetric density. The borders of the mass usually appear smooth, but the tumor can have spiculated or ill-defined margins sometimes obscured by surrounding tissue. Ultrasound reveals a well-defined hypoechoic mass (31,47). MRI often demonstrates focal or segmental clumped enhancement.

Nodules of PASH appear well demarcated, and the smooth external surfaces sometimes resemble a capsule. The tumors measure from less than 1 cm to 15 cm in greatest dimension and average about 5 cm. Postmenopausal patients tend to have smaller tumors than premenopausal patients (34). The masses usually consist of homogeneous fibrous tan, gray, or white tissue, occasionally containing cysts up to 1 cm in diameter. Hemorrhage and necrosis are not seen except in excised tumors previously subjected to NCB or needle aspiration.

The nodules are composed of intermixed stromal and epithelial elements. Abundant nonspecialized stroma separates the glandular structures. Collagenization of intralobular stroma and attenuation of ducts can create a fibroadenoma-like appearance. Nonspecific proliferative epithelial changes include mild hyperplasia of duct and lobular epithelium, often with some accentuation of myoepithelial cells, and apocrine metaplasia with or without cyst formation.

The most striking histologic finding is a complex pattern of largely empty, often anastomosing spaces in dense collagenous stroma. These slits, sufficiently large to be identified at low magnification, typically involve the perilobular nonspecialized stroma. In florid cases, the pseudoangiomatous changes come to involve the intralobular specialized stroma as well (**Fig. 20.7**). The spaces may contain a few red blood cells, and collagen fibrils may traverse the spaces. Basement membrane material is not demonstrable around the slit-like spaces. The stroma also contains genuine small blood vessels and capillaries (**Fig. 20.8**).

Myofibroblasts distributed singly and discontinuously at the margins of the spaces resemble endothelial cells. The nuclei of the myofibroblasts usually appear attenuated. They lack atypia and do not show mitotic activity. In uncommon cases,

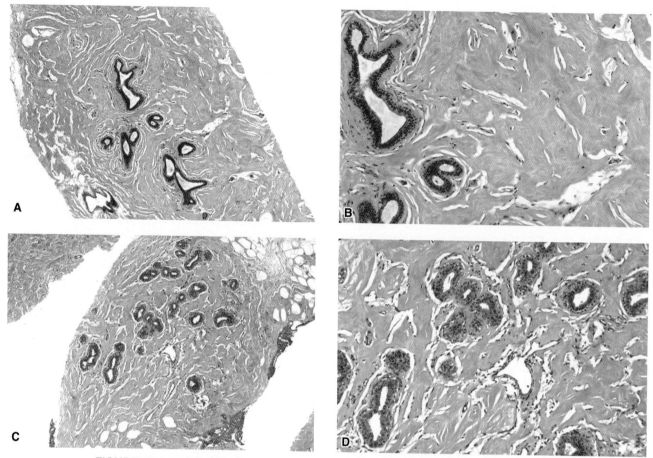

FIGURE 20.7 Pseudoangiomatous Stromal Hyperplasia. Needle core biopsy specimens from two patients are shown. **A, B:** In this specimen, the myofibroblasts appear inconspicuous, and the slit-shaped spaces are largely unconnected. Collagen fibrils traverse some of the spaces. **C, D:** This very pronounced pseudoangiomatous proliferation with connected spaces involves a lobule and the surrounding stroma.

some of these cells appear enlarged and they have noticeably hyperchromatic nuclei. Multinucleated cells may rarely line the slit-like spaces (38) **(Fig. 20.9).** One can find these cells in patients with PASH and neurofibromatosis type I (48), but the presence of multinucleated stromal giant cells is not limited to such patients (37). In an extremely unusual variant of PASH, the myofibroblasts contain cytoplasmic inclusion bodies of the type found in digital fibromas.

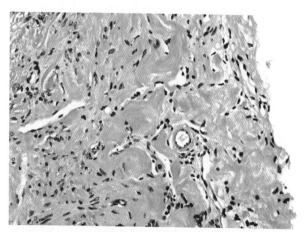

FIGURE 20.8 Pseudoangiomatous Stromal Hyperplasia. Small blood vessels are distributed among the pseudoangiomatous spaces in this needle core biopsy specimen.

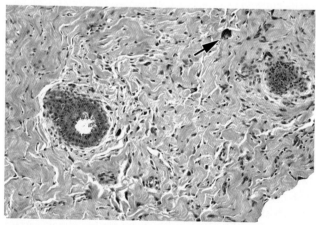

FIGURE 20.9 Pseudoangiomatous Stromal Hyperplasia. A needle core biopsy specimen demonstrates enlarged multinucleate cells (*arrow*).

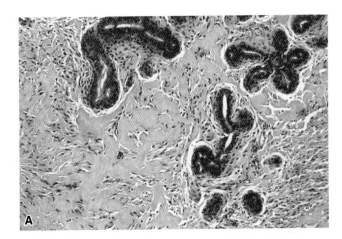

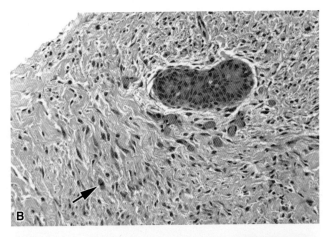

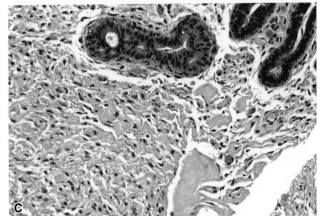

FIGURE 20.10 Atypical Pseudoangiomatous Stromal Hyperplasia, Fascicular. A–C: This needle core biopsy specimen was obtained from a 12-cm tumor in a 29-year-old woman. The stroma has occasional mitotic figures *(arrow)* and is focally very cellular. The pseudoangiomatous pattern is maintained in the cellular foci. Ductal hyperplasia is also evident.

Cytologic alterations of myofibroblasts are sometimes encountered in PASH. Pleomorphic nuclei are infrequent, but they can be found in PASH displaying conventional and fascicular patterns, sometimes accompanied by mitotic activity **(Fig. 20.10)**. Several instances of tumor-forming PASH in which the myofibroblasts demonstrate marked cytologic atypia, multinucleation, and mitotic activity have been encountered in teenage girls. These tumors appear to be examples of

myofibroblastic sarcoma arising in PASH. The literature does not contain sufficient information to characterize the clinical course of these tumors.

When myofibroblasts accumulate in distinct bundles or fascicles, they give rise to the lesion known as *fascicular PASH* **(Figs. 20.11 and 20.12)**. The presence of these bundles attests to a more robust proliferation of the myofibroblasts. Examples of fascicular PASH showing extreme myofibroblastic proliferation

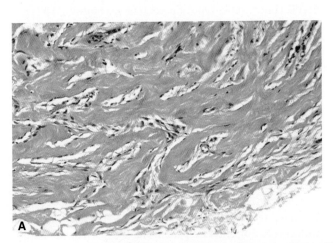

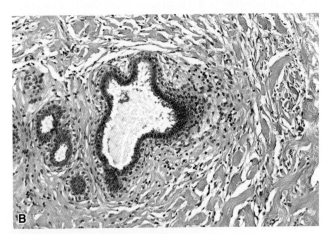

FIGURE 20.11 Pseudoangiomatous Stromal Hyperplasia, Early Fascicular Growth. A: The lesion shown in this needle core biopsy specimen has a circumscribed border. The presence of myofibroblastic nuclei in some of the spaces reflects an early phase in the development of the fascicular growth pattern. **B:** This periductal myofibroblastic proliferation also represents an early phase in the development of fascicular PASH.

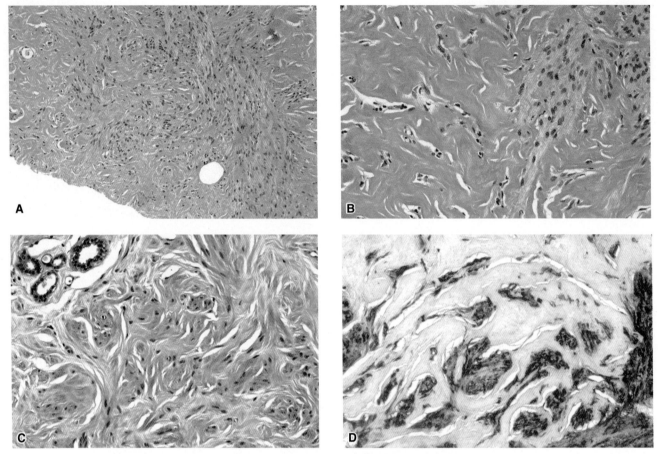

FIGURE 20.12 Pseudoangiomatous Stromal Hyperplasia, Fascicular. A: Myofibroblasts have formed distinct bundles with an interlacing pattern in this needle core biopsy specimen. **B:** Another portion of the specimen shows pseudoangiomatous and fascicular elements. **C:** A fascicular pattern with myoid differentiation is shown. **D:** The myofibroblasts are immunoreactive for actin.

display a growth pattern similar to that of myofibroblastomas. This similarity becomes especially evident when the myofibroblasts have abundant cytoplasm and grow as a localized tumor rather than a diffuse process. Myoid differentiation can occur in isolated myofibroblasts. When this phenomenon occurs in many cells, the resulting nodule comes to resemble an ill-defined leiomyoma.

The myofibroblasts lining pseudoangiomatous spaces usually stain for CD34. They exhibit strong immunoreactivity for vimentin and variable immunoreactivity for SMA, muscle-specific actin, and calponin, and they do not show immunoreactivity for cytokeratin, factor VIII-related antigen, or CD31. Fascicular and cellular variants of PASH retain immunoreactivity for CD34 and may be reactive for SMA, desmin, and calponin.

The results of studies of hormone receptor expression by the myofibroblasts in PASH have varied. Bowman et al. (34) found high rates of ER and PR immunoreactivity (79% and 63%, respectively), but most ER-positive cases showed only "occasional" positive cells. The propensity for tumorous PASH to affect premenopausal women and postmenopausal women taking hormone replacement therapy and the frequent coexistence of PASH and gynecomastia also suggest that hormonal factors contribute to the development of PASH.

The recommended treatment for tumorous PASH is local excision. Mastectomy may be necessary to control multiple recurrent tumors (35). A small number of patients have proceeded with clinical observation after a diagnosis of PASH by needle core or other type of percutaneous biopsy. Of 80 such cases with reported follow-up information, 78% had stable disease, 18% showed progression, and 4% had regression or resolution of the imaging findings (31,32). Most lesions that progressed were excised, and pathologic evaluation revealed PASH without atypical features. A few patients continued observation even after initial progression, and further follow-up demonstrated stable disease. Careful clinicopathologic correlation is required in such instances because PASH can be an incidental finding unrelated to the targeted abnormality. Isolated case reports document the response of PASH to selective ER modulators (49,50).

Most patients have remained well after excision of PASH. Ipsilateral recurrences have been reported in 2% to 30% of the patients (25,30), and rare patients have experienced multiple ipsilateral recurrences (30). Recurrent lesions do not ordinarily exhibit increased cellularity or other atypical features; moreover, examples that have recurred do not differ in their histologic attributes from those that did not recur.

PASH is not associated with an increased risk of subsequent breast carcinoma (28).

Myofibroblastoma

Myofibroblastoma is a benign tumor composed of myofibroblasts. These spindle-shaped mesenchymal cells occur in small numbers in virtually all tissues outside the central nervous system. When studied by electron microscopy, myofibroblasts, like myoepithelial cells, are found to contain cytoplasmic actin-like microfilaments 5 to 7 nm in diameter with focal dense bodies and pinocytotic vesicles; however, myofibroblasts lack the prekeratin tonofilaments and easily detected desmosomes characteristic of myoepithelial cells. Both types of cells can express actin and calponin, but only myoepithelial cells demonstrate immunoreactivity for high-molecular-weight cytokeratins and p63.

Myofibroblastomas typically afflict middle-aged to elderly patients (age range, 41–87 years; mean, seventh decade) (51–53). They are seen in younger patients only exceptionally, but one tumor presented in a 10-month-old boy (54). Although the initial description suggested a male predominance, the tumor occurs in women equally commonly.

Most patients present with a solitary, slow-growing, painless, mobile mass. Progressive enlargement of the tumor may occur over the course of years. In the case reported by Bégin (55), a 77-year-old patient experienced progressive breast enlargement over 7 years, resulting in a 6.5-cm tumor. Very rare tumors demonstrate rapid enlargement, and associated *peau d'orange* change of the skin has been described in one such case in a 65-year-old man (56). The vast majority of tumors are unilateral. Rare examples of bilateral myofibroblastomas have been reported in males. Two of the lesions described by Toker et al. (57) as "benign spindle cell breast tumors" in men are probably myofibroblastomas. One patient had two identical separate tumors in his left breast, which were treated by simple mastectomy, and 17 years later, he underwent a right mastectomy, which disclosed six foci of the same neoplastic process. A man with synchronous bilateral tumors was reported by Hamele-Bena et al. (52). Concurrent gynecomastia is reported in some patients.

Radiographically, the tumors are homogeneous, lobulated, well circumscribed, and lack microcalcifications (55,58). Mammography has detected nonpalpable myofibroblastomas (59). The findings evident by ultrasonography may suggest the diagnosis of fibroadenoma.

The average diameter of the tumors is approximately 2 cm; most are smaller than 4 cm. Size extremes include one lesion that measured 0.9 cm (52) and one 16-cm tumor (60). The excised mass has a lobulated contour and consists of homogeneous, bulging gray to pink, whorled, or lobulated tissue with a rubbery to firm consistency. An attempt at NCB in one case (61) was not successful because the tumor was "stony hard," although the excised tumor was not calcified or ossified. Cystic degeneration, necrosis, and hemorrhage have not been reported.

The classic type of myofibroblastoma is devoid of mammary ducts and lobules. The border of the tumor is usually circumscribed, and compressed breast parenchyma forms a peripheral pseudocapsule. A few examples incorporate adipocytes or small collections of glandular tissue into the periphery of the mass, a phenomenon that indicates invasion of surrounding parenchyma. Two distinctive histologic features are bundles of slender, bipolar, uniform spindle cells typically arranged in short fascicles, and intervening broad bands of hyalinized collagen (**Fig. 20.13**). The spindle cells have bland, ovoid to spindly nuclei with dispersed chromatin and small nucleoli. Nuclear grooves may be present (62). The cytoplasm is typically pale and eosinophilic, and cell borders are indistinct. Mitotic figures are sparse or undetectable. Multinucleated cells are uncommon, and pleomorphic nuclei, which are believed to represent a degenerative phenomenon are encountered only rarely (63,64). Nuclear palisading can create Verocay-like bodies, which would bring to mind the diagnosis of schwannoma (62,65). Rarely, adipocytes are dispersed separately or in small groups throughout the tumor, and certain myofibroblastomas have foci of leiomyomatous or cartilaginous differentiation (51,63,66). One can sometimes

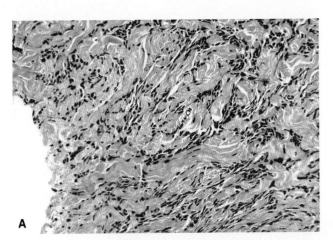
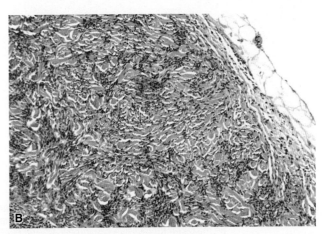

FIGURE 20.13 Myofibroblastoma. **A:** This needle core biopsy specimen shows the characteristic fascicles of myofibroblasts and intervening bands of collagen. **B:** The excised tumor has a circumscribed border.

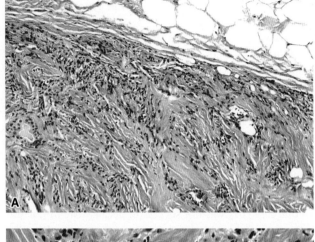

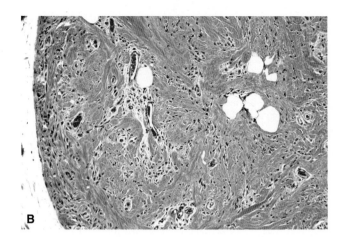

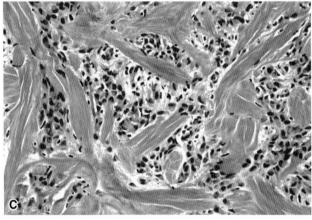

FIGURE 20.14 **Myofibroblastoma, Collagenized. A:** Bundles of myofibroblasts are distributed between prominent bands of collagen. The tumor has a circumscribed border. **B, C:** Another tumor consists of dense collagen bands and epithelioid myofibroblasts.

identify a perivascular lymphoplasmacytic infiltrate. Most tumors possess many mast cells.

The histologic features of certain myofibroblastomas deviate from those of the classic type. These variant forms exhibit a spectrum of histologic appearances. A single variant pattern may dominate in a tumor, or several variant patterns may be mixed. In the *collagenized* or *fibrous myofibroblastoma*, the spindle cells are distributed in collagenous stroma (**Fig. 20.14**). The

broad, deeply eosinophilic fibrous bands that are so prominent in a classic myofibroblastoma are absent or greatly reduced in number. Irregular slit-like spaces are formed between tumor cells. The stroma is reminiscent of PASH, and some of these tumors have a fascicular structure.

The *epithelioid variant* of myofibroblastoma features medium to large polygonal or epithelioid cells arranged in alveolar groups (**Fig. 20.15**). Nuclei are round to oval and may be

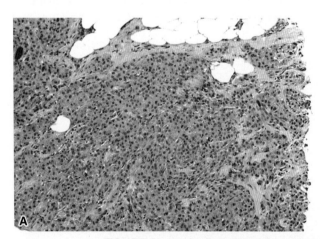

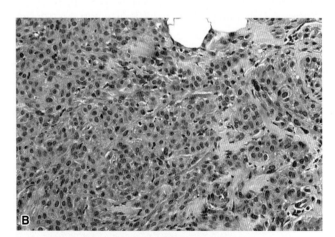

FIGURE 20.15 **Myofibroblastoma, Epithelioid. A, B:** Epithelioid myofibroblasts form alveolar clusters and small bundles in this very cellular needle core biopsy specimen. This appearance could be mistaken for invasive carcinoma. **C:** The cells are strongly immunoreactive for smooth muscle actin. **D:** The epithelioid myofibroblasts demonstrate reactivity for estrogen receptor.
E–H: This needle core biopsy sample is from a spindle and epithelioid cell myofibroblastoma with myxoid stroma. The tumor was strongly reactive for CD34 **(G)** and desmin **(H)**.

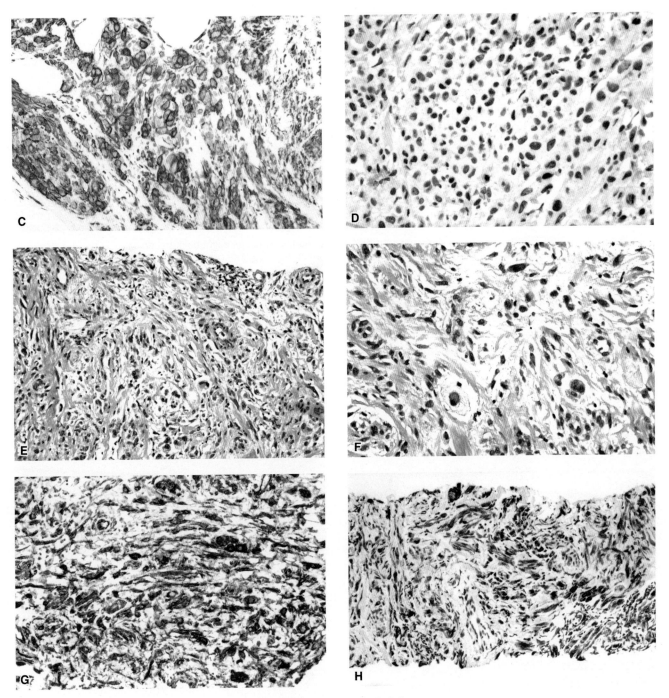

FIGURE 20.15 (continued)

eccentrically located. Mild to moderate nuclear pleomorphism can be seen, and scattered binucleated and multinucleated cells are not uncommon (67,68). Mitotic activity is absent or minimal. Epithelioid areas may be mixed with classic elements, or they can constitute the predominant growth pattern. The term *epithelioid variant* is used arbitrarily for tumors in which more than 50% of the lesion has this histologic pattern. The epithelioid cells in an epithelioid myofibroblastoma with sclerotic stroma can have a linear growth pattern that resembles the appearance of invasive lobular carcinoma. In contrast to invasive carcinoma, epithelioid myofibroblastoma usually has

well-circumscribed borders. Rare tumors composed of large cells with abundant glassy cytoplasm and vesicular nuclei have been referred to as a *"deciduoid-like" variant* (69).

A *cellular variant* of myofibroblastoma features a dense proliferation of spindle-shaped neoplastic myofibroblasts. Collagenous bands may be absent in some parts of the lesion. These tumors tend to have infiltrative borders. Rarely, cellular and collagenous or fibrous growth patterns are combined in a single tumor.

The *infiltrative variant* of myofibroblastoma is characterized by invasive growth (**Fig. 20.16**). One finds bundles of

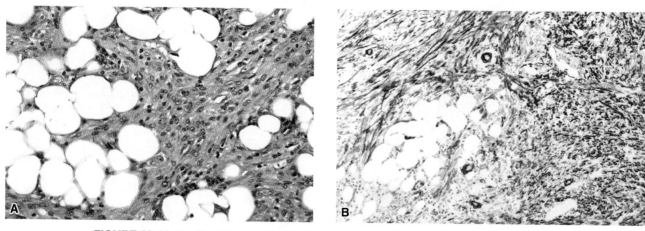

FIGURE 20.16 Myofibroblastoma, Infiltrating. A: Tumor cells in fat might be mistaken for infiltrating carcinoma in this needle core biopsy specimen. **B:** The tumor cells are strongly immunoreactive for smooth muscle actin.

relatively evenly dispersed spindle, ovoid, and epithelioid cells embedded in collagenous stroma interspersed with fat, mammary stroma, ducts, and lobules. The classic and other foregoing variants of myofibroblastoma ordinarily consist almost entirely of lesional tissue. One sometimes finds small collections of glandular tissue entrapped at the periphery of a typical myofibroblastoma, but commonplace myofibroblastomas

do not demonstrate either the abundance or the diffuse distribution of mammary tissues seen in the infiltrative types of myofibroblastoma. Certain infiltrative myofibroblastomas exhibit a peculiar tendency for the neoplastic myofibroblasts to be oriented around blood vessels.

Myxoid myofibroblastomas consist of sparse spindle cells distributed in the myxoid stroma **(Fig. 20.17)**. This variety

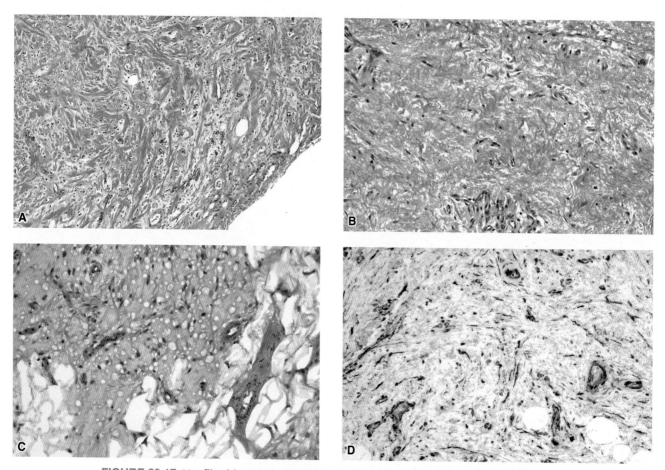

FIGURE 20.17 Myofibroblastoma, Myxoid. A: A collagenized portion of the tumor is shown. **B:** Basophilic myxoid material is evident in the tumor. **C:** Fully developed myxoid myofibroblastoma invades fat. **D:** The invasive myxoid portion of the tumor is immunoreactive for CD34.

of myofibroblastoma often exhibits an infiltrative manner of growth. Certain tumors classified as mucinosis may represent myxoid myofibroblastomas. Magro et al. (70) described a myofibroblastoma with extensive myxedematous stromal change.

Rarely, myofibroblastomas contain abundant fat suggestive of a lipomatous element. The term *lipomatous myofibroblastoma* has been suggested for this type of lesion **(Fig. 20.18)** (71,72). An example of a *pericytoma-like myofibroblastoma* has been described (73).

Most myofibroblastomas, including the epithelioid variety, are immunoreactive for vimentin, desmin, calponin, SMA, muscle actin, CD10, CD34, bcl-2, and CD99. The tumors usually stain for vimentin diffusely, whereas the other markers can show variable reactivity. The tumors do not stain for cytokeratin or factor VIII, and they stain for S-100 protein only rarely and weakly. Myofibroblasts exhibiting overt smooth muscle differentiation are strongly immunoreactive for desmin and variably reactive for actin, SMA, and h-caldesmon. The myofibroblasts often stain for ER, PR, and androgen receptor (AR), although the reactivity can be variable. Fluorescence in situ hybridization studies demonstrated a monoallelic loss of the *FOXO1*/13q14 locus in one case (65), but another tumor did not show this alteration (68).

Myofibroblastoma must be considered in the differential diagnosis of spindle cell mammary tumors. Sarcoma and metaplastic carcinoma typically display greater cellularity, atypia, and mitotic activity than do myofibroblastomas, and

sarcomas and metaplastic carcinomas often exhibit distinctive histologic features. Fasciitis and fibromatosis, which also contain myofibroblasts, tend to be stellate invasive lesions. Plump myoid cells and the inflammatory reaction of fasciitis are not seen in a myofibroblastoma. Fibromatosis exhibits abundant collagen and spindle cells arranged in broad bands rather than in short fascicles. Spindle cell lipomas commonly occur in males and sometimes may be well circumscribed. They have more abundant adipose tissue than myofibroblastomas; however, the distinction between spindle cell lipoma and myofibroblastoma (particularly the lipomatous variant) by light microscopy can be difficult (57). Molecular analysis indicates that both lesions often show loss of genes located on 13q (65,74–78). These findings suggest that the two lesions may represent related entities rather than distinct lesions. The report of a tumor showing intermixed, distinct regions of spindle cell lipoma within a myofibroblastoma adds support to this suggestion (79).

The epithelioid variant of myofibroblastoma can mimic an invasive carcinoma such as pleomorphic lobular carcinoma or apocrine carcinoma (67,68,80). The distinction can be particularly problematic in the setting of a NCB. Morphologic features that suggest the diagnosis of epithelioid myofibroblastoma include a well-circumscribed, pushing border; absent or minimal mitotic activity; associated spindle cells with typical myofibroblastic morphology; lack of glandular elements within the tumor; and dense collagenized stroma.

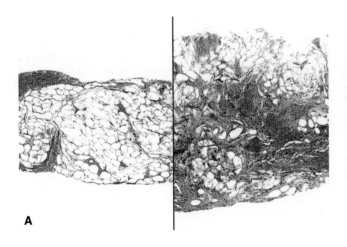

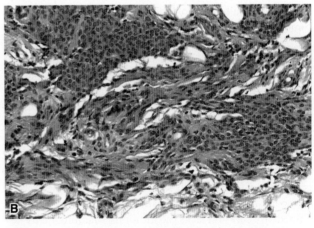

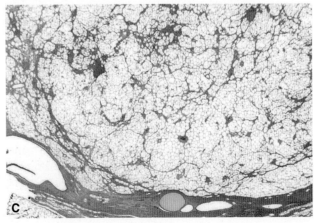

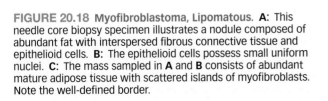

FIGURE 20.18 Myofibroblastoma, Lipomatous. **A:** This needle core biopsy specimen illustrates a nodule composed of abundant fat with interspersed fibrous connective tissue and epithelioid cells. **B:** The epithelioid cells possess small uniform nuclei. **C:** The mass sampled in **A** and **B** consists of abundant mature adipose tissue with scattered islands of myofibroblasts. Note the well-defined border.

An excision of the mass provides adequate treatment for virtually all patients, although large lesions in men have necessitated mastectomies. Complete excision is recommended when a myofibroblastoma is identified in a NCB sample. Re-excision may be considered if a myofibroblastoma is present at the margin of an excision specimen. Recurrences have not been reported after follow-up periods of 3 to 126 months after complete excision.

Granular Cell Tumor

Granular cell tumors are derived from the Schwann cells of peripheral nerves. These tumors occur throughout the body, and approximately 5% arise in the breast (81).

Granular cell tumor of the breast (GCTB) typically affects women between the ages of 30 and 50 years, but it has been described in adolescents and elderly women. The patients' ages range from 14 to 77 years. About 10% of GCTBs occur in males. In several studies, the majority of patients have been African-American, and Papalas et al. (82) reported a younger average age at presentation for African-Americans (41 years) than Caucasians (54 years).

Most patients present with a firm or hard painless mass. The left and right breasts are affected equally. GCTB may arise in any part of the breast including the axillary tail and in a subcutaneous location. Superficial lesions may cause skin retraction, and nipple inversion has been reported with subareolar tumors. In one woman, the hyperplastic skin and the underlying nests of tumor cells created a polypoid mass likened to a mulberry protruding from the breast (83). Large tumors and those that arise deep in the breast may adhere to the pectoral fascia or invade the pectoral muscle and partially encase the ribs (84). GCTB usually occurs as a solitary unilateral mass, but rare instances of multiple and bilateral tumors have been reported (85,86). Patients who have multiple granular cell tumors at various sites may have one or more lesions in the breast (82,86,87). The publication by Brown et al. (88) presents clinical, radiologic, and pathologic details of 91 cases of GCTB published between 1989 and 2008.

On mammography, GCTB is difficult to distinguish from carcinoma. GCTB typically forms a stellate mass, but circumscribed lesions occur occasionally (85,89). The mass usually has a dense core and lacks calcifications. Mammography has detected nonpalpable GCTB (90). Ultrasound often shows a solid mass with indistinct margins and posterior shadowing suggestive of carcinoma. The findings using MRI can overlap with those of carcinoma.

Granular cell tumors as large as 9 cm have been reported, but the typical example spans 2 cm or less. The mass consists of white, gray, yellow, or tan tissue, which feels firm or hard. Many tumors appear well circumscribed, but occasional examples have ill-defined infiltrative borders.

The histologic and immunohistochemical features of mammary granular cell tumors duplicate those of extramammary granular cell tumors. The tumor consists of compact nests or sheets of cells containing eosinophilic cytoplasmic granules **(Fig. 20.19)**. The cells vary from polygonal to spindly, and the cell borders appear well defined. The nuclei are round to slightly oval. They contain open chromatin and prominent nucleoli. In some cases, a modest amount of nuclear pleomorphism, occasional multinucleated cells, and rare mitoses may be found. These features should not be interpreted as evidence of malignancy. Easily seen granules usually fill the cytoplasm; however, in some lesions, the cytoplasm displays vacuolization and clearing. The cytoplasmic granules are PAS-positive and diastase-resistant. Variable amounts of collagenous stroma are present. The neoplastic cells may surround ducts and lobules and incorporate them into the mass, and these cells may penetrate into the lobules. When the neoplastic cells invade the dermis, the overlying epidermis may demonstrate pseudoepitheliomatous hyperplasia (83,84). Small nerve bundles are sometimes seen in the tumor or in close association with its peripheral extensions.

Mammary granular cell tumors typically stain for S-100 protein, carcinoembryonic antigen (CEA), and AR, and most stain for vimentin. GCTB does not stain for cytokeratin, GCDFP-15, ER, PR, or myoglobin. The cytoplasmic granules in these tumors are Luxol fast blue-positive, an observation that suggests that they contain myelin.

The differential diagnosis of GCTB includes histiocytic lesions, mammary carcinoma, and metastatic neoplasms. The superficial resemblance between the cells of GCTB and histiocytes can lead to confusion with a granulomatous inflammatory reaction or a histiocytic tumor. GCTB does not stain for histiocyte-associated antigens such as $\alpha 1$-antitrypsin, $\alpha 1$-antichymotrypsin, and muramidase, but reactivity for CD68 (KP-1) has been described in GCTB (91).

GCTB can closely resemble an invasive apocrine carcinoma. The presence of carcinoma in situ, often of the comedo type, as well as cytologic pleomorphism usually serve to identify apocrine carcinoma, but NCB specimens may not demonstrate these findings. In such situations, a confident diagnosis requires the analysis of the results of immunohistochemical staining. GCTB shows strong, diffuse immunoreactivity for S-100 protein and CEA; however, these results do not distinguish GCTB from mammary carcinoma, because some carcinomas are also S-100- and CEA-positive. A positive reaction for vimentin supports the diagnosis of GCTB, because few carcinomas express this protein. GCTB is negative for cytokeratin, GCDFP-15, ER, and PR. Apocrine carcinomas stain for epithelial markers such as cytokeratin, they often stain for epithelial membrane antigen (EMA), and they typically express AR.

GCTB must also be distinguished from metastatic neoplasms that have oncocytic or clear cell features such as renal carcinoma and malignant melanoma and from alveolar soft part sarcoma. Details of the clinical history and the results of immunohistochemical staining will establish the primary site in most cases.

NCB represents an accurate method for rendering a diagnosis of GCTB. Among the cases collated by Brown et al. (88), correct diagnosis was made in all NCB specimens.

Benign GCTB is treated by wide excision. Local recurrence may occur after incomplete excision, but it is sometimes difficult to distinguish recurrences from asynchronous multifocal

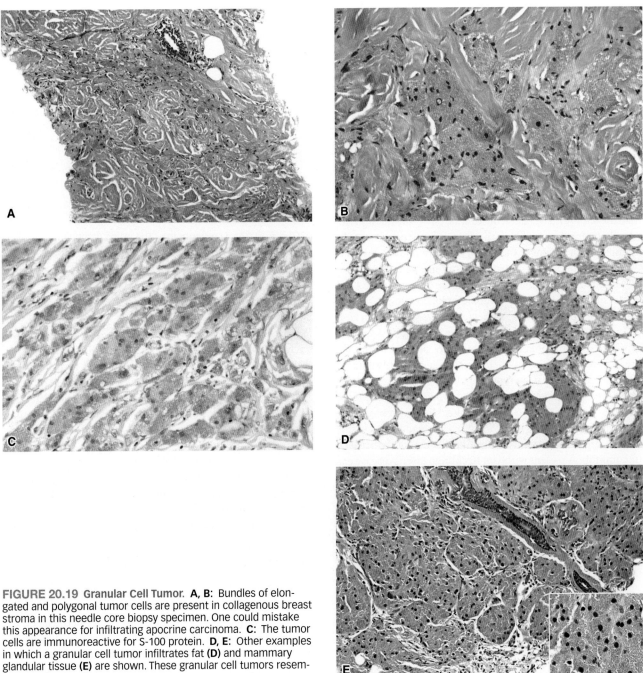

FIGURE 20.19 Granular Cell Tumor. A, B: Bundles of elongated and polygonal tumor cells are present in collagenous breast stroma in this needle core biopsy specimen. One could mistake this appearance for infiltrating apocrine carcinoma. **C:** The tumor cells are immunoreactive for S-100 protein. **D, E:** Other examples in which a granular cell tumor infiltrates fat **(D)** and mammary glandular tissue **(E)** are shown. These granular cell tumors resemble apocrine carcinoma.

lesions. Most patients with positive or close margins do not experience recurrence of their tumors.

Fewer than 1% of all granular cell tumors, including mammary lesions, are malignant. Criteria of malignancy proposed for extramammary granular cell tumors include a diameter greater than 5 cm, necrosis, spindling of the cells, nuclear pleomorphism, vesicular chromatin, prominent nucleoli, high nuclear-to-cytoplasmic ratio, increased mitotic activity (more than 2 mitotic figures per 10 HPF at 200X magnification), and the presence of metastatic foci.

Both locoregional and distant metastatic spread from GCTB have been described (92). Metastases in the breast and axillary lymph nodes from extramammary granular cell tumors have also been reported (93,94). In some instances, it may not be possible to distinguish between multifocal benign granular cell tumors and metastatic malignant granular cell tumor.

Benign Neural Neoplasms

Benign neural neoplasms commonly found in the soft tissues at various sites rarely occur in the breast. Benign nerve sheath tumors of the breast have been reported, usually diagnosed as schwannomas or as "neurilemomas." Many of these tumors occupied the mammary subcutaneous tissue (95); however, parenchymal lesions have also been described, and a schwannoma originating in the chest wall presented as a mass in the breast (96). The age range at diagnosis is 6 to 83 years, with most patients in their fourth to sixth decade of life. Although most patients have been female, benign neural neoplasms have arisen in the male breast (97).

Mammary schwannomas account for less than 3% of all schwannomas (98). Two publications (98,99) list clinical and pathologic findings of 23 cases described prior to 2007. A typical schwannoma presents as a painless, well-defined mass, which may have grown slowly (96,100) or remained stable for as long as 25 years (101). Two reports (100,102) illustrate exophytic tumors. Schwannomas involve the right breast more commonly than the left (98). The lateral quadrants, especially the superior lateral quadrant, seem like favored sites, but reports describe examples in all regions of the breast. One report (103) describes the case of a patient with two schwannomas of one breast.

Mammary neurofibroma in neurofibromatosis type 1 patients commonly involves the nipple-areolar region (104,105). The clinical appearance of cutaneous tumors ranges from large pedunculated masses to small nodules that mimic accessory nipples. Neurofibroma is less commonly situated within the breast parenchyma. Multiple parenchymal neurofibromas in a single breast have been reported (106). Neurofibromas can cause breast enlargement mimicking gynecomastia in prepubertal boys (97). Patients with von Recklinghausen's disease develop neurofibromas in the mammary subcutaneous tissues and the breast, but massive neurofibromatosis of the breast is uncommon. A patient with von Recklinghausen's disease can also develop mammary carcinoma; therefore, the appearance of a new breast mass in this setting should prompt appropriate diagnostic evaluation.

Mammography of benign neural neoplasms demonstrates well-defined masses. Using sonography, the masses appear hypoechoic and exhibit posterior enhancement. The MRI characteristics do not differ from those of other benign lesions.

The tumors usually span a few centimeters. One asymptomatic 7-mm schwannoma was detected by mammography (107), and a long-standing exophytic schwannoma measured 15 cm × 12 cm (100). The masses consist of dense, firm, gray or white tissue, which may have soft mucoid regions. Cystic degeneration, which develops only rarely, can create a multicystic mass (108).

Microscopic examination discloses the typical attributes of benign nerve sheath tumors. Schwannomas consist of spindle cells growing in bundles. Lining up of the nuclei in a palisade array gives rise to the Antoni A pattern (**Fig. 20.20**); less cellular areas containing thick-walled blood vessels represent the Antoni B pattern. One can observe vascular thrombi, hyalinized blood vessels, cells with atypical nuclei, and xanthomatous areas in sclerotic schwannomas. Neurofibromas contain delicate spindle cells with wavy, dark nuclei set in a background of ropey collagen. Myxoid change may be present.

Benign peripheral nerve sheath tumors stain for S-100, but they vary in the extent of their reactivity. Schwannomas tend to demonstrate intense staining of the entire neoplastic population, whereas neurofibromas display heterogeneous

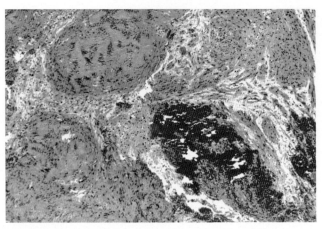

FIGURE 20.20 Schwannoma. The lesion demonstrates the Antoni A pattern. Hemorrhage marks the site of a recent needle core biopsy.

positivity for this marker. Staining for SOX-10 demonstrates similar results.

The differential diagnosis includes other spindle cell tumors such as fibroadenomas, phyllodes tumor, fibromatosis, and metaplastic carcinoma. One can usually readily differentiate these lesions when studying excision specimens, but difficulty may be encountered when examining NCB specimens. The diagnosis of schwannoma is suggested when a NCB sample demonstrates palisading spindle cells (108), but a small specimen may not demonstrate this finding. The diagnosis of a benign peripheral nerve sheath tumor is supported by the absence of glandular elements and mitotic activity, a positive immunohistochemical stain for S-100 protein, and the absence of immunostaining for actin.

Complete excision provides adequate therapy.

Hamartoma

It would seem that the diagnosis of hamartoma has been used indiscriminately in the breast literature because certain so-called hamartomas probably would be better classified using other diagnoses. *Stedman's Medical Dictionary* defines hamartoma as "a focal malformation that resembles a neoplasm, grossly and even microscopically, but results from faulty development in an organ; it is composed of an abnormal mixture of tissue elements, or an abnormal proportion of a single element normally present at that site" (109). *Churchill's Illustrated Medical Dictionary* defines the term as "a benign tumor or tumor-like lesion composed of one or more tissues, normal to the organ but abnormally mixed and overgrown" (110). Both definitions include the possibility that a hamartoma could consist of just one type of tissue intrinsic to the organ in question. According to this line of thinking, a lipoma could represent a type of mammary hamartomas, and the distinction between a hamartoma composed entirely of smooth muscle and a leiomyoma would seem arbitrary. A definition more in keeping with current thought might read, "a benign tumor composed of two or more tissues normally found in an organ that are normal in histological characteristic but appear abnormally arranged." Mammary tumors that fit this concept usually consist of disordered glandular tissue and stroma. Those composed of glands and fat have been referred to as *adenolipomas* as well as hamartomas.

When carefully categorized, hamartomas represent approximately 4% of benign breast lesions (111). These neoplasms occur most often in premenopausal women, but they have been described in teenagers and in women in their ninth decade. The mean age of the patients in several series ranges from 38 to 50 years. Several studies report a greater incidence in the left breast compared to the right, but other investigations have not duplicated this finding. An association with pregnancy has been noted in a minority of cases. A publication by Sevim et al. (112) lists clinical and pathologic findings of many cases published between 1993 and 2013.

Approximately 50% of hamartomas present as palpable painless masses; screening mammography detects the remainder. A few patients have presented with two hamartomas in the same breast (111,113). Some patients report slow growth over the course of several years, whereas others describe rapid enlargement of the tumor. Especially large hamartomas may not be palpable as distinct masses; instead, they present as unilateral macromastia or asymmetry (114,115). Multiple and bilateral hamartomas and "hamartoma-like lesions" have been described in patients with Cowden syndrome; however, most patients with mammary hamartomas do not seem to have the syndrome. One publication describes a hamartoma arising in axillary breast tissue (116).

Mammography may reveal a well-circumscribed, dense, round or oval mass surrounded by a narrow lucent zone, but some palpable tumors are not evident using this imaging modality. The borders can appear irregular, indistinct, or lobulated, and some hamartomas contain calcifications. Predominantly fatty tumors may have the lucent appearance of lipomas, whereas those with abundant glandular tissue appear dense. Ultrasonography reveals a mixed pattern of echogenic and sonolucent regions.

Gross examination discloses a well-defined, circumscribed, sometimes lobulated, mass bordered by a thin, fibrous pseudocapsule. The tumors range from less than 1 to 27 cm. They present as soft, rubbery, or firm consistency depending on the nature of the tissue composing them. Most tumors look tan-pink to white, and one can see islands of yellow adipose tissue in certain examples. Hamartomas with abundant fat resemble lipomas. Scattered cysts may be present.

On histologic study, the lesion consists of intermixed mammary glandular tissue and stroma bounded by a pseudocapsule of compressed mammary parenchyma **(Fig. 20.21)**. The glandular tissue usually consists of ducts and lobules, although the lobules may be larger or more disorganized than normal lobules. The stroma in certain hamartomas consists almost entirely of fat, whereas other hamartomas lack fat entirely. Rare examples contain brown fat ("adenohibernoma") (117). The stroma in many hamartomas demonstrates PASH (118).

Hamartomas are adequately treated by excision. Good cosmetic results have been reported even when tumors larger than a quadrant were excised. Hamartomas do not ordinarily

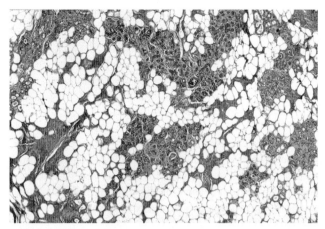

FIGURE 20.21 Adenolipoma. Lobule-like aggregates of acini are distributed in lipomatous adipose tissue.

recur, but the literature contains reports of a few exceptions to this generalization (118,119), probably resulting from incomplete excision.

The so-called *leiomyomatous (myoid) hamartoma* does not represent a type of hamartoma as defined earlier. The regrettable designation of these tumors as "hamartomas" is now so well entrenched in the literature that correction of this misnomer seems unlikely. The lesion most often develops as a tumorous form of sclerosing adenosis with leiomyomatous metaplasia of the myoepithelial cell component (120,121). Adequate sampling reveals foci of sclerosing adenosis in virtually all myoid "hamartomas," and the origin of the myoid element can be traced to myoepithelial cells (122). Associated fibrocystic changes include cystic apocrine metaplasia and duct hyperplasia.

Leiomyoma

Most leiomyomas of the breast arise from smooth muscle in the nipple and areola (123). Parenchymal leiomyomas probably arise either from smooth muscle metaplasia of myoepithelial cells or myofibroblasts or from vascular smooth muscle. The diagnosis of leiomyoma should be restricted to lesions composed entirely of smooth muscle. One should exclude fibroadenomas and sclerosing adenosis with myomatous metaplasia (myoid "hamartoma"), for example, from this category.

Leiomyomas of the nipple and those arising within the parenchyma of the breast are rare neoplasms. The literature contains approximately 30 reports of leiomyomas in each location (124–126). The ages of patients range from the third to the eighth decade. Approximately one-third of leiomyomas of the nipple arise in men, but we found only one report of an intraparenchymal leiomyoma in a male (127).

Patients with leiomyomas of the nipple frequently report pain or discomfort, but parenchymal leiomyomas do not usually cause these symptoms. The reported duration of symptoms ranges from a few weeks to more than two decades. Leiomyomas involving the nipple may cause nipple erosion and enlargement (124). One tumor situated immediately superior to the nipple was described as "cauliflower-shaped" (128), and another growing beneath the nipple caused nipple inversion

(129). A 31-year-old woman presented with bilateral nipple leiomyomas (130), and a 61-year-old man developed a leiomyoma of the nipple in the setting of spironolactone-induced gynecomastia (131). Intraparenchymal leiomyomas usually present as palpable, solitary masses. There is no predilection as to the location of parenchymal lesions. One report describes a 38-year-old woman with four synchronous parenchymal leiomyomas (132).

Mammographic studies of parenchymal leiomyomas typically reveal smoothly contoured, high-density masses without calcifications. Sonography and MRI disclose findings consistent with a benign tumor. The radiologic findings of leiomyomas of the nipple appear similar to those of parenchymal leiomyomas (124).

The tumor forms a firm, circumscribed mass composed of whorled, white-pink tissue. Tumors as large as a "small grapefruit" and another spanning 13.8 cm have been reported (125), but most leiomyomas are smaller than 5 cm.

On histologic study, leiomyomas appear circumscribed. They consist of interlacing fascicles of spindle cells with eosinophilic cytoplasm (**Fig. 20.22**). An epithelioid variant of mammary parenchymal leiomyoma was described by Roncaroli et al. (133). When examining a core biopsy specimen, one must exclude several other lesions before rendering the diagnosis of leiomyoma. Leiomyosarcoma represents the malignant neoplasm most likely to cause diagnostic confusion. Leiomyomas do not exhibit the cytologic atypia, mitotic activity, necrosis, or infiltration of parenchyma that characterize high-grade leiomyosarcoma; however, one may have difficulty distinguishing a leiomyoma from a low-grade leiomyosarcoma based on findings in a NCB specimen. By evaluating histologic findings and the results of immunohistochemical staining, one can more confidently exclude other lesions in the differential diagnosis such as myofibroblastoma, fibromatosis, PASH, low-grade spindle cell carcinoma, nodular fasciitis, myoepithelial carcinoma, and fibrosarcoma (134).

Leiomyomas stain for vimentin, desmin, SMA, h-caldesmon, ER, and PR.

Complete excision is usually recommended. This may necessitate removing the nipple if the lesion is in the subareolar region or nipple. Local recurrence has been reported rarely (123,135).

Lipoma

Lipomas of the breast usually affect women between the ages of 40 and 60 years, but they have been seen in men of similar ages (136). Many lipomas are located in the subcutaneous fat rather than the mammary parenchyma. Lipomas typically present as painless solitary masses spanning a few centimeters, but examples as large as 50 cm and weighing as much as 15,500 g have been reported (137). Patients may report slow growth of the tumor during a period of many years. In one woman, the mass grew from 2 to 32 cm over 30 years (138). Multiple lipomas may be encountered.

Mammograms sometimes disclose a radiolucent homogeneous mass with a distinct border or capsule (139). If the breast consists mostly of fat, a mammogram may not detect the presence of a lipoma. Fat necrosis within a lipoma may present as a spiculated lesion on mammography, and skin ulceration may develop in association with very large tumors (137).

Macroscopic examination demonstrates a well-defined mass of yellow glistening tissue that bulges from the surface.

Histologic study reveals that the mass consists of mature adipose tissue essentially devoid of glandular elements. It is not always possible to appreciate a pseudocapsule of compressed tissue around the mass when examining a NCB specimen. One can suggest the diagnosis of lipoma based on the presence of a mass with appropriate imaging characteristics and the finding of mature fat in the NCB specimen. Lipomas can exhibit several variant patterns, which are termed *hibernoma, osteolipoma, chondrolipoma, fibrolipoma, myolipoma, chondromyolipoma, spindle cell lipoma,* and *angiolipoma.*

Hibernomas are tumors composed of brown fat. In the mammary region, hibernomas occur in the axillary tail of the breast or in the axilla (140) (**Fig. 20.23**). They consist of

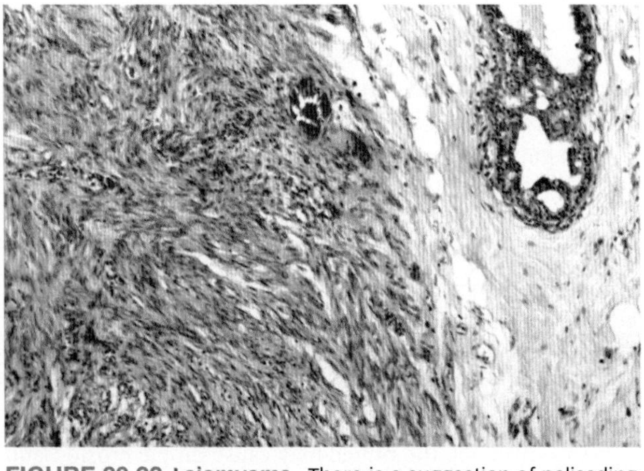

FIGURE 20.22 Leiomyoma. There is a suggestion of palisading in the arrangement of the smooth muscle cells in this circumscribed tumor. An adjacent duct shows micropapillary ductal hyperplasia.

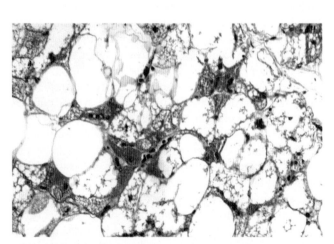

FIGURE 20.23 Hibernoma. Brown fat is present in a tumor from the axillary tail of the breast.

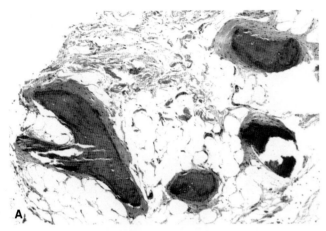
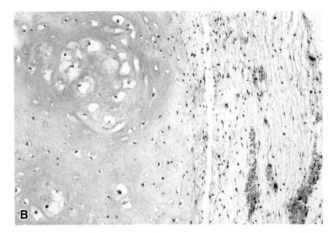

FIGURE 20.24 Osteolipoma and Chondrolipoma. A: Mature bone is evident in this needle core biopsy specimen from an osteolipoma. **B:** The presence of mature hyaline cartilage characterizes this chondrolipoma.

multivacuolated adipocytes containing small, central nuclei. The cytoplasm varies from pale to deeply eosinophilic and granular. Univacuolar adipocytes are also usually present. They may constitute such a large proportion of the tumor that it resembles a conventional lipoma. The stroma can show myxoid change or consist of spindle cells with ropey collagen and interspersed mast cells. The nuclei do not display atypia or mitotic figures. Small blood vessels traverse the mass. *Osteolipomas* consist entirely of fat with isolated foci of osseous calcification **(Fig. 20.24A)**. *Chondrolipomas* are composed of sharply defined islands of hyaline cartilage, sometimes with focal calcification, distributed in mature fat and fibrofatty mammary parenchyma **(Fig. 20.24B)** (141–144). *Fibrolipomas* are grossly well-circumscribed tumors composed of mature adipose tissue and collagenous stroma that contain prominent fibroblasts. Microscopically, the lesion may blend with glandular parenchyma. The stromal cells do not exhibit the myoid features of myofibroblasts. *Myolipomas* consist of fat, smooth muscle, and fibrous connective tissue. Those that also possess cartilage merit the diagnosis of *chondromyolipomas*.

Spindle cell lipomas occur in the breast rarely (139,145–148). One example presented as a 2.1-cm mammographically well-circumscribed hyperechoic mass (148). Biopsy reveals lipomatous tissue mixed with spindly myofibroblasts and variably collagenous stroma. CD10 and CD34 immunoreactivity can be demonstrated in the spindle cell myofibroblastic component. Loss of the 13q14 chromosomal region has been reported in both spindle cell lipomas and myofibroblastomas. This observation suggests a close relationship between the two entities.

Angiolipomas identical to those of subcutaneous tissue can arise in the breast. One 55-year-old man developed an angiolipoma (149), but other reported cases have affected women. The ages at diagnosis range from 19 to 75 years. Typical angiolipomas occur as solitary masses, which usually span 2 cm or less. Their imaging characteristics are variable, and radiologic studies may suggest the diagnosis of malignancy. On macroscopic examination, an angiolipoma forms an encapsulated yellow nodule, which may also contain focal gray or pink regions.

Histologic study reveals mature adipose tissue separated by small blood vessels that tend to form lobulated aggregates at the periphery and to contain fibrin thrombi **(Fig. 20.25)**.

Hemangiomas

The *perilobular hemangioma* is a benign vascular tumor of microscopic size detected in sections of breast tissue taken to evaluate unrelated lesions (150). Although a few have reportedly measured between 2 and 4 mm, none was clinically or mammographically evident. Perilobular hemangiomas were found in 1.3% of mastectomies performed for carcinoma (151), 4.5% of excision specimens showing benign conditions, and in 11% of women whose breast tissue was sampled in forensic autopsies (152).

Perilobular hemangiomas are not limited to a perilobular distribution. Many are partially or completely within the lobular stroma; others sit in the extralobular stroma next to ducts; and a few appear separate from any glandular tissue. Although the term "perilobular" does not accurately describe the microanatomic distribution of many of these lesions, it is widely used, and there is no compelling reason to propose an alternative.

When visible on macroscopic examination, perilobular hemangiomas look like pinpoint red spots. Multiple perilobular hemangiomas may occur in one or both breasts.

During microscopic study, one can often identify perilobular hemangiomas at low magnification because they usually contain red blood cells. In some instances, the blood vessels lack erythrocytes and contain only fluid, which may be plasma. The typical perilobular hemangioma consists of a meshwork of small, distinct blood vessels **(Fig. 20.26)**. They usually form a compact collection, but when the vessels extend into the adjacent tissue, the border appears ill defined. The calibers of the vessels vary from those of a capillary to those of ectatic, miniature cavernous channels. Anastomosing channels may be seen, but they are not conspicuous. The thin, delicate vessels consist of endothelial cells encased in inconspicuous stroma, which contains little or no smooth muscle.

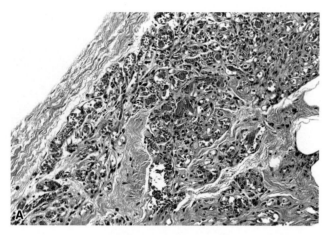
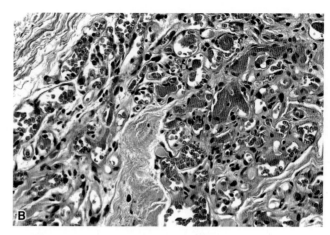

FIGURE 20.25 **Angiolipoma.** **A:** Capillaries cluster in the subcapsular region of this angiolipoma. **B:** The endothelial cells appear flat and they contain small, bland nuclei. Fibrin thrombi occlude several small vessels.

It is common to find varying numbers of lymphocytes in the stroma regardless of the presence or absence of erythrocytes within the vascular spaces.

Some microscopic vascular lesions with the general features of perilobular hemangiomas have endothelial cells with prominent, hyperchromatic nuclei (150). Interconnected channels are often present, but papillary endothelial proliferation, mitotic activity, and extensive vascular anastomoses are not seen in these *atypical perilobular hemangiomas*. Most atypical

perilobular hemangiomas have rounded, circumscribed contours and are subdivided into aggregates of vessels or vascular lobules by slender fibrous septa. A few lesions with irregular margins have been noted.

There is no evidence that angiosarcoma arises from perilobular hemangiomas, although the existence of these cytologically atypical variants leaves this issue open to speculation. Given the rarity of mammary angiosarcoma and the frequent detection of perilobular hemangiomas in "normal" breast tissue

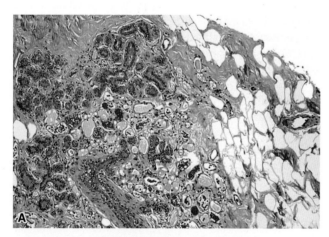
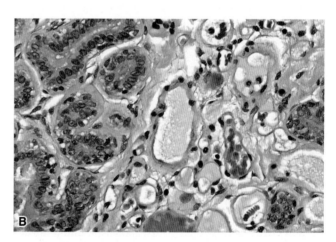

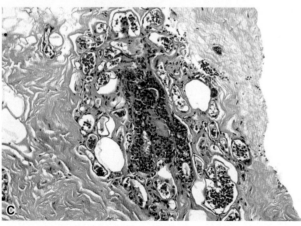

FIGURE 20.26 **Perilobular Hemangioma.** **A, B:** This vascular lesion occupying the intralobular stroma was an incidental finding in a needle core biopsy specimen obtained to sample nearby calcifications. **C:** The microscopic hemangioma in this needle core biopsy specimen is centered on a duct.

and in specimens examined for various unrelated conditions, malignant transformation of perilobular hemangiomas must be exceedingly uncommon, if it does occur.

Typical perilobular hemangiomas, whether unifocal, multiple, or bilateral, do not require treatment. Whether treated by mastectomy in the management of mammary carcinoma or by excision, no patient with an atypical perilobular hemangioma is known to have experienced recurrence of the lesion or progression to angiosarcoma. No treatment other than local excision is recommended for atypical perilobular hemangiomas.

Hemangiomas of the breast are benign vascular tumors large enough to be clinically detected. They occur in patients ranging from 18 months to 82 years of age and only rarely affect men (153). The tumors do not show a predilection to arise in a particular location within the breast. Palpable hemangiomas typically create well-defined, firm masses, but a substantial number of hemangiomas are nonpalpable and evident only by radiologic imaging.

Mammography of a hemangioma usually demonstrates a well-defined lobulated mass, which may have fine or coarse calcifications (154,155). Ultrasonography reveals a hypoechoic, lobulated, well-defined nodule oriented parallel to the skin surface. Variations in these findings have been described, and imaging fails to detect a few tumors. Multiple mammary hemangiomas were demonstrated by MRI in the breast of a 41-year-old woman with Kasabach-Merritt syndrome (156).

One can identify several types of hemangiomas, each with its particular morphologic characteristics.

Cavernous hemangioma is the most common form of mammary hemangioma. The lesion is typically described as a dark red or brown, circumscribed mass spanning a few centimeters or less, but larger examples have been reported (153,157,158). The mass may appear spongy to the unaided eye (150,159). Microscopic examination reveals dilated vessels congested with red blood cells **(Fig. 20.27)**. Small vessels of capillary dimension may be seen in portions of a cavernous hemangioma. The individual channels seem to be independent, and one sees few, if any, anastomosing vessels. The inconspicuous endothelial nuclei look flat. The vessels are supported by fibrous stroma, which tends to be more prominent toward the center of the tumor. Calcification may occur in the stroma. Extramedullary hematopoiesis (EMH) in vascular channels should be distinguished from lymphocytic reaction, which occurs mainly in the stroma. Among mammary vascular lesions,

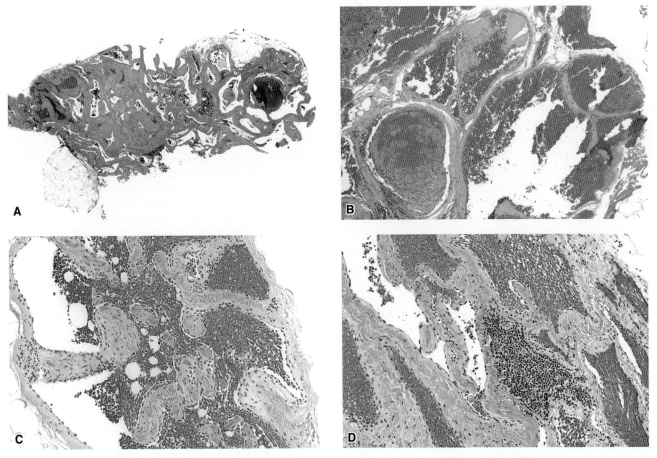

FIGURE 20.27 Cavernous Hemangioma. A: A low-magnification view of the entire needle core biopsy specimen is shown. Dilated vascular spaces are evident, some congested with red blood cells. **B:** A blood clot **(lower left)** has formed in one of the cavernous vascular channels. **C:** Flat endothelial cells with small, oval, bland nuclei line the channels of the cavernous hemangioma in another needle core biopsy specimen. **D:** A small collection of lymphocytes nestles in the stroma between the vascular channels.

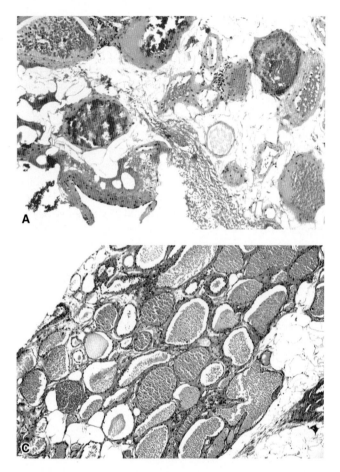
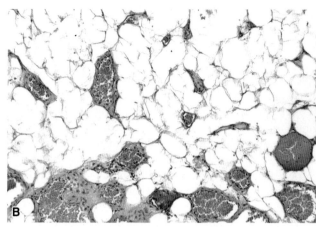

FIGURE 20.28 Cavernous Hemangioma. A: This needle core biopsy specimen shows a portion of a mass composed of dilated vascular channels in fat. **B:** Small vascular channels congested with red blood cells extend into the fat at the periphery of the excised tumor. **C:** Numerous congested round and oval vascular channels can be seen in the needle core biopsy specimen from another patient.

EMH occurs almost exclusively in hemangiomas. Thrombosis within cavernous channels sometimes elicits a lymphocytic reaction, and one may discover endothelial proliferation within the organizing clot. This phenomenon can result in papillary endothelial hyperplasia, which one should not mistake as evidence of an angiosarcoma.

There is considerable variability in the degree of microscopic circumscription. In many cavernous hemangiomas, the vascular channels become smaller at the periphery of the tumor and drift into the fatty parenchyma **(Fig. 20.28)**. This pattern duplicates the appearance of peripheral parts of certain well-differentiated angiosarcomas. Because of this similarity, one cannot distinguish a hemangioma from a low-grade angiosarcoma based on the histologic examination of a NCB sample.

Capillary hemangiomas consist of a compact collection of blood vessels of capillary dimensions. The mean size of these hemangiomas is 1.0 cm. Many are detected by mammography. Capillary hemangiomas often appear cellular. They are usually well circumscribed, but some have irregular borders. Fibrous septa frequently divide capillary hemangiomas into segments resulting in a lobulated structure that superficially resembles a pyogenic granuloma **(Fig. 20.29)**. Endothelial cells, which may have hyperchromatic nuclei, line the small vascular channels **(Fig. 20.30)**. Some examples have prominent anastomosing vascular channels or spindle cells. Papillary endothelial hyperplasia may be present at sites of organizing thrombi.

Florid papillary endothelial hyperplasia can obscure the basic angiomatous character of the lesion or even suggest the diagnosis of a well-differentiated angiosarcoma. Muscular blood vessels may be found within and at the periphery of the tumor.

Five examples of *venous hemangiomas* have been reported (160). The ages of the patients range from 24 to 59 years and average 40 years. Each presented with a palpable tumor. One patient reported that the mass had been present for 13 years; another patient became aware of the lesion after trauma to the breast. The tumors measured from 1.0 to 5.3 cm and averaged 3.2 cm. They appeared well circumscribed, firm, and darkly colored. Hemorrhagic cysts 0.5 to 1.3 cm in diameter were noted in one lesion.

Histologic diversity characterizes the microscopic appearance of venous hemangiomas. All venous hemangiomas have dilated venous channels with smooth muscle walls of varying structural completeness **(Fig. 20.31)**. Red blood cells are present in the lumina of some vascular spaces; others spaces are empty or contain fluid. Thick-walled arterial channels and capillaries are not conspicuous. Lobules and ducts are sometimes distributed in the mammary stroma between the vascular channels, and focal perivascular lymphocytic infiltrates, often accompanied by congested capillaries, are usually present in the stroma.

The dilated vascular channels are irregularly shaped, and they vary greatly in caliber. A smooth muscle layer is evident

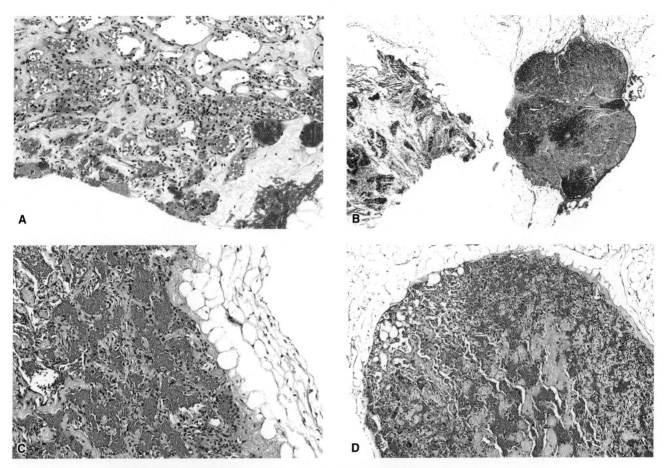

FIGURE 20.29 Capillary Hemangioma. A: Capillaries are present in this needle core biopsy specimen. **B:** The excised tumor has a lobulated configuration. **C, D:** Congested anastomosing capillaries can be seen in the needle core biopsy sample **(C)** and in the excised 5-mm tumor **(D)**.

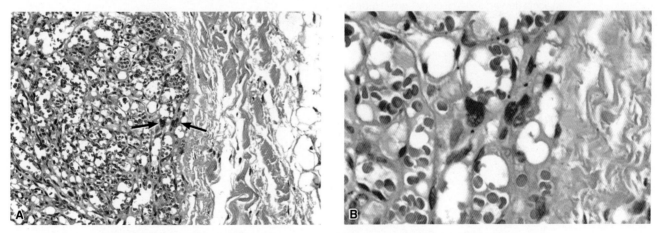

FIGURE 20.30 Capillary Hemangioma. A, B: This needle core biopsy specimen shows the circumscribed border of the tumor. A few endothelial cells have prominent hyperchromatic nuclei *(arrows)*.

in the walls of some of the tumor vessels, but often it does not encompass the entire circumference. In some areas, smooth muscle elements appear incompletely formed or absent in sections stained with H&E, an impression confirmed by the results of a trichrome stain or an immunohistochemical stain for SMA.

Complex hemangiomas consist of dilated vascular channels of varying sizes and compact, dense aggregates of capillary structures. The average size of these hemangiomas is 0.7 cm. Many have been detected by mammography. Some complex hemangiomas have conspicuous, anastomosing vascular channels **(Fig. 20.32)**.

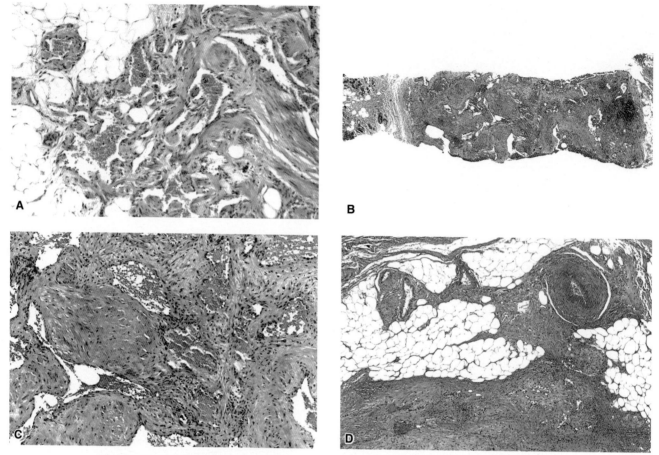

FIGURE 20.31 Venous Hemangioma. A: The lesion shown in this needle core biopsy specimen consists of vascular structures of various sizes with mural smooth muscle. **B:** Another needle core biopsy specimen contains a smoothly contoured discrete vascular tumor within the mammary parenchyma. **C:** Disorganized collagen and smooth muscle compose the walls of the neoplastic blood vessels. **D:** The excision specimen from the mass shown in **B** and **C** contains residual hemangioma **(lower)** and a "feeding" vessel **(upper right)**.

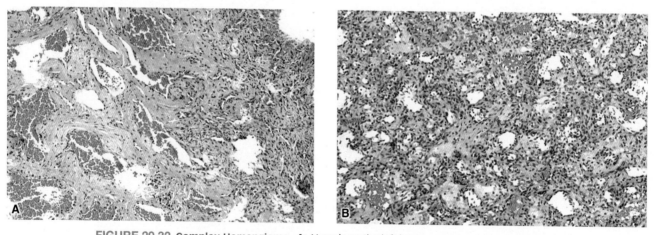

FIGURE 20.32 Complex Hemangioma. A: Vessels on the left have a cavernous appearance, whereas a cellular capillary network is evident on the right. **B:** This image depicts another hemangioma in which cellular fibrous stroma is distributed between capillaries.

One can observe the presence of a "feeding" vessel at the periphery of any type of hemangioma. These non-neoplastic vessels often display sinuous configurations and malformed or incomplete muscular layers in their walls. The close association of these "feeding" vessels and the hemangiomas suggests that the hemangiomas arose from the "feeding" vessel. It is unlikely that a "feeding" vessel can be identified in a NCB specimen, and it may require extensive sampling of the excised tumor to detect one.

Hemorrhage and infarction can occur in all types of hemangiomas and especially those subjected to NCB or needle localization excision. These phenomena should not be confused with the hemorrhagic necrosis that results in the formation of "blood lakes" characteristically found in high-grade angiosarcomas. Calcification may occur in organized thrombi, sometimes associated with endothelial hyperplasia, or in fibrous septa between vascular spaces. Marked septal fibrosis is sometimes found in hemangiomas. Mast cells are frequently present individually or in small clusters in hemangiomas.

The Ki67 immunostain is a useful adjunct in the diagnosis of the mammary hemangiomas. The nuclear Ki67-labeling index in mammary hemangiomas is very low and rarely exceeds 5%. Hemangiomas may show higher rates of labeling at sites of organizing thrombi or in tissue adjacent to a biopsy site; therefore, one should correlate the results of a Ki67 stain with the histologic findings evident on an H&E-stained section. The Ki67-labeling index of mammary angiosarcomas is greater than that of hemangiomas and typically exceeds 20% even in low-grade tumors. Because the distribution of labeling is not uniform in an angiosarcoma, it is possible to obtain a small biopsy sample with less than 5% labeling from a low-grade angiosarcoma. A robust Ki67-labeling index on a NCB sample from a mammary vascular lesion would strongly favor angiosarcoma. Very sparse labeling in such a limited sample can assist in making a diagnosis of hemangioma when correlated with the size and the H&E appearance of the lesion.

A small number of hemangiomas display mild nuclear enlargement or slight nuclear pleomorphism, anastomosing vascular channels, and microscopically invasive borders. Because of the concern that these tumors might be precursors of angiosarcoma, some of these tumors were once classified as *"atypical" hemangiomas* (**Fig. 20.33**) (150). Additional follow-up has not demonstrated that so-called "atypical" hemangiomas are borderline or low-grade variants of angiosarcoma or that "atypical" hemangiomas predispose to the development of angiosarcoma (159). Consequently, the designation of "atypical"

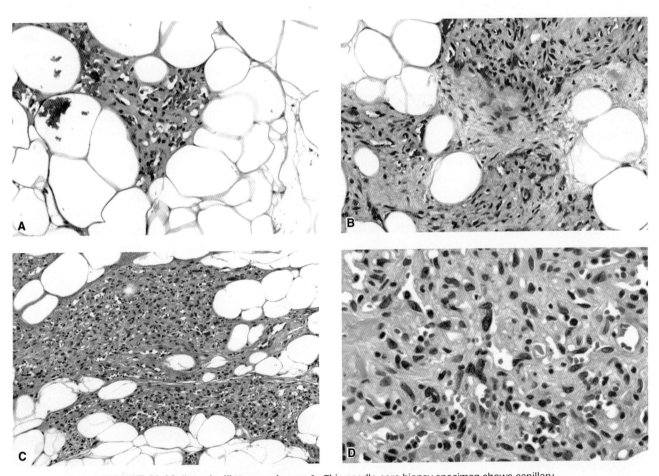

FIGURE 20.33 "Atypical" Hemangioma. A: This needle core biopsy specimen shows capillary vessels in fat. **B:** A more compact portion of the same specimen is depicted. **C, D:** The excised tumor has an invasive growth pattern. Endothelial cell nuclei in the anastomosing capillary channels are pleomorphic and hyperchromatic. Mitotic figures were not identified.

is no longer warranted in most cases, and the tumors should be classified simply as *hemangiomas* of one type or another. The designation "atypical" is now reserved for a small group of hemangiomas with clearly evident cytologic atypia or evidence of proliferative activity manifested by the presence of mitotic figures or by a Ki67-labeling index in the upper range for hemangiomas.

Complete excision of a vascular tumor is usually necessary for an accurate diagnosis. Peripheral portions of a cavernous hemangioma may be indistinguishable from low-grade angiosarcoma in the small sample obtained with a NCB. Experience derived from palpable tumors indicates that hemangiomas usually do not exceed 2.0 cm in diameter, whereas few angiosarcomas are smaller than 3.0 cm; however, one cannot rely on this experience in all settings, because smaller, nonpalpable examples of angiosarcomas have been detected by radiologic imaging. Consequently, it is prudent to perform an excision when a NCB reveals a vascular lesion. When imaging after a NCB indicates that the procedure removed most or all of a histologically benign lesion and a clip has been left at the biopsy site, follow-up by mammography can be an alternative to surgical excision. Excision of the tissue surrounding the biopsy site is indicated if it seems that a substantial portion of the lesion remains in place. Re-excision may not be necessary if only a few peripheral capillaries extend to the margin of a specimen that is clearly a hemangioma. It is often not possible to recognize residual hemangioma in the granulation tissue of a healing biopsy site. No patient with any of the foregoing types of hemangiomas has experienced a recurrence after excision. The period of follow-up in such instances averages 44 months but extends as long as 140 months.

Angiomatosis

Angiomatosis is a diffuse benign vascular lesion that produces a mass (161). The term represents a descriptive compromise reached because these tumors often consist of both hemangiomatous and lymphangiomatous channels. Angiomatosis should be distinguished from the presence of multiple perilobular hemangiomas, a condition sometimes referred to as "hemangiomatosis." Even when numerous, perilobular hemangiomas retain their typical localized capillary structure, whereas angiomatosis consists of larger, irregularly shaped channels growing in a seemingly infiltrative manner.

Four female patients have been reported (161,162). Three were adults 19 to 40 years old when the lesion was diagnosed, and the fourth had a congenital tumor. Each presented with a mass in the breast. The tumors from adults measured 9 to 11 cm and appeared spongy. When the vascular spaces contain blood, the tumor appears hemorrhagic and resembles an angiosarcoma. One tumor had a 15-cm blood-filled cyst (162).

Although angiomatosis forms a mass clinically and on macroscopic examination, it does not have the microscopically circumscribed structure that typifies mammary hemangiomas. The lesion is composed of anastomosing, large vascular channels extending diffusely in the breast parenchyma. They surround ducts and lobules but do not invade the lobular stroma. The vessels are lined by flat inconspicuous endothelium and supported by sparse mural tissue virtually devoid of smooth muscle **(Fig. 20.34)**. The vascular structures consist predominantly of hemangiomatous erythrocyte-containing channels, lymphangiomatous empty channels accompanied by lymphoid aggregates, or a mixture of the two types of vessels.

The microscopic distinction between angiomatosis and low-grade angiosarcoma may be difficult, especially in a NCB sample. Anastomosing channels that appear "empty" or contain erythrocytes occur in both lesions. When multiple areas are sampled, significant differences become apparent. The vascular channels in angiomatosis are distributed uniformly throughout the tumor with very little variation. In contrast, even the most well-differentiated angiosarcoma has a heterogeneous pattern showing numerous aggregated vessels in some regions and sparse, widely separated vessels elsewhere. The vascular structures of angiomatosis tend not to diminish in caliber at the periphery, whereas neoplastic vessels of capillary size merge with the surrounding tissue at the periphery of angiosarcomas. The vascular proliferation in angiomatosis surrounds lobules but does not invade them; however, in angiosarcomas, the

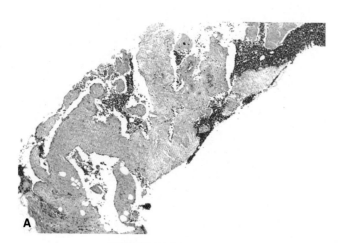
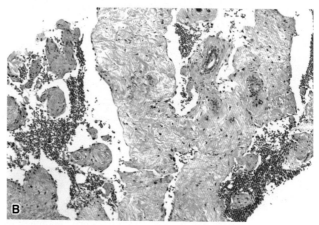

FIGURE 20.34 Angiomatosis. A, B: This needle core biopsy specimen reveals anastomosing dilated vascular spaces in fibrous breast stroma, which contains small ducts.

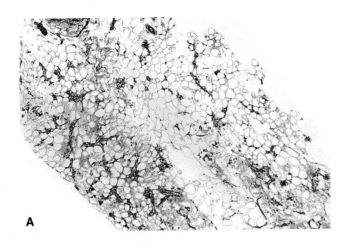

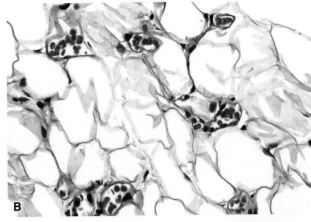

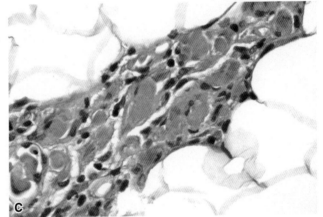

FIGURE 20.35 Nonparenchymal Angiolipoma. A, B: Capillaries are dispersed in fat in this needle core biopsy specimen. Areas with a very similar histologic appearance can be found at the periphery of angiosarcomas. **C:** One can observe microthrombi in the capillaries of this angiolipoma.

vascular channels grow into lobules, which are consequently destroyed. Finally, endothelial nuclei are histologically normal in angiomatosis, or they may be so attenuated that they may be difficult to find. Prominent, hyperchromatic endothelial nuclei are found in angiosarcomas, even when papillary endothelial proliferation is absent. Mitoses are not found in angiomatosis, and it has a very low Ki67-labeling index.

Angiomatosis of the breast is comparable to similar lesions that arise at other anatomic sites. The large size attained in the breast without the development of a histologically or clinically malignant component indicates that these are benign tumors. It may be necessary to perform a mastectomy to control a bulky lesion, but less-extensive surgery is preferable whenever possible. It may recur, sometimes after a long interval, indicating that the lesion is a chronic condition in some patients (161).

Nonparenchymal Vascular Lesions

For many years, considerable emphasis was placed on the distinction between subcutaneous and intraparenchymal vascular lesions of the breast. Virtually all of the former proved to be benign, whereas the majority of the latter were interpreted as angiosarcomas. It has become clear that location alone is not sufficient to determine the diagnosis. The existence of intraparenchymal hemangiomas is now well documented, and angiosarcoma may involve the mammary skin and subcutaneous tissue.

Nonparenchymal mammary hemangiomas occur in the mammary subcutaneous tissue (163). A lesion is classified as nonparenchymal if the neoplastic vessels do not involve the mammary glandular tissue. The distinction between a parenchymal and a nonparenchymal hemangioma cannot be made based on examination of a NCB specimen unless the lesion is seen to involve mammary glandular tissue. Breast parenchyma may be included in a biopsy specimen; however, in most cases, it contains only the tumor and surrounding fat.

Several types of nonparenchymal hemangiomas have been identified: angiolipoma (**Figs. 20.35 and 20.36**), cavernous hemangioma, hemangioma with papillary endothelial hyperplasia, capillary hemangioma, and venous hemangioma. The frequencies of these types of hemangiomas correspond roughly to their relative occurrence in the soft tissues generally. This correspondence suggests that there is no strong predilection for a particular type of hemangioma to occur in the mammary subcutaneous tissue.

Almost all patients are women, whose ages range from 20 to 76 years; the average age is 53 years. Nonparenchymal hemangiomas of the male breast have been reported (149,164). The subcutaneous tissues of the right and left breasts are involved with nearly equal frequency. Some tumors occur in the inframammary region, but most involve the subcutaneous tissue overlying the breast itself. They do not demonstrate a predilection to involve any specific region of the gland. The presenting symptom is a

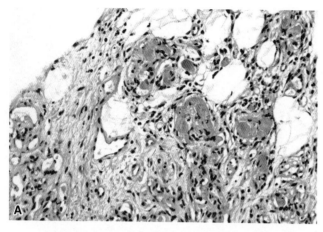

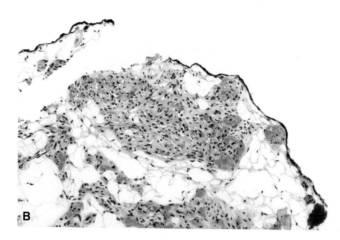

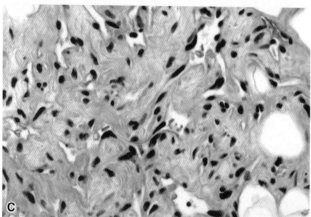

FIGURE 20.36 Nonparenchymal Angiolipoma with Atypia.
A: This needle core biopsy specimen displays a compact area of capillary proliferation. Some cells have hyperchromatic nuclei. Microthrombi characteristic of angiolipoma are present. **B:** The excised tumor extended to a margin. **C:** This part of the excised tumor resembles the needle core biopsy specimen. Prominent hyperchromatic nuclei are shown.

mass in most cases. The sizes of the tumors range from 0.8 to 3.2 cm and average 1.8 cm.

Nonpalpable lesions have been detected by screening mammography. Sonography is a useful procedure for determining whether the lesion is in the subcutaneous tissue or in the breast.

The histologic appearances of various types of hemangiomas in the mammary subcutaneous tissue do not differ from those of comparable lesions in other subcutaneous locations or in the breast parenchyma. Some hemangiomas found in mammary subcutaneous tissue feature interconnected vascular channels, sometimes with a pseudopapillary pattern. The vascular spaces can be larger toward the center than at the periphery, where they tend to spread into the subcutaneous fat producing a microscopically ill-defined margin.

The histologic features evident in a NCB specimen of a superficial vascular tumor may not permit a secure diagnosis. The sample may not allow one to determine the nature of the margin of the mass or its relationship with the mammary glandular tissue, for instance, or to exclude the possibility of an underlying low-grade angiosarcoma. Complete excision of the mass is prudent in most cases.

Nonparenchymal hemangiomas of the breast are adequately treated by local excision.

SARCOMAS

Mammary sarcomas arise only rarely. According to data from the SEER database, the annual incidence is 4.6 cases per million women (165). Several factors predispose patients to the development of mammary sarcomas. Women treated for breast carcinoma experience a slight increase in their risk for soft tissue sarcomas, and the use of irradiation further increases the risk for the development of angiosarcomas, undifferentiated pleomorphic carcinomas, and other rare types of sarcoma within the field of irradiation (166–168). The risk for the development of postirradiation sarcoma increases significantly 3 years after the diagnosis of carcinoma, peaks at approximately 10 years, and declines to approximately the risk seen in patients who did not receive irradiation after 23 years (167). Rare mammary sarcomas have developed in association with cosmetic implants or other foreign material, but the evidence does not prove a causal relationship between the presence of these substances and the development of the sarcomas.

Mammary sarcomas demonstrate morphologic characteristics identical to comparable sarcomas arising in other regions of the body. One should employ the terminology used for extramammary sarcomas when referring to their mammary counterparts. It is difficult to determine the frequencies of the various types of mammary sarcomas because authors have sometimes referred to these lesions using the all-encompassing term, *stromal sarcoma*. Despite this ambiguity, one can identify certain differences in the relative frequency of mammary sarcomas when compared with extramammary sarcomas. For example, angiosarcoma, an uncommon extramammary sarcoma, represents the most common type of mammary sarcoma.

Women make up the vast majority of patients with mammary sarcomas. Females accounted for 98.5% of the cases of sarcoma in the 19 studies tabulated by Al-Benna et al. (169), some of which included cases of malignant phyllodes tumors and metaplastic carcinomas. These data may not account for all cases affecting males because some of the tumors may have been classified as sarcomas of the chest wall rather than of the breast. Females of all ages are affected. In one series (170), the patients' ages range from 13 to 86 years, and the median age is 55 years. Using information from published studies, Al-Benna et al. (169) calculated a weighted mean age of 50.0 years.

Mammary sarcomas range from less than 1 to more than 30 cm. In most studies, the mean and median sizes fall between 4 and 7 cm. The gross appearance of the tumor is influenced in part by the histologic characteristics of the lesion, but the specimens typically consist of fleshy, moderately firm, pale tissue with varying amounts of hemorrhage and necrosis. Most sarcomas appear well circumscribed grossly, even if the border is invasive histologically.

The microscopic features of mammary sarcomas appear identical to those of sarcomas arising in other organs and depend on the nature of the neoplastic cells. Before making a diagnosis of any types of mammary sarcoma, one must exclude more common entities such as phyllodes tumor with a dominant stromal component, metaplastic carcinoma, and certain benign stromal proliferations of mesenchymal cells.

The prognosis for patients with mammary sarcomas varies depending on certain characteristics of the sarcoma. Among the histologic types of sarcomas, high-grade angiosarcomas have an especially unfavorable prognosis. The size of the sarcoma may also provide prognostic information. In a group of 83 women with primary breast sarcomas studied by Zelek et al. (165), tumor size was significantly related to 10-year disease-free survival. Adem et al. (171) reported a 5-year disease-free survival of 90% for tumors 5 cm or less and 50% for tumors larger than 5 cm. In two other studies (170,172), on the other hand, the size of the sarcoma did not correlate with the survival of the patients. Grading of mammary sarcomas is prognostically important for angiosarcoma, but its significance for other types of sarcoma is unclear. Hemangiopericytoma represents a special case, because all of these tumors reported thus far have pursued a benign clinical course regardless of size or histologic features.

Complete excision of the sarcoma represents the crucial aspect of treatment of mammary sarcomas. The surgical procedure can consist of either a mastectomy or an excision depending on the size of the mass and other surgical and personal considerations. Several studies failed to demonstrate a relationship between the type of primary surgical procedure and the survival of the patient, but the adequacy of the definitive treatment represents an influential factor in determining survival. If disease remained after the completion of initial treatment, the 10-year probability of local control and of disease-free survival was 0% for both parameters in one study (170). Several other studies detected an adverse effect of positive margins on the chance of survival. Contemporary multimodal approaches including irradiation and chemotherapy may reduce the frequency of local and systemic recurrence in extramammary sarcomas, but the results to date are inconclusive.

Axillary lymph node metastases are exceedingly uncommon at the time of primary therapy. In the series of Bousquet et al. (170), metastatic sarcoma was found in 4 of 44 (9%) patients who underwent lymph node evaluation; 3 of these patients had angiosarcomas. Axillary dissection or sentinel lymph node sampling are not ordinarily indicated in the absence of clinically involved lymph nodes.

Radiation-induced sarcomas of the breast have attracted special interest. A publication by Sheth et al. (173) lists 124 original articles describing 1,831 cases of radiation-induced mammary sarcomas. The authors did not analyze the reported histologic features of the sarcomas, but they did note that both the size and the grade of the tumor had prognostic significance. Based on the accumulated published data, the authors concluded that, "surgery with widely negative margins remains the primary treatment of [radiation-induced sarcomas]. Unfortunately, the role of adjuvant and neoadjuvant chemotherapy remains uncertain." These conclusions seem to indicate that neither the nature nor the treatment of radiation-induced sarcomas of the breast differs significantly from those of spontaneously occurring mammary sarcomas.

Angiosarcoma

Angiosarcoma arises in the breast more often than in any other organ. It occurs in two forms: sporadic angiosarcoma and post-irradiation angiosarcoma. Although these two forms exhibit many common features, the tumors differ in certain clinical, histologic, immunohistochemical, and therapeutic respects.

Sporadic angiosarcoma afflicts women almost exclusively. Only four well-documented instances of angiosarcoma in men have been reported (174–177). The age at diagnosis ranges from the teens to the tenth decade with a mean age of 34 (178) and a median of 38 to 39 years (174). Several reported patients have been pregnant, an observation that probably reflects the relative youth of women with sporadic angiosarcoma. Angiosarcomas at various extramammary sites have been associated with foreign body material retained for many years. Two reports (179,180) described angiosarcomas associated with breast implants, and a third case illustrates an angiosarcoma involving the site of silicone injection carried out many years previously for cosmetic purposes (181). The literature contains several reports of synchronous or metachronous presentations of mammary angiosarcoma and carcinoma.

Sporadic angiosarcoma usually presents as a painless mass, but rare cases lack physical findings to suggest the presence of an angiosarcoma. Patients usually report the presence of symptoms for only a short time, but symptomatic intervals as long as 5 years have been described (175). Blue or purple discoloration

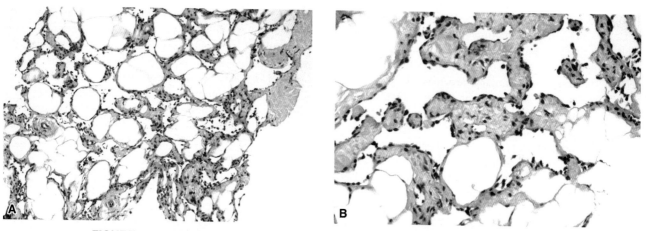

FIGURE 20.37 Angiosarcoma, Low-grade. A, B: Open, empty irregularly shaped vascular channels are distributed diffusely in this needle core biopsy specimen. The endothelial layer is flat, and the endothelial nuclei appear slightly prominent.

of the skin reflecting hemorrhage or the vascularity of the lesion accompanies large or superficial tumors. Blistering has been noted, and large angiosarcomas can present as fungating masses. The left and right breasts are involved with nearly equal frequency. Concurrent bilateral angiosarcomas are very uncommon. Contralateral breast involvement is usually evidence of metastatic spread, with often the first site of metastasis identified.

Some angiosarcomas are not visualized by mammography (182,183) but may be evident using sonography or MRI (183,184). MRI often helps to determine the extent of the tumor (184).

On macroscopic study, the size of the tumors ranges from 0.7 to 25 cm and averages between 5.5 and 7.0 cm. Very few angiosarcomas are smaller than 3 cm. There is no significant difference in the average size of high- and low-grade lesions (185). Many angiosarcomas form friable, firm, or spongy hemorrhagic masses. Those showing little or no hemorrhage are generally described as poorly defined areas of thickening.

Three histologic patterns of growth of the primary tumor have been described. These patterns, which reflect the degree of differentiation of the malignant cells, correlate with prognosis

(174,178,186). Low-grade, or type I tumors, are composed of open, anastomosing vascular channels that proliferate diffusely in mammary glandular tissue and fat (**Fig. 20.37**). Infiltration into lobules is characterized by spread of the vascular channels within the intralobular stroma, a process that leads to separation and atrophy of the lobular glandular units (**Fig. 20.38**). Endothelial cells are distributed in a flat single-cell layer around the vascular spaces. Some prominent, hyperchromatic endothelial nuclei may be found, but the endothelial cells often have inconspicuous nuclei. Papillary formations are absent or at most very infrequent. Mitotic figures are rarely seen, and the Ki67-labeling index averages 25% in low-grade angiosarcomas (187). If mitotic figures are encountered with regularity in a low-grade area in a biopsy specimen, high-grade areas are likely to be present elsewhere in the tumor, the Ki67-labeling index will be greater than is typical for low-grade angiosarcoma, and the tumor is likely to be high-grade when it recurs. The vascular lumina are usually large, open, and anastomosing in low-grade angiosarcomas. Red blood cells are typically present in small numbers, but the vessels in occasional lesions are congested.

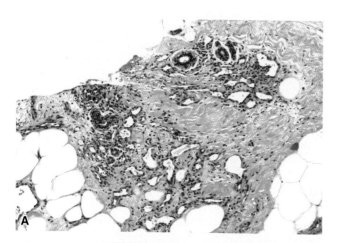
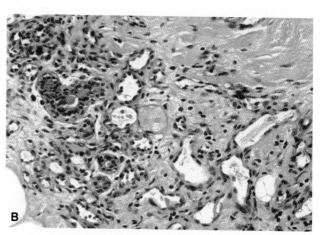

FIGURE 20.38 Angiosarcoma, Low-grade. A, B: Neoplastic vascular channels invade around and into lobules in this needle core biopsy specimen. **C, D:** Angiosarcoma has partially destroyed the lobules in this needle core biopsy specimen. In **D**, the neoplastic vessels are reactive for CD31, and residual acini are highlighted by the pale, blue–gray hematoxylin counterstain.

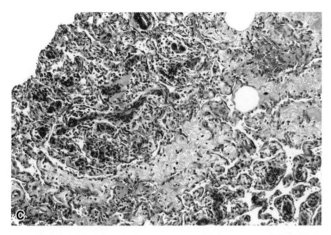

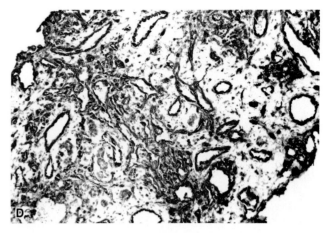

FIGURE 20.38 (*continued*)

Several unusual structural variants of low-grade angiosarcoma may be difficult to recognize in a NCB specimen. One variant is composed predominantly of capillary-like vascular spaces; another consists of small, often narrow, vascular channels without a conspicuous anastomosing structure. In a third pattern, the neoplastic vessels are dispersed in the stroma in a pattern that may be mistaken for PASH. Finally, diffusely infiltrating low-grade angiosarcoma composed predominantly of spindle cells may be mistaken for an angiolipoma.

The amount of stroma formed in low-grade angiosarcomas varies to a considerable degree. In most instances, little

stroma is formed, and the lesion consists largely of vascular channels permeating the mammary parenchyma. A minority of low-grade angiosarcomas have a focal or diffuse collagenous stroma. Despite their denser appearance, these lesions qualify as low-grade tumors if there is no endothelial proliferation and mitoses are sparse or not detectable.

Intermediate-grade (type II) angiosarcomas are distinguished from low-grade tumors by the presence of foci showing evidence of more pronounced cellular proliferation. The proliferative foci usually consist of small buds or papillary fronds of endothelial cells that project into the vascular lumina **(Fig. 20.39)**. Less

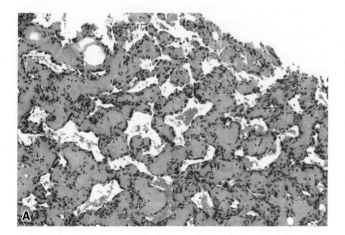

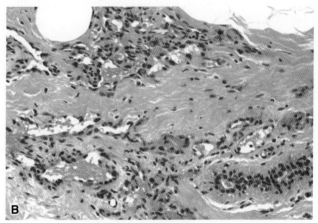

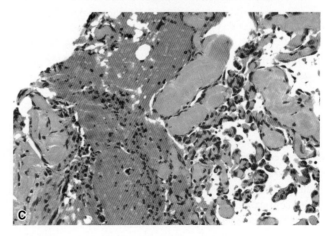

FIGURE 20.39 Angiosarcoma, Intermediate-grade.
A, B: This needle core biopsy specimen shows a low-grade area with fibrous stroma between anastomosing vascular channels.
C: This region of the specimen shows focal papillary endothelial growth and thrombosis.

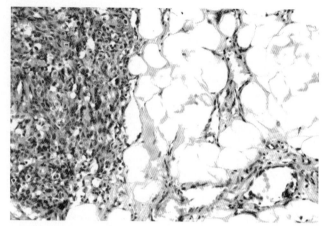

FIGURE 20.40 Angiosarcoma, Intermediate-grade. Low-grade angiosarcoma is shown on the right, and a nodule of spindle cell angiosarcoma is seen on the left in this needle core biopsy specimen. These findings are compatible with an intermediate-grade tumor if the nodular component is limited to isolated foci in the excised tumor.

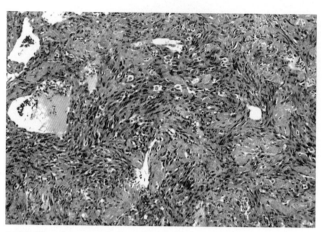

FIGURE 20.41 Angiosarcoma, High-grade. A relatively solid spindle cell area is shown.

often, the focally cellular areas feature polygonal and spindle cells, or there are foci that combine spindle cell and papillary elements **(Fig. 20.40)**. Infrequent mitoses may be found in papillary or spindle cell areas. Some spindle cell foci resemble lesions encountered in Kaposi sarcoma. Ki67-labeling is most evident in the cellular areas, whereas the remainder of the tumor exhibits labeling similar to that found in low-grade angiosarcoma. The mean Ki67-labeling index is about 40% in cellular areas (187).

Low-grade components are found in intermediate- and high-grade lesions and sometimes comprise the bulk of the tumor. This is particularly true for type II or intermediate-grade angiosarcomas. At least 75% of intermediate-grade angiosarcomas contain low-grade elements. Transitions to the intermediate-grade, cellular foci occur abruptly.

Type III, or high-grade, angiosarcoma exhibits the malignant histologic features usually attributed to angiosarcomas. Part of the lesion is composed of low- and intermediate-grade elements; however, in many cases, more than half of the tumor has high-grade malignant features. These features include prominent endothelial tufting and solid papillary formations that contain cytologically malignant endothelial cells and conspicuous solid and spindle cell areas with sparse vascular elements **(Fig. 20.41)**. Mitoses are usually identified without difficulty in the cellular components. Typically, Ki67-labeling is found in 45% or more of the tumor cells in high-grade angiosarcoma. Areas of hemorrhage, often accompanied by necrosis, have been referred to as "blood lakes" **(Fig. 20.42)**. Only high-grade angiosarcomas demonstrate necrosis and "blood lakes."

With few exceptions, angiosarcomas have infiltrative borders composed of well-formed or low-grade vascular channels. In some cases, the peripheral vascular component is so orderly that the neoplastic vessels are either structurally indistinguishable from existing capillaries in the normal parenchyma or resemble those of an angiolipoma.

Epithelioid angiosarcoma **(Fig. 20.43)** is an uncommon high-grade variant with histologic features similar to those of the type of angiosarcoma often seen in the Stewart-Treves syndrome. The lesion consists predominantly or exclusively of large, polygonal or rounded epithelioid endothelial cells lining slit-like spaces and containing abundant amphophilic or eosinophilic cytoplasm and large vesicular nuclei. Because of the epithelioid appearance of the cells, the tumor may be mistaken for mammary adenocarcinoma. The results of immunohistochemical staining for epithelial and vascular proteins will assist in distinguishing the two lesions.

Because of the varied microscopic structure of intermediate- and high-grade lesions, it is not possible to classify a tumor as low-grade angiosarcoma accurately unless it has been excised and generously sampled. The tendency for peripheral portions of an intermediate- or high-grade angiosarcoma to have a low-grade structure is likely to lead to an erroneous diagnosis if one examines only a NCB specimen or one obtained by a superficial biopsy.

Two studies of mammary angiosarcomas reported more intense staining for factor VIII-related antigen in well-differentiated than in poorly differentiated portions of the tumor (186,188). Angiosarcomas also exhibit reactivity for CD31 and CD34. These markers are especially useful for distinguishing epithelioid angiosarcoma from carcinoma and other neoplasms. Epithelioid angiosarcomas typically stain for CD31, but reactivity for CD34 varies. Reactivity for D2-40 has been reported in some angiosarcomas. Although angiosarcomas usually do not stain for keratin, two reports (177,185), including one describing an epithelioid angiosarcoma (177), noted staining for keratin in two cases. Angiosarcomas do not stain for ER or PR, and the few tested do not show evidence of *HER2* overexpression.

It is not difficult to distinguish a high-grade angiosarcoma from a hemangioma, but problems may be encountered with low-grade and intermediate-grade tumors. Some general guidelines are helpful in these situations. Hemangiomas are rarely larger than 2 cm, and few angiosarcomas measure less than 3 cm. Most hemangiomas tend to have well-circumscribed borders grossly and microscopically, whereas angiosarcomas

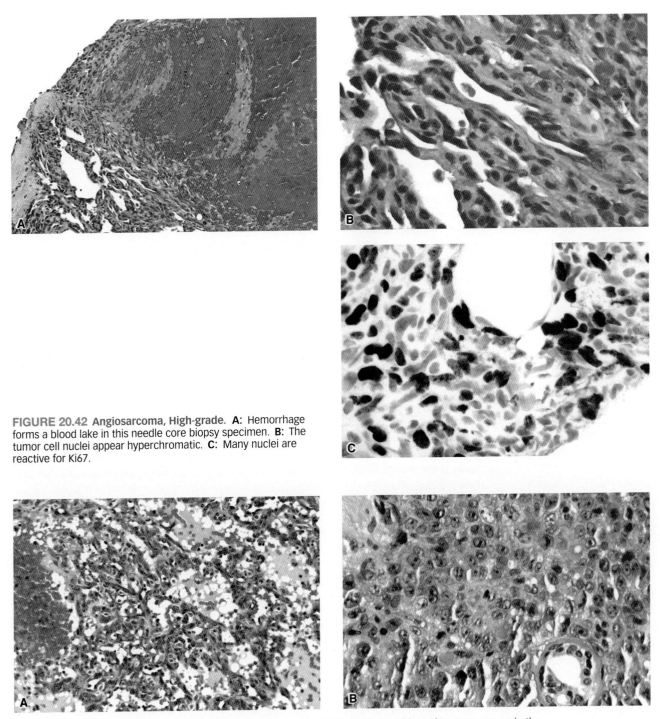

FIGURE 20.42 **Angiosarcoma, High-grade.** **A:** Hemorrhage forms a blood lake in this needle core biopsy specimen. **B:** The tumor cell nuclei appear hyperchromatic. **C:** Many nuclei are reactive for Ki67.

FIGURE 20.43 **Angiosarcoma, High-grade, Epithelioid.** **A:** This angiosarcoma arose in the breast 4 years after conservative surgery and radiotherapy. **B:** The neoplastic cells in this high-grade postirradiation angiosarcoma demonstrate an epithelioid appearance. The cells possess the characteristic vesicular nuclei and prominent nucleoli.

have invasive margins. Many hemangiomas are divided into lobules or nodules by fibrous septa, a feature not seen in angiosarcomas, which lack an internal structure. Hemangiomas usually consist of isolated, largely unconnected vascular channels such as those typically seen in cavernous hemangiomas. Anastomosing vascular spaces may be found in hemangiomas; however, except in angiomatosis, the anastomoses are not as numerous or as serpiginous as those in angiosarcomas. In the mammary parenchyma, the vascular proliferation in angiosarcomas invades into and expands lobules, whereas the vessels in hemangiomas other than perilobular hemangiomas tend to surround lobules and ducts. A thick-walled, non-neoplastic "feeding" blood vessel is sometimes found at the periphery of hemangiomas; this feature is not seen in angiosarcomas.

The Ki67-labeling index of hemangiomas is substantially lower than the labeling index of angiosarcomas (187).

Distinguishing between a contralateral mammary metastasis of an angiosarcoma and a new primary contralateral angiosarcoma is very difficult. Taking note of clinical details such as the interval between the detection of the two tumors and the presence of other metastatic foci and comparing the morphologic features of the cells in the two masses should help to distinguish the two situations.

In 1981, Donnell et al. (178) studied 40 patients with mammary angiosarcoma treated by mastectomy and found that the grade of the tumor was the most important prognostic factor. The majority of patients with orderly or low-grade lesions remained disease-free, whereas virtually all women with high-grade tumors died of recurrent sarcoma within 5 years. A later study of 87 patients confirmed the correlation between the tumor grade and prognosis, (174) and so did a study of 226 women in the SEER database (189).

Despite the relatively favorable prognosis of low-grade angiosarcoma, patients with these tumors can develop local and systemic recurrences (174,178). A patient who initially has a low-grade angiosarcoma may develop intermediate- or high-grade areas in recurrent lesions. Moreover, recurrences and metastases that originate from high-grade sarcomas can be composed in part or entirely of low-grade components.

A review by Kaklamanos et al. (190) summarizes information regarding treatment and survival culled from 10 major series that include cases of mammary angiosarcomas published prior to 2008. Total mastectomy is the recommended primary surgical therapy. Unless there is a clinically apparent nodal abnormality, axillary dissection is not indicated because metastases involve these lymph nodes in fewer than 10% of the cases. Radical mastectomy is not appropriate unless the tumor is close to or involves the deep fascia. Rarely, a small lesion might be encompassed by quadrantectomy.

The role of radiation in the primary treatment of mammary angiosarcoma has not been determined nor has the use of adjuvant systemic chemotherapy. It would seem that adjuvant radiation does not confer a survival benefit for patients with localized disease (189). Because high-grade lesions have an especially poor prognosis and most of the few long-term survivors had adjuvant chemotherapy, such treatment might be considered for these patients.

Radiation-related angiosarcomas can arise in either the chest wall after a mastectomy or the breast after a partial mastectomy. An analysis of SEER data (166) revealed that women with breast carcinoma who undergo irradiation experience a relative risk of 15.9 for the development of angiosarcoma at all sites compared to nonirradiated patients. When considering only angiosarcoma of the breast or chest wall, the comparable relative risk is 59.3.

Angiosarcoma of the irradiated breast is an infrequent complication of breast conservation therapy. The incidence averages to approximately 0.1%. A publication by Abbott and Palmieri (191) lists selected clinical details of 237 cases published prior to 2008. In almost every case, radiation was delivered using an external beam, but an angiosarcoma arose in the breast of a 74-year-old woman 4 years after receiving MammoSite balloon brachytherapy (192).

The interval between irradiation and the diagnosis of angiosarcoma ranges from 1 to more than 24 years, but most cases come to attention within 6 years after radiotherapy (193). The latent period for the appearance of postirradiation angiosarcoma tends to be shorter than that for other types of radiation-associated sarcoma and it appears inversely related to the patient's age at the time of treatment for breast carcinoma (194). Billings et al. (195) reported that for each 1-year increase in the age of the patient, the latency period decreases by 0.5 month. Studies have not discovered a relationship between that the amount of radiation delivered, the use of a radiation boost, or the presence of postirradiation edema and the development of radiation-related angiosarcoma.

With a few exceptions, women with postirradiation angiosarcoma have been older than 50 years of age when treated for mammary carcinoma. In one study (193), the median age at diagnosis of angiosarcoma is 70.6 years, and the range is 46.2 to 87.2 years. A meta-analysis of 184 published cases (191) yielded a median age of 70 years and a range of 36 to 92 years. A 98-year-old woman developed an epithelioid angiosarcoma 5 years after radiation treatment of an invasive ductal carcinoma (196).

Postirradiation angiosarcoma presents more frequently in the skin than within the breast parenchyma. The tumors usually involve the skin overlying the site of the prior carcinoma or the scar from the excision. The sarcomas can present as palpable skin or subcutaneous nodules, but equally frequently they create plaques or papules described as shades of blue, purple, or red. Certain examples cause edema, the formation of vesicles, or *peau d'orange* change, and others mimic a hematoma. Skin thickening and dimpling sometimes occur. Multiple nodules are common, and they sometimes number so many that they cover the entire breast. The formation of an exophytic mass has been described (197). In certain patients, the skin changes may be especially subtle. Many patients who present with angiosarcoma in the skin will also have parenchymal involvement.

Imaging studies in patients with postirradiation angiosarcomas do not demonstrate distinctive findings. Mammograms and CT scans sometime display thickening of the skin or enhancement of the trabecular pattern. In other respects, the imaging findings in patients with postirradiation angiosarcomas do not differ from those in patients with sporadic angiosarcomas.

The macroscopic pathologic characteristics of skin-based angiosarcomas duplicate the findings evident on clinical examination. Larger nodules and those involving the mammary parenchyma display the macroscopic features seen in angiosarcomas arising *de novo*.

Certain histologic details of postirradiation angiosarcoma of the skin, subcutaneous tissue, and breast differ from those of angiosarcomas not associated with radiotherapy (198). High-grade areas, found in the majority of these cases, consist of compact epithelioid or spindle cell foci, which may contain extravasated red blood cells or slit-like, erythrocyte-containing spaces. Hemorrhage resulting in the formation of blood lakes is typically distributed in these sarcomatous foci. Lesions with low- and intermediate-grade structural patterns exhibit variable vasoformative growth and papillary endothelial hyperplasia. In contrast to sporadic parenchymal angiosarcomas, in which nuclear grade frequently parallels structural differentiation, the malignant cells in postirradiation angiosarcoma typically have poorly differentiated nuclei, dark chromatin, prominent nucleoli, and mitotic figures. The mitotic rate varies from fewer than 1 to 35 mitotic figures per HPF with a mean of 9 per HPF. Unusual histologic variants of cutaneous angiosarcoma include a perithelial arrangement of neoplastic cells, storiform spindle cell growth, the formation of cavernous structures, and a pattern that mimics epidermotropic metastatic mammary carcinoma (199).

Like their sporadic counterparts, postirradiation angiosarcomas typically stain for vimentin and proteins found in endothelial cells such as CD31, CD34, and factor VIII. Two epithelioid angiosarcomas stained for keratin (196,200). The tumors do not stain for ER or PR.

Recent genetic studies implicate overexpression of *MYC* in the development of postirradiation mammary angiosarcomas. Of the 34 cases studied by three groups (201–203), 30 showed evidence of amplification of the *MYC* gene or overexpression of the MYC protein. In contrast, none of the 25 sporadic mammary angiosarcomas (202,204,205) exhibited amplification or overexpression.

The prognosis of angiosarcoma arising in the breast after radiotherapy does not seem to differ substantially from that of angiosarcoma unassociated with radiotherapy. A meta-analysis based on 151 cases (191) demonstrated a median overall survival of 18 months for patients with postirradiation angiosarcoma; however, studies from single institutions report higher median overall survival values. The largest single-institution study (206) includes 95 patients followed up for a median of 10.8 years. Local recurrences occurred in 48% and distant metastases in 27% of the patients. The 1-, 2-, and 5-year overall survival values were 91%, 78%, and 54%, respectively and the 1-, 2-, and 5-year disease-specific survival values were 94%, 84%, and 63%, respectively. Investigations of factors predicting the outcome of patients with postirradiation angiosarcoma have not yielded consistent findings.

As is the case with sporadic angiosarcomas, surgery constitutes the primary treatment of postirradiation angiosarcomas. The surgical procedure most often consists of a mastectomy, but surgery does not control the disease in most patients. Several studies report recurrences within a year even when the margins of the surgical specimen appeared free of the angiosarcoma. The high rate of local recurrence has led several investigators to conclude that many postirradiation angiosarcomas involve the irradiated tissue in a discontinuous, multifocal manner. Based on this belief, certain oncologists advocate excision of all irradiated skin. Two patients in the series of Seinen et al. (207) underwent mastectomy and excision of all irradiated tissue, and 12 of the 33 patients in the study of Morgan et al. (208) were treated similarly. The authors of the latter study reported: "Although this did not universally prevent recurrence, we found that patients who did not undergo resection of all irradiated breast skin trended toward a worse median [local relapse free survival] (10.0 vs. 80.8 months) and [overall survival] (29 months vs. not achieved)." Further studies will define the value of this approach.

Because angiosarcomas spread to lymph nodes uncommonly, lymph node excision is not usually carried out as a component of the primary therapy. Radiation therapy has not usually played a role in the primary treatment of postirradiation angiosarcomas, although it has been used in certain settings. Antineoplastic agents have been administered singly and in various combinations in both the adjuvant and neoadjuvant settings, but success has been limited. Therapies targeted to the VEGF receptor or c-kit may hold promise, but the literature contains only minimal information in this regard.

Postirradiation Atypical Vascular Lesions

Benign cutaneous vascular lesions can arise in the field of radiation delivered during either postmastectomy radiotherapy or breast conservation. Known in earlier days by a variety of names, these vascular lesions are now referred to by the term first proposed by Fineberg and Rosen (198), *atypical vascular lesions* (AVLs).

AVLs have developed in women between the ages of 29 and 91 years. The average age ranges from 52 years to 68 years. AVLs typically develop 2 to 5 years after radiotherapy, but intervals as long as 27 years have been reported.

The lesions present as one or more pink or brown papules in the skin of the breast, axilla, or chest wall. Plaques, vesicles, and cystic examples have been observed much less commonly. The lesions usually span 5 mm or less, although larger lesions have been reported. Only rarely do AVLs develop in the breast parenchyma. Consequently, they are not often sampled by a NCB and most often come to the attention of the pathologist in a specimen obtained by a punch biopsy or a small superficial cutaneous excision.

Histologic examination of the typical case reveals a focal proliferation of dilated, anastomosing vascular channels centered in the papillary and reticular dermis and lined by a single layer of endothelial cells **(Fig. 20.44)**. The overlying epidermis appears normal or displays mild acanthosis. The superficial vascular channels often appear large and open, whereas those in the deeper reaches of the skin look small and compressed. One can recognize two types of AVLs: lymphatic AVLs and vascular AVLs.

Lymphatic AVLs, the more common type, usually form a circumscribed collection of ectatic, thin-walled vessels lined by flat or slightly protuberant (hobnail) endothelial cells within the superficial dermis. In a minority of cases, the vessels grow in a serpiginous or somewhat infiltrative manner and extend into the deep dermis or subcutis. The neoplastic vessels can surround preexisting vessels or skin adnexa and infiltrate the arrector pili. The vascular spaces usually appear empty, but one can occasionally find lymphocytes in the nearby stroma or in the vascular lumina. Tufts of stroma typically project into the vascular lumina. One can divide lymphatic AVLs into three subtypes: a lymphangioma circumscriptum-like pattern in which dilated vessels in the superficial dermis create an

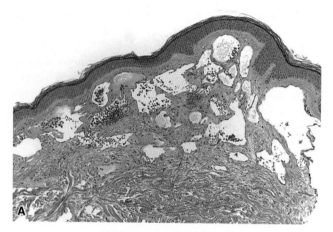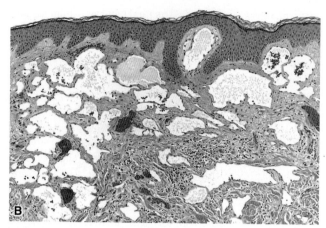

FIGURE 20.44 Atypical Vascular Lesion. A: Irregular, thin-walled vascular channels containing a few erythrocytes occupy the superficial regions of the dermis in this punch biopsy specimen. **B:** The excised nodule demonstrates the vascular structures with irregular contours. Some vascular channels contain erythrocytes; others appear devoid of cells.

exophytic bulging papule, a lymphangioendothelioma-like pattern in which narrow, slit-like vessels occupy the dermis, and a pattern in which the vessels resemble those of a hobnail hemangioma. Certain AVLs display a combination of these patterns.

Vascular type AVLs consist of irregular collections of round to linear capillaries growing in the dermis and surrounded by pericytes. In certain respects, vascular AVLs resemble capillary hemangiomas, although the former lack the lobular pattern characteristic of the latter. The vessels in the vascular type of AVL usually do not seem to communicate with each other in the manner of an angiosarcoma. The stroma often contains chronic inflammatory cells including mast cells and occasionally plasma cells. Hemorrhage and stromal hemosiderin deposition occur frequently. The background stromal cells in all types of AVL often display cellular atypia characteristic of radiation damage.

The endothelial cells lining the vessels of both lymphatic and vascular AVLs look bland. The nuclei can appear slightly hyperchromatic, but they do not demonstrate enlargement, angulation of their contours, or prominence of the nucleoli. Stratification of the endothelial cells is not usually present but may occur. Mitotic figures are rarely seen; their presence increases the possibility that low-grade angiosarcoma is present.

The endothelial cells of the lymphatic type of AVL stain for CD31 and D2-40, and they may stain for CD34; those of the vascular type of AVL stain for CD31 and CD34, but they do not stain for D2-40. Reactivity for factor VIII-related antigen has been described, but the endothelial cells do not stain for Ki67. Santi et al. (209) demonstrated immunohistochemical staining for p53 in 9 of 10 AVLs and alterations in the *p53* gene in 10 of 12 AVLs.

The differential diagnosis of AVL includes acquired progressive lymphangioma (benign lymphangioendothelioma), which rarely arises in the setting of antecedent radiotherapy, reactive angioendotheliomatosis, which usually occurs on the limbs in association with a systemic disease, and patch-stage

Kaposi sarcoma, which typically exhibits the presence of erythrocytes, hemosiderin, and plasma cells. AVLs must also be distinguished from postirradiation angiosarcomas. AVLs tend to occur earlier and to form smaller masses than angiosarcomas; however, both parameters show considerable overlap between the two entities, and the differentiation ultimately rests on histologic characteristics. None of the AVLs from 48 patients showed evidence of the amplification of *MYC* characteristic of postirradiation angiosarcomas (201–205), and only one case displayed immunoreactivity for MYC, which was seen in just a few cells (205).

Fineberg and Rosen (198) did not find evidence that AVLs evolved into angiosarcoma in patients who had been followed up for as long as 10 years; however, local recurrences of AVLs were reported in this publication and others. A few observations raise the possibility that AVLs might progress to angiosarcomas in rare circumstances. The presence of AVL-like formations in angiosarcomas, the mingling of possible AVLs with angiosarcomas, and the presence of mutations in the *p53* gene in both AVLs and angiosarcomas suggest a pathogenetic link between the two lesions. Moreover, the clinical courses in rare cases seem to demonstrate progression of AVLs to angiosarcomas (210,211).

Uncommon examples of AVLs show focal cytologic atypia or rare mitotic figures associated with otherwise entirely bland, typical AVLs. In one case studied by the Senior Editor, the patient had recurrent atypical lesions that were focally indistinguishable from low-grade angiosarcoma. The vascular proliferation was limited to the skin in the mastectomy specimen. The study of Gengler et al. (212) includes 10 patients who had AVLs with atypical features: focal nuclear hyperchromasia of endothelial cells, prominence of nucleoli, or an infiltrative pattern of growth. None of the patients developed an angiosarcoma despite incomplete excision in two cases. Patton et al. (211) noted "significant cytologic atypia" in 4 of the 10 vascular type AVLs in their study. One patient developed angiosarcoma, and one developed additional AVLs with atypical features.

Leiomyosarcoma

Leiomyosarcoma arises in the breast only very rarely; it accounts for fewer than 5% of the reported sarcomas of the breast. Fujita et al. (213) tabulated clinical features of 46 cases reported as single examples or in small series. Leiomyosarcoma probably originates from blood vessels, the smooth muscle of the nipple–areolar complex, or myofibroblasts. One leiomyosarcoma may have arisen in an ectopic areola (214). A leiomyosarcoma of uncertain origin diagnosed by NCB presented as bilateral mammary masses (215).

Most patients have been female, but leiomyosarcomas have developed in the male breast (216,217). The age at diagnosis ranges from 18 to 86 years, and the mean age is approximately 53 years. Patients present with a mass measuring from less than 1 cm to 23 cm and averaging approximately 5.5 cm. Almost one-half of the tumors are in or near the nipple–areola complex, but any quadrant may be affected. The tumors are circumscribed and firm. Fixation to the skin and ulceration can occur. Patients report pain only rarely.

Radiologic imaging reveals a dense, lobulated mass with a defined border. Calcifications are seen only infrequently.

Macroscopic examination reveals a circumscribed, firm, lobulated pale tumor. Examination of histologic sections reveals interlacing bundles of fusiform cells with the typical blunt-end nuclei characteristic of smooth muscle tumors **(Fig. 20.45)**. Cells with an epithelioid phenotype may be present. The most commonly reported malignant cytologic features include nuclear hyperchromasia and pleomorphism and the formation of multinucleated giant cells. Mitotic figures range from 2 to 50 per 10 HPF and average to 12 per 10 HPF. Focal areas of degeneration exhibit nuclear pyknosis, necrosis, and lymphocytic infiltration. Areas of hyalinized stromal fibrosis with a pattern that resembles PASH may be present. Mammary ducts and lobules, sometimes with proliferative changes, can become incorporated into the neoplasm, particularly at its periphery. This finding may lead one to consider diagnoses such as metaplastic carcinoma and phyllodes tumor. Unusual histologic findings include the presence of metaplastic bone and cartilage, rhabdomyoblastic cellular features, and osteoclast-like giant cells.

The malignant cells usually stain for desmin, SMA, and vimentin; however, some cases show only focal or weak staining, and others do not stain at all. Reactivity for h-caldesmon has been reported. Most examples do not stain for cytokeratin, S-100, or EMA, but rare examples have been weakly or focally positive for one or more of these three markers. The classification of the tumors with cytokeratin immunoreactivity remains uncertain. The few tumors tested failed to stain for ER, PR, or HER2.

The cellular features and results of immunohistochemical staining allow one to recognize the smooth muscle nature of most leiomyosarcomas easily, and the malignant properties of these sarcomas usually appear obvious. Nevertheless, pathologists have not yet established criteria to distinguish leiomyosarcomas from leiomyomas of the breast, nor have they recognized a category of mammary smooth muscle tumors with "uncertain malignant potential." The presence of noticeable mitotic activity (1–3 mitotic figures per 10 HPF) may indicate the potential for local recurrence (218). The combination of mitotic activity and ominous histologic features such as hypercellularity, cytologic atypia, and necrosis suggests the diagnosis of leiomyosarcoma.

The publication by Rane et al. (219) lists the treatment and follow-up of most cases published in the English literature. Primary treatment consisted of total mastectomy in approximately 75% of the patients. Approximately one-half the patients treated with excision alone developed recurrences. Axillary nodal metastases have not been reported. Irradiation and chemotherapy have been used in selected circumstances. Their value has not been established.

Among the nearly 50 reported cases of mammary leiomyosarcoma, approximately 20% of patients died of the disease. Outcome has not correlated well with the mitotic rate in the primary tumor. Fatalities occurred in cases with 2 or 3 mitoses per 10 HPF as well as in tumors with higher mitotic rates. Late recurrences and death from disease 15 and 20 years after initial diagnoses have occurred.

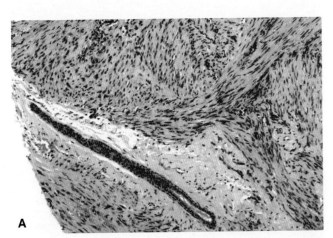
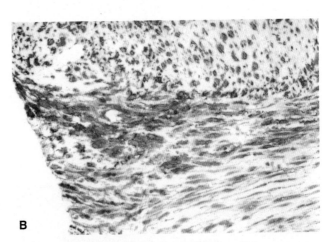

FIGURE 20.45 Leiomyosarcoma. A: A needle core biopsy specimen shows sarcoma infiltrating around a duct. **B:** The sarcoma is immunoreactive for smooth muscle actin.

Liposarcoma

Liposarcomas account for approximately 5% of the reported mammary sarcomas (220–222). The ages of the patients range from the teens to 90 years at the time of diagnosis, with an average age of 49 years. Two male patients have been described (220). The presenting symptom is a mass of variable duration occasionally accompanied by pain. Rare patients have presented with bilateral low-grade liposarcoma and bilateral multifocal liposarcoma. One woman was pregnant at the time of diagnosis, and a few others came to attention during the postpartum period (223). Pleomorphic liposarcoma of the chest wall has been reported after breast-conserving excision and irradiation and after mastectomy. Twenty-one months following resection of a myxoid liposarcoma from the thigh of a 66-year-old woman, a NCB specimen disclosed a solitary mammary metastasis (224).

The tumor is typically firm and well circumscribed, and the overlying skin is usually unaffected. Uncommon liposarcomas form ill-defined masses, and especially large examples can ulcerate. Imaging studies demonstrate a mass, which most often appears well defined and smoothly outlined. The presence of cystic and solid components may give rise to a complex echo pattern on the sonogram.

Liposarcomas span 2 to 40 cm and average approximately 8 cm. They consist of greasy yellow tissue. The presence of gray gelatinous tissue or mucoid material suggests a component of myxoid liposarcoma. Necrosis and cavitation can occur.

The histologic features of liposarcoma in the breast are identical to those of liposarcoma arising in the extremities or trunk. Among published reports, 14 (41%) were myxoid **(Fig. 20.46A)**, 9 (26%) were well differentiated, 7 (21%) were pleomorphic **(Figs. 20.46B,C)**, and 4 (12%) were poorly differentiated. The well-differentiated liposarcomas include several examples of sclerosing or fibrous liposarcomas. The cases do not demonstrate a relationship between tumor type, tumor size, and patient age at diagnosis.

Immunohistochemical staining yields the results seen in liposarcomas of other sites. The malignant cells do not stain for epithelial markers in most cases, and they typically stain for S-100. One tumor did not stain for ER or PR.

Nandipati et al. (223) tabulated the treatment and outcome of many reported cases of liposarcoma. Treatment often consisted of mastectomy; wide excision constituted the primary surgical procedure in a few cases. Axillary lymph node metastases have not been reported. In isolated cases, systemic chemotherapy and irradiation have been used for palliative purposes. With follow-up intervals ranging from less than a year to 20 years, approximately 70% of patients have remained recurrence-free, 6% were alive with systemic recurrence, and 24% died of metastatic liposarcoma. Systemic recurrences and deaths due to disease usually occurred within 2 years of diagnosis and were limited to patients with pleomorphic or high-grade tumors. The size of the tumor did not predict the patient's outcome.

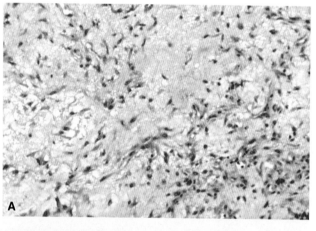

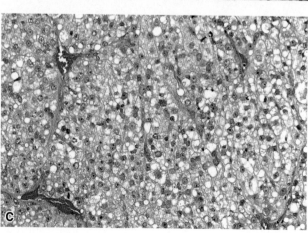

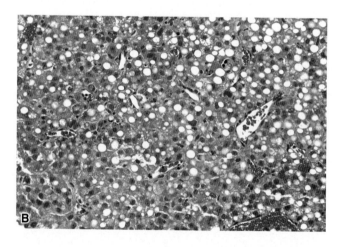

FIGURE 20.46 Liposarcoma. A: This myxoid liposarcoma exhibits the characteristic network of capillaries. **B:** The tumor in this needle core biopsy specimen shows the nuclear features of a pleomorphic liposarcoma. **C:** The excision specimen of the mass shown in **B** illustrates the presence of abundant cytoplasmic vacuoles of varying size.

Osteo- and Chondrosarcoma

Malignant tumors displaying the features of extraskeletal osteosarcomas or chondrosarcomas occasionally arise in the breast. Several authors point out that most mammary neoplasms with malignant osseous or cartilaginous differentiation represent heterologous metaplastic carcinomas or malignant phyllodes tumors. Rakha et al. (225) suggest that essentially all mammary malignancies showing osseous or chondroid features represent either matrix-producing metaplastic carcinomas or phyllodes tumors with massive stromal overgrowth. Irrespective of the pathogenesis of these malignant tumors, a body of literature describes their clinical and pathologic features.

The precise frequency of these neoplasms is difficult to determine because certain reports do not clearly exclude metaplastic carcinoma or phyllodes tumor. Publications by Silver and Tavassoli (226), Trihia et al. (227), and Pasta et al. (228) list many of the reported cases. The ages of the patients range from 16 to 96 years. The mean age in the largest series of osteosarcomas is 64.2 years (226). Origin in the male breast has been described rarely (226,229). The presenting symptom is a mass typically described as circumscribed and freely movable. A minority of the tumors are irregular or multinodular. Fixation to the skin or the chest wall and ulceration of the skin occur in a minority of the cases. Osteosarcoma has developed in the breast following breast conservation therapy, and both osteosarcoma and chondrosarcoma have arisen following postmastectomy irradiation.

Mammography reveals a dense mass, which can appear either well defined or ill defined. The mammographic appearance sometimes suggests the diagnosis of fibroadenoma. Tumors in which the osteosarcomatous component dominates appear heavily calcified and they may be positive on a technetium 99-methyl diphosphonate scan (230). Chondrosarcomatous tumors appear hyperdense and may contain calcifications.

The excised tumors have measured 1.5 to 25 cm in diameter, with an average size of 10 cm. A well-defined border is described in most cases. The mass consists of firm, gray or white tissue and often contains regions of softening, gelatinous degeneration, or necrosis. A gritty sensation is encountered when cutting areas of ossification.

Although the diagnosis of a mammary osteo- or chondrosarcoma may be suggested by the clinical findings and samples obtained by NCB (228,230,231), thorough examination of the excised tumor is necessary to ensure an accurate diagnosis. Histologic examination of the resected tumor typically reveals a spectrum of microscopic patterns (**Fig. 20.47**). The tumors have in common a prominent component of high-grade spindle cell sarcoma with a variable mitotic rate. Tumors with chondroid differentiation alone occur less frequently than those with both chondroid and osseous components. Multinucleate osteoclastic giant cells are usually present in areas of bone formation. Rarely, giant cells constitute a conspicuous element, and they may be associated with hemorrhagic cysts with a telangiectatic appearance.

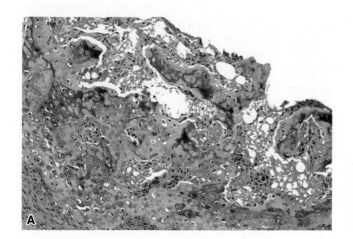

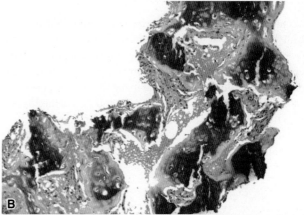

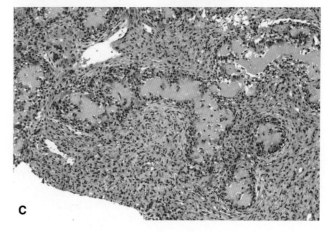

FIGURE 20.47 Osteochondrosarcoma. A: This needle core biopsy specimen shows moderately differentiated cartilage with ossification. Cytokeratin immunostains did not reveal evidence of epithelial differentiation. **B:** This part of the needle core biopsy specimen contains trabeculae of bone. **C:** Another area in the specimen consists of high-grade spindle cell sarcoma and osteoid.

Immunohistochemical staining for cytokeratins, myoepithelial proteins, and molecules found in muscle cells are negative. Lack of reactivity for cytokeratin and myoepithelial markers is essential to rule out an epithelial component and thereby exclude the diagnosis of metaplastic carcinoma. Areas with cartilaginous differentiation can be immunoreactive for EMA or S-100. None of the cases studied have expressed ER, PR, or HER2.

The series of patients studied by Silver and Tavassoli (226) provides the most detailed analysis of the treatment and clinical outcome of patients with mammary osteosarcomas. Complete excision of the sarcoma with negative margins is needed to forestall local recurrence of the tumor. Axillary staging is not necessary unless the clinical evaluation indicates otherwise. Metastases usually appear within a year from the time of diagnosis, and death ensues within a year or two from the appearance of metastases. Using the Kaplan–Meier method, the probability of overall survival is 38% at 5 years and 10% at 10 years (226). Patients with osteosarcomas smaller than 4.6 cm had a higher likelihood for survival than patients with larger tumors, and patients with the fibroblastic type of osteosarcoma had a better prognosis than patients with the osteoclastic or osteoblastic subtypes. Follow-up information provided in other reports support these observations. Irradiation and systemic chemotherapy have been administered in several cases, but the variable nature of these treatments precludes drawing secure conclusions regarding their efficacy.

Undifferentiated Pleomorphic Sarcoma (Malignant Fibrous Histiocytoma)

In contemporary parlance, the term malignant fibrous histiocytoma (MFH) has given way to the less-committal term, undifferentiated pleomorphic sarcoma (UPS). Although rare, this type of sarcoma represents a common type of mammary sarcoma. It accounts for 36% of the 240 breast sarcomas in the studies published after 1982 and tabulated by Adem et al. (171) and 24% of the 25 cases from the Mayo Clinic described in this publication.

The majority of patients have been women, but tumors of the male breast have been reported (232). Jeong et al. (233)

described the case of a 76-year-old man in whom a tumor classified as an "atypical spindle cell lesion" recurred after 1 year as an UPS. The age at diagnosis ranges from 24 to 93 years and averages 52 years. In one series, patients with low-grade tumors tended to be younger than patients with high-grade tumors (232). The initial symptom is a mass, which may be located in any portion of the breast. Reported symptomatic intervals vary from 1 month to 17 years. The tumors are usually solitary, but patients with multiple tumors have been described. The overlying skin can exhibit dimpling, induration, ecchymosis, or ulceration. Occasional patients give a history of antecedent trauma. In several case reports, irradiation for breast carcinoma preceded the presentation of the sarcoma.

The tumors measured from 1.0 to 20 cm (234). The average diameter is 7.5 cm. In a patient with multiple nodules, the two largest nodules each spanned 7.0 cm (235). The mass may have a circumscribed or an ill-defined border. The neoplasm consists of gray, tan, or white tissue that feels fleshy, firm, or hard. Hemorrhage, necrosis, mucoid change, and calcification are infrequent.

The microscopic hallmark of UPS is the storiform growth pattern in which the spindle cells are arranged in a pinwheel pattern (**Fig. 20.48**). Capillaries or small blood vessels may be found at the centers of the storiform collections. Multinucleate giant cells, myxoid change, and a chronic inflammatory cell infiltrate are variably present. Low-grade tumors have little mitotic activity, minimal pleomorphism, and scant or no necrosis. Easily identified mitoses, generally numbering more than 3 per HPF, prominent cellular pleomorphism, and necrosis characterize high-grade examples. Cellularity alone is not a reliable criterion for distinguishing between low- and high-grade tumors.

Immunohistochemical stains are not specific. The malignant cells are reactive for vimentin, occasionally for actin, and rarely for cytokeratin. All pathologic and clinical features must be given careful consideration when a tumor with storiform growth displays cytokeratin reactivity. Such lesions usually represent metaplastic carcinomas, but sarcomas can exhibit aberrant cytokeratin expression.

Treatment of most reported cases has been by mastectomy. A small minority of patients has been managed successfully

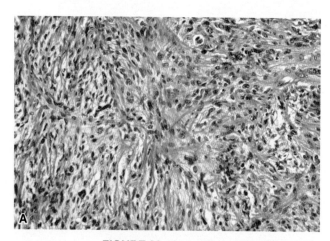
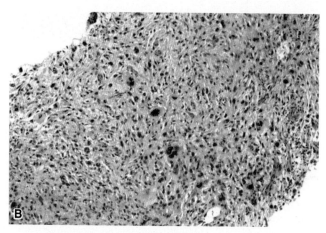

FIGURE 20.48 Undifferentiated Pleomorphic Sarcoma (Malignant Fibrous Histiocytoma). **A:** The spindle cell tumor has a typical storiform structure. No epithelial differentiation was detected. **B:** This needle core biopsy specimen from another tumor shows multinucleate giant cells.

by local excision alone. Local recurrences have developed after both mastectomy and local excision. The choice between mastectomy and local excision depends on the clinical details and must include consideration of the likelihood of obtaining complete excision with a cosmetically satisfactory result. Rare examples of MFH have metastasized to axillary lymph nodes (235), but axillary lymph node dissection is not indicated unless needed to obtain an adequate margin or the clinical findings suggest the presence of nodal metastases.

Recurrence and death due to disease have been reported in approximately 40% of the patients. Local recurrence is common among low-grade tumors. Metastases usually originate from high-grade tumors. Systemic recurrences and deaths most commonly occur within 3 years and rarely more than 5 years after diagnoses. The most frequent sites of metastases are the lungs and bones.

Fibrosarcoma

Fibrosarcoma, once a commonly used diagnosis for mammary sarcoma, has almost disappeared from use in the classification of mammary sarcomas. Bahrami and Folpe (236) reexamined 163 tumors of soft tissue classified as fibrosarcomas at the Mayo Clinic between 1960 and 2008 and confirmed the diagnosis in only 26 (16%) cases. The authors reclassified the remaining 137 tumors as 32 examples of UPS, 20 variants of fibrosarcoma, 78 mesenchymal tumors of other types, and 7 nonmesenchymal tumors. The authors concluded that "true [fibrosarcoma] is exceedingly rare…and should be diagnosed with great caution." Although the writers issued this warning in the context of tumors of soft tissues, it may apply to sarcomas of the breast equally well.

Currently proposed histologic criteria for the diagnosis of fibrosarcoma of soft tissue consist of hyperchromatic spindled cells showing no more than moderate pleomorphism, a fascicular, "herringbone" pattern of growth, the presence of interstitial collagen, the absence of morphologic features of all subtypes of fibrosarcomas (myxofibrosarcoma, low-grade fibromyxoid sarcoma, sclerosing epithelioid fibrosarcoma, and fibrosarcoma arising in dermatofibrosarcoma protruberans), and lack of expression of all markers except vimentin and very minimal SMA.

It seems reasonable to apply these criteria to sarcomas arising in the breast. Thus, mammary sarcomas composed of elongated spindle cells with hyperchromatic spindly nuclei, variably prominent nucleoli, and scant cytoplasm predominantly arranged in broad interdigitating sheets, bands, or fascicles displaying the "herringbone" pattern would be classified as fibrosarcoma. Mitotic figures are usually evident. The amount of extracellular collagen varies from sparse delicate strands to broad keloidal bands. According to the French system for grading sarcomas (FNCLCC), fibrosarcomas should fall in the grade 1 or grade 2 categories. Deviations from these characteristics should prompt consideration of another diagnosis. For example, tumors showing more than a moderate degree of cellular pleomorphism usually merit the diagnosis of UPS (MFH). The presence of large areas showing a storiform growth pattern would bring up the diagnosis of fibrosarcoma arising from a dermatofibrosarcoma protruberans (DFSP), and the presence of focal adipocytic differentiation would suggest the diagnosis of dedifferentiated liposarcoma. Tumors showing a loosely structured growth pattern without the typical "herringbone" arrangement or showing foci of osteoid formation without osteoblastic differentiation may represent a specific subtype of fibrosarcoma such as low-grade fibromyxoid sarcoma or myxofibrosarcoma. Finally, detection of proteins characteristic of stromal cells other than fibroblasts would exclude a sarcoma from the fibrosarcoma category. Staining of the tumor cells for CD34, for instance, would provoke consideration of the diagnosis of fibrosarcoma arising from either DFSP or solitary fibrous tumor.

Sarcomas such as synovial sarcoma, malignant peripheral nerve sheath tumor, solitary fibrous tumor, rhabdomyosarcoma, angiosarcoma, and epithelioid sarcoma and epithelial malignancies such as melanoma and spindle cell carcinoma sometimes display regions resembling fibrosarcomas. Immunohistochemical staining and testing for genetic alterations should allow one to exclude these possibilities in problematic cases.

These considerations suggest that one should probably consider the diagnosis of fibrosarcoma only after excluding all other possibilities. The limited information provided in published cases of mammary fibrosarcomas does not allow one to evaluate the nature of the sarcomas thoroughly; consequently, the diagnosis of fibrosarcoma remains open to question in almost every instance. Several recently reported cases (237–240) may represent a *bona fide* mammary fibrosarcomas.

The lack of well-documented cases of fibrosarcoma makes it impossible to make secure statements about the clinical behavior and optimal treatment of this type of sarcoma. Lacking well-founded information, physicians should probably evaluate and treat patients with fibrosarcomas according to the principles used for treatment of other types of mammary sarcoma.

Hemangiopericytoma (Solitary Fibrous Tumor)

In recent years, pathologists who specialize in diseases of the soft tissues have come to believe that the entity originally termed hemangiopericytoma represents a cellular variety of solitary fibrous tumors. The latter term has replaced the former when referring to this lesion in most sites, but publications still appear referring to tumors of the breast as hemangiopericytomas.

Irrespective of one's choice of terminology, this lesion is an uncommon neoplasm of the breast. Fewer than 30 cases have been reported. The publication of Kanazawa et al. (241) lists clinical and pathologic features of 25 cases reported in the English and Japanese literatures, and the report of Koukourakis et al. (242) cites several cases reported subsequently. With the exception of two children, all the other patients were adults (24 women and 4 men) between the ages of 24 and 81 years. The patients presented with enlarging painless masses, which occurred in the left and right breasts with equal frequency. The masses usually had been present for a few weeks or months, but symptomatic intervals as long as 1 year have been noted. Physicians described the masses as irregular and firm. Hemangiopericytomas (solitary fibrous tumors) originating from extramammary sites have metastasized to the breast, and a hemangiopericytoma (solitary fibrous tumor) of the pectoralis major presented as a breast mass (243).

Mammography reveals a dense mass lacking calcifications, and sonography demonstrates a solid hypoechogenic mass with heterogeneous internal echoes and posterior enhancement (244).

The diameters of these well-circumscribed round to oval tumors range from 1 (245) to 20 cm (234), and the average size is 6.5 cm. They consist of firm to hard, homogeneous pale yellow, gray, or white tissue. It may display a whorled texture with dilated vascular spaces and a nodular contour.

The histologic features of mammary hemangiopericytomas (solitary fibrous tumors) duplicate those of the examples arising in other sites. The tumor consists of regions of variable cellularity distributed in a seemingly patternless way **(Fig. 20.49)**.

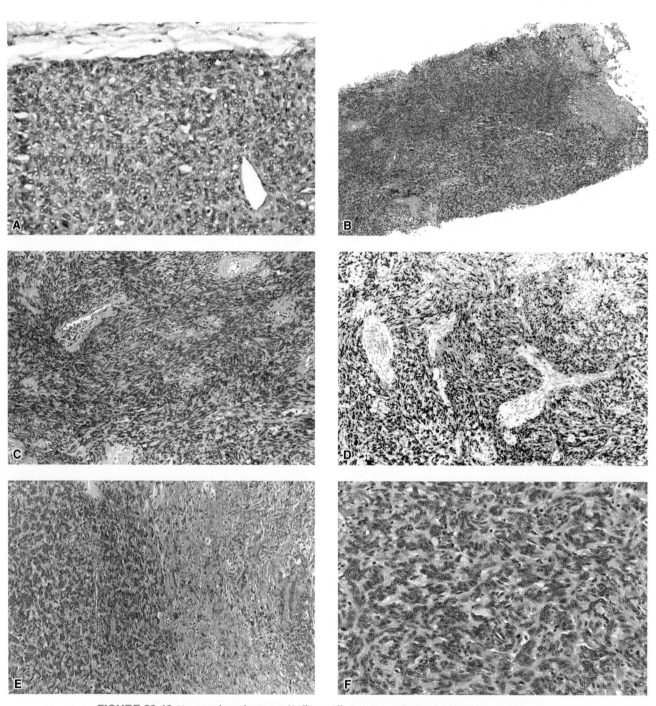

FIGURE 20.49 Hemangiopericytoma (Solitary Fibrous Tumor). A: The tumor has a circumscribed border. Numerous capillaries contain red blood cells. The dilated, empty vascular space in the lower right corner is a characteristic element. **B:** The needle core biopsy specimen from another hemangiopericytoma (solitary fibrous tumor) shows a well-defined mass. **C:** Spindle cells, collagen, and thick-walled blood vessels compose the mass shown in **B**. **D:** An immunostain for STAT6 is shown. **E, F:** The excision specimen from the mass shown in **B** to **D** displays regions of variable cellularity and aggregates of small, uniform tumor cells with bland nuclei.

The round, oval, or spindle-shaped tumor cells form sheets, bands, and trabeculae around vascular spaces. The cells possess uniform bland nuclei, and mitotic figures are infrequent. The vessels vary in caliber and typically display a branching or "staghorn" configuration. Perivascular fibrosis is variably present. Focal fibrosis may be especially prominent at the tumor margin, where atrophic breast tissue compressed by the expanding tumor tends to form a pseudocapsule. Necrosis rarely occurs in mammary hemangiopericytomas (solitary fibrous tumors). Histologic findings suggesting an aggressive nature include an infiltrative border, cytologic atypia, and noticeable mitotic activity (246).

The tumor cells typically express CD34 vimentin, CD99, STAT6 (247), and bcl-2. They do not stain for keratin. Endothelial cells lining the capillaries are immunoreactive for *Ulex europaeus* 1 lectin (UEA-1), factor VIII, CD34, and CD31.

The differential diagnosis mainly centers on other malignant tumors. Benign tumors such as myoepithelioma, myofibroblastoma, and peripheral nerve sheath tumor could have areas that superficially resemble hemangiopericytoma (solitary fibrous tumor), but these lesions do not exhibit the structural, morphologic, or immunohistochemical characteristics of a hemangiopericytoma (solitary fibrous tumor). Malignant tumors such as high-grade leiomyosarcoma and UPS may have vascular areas that resemble hemangiopericytoma (solitary fibrous tumor). These sarcomas have readily identifiable mitotic figures and exhibit other structural features that distinguish the tumors from hemangiopericytomas (solitary fibrous tumors). Metastatic sarcomatous renal carcinoma may mimic mammary hemangiopericytoma (solitary fibrous tumor), and rarely hemangiopericytoma (solitary fibrous tumor) originating at another site may spread to the breast. Staining for STAT6 may prove especially useful in resolving the diagnosis in problematic cases.

Reported follow-up varies from less than 12 months to 276 months. Approximately equal numbers of patients have been treated by mastectomy and local excision. No patient had metastases detected in axillary lymph nodes. None of the patients described in published reports has developed a local recurrence whether treated by local excision or mastectomy, with follow-up as long as 23 years and averaging 5 years. One patient treated with a modified radical mastectomy for a 5.5-cm malignant hemangiopericytoma (solitary fibrous tumor) apparently confined to the breast succumbed to disease involving the bones, brain, lungs, pleura, skin, and liver 14 months from the time of diagnosis (248). It seems that mammary hemangiopericytomas (solitary fibrous tumors) that lack high-grade features such as necrosis or numerous mitoses should be considered low-grade neoplasms. Treatment can be conservative, with emphasis on wide local excision rather than mastectomy if an adequate margin can be achieved with an acceptable cosmetic result. Axillary dissection is not indicated.

Other Sarcomas

Other sarcomas described in the breast include primary and metastatic *rhabdomyosarcoma* (249), *malignant peripheral nerve sheath tumor* (250), primary and metastatic *primitive neuroectodermal tumor* (EFT) (251,252), primary and metastatic *alveolar soft part sarcoma* (253,254), *synovial sarcoma* (255), *myofibroblastic sarcoma* (256), Kaposi sarcoma (257), myxoid variant of follicular dendritic cell sarcoma (258), and angioblastic sarcoma.

REFERENCES

Benign Mesenchymal Lesions

1. Rosen PP, Ernsberger D. Mammary fibromatosis: a benign spindle-cell tumor with significant risk for local recurrence. *Cancer.* 1989;63:1363–1369.
2. Wargotz ES, Norris HJ, Austin RM, et al. Fibromatosis of the breast: a clinical and pathological study of 28 cases. *Am J Surg Pathol.* 1987;11:38–45.
3. Gump FE, Sternschein MJ, Wolff M. Fibromatosis of the breast. *Surg Gynecol Obstet.* 1981;153:57–60.
4. Haggitt RC, Booth JL. Bilateral fibromatosis of the breast in Gardner's syndrome. *Cancer.* 1970;25:161–166.
5. Needelman P, Leibman AJ, Capasse J. Fibromatosis of the axillary breast in a young patient. *Breast Dis.* 1996;9:171–175.
6. Mátrai Z, Tóth L, Gulyás G, et al. A desmoid tumor associated with a ruptured silicone breast implant. *Plast Reconstr Surg.* 2011;127:1e–4e.
7. Balzer BL, Weiss SW. Do biomaterials cause implant-associated mesenchymal tumors of the breast? Analysis of 8 new cases and review of the literature. *Hum Pathol.* 2009;40:1564–1570.
8. Plaza MJ, Yepes M. Breast fibromatosis response to tamoxifen: dynamic MRI findings and review of the current treatment options. *J Radiol Case Rep.* 2012;6:16–23.
9. Abraham SC, Reynolds C, Lee JH, et al. Fibromatosis of the breast and mutations involving the APC/beta-catenin pathway. *Hum Pathol.* 2002;33:39–46.
10. Neuman HB, Brogi E, Ebrahim A, et al. Desmoid tumors (fibromatoses) of the breast: a 25-year experience. *Ann Surg Oncol.* 2008;15:274–280.
11. Kim T, Jung EA, Song JY, et al. Prevalence of the CTNNB1 mutation genotype in surgically resected fibromatosis of the breast. *Histopathology.* 2012;60:347–356.
12. Pettinato G, Manivel JC, Gould EW, et al. Inclusion body fibromatosis of the breast: two cases with immunohistochemical and ultrastructural findings. *Am J Clin Pathol.* 1994;101:714–718.
13. Lacroix-Triki M, Geyer FC, Lambros MB, et al. Beta-catenin/Wnt signalling pathway in fibromatosis, metaplastic carcinomas and phyllodes tumours of the breast. *Mod Pathol.* 2010;23:1438–1448.
14. Brown V, Carty NJ. A case of nodular fasciitis of the breast and review of the literature. *Breast.* 2005;14:384–387.
15. Samardzic D, Chetlen A, Malysz J. Nodular fasciitis in the axillary tail of the breast. *J Radiol Case Rep.* 2014;8:16–26.
16. Maly B, Maly A. Nodular fasciitis of the breast: report of a case initially diagnosed by fine needle aspiration cytology. *Acta Cytol.* 2001;45:794–796.
17. Green JS, Crozier AE, Walker RA. Case report: nodular fasciitis of the breast. *Clin Radiol.* 1997;52:961–962.
18. Squillaci S, Tallarigo F, Patarino R, Bisceglia M. Nodular fasciitis of the male breast: a case report. *Int J Surg Pathol.* 2007;15:69–72.
19. Iwatani T, Kawabata H, Miura D, et al. Nodular fasciitis of the breast. *Breast Cancer.* 2012;19:180–182.
20. Stanley MW, Skoog L, Tani EM, et al. Nodular fasciitis: spontaneous resolution following diagnosis by fine-needle aspiration. *Diagn Cytopathol.* 1993;9:322–324.
21. Puente JL, Potel J. Fibrous tumor of the breast. *Arch Surg.* 1974;109:391–394.
22. Rosen EL, Soo MS, Bentley RC. Focal fibrosis: a common breast lesion diagnosed at imaging-guided core biopsy. *AJR Am J Roentgenol.* 1999;173:1657–1662.
23. Harvey SC, Denison CM, Lester SC, et al. Fibrous nodules found at large-core needle biopsy of the breast: imaging features. *Radiology.* 1999;211:535–540.
24. Chowdhury N, Bhat RV, Barman PP. Fibrous tumor of the breast: case report of an underrecognized entity. *Patholog Res Int.* 2011;2010:847594.

25. Vuitch MF, Rosen PP, Erlandson RA. Pseudoangiomatous hyperplasia of mammary stroma. *Hum Pathol.* 1986;17:185–191.

26. Asioli S, Eusebi V, Gaetano L, et al. The pre-lymphatic pathway, the rooths of the lymphatic system in breast tissue: a 3D study. *Virchows Arch.* 2008;453:401–406.

27. Ibrahim RE, Sciotto CG, Weidner N. Pseudoangiomatous hyperplasia of mammary stroma: some observations regarding its clinicopathologic spectrum. *Cancer.* 1989;63:1154–1160.

28. Degnim AC, Frost MH, Radisky DC, et al. Pseudoangiomatous stromal hyperplasia and breast cancer risk. *Ann Surg Oncol.* 2010;17:3269–3277.

29. Anderson C, Ricci A Jr, Pedersen CA, et al. Immunocytochemical analysis of estrogen and progesterone receptors in benign stromal lesions of the breast: evidence for hormonal etiology in pseudoangiomatous hyperplasia of mammary stroma. *Am J Surg Pathol.* 1991;15:145–149.

30. Powell CM, Cranor ML, Rosen PP. Pseudoangiomatous stromal hyperplasia (PASH): a mammary stromal tumor with myofibroblastic differentiation. *Am J Surg Pathol.* 1995;19:270–277.

31. Mercado CL, Naidrich SA, Hamele-Bena D, et al. Pseudoangiomatous stromal hyperplasia of the breast: sonographic features with histopathologic correlation. *Breast J.* 2004;10:427–432.

32. Ferreira M, Albarracin CT, Resetkova E. Pseudoangiomatous stromal hyperplasia tumor: a clinical, radiologic and pathologic study of 26 cases. *Mod Pathol.* 2008;21:201–207.

33. Shehata BM, Fishman I, Collings MH, et al. Pseudoangiomatous stromal hyperplasia of the breast in pediatric patients: an underrecognized entity. *Pediatr Dev Pathol.* 2009;12:450–454.

34. Bowman E, Oprea G, Okoli J, et al. Pseudoangiomatous stromal hyperplasia (PASH) of the breast: a series of 24 patients. *Breast J.* 2012;18:242–247.

35. Singh KA, Lewis MM, Runge RL, et al. Pseudoangiomatous stromal hyperplasia: a case for bilateral mastectomy in a 12-year-old girl. *Breast J.* 2007;13:603–606.

36. Milanezi MF, Saggioro FP, Zanati SG, et al. Pseudoangiomatous hyperplasia of mammary stroma associated with gynaecomastia. *J Clin Pathol.* 1998;51:204–206.

37. Pižem J, Velikonja M, Matjašič A, et al. Pseudoangiomatous stromal hyperplasia with multinucleated stromal giant cells is neither exceptional in gynecomastia nor characteristic of neurofibromatosis type 1. *Virchows Arch.* 2015;466:465–472.

38. Badve S, Sloane JP. Pseudoangiomatous hyperplasia of male breast. *Histopathology.* 1995;26:463–466.

39. Mizutou A, Nakashima K, Moriya T. Large pseudoangiomatous stromal hyperplasia complicated with gynecomastia and lobular differentiation in a male breast. *SpringerPlus.* 2015;4:282.

40. Vega RM, Pechman D, Ergonul B, et al. Bilateral pseudoangiomatous stromal hyperplasia tumors in axillary male gynecomastia: report of a case. *Surg Today.* 2015;45:105–109.

41. Seidman JD, Borkowski A, Aisner SC, et al. Rapid growth of pseudoangiomatous hyperplasia of mammary stroma in axillary gynecomastia in an immunosuppressed patient. *Arch Pathol Lab Med.* 1993;117:736–738.

42. Kollias J, Gill PG, Leong AS, et al. Gynaecomastia presenting as fibroadenomatoid tumours of the breast arising in a renal transplant recipient associated with cyclosporin treatment. *ANZ J Surg.* 1998;68:679–681.

43. Larbcharoensub N, Wattanatranon D, Sanpaphant S, et al. Bilateral pseudoangiomatous stromal hyperplasia in a human immunodeficiency viral-infected patient. *Indian J Pathol Microbiol.* 2015;58:356–358.

44. Iancu D, Nochomovitz LE. Pseudoangiomatous stromal hyperplasia: presentation as a mass in the female nipple. *Breast J.* 2001;7:263–265.

45. Jordan AC, Jaffer S, Mercer SE. Massive nodular pseudoangiomatous stromal hyperplasia (PASH) of the breast arising simultaneously in the axilla and vulva. *Int J Surg Pathol.* 2011;19:113–116.

46. Almohawes E, Khoumais N, Arafah M. Pseudoangiomatous stromal hyperplasia of the breast: a case report of a 12-year-old girl. *Radiol Case Rep.* 2015;10:1–4.

47. Cohen MA, Morris EA, Rosen PP, et al. Pseudoangiomatous stromal hyperplasia: mammographic, sonographic, and clinical patterns. *Radiology.* 1996;198:117–120.

48. Damiani S, Eusebi V. Gynecomastia in type-1 neurofibromatosis with features of pseudoangiomatous stromal hyperplasia with giant cells: report of two cases. *Virchows Arch.* 2001;438:513–516.

49. Pruthi S, Reynolds C, Johnson RE, et al. Tamoxifen in the management of pseudoangiomatous stromal hyperplasia. *Breast J.* 2001;7:434–439.

50. Seltzer MH, Kintiroglou M. Pseudoangiomatous stromal hyperplasia and response to tamoxifen therapy. *Breast J.* 2003;9:344.

51. Wargotz ES, Weiss SW, Norris HJ. Myofibroblastoma of the breast: sixteen cases of a distinctive benign mesenchymal tumor. *Am J Surg Pathol.* 1987;11:493–502.

52. Hamele-Bena D, Cranor ML, Sciotto C, et al. Uncommon presentation of mammary myofibroblastoma. *Mod Pathol.* 1996;9:786–790.

53. Magro G, Bisceglia M, Michal M, et al. Spindle cell lipoma-like tumor, solitary fibrous tumor and myofibroblastoma of the breast: a clinico-pathological analysis of 13 cases in favor of a unifying histogenetic concept. *Virchows Arch.* 2002;440:249–260.

54. Soyer T, Ayva S, Senyucel MF, et al. Myofibroblastoma of breast in a male infant. *Fetal Pediatr Pathol.* 2012;31:164–168.

55. Bégin LR. Myogenic stromal tumor of the male breast (so-called myofibroblastoma). *Ultrastruct Pathol.* 1991;15:613–622.

56. Abeysekara AM, Siriwardana HP, Abbas KF, et al. An unusually large myofibroblastoma in a male breast: a case report. *J Med Case Rep.* 2008;2:157.

57. Toker C, Tang CK, Whitely JF, et al. Benign spindle cell breast tumor. *Cancer.* 1981;48:1615–1622.

58. Rebner M, Raju U. Myofibroblastoma of the male breast. *Breast Dis.* 1993;6:157–160.

59. Greenberg JS, Kaplan SS, Grady C. Myofibroblastoma of the breast in women: imaging appearances. *AJR Am J Roentgenol.* 1998;171:71–72.

60. Kataria K, Srivastava A, Singh L, et al. Giant myofibroblastoma of the male breast: a case report and literature review. *Malays J Med Sci.* 2012;19:74–76.

61. Bharathi K, Chandrasekar VA, Hemanathan G, et al. Myofibroblastoma of female breast masquerading as schirrous malignancy—a rare case report with review of literature. *J Clin Diagn Res.* 2014;8:ND10–ND11.

62. Ali S, Teichberg S, DeRisi DC, et al. Giant myofibroblastoma of the male breast. *Am J Surg Pathol.* 1994;18:1170–1176.

63. Fukunaga M, Ushigome S. Myofibroblastoma of the breast with diverse differentiations. *Arch Pathol Lab Med.* 1997;121:599–603.

64. Magro G, Amico P, Gurrera A. Myxoid myofibroblastoma of the breast with atypical cells: a potential diagnostic pitfall. *Virchows Arch.* 2007;450:483–485.

65. Magro G, Foschini MP, Eusebi V. Palisaded myofibroblastoma of the breast: a tumor closely mimicking schwannoma: report of 2 cases. *Hum Pathol.* 2013;44:1941–1946.

66. Thomas TM, Myint A, Mak CK, et al. Mammary myofibroblastoma with leiomyomatous differentiation. *Am J Clin Pathol.* 1997;107:52–55.

67. Magro G. Epithelioid-cell myofibroblastoma of the breast: expanding the morphologic spectrum. *Am J Surg Pathol.* 2009;33:1085–1092.

68. Magro G, Vecchio GM, Michal M, et al. Atypical epithelioid cell myofibroblastoma of the breast with multinodular growth pattern: a potential pitfall of malignancy. *Pathol Res Pract.* 2013;209:463–466.

69. Magro G, Gangemi P, Greco P. Deciduoid-like myofibroblastoma of the breast: a potential pitfall of malignancy. *Histopathology.* 2008;52:652–654.

70. Magro G, Salvatorelli L, Spadola S, et al. Mammary myofibroblastoma with extensive myxoedematous stromal changes: a potential diagnostic pitfall. *Pathol Res Pract.* 2014;210:1106–1111.

71. Magro G, Michal M, Vasquez E, et al. Lipomatous myofibroblastoma: a potential diagnostic pitfall in the spectrum of the spindle cell lesions of the breast. *Virchows Arch.* 2000;437:540–544.

72. Magro G, Longo FR, Salvatorelli L, et al. Lipomatous myofibroblastoma of the breast: case report with diagnostic and histogenetic considerations. *Pathologica.* 2014;106:36–40.

73. Magro G, Fraggetta F, Torrisi A, et al. Myofibroblastoma of the breast with hemangiopericytoma-like pattern and pleomorphic lipoma-like areas: report of a case with diagnostic and histogenetic considerations. *Pathol Res Pract.* 1999;195:257–262.

74. Fritchie KJ, Carver P, Sun Y, et al. Solitary fibrous tumor: is there a molecular relationship with cellular angiofibroma, spindle cell lipoma, and mammary-type myofibroblastoma? *Am J Clin Pathol.* 2012;137:963–970.

75. Pauwels P, Sciot R, Croiset P, et al. Myofibroblastoma of the breast: genetic link with spindle cell lipoma. *J Pathol.* 2000;191:282–285.

76. Trepant AL, Sibille C, Frunza AM, et al. Myofibroblastoma of the breast with smooth muscle differentiation showing deletion of 13q14 region: report of a case. *Pathol Res Pract.* 2014;210:389–391.

77. Magro G, Righi A, Casorzo L, et al. Mammary and vaginal myofibroblastomas are genetically related lesions: fluorescence in situ hybridization analysis shows deletion of 13q14 region. *Hum Pathol.* 2012;43:1887–1893.

78. Dal Cin P, Sciot R, Polito P, et al. Lesions of 13q may occur independently of deletion of 16q in spindle cell/pleomorphic lipomas. *Histopathology.* 1997;31:222–225.

79. Ibrahim HA, Shousha S. Myofibroblastoma of the female breast with admixed but distinct foci of spindle cell lipoma: a case report. *Case Rep Pathol.* 2013;2013:738014.

80. Wahbah MM, Gilcrease MZ, Wu Y. Lipomatous variant of myofibroblastoma with epithelioid features: a rare and diagnostically challenging breast lesion. *Ann Diagn Pathol.* 2011;15:454–458.

81. Turnbull AD, Huvos AG, Ashikari R, et al. Granular-cell myoblastoma of breast. *N Y State J Med.* 1971;71:436–438.

82. Papalas JA, Wylie JD, Dash RC. Recurrence risk and margin status in granular cell tumors of the breast: a clinicopathologic study of 13 patients. *Arch Pathol Lab Med.* 2011;135:890–895.

83. Desimone RA, Ginter PS, Chen YT. Granular cell tumor of the breast eliciting exuberant pseudoepitheliomatous hyperplasia. *Int J Surg Pathol.* 2014;22:156–157.

84. Coates SJ, Mitchell K, Olorunnipa OB, et al. An unusual breast lesion: granular cell tumor of the breast with extensive chest wall invasion. *J Surg Oncol.* 2014;110:345–347.

85. Gibbons D, Leitch M, Coscia J, et al. Fine needle aspiration cytology and histologic findings of granular cell tumor of the breast: review of 19 cases with clinical/radiologic correlation. *Breast J.* 2000;6:27–30.

86. Adeniran A, Al-Ahmadie H, Mahoney MC, et al. Granular cell tumor of the breast: a series of 17 cases and review of the literature. *Breast J.* 2004;10:528–531.

87. Patel HB, Leibman AJ. Granular cell tumor in a male breast: mammographic, sonographic, and pathologic features. *J Clin Ultrasound.* 2013;41:119–121.

88. Brown AC, Audisio RA, Regitnig P. Granular cell tumour of the breast. *Surg Oncol.* 2011;20:97–105.

89. Mátrai Z, Langmár Z, Szabó E, et al. Granular cell tumour of the breast: case series and review of the literature. *Eur J Gynaecol Oncol.* 2010;31:636–640.

90. Tai G, D'Costa H, Lee D, et al. Case report: coincident granular cell tumour of the breast with invasive ductal carcinoma. *Br J Radiol.* 1995;68:1034–1036.

91. Rekhi B, Jambhekar NA. Morphologic spectrum, immunohistochemical analysis, and clinical features of a series of granular cell tumors of soft tissues: a study from a tertiary referral cancer center. *Ann Diagn Pathol.* 2010;14:162–167.

92. Akahane K, Kato K, Ogiso S, et al. Malignant granular cell tumor of the breast: case report and literature review. *Breast Cancer.* 2015;22(3):317–323. doi:10.1007/s12282-120-0362-1.

93. Uzoaru I, Firfer B, Ray V, et al. Malignant granular cell tumor. *Arch Pathol Lab Med.* 1992;116:206–208.

94. Chen J, Wang L, Xu J, et al. Malignant granular cell tumor with breast metastasis: a case report and review of the literature. *Oncol Lett.* 2012;4:63–66.

95. Fujii T, Yajima R, Morita H, et al. A rare case of anterior chest wall schwannoma masquerading as a breast tumor. *Int Surg.* 2014;99:196–199.

96. Datta S, Pal A, Maiti M, et al. Rare case of chest wall schwannoma with destruction of rib, masquerading as a breast mass. *J Clin Diagn Res.* 2014;8:FD01–FD02.

97. Cho YR, Jones S, Gosain AK. Neurofibromatosis: a cause of prepubertal gynecomastia. *Plast Reconstr Surg.* 2008;121:34e–40e.

98. Bellezza G, Lombardi T, Panzarola P, et al. Schwannoma of the breast: a case report and review of the literature. *Tumori.* 2007;93:308–311.

99. Uchida N, Yokoo H, Kuwano H. Schwannoma of the breast: report of a case. *Surg Today.* 2005;35:238–242.

100. Thejaswini M, Padmaja K, Srinivasamurthy V, et al. Solitary intramammary schwannoma mimicking phylloides tumor: cytological clues in the diagnosis. *J Cytol.* 2012;29:258–260.

101. Salihoglu A, Esatoglu SN, Eskazan AE, et al. Breast schwannoma in a patient with diffuse large B-cell lymphoma: a case report. *J Med Case Rep.* 2012;6:423.

102. Lee EK, Kook SH, Kwag HJ, et al. Schwannoma of the breast showing massive exophytic growth: a case report. *Breast.* 2006;15:562–566.

103. Galant C, Mazy S, Berliere M, et al. Two schwannomas presenting as lumps in the same breast. *Diagn Cytopathol.* 1997;16:281–284.

104. Bongiorno MR, Doukaki S, Arico M. Neurofibromatosis of the nipple-areolar area: a case series. *J Med Case Rep.* 2010;4:22.

105. Friedrich RE, Hagel C. Appendices of the nipple and areola of the breast in Neurofibromatosis type 1 patients are neurofibromas. *Anticancer Res.* 2010;30:1815–1817.

106. Gokalp G, Hakyemez B, Kizilkaya E, et al. Myxoid neurofibromas of the breast: mammographical, sonographical and MRI appearances. *Br J Radiol.* 2007;80:e234–e237.

107. Gultekin SH, Cody HS III, Hoda SA. Schwannoma of the breast. *South Med J.* 1996;89:238–239.

108. Casey P, Stephens M, Kirby RM. A rare cystic breast lump—schwannoma of the breast. *Breast J.* 2012;18:491–492.

109. *Stedman's Medical Dictionary.* 28th ed. Baltimore, MD: Lippincott Williams & Wilkins; 1982.

110. *Churchill's Illustrated Medical Dictionary.* New York, NY: Churchill Livingstone; 1989.

111. Herbert M, Sandbank J, Liokumovich P, et al. Breast hamartomas: clinicopathological and immunohistochemical studies of 24 cases. *Histopathology.* 2002;41:30–34.

112. Sevim Y, Kocaay AF, Eker T, et al. Breast hamartoma: a clinicopathologic analysis of 27 cases and a literature review. *Clinics (Sao Paulo).* 2014;69:515–523.

113. Wahner-Roedler DL, Sebo TJ, Gisvold JJ. Hamartomas of the breast: clinical, radiologic, and pathologic manifestations. *Breast J.* 2001;7:101–105.

114. Birrell AL, Warren LR, Birrell SN. Misdiagnosis of massive breast asymmetry: giant hamartoma. *ANZ J Surg.* 2012;82:941–942.

115. Weinzweig N, Botts J, Marcus E. Giant hamartoma of the breast. *Plast Reconstr Surg.* 2001;107:1216–1220.

116. Desai A, Ramesar K, Allan S, et al. Breast hamartoma arising in axillary ectopic breast tissue. *Breast J.* 2010;16:433–434.

117. Kapucuoglu N, Percinel S, Angelone A. Adenohibernoma of the breast. *Virchows Arch.* 2008;452:351–352.

118. Tse GM, Law BK, Ma TK, et al. Hamartoma of the breast: a clinicopathological review. *J Clin Pathol.* 2002;55:951–954.

119. Daya D, Trus T, D'Souza TJ, et al. Hamartoma of the breast, an under-recognized breast lesion: a clinicopathologic and radiographic study of 25 cases. *Am J Clin Pathol.* 1995;103:685–689.

120. Eusebi V, Cunsolo A, Fedeli F, et al. Benign smooth muscle cell metaplasia in breast. *Tumori.* 1980;66:643–653.

121. Stafyla V, Kotsifopoulos N, Grigoriadis K, et al. Myoid hamartoma of the breast: a case report and review of the literature. *Breast J.* 2007;13:85–87.

122. Davies JD, Riddell RH. Muscular hamartomas of the breast. *J Pathol.* 1973;111:209–211.

123. Nascimento AG, Karas M, Rosen PP, et al. Leiomyoma of the nipple. *Am J Surg Pathol.* 1979;3:151–154.

124. Cho HJ, Kim SH, Kang BJ, et al. Leiomyoma of the nipple diagnosed by MRI. *Acta Radiol Short Rep.* 2012;1(9). pii:arsr.2012.120025.

125. Minami S, Matsuo S, Azuma T, et al. Parenchymal leiomyoma of the breast: a case report with special reference to magnetic resonance imaging findings and an update review of literature. *Breast Cancer.* 2011;18:231–236.

126. Granic M, Stefanovic-Radovic M, Zdravkovic D, et al. Intraparenchimal leiomyoma of the breast. *Arch Iran Med.* 2015;18:608–612.

127. Strader LA, Galan K, Tenofsky PL. Intraparenchymal leiomyoma of the male breast. *Breast J.* 2013;19:675–676.

128. Pavlidis L, Vakirlis E, Spyropoulou GA, et al. A 35-year-old woman presenting with an unusual post-traumatic leiomyoma of the nipple: a case report. *J Med Case Rep.* 2013;7:49.

129. Wang H, Luo B, Li F. Nipple inversion caused by a breast leiomyoma. *Breast J.* 2012;18:376–377.

130. Deveci U, Kapakli MS, Altintoprak F, et al. Bilateral nipple leiomyoma. *Case Rep Surg.* 2013;2013:475215.

131. Nakamura S, Hashimoto Y, Takeda K, et al. Two cases of male nipple leiomyoma: idiopathic leiomyoma and gynecomastia-associated leiomyoma. *Am J Dermatopathol.* 2012;34:287–291.

132. Alawad AA. Multiple parenchymal leiomyomas of the breast in a Sudanese female. *Breast Dis.* 2014;34:165–167.

133. Roncaroli F, Rossi R, Severi B, et al. Epithelioid leiomyoma of the breast with granular cell change: a case report. *Hum Pathol.* 1993;24:1260–1263.

134. Vecchio GM, Cavaliere A, Cartaginese F, et al. Intraparenchymal leiomyoma of the breast: report of a case with emphasis on needle core biopsy-based diagnosis. *Pathologica.* 2013;105:122–127.

135. Boscaino A, Ferrara G, Orabona P, et al. Smooth muscle tumors of the breast: clinicopathologic features of two cases. *Tumori.* 1994;80:241–245.

136. Groh O, In't Hof K. Giant lipoma of the male breast: case report and review of literature. *Eur J Plast Surg.* 2012;35:407–409.

137. Schmidt J, Schelling M, Lerf B, et al. Giant lipoma of the breast. *Breast J.* 2009;15:107–108.

138. Li YF, Lv MH, Chen LF, et al. Giant lipoma of the breast: a case report and review of the literature. *Clin Breast Cancer.* 2011;11:420–422.

139. Pui MH, Movson IJ. Fatty tissue breast lesions. *Clin Imaging.* 2003;27:150–155.

140. Riley MP, Karamchandani DM. Mammary hibernoma: a rare entity. *Arch Pathol Lab Med.* 2015;139:1565–1567.

141. Kaplan L, Walts AE. Benign chondrolipomatous tumor of the human female breast. *Arch Pathol Lab Med.* 1977;101:149–151.

142. Lugo M, Reyes JM, Putong PB. Benign chondrolipomatous tumors of the breast. *Arch Pathol Lab Med.* 1982;106:691–692.

143. Marsh WL Jr, Lucas JG, Olsen J. Chondrolipoma of the breast. *Arch Pathol Lab Med.* 1989;113:369–371.

144. Banev SG, Filipovski VA. Chondrolipoma of the breast—case report and a review of literature. *Breast.* 2006;15:425–426.

145. Hansen PE, Williamson EO. Lipoma with central fat necrosis: is core biopsy a good way to diagnose fat necrosis of the breast? *Breast J.* 1999;5:202–203.

146. Chan KW, Ghadially FN, Alagaratnam TT. Benign spindle cell tumour of breast—a variant of spindled cell lipoma or fibroma of breast? *Pathology.* 1984;16:331–336.

147. Lew WY. Spindle cell lipoma of the breast: a case report and literature review. *Diagn Cytopathol.* 1993;9:434–437.

148. Smith DN, Denison CM, Lester SC. Spindle cell lipoma of the breast: a case report. *Acta Radiol.* 1996;37:893–895.

149. Noel JC, Van Geertruyden J, Engohan-Aloghe C. Angiolipoma of the breast in a male: a case report and review of the literature. *Int J Surg Pathol.* 2011;19:813–816.

150. Jozefczyk MA, Rosen PP. Vascular tumors of the breast: II: perilobular hemangiomas and hemangiomas. *Am J Surg Pathol.* 1985;9:491–503.

151. Rosen PP, Ridolfi RL. The perilobular hemangioma: a benign microscopic vascular lesion of the breast. *Am J Clin Pathol.* 1977;68:21–23.

152. Lesueur GC, Brown RW, Bhathal PS. Incidence of perilobular hemangioma in the female breast. *Arch Pathol Lab Med.* 1983;107:308–310.

153. Vourtsi A, Zervoudis S, Pafiti A, et al. Male breast hemangioma—a rare entity: a case report and review of the literature. *Breast J.* 2006;12:260–262.

154. Glazenbrook KN, Morton MJ, Reynolds C. Vascular tumors of the breast: mammographic, sonographic, and MRI appearances. *AJR Am J Roentgenol.* 2005;184:331–338.

155. Mesurolle B, Sygal V, Lalonde L, et al. Sonographic and mammographic appearances of breast hemangioma. *AJR Am J Roentgenol.* 2008;191:W17–W22.

156. Courcoutsakis NA, Hill SC, Chow CK, et al. Breast hemangiomas in a patient with Kasabach-Merritt syndrome: imaging findings. *AJR Am J Roentgenol.* 1997;169:1397–1399.

157. Gopal SV, Nayak P, Dharanipragada K, et al. Breast hemangioma simulating an inflammatory carcinoma. *Breast J.* 2005;11:498–499.

158. Ma W, Jin F, Wu Y. Capillary hemangioma of the breast—a rare type of benign breast tumor. *Breast J.* 2016;22(3):355–356.

159. Hoda SA, Cranor ML, Rosen PP. Hemangiomas of the breast with atypical histological features: further analysis of histological subtypes confirming their benign character. *Am J Surg Pathol.* 1992;16:553–560.

160. Rosen PP, Jozefczyk MA, Boram LH. Vascular tumors of the breast: IV: the venous hemangioma. *Am J Surg Pathol.* 1985;9:659–665.

161. Rosen PP. Vascular tumors of the breast: III: angiomatosis. *Am J Surg Pathol.* 1985;9:652–658.

162. Morrow M, Berger D, Thelmo W. Diffuse cystic angiomatosis of the breast. *Cancer.* 1988;62:2392–2396.

163. Rosen PP. Vascular tumors of the breast: V: nonparenchymal hemangiomas of mammary subcutaneous tissues. *Am J Surg Pathol.* 1985;9:723–729.

164. Franco RL, de Moraes Schenka NG, Schenka AA, et al. Cavernous hemangioma of the male breast. *Breast J.* 2005;11:511–512.

Sarcomas

165. Zelek L, Llombart-Cussac A, Terrier P, et al. Prognostic factors in primary breast sarcomas: a series of patients with long-term follow-up. *J Clin Oncol.* 2003;21:2583–2588.

166. Huang J, Mackillop WJ. Increased risk of soft tissue sarcoma after radiotherapy in women with breast carcinoma. *Cancer.* 2001;92:172–180.

167. Mery CM, George S, Bertagnolli MM, et al. Secondary sarcomas after radiotherapy for breast cancer: sustained risk and poor survival. *Cancer.* 2009;115:4055–4063.

168. Yap J, Chuba PJ, Thomas R, et al. Sarcoma as a second malignancy after treatment for breast cancer. *Int J Radiat Oncol Biol Phys.* 2002;52:1231–1237.

169. Al-Benna S, Poggemann K, Steinau HU, et al. Diagnosis and management of primary breast sarcoma. *Breast Cancer Res Treat.* 2010;122:619–626.

170. Bousquet G, Confavreux C, Magné N, et al. Outcome and prognostic factors in breast sarcoma: a multicenter study from the rare cancer network. *Radiother Oncol.* 2007;85:355–361.

171. Adem C, Reynolds C, Ingle JN, et al. Primary breast sarcoma: clinicopathologic series from the Mayo Clinic and review of the literature. *Br J Cancer.* 2004;91:237–241.

172. Blanchard DK, Reynolds CA, Grant CS, et al. Primary nonphylloides breast sarcomas. *Am J Surg.* 2003;186:359–361.

173. Sheth GR, Cranmer LD, Smith BD, et al. Radiation-induced sarcoma of the breast: a systematic review. *Oncologist.* 2012;17:405–418.

174. Rosen PP, Kimmel M, Ernsberger D. Mammary angiosarcoma: the prognostic significance of tumor differentiation. *Cancer.* 1988;62:2145–2151.

175. Rainwater LM, Martin JK Jr, Gaffey TA, et al. Angiosarcoma of the breast. *Arch Surg.* 1986;121:669–672.

176. Shackelford RT. Surgical disorders of the breast. In: *Diagnosis of Surgical Disease.* Philadelphia, PA: W. B. Saunders; 1968.

177. Wang ZS, Zhan N, Xiong CL, et al. Primary epithelioid angiosarcoma of the male breast: report of a case. *Surg Today.* 2007;37:782–786.

178. Donnell RM, Rosen PP, Lieberman PH, et al. Angiosarcoma and other vascular tumors of the breast. *Am J Surg Pathol.* 1981;5:629–642.

179. Kotton DN, Muse VV, Nishino M. Case records of the Massachusetts General Hospital: case 2-2012: a 63-year-old woman with dyspnea and rapidly progressive respiratory failure. *N Engl J Med.* 2012;366:259–269.

180. Cuesta-Mejías T, de León-Bojorge B, Abel de la Peña J, et al. Angiosarcoma de la mama en paciente con cirugias multiples e implante mamario: informe de un caso. *Ginecol Obstet Mex.* 2002;70:76–81.

181. Takenaka M, Tanaka M, Isobe M, et al. Angiosarcoma of the breast with silicone granuloma: a case report. *Kurume Med J.* 2009;56:33–37.

182. Liberman L, Dershaw DD, Kaufman RJ, et al. Angiosarcoma of the breast. *Radiology.* 1992;183:649–654.

183. Yang WT, Hennessy BT, Dryden MJ, et al. Mammary angiosarcomas: imaging findings in 24 patients. *Radiology.* 2007;242:725–734.

184. Glazebrook KN, Magut MJ, Reynolds C. Angiosarcoma of the breast. *AJR Am J Roentgenol.* 2008;190:533–538.

185. Nascimento AF, Raut CP, Fletcher CD. Primary angiosarcoma of the breast: clinicopathologic analysis of 49 cases, suggesting that grade is not prognostic. *Am J Surg Pathol.* 2008;32:1896–1904.

186. Merino MJ, Carter D, Berman M. Angiosarcoma of the breast. *Am J Surg Pathol.* 1983;7:53–60.

187. Shin SJ, Lesser M, Rosen PP. Hemangiomas and angiosarcomas of the breast: diagnostic utility of cell cycle markers with emphasis on Ki-67. *Arch Pathol Lab Med.* 2007;131:538–544.

188. Guarda LA, Ordonez NG, Smith JL Jr, et al. Immunoperoxidase localization of factor VIII in angiosarcomas. *Arch Pathol Lab Med.* 1982;106:515–516.

189. Pandey M, Sutton GR, Giri S, et al. Grade and prognosis in localized primary angiosarcoma. *Clin Breast Cancer.* 2015;15(4):266–269. doi:10.1016/j.clbc.2014.12.009.

190. Kaklamanos IG, Birbas K, Syrigos KN, et al. Breast angiosarcoma that is not related to radiation exposure: a comprehensive review of the literature. *Surg Today.* 2011;41:163–168.

191. Abbott R, Palmieri C. Angiosarcoma of the breast following surgery and radiotherapy for breast cancer. *Nat Clin Pract Oncol*. 2008;5:727–736.

192. Andrews S, Wilcoxon R, Benda J, et al. Angiosarcoma following MammoSite partial breast irradiation. *Breast Cancer Res Treat*. 2010;124:279–282.

193. Vorburger SA, Xing Y, Hunt KK, et al. Angiosarcoma of the breast. *Cancer*. 2005;104:2682–2688.

194. Strobbe LJ, Peterse HL, van Tinteren H, et al. Angiosarcoma of the breast after conservation therapy for invasive cancer, the incidence and outcome: an unforseen sequela. *Breast Cancer Res Treat*. 1998;47:101–109.

195. Billings SD, McKenney JK, Folpe AL, et al. Cutaneous angiosarcoma following breast-conserving surgery and radiation: an analysis of 27 cases. *Am J Surg Pathol*. 2004;28:781–788.

196. Mobini N. Cutaneous epithelioid angiosarcoma: a neoplasm with potential pitfalls in diagnosis. *J Cutan Pathol*. 2009;36:362–369.

197. Poellinger A, Landt S, Diekmann F, et al. Rapid growth of an exophytic angiosarcoma of the breast. *Breast J*. 2006;12:80–82.

198. Fineberg S, Rosen PP. Cutaneous angiosarcoma and atypical vascular lesions of the skin and breast after radiation therapy for breast carcinoma. *Am J Clin Pathol*. 1994;102:757–763.

199. Liu YC, Fung MA. Angiosarcoma with pseudoepidermotropism in a patient with breast cancer: a mimic of epidermotropic metastatic adenocarcinoma. *Am J Dermatopathol*. 2011;33:400–402.

200. Seo IS, Min KW. Postirradiation epithelioid angiosarcoma of the breast: a case report with immunohistochemical and electron microscopic study. *Ultrastruct Pathol*. 2003;27:197–203.

201. Fernandez AP, Sun Y, Tubbs RR, et al. FISH for MYC amplification and anti-MYC immunohistochemistry: useful diagnostic tools in the assessment of secondary angiosarcoma and atypical vascular proliferations. *J Cutan Pathol*. 2012;39:234–242.

202. Ginter PS, Mosquera JM, MacDonald TY, et al. Diagnostic utility of MYC amplification and anti-MYC immunohistochemistry in atypical vascular lesions, primary or radiation-induced mammary angiosarcomas, and primary angiosarcomas of other sites. *Hum Pathol*. 2014;45:709–716.

203. Cornejo KM, Deng A, Wu H, et al. The utility of MYC and FLT4 in the diagnosis and treatment of postradiation atypical vascular lesion and angiosarcoma of the breast. *Hum Pathol*. 2015;46:868–875.

204. Guo T, Zhang L, Chang NE, et al. Consistent MYC and FLT4 gene amplification in radiation-induced angiosarcoma but not in other radiation-associated atypical vascular lesions. *Genes Chromosomes Cancer*. 2011;50:25–33.

205. Mentzel T, Schildhaus HU, Palmedo G, et al. Postradiation cutaneous angiosarcoma after treatment of breast carcinoma is characterized by MYC amplification in contrast to atypical vascular lesions after radiotherapy and control cases: clinicopathological, immunohistochemical and molecular analysis of 66 cases. *Mod Pathol*. 2012;25:75–85.

206. Torres KE, Ravi V, Kin K, et al. Long-term outcomes in patients with radiation-associated angiosarcomas of the breast following surgery and radiotherapy for breast cancer. *Ann Surg Oncol*. 2013;20:1267–1274.

207. Seinen JM, Styring E, Verstappen V, et al. Radiation-associated angiosarcoma after breast cancer: high recurrence rate and poor survival despite surgical treatment with R0 resection. *Ann Surg Oncol*. 2012;19:2700–2706.

208. Morgan EA, Kozono DE, Wang Q, et al. Cutaneous radiation-associated angiosarcoma of the breast: poor prognosis in a rare secondary malignancy. *Ann Surg Oncol*. 2012;19:3801–3808.

209. Santi R, Cetica V, Franchi A, et al. Tumour suppressor gene TP53 mutations in atypical vascular lesions of breast skin following radiotherapy. *Histopathology*. 2011;58:455–466.

210. Brenn T, Fletcher CD. Radiation-associated cutaneous atypical vascular lesions and angiosarcoma: clinicopathologic analysis of 42 cases. *Am J Surg Pathol*. 2005;29:983–996.

211. Patton KT, Deyrup AT, Weiss SW. Atypical vascular lesions after surgery and radiation of the breast: a clinicopathologic study of 32 cases analyzing histologic heterogeneity and association with angiosarcoma. *Am J Surg Pathol*. 2008;32:943–950.

212. Gengler C, Coindre JM, Leroux A, et al. Vascular proliferations of the skin after radiation therapy for breast cancer: clinicopathologic analysis of a series in favor of a benign process: a study from the French Sarcoma Group. *Cancer*. 2007;109:1584–1598.

213. Fujita N, Kimura R, Yamamura J, et al. Leiomyosarcoma of the breast: a case report and review of the literature about therapeutic management. *Breast*. 2011;20:389–393.

214. Alessi E, Sala F. Leiomyosarcoma in ectopic areola. *Am J Dermatopathol*. 1992;14:165–169.

215. Vasan N, Saglam O, Killelea BK. Metastatic leiomyosarcoma presenting as bilateral, multifocal breast masses. *BMJ Case Rep*. 2012;2012. doi:10.1136/bcr-2012-007188.

216. Hernandez FJ. Leiomyosarcoma of male breast originating in the nipple. *Am J Surg Pathol*. 1978;2:299–304.

217. Visfeldt J, Scheike O. Male breast cancer: histologic typing and grading of 187 Danish cases. *Cancer*. 1973;32:985–990.

218. Boscaino A, Ferrara G, Orabona P, et al. Smooth muscle tumors of the breast: clinicopathologic features of two cases. *Tumori*. 1994;80:241–245.

219. Rane SU, Batra C, Saikia UN. Primary leiomyosarcoma of breast in an adolescent girl: a case report and review of the literature. *Case Rep Pathol*. 2012;2012:491984.

220. Austin RM, Dupree WB. Liposarcoma of the breast: a clinicopathologic study of 20 cases. *Hum Pathol*. 1986;17:906–913.

221. Odom JW, Mikhailova B, Pryce E, et al. Liposarcoma of the breast: report of a case and review of the literature. *Breast Dis*. 1991;4:293–298.

222. Pollard SG, Marks PV, Temple LN, et al. Breast sarcoma: a clinicopathologic review of 25 cases. *Cancer*. 1990;66:941–944.

223. Nandipati KC, Nerkar H, Satterfield J, et al. Pleomorphic liposarcoma of the breast mimicking breast abscess in a 19-year-old postpartum female: a case report and review of the literature. *Breast J*. 2010;16:537–540.

224. Yokouchi M, Nagano S, Kijima Y, et al. Solitary breast metastasis from myxoid liposarcoma. *BMC Cancer*. 2014;14:482. doi:410.1186/1471-2407-1114-1482.

225. Rakha EA, Tan PH, Shaaban A, et al. Do primary mammary osteosarcoma and chondrosarcoma exist? A review of a large multi-institutional series of malignant matrix-producing breast tumours. *Breast*. 2013;22:13–18.

226. Silver SA, Tavassoli FA. Primary osteogenic sarcoma of the breast: a clinicopathologic analysis of 50 cases. *Am J Surg Pathol*. 1998;22:925–933.

227. Trihia H, Valavanis C, Markidou S, et al. Primary osteogenic sarcoma of the breast: cytomorphologic study of 3 cases with histologic correlation. *Acta Cytol*. 2007;51:443–450.

228. Pasta V, Sottile D, Urciuoli P, et al. Rare chondrosarcoma of the breast treated with quadrantectomy instead of mastectomy: a case report. *Oncol Lett*. 2015;9:1116–1120.

229. Badyal RK, Kataria AS, Kaur M. Primary chondrosarcoma of male breast: a rare case. *Indian J Surg*. 2012;74:418–419.

230. Krishnamurthy A. Primary breast osteosarcoma: a diagnostic challenge. *Indian J Nucl Med*. 2015;30:39–41.

231. Kallianpur AA, Gupta R, Muduly DK, et al. Osteosarcoma of breast: a rare case of extraskeletal osteosarcoma. *J Cancer Res Ther*. 2013;9:292–294.

232. Jones MW, Norris HJ, Wargotz ES, et al. Fibrosarcoma-malignant fibrous histiocytoma of the breast: a clinicopathological study of 32 cases. *Am J Surg Pathol*. 1992;16:667–674.

233. Jeong YJ, Oh HK, Bong JG. Undifferentiated pleomorphic sarcoma of the male breast causing diagnostic challenges. *J Breast Cancer*. 2011;14:241–246.

234. Callery CD, Rosen PP, Kinne DW. Sarcoma of the breast: a study of 32 patients with reappraisal of classification and therapy. *Ann Surg*. 1985;201:527–532.

235. van Niekerk JL, Wobbes T, Holland R, et al. Malignant fibrous histiocytoma of the breast with axillary lymph node involvement. *J Surg Oncol*. 1987;34:32–35.

236. Bahrami A, Folpe AL. Adult-type fibrosarcoma: a reevaluation of 163 putative cases diagnosed at a single institution over a 48-year period. *Am J Surg Pathol*. 2010;34:1504–1513.

237. Lee JY, Kim DB, Kwak BS, et al. Primary fibrosarcoma of the breast: a case report. *J Breast Cancer*. 2011;14:156–159.

238. Jiao Q, Wu A, Liu P, et al. A young woman with a giant breast fibrosarcoma: a case report. *J Thorac Dis*. 2013;5:E199–E202.

239. Shukla S, Chauhan R, Jyotsna PL, et al. Primary fibrosarcoma of male breast: a rare entity. *J Clin Diagn Res*. 2014;8:FD11–FD12.

240. Yadav SK, Yadav J, Abhinav A, et al. Ulcerated primary fibrosarcoma of breast: case report and review of literature. *Breast Dis*. 2015;35:41–44.

241. Kanazawa N, Ono A, Nitou G, et al. Primary malignant hemangiopericytoma of the breast: report of a case. *Surg Today.* 1999;29:939–944.

242. Koukourakis G, Filopoulos E, Kapatou K, et al. Hemangiopericytoma of the breast: a case report and a review of the literature. *Case Rep Oncol Med.* 2015;2015:210643.

243. Dragoumis D, Desiris K, Kyropoulou A, et al. Hemangiopericytoma/solitary fibrous tumor of pectoralis major muscle mimicking a breast mass. *Int J Surg Case Rep.* 2013;4:338–341.

244. van Kints MJ, Tham RT, Klinkhamer PJ, et al. Hemangiopericytoma of the breast: mammographic and sonographic findings. *AJR Am J Roentgenol.* 1994;163:61–63.

245. Mittal KR, Gerald W, True LD. Hemangiopericytoma of breast: report of a case with ultrastructural and immunohistochemical findings. *Hum Pathol.* 1986;17:1181–1183.

246. Yang LH, Dai SD, Li QC, et al. Malignant solitary fibrous tumor of breast: a rare case report. *Int J Clin Exp Pathol.* 2014;7:4461–4466.

247. Cheah AL, Billings SD, Goldblum JR, et al. STAT6 rabbit monoclonal antibody is a robust diagnostic tool for the distinction of solitary fibrous tumour from its mimics. *Pathology.* 2014;46:389–395.

248. Ruhland B, Dittmer C, Thill M, et al. Metastasized hemangiopericytoma of the breast: a rare case. *Arch Gynecol Obstet.* 2009;280:491–494.

249. Hays DM, Donaldson SS, Shimada H, et al. Primary and metastatic rhabdomyosarcoma in the breast: neoplasms of adolescent females, a report from the Intergroup Rhabdomyosarcoma Study. *Med Pediatr Oncol.* 1997;29:181–189.

250. Catania S, Pacifico E, Zurrida S, et al. Malignant schwannoma of the breast. *Eur J Surg Oncol.* 1992;18:80–81.

251. Chuthapisith S, Prasert W, Warnnissorn M, et al. Ewing's sarcoma and primitive neuroectodermal tumour (ES/PNET) presenting as a breast mass. *Oncol Lett.* 2012;4:67–70.

252. Kwak JY, Kim EK, You JK, et al. Metastasis of primitive neuroectodermal tumor to the breast. *J Clin Ultrasound.* 2002;30:374–377.

253. Wu J, Brinker DA, Haas M, et al. Primary alveolar soft part sarcoma (ASPS) of the breast: report of a deceptive case with xanthomatous features confirmed by TFE3 immunohistochemistry and electron microscopy. *Int J Surg Pathol.* 2005;13:81–85.

254. Hanna NN, O'Donnell K, Wolfe GR. Alveolar soft part sarcoma metastatic to the breast. *J Surg Oncol.* 1996;61:159–162.

255. Yoshitani K, Kido A, Honoki K, et al. Pelvic metastasis of breast synovial sarcoma. *J Orthop Sci.* 2009;14:219–223.

256. Lučin K, Mustać E, Jonjić N. Breast sarcoma showing myofibroblastic differentiation. *Virchows Arch.* 2003;443:222–224.

257. Ng CS, Taylor CB, O'Donnell PJ, et al. Case report: mammographic and ultrasound appearances of Kaposi's sarcoma of the breast. *Clin Radiol.* 1996;51:735–736.

258. Fisher C, Magnusson B, Hardarson S, et al. Myxoid variant of follicular dendritic cell sarcoma arising in the breast. *Ann Diagn Pathol.* 1999;3:92–98.

Lymphoid and Hematopoietic Tumors

JUDITH A. FERRY

LYMPHOMAS OF THE BREAST

Primary lymphoma of the breast is defined as lymphoma involving one or both breasts with or without ipsilateral axillary lymph node involvement, without evidence of disease elsewhere at presentation, in a patient without a prior history of lymphoma (1). Some authorities also accept cases with more distant lymph node or bone marrow involvement, so long as clinically the primary or major manifestation of the lymphoma is the breast (2). The breast is a very uncommon primary site for lymphoma, accounting for 0.1% to 0.15% (2–5) of all malignant neoplasms of the breast, for 0.34% to 0.85% of all non-Hodgkin lymphomas (2,4,6–8) and for <2% of all extranodal non-Hodgkin lymphomas (2).

Establishing a diagnosis based on a needle biopsy specimen presents special challenges in the diagnosis of lymphoma. For high-grade lymphomas with obvious cytologic atypia, needle biopsies are often adequate to establish a diagnosis. For low-grade lymphomas such as follicular lymphoma and extranodal marginal zone lymphoma (MALT lymphoma) that often have features overlapping with those of reactive, chronic inflammatory lymphoid proliferations, establishing a diagnosis on a needle biopsy may be difficult. In such instances, ancillary studies play a key role in diagnosis. Obtaining a larger specimen may also be required.

Clinical Features

Most patients are middle-aged to elderly women, although occasionally younger females and rarely males are affected (1,3–6,8–23). They typically present with a palpable breast mass, with or without ipsilateral axillary lymphadenopathy (4,6,15,17,20,21,23). A few patients have had the lymphoma detected by mammography; lymphomas detected initially by routine mammography are typically low-grade lymphomas (4,10,11,13). Constitutional symptoms are uncommon, being found in 0% (6,13,15,17,24) to 4% (19) of patients in different series. In some series, right-sided lymphoma was more common than left-sided lymphoma (23,25). Approximately 10% of primary breast lymphomas are bilateral (1,3,5,7,8,16,17,19,22–24,26). A few patients have a history of autoimmune disease, diabetes mellitus, mastitis (2,4,5,15), or HIV infection (27). However,

most patients have no underlying illness, and specific factors predisposing to lymphoma of the breast are not identified (8,21,26). On physical examination, patients usually have discrete, mobile masses. The overlying skin is involved infrequently; it may be thickened (20), erythematous, or inflamed (3,28) mimicking inflammatory carcinoma. Skin retraction and nipple discharge are virtually never found. The proportion of cases with ipsilateral axillary lymphadenopathy varies widely among series from 11% (10) to about 50%.

Pathologic Features and Clinicopathologic Correlates

The specimen obtained must yield sufficient tissue to firmly establish a diagnosis (29). Excision is not required if a smaller biopsy is diagnostic. A diagnosis of lymphoma may be established by fine needle aspiration biopsy, but tissue for histopathology or at least a cell block is typically required to establish a complete diagnosis with subclassification (30). In most series, diffuse large B-cell lymphoma is the most common type, accounting for approximately 60% of the cases (3–7,12,13,17,18,21,31,32). The remainder are mainly low-grade lymphomas (MALT lymphoma or follicular lymphoma). Burkitt lymphoma is uncommon. T-cell lymphoma is very rare (11,21). The breast is rarely involved by post-transplant lymphoproliferative disorders, which are usually high-grade B-lineage lymphomas (33).

Diffuse Large B-cell Lymphoma

Diffuse large B-cell lymphoma affects women (and a few men) across a wide age range (4,12,15,19,22,29), with a median age in the sixth decade (32). Lesions range from 1 to 20 cm in greatest dimension, with a median size of 4 to 5 cm. A few patients have diffuse breast enlargement (7,8,15,17,19,22,32). The tumors have been described as discrete, hard, rubbery (16), soft or fleshy masses (3) that are sometimes rapidly enlarging (1,16,28).

The lymphomas are composed of a diffuse infiltrate of large lymphoid cells. Histologic and immunophenotypic features overlap with those seen in other sites (**Table 21.1**) (3,18,21,34). The lymphomas are CD45+, CD20+, with rare CD5+ cases

413

TABLE 21.1

Hematolymphoid Neoplasms of the Breast: Principal Features

Type of Neoplasm	Patients Affected	Histology	Neoplastic Cells, Usual Immunophenotype	Genetic, Cytogenetic Features	Clinical Behavior
Diffuse large B-cell lymphoma	Adults, females >> males, broad age range; few pregnant	Diffuse proliferation of large lymphoid cells; CB more common than IB	CD45+, CD20+, CD10 usually −, BCL6+/−, BCL2 and MUM1/IRF4 usually +, Ki67 high; non-GC > GC	Rare *MALT1* rearrangements; trisomy 18 in some; NFκB activation in some	Aggressive; CNS, opposite breast: common sites of relapse; best outcomes with R-CHOP or R-CHOP-like chemo +/− RT
Extranodal marginal zone Lymphoma (MALT lymphoma)	Middle-aged and older adults; females >> males	Marginal zone B-cells, plasma cells variable, reactive follicles may be present. LELs often not prominent.	CD45+, CD20+, CD5−, CD10−, CD23−, CD43+/−, BCL2+/−, cyclin D1−, cIg+/−	Rare *MALT1* rearrangements; minority of cases: trisomy 3, 12 and/or 18	Good prognosis. Localized extranodal relapses may occur. Few have large cell transformation. Few die of lymphoma.
Follicular lymphoma (FL)	Middle-aged and older women	Similar to lymph nodal follicular lymphoma	CD45+, CD20+, CD10+, BCL6+, CD5−, CD23−, CD43−, BCL2+, cyclin D1−, sIg+, occasionally BCL2−		Prognosis less good than MALT lymphoma. Behavior similar to nodal FL.
Burkitt Lymphoma	Young to middle-aged, few older women, some pregnant or lactating	Diffuse infiltrate of medium-sized round cells, many mitoses, starry sky	CD45+, CD20+, CD10+, BCL6+, BCL2−, Ki67 ~ 100%[a]	Translocation of *MYC* with IGH [t(8;14)], less often with *IGK* or *IGL*[a]	Very aggressive; disease is often widespread
B- and T-lymphoblastic lymphoma/leukemia	Mostly adolescents and young adults, often with concurrent acute lymphoblastic leukemia	Diffuse infiltrate of small- to medium-sized cells with oval or irregular nuclei, fine chromatin, small nucleoli, and scant cytoplasm	B-lineage: CD19+, CD20−, CD10+, TdT+[a] T-lineage: Variable expression of T-cell markers, but often CD3+, CD7+, CD4+/CD8+ (double+), CD1a+, TdT+[a]	Variable	Aggressive disease with relatively good prognosis depending on underlying genetic abnormalities, if optimally treated
Anaplastic large cell lymphoma, ALK−, associated with implant	Women with saline or silicone implants, for cosmetic purposes or following mastectomy; lymphoma occurs years after implant; seroma rather than discrete mass	Large atypical, pleomorphic cells in a background of fibrosis, debris, and sometimes chronic inflammation	CD30+, Alk1−, CD45+/−, CD4+/−, CD43+/−, CD3−/+, CD5−/+, CD8−, EMA+/−, TIA1+/−, granzyme B+/−, EBV−, HHV8−	TCR: clonal IGH: polyclonal	Very good prognosis in absence of a discrete mass or spread beyond capsule
Chronic Hodgkin lymphoma (CHL)	Rare; breast involvement virtually always secondary to lymph nodal disease	Reed–Sternberg cells and variants in a reactive background	CD15+, CD30+, CD45−, Pax5 dim+, CD20−, CD3−, Alk1−	TCR: polyclonal IGH: polyclonal	Outcome likely similar to other CHL of same stage
Plasmacytoma	Rare; usually in setting of plasma cell myeloma; rarely isolated	Sheets of mature and/or immature plasma cells	CD138+, cIg+, EMA+/−, CD45−/+, Keratin−		Relatively poor in setting of myeloma

CB, centroblastic; cIg, monotypic cytoplasmic immunoglobulin; R-CHOP, rituximab-cytoxan, adriamycin, vincristine, prednisone; GC, germinal center immunophenotype; IB, immunoblastic; IGH, immunoglobulin heavy chain gene; IGK, immunoglobulin kappa light chain gene; IGL, immunoglobulin lambda light chain gene; LELs, lymphoepithelial lesions; non-GC, nongerminal center immunophenotype; RT, radiation therapy; sIg, monotypic surface immunoglobulin; TCR, T-cell receptor genes; CHL, chronic Hodgkin lymphoma.
[a]Based in part on data on same types of lymphoma in other sites.

(22) and a relatively high proliferation index (60%–95% in one series) (22). The majority of cases has a nongerminal center B-cell (non-GCB) immunophenotype (CD10–, BCL6+, MUM1/IRF4+, or CD10–, BCL6–) **(Fig. 21.1)**, while a minority has a germinal center B-cell (GCB) phenotype (CD10+, BCL6+ or CD10–, BCL6+, MUM1/IRF4–) (21,29). In recent large series, 77% of the cases (32) and 95% of the cases (35) had a non-GCB immunophenotype. Immunostaining for p50 and p65 has shown nuclear localization of p50 in a minority, suggesting NFκB activation in a subset of cases (34). In situ hybridization for Epstein–Barr virus (EBV) using a probe for EBER is typically negative (22). As is true of other nongerminal center/activated B-cell type diffuse large B-cell lymphomas, primary breast diffuse large B-cell lymphomas often have mutations of *MYD88* (MYD88 L265) and *CD79B*, resulting in activation of the NFκB pathway, contributing to lymphomagenesis (36). Translocations of *BCL2, BCL6,* and *MYC* are absent or rare (36).

Extranodal Marginal Zone Lymphoma of Mucosa-Associated Lymphoid Tissue (MALT Lymphoma)

MALT lymphoma mainly affects middle-aged and older women and rarely men (2–4,6,10,25,31,37,38), with a median age of 68 years in one large series (39). Patients with MALT lymphoma of the breast typically have no recognized factors predisposing to lymphoma. Patients present with a lesion that is typically unilateral, and that may be detected by physical examination or by mammography. Constitutional symptoms are almost never present (39).

The lymphomas range from <1 to 20 cm, with a median size of approximately 3 cm (3,6,10,31,37–39). Their histologic features are similar to those of MALT lymphomas in other sites. The lymphomas have a vaguely nodular to diffuse appearance on low-power microscopic examination. They are composed of small- to medium-sized cells with slightly irregular nuclei and a scant-to-abundant quantity of pale cytoplasm. Reactive follicles, sometimes with follicular colonization (infiltration and partial-to-complete replacement by neoplastic marginal zone cells), and plasmacytic differentiation, sometimes accompanied by Dutcher bodies (intranuclear protrusions of cytoplasm containing immunoglobulin), are found in some cases. Mitotic activity is low, except in residual reactive follicles **(Fig. 21.2)**. Necrosis and sclerosis are typically absent. Well-formed lymphoepithelial lesions are found less often than in MALT lymphomas involving some other sites (4,10,21,34). Rare MALT lymphomas with plasmacytic differentiation are associated with localized deposition of amyloid (3,40).

The neoplastic cells are typically CD45+, CD20+, CD5–, CD10–, CD23–, CD43+/–, BCL2+/–, and cyclin D1–, with monotypic cytoplasmic immunoglobulin in those cases with plasmacytic differentiation (5,25,37). The proliferation index is low. If there are remnants of reactive follicles, the germinal center cells are CD10+, BCL6+, and BCL2–, with a high proliferation index. Markers of follicular dendritic cells (CD21, CD23) typically show underlying follicular dendritic meshwork, which are often expanded and disrupted. The presence of follicular dendritic cell meshwork tends to correlate with a vaguely nodular growth pattern in MALT lymphomas.

Chromosomal translocations that involve the *MALT1* gene, including t(11;18), involving *API2* and *MALT1*, and t(14;18) involving *IGH* and *MALT1* are rare (34,41,42). Trisomies of chromosomes 3, 12, and 18 are uncommon (41). The absence of nuclear p50 and p65 expression is reported, which suggests lack of NFκB activation (34). The genetic defects leading to the development of MALT lymphoma of the breast are not well understood.

Follicular Lymphoma

Follicular lymphoma mainly affects middle-aged and older women (6,10,31), and rarely men (39). Patients present with lesions that are unilateral in approximately 95% of the cases, typically unaccompanied by constitutional symptoms (39). The tumors appear to range from <1 to 9 cm, with a median size of about 2 to 3 cm (6,10,31,39). Histologic and immunophenotypic features are similar to those of nodal follicular lymphomas. The lymphomas are sometimes associated with

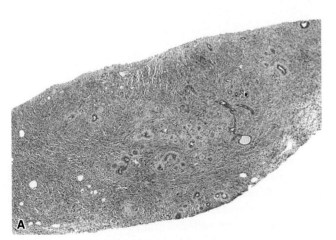

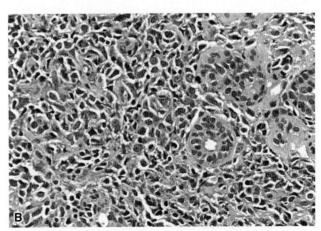

FIGURE 21.1 Diffuse Large B-cell Lymphoma. A: This needle core biopsy shows a dense, diffuse infiltrate of lymphoid cells. **B:** High power shows closely packed large atypical lymphoid cells surrounding lobular glands.

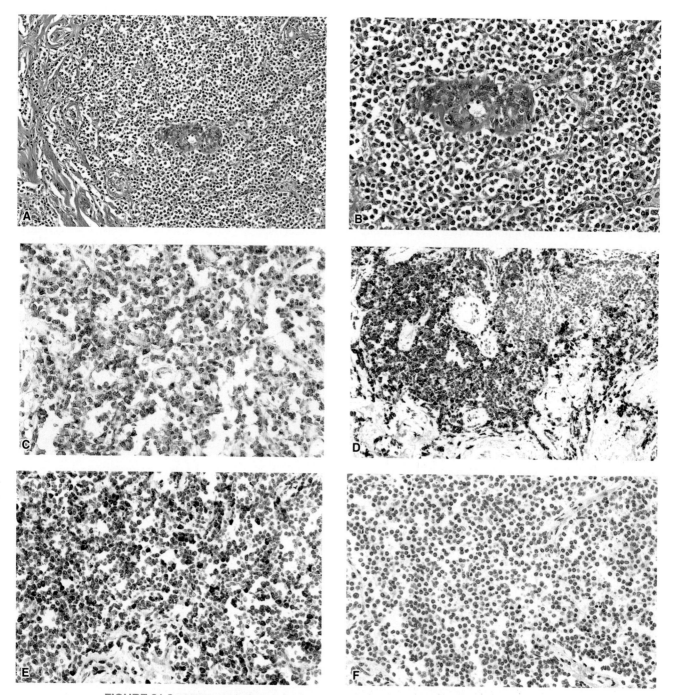

FIGURE 21.2 MALT Lymphoma. A, B: The lymphomatous infiltrate around a mammary duct consists of small cells with clear cytoplasm and scattered plasma cells. **C:** The tumor cells are reactive for CD43. **D:** Immunoreactivity for CD79 is shown. **E:** Immunoreactivity for kappa is shown. **F:** There was no reactivity for lambda.

sclerosis. Follicular lymphomas of all grades (1–3) have been reported **(Fig. 21.3)** (10,11,15,17). Neoplastic follicles are typically CD45+, CD20+, CD10+, CD5–, CD23–, CD43–, BCL2+ or BCL2–, and cyclin D1–.

Burkitt Lymphoma

Burkitt lymphoma occurs in one of three clinical settings: endemic Burkitt lymphoma, occurring mainly in equatorial Africa, where malaria is endemic; sporadic Burkitt lymphoma, occurring worldwide in individuals without immunodeficiency; and immunodeficiency-associated Burkitt lymphoma, occurring in immunodeficient individuals. The most common cause of immunodeficiency in the third scenario is HIV infection (43). The breast can be affected in any of these clinical settings.

Burkitt lymphoma mainly affects young to middle-aged females (4,17,18,44); some have been pregnant or postpartum at the time of diagnosis (4,17,18). Cases of endemic Burkitt

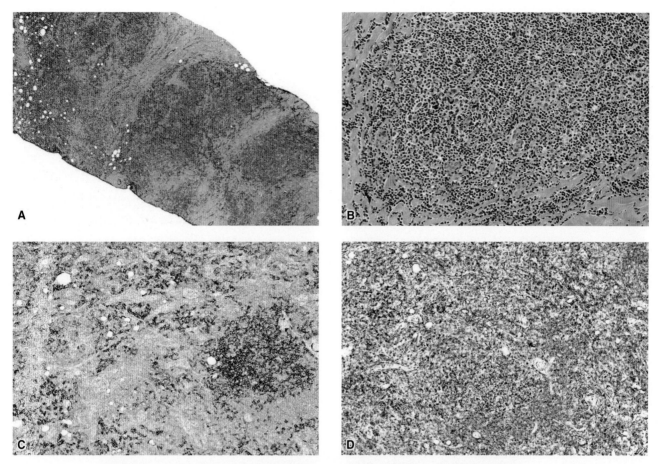

FIGURE 21.3 Follicular Lymphoma, Follicular, and Diffuse Pattern, Grade 1 to 2 of 3. **A:** The needle core biopsy shows ill-defined follicles and a patchy interfollicular lymphoid infiltrate. **B:** High magnification shows one poorly delineated follicle composed of centrocytes and occasional centroblasts in a background of small lymphocytes. **C:** The atypical cells were also CD20+ and BCL6+ (not shown); CD10 highlights atypical cells in a follicular and diffuse pattern. **D:** The atypical B-cells co-express BCL2.

lymphoma resulting in dramatic, bilateral mammary enlargement in African females who were sometimes pregnant or lactating were recognized by Burkitt (45). Premenarchal girls are rarely affected (46).

Burkitt lymphoma is typically composed of a dense, diffuse proliferation of uniform, medium-sized cells with round nuclei, clumped chromatin, several nucleoli, and a scant to moderate amount of cytoplasm that is deeply basophilic on a Giemsa stain. The proliferation is highly cellular with minimal intervening stroma. The mitotic rate is very high, and there is abundant apoptotic debris. Burkitt lymphoma has many interspersed pale tingible body macrophages containing apoptotic debris in a background of deeply stained neoplastic cells creating the characteristic starry sky pattern **(Fig. 21.4)** (43).

Burkitt lymphoma also has a characteristic immunophenotype: the neoplastic cells are uniformly CD20+, CD10+, BCL6+, BCL2−, monotypic surface immunoglobulin (IgM)+, with virtually all cells positive for Ki67 (proliferation). The underlying genetic event is a translocation involving *MYC* on chromosome 8 and *IGH* on chromosome 14 and less often the gene for κ or λ light chain rather than the *IGH*. The neoplastic cells almost always harbor EBV in endemic cases; sporadic

and immunodeficiency-associated Burkitt lymphoma are each EBV-associated in about one-third of the cases (43).

T-Cell Lymphomas

Primary breast lymphoma of T-lineage is rare, accounting for only about 2% to 3% of the cases (4,16,21). ALK-negative anaplastic large cell lymphomas (ALCLs) arising in association with breast implants is a distinct entity (see the section on Lymphoma of the Breast in Association with Implants). Other T-cell lymphomas arise sporadically; they include ALK+ ALCL, peripheral T-cell lymphoma, not otherwise specified, including both CD4+ and CD8+ cases, subcutaneous panniculitis-like T-cell lymphoma, and T-lymphoblastic lymphoma (4,21,31,47–52). T-cell lymphomas involving the breast in the setting of widespread disease are more common than primary T-lineage breast lymphoma (52). These secondary lymphomas are also of a variety of types (52). Cases of adult T-cell leukemia/lymphoma occurring in patients from an area endemic for HTLV1, involving the breasts unilaterally and bilaterally, have been reported (52).

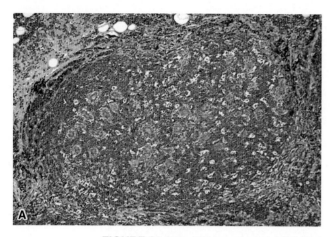
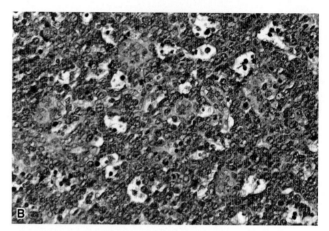

FIGURE 21.4 Burkitt Lymphoma, with Bilateral Breast Involvement in a Young Woman.
A: A lobule is surrounded and infiltrated by a dense infiltrate of deeply basophilic, atypical lymphoid cells, with scattered tingible body macrophages creating a "starry sky" pattern.
B: High magnification shows numerous medium-sized lymphoid cells with occasional distinct nucleoli, as well as frequent mitoses and scattered tingible body macrophages.

Hodgkin Lymphoma

Rare cases of Hodgkin lymphoma, most often the nodular sclerosis classic Hodgkin lymphoma, have involved the breast at the time of presentation or at relapse (21,53–55). Typically, Hodgkin lymphoma involves the breast in the setting of concurrent lymph node involvement, and sometimes widespread disease. Relapse in the form of isolated breast involvement is very rare but has been described (55). Primary Hodgkin lymphoma of the breast is vanishingly rare, and when breast involvement occurs it is generally secondary (21). There are very rare instances in which Hodgkin lymphoma presents first in the breast (54). Breast involvement is usually unilateral but occasionally bilateral (53). As in other sites, Hodgkin lymphoma in the breast takes the form of a mixed infiltrate of reactive cells in varying proportions (lymphocytes, histiocytes, eosinophils, plasma cells, and/or neutrophils) with scattered large atypical uninucleate, binucleated, or multinucleated Reed–Sternberg cells and variants with large oval or irregular

nuclei, inclusion-like reddish nucleoli, paranucleolar haloes, and scant to moderate quantity of pale cytoplasm **(Fig. 21.5)**. The neoplastic cells typically are CD15+, CD30+, Pax5 dim+, CD20–, CD3–, and ALK1–. Because of the rarity of Hodgkin lymphoma involving the breast, the diagnosis should be made with extreme caution, particularly in the absence of concurrent lymph nodal involvement by Hodgkin lymphoma, or in the absence of a history of Hodgkin lymphoma.

Lymphoma of the Breast in Association with Implants

Lymphoma has rarely arisen adjacent to breast implants used for both cosmetic purposes and reconstruction after mastectomy for carcinoma (31,52,56–60). In contrast to the marked preponderance of B-cell lymphomas among breast lymphomas, the vast majority of lymphomas arising in patients with implants have almost all been ALK-negative ALCLs.

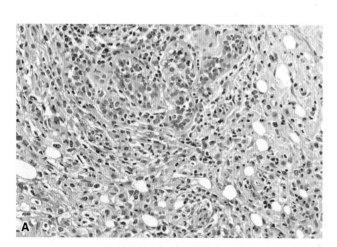
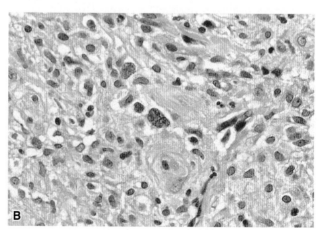

FIGURE 21.5 Hodgkin Lymphoma. A, B: Breast involvement in a patient with a diagnosis previously established in a cervical lymph node. Large atypical cells are present in small numbers in a background of sclerosis with scattered reactive cells.

These lymphomas account for a small proportion of all lymphomas of the breast; only 2% of cases in each of two large series of lymphoma involving the breast arose in association with an implant (21,31).

There appears to be a slightly increased risk of developing ALCL in association with breast implants. In one study, the risk of developing an implant-associated ALCL was estimated to be 0.1 to 0.3 per 100,000 individuals per year, with an odds ratio of 18.2 for developing implant-associated ALCL (44).

Affected patients are adults, over a broad age range. The implants have been of saline and silicone types; however, even the saline implants typically have a silicone capsule, leading to speculation about a role for silicone or its breakdown products in the pathogenesis of lymphoma through an immunologic mechanism (56,57,61–65). The interval from insertion of the implant to diagnosis of lymphoma has ranged from 1 to 32 years, with a median ranging from 7 to 11 years in larger series (31,44,51,56,65–72). Most patients present with a unilateral swelling related to a fluid collection ("seroma") developing between the implant and the fibrous capsule surrounding the implant, without a discrete mass (31,56–59,66–70,72). A minority of patients have a discrete mass, with disease not confined by the fibrous capsule around the implant (65). Patients usually present with localized disease (56,57,68).

Microscopic examination reveals large, atypical, pleomorphic, mitotically active cells with oval or indented nuclei, prominent nucleoli, and moderately abundant cytoplasm often accompanied by a mixed inflammatory infiltrate composed of lymphocytes, plasma cells, histiocytes, and sometimes eosinophils, neutrophils and giant cells. The neoplastic cells typically form a thin, discontinuous layer along the inner aspect of the fibrous capsule, sometimes with nodular foci of more abundant tumor cells, present in a background of necrotic debris or fibrinoid material **(Fig. 21.6)** (57). The neoplastic cells infrequently invade the fibrous capsule (58,70); but in most cases, they do not come into contact with breast parenchyma (66). A cell block prepared from the fluid is very useful for visualizing the abnormal cellular population. Cytologic examination of fluid from the seroma may reveal large numbers of neoplastic cells.

In a minority of cases, there is deviation from this classic scenario. In these instances, patients have a discrete mass in addition to an effusion, and the mass may penetrate the capsule and involve breast tissue (51,66).

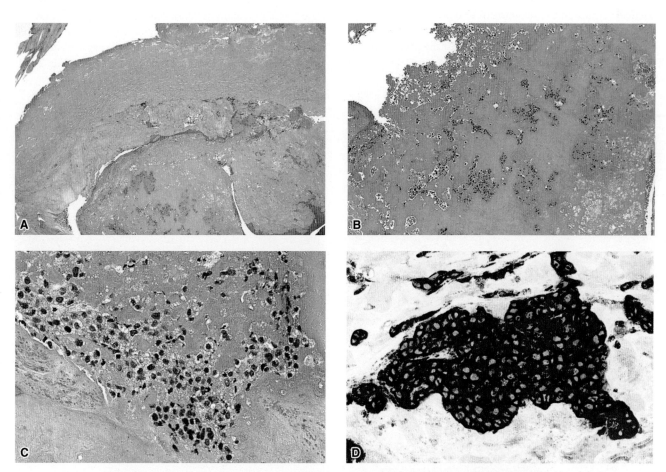

FIGURE 21.6 Anaplastic Large Cell Lymphoma, ALK-Negative, Arising in Association with a Breast Implant. A: Low power shows a hypocellular fibrous pseudocapsule **(top of image)** overlying an area with hyaline material with a few clusters of cells. **B:** Clusters of atypical cells are scattered in a background of hyalinized collagen and amorphous debris. **C:** High magnification shows large atypical cells with oval and irregular nuclei in a background of debris. **D:** The large atypical cells are intensely positive for CD30.

The ALCLs are typically CD30+, ALK−, CD45+/−, and EMA+, with variable expression of T-cell antigens. CD4, CD43, and cytotoxic granule proteins (e.g., TIA1 and granzyme B) are usually positive, whereas CD3, CD5, CD7, and CD8 are often negative. EBV and human herpes virus 8 (HHV8) are absent (56–59,66,67,69–72). The proliferation index is high (71). Clonal rearrangement of the T-cell receptor γ chain gene can typically be demonstrated, whereas clonal B-cells are not found (56,57,66,67,70).

Patients presenting with the classical picture: ALK-ALCL associated with an effusion without a discrete mass, and with localized disease, appear to have an excellent prognosis. It is likely that excision of the implant and capsulectomy, with close follow-up to monitor for recurrence, would constitute sufficient therapy for these patients (73). Patients with more aggressive disease, in a few cases resulting in death (66,71), correspond to those who present with lymphoma that has penetrated the fibrous capsule to form a discrete mass (65).

Establishing a diagnosis may be problematic. The manner of presentation can lead to a clinical impression of inflammation, infection, or leaking implant. The associated inflammation may obscure the neoplastic population. The neoplastic lymphoid cells may be mistaken for carcinoma, particularly in women previously treated for breast carcinoma. Familiarity with the rare occurrence of ALCL arising in association with a breast implant will assist the pathologist in establishing a diagnosis.

Differential Diagnosis of Mammary Lymphoma

The diagnosis of lymphoma of the breast is almost never suspected preoperatively. The clinical impression is typically carcinoma but may also be fibroadenoma or phyllodes tumor (28). On an average, lymphoma forms a larger mass than carcinoma, with lymphomas having a mean or median diameter of about 4 cm (23,32). Occasionally, lymphomas can present with a clinical picture that mimics inflammatory carcinoma (74) or mastitis (75,76). Evaluation of histologic and immunophenotypic features, in conjunction with familiarity of the range of types of lymphoma that can involve the breast, typically allows a diagnosis to be established.

PLASMA CELL NEOPLASMS

Breast involvement by a plasmacytoma is much less common than involvement by lymphoma and usually occurs in patients with plasma cell myeloma. Patients are mostly middle-aged and older women (77–82), with rare cases affecting the male breast (81). Patients present with painless or painful nodules within the breast; usually the nodules are multiple and bilateral (80). Plasmacytoma of the breast rarely presents as an isolated lesion, which usually (79,83), but not always, progresses to myeloma (84–86). The histologic and immunophenotypic features of the breast lesions in plasma cell myeloma and solitary plasmacytoma are similar (see **Table 21.1 and Fig. 21.7**).

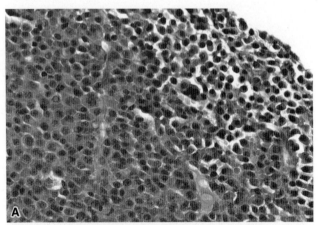

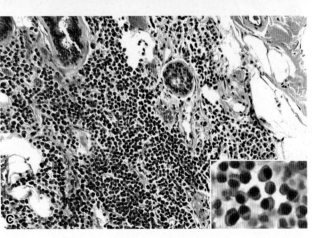

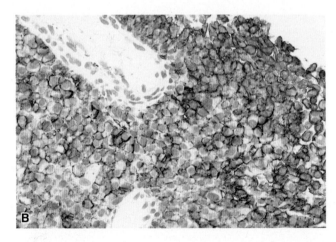

FIGURE 21.7 Plasmacytoma of the Breast in a Patient with Plasma Cell Myeloma. A: Numerous mature to slightly immature plasma cells are present. **B:** Plasma cells are CD138+. **C:** The plasma cells infiltrate breast glandular tissue. The inset shows detail.

MYELOID SARCOMA

Myeloid sarcoma is a mass-forming neoplasm composed of myeloid blasts with or without maturation occurring at a site other than the bone marrow (87,88). Myeloid sarcoma involving the breast is rare. It can occur in the breast as an isolated finding in a patient with no history of a myeloid neoplasm; this accounts for a minority of the cases (89,90). It is more commonly found in a patient with concurrent acute myeloid leukemia (AML) or concurrent myeloid sarcoma in other sites, or as a relapse of AML in a patient previously treated for AML (90–94). Myeloid sarcoma may also arise in patients with other myeloid neoplasms such as myeloproliferative neoplasms or myelodysplastic syndrome (90). When myeloid sarcomas occur in this setting, they may represent the first sign of progression to AML/blast crisis.

Irrespective of the clinical scenario, myeloid sarcoma of the breast shows a marked female preponderance, with men accounting for only about 5% of the cases (92). Patients are affected over a wide age range; many are adolescents or young adults (92). Patients present with a mass lesion or swelling of the breast unassociated with nipple discharge or retraction of overlying skin. Lesions are usually unilateral but may be bilateral (92,94). Most are in the range of 1 to 6 cm (88–91,93,94). Concurrent ipsilateral axillary lymph node involvement is common (90,92,94). Among patients with sites of extramedullary disease other than the breast, including disease occurring before, concurrent with or after the diagnosis of myeloid sarcoma of the breast, the most common sites are skin and subcutaneous tissue, female genital tract, central nervous system, and lymph nodes (axillary and nonaxillary) (92).

Outcome has been variable. Patients who present with isolated breast myeloid sarcoma appear to have a favorable outcome, particularly if they receive systemic chemotherapy (89,90). Those patients with widespread disease have a guarded prognosis (88–90), although outcome is strongly dependent on the underlying molecular genetic and cytogenetic abnormalities of the associated AML.

Myeloid sarcomas are composed of primitive myeloid and/or monocytic cells. In a subset of cases, there is some maturation of the neoplastic clone to more mature myeloid forms. On microscopic examination, the tumors typically have a diffuse pattern, although typically with sparing of mammary epithelial structures. In some instances, the neoplastic cells infiltrate stroma and mimic carcinoma. This occurs when a string of single cells take on an "Indian file" appearance or surround non-neoplastic ducts and lobules in a "targetoid" pattern. Mitoses are usually easily found (89,90,93). The neoplastic cells are discohesive, with round, oval, irregular or reniform, medium-sized nuclei with finely dispersed chromatin and variably prominent nucleoli. The cytoplasm ranges from scant in primitive cells to moderately abundant, sometimes with a distinct eosinophilic color owing to the presence of granules, if there is some maturation of the blasts **(Fig. 21.8)**. There may be admixed eosinophils and their precursors.

With immunohistochemistry, the neoplastic cells are usually positive for myeloperoxidase, lysozyme, CD117, and CD43. CD45 (leukocyte common antigen) is often expressed but may be dim. Myeloid sarcomas composed exclusively of monocytes and their precursors (monocytic sarcoma) are CD68+ and lysozyme+ but are negative for myeloperoxidase and often negative for CD34 and CD117. Tumor cells are negative for CD20, CD3, and keratins. In a few cases, there may be expression of one or more lymphoid-associated antigens, such as TdT, CD79a, or Pax5; a broad panel of immunostains including myeloid markers will help avoid misinterpretation of such cases as lymphoblastic lymphoma (89,90,93).

The main entity in the differential diagnosis of myeloid sarcoma is lymphoma, especially diffuse large B-cell lymphoma. On routinely stained sections, large lymphoid cells typically have slightly larger nuclei, with either more vesicular or more coarsely clumped chromatin, and less delicate nuclear membranes than the neoplastic cells of myeloid sarcoma. Differentiation into recognizable maturing myeloid elements, when present, helps to identify a neoplasm as myeloid sarcoma. Immunophenotyping with an appropriate panel of lymphoid and myeloid antigens will confirm the diagnosis.

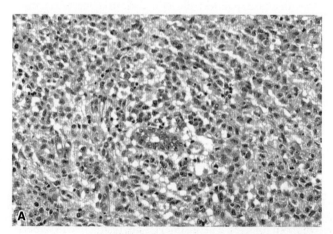
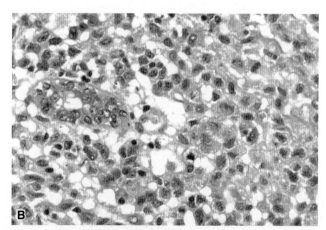

FIGURE 21.8 Myeloid Sarcoma. A, B: This periductal infiltrate of undifferentiated granulocytic cells could be mistaken for carcinoma. **C:** A few tumor cells are reactive (red) with naphthol-ASD-chloroacetate esterase stain. Undifferentiated cells are not stained. **D:** Many primitive cells are positive with the immunostain for muramidase (lysozyme).

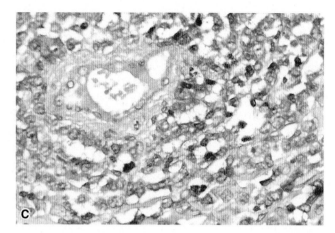

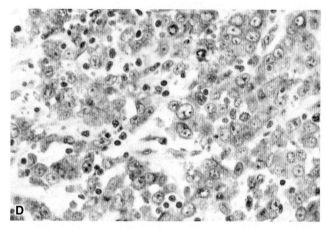

FIGURE 21.8 (continued)

When myeloid sarcoma grows in an Indian file or targetoid pattern, it can mimic carcinoma, particularly lobular carcinoma. The presence of in situ carcinoma makes myeloid sarcoma less likely (90). Areas with cohesive neoplastic cells and the formation of tubules or lumina support carcinoma. A history of a myeloid neoplasm should prompt consideration of myeloid sarcoma. Of note, a small subset of patients treated for breast carcinoma with chemotherapy develop therapy-related AML, so that a history of carcinoma does not exclude the possibility of AML/myeloid sarcoma.

The differential diagnosis also includes extramedullary hematopoiesis, or myeloid metaplasia, which rarely involves the breast, usually in association with an underlying hematologic disorder. Breast masses formed by extramedullary hematopoiesis are rare but have been reported in middle-aged and elderly female patients, most of whom carry a diagnosis of a chronic myeloproliferative neoplasm, most often primary myelofibrosis (formerly known as chronic idiopathic myelofibrosis and as myelofibrosis with myeloid metaplasia). Extramedullary hematopoiesis also occurs rarely in the breast in women with no prior hematologic disorder (95–99). Microscopic examination reveals a diffuse infiltrate of mature and maturing hematopoietic cells, including megakaryocytes **(Fig. 21.9)**. There is a

variable admixture of cells of myeloid and erythroid lines, with predominance of myeloid elements described in some cases. In patients with primary myelofibrosis, the megakaryocytes are often large, hyperchromatic, and atypical or even bizarre (99,100). The presence of more than one cell line, full maturation, and fewer blasts exclude myeloid sarcoma.

HISTIOCYTIC PROLIFERATIONS OF THE BREAST

Rosai–Dorfman Disease

Rosai–Dorfman disease (sinus histiocytosis with massive lymphadenopathy) is an uncommon disorder of unknown etiology that typically presents with lymphadenopathy and less often with extranodal involvement. Breast involvement by Rosai–Dorfman disease is very unusual. Most patients with Rosai–Dorfman disease involving the breast are adults, with rare occurrence during adolescence. Patients range from 15 to 84 years of age, with a median age in the early 50s at presentation (101–104). There is a marked female preponderance, with a M:F ratio of about 1:10 (102,103,105). Patients often present with a firm, painless, ill-defined, or irregular breast mass (101,103). In rare instances, retraction and inflammation of skin overlying the lesion has been described (101). The lesions range in size from 1 to 6.5 cm (median, 3 cm) (102). They are usually single and unilateral, but a few cases with multifocal or bilateral breast involvement are described (101–103,105). Most patients have Rosai–Dorfman disease confined to the breast, but a minority have axillary lymph node involvement (101,106), or more widespread disease (101). Patients with bilateral breast involvement appear more likely to have spread of Rosai–Dorfman disease beyond the breast than those with unilateral involvement (101,103).

Microscopic examination of the lesions reveals a dense infiltrate of lymphocytes, plasma cells, histiocytes, and sometimes lymphoid follicles. The histiocytes are distinctive in appearance: they are large with large oval nuclei, open chromatin, distinct nucleoli, and abundant cytoplasm. Some of these large histiocytes show emperipolesis, which may be translated as

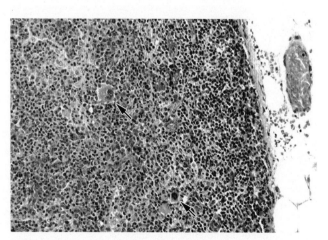

FIGURE 21.9 Intramammary Lymph Node with Extramedullary Hematopoiesis. Megakaryocytes *(arrows)* are evident in this intramammary lymph node from a patient with myelofibrosis.

"inside round about wandering" in which intact cells, usually lymphocytes, but sometimes plasma cells, red blood cells, and neutrophils, are present within the cytoplasm. A clear halo may surround the engulfed cells. Although the large nuclei of the histiocytes give them an atypical appearance, mitoses and necrosis are absent. Eosinophils are very infrequent. Abscess formation and granulomas are absent. In lymph nodes, the large histiocytes are mainly confined to expanded sinuses (sinus histiocytosis with massive lymphadenopathy). Emperipolesis may be more difficult to identify in extranodal sites than in lymph nodes. Examination of touch preps may help with identification of emperipolesis. Extranodal lesions may be associated with fibrosis, which may become prominent, and may be band-like. The distinctive histiocytes are positive for S-100 and for histiocytic markers such as CD68, and are negative for CD1a. The S-100 stain can be helpful in highlighting cells with emperipolesis (**Fig. 21.10**) (101–103,105,106).

When follow-up is available, patients have typically been alive and well (102,103). The breast lesions may persist for months to years if not excised, however (104,106). Recurrence after excision has also been reported (104,106). Rare patients with disease involving the breast and other sites at presentation have had persistent or progressive disease. One death due to widespread Rosai–Dorfman disease that involved the breast has been reported (101).

Erdheim–Chester Disease

Erdheim–Chester disease is a rare non-Langerhans cell histiocytosis characterized by xanthomatous features. Nearly all cases show involvement of long bones of the lower extremities associated with characteristic radiographic features. About half of the patients have extraskeletal involvement that may include skin, orbit, lung, and other sites. Breast involvement is very rare, but when it occurs it can take the form of mass lesions clinically mimicking carcinoma. Histologic examination shows CD68+ xanthomatous histiocytes, scattered Touton-type giant cells, admixed lymphocytes, and fibrosis (107).

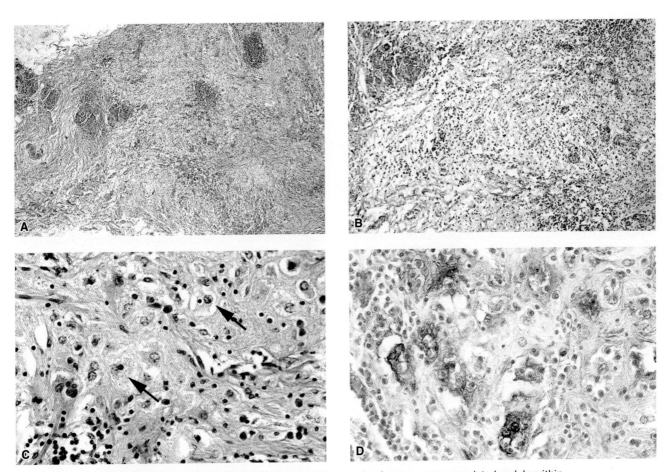

FIGURE 21.10 Rosai–Dorfman Disease. A: The lesion forms an unencapsulated nodule within breast tissue. A few lobules are present in the upper left portion of the lesion. **B:** Medium magnification shows a proliferation of histiocytes with abundant pale cytoplasm and a patchy infiltrate of lymphocytes and plasma cells. A lobule is present in the upper left corner of the image. **C:** High power shows scattered large histiocytes with large, somewhat atypical nuclei, vesicular chromatin, small nucleoli, and abundant pale finely fibrillar cytoplasm. Occasional histiocytes appear to have intracytoplasmic lymphocytes *(arrow)*. **D:** S-100 protein highlights the characteristic histiocytes and facilitates identification of intracytoplasmic lymphocytes, many of which are surrounded by a clear halo.

Langerhans Cell Histiocytosis

Langerhans cell histiocytosis, formerly called histiocytosis X, is a clonal proliferation of Langerhans cells that affects children more than adults and can present as unifocal or multifocal disease in one of three clinical patterns: (1) unifocal disease (previously referred to as eosinophilic granuloma), (2) multifocal disease (formerly referred to as Hand–Schüller–Christian disease), or (3) multifocal disease with disseminated or visceral involvement (formerly called Letterer–Siwe disease) (108). Breast involvement by Langerhans cell histiocytosis is rare. Biopsy shows an infiltrate of large pale Langerhans cells with large pale nuclei with longitudinal or complex folds and moderately abundant pale cytoplasm. The Langerhans cells are CD1a+, S-100+, Langerin+, and in a subset, BRAF+ (108,109). There is a background inflammatory cell infiltrate of eosinophils and small lymphocytes. Langerhans cell histiocytosis is rarely found in association with Hodgkin or non-Hodgkin lymphoma. A case of follicular lymphoma involving the breast with nodules of Langerhans cells present within the lymphoma has been reported (110).

INTRAMAMMARY LYMPH NODES

The differential diagnosis of lymphoid tissue obtained in a biopsy specimen includes intramammary lymph nodes that may be single or multiple. Differentiating an intramammary lymph node from a lymphoid infiltrate involving the breast parenchyma itself is important, and can occasionally be difficult, particularly on a small biopsy. The area with the lymphoid infiltrate should be examined for evidence of an underlying lymph node, such as a discrete capsule or patent sinuses, confirming the presence of a lymph node, whereas finding the infiltrate in continuity with ducts or lobules indicates breast parenchymal involvement. Mammographic examination usually reveals a well-circumscribed mass that may have a lucent center and a peripheral notch corresponding to the hilus of the lymph node (111). Lymph nodes measuring 3 to 15 mm have been described (112,113). Lymph nodes larger than 1 cm are considered abnormal (113) and warrant further investigation. Enlargement of intramammary lymph nodes may be caused by lymphoid hyperplasia, including sinus histiocytosis, involvement by or reaction to inflammatory conditions, HIV-associated lymphadenopathy, and neoplasms such as metastatic tumor or lymphoma (114–117). Reactive lymph nodes sampled by fine needle aspiration (FNA) show a range of findings. Some show a polymorphous admixture of germinal center cells, small lymphocytes, plasma cells, and immunoblasts, whereas others may show mainly small lymphocytes with some plasma cells and few immunoblasts (113). Flow cytometry shows a mixture of phenotypically normal T-cells and polytypic B-cells in such cases.

A number of studies have focused on involvement of intramammary lymph nodes by breast carcinoma. In one study of 1,655 retrospectively reviewed mammograms from patients with breast carcinoma, 16 (0.9%) had metastatic carcinoma in an intramammary lymph node detected radiologically (118). All lymph nodes with carcinoma were larger than 1.0 cm, and one had calcifications. Predictors of intramammary nodal metastases are tumor size greater than 1 cm, high-grade tumor, and positive axillary lymph nodes (119). Rampaul et al. (120) studied completion mastectomy specimens from 157 women who were not candidates for conservation therapy after wide local excision for invasive carcinoma because of findings such as extensive intraductal carcinoma or multifocal invasion. Intramammary lymph nodes were found in 44 of 70 (63%) women with negative axillary lymph nodes. 10 (14%) had a positive intramammary lymph node and were consequently converted from stage I to stage II.

Shen et al. (121) reported that the presence of metastatic carcinoma in an intramammary lymph node was usually associated with concurrent axillary nodal metastases. However, 2 (5%) of the 36 patients with positive intramammary lymph nodes had negative axillary lymph nodes. In another review, 71% of patients with a positive intramammary lymph node had a positive axillary sentinel node (122). The presence of metastatic carcinoma in an intramammary lymph node has been associated with a significantly less-favorable prognosis when compared with patients with a negative intramammary lymph node (121). Nassar et al. (119) found that the presence of positive intramammary lymph nodes was a predictor of poor prognosis in univariate analysis, but it was not an independent prognostic factor in multivariate analysis. For the minority of patients with a positive intramammary lymph node and negative axillary sentinel lymph node, completion axillary lymph node dissection is almost always negative for carcinoma (122), so that full axillary dissection may not be warranted in patients with a negative sentinel node, despite intramammary lymph nodal involvement.

The distinction between breast carcinoma with a dense lymphoid infiltrate and metastatic carcinoma in an intramammary lymph node is sometimes difficult and may not always be made with confidence in a needle core biopsy (NCB) sample. This issue can arise in the breast proper and in the axillary region. The presence of a capsule and sinusoidal structure is the best evidence of a lymph node. Germinal centers suggest a lymph node, but they are present rarely at sites of extranodal carcinoma. Intramammary lymph nodes are rarely the site of metastasis from a carcinoma arising outside the breast (123).

Nevus cell aggregates that occur in the capsule (**Fig. 21.11**) or rarely in the parenchyma of axillary or intramammary lymph nodes may be mistakenly interpreted as metastatic carcinoma (124,125). This possibility should be considered when examining a NCB sample from a mammary parenchymal lymph node.

TISSUE PROCESSING AND ANCILLARY STUDIES

Several different types of specimens may be submitted for pathologic evaluation, and depending on the quantity of tissue, triage for routine processing and ancillary studies varies. When relatively large amount of tissue is obtained and there is clinical

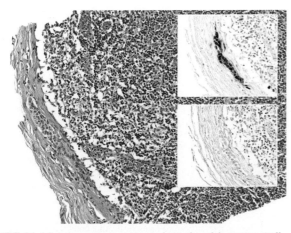

FIGURE 21.11 Intramammary Lymph Node with Nevus Cell Aggregate. The capsule of the lymph node contains an elongate aggregate of cytologically bland, cohesive cells that are positive for S-100 **(inset, upper right)** and negative for cytokeratin **(inset, lower right)**.

suspicion for lymphoma (an uncommon scenario), tissue should be submitted fresh to the Pathology Laboratory. A frozen section should be performed, and if the features are suspicious for lymphoma, separate tissue samples should be fixed for routine sections, submitted for flow cytometry, and, particularly if features suggest a high-grade lymphoma, tissue should be submitted for cytogenetic analysis. However, ensuring that ample tissue remains for routinely stained sections is paramount.

In most cases in which only NCBs are obtained, tissue should all be fixed for routine sections. If the needle cores are large and multiple, and submitted fresh, triaging tissue for flow cytometry in addition to tissue for routine sections can be considered if lymphoma is known to be a concern.

For cases in which the specimen is a FNA biopsy, if a rapid read discloses suspicion of lymphoma, freshly aspirated material can be submitted for flow cytometry to aid in establishing a diagnosis.

In most cases, there is no prebiopsy suspicion for a diagnosis of lymphoma, and material is not obtained for flow cytometry or cytogenetics. In such cases, particularly for low-grade lymphomas, a differential diagnosis of lymphoma and a reactive lymphoid infiltrate may remain, even after careful study of H&E- and immunostained sections. Sending paraffin-embedded tissue for molecular genetic studies to evaluate clonality using polymerase chain reaction (PCR) may be useful in these cases. For high-grade lymphomas in which the differential diagnosis includes entities such as diffuse large B-cell lymphoma, Burkitt lymphoma, and others, sending paraffin sections for fluorescence in situ hybridization (FISH) to investigate the presence of rearrangements of *MYC*, *IGH*, and *BCL2* can be helpful. FISH can also be helpful in investigating the presence of a *BCL2* rearrangement in follicular lymphoma.

REFERENCES

1. Wiseman C, Liao K. Primary lymphoma of the breast. *Cancer.* 1972;29:1705–1712.
2. Hugh J, Jackson F, Hanson J, et al. Primary breast lymphoma—an immunohistologic study of 20 new cases. *Cancer.* 1990;66:2602–2611.
3. Lamovec J, Jancar J. Primary malignant lymphoma of the breast—lymphoma of the mucosa-associated lymphoid tissue. *Cancer.* 1987;60:3033–3041.
4. Domchek SM, Hecht JL, Fleming MD, et al. Lymphomas of the breast: primary and secondary involvement. *Cancer.* 2002;94:6–13.
5. Farinha P, Andre S, Cabecadas J, et al. High frequency of MALT lymphoma in a series of 14 cases of primary breast lymphoma. *Appl Immunohistochem Mol Morphol.* 2002;10:115–120.
6. Cabras MG, Amichetti M, Nagliati M, et al. Primary non-Hodgkin's lymphoma of the breast: a report of 11 cases. *Haematologica.* 2004;89:1527–1528.
7. Lin Y, Guo XM, Shen KW, et al. Primary breast lymphoma: long-term treatment outcome and prognosis. *Leuk Lymphoma.* 2006;47:2102–2109.
8. Vigliotti ML, Dell'olio M, La Sala A, et al. Primary breast lymphoma: outcome of 7 patients and a review of the literature. *Leuk Lymphoma.* 2005;46:1321–1327.
9. Liu M, Hsieh C, Wang A, et al. Primary breast lymphoma: a pooled analysis of prognostic factors and survival in 93 cases. *Ann Saudi Med.* 2005;25:288–293.
10. Mattia A, Ferry J, Harris N. Breast lymphoma: a B-cell spectrum including the low grade B-cell lymphoma of mucosa associated lymphoid tissue. *Am J Surg Pathol.* 1993;17:574–587.
11. Wang LA, Harris NL, Ferry JA. Lymphoma of the breast and the role of mammography in the detection of low-grade lymphomas. *Mod Pathol.* 2004;17:276A.
12. Lin YC, Tsai CH, Wu JS, et al. Clinicopathologic features and treatment outcome of non-Hodgkin lymphoma of the breast—a review of 42 primary and secondary cases in Taiwanese patients. *Leuk Lymphoma.* 2009;50:918–924.
13. Lyons J, Myles J, Pohlman B, et al. Treatment and prognosis of primary breast lymphoma—a review of 13 cases. *Am J Clin Oncol.* 2000;23:334–336.
14. Aviles A, Delgado S, Nambo MJ, et al. Primary breast lymphoma: results of a controlled clinical trial. *Oncology.* 2005;69:256–260.
15. Fruchart C, Denoux Y, Chasle J, et al. High grade primary breast lymphoma: is it a different clinical entity? *Breast Cancer Res Treat.* 2005;93:191–198.
16. Uesato M, Miyazawa Y, Gunji Y, et al. Primary non-Hodgkin's lymphoma of the breast: report of a case with special reference to 380 cases in the Japanese literature. *Breast Cancer (Tokyo, Japan).* 2005;12:154–158.
17. Vignot S, Ledoussal V, Nodiot P, et al. Non-Hodgkin's lymphoma of the breast: a report of 19 cases and a review of the literature. *Clin Lymphoma.* 2005;6:37–42.
18. Ribrag V, Bibeau F, El Weshi A, et al. Primary breast lymphoma: a report of 20 cases. *Br J Haematol.* 2001;115:253–256.
19. Ryan G, Martinelli G, Kuper-Hommel M, et al. Primary diffuse large B-cell lymphoma of the breast: prognostic factors and outcomes of a study by the International Extranodal Lymphoma Study Group. *Ann Oncol.* 2008;19:233–241.
20. Sabate JM, Gomez A, Torrubia S, et al. Lymphoma of the breast: clinical and radiologic features with pathologic correlation in 28 patients. *Breast J.* 2002;8:294–304.
21. Talwalkar SS, Miranda RN, Valbuena JR, et al. Lymphomas involving the breast: a study of 106 cases comparing localized and disseminated neoplasms. *Am J Surg Pathol.* 2008;32:1299–1309.
22. Yoshida S, Nakamura N, Sasaki Y, et al. Primary breast diffuse large B-cell lymphoma shows a non-germinal center B-cell phenotype. *Mod Pathol.* 2005;18:398–405.
23. Brustein S, Filippa DA, Kimmel M, et al. Malignant lymphoma of the breast: a study of 53 patients. *Ann Surg.* 1987;205:144–150.
24. Pisani F, Romano A, Anticoli Borza P, et al. Diffuse large B-cell lymphoma involving the breast: a report of four cases. *J Exp Clin Cancer Res.* 2006;25:277–281.
25. Liguori G, Cantile M, Cerrone M, et al. Breast MALT lymphomas: a clinicopathological and cytogenetic study of 9 cases. *Oncol Rep.* 2012;28:1211–1216.
26. Aozasa K, Ohsawa M, Saeki K, et al. Malignant lymphoma of the breast: immunologic type and association with lymphocytic mastopathy. *Am J Clin Pathol.* 1992;97:699–704.
27. Chanan-Khan A, Holkova B, Goldenberg AS, et al. Non-Hodgkin's lymphoma presenting as a breast mass in patients with HIV infection: a report of three cases. *Leuk Lymphoma.* 2005;46:1189–1193.

28. Jeon H, Akagi T, Hoshida Y, et al. Primary non-Hodgkin's malignant lymphoma of the breast. *Cancer.* 1992;70:2451–2459.

29. Aviv A, Tadmor T, Polliack A. Primary diffuse large B-cell lymphoma of the breast: looking at pathogenesis, clinical issues and therapeutic options. *Ann Oncol.* 2013;24:2236–2244.

30. Arora S, Gupta N, Srinivasan R, et al. Non-Hodgkin's lymphoma presenting as breast masses: a series of 10 cases diagnosed on FNAC. *Diagn Cytopathol.* 2011;41:53–59.

31. Gualco G, Bacchi CE. B-cell and T-cell lymphomas of the breast: clinical, pathological features of 53 cases. *Int J Surg Pathol.* 2008;16: 407–413.

32. Aviles A, Neri N, Nambo MJ. The role of genotype in 104 cases of diffuse large B-cell lymphoma primary of breast. *Am J Clin Oncol.* 2012;35:126–129.

33. Law MF, Chan HN, Leung C, et al. Burkitt-like post-transplant lymphoproliferative disorder (PTLD) presenting with breast mass in a renal transplant recipient: a report of a rare case. *Ann Hematol.* 2014;93:2083–2085.

34. Talwalkar SS, Valbuena JR, Abruzzo LV, et al. MALT1 gene rearrangements and NF-kB activation involving p65 and p50 are absent or rare in primary MALT lymphomas of the breast. *Mod Pathol.* 2006;19:1402–1408.

35. Yhim HY, Kim JS, Kang HJ, et al. Matched-pair analysis comparing the outcomes of primary breast and nodal diffuse large B-cell lymphoma in patients treated with rituximab plus chemotherapy. *Int J Cancer.* 2012;131:235–243.

36. Taniguchi K, Takata K, Chuang SS, et al. Frequent MYD88 L265P and CD79B mutations in primary breast diffuse large B-cell lymphoma. *Am J Surg Pathol.* 2016;40:324–334.

37. Duman BB, Sahin B, Guvenc B, et al. Lymphoma of the breast in a male patient. *Med Oncol.* 2011;28(suppl 1):S490–S493.

38. Ghetu D, Membrez V, Bregy A, et al. Expect the unexpected: primary breast MALT lymphoma. *Arch Gynecol Obstet.* 2011;284:1323–1324.

39. Martinelli G, Ryan G, Seymour JF, et al. Primary follicular and marginal-zone lymphoma of the breast: clinical features, prognostic factors and outcome: a study by the International Extranodal Lymphoma Study Group. *Ann Oncol.* 2009;20:1993–1999.

40. Kambouchner M, Godmer P, Guillevin L, et al. Low grade marginal zone B-cell lymphoma of the breast associated with localised amyloidosis and corpora amylacea in a woman with long standing primary Sjogren's syndrome. *J Clin Pathol.* 2003;56:74–77.

41. Joao C, Farinha P, da Silva MG, et al. Cytogenetic abnormalities in MALT lymphomas and their precursor lesions from different organs: a fluorescence in situ hybridization (FISH) study. *Histopathology.* 2007;50:217–224.

42. Mulligan S, Hu P, Murphy A, et al. Variations in MALT1 gene disruptions detected by FISH in 109 MALT lymphomas occurring in different primary sites. *J Assoc Genet Technol.* 2011;37:76–79.

43. Leoncini L, Raphael M, Stein H, et al. Burkitt lymphoma. In: Swerdlow S, Campo E, Harris N, et al, eds. *WHO Classification Tumours of Haematopoietic and Lymphoid Tissues.* 4th ed. Lyon, France: IARC; 2008:262–264.

44. de Jong D, Vasmel WL, de Boer JP, et al. Anaplastic large-cell lymphoma in women with breast implants. *JAMA.* 2008;300:2030–2035.

45. Burkitt D, Wright D. *Burkitt's Lymphoma.* 1st ed. Edinburgh and London, UK: E & S Livingstone; 1970.

46. Lingohr P, Eidt S, Rheinwalt KP. A 12-year-old girl presenting with bilateral gigantic Burkitt's lymphoma of the breast. *Arch Gynecol Obstet.* 2009;279:743–746.

47. Kebudi A, Coban A, Yetkin G, et al. Primary T-lymphoma of the breast with bilateral involvement, unusual presentation. *Int J Clin Pract.* 2005;59(suppl 147):95–98.

48. Vakiani E, Savage DG, Pile-Spellman E, et al. T-cell lymphoblastic lymphoma presenting as bilateral multinodular breast masses: a case report and review of the literature. *Am J Hematol* 2005;80:216–222.

49. Aguilera NS, Tavassoli FA, Chu WS, et al. T-cell lymphoma presenting in the breast: a histologic, immunophenotypic and molecular genetic study of four cases. *Mod Pathol.* 2000;13:599–605.

50. Briggs JH, Algan O, Stea B. Primary T-cell lymphoma of the breast: a case report. *Cancer Invest.* 2003;21:68–72.

51. Popplewell L, Thomas SH, Huang Q, et al. Primary anaplastic large-cell lymphoma associated with breast implants. *Leuk Lymphoma.* 2011;52:1481–1487.

52. Gualco G, Chioato L, Harrington WJ Jr, et al. Primary and secondary T-cell lymphomas of the breast: clinico-pathologic features of 11 cases. *Appl Immunohistochem Mol Morphol.* 2009;17:301–306.

53. Ergul N, Guner SI, Sager S, et al. Bilateral breast involvement of Hodgkin lymphoma revealed by FDG PET/CT. *Med Oncol.* 2012;29:1105–1108.

54. Hoimes CJ, Selbst MK, Shafi NQ, et al. Hodgkin's lymphoma of the breast. *J Clin Oncol.* 2010;28:e11–e13.

55. Park J, Rizzo M, Jackson S, et al. Reed–Sternberg cells in breast FNA of a patient with left breast mass. *Diagn Cytopathol.* 2010;38:663–668.

56. Roden AC, Macon WR, Keeney GL, et al. Seroma-associated primary anaplastic large-cell lymphoma adjacent to breast implants: an indolent T-cell lymphoproliferative disorder. *Mod Pathol.* 2008;21:455–463.

57. Wong AK, Lopategui J, Clancy S, et al. Anaplastic large cell lymphoma associated with a breast implant capsule: a case report and review of the literature. *Am J Surg Pathol.* 2008;32:1265–1268.

58. Farkash EA, Ferry JA, Harris NL, et al. Rare lymphoid malignancies of the breast: a report of two cases illustrating potential diagnostic pitfalls. *J Hematop.* 2009;2:237–244.

59. Miranda RN, Lin L, Talwalkar SS, et al. Anaplastic large cell lymphoma involving the breast: a clinicopathologic study of 6 cases and review of the literature. *Arch Pathol Lab Med.* 2009;133:1383–1390.

60. Keech JA Jr, Creech BJ. Anaplastic T-cell lymphoma in proximity to a saline-filled breast implant. *Plast Reconstr Surg.* 1997;100:554–555.

61. Cook PD, Osborne BM, Connor RL, et al. Follicular lymphoma adjacent to foreign body granulomatous inflammation and fibrosis surrounding silicone breast prosthesis. *Am J Surg Pathol.* 1995;19:712–717.

62. Duvic M, Moore D, Menter A, et al. Cutaneous T-cell lymphoma in association with silicone breast implants. *J Am Acad Dermatol.* 1995;32:939–942.

63. Kraemer DM, Tony HP, Gattenlohner S, et al. Lymphoplasmacytic lymphoma in a patient with leaking silicone implant. *Haematologica.* 2004;89:ELT01.

64. Sendagorta E, Ledo A. Sezary syndrome in association with silicone breast implant. *J Am Acad Dermatol.* 1995;33:1060–1061.

65. Miranda RN, Aladily TN, Prince HM, et al. Breast implant-associated anaplastic large-cell lymphoma: long-term follow-up of 60 patients. *J Clin Oncol.* 2014;32:114–120.

66. Aladily TN, Medeiros LJ, Amin MB, et al. Anaplastic large cell lymphoma associated with breast implants: a report of 13 cases. *Am J Surg Pathol.* 2012;36:1000–1008.

67. Gaudet G, Friedberg JW, Weng A, et al. Breast lymphoma associated with breast implants: two case-reports and a review of the literature. *Leuk Lymphoma.* 2002;43:115–119.

68. Newman MK, Zemmel NJ, Bandak AZ, et al. Primary breast lymphoma in a patient with silicone breast implants: a case report and review of the literature. *J Plast Reconstr Aesthet Surg.* 2008;61:822–825.

69. Olack B, Gupta R, Brooks GS. Anaplastic large cell lymphoma arising in a saline breast implant capsule after tissue expander breast reconstruction. *Ann Plast Surg.* 2007;59:56–57.

70. Sahoo S, Rosen PP, Feddersen RM, et al. Anaplastic large cell lymphoma arising in a silicone breast implant capsule: a case report and review of the literature. *Arch Pathol Lab Med.* 2003;127:e115–e118.

71. Carty MJ, Pribaz JJ, Antin JH, et al. A patient death attributable to implant-related primary anaplastic large cell lymphoma of the breast. *Plast Reconstr Surg.* 2011;128:e112–e118.

72. Taylor KO, Webster HR, Prince HM. Anaplastic large cell lymphoma and breast implants: five Australian cases. *Plast Reconstr Surg.* 2012;129:e610–e617.

73. Clemens MW, Medeiros LJ, Butler CE, et al. Complete surgical excision is essential for the management of patients with breast implant-associated anaplastic large-cell lymphoma. *J Clin Oncol.* 2016;34:160–168.

74. Anne N, Pallapothu R. Lymphoma of the breast: a mimic of inflammatory breast cancer. *World J Surg Oncol.* 2011;9:125.

75. Antoniou SA, Antoniou GA, Makridis C, et al. Bilateral primary breast lymphoma masquerading as lactating mastitis. *Eur J Obstet Gynecol Reprod Biol.* 2010;152:111–112.

76. Sun LM, Huang EY, Meng FY, et al. Primary breast lymphoma clinically mimicking acute mastitis: a case report. *Tumori.* 2011;97:233–235.

77. Pasquini E, Rinaldi P, Nicolini M, et al. Breast involvement in immuno-lymphoproliferative disorders: report of two cases of multiple myeloma of the breast. *Ann Oncol.* 2000;11:1353–1359.

78. Ross JS, King TM, Spector JI, et al. Plasmacytoma of the breast: an unusual case of recurrent myeloma. *Arch Intern Med.* 1987;147:1838–1840.

79. Kumar PV, Vasei M, Daneshbod Y, et al. Breast myeloma: a report of 3 cases with fine needle aspiration cytologic findings. *Acta Cytol.* 2005;49:445–448.

80. Escobar PF, Patrick RJ, Hicks D, et al. Myeloma of the breast. *Breast J.* 2006;12:387–388.

81. Daneshbod Y, Bagheri MH, Zakernia M, et al. Multiple myeloma recurrence presenting as bilateral breast masses. *Breast J.* 2007;13:310–311.

82. Fayyaz A, Ghani UF. Multiple breast masses in a case of multiple myeloma. *J Coll Physicians Surg Pak.* 2009;19:529–530.

83. Ben-Yehuda A, Steiner-Saltz D, Libson E, et al. Plasmacytoma of the breast: unusual initial presentation of myeloma: report of two cases and review of the literature. *Blut.* 1989;58:169–170.

84. Innes J, Newall J. Myelomatosis. *Lancet.* 1961;1:239–245.

85. Proctor NS, Rippey JJ, Shulman G, et al. Extramedullary plasmacytoma of the breast. *J Pathol.* 1975;116:97–100.

86. Cao S, Kang HG, Liu YX, et al. Synchronous infiltrating ductal carcinoma and primary extramedullary plasmacytoma of the breast. *World J Surg Oncol.* 2009;7:43.

87. Pileri S, Orazi A, Falini B. Myeloid sarcoma. In: Swerdlow S, Campo E, Harris N, et al, eds. *WHO Classification Tumours of Haematopoietic and Lymphoid Tissues.* Lyon, France: IARC; 2008:140–141.

88. Jelic-Puskaric B, Ostojic-Kolonic S, Planinc-Peraica A, et al. Myeloid sarcoma involving the breast. *Coll Antropol.* 2010;34:641–644.

89. Azim HA Jr, Gigli F, Pruneri G, et al. Extramedullary myeloid sarcoma of the breast. *J Clin Oncol.* 2008;26:4041–4043.

90. Valbuena JR, Admirand JH, Gualco G, et al. Myeloid sarcoma involving the breast. *Arch Pathol Lab Med.* 2005;129:32–38.

91. Choschzick M, Bacher U, Ayuk F, et al. Immunohistochemistry and molecular analyses in myeloid sarcoma of the breast in a patient with relapse of NPM1-mutated and FLT3-mutated AML after allogeneic stem cell transplantation. *J Clin Pathol.* 2010;63:558–561.

92. Cunningham I. A clinical review of breast involvement in acute leukemia. *Leuk Lymphoma.* 2006;47:2517–2526.

93. Lim HS, Park MH, Heo SH, et al. Myeloid sarcoma of the breast mimicking hamartoma on sonography. *J Ultrasound Med.* 2008;27:1777–1780.

94. Toumeh A, Phinney R, Kobalka P, et al. Bilateral myeloid sarcoma of the breast and cerebrospinal fluid as a relapse of acute myeloid leukemia after stem-cell transplantation: a case report. *J Clin Oncol.* 2012;30:e199–e201.

95. Brooks JJ, Krugman DT, Damjanov I. Myeloid metaplasia presenting as a breast mass. *Am J Surg Pathol.* 1980;4:281–285.

96. Glew RH, Haese WH, McIntyre PA. Myeloid metaplasia with myelofibrosis: the clinical spectrum of extramedullary hematopoiesis and tumor formation. *Johns Hopkins Med J.* 1973;132:253–270.

97. Martinelli G, Santini D, Bazzocchi F, et al. Myeloid metaplasia of the breast: a lesion which clinically mimics carcinoma. *Virchows Arch A Pathol Anat Histopathol.* 1983;401:203–207.

98. Zonderland HM, Michiels JJ, ten Kate FJ. Case report: mammographic and sonographic demonstration of extramedullary haematopoiesis of the breast. *Clin Radiol.* 1991;44:64–65.

99. Cufer T, Bracko M. Myeloid metaplasia of the breast. *Ann Oncol.* 2001;12:267–270.

100. Al-Nafussi A, Al-Okati D, Alsewan M. Extramedullary haematopoietic tumour of the breast: a case report in a woman with secondary myelofibrosis following essential thrombocythaemia. *Histopathol.* 2004;44:625–626.

101. Green I, Dorfman RF, Rosai J. Breast involvement by extranodal Rosai–Dorfman disease: report of seven cases. *Am J Surg Pathol.* 1997;21:664–668.

102. Morkowski JJ, Nguyen CV, Lin P, et al. Rosai–Dorfman disease confined to the breast. *Ann Diagn Pathol.* 2010;14:81–87.

103. Bansal P, Chakraborti S, Krishnanand G, et al. Rosai–Dorfman disease of the breast in a male: a case report. *Acta Cytol.* 2010;54:349–352.

104. Wu YC, Hsieh TC, Kao CH, et al. A mimic of breast lymphoma: extranodal Rosai–Dorfman disease. *Am J Med Sci.* 2010;339:282–284.

105. Baladandapani P, Hu Y, Kapoor K, et al. Rosai–Dorfman disease presenting as multiple breast masses in an otherwise asymptomatic male patient. *Clin Radiol.* 2012;67:393–395.

106. Tenny SO, McGinness M, Zhang D, et al. Rosai–Dorfman disease presenting as a breast mass and enlarged axillary lymph node mimicking malignancy: a case report and review of the literature. *Breast J.* 2011;17:516–520.

107. Provenzano E, Barter SJ, Wright PA, et al. Erdheim–Chester disease presenting as bilateral clinically malignant breast masses. *Am J Surg Pathol.* 2010;34:584–588.

108. Jaffe E, Weiss L, Facchetti F. Tumours derived from Langerhans cells. In: Swerdlow S, Campo E, Harris N, et al, eds. *WHO Classification of Tumours of Haematopoietic and Lymphoid Tissues.* 4th ed. Lyon, France: IARC; 2008:358–360.

109. Roden AC, Hu X, Kip S, et al. BRAF V600E expression in Langerhans cell histiocytosis: clinical and immunohistochemical study on 25 pulmonary and 54 extrapulmonary cases. *Am J Surg Pathol.* 2014;38:548–551.

110. Adu-Poku K, Thomas DW, Khan MK, et al. Langerhans cell histiocytosis in sequential discordant lymphoma. *J Clin Pathol.* 2005;58:104–106.

111. Kopans DB, Meyer JE, Murphy GF. Benign lymph nodes associated with dermatitis presenting as breast masses. *Radiology.* 1980;137:15–19.

112. McSweeney MB, Egan RL. Prognosis of breast cancer related to intramammary lymph nodes. *Recent Results Cancer Res.* 1984;90:166–172.

113. Vigliar E, Cozzolino I, Fernandez LV, et al. Fine-needle cytology and flow cytometry assessment of reactive and lymphoproliferative processes of the breast. *Acta Cytol.* 2012;56:130–138.

114. Arnaout AH, Shousha S, Metaxas N, et al. Intramammary tuberculous lymphadenitis. *Histopathology.* 1990;17:91–93.

115. Kinoshita T, Yashiro N, Yoshigi J, et al. Inflammatory intramammary lymph node mimicking the malignant lesion in dynamic MRI: a case report. *Clin Imaging.* 2002;26:258–262.

116. Konstantinopoulos PA, Dezube BJ, March D, et al. HIV-associated intramammary lymphadenopathy. *Breast J.* 2007;13:192–195.

117. Lindfors KK, Kopans DB, Googe PB, et al. Breast cancer metastasis to intramammary lymph nodes. *AJR Am J Roentgenol.* 1986;146:133–136.

118. Gunhan-Bilgen I, Memis A, Ustun EE. Metastatic intramammary lymph nodes: mammographic and ultrasonographic features. *Eur J Radiol.* 2001;40:24–29.

119. Nassar A, Cohen C, Cotsonis G, et al. Significance of intramammary lymph nodes in the staging of breast cancer: correlation with tumor characteristics and outcome. *Breast J.* 2008;14:147–152.

120. Rampaul RS, Dale OT, Mitchell M, et al. Incidence of intramammary nodes in completion mastectomy specimens after axillary node sampling: implications for breast conserving surgery. *Breast (Edinburgh, Scotland).* 2008;17:195–198.

121. Shen J, Hunt KK, Mirza NQ, et al. Intramammary lymph node metastases are an independent predictor of poor outcome in patients with breast carcinoma. *Cancer.* 2004;101:1330–1337.

122. Diaz R, Degnim AC, Boughey JC, et al. A positive intramammary lymph node does not mandate a complete axillary node dissection. *Am J Surg.* 2012;203:151–155.

123. Maffini F, Bozzini A, Casadio C, et al. Ovarian serous papillary carcinoma, metastatic to intramammary lymph-node mimic a primary breast carcinoma on RX mammography. *Breast J.* 2012;18:484–485.

124. Biddle DA, Evans HL, Kemp BL, et al. Intraparenchymal nevus cell aggregates in lymph nodes: a possible diagnostic pitfall with malignant melanoma and carcinoma. *Am J Surg Pathol.* 2003;27:673–681.

125. Ridolfi RL, Rosen PP, Thaler H. Nevus cell aggregates associated with lymph nodes: estimated frequency and clinical significance. *Cancer.* 1977;39:164–171.

22

Metastases in the Breast from Nonmammary Malignant Neoplasms

SYED A. HODA

The preoperative clinical workup of an apparently healthy patient with a breast mass can be cursory and is unlikely to exclude a metastasis from a clinically inapparent (that is, "occult") nonmammary malignant neoplasm (NMMN). Even if a history of a previously treated NMMN is known to the clinician when a needle core biopsy (NCB) is obtained, this information may not be conveyed to the pathologist. Thus, when faced with a mammary neoplasm that has unusual clinical, radiologic, or histologic features, it is important to consider metastasis in the differential diagnosis.

CLINICAL FEATURES

Metastases from NMMN are rare and account for less than 1% of all mammary malignant neoplasms in clinical series, and up to 5% of autopsies of patients who die as a result of NMMN (1). Such tumors are relatively more common in females. The interval between initial diagnosis of a NMMN and mammary metastases is usually about 2 years—but it can vary from a few weeks to several years. In approximately one-third of the cases, the metastasis in the breast is the first presentation of the NMMN. Usually, there have already been metastases at other sites, or the tumors are detected at various sites synchronously (2,3).

Metastatic foci in breast often present initially as solitary masses (2). Upon disease progression, such tumors can become multiple and bilateral (3). Metastases have been described in the ipsilateral axillary lymph nodes in a substantial proportion of patients with metastases in the breast (2).

Hematopoietic and lymphoid neoplasms involving the breast are sometimes listed under the rubric of breast "metastases," but they are best regarded as either primary breast neoplasms or as a manifestation of a systemic condition, depending upon the extent of organ involvement. If hematopoietic and lymphoid neoplasms are excluded, the most common NMMNs that secondarily involve the breast include carcinomas of the lung, ovary, stomach, kidney, and cutaneous melanoma. Metastasis from the contralateral breast is a diagnostic consideration when there is bilateral involvement

(or history thereof), the histologic appearances of the tumors in the breasts are similar, and there is no evidence of in situ carcinoma in the contralateral breast. In the pediatric population, lymphoma and rhabdomyosarcoma are the most common sources of NMMN in the breast.

RADIOLOGIC FEATURES

On *mammography*, metastatic tumors tend to present as discrete, solitary, or multiple round masses without spiculation (3). As a result, metastatic tumors cannot be distinguished radiologically from circumscribed primary breast carcinomas, particularly those of the papillary, medullary, or mucinous types. Calcific deposits are uncommon in metastases from NMMN but may occur in metastatic mullerian (tubal, ovarian, or peritoneal) carcinomas (4,5). *Ultrasonography* typically shows the lesions to be hypoechoic without spiculations (6). Radiologic techniques such as *MRI* (magnetic resonance imaging) and *FDG-PET/CT* (fluorodeoxyglucose-positron emission tomography–computed tomography) have also detected metastases in the breast from carcinoma of the thyroid (7), ovary (8), and soft tissue liposarcoma (9). In the latter two instances, the diagnosis of a metastatic NMMN was confirmed by a NCB.

HISTOPATHOLOGIC EVALUATION

The histopathologic appearance of NMMN in the breast is seldom specifically indicative of the site of origin. A notable exception is pigmented metastatic melanoma, although pigmented melanocytic differentiation can occur in metaplastic mammary carcinoma (10). Melanoma arising in the breast is usually a form of metaplastic carcinoma, and it may therefore express cytokeratin. Noncytokeratin expressing primary melanoma of the breast is neurogenic in origin and cytokeratin-negative. Nonetheless, primary melanocytic lesions of the breast are exceedingly less common than metastatic melanocytic neoplasms.

Among the metastatic carcinomas in the breast that are most likely to be mistaken for a breast primary are those arising in the lung, ovary, mullerian system, and bowel. Included in this group are mucinous, signet ring cell, clear cell, and poorly differentiated non–small cell carcinomas of various organs, as well as malignant melanoma (11). Some types of breast tumors such as small cell, adenoid cystic, and mucoepidermoid carcinomas can occur in other organs, and appropriate clinical workup is prudent in these cases. Metastatic neuroendocrine carcinomas of various organs generally share histologic features with primary mammary carcinoma (12).

Histopathologic evaluation of the limited material obtained in NCB samples is unlikely to provide all of the information that would help to distinguish between a primary and a metastatic tumor. The presence of in situ carcinoma that is histologically similar to the invasive lesion rules out a metastatic NMMN. On the other hand, the absence of in situ carcinoma in association with invasive carcinoma is supportive (but not diagnostic) of metastatic rather than a primary breast carcinoma. Metastatic tumor often surrounds and displaces histologically unremarkable breast glandular parenchyma. This phenomenon is less frequent in primary mammary ductal carcinoma, but it is encountered in invasive lobular carcinoma. The latter typically shows little or no hyperplasia. A peripheral lymphocytic infiltrate and stromal reaction are not unusual at the site of metastatic tumor in the breast as well as in primary breast carcinomas. The finding of more than two grossly evident tumor nodules should lead one to consider metastatic tumor, especially if the histologic pattern is unusual. Lymphovascular tumor emboli may result from metastases in the breast as well as from primary breast carcinomas. Diffuse lymphatic spread of metastatic tumor within the breast can occur, and rarely it produces the clinical appearance of inflammatory carcinoma (13).

An unusual histologic pattern and clinical information about a prior neoplasm are the best clues for identifying a metastatic tumor in the breast. It is important to be sensitive to histopathologic patterns that are not typical for breast carcinoma.

COMMON SOURCES OF NMMN INVOLVING THE BREAST

Carcinoma of the Lung and Mesothelioma

Non–small cell carcinoma of the lung is among the most common NMMN to metastasize to the breast (14–17). Pulmonary adenocarcinoma has diverse histologic appearances some of which resemble mammary carcinoma (**Fig. 22.1**). Knowledge of any synchronously or metachronously occurring carcinoma of the lung as well as comparative histopathologic review of the concurrent or prior lung tumor are vital aides in this circumstance (18).

About 75% of pulmonary carcinomas are positive for thyroid transcription factor (TTF1). Although TTF1 immunoreactivity has been reported in mammary carcinomas, the main factor influencing the purported prevalence of TTF1 expression in tumors other than those of pulmonary and thyroid origin is the type of clone used. It has been reported that clone SPT24 (Leica/Novocastra) is more sensitive but less specific than clone 8G7G3/1 (Dakocytomation) (19). Napsin A can be confirmatory of lung primary (20).

Small cell carcinoma can be primary or metastatic in the breast. The diagnosis of primary small cell carcinoma of the breast is supported by the concurrent presence of a conventional ductal type of invasive and/or in situ carcinoma. The diagnosis of metastatic small cell carcinoma in the breast from another organ including lung can be rendered by the exclusion of a mammary primary and comparative histopathologic review of the nonmammary primary tumor. Immunohistochemical stains are unhelpful in this regard since most nonpulmonary (including mammary) small cell carcinomas are ER (−), PR (−), and TTF1 (+). Metastatic small carcinoma is more often multifocal and multicentric.

An exceedingly rare source of metastatic tumor in the breast is *mesothelioma*, especially the epithelioid variant that may mimic a mammary primary. Immunoreactivity for D2-40 (podoplanin) and calretinin strongly favors mesothelioma

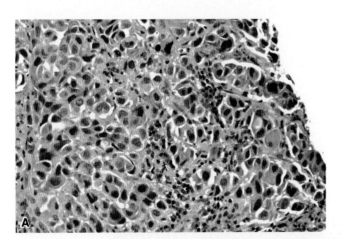
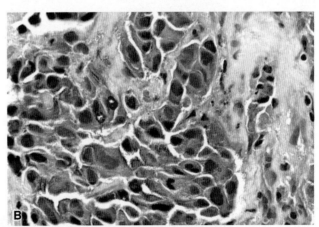

FIGURE 22.1 Metastatic Pulmonary Adenocarcinoma. A: Adenocarcinoma in a needle core biopsy specimen of the breast. Without a clinical history of pulmonary carcinoma, this tumor might be interpreted as mammary carcinoma. **B:** Intracytoplasmic mucin appears magenta with the mucicarmine stain. A histologically similar adenocarcinoma of lung had been previously diagnosed and treated.

over carcinoma (21). Other stains that are helpful to confirm the diagnosis of mesothelioma include claudin-4, CD15, and MOC-31 (21–24).

Malignant Melanoma

Metastatic malignant melanoma presenting clinically as a breast tumor may be difficult to recognize if the primary (cutaneous or ocular) lesion is occult or if the pathologist is uninformed of the clinical history **(Fig. 22.2)** (25). Metastatic melanoma has been reported in the male breast, and it may also involve axillary lymph nodes (2). As stated earlier, exceedingly rare examples of metaplastic mammary carcinoma display melanocytic differentiation (10).

Gastrointestinal Neoplasms

Adenocarcinomas originating in the gastrointestinal tract, especially in the colon and rectum, are rarely the source of metastatic carcinoma in the breast, despite their relatively higher prevalence (26–28). In this setting, nuclear immunoreactivity

for CDX2 is supportive of the diagnosis of metastatic colorectal adenocarcinoma **(Fig. 22.3)** (29).

Neuroendocrine ("carcinoid") tumors of the gastrointestinal tract are a surprisingly frequent source of metastases in one or both breasts (12,30,31). Without knowledge of an extramammary primary, a metastatic neuroendocrine tumor in the breast can be mistaken for a mammary carcinoma with neuroendocrine differentiation (32), or for invasive lobular carcinoma.

Neoplasms of Gynecological Organs

Serous carcinomas of mullerian (that is, tubo-ovarian or peritoneal) origin usually display a papillary appearance with abundant psammoma bodies **(Fig. 22.4)**. The typical immunoprofile of these neoplasms is CK7 (+), CK20 (−), CA125 (+), WT1 (+), and PAX8 (+). The final diagnosis depends on clinical and radiologic correlation (4,33–35). Clinically, occult serous carcinomas of tubal origin can present with axillary lymph nodal involvement (36). Mullerian carcinomas in the breast have generally been serous rather than mucinous. Metastatic endometrial carcinoma with a solid growth pattern

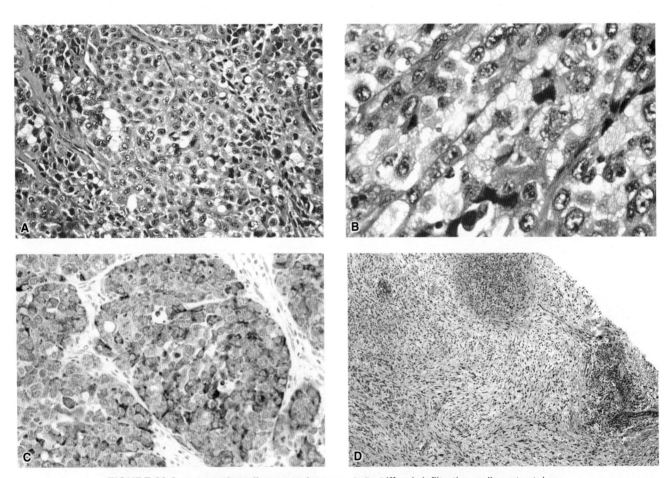

FIGURE 22.2 Metastatic Malignant Melanoma. A, B: Diffusely infiltrating malignant cytokeratin-negative (not shown) cells with an epithelioid appearance. **C:** The tumor cells are immunoreactive for HMB-45. **D–E:** Metastatic spindle and epithelioid melanoma in another needle core breast biopsy sample. The spindle cell component is reactive for S-100 protein **(F)**. There was no reactivity for HMB-45 or Melan-A (not shown). **G–H:** Histopathologic diversity of metastatic melanoma is evident in two additional needle core biopsy specimens of the breast. The melanoma cells appear epithelioid and relatively cohesive in **(G)**, and are discohesive and pigmented in **(H)**.

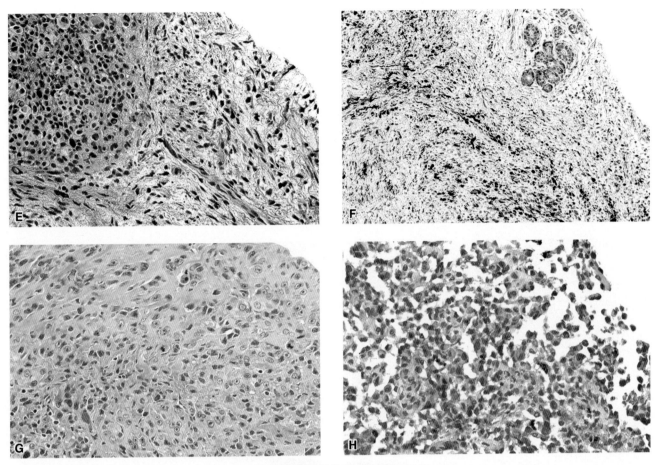

FIGURE 22.2 *(continued)*

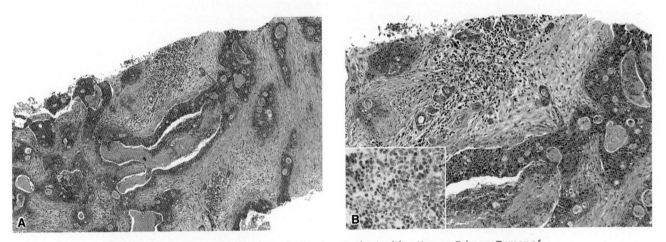

FIGURE 22.3 Metastatic Adenocarcinoma in a Patient with a Known Primary Tumor of Sigmoid Colon. A, B: This needle core biopsy of the breast shows adenocarcinoma. A cluster of native benign inactive breast glands is evident **(top center)**. The tumor cells are immunoreactive with CDX2 (inset in **B**)—a result that is supportive of the diagnosis of metastatic colonic carcinoma. (Courtesy of Drs. S. Titi and A. Ahmad.)

may mimic poorly differentiated or solid papillary mammary carcinoma **(Fig. 22.5)** (37).

The immunostain for *WT1* (Wilms tumor suppressor gene 1), a nuclear marker associated with mullerian (that is, tubo-ovarian and peritoneal) serous papillary carcinomas, has not been reported to be reactive in mammary carcinomas

(35,38,39), with the exception of rare cases of invasive micro-papillary carcinoma (40,41). This is of interest because of the reported upregulation of the *WT1* gene in breast carcinomas (42,43), and the observation that higher WT1 messenger ribonucleic acid (mRNA) levels were associated with a relatively poor prognosis in a series of 99 breast carcinoma patients with

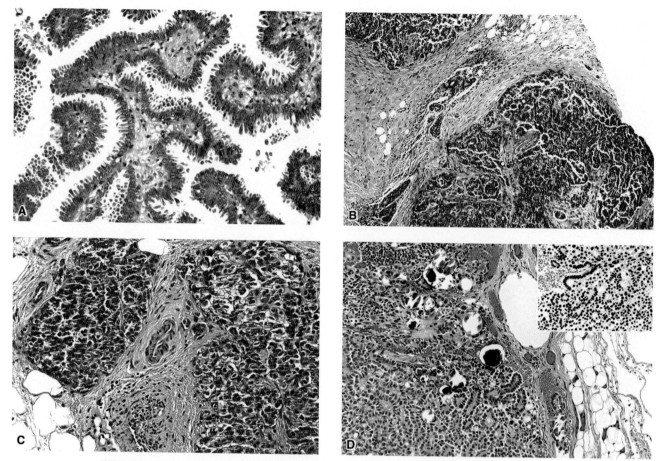

FIGURE 22.4 Metastatic Ovarian Carcinoma. A: Part of needle core biopsy of the breast with metastatic papillary serous ovarian carcinoma. **B, C:** This needle core biopsy sample of the breast shows metastatic poorly differentiated ovarian carcinoma with a solid architecture that resembles mammary carcinoma. **D:** This biopsy of an axillary lymph node shows metastatic papillary serous carcinoma of the ovary with calcifications. PAX8 positivity is shown in inset.

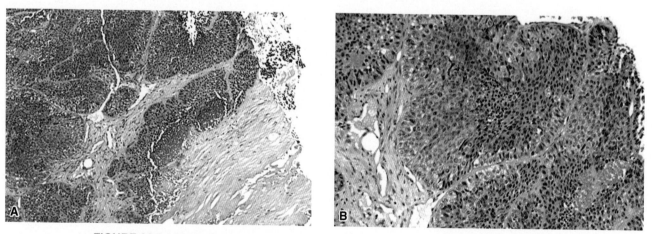

FIGURE 22.5 Metastatic Endometrial Carcinoma. A, B: The solid growth pattern divided into alveolar nests in this needle core biopsy of metastatic endometrial carcinoma resembles the structure of solid papillary mammary carcinoma.

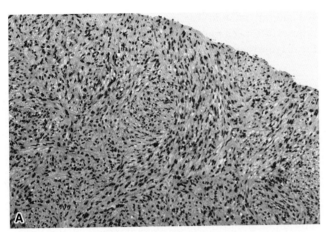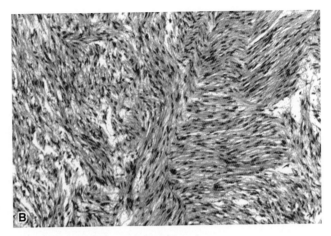

FIGURE 22.6 Metastatic Leiomyosarcoma. A: This needle core biopsy shows a dense tumor composed of interlacing spindle cells with eosinophilic cytoplasm. The tumor cells were immunoreactive for smooth muscle actin (not shown). **B:** The source of the metastasis was a primary leiomyosarcoma of the groin which had been resected 1-year earlier.

a median follow-up of 48 months (44). Focal cytoplasmic reactivity for WT1 in breast carcinomas noted in one report (42) is not considered to be a positive result. Because the majority of mullerian carcinomas are CA125-positive and WT1 is negative in most mammary carcinomas, nuclear reactivity for WT1 and cytoplasmic reactivity for CA125 strongly favors metastatic mullerian carcinoma over primary mammary carcinoma (14,40).

PAX8 is a key transcription factor for organogenesis of the thyroid gland, kidney, and Müllerian system. Nonaka et al. (45) studied 124 ovarian carcinomas (84 serous papillary, 18 endometrioid, 12 mucinous, 10 clear cell) and 243 invasive breast carcinomas (178 ductal, 65 lobular) by immunostaining for PAX8 and WT1 in tissue microarrays. PAX8 reactivity was found in 108 of 124 ovarian carcinomas (87.1%), whereas WT1 expression was observed in 78 of 124 ovarian carcinomas (62.9%). All mammary carcinomas were negative for PAX8, but WT1 expression was seen in 5 of 243 cases (2.1%). In this study, PAX8 was found to be a useful marker in the differential diagnosis of ovarian and breast carcinomas, and superior to WT1 for the diagnosis of all types of nonmucinous ovarian carcinomas, especially clear cell and endometrioid types wherein WT1 expression is generally negative or only focal.

Leiomyosarcomas metastatic to the breast, originating in gynecological organs, have been reported (**Fig. 22.6**) (2).

UNCOMMON SOURCES OF BREAST METASTASES FROM NMMN

Metastatic medullary carcinoma of the thyroid gland growing in the breast with a pattern of invasive lobular carcinoma has been described (46). Papillary and follicular carcinomas of the thyroid gland may rarely metastasize to the breast (47). Papillary carcinoma of the thyroid and lung can produce cystic papillary metastases that mimic primary papillary carcinoma of the breast. A primary breast tumor that resembles the tall cell variant of papillary thyroid carcinoma has also been reported

(48). Thyroid carcinoma will be immunoreactive for TTF1 and thyroglobulin, two markers typically not expressed in mammary carcinoma (49,50).

Among sarcomas metastatic to the breast, solitary fibrous tumor (erstwhile hemangiopericytoma), leiomyosarcoma, and pleomorphic sarcoma (formerly malignant fibrous histiocytoma) and liposarcoma may be difficult to distinguish from primary mammary sarcomas (including malignant phyllodes tumors) and spindle cell metaplastic mammary carcinomas (9,51).

Instances of mammary metastases of extremely uncommon tumors, such as esthesioneuroblastoma, have been recorded (52). Mammary metastases from various small, blue, round cell tumors such as medulloblastoma, rhabdomyosarcoma, and neuroblastoma can occur in children and adults (**Fig. 22.7**) (53–56).

At least one case of tumor-to-tumor metastasis (specifically a renal cell carcinoma metastatic to invasive ductal carcinoma) has been reported in the breast (57). This "collision tumor" was evident only on the excisional biopsy. The initial NCB showed only ductal carcinoma in situ—illustrating the sampling issues inherent with limited technique.

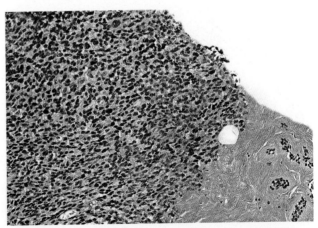

FIGURE 22.7 Metastatic Embryonal Rhabdomyosarcoma. The needle core biopsy specimen showing a small blue round cell tumor is from a breast mass in a female child. The patient had a history of embryonal rhabdomyosarcoma.

OCCULT PRIMARY NEOPLASMS

A review of records over a 92-year period at Royal London Hospital revealed that about one-third of metastatic NMMN originated from an occult primary tumor (17). A surprising proportion of occult lung tumors that have presented with breast metastases have been small cell carcinomas (15–17). Other sites of occult neoplasms include kidney, stomach, and ovary-tube (34), as well as those originating from the intestinal neuroendocrine system (erstwhile "carcinoid" tumors) (30,58).

METASTATIC PROSTATIC CARCINOMA

When a breast mass is discovered in a man known to have prostate carcinoma, comparative histopathologic review of the two tumors is essential. Stains for prostate-specific antigen (PSA), prostate acid phosphatase (PSAP), and NKX3 should be performed in equivocal cases (59,60). Because PSA has been detected by immunostaining in breast carcinomas from men and women, a positive result is not by itself diagnostic of metastatic prostate carcinoma (61). Estrogen receptor (ER) and androgen receptor (AR) immunoreactivity may not be helpful in this regard, because prostate carcinomas can be ER (+) and AR (+) (62). The extent, if any, of GCDFP-15, GATA3, and NY-BR1 expression in prostatic carcinoma remains to be determined.

A "collision" tumor consisting of metastatic prostatic carcinoma in a primary solid papillary carcinoma of the male breast has been described (63).

LATE PRESENTATION OF METASTATIC NMMN IN THE BREAST

Previously diagnosed neoplasms that have given rise to breast metastases later in the clinical course of the disease include malignant melanoma, sarcoma, lung carcinoma, intestinal "carcinoid," bladder (urothelial) carcinoma, and renal (clear cell and sarcomatoid) carcinoma **(Fig. 22.8)** (3,64–66). Metastases have been found in the breast as long as 16 years after the diagnosis of the primary neoplasm (2).

AXILLARY LYMPH NODE METASTASES FROM NMMN

Metastatic carcinoma in axillary lymph nodes without an apparent ipsilateral or contralateral breast primary is a well-recognized clinical scenario. An occult mammary primary should be the primary consideration in the differential diagnosis, and initial evaluation should be guided by this concept. Mammography, ultrasound, and MRI examinations are helpful in this regard. Apocrine carcinomas of the breast have a predilection to present either as occult mammary primaries or axillary nodal metastases. Most of these tumors are CK (+), ER (−), PR (−), AR (+), and HER2 (−). This immunoprofile will distinguish apocrine carcinoma from metastatic melanoma, which it can resemble.

Axillary nodal involvement by metastatic NMMN is usually accompanied by coincidental metastatic spread to one or both breasts (2). However, NMMN may involve axillary lymph nodes without clinically evident metastases in either breast. Delair (2) studied 85 patients with breast and/or axillary lymph node by metastatic NMMN. Axillary involvement alone occurred in 6/85 (79%) cases, with the most frequent primary lesion being cutaneous malignant melanoma. The authors did not indicate how many of the primary lesions were contiguous to the axillary metastasis. Nonmelanomatous primary sites of axillary nodal involvement by NMMN in the absence of breast metastases includes serous papillary ovarian carcinoma (67), large cell neuroendocrine carcinoma of the lung (68), and squamous cell carcinoma of the tonsil (69).

A benign squamous epithelium-lined inclusion cyst in an axillary lymph node can be mistaken for metastatic squamous cell carcinoma on NCB sampling (70). Endosalpingiosis is a unique type of benign glandular inclusion in axillary lymph

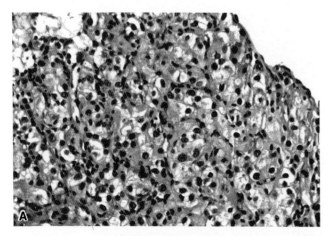
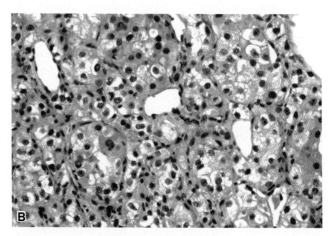

FIGURE 22.8 Metastatic Renal Carcinoma. A: A needle core biopsy of the breast showing metastatic renal clear cell carcinoma in a patient with a remote history of histologically similar renal carcinoma. **B:** The tumor shows an alveolar structure and cytoplasmic clearing that resemble mammary apocrine carcinoma with clear cell change.

nodes (71), which can simulate metastatic well-differentiated adenocarcinoma (72). High-power microscopic examination reveals the epithelial lining to be of the ciliated type with interspersed "peg" cells.

"IMPLANTATION METASTASES" IN THE BREAST

The development of secondary tumor deposit along the healing biopsy tract of a needle biopsy procedure has been called "implantation metastasis." Several cases have been reported in the breast. In some instances, the tract of the fine needle aspiration (FNA) biopsy procedure traversed breast tissues *en route* to and from the targeted lesion in the lung.

In one such case, a 57-year-old woman developed an "implant metastasis" in the breast 3 months after a CT-guided FNA of the ipsilateral lung with a 20-gauge needle. The tumor deposit involved breast tissue as well as skin (73). In another notable case, a 52-year-old woman developed an "implant metastasis" in the skin and subcutaneous tissue of the breast

4 months after a CT-guided FNA of the ipsilateral lung with a 22-gauge needle (74) **(Fig. 22.9)**.

An unusual case of "implantation metastasis" was reported in a 38-year-old woman who had been treated by skin-sparing mastectomy for microinvasive carcinoma associated with high-grade ductal carcinoma in situ (75). The ipsilateral breast underwent immediate autologous reconstruction. Three years later, Paget disease of the skin occurred at the puncture site of the original NCB site.

An implantation metastasis can mimic primary breast carcinoma. The clinical history, a comparative review of the primary and secondary tumors, and immunohistochemical studies will usually clarify the diagnosis.

USE OF IMMUNOSTAINS IN THE DIAGNOSIS OF METASTASES IN THE BREAST

Typically, a panel of immunostains ought to be employed in this setting as no single marker is completely sensitive or specific.

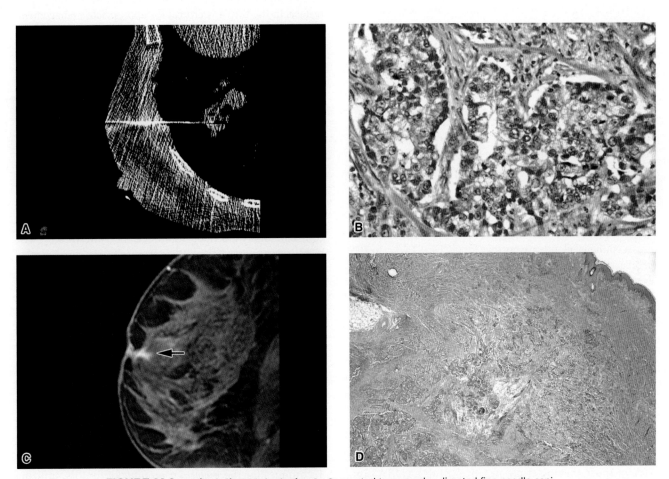

FIGURE 22.9 Implantation Metastasis. A: Computed tomography–directed fine needle aspiration (FNA) of the right lung shows passage of the needle through the right breast and anterior chest wall. Cytologic examination of the FNA showed malignant cells (not shown). **B:** The subsequent lobectomy showed adenocarcinoma of the lung. **C:** Computed tomography of the "tumor in the breast," 14 months after the FNA, shows a superficial tumor mass. **D, E:** Implantation metastasis in the skin and subcutaneous tissue of the breast. The tumor is similar to the previously diagnosed adenocarcinoma of the lung (seen in **B**), and is positive for thyroid transcription factor-1 **(F)**.

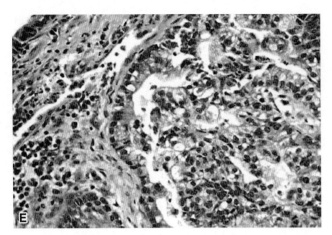

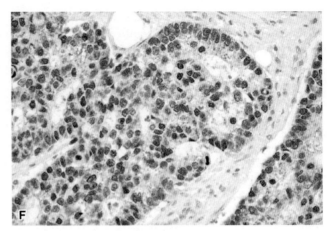

FIGURE 22.9 (*continued*)

The use of several immunostains has been mentioned in the foregoing discussions.

Most breast carcinomas are CK7 (+), CK20 (−), mammaglobin (+), GCDFP15 (+), NY-BR-1 (+), and GATA3 (+). Approximately 70% of breast carcinomas are ER (+) and PR (+). A panel utilizing some, if not all, of these markers can be helpful in confirming mammary origin of a tumor, which is deemed to be of uncertain origin.

Mammaglobin is an epithelial intracytoplasmic secretory glycoprotein of mammary epithelial cells. Mammary carcinomas of all grades may be positive for mammaglobin, whereas normal epithelial cells are typically not immunoreactive. The sensitivity of mammaglobin for breast carcinoma is around 77%, but it lacks the specificity of GCDFP-15 (76,77). Carcinomas of cutaneous adnexal glands as well as salivary glands may also be mammaglobin-positive.

GCDFP-15 (BRST-2) is a secretory product of mammary cells that can be demonstrated via immunostains in mammary and extramammary apocrine epithelia. Only rare cells in normal breast epithelial glands are positive for GCDFP-15. Up to 70% of breast carcinomas are positive for GCDFP-15 (76,77). Rare examples of pulmonary adenocarcinoma (approximately 5%) can be positive for GCDFP-15 (78).

NY-BR-1 is a mammary differentiation antigen that is expressed in benign and malignant mammary epithelial tissue. About 50% of breast carcinomas can be positive for NY-BR-1 (79); and about 5% of carcinomas of mullerian origin may also be positive, albeit weakly (80).

GATA3, a transcription factor that mainly regulates differentiation of mammary and urothelial epithelia, can be useful in confirming mammary origin of a tumor. Immunohistochemical expression of GATA3 can be found in more than 90% of mammary carcinomas, including about 70% of those that are triple-negative (81,82). GATA3 immunoreactivity is encountered in the majority of urothelial carcinomas, and it has also been reported in cutaneous basal cell carcinomas as well as trophoblastic and yolk sac tumors. GATA3 expression has been reported in 69% of ER-negative breast carcinomas (83,84).

MANAGEMENT OF BREAST METASTASES FROM NMMN

The distinction between a primary breast tumor and a metastasis in the breast is critical for appropriate management. A multidisciplinary integrated approach among pathologists, oncologists, surgeons, and radiologists (85) is important. It is vital that comparative histopathological review of the primary nonmammary and mammary tumors be performed whenever possible. When an occult extramammary neoplasm presents with a breast metastasis, the diagnostic workup of the patient will be largely influenced by morphologic features of the tumor that may suggest one or more particular primary sites. Advances in immunohistochemistry and other techniques can enable the identification of primary site of tumor facilitating site-specific therapy.

In most cases, mastectomy is not appropriate for metastatic tumor in the breast, but it may be performed to obtain local control of bulky ulcerated, multifocal, necrotic, or otherwise highly symptomatic lesions. Wide excision can be supplemented by radiation therapy to the breast for appropriately selected neoplasms, and axillary dissection should be performed if the lymph nodes therein are involved. Emphasis should necessarily be placed on systemic treatment appropriate to the primary lesion. Metastatic involvement of the breast is a manifestation of generalized metastases in virtually all cases, and the prognosis depends on the clinical characteristics of the particular primary neoplasm. Median survival was 15 months after the diagnosis of breast or axillary metastases in 55 patients in one series (2).

FUTURE DIRECTIONS

Techniques for the *molecular profiling* of tumors, utilizing various platforms including RT-PCR, cDNA microarray, and microRNA profiling, have become increasingly available in recent years. When a metastatic NMMN is suspected, the aim of such profiling is to reliably establish the primary site, thus enabling site-specific chemotherapy. The latter, when initiated

TABLE 22.1

Immunohistochemical Approach to Establish Possible Primary Site of a Suspected Metastatic Malignant Neoplasms in the Breast

To Determine...	Diagnosis	Immunohistochemical Marker
Lineage	Carcinoma	Cytokeratin
	Lymphoma	CD45
	Melanoma	A103, HMB45, MITF, S100p
	Sarcoma[a]	Vimentin
Type of carcinoma	Adenocarcinoma	CK7 or CK20
	Germ cell tumor	PLAP, OCT4, AFP, B-HCG
	Hepatocellular	HEPPAR1, pCEA, CD10, CD13
	Renal cell	RCC, CD10, PAX2, PAX8
	Squamous cell	CK5/6, p63
	Neuroendocrine	Chromogranin, synaptophysin, CD56
	Urothelial	GATA3
Site	Colorectal	CDX2, CK7(−), CK20(+)
	Lung	TTF1, Napsin A, CK7(+), CK20(-)
	Ovary	ER, CA125, WT1, PAX2, PAX8
	Pancreatobiliary	CDX2, CK7(+), CK20(+), SMAD4 inactivation
	Prostate	PSA, PrAP
	Thyroid	TTF1, thyroglobulin

AFP, alpha fetoprotein; B-HCG, beta human chorionic gonadotrophin; ca, carcinoma; CD, cluster designation; CDX2, caudal type homeobox transcription factor-2; CK, cytokeratin; ER, estrogen receptor; GATA3, GATA binding protein 3 to DNA sequence [A/T]GATA[A/G]; HEPPAR1, hepatocyte paraffin-1; HMB45, human melanoma black 45; MITF, microphthalmic transcription factor; OCT4, octamer binding transcription factor-4; PAX8, paired-box gene-8; PLAP, placental alkaline phosphatase; pCEA, polyclonal carcinoembryonic antigen; PrAP, prostate acid phosphatase; PSA, prostate-specific antigen; RCC, renal cell carcinoma; S100p, S100 protein; TTF1, thyroid transcription factor-1; WT1, Wilms tumor-1.
[a]In tumors negative for carcinoma, lymphoma, and melanoma markers, and with appropriate histologic appearance.
Modified from Kim KW, Krajewski KM, Jagannathan JP, et al. Cancer of unknown primary sites: what radiologists need to know and what oncologists want to know. *AJR Am J Roentgenol.* 2013;200:484–492.

on the basis of either immunohistochemistry or molecular profiling, can be more effective than empiric chemotherapy (86).

Several commercial *molecular test kits* for the identification of primary site in tumors of unknown primary are available, and their accuracy rate ranges from 33% to 93% (87,88). Most of these assays are based on processes that have been developed by utilizing better-differentiated examples of various tumor types, and their utility in yielding "actionable" information in poorly differentiated tumors may be of dubious value. At this time, it is possible that a well-designed immunohistochemical panel **(Table 22.1)** may be more informative in this regard.

The identification of key *gene mutations* such as *HER2, ALK, EGFR, KRAS*, etc., is another emerging application of molecular profiling. Upon detection, such mutations may be "actionable," that is, be targets for therapy. It is likely that molecular profiling of primary or metastatic tumors in the breast (including those that are diagnosed on the limited samples procured in NCBs) will be increasingly performed (89).

It is also likely that *massively parallel sequencing* will prove to be a useful tool to define the relationship, clonality, and intratumoral genetic heterogeneity between the primary malignant neoplasms and metastatic deposits in patients with multiple primary neoplasms and synchronous metastases (90).

REFERENCES

1. Abrams HL, Spiro R, Goldstein N. Metastases in carcinoma: analysis of 1,000 autopsied cases. *Cancer.* 1950;3:74–85.
2. DeLair DF, Corben AD, Catalano JP, et al. Non-mammary metastases to the breast and axilla: a study of 85 cases. *Mod Pathol.* 2013;26:343–349.
3. Toombs BD, Kalisher L. Metastatic disease to the breast: clinical, pathologic, and radiographic features. *AJR Am J Roentgenol.* 1977;129:673–676.
4. Recine MA, Deavers MT, Middleton LP, et al. Serous carcinoma of the ovary and peritoneum with metastases to the breast and axillary lymph nodes: a potential pitfall. *Am J Surg Pathol.* 2004;28:1646–1651.
5. Goldstein NS, Uzieblo A. WT1 immunoreactivity in uterine papillary serous carcinomas is different from ovarian serous carcinomas. *Am J Clin Pathol.* 2002;117:541–545.
6. Mun SH, Ko EY, Han BK, et al. Breast metastases from extramammary malignancies: typical and atypical ultrasound features. *Korean J Radiol.* 2014;15:20–28.
7. Formicola F, Riccardi A, Vigliar E, et al. Multimetastatic medullary thyroid carcinoma to the breast: PET/CT-mammographic-US and MR findings. *Breast J.* 2014;20:653–654.
8. Gayer G, Ben-Haim S. Ovarian carcinoma metastasis to breast: role of PET/CT. *Isr Med Assoc J.* 2013;15:784.
9. Yokouchi M, Nagano S, Kijima Y, et al. Solitary breast metastasis from myxoid liposarcoma. *BMC Cancer.* 2014;14:482.
10. Ruffolo EF, Koerner FC, Maluf HM. Metaplastic carcinoma of the breast with melanocytic differentiation. *Mod Pathol.* 1997;10:592–596.
11. Boutis AL, Andreadis C, Patakiouta F, et al. Gastric signet-ring adenocarcinoma presenting with breast metastasis. *World J Gastroenterol.* 2006;12:2958–2961.

12. Perry KD, Reynolds C, Rosen DG, et al. Metastatic neuroendocrine tumour in the breast: a potential mimic of in situ and invasive mammary carcinoma. *Histopathology.* 2011;59:619–630.

13. Njiaju UO, Truica CI. Metastatic prostatic adenocarcinoma mimicking inflammatory breast carcinoma: a case report. *Clin Breast Cancer.*2010;10:E3–E5.

14. Lee AHS. The histological diagnosis of metastases to the breast from extramammary malignancies. *J Clin Pathol.* 2007;60:1333–1341.

15. Kelly C, Henderson D, Corris P. Breast lumps: rare presentation of oat cell carcinoma of lung. *J Clin Pathol.* 1988;41:171–172.

16. McCrea ES, Johnston C, Haney PJ. Metastases to the breast. *AJR Am J Roentgenol.* 1983;141:685–690.

17. Georgiannos SN, Chin J, Goode AW, et al. Secondary neoplasms of the breast: a survey of the 20th century. *Cancer.* 2001;92:2259–2266.

18. Mirrielees JA, Kapur JH, Szalkucki LM, et al. Metastasis of primary lung carcinoma to the breast: a systematic review of the literature. *J Surg Res.* 2014;188:419–431.

19. Masood S, Davis C, Kubik MJ. Changing the term "breast tumor resembling the tall cell variant of papillary thyroid carcinoma" to "tall cell variant of papillary breast carcinoma." *Adv Anat Pathol.* 2012;19:108–110.

20. Turner BM, Cagle PT, Sainz IM, et al. Napsin A: a new marker for lung adenocarcinoma, is complementary and more sensitive and specific than thyroid transcription factor 1 in the differential diagnosis of primary pulmonary carcinoma: evaluation of 1674 cases by tissue microarray. *Arch Pathol Lab Med.* 2012;136:163–171.

21. Ordóñez NG. Immunohistochemical diagnosis of epithelioid mesothelioma: an update. *Arch Pathol Lab Med.* 2005;129:1407–1414.

22. Hyun TS, Barnes M, Tabatabai ZL. The diagnostic utility of D2-40, calretinin, CK5/6, desmin and MOC-31 in the differentiation of mesothelioma from adenocarcinoma in pleural effusion cytology. *Acta Cytol.* 2012;56:527–532.

23. Mohammad T, Garratt J, Torlakovic E, et al. Utility of a CEA, CD15, calretinin, and CK5/6 panel for distinguishing between mesotheliomas and pulmonary adenocarcinomas in clinical practice. *Am J Surg Pathol.* 2012;36:1503–1508.

24. Ordóñez NG. Application of immunohistochemistry in the diagnosis of epithelioid mesothelioma: a review and update. *Hum Pathol.* 2013;44:1–19.

25. Ravdel L, Robinson WA, Lewis K, et al. Metastatic melanoma in the breast: a report of 27 cases. *J Surg Oncol.* 2006;94:101–104.

26. Ho YY, Lee WK. Metastasis to the breast from an adenocarcinoma of the colon. *J Clin Ultrasound.* 2009;37:239–241.

27. Noh KT, Oh B, Sung SH, et al. Metastasis to the breast from colonic adenocarcinoma. *J Korean Surg Soc.* 2011;81:S43–S46.

28. Alexander HR, Turnbull AD, Rosen PP. Isolated breast metastases from gastrointestinal carcinomas: report of two cases. *J Surg Oncol.* 1989;42:264–266.

29. Ahmad A, Baiden-Amissah K, Oyegade A, et al. Primary sigmoid adenocarcinoma metastasis to the breast in a 28-year-old female: a case study and a review of literature. *Korean J Pathol.* 2014;48:58–61.

30. Geyer HL, Viney J, Karlin N. Metastatic carcinoid presenting as a breast lesion. *Curr Oncol.* 2010;17:73–77.

31. Upalakalin JN, Collins LC, Tawa N, et al. Carcinoid tumors in the breast. *Am J Surg.* 2006;191:799–805.

32. Mosunjac MB, Kochhar R, Mosunjac MI, et al. Primary small bowel carcinoid tumor with bilateral breast metastases: report of 2 cases with different clinical presentations. *Arch Pathol Lab Med.* 2004;128:292–297.

33. Laury AR, Perets R, Piao H, et al. A comprehensive analysis of PAX8 expression in human epithelial tumors. *Am J Surg Pathol.* 2011;35:816–826.

34. Elit LM, Cunnane MF. Breast metastasis from ovarian carcinoma: report of two cases and literature review. *Acta Obstet Gynecol Scand.* 1992;71:81–83.

35. Abehsera D, Hernández A, Santisteban J, et al. Ovarian serous cystadenocarcinoma metastasizing to the breast. *J Obstet Gynaecol.* 2013;33:215–216.

36. Atallah C, Altinel G, Fu L, et al. Axillary metastasis from an occult tubal serous carcinoma in a patient with ipsilateral breast carcinoma: a potential diagnostic pitfall. *Case Rep Pathol.* 2014;2014:534034.

37. Moore DH, Wilson DK, Hurteau JA, et al. Gynecologic cancers metastatic to the breast. *J Am Coll Surg.* 1998;187:178–181.

38. Tornos C, Soslow R, Chen S, et al. Expression of WT1, CA 125, and GCDFP-15 as useful markers in the differential diagnosis of primary ovarian carcinomas versus metastatic breast cancer to the ovary. *Am J Surg Pathol.* 2005;29:1482–1489.

39. Hedley C, Sriraksa R, Showeil R, et al. The frequency and significance of WT-1 expression in serous endometrial carcinoma. *Hum Pathol.* 2014;45:1879–1884.

40. Domfeh AB, Carley AL, Striebel JM, et al. WT1 immunoreactivity in breast carcinoma: selective expression in pure and mixed mucinous subtypes. *Mod Pathol.* 2008;21:1217–1223.

41. Lee AH, Paish EC, Marchio C, et al. The expression of Wilms' tumour-1 and Ca125 in invasive micropapillary carcinoma of the breast. *Histopathology.* 2007;51:824–828.

42. Silberstein GB, Van Horn K, Strickland P, et al. Altered expression of the WT1 Wilms tumor suppressor gene in human breast cancer. *Proc Natl Acad Sci U S A.* 1997;94:8132–8137.

43. Loeb DM, Evron E, Patel CB, et al. Wilms' tumor suppressor gene (WT1) is expressed in primary breast tumors despite tumor-specific promoter methylation. *Cancer Res.* 2001;61:921–925.

44. Miyoshi Y, Ando A, Egawa C, et al. High expression of Wilms' tumor suppressor gene predicts poor prognosis in breast cancer patients. *Clin Cancer Res.* 2002;8:1167–1171.

45. Nonaka D, Chiriboga L, Soslow RA. Expression of PAX8 as a useful marker in distinguishing ovarian carcinomas from mammary carcinomas. *Am J Surg Pathol.* 2008;32:1566–1571.

46. Ali SZ, Teichberg S, Attie JN, et al. Medullary thyroid carcinoma metastatic to breast masquerading as infiltrating lobular carcinoma. *Ann Clin Lab Sci.* 1994;24:441–447.

47. Loureiro MM, Leite VH, Boavida JM, et al. An unusual case of papillary carcinoma of the thyroid with cutaneous and breast metastases only. *Eur J Endocrinol.* 1997;137:267–269.

48. Tosi AL, Ragazzi M, Asioli S, et al. Breast tumor resembling the tall cell variant of papillary thyroid carcinoma: report of 4 cases with evidence of malignant potential. *Int J Surg Pathol.* 2007;15:14–19.

49. Robens J, Goldstein L, Gown AM, et al. Thyroid transcription factor-1 expression in breast carcinomas. *Am J Surg Pathol.* 2010;34:1881–1885.

50. Bisceglia M, Galliani C, Rosai J. TTF-1 expression in breast carcinoma-the chosen clone matters. *Am J Surg Pathol.* 2011;35:1087–1088.

51. Ruhland B, Dittmer C, Thill M, et al. Metastasized hemangiopericytoma of the breast: a rare case. *Arch Gynecol Obstet.* 2009;280:491–494.

52. Larbcharoensub N, Kanoksil W, Cheewaruangroj W, et al. Esthesioneuroblastoma metastasis to the breast: a case report and review of the literature. *Oncol Lett.* 2014;8:1505–1508.

53. Kapila K, Sarkar C, Verma K. Detection of metastatic medulloblastoma in a fine needle breast aspirate. *Acta Cytol.* 1996;40:384–385.

54. Merced C, Rubio IT, Rodríguez J, et al. Breast metastasis from rhabdomyosarcoma of the nasal septum in a pregnant adult woman. *Breast J.* 2011;17:420–421.

55. Jung SP, Lee Y, Han KM, et al. Breast metastasis from rhabdomyosarcoma of the anus in an adolescent female. *J Breast Cancer.* 2013;16:345–348.

56. Yaren A, Guclu A, Sen N, et al. Breast metastasis in a pregnant woman with alveolar rhabdomyosarcoma of the upper extremity. *Eur J Obstet Gynecol Reprod Biol.* 2008;140:131–133.

57. Chen TD, Lee LY. A case of renal cell carcinoma metastasizing to invasive ductal breast carcinoma. *J Formos Med Assoc.* 2014;113:133–136.

58. Kashlan RB, Powell RW, Nolting SF. Carcinoid and other tumors metastatic to the breast. *J Surg Oncol.* 1982;20:25–30.

59. Green LK, Klima M. The use of immunohistochemistry in metastatic prostatic adenocarcinoma to the breast. *Hum Pathol.* 1991;22:242–246.

60. Gurel B, Ali TZ, Montgomery EA, et al. NKX3.1 as a marker of prostatic origin in metastatic tumors. *Am J Surg Pathol.* 2010;34:1097–1105.

61. Yu H, Levesque MA, Clark GM, et al. Enhanced prediction of breast cancer prognosis by evaluating expression of p53 and prostate-specific antigen in combination. *Br J Cancer.* 1999;81:490–495.

62. Asgari M, Morakabati A. Estrogen receptor beta expression in prostate adenocarcinoma. *Diagn Pathol.* 2011;6:61.

63. Sahoo S, Smith RE, Potz JL, et al. Metastatic prostatic adenocarcinoma within a primary solid papillary carcinoma of the male breast. *Arch Pathol Lab Med.* 2001;125:1101–1103.

64. Belton AL, Stull MA, Grant T, et al. Mammographic and sonographic findings in metastatic transitional cell carcinoma of the breast. *AJR Am J Roentgenol.* 1997;168:511–512.

65. Vassalli L, Ferrari VD, Simoncini E, et al. Solitary breast metastases from a renal cell carcinoma. *Breast Cancer Res Treat.* 2001;68:29–31.

66. Ding GT, Hwang JS, Tan PH. Sarcomatoid renal cell carcinoma metastatic to the breast: report of a case with diagnosis on fine needle aspiration cytology. *Acta Cytol.* 2007;51:451–455.

67. Sibio S, Sammartino P, Accarpio F, et al. Axillary lymph node metastasis as first presentation of peritoneal carcinomatosis from serous papillary ovarian cancer: case report and review of the literature. *Eur J Gynaecol Oncol.* 2014;35:170–173.

68. Terada T. Pathologic diagnosis of large cell neuroendocrine carcinoma of the lung in an axillary lymph node: a case report with immunohistochemical and molecular genetic studies. *Int J Clin Exp Pathol.* 2013;6:1177–1179.

69. Cheng CY, Su TF, Lin YH, et al. Rare axillary metastasis from squamous cell carcinoma of the tonsil. *Clin Nucl Med.* 2013;38:e304–e305.

70. Zhang C, Xiong J, Quddus MR, at al. A rapidly enlarging squamous inclusion cyst in an axillary lymph node following core needle biopsy. *Case Rep Pathol.* 2012;2012:418070.

71. Carney E, Cimino-Mathews A, Argani C, et al. A subset of nondescript axillary lymph node inclusions have the immunophenotype of endosalpingiosis. *Am J Surg Pathol.* 2014;38:1612–1617.

72. Salehi AH, Omeroglu G, Kanber Y, et al. Endosalpingiosis in axillary lymph nodes simulating metastatic breast carcinoma: a potential diagnostic pitfall. *Int J Surg Pathol.* 2013;21:610–612.

73. Sacchini V, Galimberti V, Marchini S, et al. Percutaneous transthoracic needle aspiration biopsy: a case report of implantation metastasis. *Eur J Surg Oncol.* 1989;15:179–183.

74. Schreiner AM, Jones JG, Swistel AJ, et al. Transthoracic fine needle aspiration resulting in implantation metastasis in the superficial tissues of the breast. *Cytopathology.* 2013;24:58–60.

75. Calvillo KZ, Guo L, Brostrom V, et al. Recurrence of breast carcinoma as Paget disease of the skin at a prior core needle biopsy site: case report and review of the literature. *Int J Surg Case Rep.* 2015;15:152–156.

76. Bhargava R, Beriwal S, Dabbs DJ. Mammaglobin versus GCDFP-15: an immunohistologic validation survey for sensitivity and specificity. *Am J Clin Pathol.* 2007;127:103–113.

77. Lewis GH, Subhawong AP, Nassar H, et al. Relationship between molecular subtype of invasive breast carcinoma and expression of gross cystic disease fluid protein 15 and mammaglobin. *Am J Clin Pathol.* 2011;135:587–591.

78. Striebel JM, Dacic S, Yousem SA. Gross cystic disease fluid protein-(GCDFP-15): expression in primary lung adenocarcinoma. *Am J Surg Pathol.* 2008;32:426–432.

79. Balafoutas D, zur Hausen A, Mayer S, et al. Cancer testis antigens and NY-BR-1 expression in primary breast cancer: prognostic and therapeutic implications. *BMC Cancer.* 2013;13:271. doi:10.1186/1471-2407-13-271.

80. Woodard AH, Yu J, Dabbs DJ, et al. NY-BR-1 and PAX8 immunoreactivity in breast, gynecologic tract, and other CK7+ carcinomas: potential use for determining site of origin. *Am J Clin Pathol.* 2011;136:428–435.

81. Clark BZ, Beriwal S, Dabbs DJ, et al. Semiquantitative GATA-3 immunoreactivity in breast, bladder, gynecologic tract, and other cytokeratin 7-positive carcinomas. *Am J Clin Pathol.* 2014;142:64–71.

82. Cimino-Mathews A, Subhawong AP, Illei PB, et al. GATA3 expression in breast carcinoma: utility in triple-negative, sarcomatoid, and metastatic carcinomas. *Hum Pathol.* 2013;44:1341–1349.

83. Miettinen M, McCue PA, Sarlomo-Rikala M, et al. GATA3: a multispecific but potentially useful marker in surgical pathology: a systematic analysis of 2500 epithelial and nonepithelial tumors. *Am J Surg Pathol.* 2014;38:13–22.

84. Liu H, Shi J, Prichard JW, et al. Immunohistochemical evaluation of GATA-3 expression in ER-negative breast carcinomas. *Am J Clin Pathol.* 2014;141:648–655.

85. Abbas J, Wienke A, Spielmann RP, et al. Intramammary metastases: comparison of mammographic and ultrasound features. *Eur J Radiol.* 2013;82:1423–1430.

86. Kim KW, Krajewski KM, Jagannathan JP, et al. Cancer of unknown primary sites: what radiologists need to know and what oncologists want to know. *AJR Am J Roentgenol.* 2013;200:484–492.

87. Varadhachary GR, Talantov D, Raber MN, et al. Molecular profiling of carcinoma of unknown primary and correlation with clinical evaluation. *J Clin Oncol.* 2008;26:4442–4448.

88. Pavlidis N, Pentheroudakis G. Cancer of unknown primary site. *Lancet.* 2012;379:1428–1435.

89. Drubin D, Smith JS, Liu W, et al. Comparison of cryopreservation and standard needle biopsy for gene expression profiling of human breast cancer specimens. *Breast Cancer Res Treat.* 2005;90:93–96.

90. De Mattos-Arruda L, Bidard FC, Won HH, et al. Establishing the origin of metastatic deposits in the setting of multiple primary malignancies: the role of massively parallel sequencing. *Mol Oncol.* 2014;8:150–158.

23

Pathologic Effects of Therapy

FREDERICK C. KOERNER

IRRADIATION

Radiation and Hodgkin Lymphoma

The breasts may be secondarily exposed to radiation during diagnostic procedures such as mammography and fluoroscopy (1), or in the course of irradiation administered to another organ such as mediastinal radiotherapy for Hodgkin lymphoma (2–5). The radiation exposure in these situations has been associated with an increased risk for the development of breast carcinoma (2,6–9). Wendland et al. (10) reported that the standard incidence ratio (SIR) for breast carcinoma among Hodgkin lymphoma patients who received radiotherapy was 3.17 when compared to the general population, and Schaapveld et al. (11) recorded an SIR of 4.7. The SIR for breast carcinoma in irradiated Hodgkin lymphoma patients was 1.90 when compared to nonirradiated patients, and the SIR in nonirradiated Hodgkin lymphoma patients was 1.67 when compared to the general population. These findings indicate that women treated for Hodgkin lymphoma have an elevated risk for breast carcinoma compared to the general population and that irradiation further increases this risk. Girls irradiated between the ages of 9 and 16 years face an especially high likelihood of developing breast carcinoma (9,12,13). This risk declines gradually during later adolescence and early adulthood. These results suggest greater susceptibility to breast carcinoma when radiation exposure is near puberty. The cumulative probability of developing breast carcinoma by 40 years of age has been reported to be 30% to 35% (3,13).

Most studies report breast carcinoma after irradiation for Hodgkin lymphoma in women, but in rare instances breast carcinoma may also occur in men (14). Data from several studies (15–17) include 189 patients who developed 214 breast carcinomas after radiotherapy for Hodgkin lymphoma. The median age at the time of diagnosis of Hodgkin lymphoma was 25 years. The median age at the time of diagnosis of breast carcinoma was 42 years, and the median interval was 18.6 years. The frequency of bilaterality was 13.2%; most contralateral tumors were metachronous. Axillary lymph node metastases occurred in 32% of the invasive carcinomas for which axillary lymph nodes were examined.

Patients who received supradiaphragmatic radiotherapy for the treatment of Hodgkin lymphoma are candidates for radiologic surveillance. In the absence of randomized controlled clinical trials, the efficacy of various imaging techniques has not been established for this situation. Mammography is reported to have high sensitivity for detecting carcinomas in the breast of women irradiated for Hodgkin lymphoma, especially when calcifications are present (18–21). Ultrasonography may be employed as an adjunct to mammography, but one cannot rely on this technique as a primary screening modality because of a relatively high frequency of false-positive findings (22). Magnetic resonance imaging (MRI) is effective for detecting tumor-forming, largely invasive carcinomas in women with genetic and other high-risk predispositions to breast carcinoma, but it has less sensitivity than mammography for detecting ductal carcinoma in situ (DCIS) (23).

Macroscopic examination of the irradiated breast does not disclose distinctive alterations, and the carcinomas arising in such breasts do not display distinctive macroscopic features. Microscopic study does not reveal structural changes attributable to irradiation in the underlying mammary tissue. Approximately 15% of the carcinomas detected in this setting are DCIS. Invasive carcinomas tend to be poorly differentiated; otherwise, they do not differ significantly in their morphologic characteristics from tumors in women without prior irradiation (5,24). Nearly all carcinomas have been ductal carcinomas of the NOS variety; however, special types of ductal carcinoma such as mucinous carcinoma have been encountered rarely, and so have invasive lobular carcinomas (14,16,17). The carcinomas are more likely to be bilateral and to occur in the medial regions of the breasts (20,25). Both synchronous and metachronous bilateral carcinomas have been reported (17,20,25). Carcinomas arising after irradiation for Hodgkin lymphoma display the "triple-negative" receptor panel more frequently than do sporadic breast carcinomas (26).

Mastectomy represents the most common primary surgical treatment of patients in this setting. Deutsch et al. (27) described 12 patients successfully treated with lumpectomy and radiation with "good to excellent cosmetic results" and "no significant acute adverse reactions and no late sequelae" after a median follow-up of 46 months.

Radiation and Breast-Conservation Therapy

Irradiation of the breast most commonly occurs as a component breast-conservation therapy for breast carcinoma. A small percentage of patients treated with breast-conserving therapy develop carcinoma in the treated breast. Recurrences most often occur 2 to 6 years after the completion of breast-conserving treatment and typically sit near the site of prior mass, whereas new primary carcinomas tend to develop more than 10 years

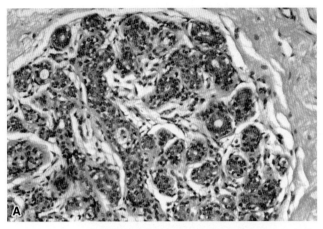
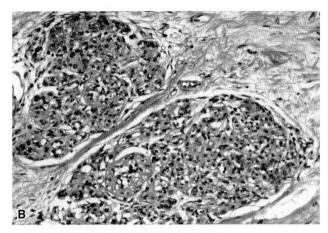

FIGURE 23.1 Radiation Atrophy of Lobules. A: This image depicts a normal lobule in the breast of a 35-year-old woman before the start of radiotherapy for invasive ductal carcinoma. **B:** A needle core biopsy was performed 3 years after irradiation. The posttreatment lobules exhibit moderate radiation atrophy, thickening of basement membranes, atrophy of epithelial cells, and clearing of the cytoplasm of the myoepithelial cells.

following treatment and most often involve tissue distant from the excision site (28). Imaging studies often disclose parenchymal distortion, scarring, fat necrosis, and scattered coarse calcifications in the treated breast. Cases exhibiting a new mass, a suspicious area of enhancement on MRI, a change in the features of a postoperative scar, or the appearance of

new, pleomorphic calcifications warrant a biopsy to investigate the possibility of recurrent carcinoma.

The histologic alterations associated with irradiation of underlying mammary tissue appear most obvious in terminal duct–lobular units (29–31) **(Figs. 23.1–23.3)**. The changes include collagenization of intralobular stroma, thickening of

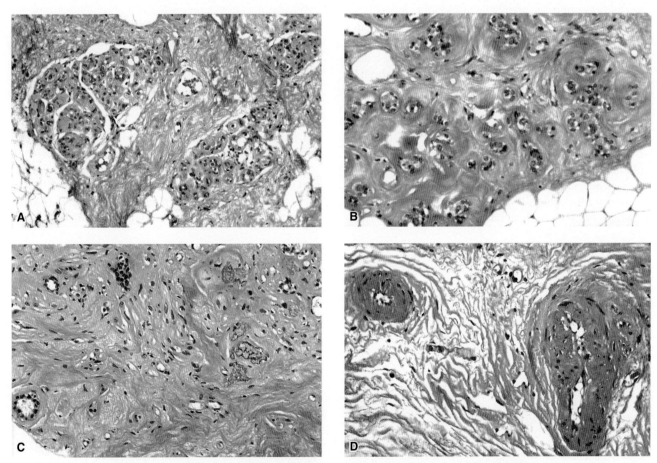

FIGURE 23.2 Radiation Atrophy of Lobules and Vascular Changes. A: Despite the marked atrophy, the structure of these lobules persists. **B:** A lobule shows nearly complete effacement. Thick basement membranes surround the glands. **C:** Severe lobular atrophy and calcification can be seen. **D:** Small arteries display mild sclerosis. **E:** These arteries demonstrate postirradiation arteritis.

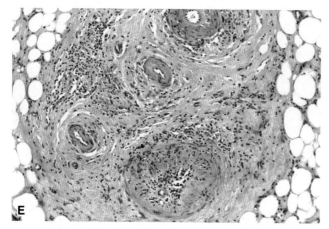

FIGURE 23.2 (*continued*)

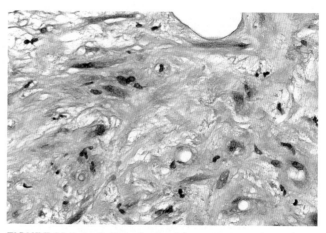

FIGURE 23.4 Radiation Atypia of Stromal Fibroblasts. Seven months after the completion of partial breast irradiation, this patient underwent a needle core biopsy to evaluate the presence of cutaneous erythema. Several fibroblasts appear enlarged and they contain large, pleomorphic nuclei.

periacinar and periductular basement membranes, atrophy of acinar and ductular epithelium, cytologic atypia of epithelial cells, and relative prominence of acinar myoepithelial cells, which seem to be preserved to a greater extent than the epithelial cells (32). Generally, the effects in larger ducts appear less pronounced than those in terminal duct–lobular units. Apocrine epithelium is susceptible to developing severe cytologic atypia after therapeutic radiotherapy, especially in hyperplastic foci. When evaluating a posttreatment biopsy, it is useful to examine the pretreatment specimen for evidence of apocrine metaplasia. Atypical fibroblasts can be found in a minority of specimens (**Fig. 23.4**).

In any one patient, most of the glandular tissue responds in a relatively uniform fashion if the entire breast has been irradiated; however, one can observe substantial variation in the severity of changes from one patient to another. The changes occasionally may be so slight as to be virtually indistinguishable from physiologic atrophy. In one study, differences in radiation effects among individual patients did not correlate with the radiation dose, patient age, posttreatment interval, or the use of adjuvant chemotherapy (29). Once established, the effects of irradiation do not seem to regress. After studying 120 breast specimens obtained at intervals ranging from less than

1 year to more than 6 years after radiotherapy, Moore et al. (31) did not observe significant variation in the appearance of the radiation-related alterations.

When a radioactive implant or an external "boost" has been used, histologic changes in the adjacent area may be more severe than those in the distant regions of the breast. Epithelial atypia may occur in larger ducts and it may be superimposed on existing hyperplasia or apocrine metaplasia (**Fig. 23.5**). Fat necrosis and atypia of stromal fibroblasts are more common in proximity to such areas (30,33,34). Radiation-induced vascular changes, which are not ordinarily seen after external beam radiotherapy, may be seen in this setting. Small- and medium-sized arteries may show sclerosis, fragmentation of elastica, endothelial atypia, and myointimal proliferation leading to narrowing of the vascular lumina. Prominent, cytologically atypical endothelial cells are also apparent in capillaries.

In situ lobular and ductal carcinomas persisting after radiation therapy are largely intact; consequently, the affected lobules and ducts appear filled and, often, expanded by the neoplastic population. Frequently, little or no microscopic change

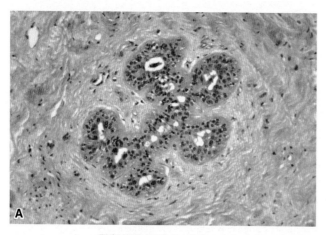

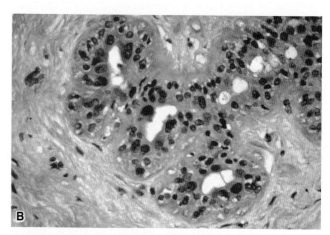

FIGURE 23.3 Radiation Atypia in a Small Duct. A, B: Isolated luminal epithelial cells possess enlarged hyperchromatic nuclei. The basement membrane appears thick.

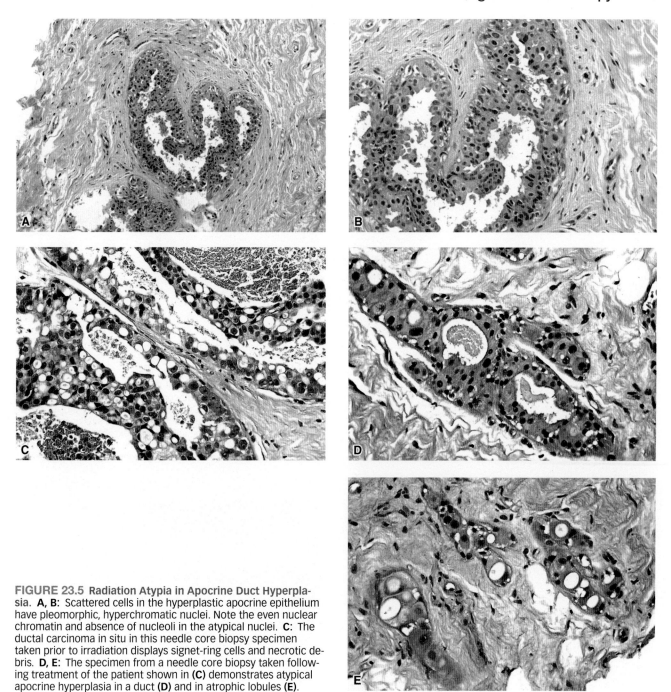

FIGURE 23.5 Radiation Atypia in Apocrine Duct Hyperplasia. A, B: Scattered cells in the hyperplastic apocrine epithelium have pleomorphic, hyperchromatic nuclei. Note the even nuclear chromatin and absence of nucleoli in the atypical nuclei. **C:** The ductal carcinoma in situ in this needle core biopsy specimen taken prior to irradiation displays signet-ring cells and necrotic debris. **D, E:** The specimen from a needle core biopsy taken following treatment of the patient shown in **(C)** demonstrates atypical apocrine hyperplasia in a duct **(D)** and in atrophic lobules **(E)**.

attributable to treatment is evident when pre- and postirradiation samples of in situ carcinoma are compared **(Figs. 23.6 and 23.7)**. Greater cytologic atypia after treatment is encountered in a minority of cases **(Fig. 23.8)**. In one study (35), the grade of the pretreatment DCIS matched that of the recurrent DCIS in 95 (84%) of 113 cases. Recurrent invasive carcinomas also resemble their pretreatment counterparts in their histologic type, grade, and receptor expression **(Fig. 23.9)**, whereas the histologic characteristics of the new primary carcinomas tend to differ from those of the pretreatment carcinomas (36). Irradiated invasive carcinoma cells occasionally contain multiple hyperchromatic nuclei or display focal necrosis not evident

in the pretreatment tissue. These findings suggest that the cells represent residual carcinoma showing radiation effects.

Differentiating irradiated glandular tissue from carcinoma can pose diagnostic problems, especially when examining needle core biopsy (NCB) specimens. The cytologic atypia produced by irradiation resembles the neoplastic atypia seen in high-grade carcinoma cells, and the glandular atrophy and scarring seen after surgery and irradiation can give rise to irregular clusters of atypical cells that resemble invasive carcinoma. Comparison of the features of a posttreatment biopsy sample with the histologic appearance of the tumor and noncarcinomatous tissue prior to treatment will usually

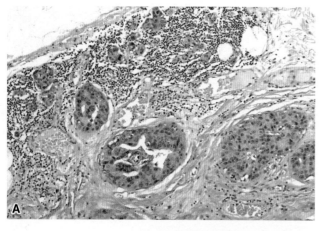
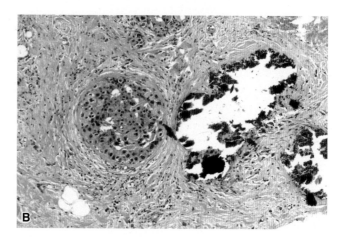
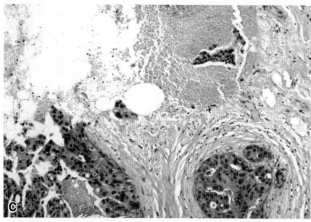

FIGURE 23.6 Recurrent Ductal Carcinoma In Situ After Radiotherapy. A: This needle core biopsy specimen obtained before treatment contains DCIS. **B:** The needle core biopsy specimen taken 4 years after irradiation shows DCIS similar to that in **(A)**. **C:** The carcinoma in the subsequent excision appears very similar to the pretreatment carcinoma. One can see a tissue defect caused by the needle core biopsy in the upper left corner.

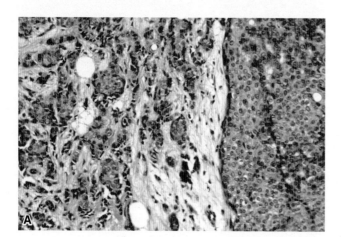
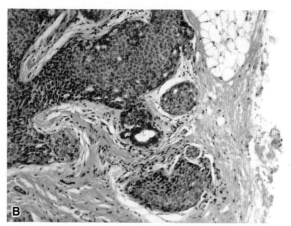

FIGURE 23.7 Recurrent Carcinoma After Radiotherapy. A: This image illustrates in situ and invasive poorly differentiated ductal carcinoma in a specimen collected before radiotherapy. **B:** This specimen from a needle core biopsy performed 1 year after radiotherapy shows ductal carcinoma in situ identical to that on the right in **(A)**.

help to clarify the nature of the atypical epithelial cells. One would not ordinarily confuse irradiated benign glandular cells with those of recurrent low-grade carcinoma, but the former can resemble high-grade carcinoma cells to a worrisome extent. To differentiate epithelial cells altered by irradiation from high-grade carcinoma, one should look for evidence of cellular proliferation: stratification of cells, filling of glandular

lumina, distention of glands, and mitotic figures. The presence of these features, especially if associated with necrosis, offers persuasive evidence to support the diagnosis of malignancy. Attention to the presence of apocrine metaplasia in the underlying glandular tissue will also help to avoid mistaking irradiated benign glandular cells for carcinoma cells. Staining for myoepithelial cells will usually allow one to recognize

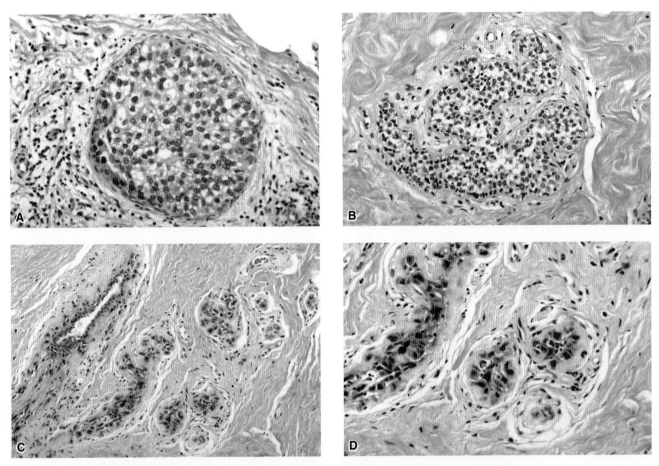

FIGURE 23.8 Radiation Atypia in Terminal Ducts with Atypical Lobular Hyperplasia.
A, B: Tissue excised prior to irradiation shows ductal carcinoma in situ in **(A)** and atypical lobular hyperplasia (ALH) in **(B)**. **C, D:** A needle core biopsy performed 2 years later revealed marked cytologic atypia in these terminal ducts. The atypical cells probably represent foci of ALH like those shown in **(B)**, which were present prior to treatment.

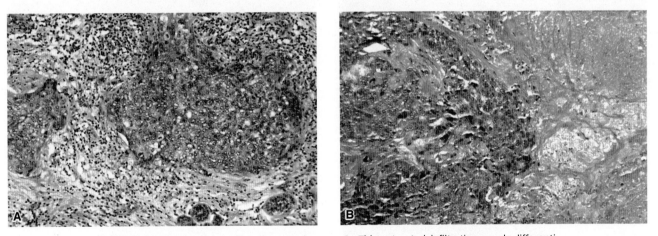

FIGURE 23.9 Recurrent Infiltrating Carcinoma. A: This untreated, infiltrating, poorly differentiated ductal carcinoma has a prominent lymphocytic reaction. **B:** One year after lumpectomy and radiotherapy, the recurrent, partially necrotic carcinoma lacks a lymphocytic reaction but otherwise looks similar to the pretreatment tumor.

foci of invasive carcinoma, but irradiated myoepithelial cells sometimes fail to stain for the usual myoepithelial markers (32). As always, one must integrate the immunohistochemical findings with those evident on H&E-stained sections.

Therapeutic or adjuvant irradiation of the breast does not seem to increase the risk of contralateral breast carcinoma significantly (37), but it has been associated with significantly increased risks for the development of carcinomas of the esophagus and lung (38,39). Locoregional irradiation for breast carcinoma leads to a small increased risk for acute myeloid leukemia, which is enhanced by chemotherapy (40). The incidence of such neoplasms appears to be low. Approximately 160 such cases developed in a cohort of 33,763 women with breast carcinoma who had radiotherapy (38). The relationship between breast irradiation and the development of angiosarcoma is discussed in Chapter 20.

CHEMOTHERAPY

Treatment-related histologic changes may be detected in mammary carcinomas and non-neoplastic mammary tissues following administration of neoadjuvant chemotherapy. In earlier times, neoadjuvant chemotherapy was mostly used to treat locally advanced breast carcinomas, but use of this form of therapy has broadened to include the treatment of earlier stages of breast carcinoma (41).

Mammography may suggest a response in patients treated with neoadjuvant chemotherapy, but this procedure is not reliable for predicting the pathologic response to the treatment. Yeh et al. (42) reported that agreement as to the quality of postchemotherapy response when compared to pathology findings was 19%, 26%, 35%, and 71% for clinical examination, mammography, sonography, and MRI, respectively. Positron emission tomography (PET) appears to be a specific but less-sensitive method for identifying patients with complete pathologic responses early in the course of chemotherapy treatment (43).

Comparing samples taken before and after treatment allows one to identify treatment effects most easily. The most noticeable changes affecting invasive carcinomas are a decrease in tumor cellularity accompanied by chronic inflammation, histiocyte accumulation, stromal fibrosis, and elastosis (**Figs. 23.10 and 23.11**). Rajan et al. (44) observed a decrease in median tumor cellularity from 40% in pretreatment core biopsy specimens to 10% in samples resected after neoadjuvant chemotherapy. There was considerable variation in changes in cellularity among clinical-response categories. Many tumors had a pronounced decrease in cellularity but only minimal reduction in size.

In the most favorable situation, no residual carcinoma is detected, an occurrence reported in 6.7% (45) and 13% (46) of the cases in cohorts with mixed subtypes of carcinoma. Breast carcinoma cohorts that are enriched for certain subtypes and treatments can show much higher rates of pathologic complete

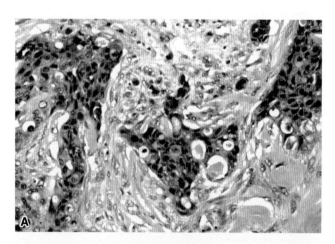

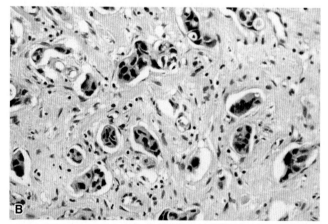

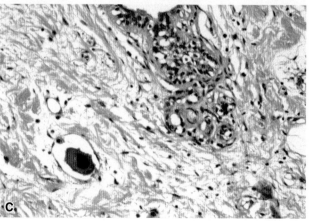

FIGURE 23.10 Chemotherapy Effect. A: The patient with this poorly differentiated invasive ductal carcinoma received neoadjuvant chemotherapy. **B:** The needle core biopsy sample obtained after the patient experienced a partial clinical response contains small nests of carcinoma cells with pleomorphic hyperchromatic nuclei growing in collagenous stroma. Shrinkage of the clusters of carcinoma cells has created an appearance that suggests the presence of lymphatic invasion. **C:** A markedly enlarged hyperchromatic cell in a lymphatic space near an atrophic lobule is shown. The cytologic changes in the carcinoma are largely attributable to the chemotherapy.

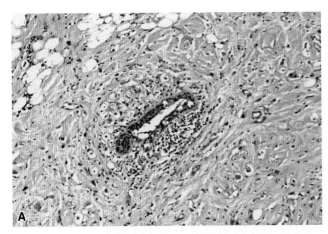 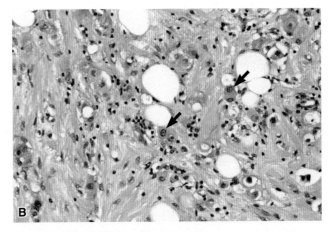

FIGURE 23.11 Chemotherapy Effect in the Breast. A, B: This needle core biopsy sample was obtained after a partial clinical response to chemotherapy. Isolated residual carcinoma cells *(arrows)* accompanied by scattered lymphocytes are dispersed in the fibrotic stroma.

response (pCR). For example, the pCR rate of HER2-positive breast carcinomas treated with trastuzumab and chemotherapy was 65% in the study by Buzdar et al. (47). If the breast of a patient who has a complete histologic and clinical response is examined histologically soon after treatment, residual degenerated and infarcted necrotic invasive carcinoma may be recognized by the loss of normal staining properties and decreased architectural detail. With the passage of time, the degenerated invasive carcinoma is absorbed. Healed sites of previous infiltrating carcinoma may be appreciated because of architectural distortion characterized by fibrosis, stromal edema, increased vascularity composed largely of thin-walled vessels, and a chronic inflammatory cell infiltrate **(Fig. 23.11)** (48).

Residual invasive carcinoma cells can appear morphologically unaltered after neoadjuvant therapy, but in most cases they exhibit cytologic changes attributable to the treatment (46,48–51). Aneuploid carcinomas are more likely than diploid tumors to exhibit histologic and cytologic changes from chemotherapy (49). The alterations may appear more pronounced after combined chemoradiotherapy than following treatment with the same agents individually. The invasive carcinoma cells usually appear enlarged. They possess increased amounts of cytoplasm, which often contains vacuoles or eosinophilic granules (52). Cell borders are typically well defined, and the cells tend to shrink from the stroma (51) **(see Fig. 23.10)**. The cells contain large, hyperchromatic, and pleomorphic nuclei. Multinucleated cells and abnormal mitotic figures may be encountered (53). The altered carcinoma cells can mimic histiocytes, especially when present individually, but they retain immunohistochemical reactivity for cytokeratin and epithelial membrane antigen (EMA). In certain cases, the residual invasive carcinoma cells appear smaller than those in the pretreatment specimen. Such cells contain scant eosinophilic cytoplasm and small collapsed nuclei.

An analysis comparing the components of histologic grading in a small series of pre- and postchemotherapy specimens did not reveal significant differences in nuclear pleomorphism, tubule formation, or mitotic count (46); however, others (48) reported that nuclear grade was increased in 32% of the cases.

In the majority of cases, it is feasible to determine histologic grade in residual carcinoma after neoadjuvant chemotherapy.

The effect of chemotherapy on tumor cell proliferation as measured with the Ki67 antibody or mitotic counts is variable. Proliferative rates may be increased, decreased, or unchanged in the course of neoadjuvant chemotherapy. Although some studies indicate changes in receptor and HER2 status before and after neoadjuvant chemotherapy, larger series indicate that most breast carcinomas maintain the pretreatment profile. Burcombe et al. (54) examined breast carcinomas from 118 patients and observed a change in estrogen receptor (ER) or progesterone receptor (PR) classification in 8% of the cases. Immunohistochemical expression of HER2 was maintained in all cases, but changes between 2+ and 3+ HER2 scores occurred in 8% of the cases.

In a minority of instances, the residual carcinoma found after neoadjuvant chemotherapy consists only of DICS, lymphatic tumor emboli, or both **(Fig. 23.12)**. Sharkey et al. (48)

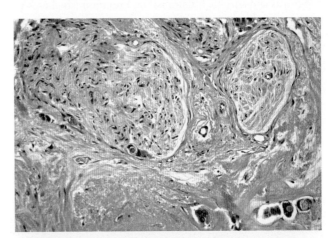

FIGURE 23.12 Chemotherapy Effect Involving Lymphatic Tumor Emboli. The clusters of carcinoma cells in a nerve and in lymphatic channels show cytologic changes related to chemotherapy. The patient had a complete clinical response, and this was the extent of the histologically detectable residual carcinoma.

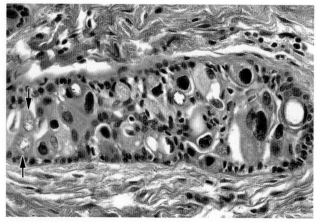

FIGURE 23.13 Chemotherapy Effect Involving Ductal Carcinoma In Situ. Neoplastic ductal cells showing marked nuclear pleomorphism overlie a layer of prominent myoepithelial cells. Intracellular mucin vacuoles are evident *(arrows)*.

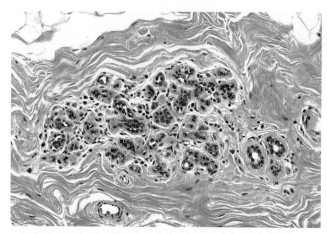

FIGURE 23.15 Chemotherapy Effect Involving a Normal Terminal–Duct Lobular Unit. This specimen comes from a 34-year-old woman treated with neoadjuvant chemotherapy. The acini have small calibers, and their lumina appear inconspicuous. The basement membranes look thick.

reported finding "unusually prominent intraductal and/or intralymphatic tumor" in 40% of specimens obtained after preoperative doxorubicin/cyclophosphamide administration. Residual DCIS sometimes demonstrates marked cellular enlargement and extreme nuclear pleomorphism **(Fig. 23.13)**. These bizarre cells can form confluent collections overlying a layer of easily recognized myoepithelial cells, or they can persist as individual cells and small clusters scattered among benign cells in the epithelium of ducts and lobules. Rabban et al. (55) observed intralymphatic carcinoma in the breasts of 11 of 146 (7.5%) patients treated with neoadjuvant chemotherapy. In six of these patients (4%), the only residual carcinoma was within the lymphatic vessels.

Chemotherapy effects in axillary nodal metastases are similar to those affecting the primary tumor. Metastatic carcinoma can disappear completely leaving behind only areas of scarring and lymphohistiocytic infiltration (48,52,56) **(Fig. 23.14)**. Small clusters of carcinoma cells may remain embedded in regions of fibrosis and chronic inflammation. Immunohistochemical

staining for cytokeratin will facilitate the detection of minimal residual metastatic carcinoma. Regressive changes may also be found in the uninvolved lymph nodes (48).

Non-neoplastic breast parenchyma is also altered following cytotoxic chemotherapy, but the changes are subtler than those induced in the tumor. The glandular elements undergo diffuse atrophy causing a reduction in the size of existing lobules, loss of acinar luminal cells, shrinkage of the acini, and condensation of the basement membrane **(Fig. 23.15)** (48,52,57). Cytologic atypia may be seen in ductal and lobular epithelial cells; however, in many cases, these changes are not specifically attributable to chemotherapy. Comparison with a pretreatment specimen is particularly helpful in this situation.

The histopathologic effects of systemic chemotherapy often correlate with the extent of clinical response. The greatest alterations are usually found in patients who clinically appear to have complete resolution of their carcinomas (44,45,49); however, oncologists may report that the patient experienced a

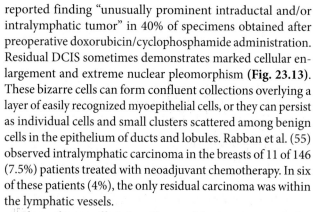

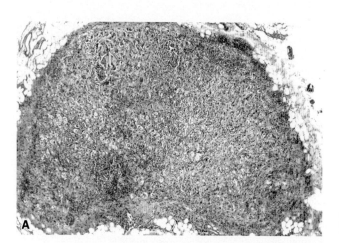

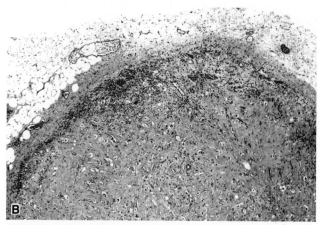

FIGURE 23.14 Chemotherapy Effect in a Lymph Node with Metastatic Carcinoma.
A: Before chemotherapy, carcinoma diffusely involved a lymph node. **B:** After chemotherapy, the tumor is largely necrotic, and the background tissue shows fibrosis and lymphoid atrophy.

complete clinical response, but histologic examination reveals residual carcinoma.

Although the findings present in a NCB specimen do not allow one to predict a patient's response to neoadjuvant chemotherapy in most circumstances, one can make a few general statements. For example, tumors with high-grade nuclei responded better to neoadjuvant chemotherapy than those with intermediate- or low-grade nuclei (58), and the use of anti-HER2 therapy often leads to a pCR of HER2-amplified carcinomas (47). On the other hand, patients with invasive lobular carcinoma rarely experience a pCR when treated with anti-estrogen adjuvant therapy (59). Pu et al. (60) reported that 80% of patients with pCRs had tumor necrosis in their NCB samples, whereas only 17% of nonresponders demonstrated the same finding. In one study (61), Ki67 and apoptotic indices were not predictive of response to the neoadjuvant chemotherapy.

ABLATION METHODS

Researchers have investigated the use of several techniques to ablate unresected carcinomas in the breast: interstitial laser therapy, radiofrequency ablation, microwave ablation, high-intensity focused ultrasound ablation, cryoablation, and irreversible electroporation (62). At present, these methods are considered investigational for the treatment of breast carcinoma. Except for high-intensity focused ultrasound ablation, these procedures use a probe placed in the lesion to damage it irreversibly. The most commonly used therapies heat the target tissue using electromagnetic (interstitial laser therapy, radiofrequency ablation, and microwave ablation) or sonic (high-intensity focused ultrasound ablation) energy; cryoablation freezes it; and electroporation opens nanoscale pores in cell membranes. Histologic changes associated with these procedures appear limited to the target and the immediately surrounding tissue.

Bloom et al. (63) studied the pathologic changes associated with laser tumor ablation after delayed excision and observed a series of concentric rings around the laser probe tract. Tissue in zone 1, immediately around the defect produced by the probe, appeared charred. Zone 2 surrounding the charred surface of the cavity exhibited coagulative necrosis with "wind swept" nuclei like those seen in typical surgical cautery artifact. The third zone consisted of carcinoma that appeared histologically intact without necrosis or inflammation. A fourth zone consisted of necrotic tumor that appeared infarcted causing "conventional tinctorial affinities to be erased." The outermost zone, 5, showed vascular proliferation with thrombosis, inflammation, and fat necrosis in parenchyma outside the carcinoma. The authors concluded that two mechanisms contributed to the destruction of the carcinoma—direct thermal damage in the center, and peripheral infarction resulting from thrombosis of peripheral blood vessels. The size of zone 3 decreased with the passage of time, whereas that of zone 4 increased. These findings suggest that the zone 3 carcinoma that appeared histologically intact had been rendered nonviable by the laser and

that the malignant cells underwent progressive degeneration and incorporation into the necrotic zone 4.

Histologic examination immediately after radiofrequency ablation of carcinomas revealed "central charring of the tumor and needle track with a surrounding area of yellow, coagulated, adipose, and breast tissue" (64). The margin of the treated tissue appeared poorly defined. Microscopic examination demonstrated thrombosis of blood vessels and coagulative necrosis of the targeted tissue. The damaged cells did not stain for NADH-diaphorase. When examined 1 to 2 weeks following radiofrequency ablation, an erythematosus halo demarcated the ablated tissue from the viable parenchyma (65). The target tissue appeared "gray–yellow" and felt firm. Histologic study showed necrosis of the ablated tissue, and lack of staining for NADH-diaphorase (65) or CK8/18 (66) confirmed the death of the damaged cells.

High-intensity focused ultrasound causes necrosis of the targeted tissue accompanied by hemorrhage and inflammation. After a few days, the affected region appears distinct and well defined, and it does not display the zonal pattern seen following radiofrequency ablation (67). Reactivity for CK18 in morphologically damaged tissue often disappears, but it may persist for several days.

The histologic effects of cryoablation are well established 7 days after treatment. The affected tissue displays coagulative necrosis surrounded by a zone of fat necrosis and scar formation (68). Residual in situ or invasive carcinoma may be found beyond the perimeter of the necrotic tissue. Cryoprobe-assisted lumpectomy is a procedure in which freezing is used to convert a nonpalpable ultrasound-detected lesion into a palpable target ("ice ball"), which can be excised without the need for wire localization (69). In a study of six specimens obtained in this way, Sahoo et al. (70) observed retraction artifact, shrinkage of cells, smudging of the nuclei, and cytoplasmic eosinophilia. Ki67 staining was not appreciably altered by freezing, but staining for ER and PR diminished after freezing. These alterations compromised grading of carcinomas, distinguishing the in situ and invasive components, assessing mitoses, detecting vascular invasion, and testing for hormone receptors. Cryoablation without surgical removal has been reported for fibroadenomas and for breast carcinoma in patients who were not good surgical candidates (71,72).

The tissue changes associated with electroporation have not been established.

REFERENCES

1. Yaffe MJ, Mainprize JG. Risk of radiation-induced breast cancer from mammographic screening. *Radiology.* 2011;258:98–105.
2. Anderson N, Lokich J. Bilateral breast cancer after cured Hodgkin's disease. *Cancer.* 1990;65:221–223.
3. Bhatia S, Robison LL, Oberlin O, et al. Breast cancer and other second neoplasms after childhood Hodgkin's disease. *N Engl J Med.* 1996;334:745–751.
4. O'Brien PC, Barton MB, Fisher R; Australasian Radiation Oncology Lymphoma Group (AROLG). Breast cancer following treatment for Hodgkin's disease: the need for screening in a young population. *Australas Radiol.* 1995;39:271–276.
5. Yahalom J, Petrek JA, Biddinger PW, et al. Breast cancer in patients irradiated for Hodgkin's disease: a clinical and pathologic analysis of 45 events in 37 patients. *J Clin Oncol.* 1992;10:1674–1681.

6. Boice JD Jr, Monson RR. Breast cancer in women after repeated fluoro-scopic examinations of the chest. *J Natl Cancer Inst.* 1977;59:823–832.

7. Hildreth NG, Shore RE, Dvoretsky PM. The risk of breast cancer after irradiation of the thymus in infancy. *N Engl J Med.* 1989;321:1281–1284.

8. Little MP, Boice JD Jr. Comparison of breast cancer incidence in the Massachusetts tuberculosis fluoroscopy cohort and in the Japanese atomic bomb survivors. *Radiat Res.* 1999;151:218–224.

9. Swerdlow AJ, Cooke R, Bates A, et al. Breast cancer risk after supradia-phragmatic radiotherapy for Hodgkin's lymphoma in England and Wales: a National Cohort Study. *J Clin Oncol.* 2012;30:2745–2752.

10. Wendland MM, Tsodikov A, Glenn MJ, et al. Time interval to the development of breast carcinoma after treatment for Hodgkin disease. *Cancer.* 2004;101:1275–1282.

11. Schaapveld M, Aleman BM, van Eggermond AM, et al. Second cancer risk up to 40 years after treatment for Hodgkin's lymphoma. *N Engl J Med.* 2015;373:2499–2511.

12. Hancock SL, Tucker MA, Hoppe RT. Breast cancer after treatment of Hodgkin's disease. *J Natl Cancer Inst.* 1993;85:25–31.

13. Schellong G, Riepenhausen M, Ehlert K, et al. Breast cancer in young women after treatment for Hodgkin's disease during childhood or adolescence—an observational study with up to 33-year follow-up. *Dtsch Arztebl Int.* 2014;111:3–9.

14. Ninkovic S, Azanjac G, Knezevic M, et al. Lobular breast cancer in a male patient with a previous history of irradiation due to Hodgkin's disease. *Breast Care (Basel).* 2012;7:315–318.

15. Cutuli B. Radiation-induced breast cancer after treatment for Hodgkin's disease. *J Clin Oncol.* 1998;16:2285–2287.

16. Cutuli B, Dhermain F, Borel C, et al. Breast cancer in patients treated for Hodgkin's disease: clinical and pathological analysis of 76 cases in 63 patients. *Eur J Cancer.* 1997;33:2315–2320.

17. Cutuli B, Kanoun S, Tunon De Lara C, et al. Breast cancer occurred after Hodgkin's disease: clinico-pathological features, treatments and outcome: analysis of 214 cases. *Crit Rev Oncol Hematol.* 2012;81:29–37.

18. Dershaw DD, Yahalom J, Petrek JA. Breast carcinoma in women previously treated for Hodgkin disease: mammographic evaluation. *Radiology.* 1992;184:421–423.

19. Diller L, Medeiros Nancarrow C, Shaffer K, et al. Breast cancer screening in women previously treated for Hodgkin's disease: a prospective cohort study. *J Clin Oncol.* 2002;20:2085–2091.

20. Tardivon AA, Garnier ML, Beaudre A, et al. Breast carcinoma in women previously treated for Hodgkin's disease: clinical and mammographic findings. *Eur Radiol.* 1999;9:1666–1671.

21. Howell SJ, Searle C, Goode V, et al. The UK national breast cancer screening programme for survivors of Hodgkin lymphoma detects breast cancer at an early stage. *Br J Cancer.* 2009;101:582–588.

22. Teh W, Wilson AR. The role of ultrasound in breast cancer screening: a consensus statement by the European Group for Breast Cancer Screening. *Eur J Cancer.* 1998;34:449–450.

23. Neubauer H, Li M, Kuehne-Heid R, et al. High grade and non-high grade ductal carcinoma in situ on dynamic MR mammography: characteristic findings for signal increase and morphological pattern of enhancement. *Br J Radiol.* 2003;76:3–12.

24. Elkin EB, Klem ML, Gonzales AM, et al. Characteristics and outcomes of breast cancer in women with and without a history of radiation for Hodgkin's lymphoma: a multi-institutional, matched cohort study. *J Clin Oncol.* 2011;29:2466–2473.

25. Cutuli B, Borel C, Dhermain F, et al. Breast cancer occurred after treatment for Hodgkin's disease: analysis of 133 cases. *Radiother Oncol.* 2001;59:247–255.

26. Horst KC, Hancock SL, Ognibene G, et al. Histologic subtypes of breast cancer following radiotherapy for Hodgkin lymphoma. *Ann Oncol.* 2014;25:848–851.

27. Deutsch M, Gerszten K, Bloomer WD, et al. Lumpectomy and breast irradiation for breast cancer arising after previous radiotherapy for Hodgkin's disease or lymphoma. *Am J Clin Oncol.* 2001;24:33–34.

28. Chansakul T, Lai KC, Slanetz PJ. The postconservation breast: part 2: imaging findings of tumor recurrence and other long-term sequelae. *AJR Am J Roentgenol.* 2012;198:331–343.

29. Schnitt SJ, Connolly JL, Harris JR, et al. Radiation-induced changes in the breast. *Hum Pathol.* 1984;15:545–550.

30. Girling AC, Hanby AM, Millis RR. Radiation and other pathological changes in breast tissue after conservation treatment for carcinoma. *J Clin Pathol.* 1990;43:152–156.

31. Moore GH, Schiller JE, Moore GK. Radiation-induced histopathologic changes of the breast: the effects of time. *Am J Surg Pathol.* 2004;28:47–53.

32. Anderson K, Williams EM, Kaplan J, et al. Utility of immunohistochemical markers in irradiated breast tissue: an analysis of the role of myoepithelial markers, p53, and Ki-67. *Am J Surg Pathol.* 2014;38:1128–1137.

33. Piroth MD, Fischedick K, Wein B, et al. Fat necrosis and parenchymal scarring after breast-conserving surgery and radiotherapy with an intra-operative electron or fractionated, percutaneous boost: a retrospective comparison. *Breast Cancer.* 2012;21(4):409–414.

34. Rivera R, Smith-Bronstein V, Villegas-Mendez S, et al. Mammographic findings after intraoperative radiotherapy of the breast. *Radiol Res Pract.* 2012;2012:758371.

35. Millis RR, Pinder SE, Ryder K, et al. Grade of recurrent in situ and invasive carcinoma following treatment of pure ductal carcinoma in situ of the breast. *Br J Cancer.* 2004;90:1538–1542.

36. Sigal-Zafrani B, Bollet MA, Antoni G, et al. Are ipsilateral breast tumour invasive recurrences in young (< or =40 years) women more aggressive than their primary tumours? *Br J Cancer.* 2007;97:1046–1052.

37. Obedian E, Fischer DB, Haffty BG. Second malignancies after treatment of early-stage breast cancer: lumpectomy and radiation therapy versus mastectomy. *J Clin Oncol.* 2000;18:2406–2412.

38. Roychoudhuri R, Evans H, Robinson D, et al. Radiation-induced malignancies following radiotherapy for breast cancer. *Br J Cancer.* 2004;91:868–872.

39. Zablotska LB, Neugut AI. Lung carcinoma after radiation therapy in women treated with lumpectomy or mastectomy for primary breast carcinoma. *Cancer.* 2003;97:1404–1411.

40. Curtis RE, Boice JD Jr, Stovall M, et al. Risk of leukemia after chemotherapy and radiation treatment for breast cancer. *N Engl J Med.* 1992;326:1745–1751.

41. Thompson AM, Moulder-Thompson SL. Neoadjuvant treatment of breast cancer. *Ann Oncol.* 2012;23(Suppl 10):x231–x236.

42. Yeh E, Slanetz P, Kopans DB, et al. Prospective comparison of mammography, sonography, and MRI in patients undergoing neoadjuvant chemotherapy for palpable breast cancer. *AJR Am J Roentgenol.* 2005;184:868–877.

43. Tateishi U, Miyake M, Nagaoka T, et al. Neoadjuvant chemotherapy in breast cancer: prediction of pathologic response with PET/CT and dynamic contrast-enhanced MR imaging—prospective assessment. *Radiology.* 2012;263:53–63.

44. Rajan R, Poniecka A, Smith TL, et al. Change in tumor cellularity of breast carcinoma after neoadjuvant chemotherapy as a variable in the pathologic assessment of response. *Cancer.* 2004;100:1365–1373.

45. Feldman LD, Hortobagyi GN, Buzdar AU, et al. Pathological assessment of response to induction chemotherapy in breast cancer. *Cancer Res.* 1986;46:2578–2581.

46. Frierson HF Jr, Fechner RE. Histologic grade of locally advanced infiltrating ductal carcinoma after treatment with induction chemotherapy. *Am J Clin Pathol.* 1994;102:154–157.

47. Buzdar AU, Ibrahim NK, Francis D, et al. Significantly higher pathologic complete remission rate after neoadjuvant therapy with trastuzumab, paclitaxel, and epirubicin chemotherapy: results of a randomized trial in human epidermal growth factor receptor 2-positive operable breast cancer. *J Clin Oncol.* 2005;23:3676–3685.

48. Sharkey FE, Addington SL, Fowler LJ, et al. Effects of preoperative chemotherapy on the morphology of resectable breast carcinoma. *Mod Pathol.* 1996;9:893–900.

49. Briffod M, Spyratos F, Tubiana-Hulin M, et al. Sequential cytopunctures during preoperative chemotherapy for primary breast carcinoma: cytomorphologic changes, initial tumor ploidy, and tumor regression. *Cancer.* 1989;63:631–637.

50. McCready DR, Hortobagyi GN, Kau SW, et al. The prognostic significance of lymph node metastases after preoperative chemotherapy for locally advanced breast cancer. *Arch Surg.* 1989;124:21–25.

51. Sahoo S, Lester SC. Pathology of breast carcinomas after neoadjuvant chemotherapy: an overview with recommendations on specimen processing and reporting. *Arch Pathol Lab Med.* 2009;133:633–642.

52. Aktepe F, Kapucuoglu N, Pak I. The effects of chemotherapy on breast cancer tissue in locally advanced breast cancer. *Histopathology.* 1996;29:63–67.

53. Rasbridge SA, Gillett CE, Seymour AM, et al. The effects of chemotherapy on morphology, cellular proliferation, apoptosis and oncoprotein expression in primary breast carcinoma. *Br J Cancer.* 1994;70:335–341.

54. Burcombe RJ, Makris A, Richman PI, et al. Evaluation of ER, PgR, HER-2 and Ki-67 as predictors of response to neoadjuvant anthracycline chemotherapy for operable breast cancer. *Br J Cancer.* 2005;92:147–155.

55. Rabban JT, Glidden D, Kwan ML, et al. Pure and predominantly pure intralymphatic breast carcinoma after neoadjuvant chemotherapy: an unusual and adverse pattern of residual disease. *Am J Surg Pathol.* 2009;33:256–263.

56. Pinder SE, Provenzano E, Earl H, et al. Laboratory handling and histology reporting of breast specimens from patients who have received neoadjuvant chemotherapy. *Histopathology.* 2007;50:409–417.

57. Kennedy S, Merino MJ, Swain SM, et al. The effects of hormonal and chemotherapy on tumoral and nonneoplastic breast tissue. *Hum Pathol.* 1990;21:192–198.

58. Fisher B, Bryant J, Wolmark N, et al. Effect of preoperative chemotherapy on the outcome of women with operable breast cancer. *J Clin Oncol.* 1998;16:2672–2685.

59. Cristofanilli M, Gonzalez-Angulo A, Sneige N, et al. Invasive lobular carcinoma classic type: response to primary chemotherapy and survival outcomes. *J Clin Oncol.* 2005;23:41–48.

60. Pu RT, Schott AF, Sturtz DE, et al. Pathologic features of breast cancer associated with complete response to neoadjuvant chemotherapy: importance of tumor necrosis. *Am J Surg Pathol.* 2005;29:354–358.

61. Burcombe R, Wilson GD, Dowsett M, et al. Evaluation of Ki-67 proliferation and apoptotic index before, during and after neoadjuvant chemotherapy for primary breast cancer. *Breast Cancer Res.* 2006;8:R31.

62. Fornage BD, Hwang RF. Current status of imaging-guided percutaneous ablation of breast cancer. *AJR Am J Roentgenol.* 2014;203:442–448.

63. Bloom KJ, Dowlat K, Assad L. Pathologic changes after interstitial laser therapy of infiltrating breast carcinoma. *Am J Surg.* 2001;182: 384–388.

64. Izzo F, Thomas R, Delrio P, et al. Radiofrequency ablation in patients with primary breast carcinoma: a pilot study in 26 patients. *Cancer.* 2001;92:2036–2044.

65. Hayashi AH, Silver SF, van der Westhuizen NG, et al. Treatment of invasive breast carcinoma with ultrasound-guided radiofrequency ablation. *Am J Surg.* 2003;185:429–435.

66. Burak WE Jr, Agnese DM, Povoski SP, et al. Radiofrequency ablation of invasive breast carcinoma followed by delayed surgical excision. *Cancer.* 2003;98:1369–1376.

67. Knuttel FM, Waaijer L, Merckel LG, et al. Histopathology of breast cancer after magnetic resonance-guided high intensity focused ultrasound and radiofrequency ablation. *Histopathology.* 2016;69(2):250–259.

68. Roubidoux MA, Sabel MS, Bailey JE, et al. Small (<2.0-cm) breast cancers: mammographic and US findings at US-guided cryoablation—initial experience. *Radiology.* 2004;233:857–867.

69. Tafra L, Smith SJ, Woodward JE, et al. Pilot trial of cryoprobe-assisted breast-conserving surgery for small ultrasound-visible cancers. *Ann Surg Oncol.* 2003;10:1018–1024.

70. Sahoo S, Talwalkar SS, Martin AW, et al. Pathologic evaluation of cryoprobe-assisted lumpectomy for breast cancer. *Am J Clin Pathol.* 2007;128:239–244.

71. Nurko J, Mabry CD, Whitworth P, et al. Interim results from the FibroAdenoma Cryoablation Treatment Registry. *Am J Surg.* 2005;190:647–651; discussion 651–652.

72. Littrup PJ, Jallad B, Chandiwala-Mody P, et al. Cryotherapy for breast cancer: a feasibility study without excision. *J Vasc Interv Radiol.* 2009;20:1329–1341.

24

Men and Children

EDI BROGI

BREAST LESIONS IN MALES

Lesions of the breast are rare in men, and they are sampled with fine needle aspiration (FNA) more often than with needle core biopsy (NCB). A pathology group servicing several community hospitals in the Netherlands received only 26 NCB specimens of the male breast between 1993 and the end of 2002, or 2.6 specimens per year (1). Between 2011 and 2013, 539 men underwent mammographic evaluation of a breast mass at a center in Norway (2). FNA was performed in 62% of patients and NCB in 2.2%.

Gynecomastia

Gynecomastia is the most common clinical and pathologic abnormality in the breast of males.

Age
In a recent study (2), the mean age of men with mammographic diagnosis of gynecomastia was 55 years (median age 60 years; range 15–91).

Predisposing Factors
Prepubertal gynecomastia is uncommon, except as a transient phenomenon in newborn male infants exposed to maternal estrogens. Approximately 30% to 40% of pubertal males develop physiologic gynecomastia, which usually regresses spontaneously in a few months. Adult males can develop gynecomastia secondary to systemic metabolic, and/or hormonal imbalances (that is, hyperthyroidism, hepatic cirrhosis, chronic renal failure, chronic pulmonary disease, and hypogonadism), use of hormones (namely, estrogens, androgens, anabolic steroids, finasteride), and other drugs (namely, digitalis, cimetidine, spironolactone, marijuana, tricyclic antidepressants, 3-hydroxy-3-methyl-glutaryl-CoA Acetyl reductase inhibitors for the control of cholesterol level (3,4), imatinib mesylate for the treatment of chronic myeloid leukemia or gastrointestinal stromal tumors (5,6), and antiretroviral therapy in HIV-positive men) (7,8). Gynecomastia secondary to paraneoplastic hormone production has been reported in patients with pulmonary carcinoma and testicular germ cell tumors (9). An association with Klinefelter syndrome is documented (10).

Imaging Studies
Mammographically, gynecomastia has different appearances. In its earliest phase, it appears as a nodular fan-shaped subareolar density. The dendritic phase is characterized by a "flame-shaped" subareolar density with prominent radial extensions; this phase correlates histologically with the onset of stromal fibrosis. Diffuse glandular gynecomastia is characterized by heterogenous breast density, with combination of nodular and dendritic patterns (11). The combined use of mammography and ultrasonography is considered the optimal approach to rule out carcinoma in a patient who presents with clinical findings of gynecomastia (12–14). Between 2011 and 2013, 65% of men who underwent mammographic evaluation of a breast mass at a medical center in Norway (2) had gynecomastia with diagnostic mammographic features; 90% of patients also underwent sonographic evaluation. FNA of the lesion was performed in 75% of patients, and only 1% underwent NCB. The diagnosis of gynecomastia was confirmed in all cases.

Symptoms
Symptoms include breast enlargement or a palpable, ill-defined mass in the central and subareolar breast. Mass-forming gynecomastia spans 2 to 6 cm clinically, but it can be larger. Lesions of recent onset may be tender or painful. Gynecomastia usually is bilateral and synchronous, but asynchronous lesions can occur. Unilateral gynecomastia is more likely to produce a discrete mass. Nipple alterations are uncommon. Invasive carcinoma arising in gynecomastia usually manifests as a localized, asymmetric area of firmness.

Microscopic Pathology
The histologic changes of gynecomastia are similar regardless of its etiologic factors. *Florid gynecomastia* is common in the first year of onset. The ducts are lined by micropapillary and/or flat usual ductal epithelial hyperplasia (**Fig. 24.1**). Scattered epithelial mitoses may be encountered. Coexisting myoepithelial hyperplasia is common. The periductal stroma shows increased cellularity, prominent vascularity, edema, and a slight chronic inflammatory cell infiltrate. *Intermediate gynecomastia* shows both florid and fibrous components, and tends to be present for 6 months or less (**Fig. 24.2**). *Fibrous (inactive) gynecomastia* is usually seen in long-standing lesions (12 months or longer). The epithelial proliferation is less conspicuous than that in the florid phase; the stroma is more collagenous with less edema, reduced vascularity, and inconspicuous inflammation (**Fig. 24.3**). Pseudoangiomatous stromal hyperplasia (PASH) can be present in any phase of gynecomastia, but it is more pronounced in the active and intermediate stages (**Fig. 24.1**).

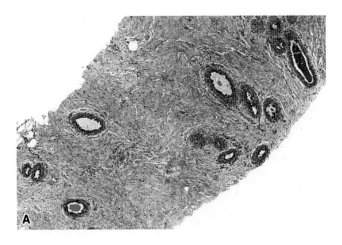

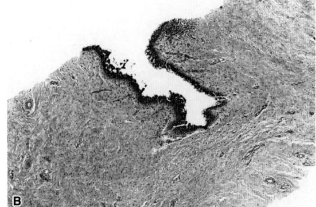

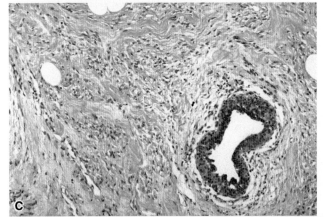

FIGURE 24.1 Gynecomastia, Florid. A, B: The ducts show micropapillary usual ductal hyperplasia. The periductal stroma has increased cellularity and prominent vascularity. **C:** Pseudoangiomatous hyperplasia of the stroma surrounds a duct with myoepithelial hyperplasia.

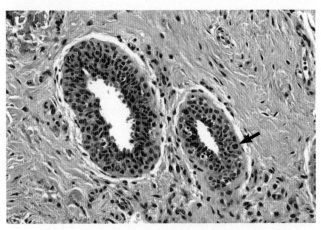

FIGURE 24.2 Gynecomastia, Intermediate. An intermediate phase lesion with compact epithelial and myoepithelial hyperplasia. An epithelial mitotic figure is present *(arrow)*. Note the periductal edema and hypervascularity.

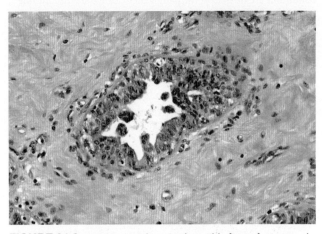

FIGURE 24.3 Gynecomastia, Inactive. This focus features micropapillary epithelial hyperplasia and a mild increase in periductal vascularity. The periductal stroma is collagenized.

Gynecomastia-like hyperplasia sometimes occurs in the breast of adolescent females.

Additional epithelial changes include lobule formation **(Fig. 24.4)**, focal squamous metaplasia **(Fig. 24.5)**, and apocrine metaplasia. Atypical ductal hyperplasia (ADH) sometimes occurs in gynecomastia (15), and morphologically resembles ADH in the female breast **(Fig. 24.6)**. The ducts with ADH (and also the ducts with ductal carcinoma in situ [DCIS]) usually lack the periductal fibrosis and increased stromal vascularity characteristic of gynecomastia.

Immunohistochemistry

The epithelium of gynecomastia consists of three cell layers (16). The myoepithelial cells express CK5, CK14, and p63 but are negative for estrogen receptor (ER), progesterone receptor (PR), and androgen receptor (AR). The intermediate layer

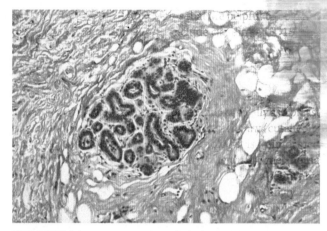

FIGURE 24.4 Gynecomastia. Lobule formation in a male breast.

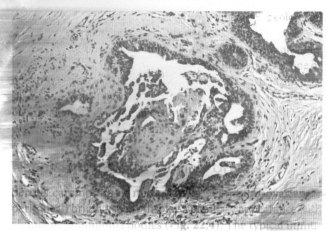

FIGURE 24.5 Gynecomastia. Florid gynecomastia with squamous metaplasia in hyperplastic duct epithelium. Note mild periductal inflammation.

consists of cuboidal or columnar ductal cells immunoreactive for ER, PR, and AR but negative for CK5 and CK14. The epithelium lining the ductal lumen consists of flattened cells that are reactive for CK5, and CK14, but only weakly positive for ER, PR, and AR. The use of immunohistochemical stains for ER and CK5/6 may be helpful to document foci of ADH in the background of gynecomastia (see also Chapter 8).

Treatment and Prognosis

Early gynecomastia sometimes may regress when the underlying conditions are treated, or the pathogenetic drugs are discontinued, but in most cases breast enlargement persists. Most patients with gynecomastia receive no specific treatment. The use of radiation (17) and tamoxifen (18) to prevent gynecomastia in men with prostatic carcinoma treated with bicalutamide is a subject of debate. Surgical excision of gynecomastia is indicated clinically only to exclude carcinoma, but sometimes it is performed for cosmetic reasons. Ultrasound-assisted liposuction may be considered in overweight or obese men,

when adipose tissue is thought to contribute to the mass (19). Liposuction can result in epithelial displacement that mimics invasive carcinoma (20). A conservative approach is adopted in children with gynecomastia, as the lesions usually resolve without treatment; the use of tamoxifen is discouraged. In a study of men younger than 21 years of age who underwent surgery for gynecomastia (10), the average age at the time of the procedure was 16.2 years, and most patients were overweight or obese. Although carcinoma may rarely arise in conjunction with gynecomastia (15), gynecomastia is not associated with an increased risk of subsequent mammary carcinoma (21).

Intraductal Papilloma

Age and Symptoms

Intraductal papillomas can occur at any age, including in adolescence (22). Nipple discharge is a common presenting symptom. Large or cystic lesions may be palpable. No predisposing factors are known.

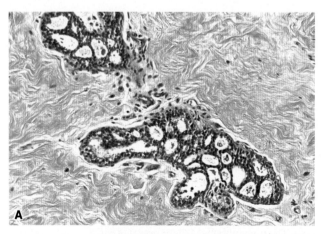

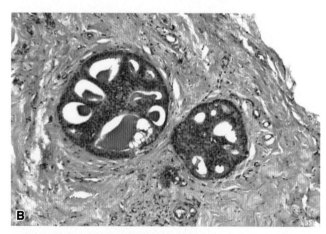

FIGURE 24.6 Gynecomastia with Atypical Duct Hyperplasia. A: The proliferation is almost entirely epithelial with a minimal myoepithelial component. **B:** Atypical cribriform duct hyperplasia.

Imaging Studies

The mammographic and sonographic appearance of papillomas of the male breast does not differ significantly from that of similar tumors in females (11,22).

Microscopic Features

Papillomas of the male breast are histologically similar to those occurring in females. Multiple papillomas can occur. Because papillary carcinomas of the male breast are relatively more common than papillomas, careful evaluation of the epithelial component is required to rule out atypia or carcinoma (see also discussion in Chapters 4 and 11).

Immunohistochemistry

Myoepithelium lines the fibrovascular cores of papillomas, atypical papillomas, and papillomas involved by DCIS. The absence of myoepithelium in the fibrovascular cores of a papillary lesion supports the diagnosis of papillary carcinoma but does not distinguish between papillary DCIS, encapsulated papillary carcinoma, and invasive papillary carcinoma. CK5/6 immunostain highlights the myoepithelium and also decorates usual ductal hyperplasia (UDH) with a characteristic "checkerboard" pattern, whereas atypical and neoplastic ductal epithelium are usually CK5/6-negative.

Treatment and Prognosis

The need for surgical excision of papillomas without atypia diagnosed at NCB with radiologic and pathologic concordant findings in females is currently subject of investigation (see also Chapter 4). Papillary lesions in the breast of males, including papillomas without epithelial atypia, usually undergo surgical excision. Complete evaluation of the lesion is recommended to rule out the possibility of papillary carcinoma, as the latter is relatively more frequent in males.

Fibroepithelial Lesions

Age

The age of men with fibroadenomas (FAs) in one series (23) ranged from 37 to 71 years; a 20-year-old man had a benign (low grade) phyllodes tumor (PT). A 15-year-old boy with unilateral gynecomastia reportedly had a 7-cm benign fibroepithelial tumor (24).

Predisposing Factors

Fibroepithelial lesions (FELs) usually arise in the context of gynecomastia (23,25–28), particularly in patients treated with estrogens or antiandrogen therapy, which can result in lobule formation. Other drugs associated with FA and/or fibroadenomatoid alterations include spironolactone, methyldopa, and chlordiazepoxide (23).

Microscopic Pathology

The morphology of FELs in men resembles that of equivalent lesions in females. Some lesions clinically regarded as FAs may just represent nodular foci of gynecomastia. PASH is common in the stroma of gynecomastia, and can be mass-forming (29).

Treatment and Prognosis

The treatment of PTs in men is similar to that of equivalent tumors in females. Most PTs in men are clinically benign.

Proliferative Fibrocystic Changes

Age and Predisposing Factors

Proliferative fibrocystic changes (FCCs) in the male breast are extremely rare. Most men with proliferative FCCs were under 50 years of age at the time of diagnosis (30–33). At least two men were described as karyotypically and phenotypically normal (30,31). Hormonal imbalance is usually the predisposing factor.

Microscopic Pathology

Proliferative FCCs in men include apocrine cysts, papillary apocrine metaplasia, UDH, and duct stasis with mastitis. The microscopic features in some lesions can resemble those of juvenile papillomatosis (JP) (32).

Treatment

FCCs without epithelial atypia do not require surgical treatment, but excision of a mass lesion might be considered. The diagnosis of FCCs in the male breast should prompt the assessment of systemic metabolic and/or hormonal imbalances, as well as evaluation of the use of hormones and drugs with hormonal side effects.

Carcinoma of the Male Breast

Incidence and Ethnicity

The standardized incidence rate of breast carcinoma in men is 0.4 per 100,000 person-years (34), and it is highest in men aged 85 years or older (35). A rise in the incidence of breast carcinoma in males has been observed recently across all racial and ethnic groups (36,37). In a California-based population study (37), 70% of men with breast carcinoma were non-Hispanic white. Race and ethnicity did not affect patient survival.

Age

The median age at diagnosis of invasive carcinoma is 68 years (37), but carcinoma can occur at any age, including rare cases in boys. Younger men have significantly more HER2-positive carcinomas (37). The median age of men with DCIS was 58 years in one study (38) and 65 years in another (39).

Predisposing Factors

Hormonal imbalance (namely, testicular dysfunction, hyperprolactinemia, prolonged estrogen or anabolic steroid treatment, hepatic insufficiency, etc.) is one of the most common predisposing factors. The association with prostatic carcinoma is partly due to hormonal treatment but may also reflect a genetic predisposition (40,41). Most men with familial breast carcinoma are *BRCA2* germline mutation carriers; *BRCA1* germline mutations are less common (42,43). The mean age at diagnosis in men with *BRCA2*-associated breast carcinoma is 59 years, and about 25% have prostate carcinoma and/or contralateral breast carcinoma. HER2 positivity in male breast carcinoma is significantly associated with *BRCA2* germline mutation carrier status (43). Klinefelter syndrome is also a predisposing genetic condition. Men with prior diagnosis of breast carcinoma have a 30-fold increased risk of developing a contralateral breast carcinoma; the risk is 110-fold higher if breast carcinoma was diagnosed before the age of 50 years (44). Radiation exposure and exposure to high environmental temperatures have also been implicated as possible risk factors. Gynecomastia is neither a predisposing factor nor a morphologic precursor of breast carcinoma.

Presenting Symptoms

The most common presenting symptom is a painless retroareolar mass. The mean duration of symptoms prior to clinical consultation ranges between 6 months and 1 year. Synchronous bilateral carcinomas are uncommon.

Imaging Studies

Mammography and ultrasonography of invasive carcinoma typically reveal a mass with irregular margins (11). Concurrent gynecomastia may occasionally obscure a carcinoma, but ultrasonography usually distinguishes the two lesions. Encapsulated papillary carcinoma appears as a discrete mass with a regular contour, and may contain calcifications. Ultrasound examination documents a cystic lesion with an internal papillary component. The presence of an irregular border may be

evidence of invasion. Microcalcifications are detected in 10% to 30% of male breast carcinomas, including DCIS, encapsulated papillary carcinoma, and invasive carcinoma. At present, there are no guidelines recommending mammographic screening for men, even in individuals with known genetic predisposition. The MRI findings of breast carcinomas in males resemble those of similar tumors in females.

Microscopic Pathology
Invasive Carcinoma

Approximately 90% of carcinomas in men are invasive ductal carcinomas, and most are moderately or poorly differentiated (37,43,45–50) **(Fig. 24.7)**. Apocrine differentiation can be present. A small percentage of invasive carcinomas have tubular, cribriform, mucinous, micropapillary, secretory, and adenoid cystic morphology (37,43,45–49). In a series of men with familial breast carcinoma, invasive micropapillary morphology showed a trend for association with *BRCA2* germline mutation status (42).

Secretory carcinoma in men harbors the characteristic ETV6-NTRK3 gene fusion (51). A carcinoma with osteoclast-like giant cells has also been reported (50). Invasive lobular carcinoma is rare. Rare examples of invasive pleomorphic lobular carcinoma (52,53) and E-cadherin-negative histiocytoid lobular carcinoma (54) are reported (see Chapter 19).

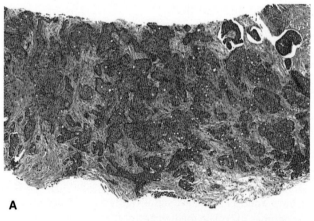

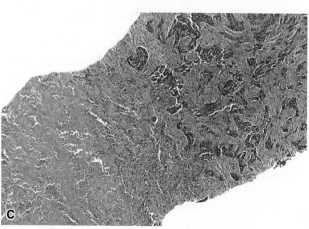

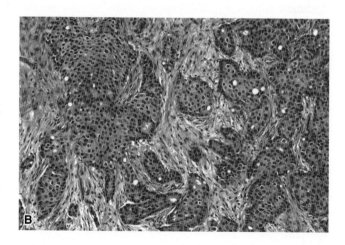

FIGURE 24.7 Male Breast, Invasive Ductal Carcinoma.
A, B: The patient was an 85-year-old man with a palpable tumor. The needle core biopsy specimen reveals **(A)** invasive ductal carcinoma, moderately differentiated. Gland formation is evident **(B)**. The invasive carcinoma was positive for estrogen receptor (ER) in 95% of the cells (not shown). **C:** The needle core biopsy specimen from a palpable mass in the breast of a 51-year-old male reveals poorly differentiated invasive ductal carcinoma with an area of necrosis. The carcinoma is associated with stromal desmoplasia. This carcinoma was also strongly and diffusely positive for ER (not shown).

Solid Papillary Carcinoma (SPC)

Overall, carcinomas with papillary morphology constitute 3% to 5% of all breast carcinomas in men, and are relatively more common in males than in females (47). Some cases previously classified as papillary DCIS likely represented solid papillary carcinomas. The neoplastic cells of EPC show low to moderate nuclear atypia, and may raise the differential diagnosis of florid hyperplasia in a papilloma. The diagnosis of papillary lesions of the male breast in NCB samples relies on the histologic and immunohistochemical criteria used to evaluate papillary proliferations of the female breast (see Chapters 4 and 11). In many cases, the NCB sample of an SPC yields only detached papillary fragments of carcinoma devoid of myoepithelium **(Fig. 24.8)**. In the absence of stromal desmoplasia or reactive changes, the absence of myoepithelium around a low-grade papillary carcinoma should not be interpreted as evidence of stromal invasion. In these cases, the assessment of stromal invasion requires examination of the entire tumor and of its interface with the surrounding stroma.

Intraductal Carcinoma

DCIS accounts for 6% (47) to 13% (55) of breast carcinomas in males, and morphologically duplicates the appearance of DCIS in women. Cribriform architecture is the most common; solid DCIS and DCIS with comedo-necrosis are rare. Some lesions previously reported as papillary DCIS may have been SPC. Micropapillary DCIS is the least common morphologic pattern. Most intraductal micropapillary epithelial proliferations

occurring in the male breast are hyperplastic, especially in the context of gynecomastia. Calcifications are more common in DCIS than in hyperplastic epithelium. Intraepidermal adenocarcinoma (Paget disease of the nipple) can also occur.

Immunohistochemistry

Approximately 90% of invasive carcinomas in the male breast are ER-positive (56–58). AR is expressed in 65% (58) to 95% (59) of the cases. HER2-positive/amplified invasive carcinoma is extremely rare but represents approximately 10% of familial cases (42), and it is significantly associated with *BRCA2* germline mutation carrier status (43). Triple-negative breast carcinoma is exceedingly rare in men.

Differential Diagnosis in Needle Core Biopsy Material

In men, the differential diagnosis of primary mammary carcinoma includes *metastases from an extramammary site*, such as lung, thyroid, kidney, and prostate; metastatic melanoma can also simulate breast carcinoma (60). Metastatic disease often involves both breasts, but it can be unilateral and unifocal (60). Accurate clinical information is very important to formulate the appropriate differential diagnosis and diagnostic workup. The identification of DCIS favors a primary mammary carcinoma. Morphologically, metastatic prostate carcinoma can closely resemble invasive ductal carcinoma of the breast and EPC. Tubular, mucinous, and micropapillary morphology

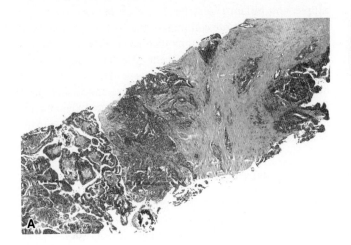

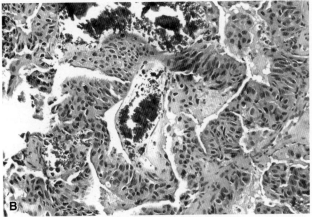

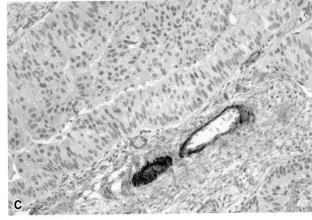

FIGURE 24.8 Papillary Carcinoma. A–C: This needle core biopsy sample is from a mass lesion in the breast of a 67-year-old man. **A:** Cystic papillary carcinoma is shown at both ends of the sample with invasive carcinoma in the center. **B:** Part of the cystic papillary carcinoma in **(A)** with calcifications. **C:** Actin reactivity is absent from the papillary carcinoma. Only vascular structures are actin-positive.

are uncommon in prostate carcinoma; intracellular mucin also supports mammary origin. Most metastatic prostatic adenocarcinomas express AR, but they can also express ER, and immunohistochemical stains for these markers are not always contributory. Most primary prostate carcinomas express prostate specific antigen (PSA), prostate specific associated protein (PSAP), racemase, and ETS-related gene (ERG), but these antigens tend to be reduced in the metastases. PSA is also expressed in breast carcinomas from men and women. Prostatic carcinoma treated with hormonal therapy for many years can acquire poorly differentiated and/or neuroendocrine morphology, and/or lose immunoreactivity for AR and prostatic markers **(Fig. 24.9)**. For these reasons, the diagnosis of primary mammary carcinoma with triple-negative immunophenotype in a man with a long-standing history of prostate carcinoma should always be rendered with extreme caution. GATA3 is a nuclear antigen expressed in most breast carcinoma in females but only in less than 7% of prostate carcinomas (61). The utility of GATA3 in the differential diagnosis of mammary versus prostatic carcinoma has not yet been studied.

Treatment and Prognosis

Men tend to present with higher-stage disease than women. In one study (47), 42% of males had lymph node (LN) metastases at diagnosis. Sentinel lymph node (SLN) biopsy is used to assess axillary LN status in clinically node-negative patients. Most men with DCIS and invasive carcinoma undergo mastectomy. A study (62) found no differences in overall survival (OS), but a significantly improved local relapse-free survival (RFS) in men with invasive carcinoma treated with postmastectomy radiation therapy was seen. Another study (63), however, reported no significant gender-related differences in locoregional RFS, breast cancer–specific survival, and OS in patients treated with mastectomy, when known prognostic factors and radiotherapy were accounted for. Treatment recommendations for men with breast carcinoma follow the guidelines established for female patients with carcinoma of similar TNM staging, and include adjuvant hormonal therapy and chemotherapy. In men, tamoxifen treatment appears to be more beneficial than treatment with aromatase inhibitors (64). HER2-targeted therapy is prescribed if the carcinoma qualifies as HER2-positive/amplified according to the ASCO-CAP recommendations.

The prognosis of male breast carcinoma is related to stage at diagnosis and receptor status. Earlier studies reported similar prognosis in male and female patients with the same stage of disease, but a recent series (47) documented significantly lower OS for males with stage I and stage II disease compared to stage-matched women. The OS of men with node-negative disease was also significantly lower than that for women (6.1 years vs. 14.6 years, respectively). In another series (46), disease-specific survival for all male patients was 75.2% at 5 years, and 52.5% at 10 years (46).

BREAST LESIONS IN CHILDREN AND ADOLESCENTS

Mass-forming lesions in the breast of children and adolescents are rare, vary according to age (65), and most are benign. Transient bilateral breast swelling in the newborn is secondary to maternal hormones. Bilateral breast enlargement in a child usually indicates a systemic hormonal imbalance. Most breast lesions in children under 18 years of age develop around the time of puberty: the most common are gynecomastia in boys and FAs in girls. Accessory breast tissue, supernumerary nipple, and inflammatory lesions, such as mastitis and fat necrosis, are also more common in the 10 to 15 years old age group. Non-neoplastic lesions such as juvenile hypertrophy and JP occur mainly in adolescent girls and young women. Other mass-forming lesions not exclusive to the breast include lipomas, vascular tumors (including angiosarcoma), metastatic extramammary malignant neoplasms, and malignant lymphoma. Primary mammary fibromatosis and metastatic alveolar rhabdomyosarcoma also can involve the breast of teenage girls.

Imaging Studies

Sonographic examination is the preferred technique for evaluation of a mass in the breast of a child or adolescent. Most solid masses in the breast of adolescent girls are FAs (66).

Risk of Subsequent Carcinoma

Most benign mass-forming lesions occurring in the breast in the first two decades of life are not associated with an increased risk of subsequent breast carcinoma.

Juvenile Papillomatosis

Age and Gender

JP usually presents in women younger than 30 years of age and is uncommon prior to puberty (67,68). There is no specific data on the incidence of JP in adolescents. JP rarely occurs in young men (32).

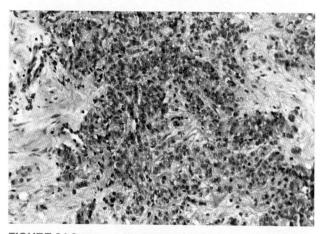

FIGURE 24.9 Metastatic Prostatic Carcinoma. This needle core biopsy sample is from a rapidly growing mass in the breast of an 85-year-old man with a long-standing history of prostatic carcinoma metastatic to bone treated with antiandrogen therapy. The patient developed rapidly progressive hormone-refractory metastatic disease. The carcinoma involving the breast was negative for ER, PR, and HER2, and focally positive for PSA (not shown).

Predisposing Factors

The reported frequency of family history for breast carcinoma in patients with JP was similar to (69,70) or higher (71) than the reported frequency in patients with mammary carcinoma. No contemporary series has investigated the relationship between JP and breast carcinoma.

Presenting Symptoms

JP typically presents as a solitary, firm, discrete unilateral tumor that clinically mimics a FA (68). Bilateral lesions are rare.

Imaging Studies

Information on the imaging findings of JP is limited (72). Mammographically, JP tends to present as a localized area of increased density not as well defined as a FA. Sonographically, JP presents as an ill-defined or discrete inhomogeneous, hypoechoic mass with multiple cysts (72). By MRI (72,73), JP can be a mass-forming lesion with a complex solid and cystic pattern, multiple small cysts on T2-weighted images, and continuous or clumped enhancement.

Microscopic Pathology

JP consists of nodular proliferative FCCs, with cysts and florid ductal hyperplasia. Cribriform or micropapillary ADH with necrosis can be found. In one series, atypia was present in 40% of JP cases, and intraductal necrosis was seen in 15% of the cases (71). Apocrine metaplasia is common **(Fig. 24.10)**. Other findings include sclerosing adenosis (SA), lobular hyperplasia, fibroadenomatoid hyperplasia, and dense stromal sclerosis.

Differential Diagnosis in Needle Core Biopsy Material

A definitive diagnosis of JP requires evaluation of the entire lesion. JP can be suspected when a NCB sample shows proliferative FCCs and the imaging findings are suggestive of FA. The differential diagnosis of JP in NCB material includes florid FCCs, papilloma, complex FA, and a complex sclerosing lesion.

Treatment and Prognosis

Although no specific data is available, in the absence of cytologic atypia, surgical excision of a lesion suggestive of JP does not appear to be required in cases with radiologic–pathologic concordant findings, and the decision to excise will depend on clinical evaluation and patient's preference. If no carcinoma or atypia is identified in JP in a surgical excision specimen, no further treatment is necessary. Local recurrence is rare. Based on the limited available data, JP does not appear to be a precancerous lesion.

Papilloma

Age, Gender, and Symptoms

Most young patients with papillomas are female, ranging between 15 and 25 years of age. Young males are rarely affected.

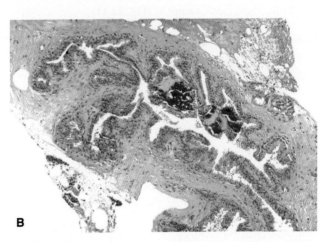

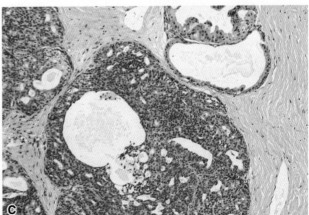

FIGURE 24.10 Juvenile Papillomatosis. A–C: This needle core biopsy specimen is from a 2-cm breast tumor in an 18-year-old girl. The diagnostic features are cysts, cystic and papillary apocrine metaplasia, duct hyperplasia, and stasis with accumulation of histiocytes. Calcifications are present in the papillary epithelium in **(B)**.

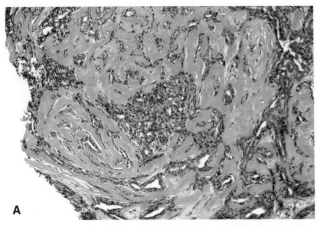
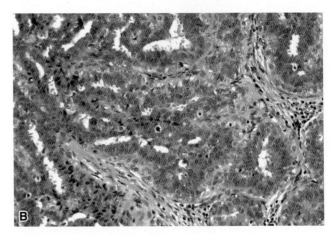

FIGURE 24.11 Sclerosing Papilloma. A: This needle core biopsy specimen from a breast tumor in a 19-year-old girl shows areas of dense sclerosis with epithelium compressed into slender cords. **B:** A portion of the lesion with florid duct hyperplasia.

The most frequent presenting symptom is a retroareolar and/or subareolar mass. Nipple discharge or bleeding can occur.

Imaging Studies

Sonographic examination is the preferred method of preoperative evaluation in children and adolescents. It usually shows a papillary mass within an anechoic or hypoechoic cystic cavity.

Microscopic Pathology

Papillomas in children and adolescents resemble equivalent lesions in adults (see Chapter 4) **(Fig. 24.11)**.

Treatment and Prognosis

Most patients with papilloma are managed by excisional biopsy. Papillomas do not appear to predispose children and young women to develop subsequent breast carcinoma.

Juvenile Atypical Ductal Hyperplasia

Age and Symptoms

Juvenile ADH was described in females with mean age of 21 years (range 18–26) (74). Rarely, ADH occurs in the breast of an adolescent male, usually in the context of gynecomastia.

Microscopic Pathology

Juvenile ADH usually constitutes an incidental finding. The morphology of juvenile ADH is similar to that of ADH in adult females **(Figs. 24.12–24.14)**.

Treatment and Prognosis

The identification of ADH in a NCB sample should prompt follow-up excision. In the absence of a more serious lesion in the surgical excision specimen, the clinical significance of juvenile ADH has not been fully evaluated in studies with long-term follow-up.

Gynecomastia in Children and Adolescents

See discussion of gynecomastia at the beginning of this chapter.

Fibroepithelial Lesions in Children and Adolescents

FELs are the most common tumors in the breast of adolescent females. The median age at diagnosis in two recent series was 14 years (75) and 16 years (76). Most FELs occur after menarche (76). FELs tend to be relatively more common in African-American girls.

Fibroadenoma

Age

In one series (76), the mean age of patients with usual/adult-type FAs was 17 years, and the mean age of patients with juvenile FAs was 15 years. The mean age at menarche of patients with either lesion was 12 years, but the mean time from menarche to diagnosis was 72 months for adult-type FAs, and 36 months for juvenile FAs.

Presenting Symptoms

FA usually present as a discrete, rubbery, ovoid, and mobile mass. Pain and nipple discharge are exceedingly rare. An

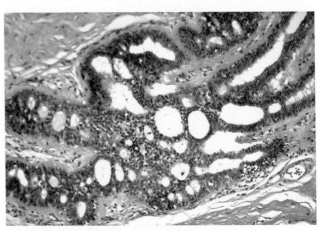

FIGURE 24.12 Juvenile Atypical Ductal Hyperplasia. Cribriform hyperplasia is present in this biopsy from an area of breast-thickening in a 21-year-old woman.

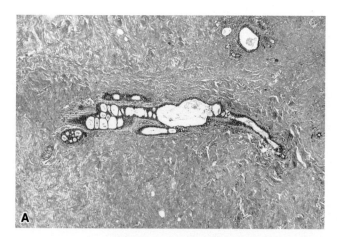
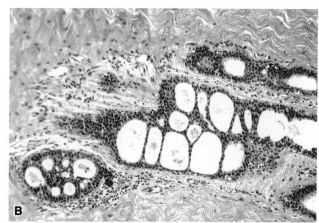

FIGURE 24.13 Juvenile Atypical Ductal Hyperplasia. A, B: This specimen was obtained from a reduction mammoplasty performed for juvenile hypertrophy in a 23-year-old woman. Cribriform hyperplasia is a focal abnormality in the duct. Note the broad expanse of collagenous stroma.

infarcted FA is usually asymptomatic; rarely it is painful or may cause bloody discharge.

Imaging Studies

Ultrasound examination is the most common imaging modality. It reveals a solid and hypoechoic lobulated mass, with smooth and circumscribed edges. FAs account for at least 75% of all solid masses in the breasts of adolescent females (66).

Size

FAs in young females can reach a considerable size, and show relatively rapid growth. The mean size of FAs (any type) was 2.9 cm in one series (76) and 3.6 cm in another (75). FAs have a benign clinical course, independent of size (75,76).

Microscopic Pathology

Usual FAs constitute 30% (76) to 40% (75) of all FAs in young females. Approximately half (75) to two-thirds (76) of FAs in adolescents are juvenile FAs. Epithelial hyperplasia is detected in 18% of usual FAs and in 30% juvenile FAs (76). A modest mitotic rate can be found in FAs in adolescents, especially in

juvenile FAs (75,76); this finding needs to be interpreted with caution in the absence of other features of PT (see Chapter 7 for detailed discussion of FAs).

Differential Diagnosis in Needle Core Biopsy Material

The diagnosis of usual FA is generally straightforward, but some lesions may show slightly cellular stroma. FAs with cellular stroma, including juvenile FAs, often raise the differential diagnosis of benign PTs **(Figs. 24.15 and 24.16)**. Complex FAs may raise the differential diagnosis of JP; the elongated ducts characteristic of FA are typically absent in JP.

Phyllodes Tumor
Symptoms

PTs present clinically as mass lesions, often with rapid growth.

Microscopic Pathology

PTs in children and adolescents have the same histologic characteristics as comparable tumors in adults (see Chapter 7).

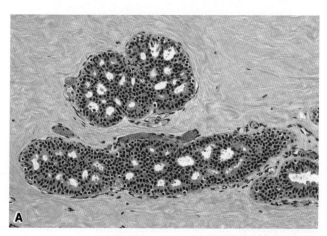
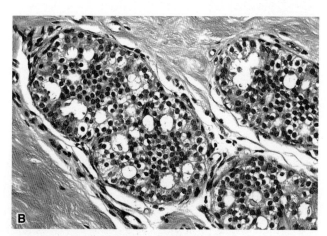

FIGURE 24.14 Juvenile Atypical Ductal Hyperplasia, Male. A: This specimen is from a 14-year-old boy who presented with bilateral breast enlargement. The stroma lacks the cellularity of gynecomastia. **B:** Atypical cribriform ductal hyperplasia in a 19-year-old boy with bilateral breast enlargement.

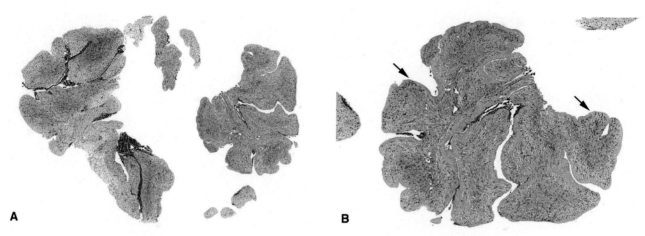

FIGURE 24.15 Benign Fibroepithelial Lesion, Excision Yielded a Juvenile Fibroadenoma. This needle core biopsy specimen was obtained from a breast mass in a 17-year-old female. **A:** Multiple detached fragments of fibroadenomatous stroma with a few elongated ducts. **B:** The stroma shows increased cellularity and slight condensation under the basement membrane layer *(arrows)*. The epithelium of these fragments has been stripped. The surgical excision specimen yielded a 3.3-cm juvenile fibroadenoma (not shown).

Treatment and Prognosis

Most PTs in children follow a benign clinical course after excision (75,76), but rare instances of local recurrence and malignant tumors with systemic metastases are reported (see Chapter 7 for a detailed discussion of PTs).

Pseudoangiomatous Stromal Hyperplasia

Pseudoangiomatous stromal hyperplasia (PASH) is often present in the stroma of pediatric FELs, in gynecomastia, and in adolescent macromastia. It can also present as a discrete

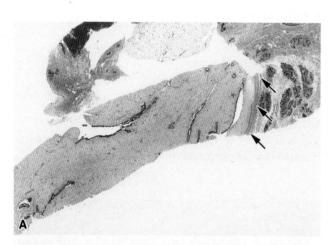

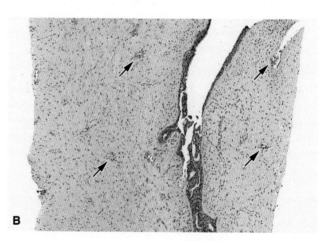

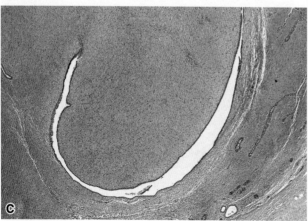

FIGURE 24.16 Benign Fibroepithelial Lesion, Excision Yielded a Benign Phyllodes Tumor. A, B: This needle core biopsy specimen was obtained from a breast mass in a 19-year-old female. **A:** The stroma is expanded and shows slightly increased cellularity. Elongated and clefted ducts are shown. The interface with the adjacent breast parenchyma is focally represented *(arrows)*. **B:** A magnified view shows slight periductal condensation of the stroma, with minimally enlarged stromal nuclei and increased vascularity *(arrows)*. **C:** The surgical excision specimen yielded a benign phyllodes tumor.

tumor indistinguishable clinically from a FA in girls and in the breast of pubertal boys with gynecomastia (77). Surgical excision of a breast mass yielding only PASH at NCB depends on the clinical and radiologic characteristics of the lesion. Peripheral and/or incomplete sampling of a PT is a possible consideration in some cases (see Chapter 20 for a detailed discussion of PASH).

Carcinoma in Children and Adolescents

Incidence, Age, and Presenting Symptoms
Primary carcinoma of the breast is extremely unusual in children and adolescents, and accounts for less than 1% of all pediatric breast lesions (65). Most patients are females, with an average age of about 13 years. The presenting symptom is usually a mass.

Predisposing Factors
Prior irradiation is a predisposing factor in some instances.

Microscopic Pathology
The morphologic spectrum of breast carcinomas in children and adolescents includes invasive ductal carcinoma, poorly differentiated and pleomorphic carcinoma, secretory carcinoma (78–80), and ACC (81–83). DCIS is also reported (84–86). The aforementioned carcinomas are morphologically similar to carcinomas of the same type occurring in adults. A secretory carcinoma in a 9-year-old girl showed the characteristic ETV6-TRK3 fusion gene and reportedly was ER-positive (79). ACC is described in adolescents, including males (81,82). No examples of ACC with solid and basaloid morphology have yet been reported. Primary breast carcinoma with small-cell morphology is exceedingly rare in children. The differential diagnosis includes high-grade lymphoma, embryonal rhabdomyosarcoma, and primitive neuroectodermal tumor (PNET). Immunoreactivity for CK is usually detectable, and the cells are not reactive with markers for lymphoma or rhabdomyosarcoma.

Nonepithelial Malignant Neoplasms

Primary mammary sarcoma is exceedingly uncommon in children and adults. Rare cases of primary mammary angiosarcoma occurred in the second decade of life (87,88). Metastases from sarcomas arising at other sites have been reported. In particular, alveolar type rhabdomyosarcoma tends to metastasize to the breast in adolescent girls (89), with most tumors originating in the extremities or buttocks. Systemic diseases such as lymphoma or leukemia can involve the breast. For further discussion of these topics, see relevant chapters elsewhere in this volume.

REFERENCES

Breast Lesions in Males
1. Westenend PJ. Core needle biopsy in male breast lesions. *J Clin Pathol.* 2003;56:863–865.
2. Tangerud A, Potapenko I, Skjerven HK, et al. Radiologic evaluation of lumps in the male breast. *Acta Radiol.* 2016;57(7):809–814.
3. Roberto G, Biagi C, Montanaro N, et al. Statin-associated gynecomastia: evidence coming from the Italian spontaneous ADR reporting database and literature. *Eur J Clin Pharmacol.* 2012;68:1007–1011.
4. Oteri A, Catania MA, Travaglini R, et al. Gynecomastia possibly induced by rosuvastatin. *Pharmacotherapy.* 2008;28:549–551.
5. Tanriverdi O, Unubol M, Taskin F, et al. Imatinib-associated bilateral gynecomastia and unilateral testicular hydrocele in male patient with metastatic gastrointestinal stromal tumor: a literature review. *J Oncol Pharm Pract.* 2012;18:303–310.
6. Liu H, Liao G, Yan Z. Gynecomastia during imatinib mesylate treatment for gastrointestinal stromal tumor: a rare adverse event. *BMC Gastroenterol.* 2011;11:116.
7. Schinina V, Busi Rizzi E, Zaccarelli M, et al. Gynecomastia in male HIV patients MRI and US findings. *Clin Imaging.* 2002;26:309–313.
8. Pantanowitz L, Sen S, Crisi GM, et al. Spectrum of breast disease encountered in HIV-positive patients at a community teaching hospital. *Breast.* 2011;20:303–308.
9. Williams MJ. Gynecomastia: its incidence, recognition and host characterization in 447 autopsy cases. *Am J Med.* 1963;34:103–112.
10. Koshy JC, Goldberg JS, Wolfswinkel EM, et al. Breast cancer incidence in adolescent males undergoing subcutaneous mastectomy for gynecomastia: is pathologic examination justified? A retrospective and literature review. *Plast Reconstr Surg.* 2011;127:1–7.
11. Nguyen C, Kettler MD, Swirsky ME, et al. Male breast disease: pictorial review with radiologic-pathologic correlation. *Radiographics.* 2013;33:763–779.
12. Munoz Carrasco R, Alvarez Benito M, Munoz Gomariz E, et al. Mammography and ultrasound in the evaluation of male breast disease. *Eur Radiol.* 2010;20:2797–2805.
13. Iuanow E, Kettler M, Slanetz PJ. Spectrum of disease in the male breast. *AJR Am J Roentgenol.* 2011;196:W247–W259.
14. Rahmani S, Turton P, Shaaban A, et al. Overview of gynecomastia in the modern era and the Leeds Gynaecomastia Investigation algorithm. *Breast J.* 2011;17:246–255.
15. Wells JM, Liu Y, Ginter PS, et al. Elucidating encounters of atypical ductal hyperplasia arising in gynaecomastia. *Histopathology.* 2015;66:398–408.
16. Kornegoor R, Verschuur-Maes AH, Buerger H, et al. The 3-layered ductal epithelium in gynecomastia. *Am J Surg Pathol.* 2012;36(5):762–768.
17. Van Poppel H, Tyrrell CJ, Haustermans K, et al. Efficacy and tolerability of radiotherapy as treatment for bicalutamide-induced gynaecomastia and breast pain in prostate cancer. *Eur Urol.* 2005;47:587–592.
18. Fradet Y, Egerdie B, Andersen M, et al. Tamoxifen as prophylaxis for prevention of gynaecomastia and breast pain associated with bicalutamide 150 mg monotherapy in patients with prostate cancer: a randomised, placebo-controlled, dose-response study. *Eur Urol.* 2007;52:106–114.
19. Li CC, Fu JP, Chang SC, et al. Surgical treatment of gynecomastia: complications and outcomes. *Ann Plast Surg.* 2012;69:510–515.
20. McLaughlin CS, Petrey C, Grant S, et al. Displaced epithelium after liposuction for gynecomastia. *Int J Surg Pathol.* 2011;19:510–513.
21. Olsson H, Bladstrom A, Alm P. Male gynecomastia and risk for malignant tumours—a cohort study. *BMC Cancer.* 2002;2:26.
22. Durkin ET, Warner TF, Nichol PF. Enlarging unilateral breast mass in an adolescent male: an unusual presentation of intraductal papilloma. *J Pediatr Surg.* 2011;46:e33–e35.
23. Ansah-Boateng Y, Tavassoli FA. Fibroadenoma and cystosarcoma phyllodes of the male breast. *Mod Pathol.* 1992;5:114–116.
24. Hilton DA, Jameson JS, Furness PN. A cellular fibroadenoma resembling a benign phyllodes tumour in a young male with gynaecomastia. *Histopathology.* 1991;18:476–477.
25. Gupta P, Foshee S, Garcia-Morales F, et al. Fibroadenoma in male breast: case report and literature review. *Breast Dis.* 2011;33:45–48.
26. Kanhai RC, Hage JJ, Bloemena E, et al. Mammary fibroadenoma in a male-to-female transsexual. *Histopathology.* 1999;35:183–185.
27. Lemmo G, Garcea N, Corsello S, et al. Breast fibroadenoma in a male-to-female transsexual patient after hormonal treatment. *Eur J Surg Suppl.* 2003;69–71.
28. Shin SJ, Rosen PP. Bilateral presentation of fibroadenoma with digital fibroma-like inclusions in the male breast. *Arch Pathol Lab Med.* 2007;131:1126–1129.

29. Bowman E, Oprea G, Okoli J, et al. Pseudoangiomatous stromal hyperplasia (PASH) of the breast: a series of 24 patients. *Breast J*. 2012;18:242–247.

30. Banik S, Hale R. Fibrocystic disease in the male breast. *Histopathology*. 1988;12:214–216.

31. McClure J, Banerjee SS, Sandilands DG. Female type cystic hyperplasia in a male breast. *Postgrad Med J*. 1985;61:441–443.

32. Sund BS, Topstad TK, Nesland JM. A case of juvenile papillomatosis of the male breast. *Cancer*. 1992;70:126–128.

33. Robertson KE, Kazmi SA, Jordan LB. Female-type fibrocystic disease with papillary hyperplasia in a male breast. *J Clin Pathol*. 2010;63:88–89.

34. Miao H, Verkooijen HM, Chia KS, et al. Incidence and outcome of male breast cancer: an international population-based study. *J Clin Oncol*. 2011;29(33):4381–4386.

35. Hodgson NC, Button JH, Franceschi D, et al. Male breast cancer: is the incidence increasing? *Ann Surg Oncol*. 2004;11:751–755.

36. Giordano SH, Cohen DS, Buzdar AU, et al. Breast carcinoma in men: a population-based study. *Cancer*. 2004;101:51–57.

37. Chavez-Macgregor M, Clarke CA, Lichtensztajn D, et al. Male breast cancer according to tumor subtype and race: a population-based study. *Cancer*. 2013;19(9):1611–1617.

38. Cutuli B, Lacroze M, Dilhuydy JM, et al. Male breast cancer: results of the treatments and prognostic factors in 397 cases. *Eur J Cancer*. 1995;31A:1960–1964.

39. Hittmair AP, Lininger RA, Tavassoli FA. Ductal carcinoma in situ (DCIS) in the male breast: a morphologic study of 84 cases of pure DCIS and 30 cases of DCIS associated with invasive carcinoma—a preliminary report. *Cancer*. 1998;83:2139–2149.

40. Leibowitz SB, Garber JE, Fox EA, et al. Male patients with diagnoses of both breast cancer and prostate cancer. *Breast J*. 2003;9:208–212.

41. Kiluk JV, Lee MC, Park CK, et al. Male breast cancer: management and follow-up recommendations. *Breast J*. 2011;17:503–509.

42. Deb S, Jene N, Investigators K, et al. Genotypic and phenotypic analysis of familial male breast cancer shows under representation of the HER2 and basal subtypes in BRCA-associated carcinomas. *BMC Cancer*. 2012;12:510.

43. Ottini L, Silvestri V, Rizzolo P, et al. Clinical and pathologic characteristics of BRCA-positive and BRCA-negative male breast cancer patients: results from a collaborative multicenter study in Italy. *Breast Cancer Res Treat*. 2012;134(1):411–418.

44. Auvinen A, Curtis RE, Ron E. Risk of subsequent cancer following breast cancer in men. *J Natl Cancer Inst*. 2002;94:1330–1332.

45. Nilsson C, Johansson I, Ahlin C, et al. Molecular subtyping of male breast cancer using alternative definitions and its prognostic impact. *Acta Oncol*. 2013;52:102–109.

46. Tural D, Selcukbiricik F, Aydogan F, et al. Male breast cancers behave differently in elderly patients. *Jpn J Clin Oncol*. 2013;43:22–27.

47. Nahleh ZA, Srikantiah R, Safa M, et al. Male breast cancer in the veterans affairs population: a comparative analysis. *Cancer*. 2007;109:1471–1477.

48. Arslan UY, Oksuzoglu B, Ozdemir N, et al. Outcome of non-metastatic male breast cancer: 118 patients. *Med Oncol*. 2012;29:554–560.

49. Kornegoor R, Verschuur-Maes AH, Buerger H, et al. Molecular subtyping of male breast cancer by immunohistochemistry. *Mod Pathol*. 2011;25(3):398–404.

50. Burga AM, Fadare O, Lininger RA, et al. Invasive carcinomas of the male breast: a morphologic study of the distribution of histologic subtypes and metastatic patterns in 778 cases. *Virchows Arch*. 2006;449:507–512.

51. Diallo R, Schaefer KL, Bankfalvi A, et al. Secretory carcinoma of the breast: a distinct variant of invasive ductal carcinoma assessed by comparative genomic hybridization and immunohistochemistry. *Hum Pathol*. 2003;34:1299–1305.

52. Maly B, Maly A, Pappo I, et al. Pleomorphic variant of invasive lobular carcinoma of the male breast. *Virchows Arch*. 2005;446:344–345.

53. Rohini B, Singh PA, Vatsala M, et al. Pleomorphic lobular carcinoma in a male breast: a rare occurrence. *Patholog Res Int*. 2010;2010:871369.

54. Hutchinson CB, Geradts J. Histiocytoid carcinoma of the male breast. *Ann Diagn Pathol*. 2011;15:190–193.

55. Flynn LW, Park J, Patil SM, et al. Sentinel lymph node biopsy is successful and accurate in male breast carcinoma. *J Am Coll Surg*. 2008;206:616–621.

56. Greif JM, Pezzi CM, Klimberg VS, et al. Gender differences in breast cancer: analysis of 13,000 breast cancers in men from the National Cancer Data Base. *Ann Surg Oncol*. 2012;19:3199–3204.

57. Ottini L, Rizzolo P, Zanna I, et al. BRCA1/BRCA2 mutation status and clinical-pathologic features of 108 male breast cancer cases from Tuscany: a population-based study in central Italy. *Breast Cancer Res Treat*. 2009;116:577–586.

58. Shaaban AM, Ball GR, Brannan RA, et al. A comparative biomarker study of 514 matched cases of male and female breast cancer reveals gender-specific biological differences. *Breast Cancer Res Treat*. 2012;133:949–958.

59. Rayson D, Erlichman C, Suman VJ, et al. Molecular markers in male breast carcinoma. *Cancer*. 1998;83:1947–1955.

60. DeLair DF, Corben AD, Catalano JP, et al. Non-mammary metastases to the breast and axilla: a study of 85 cases. *Mod Pathol*. 2013;26:343–349.

61. Miettinen M, McCue PA, Sarlomo-Rikala M, et al. GATA3: a multispecific but potentially useful marker in surgical pathology: a systematic analysis of 2500 epithelial and nonepithelial tumors. *Am J Surg Pathol*. 2014;38:13–22.

62. Yu E, Suzuki H, Younus J, et al. The impact of post-mastectomy radiation therapy on male breast cancer patients—a case series. *Int J Radiat Oncol Biol Phys*. 2012;82:696–700.

63. Macdonald G, Paltiel C, Olivotto IA, et al. A comparative analysis of radiotherapy use and patient outcome in males and females with breast cancer. *Ann Oncol*. 2005;16:1442–1448.

64. Eggemann H, Ignatov A, Smith BJ, et al. Adjuvant therapy with tamoxifen compared to aromatase inhibitors for 257 male breast cancer patients. *Breast Cancer Res Treat*. 2013;137:465–470.

Breast Lesions in Children and Adolescents

65. Pettinato G, Manivel JC, Kelly DR, et al. Lesions of the breast in children exclusive of typical fibroadenoma and gynecomastia: a clinicopathologic study of 113 cases. *Pathol Annu*. 1989;24(pt 2):296–328.

66. Sanchez R, Ladino-Torres MF, Bernat JA, et al. Breast fibroadenomas in the pediatric population: common and uncommon sonographic findings. *Pediatr Radiol*. 2010;40:1681–1689.

67. Rosen PP, Cantrell B, Mullen DL, et al. Juvenile papillomatosis (Swiss cheese disease) of the breast. *Am J Surg Pathol*. 1980;4:3–12.

68. Rosen PP, Holmes G, Lesser ML, et al. Juvenile papillomatosis and breast carcinoma. *Cancer*. 1985;55:1345–1352.

69. Rosen PP, Lyngholm B, Kinne DW, et al. Juvenile papillomatosis of the breast and family history of breast carcinoma. *Cancer*. 1982;49:2591–2595.

70. Bazzocchi F, Santini D, Martinelli G, et al. Juvenile papillomatosis (epitheliosis) of the breast: a clinical and pathologic study of 13 cases. *Am J Clin Pathol*. 1986;86:745–748.

71. Rosen PP, Kimmel M. Juvenile papillomatosis of the breast: a follow-up study of 41 patients having biopsies before 1979. *Am J Clin Pathol*. 1990;93:599–603.

72. Sabate JM, Clotet M, Torrubia S, et al. Radiologic evaluation of breast disorders related to pregnancy and lactation. *Radiographics*. 2007;27(suppl 1):S101–S124.

73. Durur-Subasi I, Alper F, Akcay MN, et al. Magnetic resonance imaging findings of breast juvenile papillomatosis. *Jpn J Radiol*. 2013;31:419–423.

74. Eliasen CA, Cranor ML, Rosen PP. Atypical duct hyperplasia of the breast in young females. *Am J Surg Pathol*. 1992;16:246–251.

75. Tay TK, Chang KT, Thike AA, et al. Paediatric fibroepithelial lesions revisited: pathological insights. *J Clin Pathol*. 2015;68:633–641.

76. Ross DS, Giri D, Akram M, et al. Fibroepithelial lesions in the breast of adolescent females: a clinicopathological study of 54 cases. *Breast J*. In press.

77. Shehata BM, Fishman I, Collings MH, et al. Pseudoangiomatous stromal hyperplasia of the breast in pediatric patients: an underrecognized entity. *Pediatr Dev Pathol*. 2009;12:450–454.

78. Buchino JJ, Moore GD, Bond SJ. Secretory carcinoma in a 9-year-old girl. *Diagn Cytopathol*. 2004;31:430–431.

79. Yorozuya K, Takahashi E, Kousaka J, et al. A case of estrogen receptor positive secretory carcinoma in a 9-year-old girl with ETV6-NTRK3 fusion gene. *Jpn J Clin Oncol*. 2012;42:208–211.

80. Kavalakat AJ, Covilakam RK, Culas TB. Secretory carcinoma of breast in a 17-year-old male. *World J Surg Oncol*. 2004;2:17.

81. Miliauskas JR, Leong AS. Adenoid cystic carcinoma in a juvenile male breast. *Pathology.* 1991;23:298–301.

82. Tang P, Yang S, Zhong X, et al. Breast adenoid cystic carcinoma in a 19-year-old man: a case report and review of the literature. *World J Surg Oncol.* 2015;13:19.

83. Delanote S, Van den Broecke R, Schelfhout VR, et al. Adenoid cystic carcinoma of the breast in a 19-year-old girl. *Breast.* 2003;12:75–77.

84. Chang HL, Kish JB, Smith BL, et al. A 16-year-old male with gynecomastia and ductal carcinoma in situ. *Pediatr Surg Int.* 2008;24:1251–1253.

85. Wadie GM, Banever GT, Moriarty KP, et al. Ductal carcinoma in situ in a 16-year-old adolescent boy with gynecomastia: a case report. *J Pediatr Surg.* 2005;40:1349–1353.

86. Sato T, Muto I, Hasegawa M, et al. Ductal carcinoma in situ with isolated tumor cells in the sentinel lymph node in a 17-year-old adolescent girl. *Breast Cancer.* 2013;20(3):271–274.

87. Yang WT, Hennessy BT, Dryden MJ, et al. Mammary angiosarcomas: imaging findings in 24 patients. *Radiology.* 2007;242:725–734.

88. van Geel AN, den Bakker MA. Bilateral angiosarcoma of the breast in a fourteen-year-old child. *Rare Tumors.* 2009;1:e38.

89. D'Angelo P, Carli M, Ferrari A, et al. Breast metastases in children and adolescents with rhabdomyosarcoma: experience of the Italian Soft Tissue Sarcoma Committee. *Pediatr Blood Cancer.* 2010;55:1306–1309.

Pathologic Changes and Clinical Complications Associated with Needling Procedures

SYED A. HODA

The objective of a needle core biopsy (NCB) procedure is adequate sampling of the target lesion. An efficacious core biopsy sampling may remove a portion, or all, of the target. The latter is almost always a nonpalpable radiologically detected (mammographic, sonographic, or MR-detected) lesion or a discrete mass. The procedure inevitably results in disruption of lesional and/or perilesional tissue. NCB-induced tissue disruption varies widely and depends mainly upon the gauge of needle used and volume of sample obtained. In recent years, the trend is toward obtaining bulkier sampling by utilizing larger gauge needles and procuring multiple samples, which results in greater tissue damage (1). The latter is evident in the subsequently performed excisional biopsy and is the main topic of this chapter. Other needling procedures such as fine needle aspirations (FNAs), needle localization procedures, and even liposuctions can cause similar disruption (2–4).

Automated NCB procedures that are typically used for targeting masses are more frequently associated with epithelial displacement than vacuum-assisted NCB procedures (5). The latter are generally used for targeting radiographically detected lesions, and are more commonly used. In the automated procedure, the needle is pushed into the target, and the sample is then directly acquired. In the vacuum-assisted procedure, the tissue sample is acquired by firing of the needle once the probe is adjacent to the target lesion, and the acquired samples are then suctioned into the probe. Direct mechanical sampling causes relatively more trauma to the lesional epithelium than vacuum-assisted acquisition.

HISTOPATHOLOGIC CHANGES CAUSED BY NEEDLE CORE BIOPSY

Long-standing or significant effects of the NCB procedure on perilesional tissue, beyond that of hemorrhage, organizing fat necrosis and subsequent scarring, are usually not apparent in imaging studies. In 24 patients studied by Kaye et al. (6), follow-up mammography performed 6 months after stereotactic

14-gauge biopsy revealed no mammographically detectable architectural distortion attributable to the procedure. In two instances, there were fewer calcifications in postbiopsy mammograms, and a 6-mm fibroadenoma contained a 3-mm defect. Lamm and Jackman (7) reported the formation of a "small" (mean size: 8 mm) mammographic density in 6 to 8 months at the biopsy site when larger (11-gauge) needles were utilized. These as well as multiple recent reports indicate that in general the performance of NCBs does not inflict notable effect on subsequent radiographic (including ultrasound, mammographic, and MRI) studies.

Nonetheless, *procedural trauma–induced changes* in and around the NCB site can affect the histopathologic interpretation of the subsequently performed excisional biopsy—an observation noted more than two decades ago (8,9). Evidence of previous NCB track (or, less accurately, tract), for example, hemorrhage, granulation tissue formation, and fibroplasia, should be sought in excisional biopsies, as evidence that the target lesion has been sampled (8,9). The presence of fresh blood or of hemosiderin within the lumina of glands in the vicinity of the target lesion as well as in lesional glands is a frequent manifestation of prior needling procedures, including needle-localizing techniques **(Fig. 25.1)**. Fragments of epidermis may be dislodged into breast tissue by the needle if a cutaneous incision was not made before inserting the needle. An epidermal inclusion cyst may form from the displaced skin epithelium (10) **(Fig. 25.2)**. Considerable diagnostic difficulties can ensue as a result of displacement of neoplastic or non-neoplastic epithelium along the healing biopsy track (vide infra) (11,12).

The healing NCB site initially develops granulation tissue (i.e., proliferating fibroblasts and capillaries amid inflammatory cells), and eventually forms a **scar**. The maturity of the scar depends on the time period that has elapsed between the initial NCB and the subsequent excisional procedure. In some cases, the reactive process displays exuberant myofibroblastic or histiocytic hyperplasia with mitotic activity (13) to a degree that it forms a "pseudotumor" (14) or appears "pseudosarcomatous"

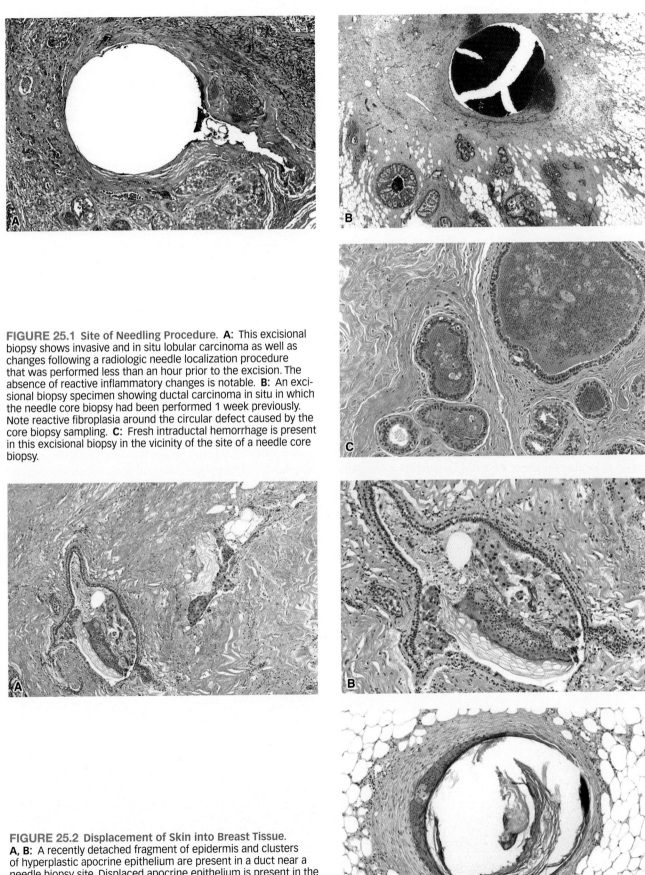

FIGURE 25.1 Site of Needling Procedure. A: This excisional biopsy shows invasive and in situ lobular carcinoma as well as changes following a radiologic needle localization procedure that was performed less than an hour prior to the excision. The absence of reactive inflammatory changes is notable. **B:** An excisional biopsy specimen showing ductal carcinoma in situ in which the needle core biopsy had been performed 1 week previously. Note reactive fibroplasia around the circular defect caused by the core biopsy sampling. **C:** Fresh intraductal hemorrhage is present in this excisional biopsy in the vicinity of the site of a needle core biopsy.

**FIGURE 25.2 Displacement of Skin into Breast Tissue.
A, B:** A recently detached fragment of epidermis and clusters of hyperplastic apocrine epithelium are present in a duct near a needle biopsy site. Displaced apocrine epithelium is present in the biopsy track **(A)**. **C:** Another excisional biopsy specimen in which displaced epidermis has formed a cyst and become encapsulated amid reactive fibroplasia. The needle core biopsy had been performed approximately 3 weeks previously.

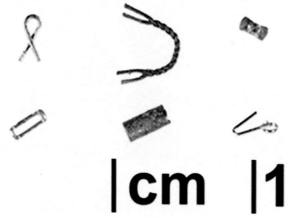

FIGURE 25.3 **A Collection of Commonly Used, Commercially Available, Clips.** These clips are utilized to mark the site of a targeted lesion after the performance of a needle core biopsy. "Extraction" of the clips at the time of gross examination of the subsequently performed excisional biopsy may cause damage to lesional tissue. It is important that the presence of one or more clips be documented in the excisional biopsy by the pathologist. Specimen radiography is helpful in localizing the clip(s) in most cases.

(15). Association with a healing biopsy track and comparative histopathologic review with findings in the NCB can be helpful in rendering the appropriate diagnoses.

It is now routine practice to place a *clip at the site of a targeted lesion* after the performance of a NCB. Clip placement primarily serves to localize the site of the lesion by spatially guiding the subsequent surgical procedure and helps optimize the volume of tissue excised. Clips also serve to mark a malignant neoplasm prior to neoadjuvant chemotherapy, indicate the edges of extensive carcinoma, and facilitate radiologic follow-up of presumed benign lesions. Clips can be placed to mark targets sampled via biopsies that are stereotactic, sonographic, or MRI-guided, and multiple clips of different shapes or sizes can mark several targets sampled either synchronously or metachronously

(16–19). The finding of the clip during gross examination of an excisional biopsy specimen ensures, at a minimum, that the vicinity of the lesion that was previously sampled by NCB has been removed. In mastectomy specimens, the clip can be particularly helpful in directing tissue sampling.

A wide variety of clips are commercially available, including those that are composed principally of stainless steel, ceramic, or titanium (**Fig. 25.3**). Clips have to be removed at the time of gross pathologic evaluation to enable complete inspection of the specimen, document its presence, and ensure that the subsequently prepared tissue block does not inadvertently contain the clip. The latter could potentially damage the microtome during sectioning of the tissue block and also compromise the quality of histologic sections. Minute sharp hooks serve to anchor the clip into the soft tissues, and the removal of clips at the time of gross pathologic examination can inflict physical injury on the pathologist.

Diligent efforts at the time of gross examination may be required to find the clip within the specimen. These efforts include serial "thin" (approximately 2 mm) sectioning and specimen radiography. Rarely, despite a concerted effort, the clip cannot be found in the excisional biopsy or mastectomy, and the most likely explanation is loss incurred either through the intraoperative use of a suction device with a 4-mm aperture (most clips span 2–3 mm) or through careless specimen procurement, transport, and handling (20,21).

Various types of *bioresorbable embedding material* such as bovine collagen (Avitene), polylactic acid/polyglycolic acid pellets, starch pellets, polyglycolic acid pads, polyethelene-glycol hydrogel, etc. are inserted along with the clip at the biopsy site to prevent displacement ("migration") of the clip and improve hemostasis by filling of the newly created cavity. Each embedding material has a distinctive histologic appearance (**Fig. 25.4**), and some of these may be mistaken by the uninitiated for amyloid, osteoid, or other foreign material (22,23). Although these materials do not typically elicit a reactive inflammatory reaction, occasionally a prominent reaction might be evident.

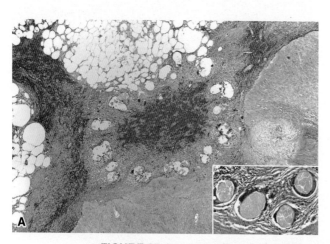
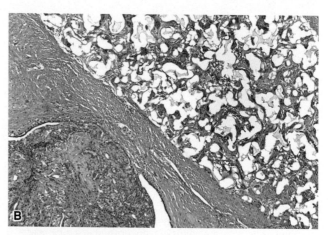

FIGURE 25.4 **Reaction to Various "Plugs" Used to Anchor the Clip into Breast Tissue.**
A–F: Various embedding materials have distinctive histologic appearances. Some of these "plugs" may be mistaken by the uninitiated for amyloid, osteoid, or other foreign material. All figures show various degrees of giant cell reaction against the "plug." Inset in **A** shows detail at the healing needle core biopsy site. A pronounced inflammatory reaction is evident in **D–F**.

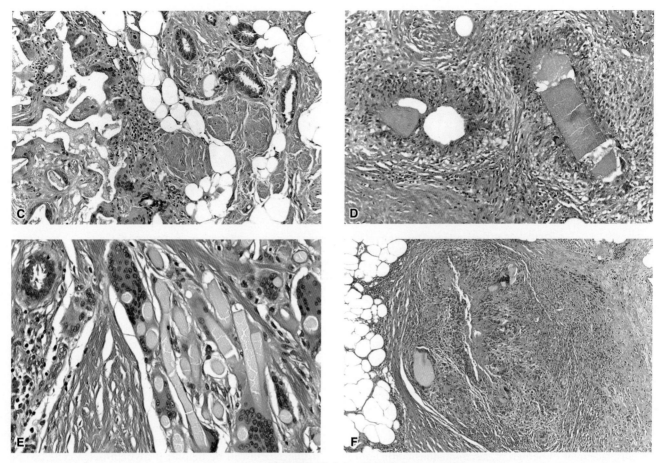

FIGURE 25.4 (*continued*)

Tissue disruption may result in *displacement of lesional epithelial cells* into the healing needle track and into stroma in the lesional area. This can produce a pattern that simulates invasive carcinoma (2,24,25) **(Figs. 25.5 and 25.6)**. Youngson et al. (8,9) were among the first to report finding displaced epithelium in excisional biopsies of breast with various types of lesions after the performance of NCBs. The average interval between the needling procedure and excisional biopsy was 10 days. Fragments of benign or malignant epithelium were present within lymphovascular channels in seven cases, six of which also had stromal displacement. One of these women, who had extensive intraductal carcinoma associated with stromal

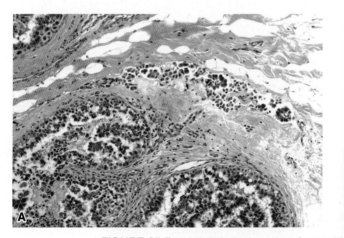

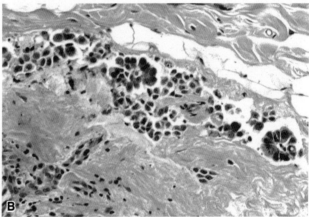

FIGURE 25.5 Epithelial Displacement in Postbiopsy Excision. A, B: Displaced fragments of intraductal carcinoma are shown in the stroma near the site of a needle core biopsy procedure performed 7 days previously. Note the absence of reactive changes in the stroma and the well-preserved cytologic appearance of the displaced tumor cells.

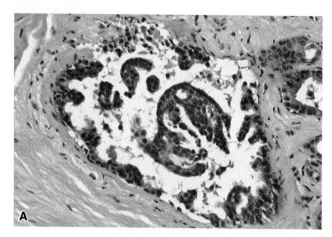
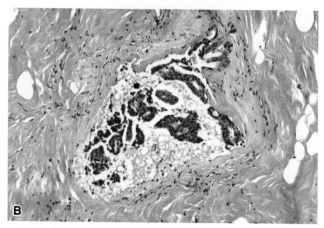

FIGURE 25.6 Disruption of Intraductal Carcinoma in Postbiopsy Excision. A: Portions of the intraductal carcinoma have been dislodged from the basement membrane and are displaced into the duct lumen after a needle core biopsy procedure. **B:** Another area in the specimen shown in **A** with severe disruption of intraductal carcinoma. The detached epithelial fragments have remained within the confines of the basement membrane.

displacement and lymphovascular tumor emboli in the breast, also had clusters of carcinoma cells in the subcapsular sinuses of two axillary lymph nodes. Hoorntje et al. (26) reported finding displaced carcinoma cells in 11 of 22 (50%) needle tracts after 14-gauge needle biopsy procedures. Prospectively, these authors found displaced carcinoma in 7 or 11 (64%) needle tracks examined 7 to 35 days (median interval, 25 days) after 14-gauge needle biopsy.

Displacement of benign or carcinomatous epithelium is suggested by the finding of scattered, isolated, clusters of epithelium in iatrogenically created minuscule cystic spaces within the healing biopsy track—generally in a linear distribution. Depending upon the time elapsed since the procedure, the displaced epithelium is accompanied by hemorrhage, hemosiderin-laden macrophages, fat necrosis, an inflammatory cell infiltrate or granulation tissue, and scarring **(Fig. 25.7)**. Displaced epithelium that is not in the immediate vicinity of the

biopsy site may not be accompanied by any significant degree of stromal reaction. This may lead to the mistaken diagnosis of invasive carcinoma even in a benign lesion. It is not unusual to find fragments of displaced epithelium within lumina of benign glands. Rarely, portions of intraductal carcinoma that is entirely dislodged into the lumen of an atrophic duct may simulate lymphatic invasion.

Immunostains for confirming the presence of epithelial displacement can be helpful if myoepithelial cells can be demonstrated via p63, p40, myosin, etc. around the extralesional epithelial cells **(Fig. 25.8)**. Coincidentally, it must be possible to immunohistochemically detect myoepithelial cells in the target lesion sampled by the NCB. Myoepithelial cells are almost certainly present if the primary lesion is benign (e.g., papillary ductal hyperplasia and intraductal papilloma), but they can also be found in in situ carcinomas. Failure to find myoepithelial cells in association with the extralesional

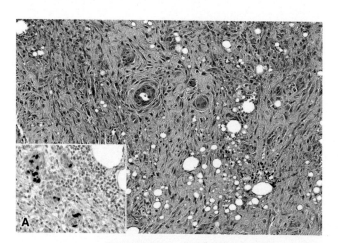
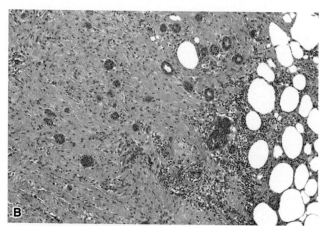

FIGURE 25.7 Displaced Epithelium in Postbiopsy Scars. A: This patient underwent a needle core biopsy procedure that showed a sclerosing papilloma. This image is from the subsequent excisional biopsy specimen performed 1 week after the needle biopsy procedure. Myoepithelial cells display nuclear p63 reactivity *(inset)* around some displaced epithelial cell fragments. **B:** Displaced epithelial fragments in fibrous scar tissue at the needle core biopsy site. The needle core biopsy had been performed 3 weeks previously.

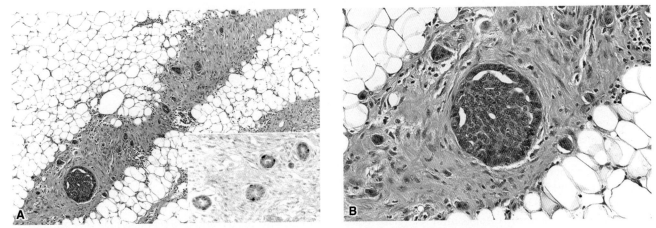

FIGURE 25.8 Epithelial Displacement along the Healing Needle Core Biopsy Track.
A, B: Clusters of disrupted epithelial cells appear along the linear healing biopsy track in an excisional biopsy specimen. Myoepithelial cells display nuclear p63 reactivity (*inset* in **A**) around some displaced epithelial cell clusters.

epithelium is not by itself diagnostic of invasive carcinoma, even if the target lesion contains myoepithelial cells, because displaced epithelial cells derived from a benign lesion may not adhere to myoepithelial cells. When p63-positive cells can be demonstrated as evidence of epithelial displacement, they are usually associated with a minor proportion of the displaced epithelial clusters. Epithelial displacement can be difficult to distinguish from invasive carcinoma and also lymphovascular channel involvement **(Fig. 25.9)** when intraductal carcinoma is present and epithelial clusters are devoid of myoepithelial cells.

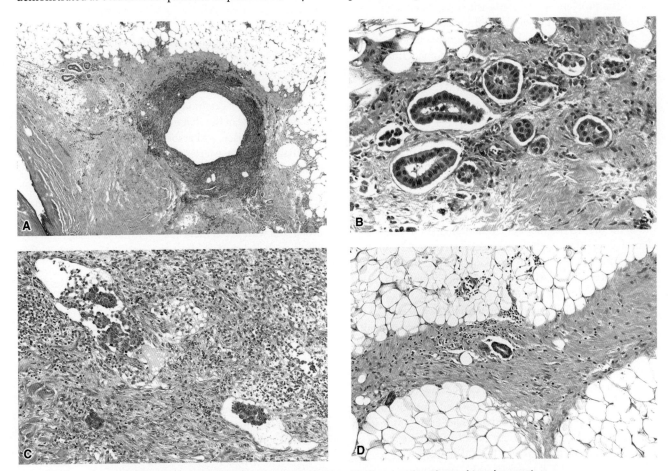

FIGURE 25.9 Epithelial Disruption Simulating Lymphovascular Channel Involvement.
A: Hyperplastic epithelial clusters have been dislodged and simulate carcinomatous involvement within lymphovascular channels (upper left). **B:** Magnified view of displaced epithelium in **A**.
C: Another excisional biopsy in which the displaced epithelial fragments are in lacunae in granulation tissue. The needle core biopsy had been performed 1 week previously. **D:** Another example of disrupted epithelial clusters simulating lymphovascular channel involvement. The needle core biopsy had been performed 4 weeks previously.

The identification of unequivocal lymphovascular channel invasion by carcinoma cells can be facilitated by the use of immunostains for endothelial cells (27,28). These markers include CD31, D2-40 (podoplanin), ERG, factor VIII, etc. ERG (i.e., avian v-ets erythroblastosis virus E26 oncogene homologue, a member of the ETS family of transcription factors) and factor VIII. CD31, D2-40 and factor VIII are immunoreactive in the cytoplasm of the endothelial cells; however, all three markers either show cross reactivity with other cell types or display background stromal reactivity. ERG marks endothelial cell nuclei and does not cross react with nuclei of other cell types; however, nuclear immunoreactivity may be difficult to visualize in minute lymphovascular channels. D2-40 is purportedly reactive in the cytoplasm of lymphatic cells, whereas the other markers are regarded as "pan-endothelial." As always, immunostains should be interpreted with caution, as the results can be misleading when "floaters" or artifactually displaced malignant cells fortuitously occupy the lumen of a vascular channel.

The *frequency of epithelial displacement* in the needle track has been substantially reduced since the introduction of vacuum-assisted stereotactic biopsy (29). Nonetheless, epithelial displacement following NCBs remains a ubiquitous diagnostic problem, particularly when papillary lesions are targeted (25,30,31). Lee et al. (2) drew attention to epithelial displacement in granulation tissue adjacent to a benign papillary tumor simulating invasive carcinoma. Others have encountered the same problem around noninvasive papillary carcinomas that were excised after a NCB (25,30).

De novo intralesional hemorrhage in a benign proliferative epithelial lesion, particularly in a cystic papillary neoplasm, may simulate changes secondary to NCB. Organization of hemorrhage with fibroplasia can entrap portions of the benign epithelia, and simulate invasive carcinoma within the lesion or at its periphery. In these cases, eliciting a history of a previous needling procedure may help prevent an incorrect interpretation.

The *long-term viability of displaced epithelium* at the biopsy site in the breast, whether benign or malignant, is uncertain. Diaz et al. (32) found epithelial displacement in 32% of excisions performed after a NCB procedure. Displacement was less frequent after vacuum-assisted biopsy than when an automated gun device was used. The observation that the incidence of detectable epithelial displacement was inversely related to the post–core biopsy interval led these investigators to conclude that displaced epithelium underwent degenerative changes in some instances.

Local recurrence arising from carcinomatous epithelial displacement is a concern after conservation surgery and radiotherapy is of obvious concern. Tumor seeding of the dermis overlying the breast was reported by Stolier et al. (33), leading to local recurrence at the biopsy site in one case. Chao et al. (34) described two patients who had subcutaneous recurrence of carcinoma in a NCB track 12 and 17 months post biopsy. A third patient was found to have carcinoma in the skin in a mastectomy specimen. The risk of cutaneous recurrence can be substantially reduced if the biopsy site in the skin can be included in the subsequent surgical excision.

Thurfjell et al. (35) studied 303 consecutive women with nonpalpable carcinomas treated by excision. The majority had undergone a preoperative NCB procedure (71%) and postoperative radiotherapy (82%). Overall, 33 or 11% of the women developed local recurrence after median follow-up of 5.4 years. On the basis of the location of the recurrence and the position of the needle track, it was considered likely that recurrences were attributable to epithelial displacement in three women who did not receive radiotherapy. Chen et al. (36) investigated the role of epithelial displacement in local recurrence by comparing women who underwent NCB before excision and those who had a needle localization biopsy as the diagnostic procedure. In a series of 551 consecutive patients treated with conservation surgery and radiotherapy, the frequency of local recurrence after a mean follow-up of 4.9 years in the NCB group (2.3%) was not significantly different from the needle localization group (5.4%).

Excising the skin puncture site with an "adequate margin" of skin at the time of breast conservation surgery reduces the risk of local recurrence in the skin (37,38). However, it is not always practical or cosmetically beneficial to excise the skin or the entire parenchymal biopsy track, and it has been suggested that postoperative radiotherapy can be relied on to eliminate displaced carcinoma cells in most cases (26).

Retraction artifact around clusters or nests of displaced carcinoma cells can simulate lymphovascular channel involvement in NCBs, as it does in excisional biopsies. In general, the established diagnostic criteria for identifying lymphovascular involvement are helpful in both types of specimens. These criteria include: presence of carcinoma within endothelial-lined space, nonconformance of the shape of the carcinoma cluster to the contour of the space, and association of other unequivocally identifiable veins or arteries in the vicinity (39). Interestingly, it has been suggested that retraction artifact may not be a "random artifactual phenomenon" when it is associated with an invasive carcinoma exhibiting micropapillary architectural features, and in this setting these findings have "a significant association with nodal metastasis" (40). It is notable that displaced epithelial clusters along the healing biopsy track often display micropapillary features.

Parenthetically, it is notable that a significant degree of retraction artifact occurs much more often around invasive carcinoma than around in situ carcinoma—and this observation may be helpful in situations wherein the differential diagnosis lies between invasive carcinoma and in situ carcinoma. In this particular context, the finding of retraction artifact has been termed as "the pathologist's friend" (41).

Rarely, displaced clusters of carcinoma cells can be present within lymphovascular channels in NCBs that show only ductal carcinoma in situ (DCIS) **(Fig. 25.10)**. In the series reported by Koo et al. (42), epithelial displacement was found in 3.2% (7 of 218) of DCIS cases on NCBs. The diagnosis of true lymphovascular invasion by carcinoma cells in NCBs can be questioned when invasive carcinoma cannot be identified in the NCB or in the subsequently performed excisional biopsy. In Koo's series, the phenomenon of displaced clusters of carcinoma cells in lymphovascular channels was encountered

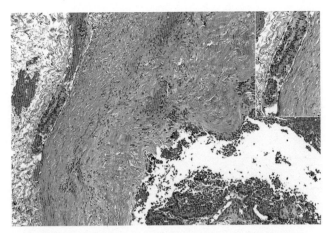

FIGURE 25.10 Displaced Epithelial Clusters of Carcinoma Cells in a Lymphovascular Channel in a Needle Core Biopsy. The needle core biopsy and the excision showed only intraductal papillary carcinoma. Inset shows detail of displaced epithelial clusters within a lymphovascular channel (left).

with biopsies acquired utilizing "automated" rather than "vacuum-assisted" techniques.

Displaced carcinomatous epithelium in lymphovascular spaces is sometimes indistinguishable from intrinsic lymphovascular invasion (8,9) **(Fig. 25.11)**, although displaced epithelial clusters are typically larger than bona fide tumor emboli. The significance of carcinomatous lymphovascular emboli in the setting of epithelial displacement remains uncertain. Until unequivocal evidence to the contrary comes to the fore, the finding of lymphovascular tumor emboli can be considered as a risk factor for the transport of carcinoma cells to axillary lymph nodes even when conventional stromal invasion cannot be identified. Carter et al. (43) introduced the term benign transport to describe instances that they concluded were iatrogenic displacement of carcinoma cells to axillary lymph nodes. It was suggested that benign transport could be recognized by the absence of reactive changes indicative of tumor growth at the site of carcinomatous nodal involvement and the presence of foamy histiocytes, presumably concurrently displaced, associated with the carcinoma.

Radiographic wire localization immediately before surgical resection is the accepted standard of care for preoperative localization of nonpalpable breast lesions. This procedure can fail owing to initial mislocalization of the wire; subsequent inadvertent wire displacement during patient transfer, or surgical positioning, or during postprocedure mammography; and, rarely, breakage of the wire. Another limitation of the wire localization procedure is the need for same-day scheduling of the two procedures to reduce the risk of wire migration. Preoperative localization with I^{125} radioactive seed localization (RSL) has the potential to mitigate the major limitations of wire localization resulting in greater patient satisfaction, better coordination between various specialties, ease of excision, and potential improvement in positive surgical margin rates, and enhanced cosmesis (44). The radioactive seed, about the size of a sesame seed **(Fig. 25.12)**, is composed of titanium and entails minimal risk of radiation to the patient and to the personnel involved. The radioactive seed is inserted through a hollow needle with sonographic or mammographic guidance. After seed placement, the position of the seed is confirmed using mammography. The seed is then localized intraoperatively with a handheld probe. Because the signal emitted from the seed is different from the signal emitted from ^{99m}Tc, used for sentinel lymph node identification, removal of both the tumor and lymph nodes can be performed simultaneously. The preoperative placement of the radioactive seed has the potential to inflict tissue damage similar to that caused by other needling procedures.

At present, there is no objective method for determining with certainty whether a deposit of epithelial cells in a sentinel

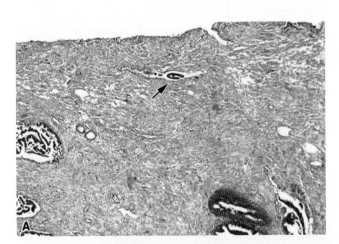

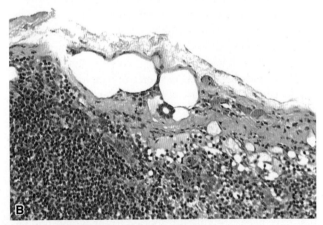

FIGURE 25.11 Intraductal Carcinoma with Lymphatic Tumor Emboli and Lymph Node Metastasis. A, B: This excisional biopsy specimen is from a procedure performed 8 days after a needle core biopsy sampling of mammographically detected calcifications revealed intraductal carcinoma. There is a U-shaped group of carcinoma cells in the lymphatic space near the upper border of the tissue *(arrow)*. Ducts with disrupted ductal carcinoma in situ (DCIS) are depicted on the left, and intact micropapillary DCIS is shown on the right. **B:** Metastatic carcinoma that formed a ring in the subcapsular sinus of a lymph node obtained in an axillary lymph node dissection performed because lymphatic tumor emboli were demonstrated in the excisional biopsy specimen shown in **A**.

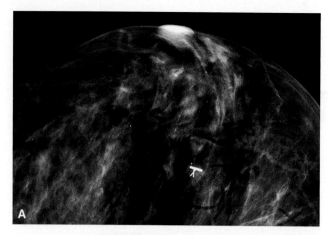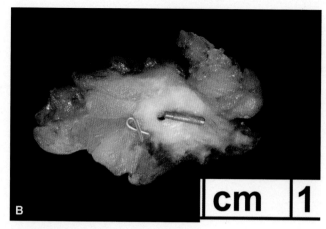

FIGURE 25.12 Preoperative Localization with I^{125} Radioactive Seed Localization (RSL).
A: The preoperative mammogram is shown with the "seed" and "clip" in place. **B:** Cut section of the subsequently performed excisional biopsy shows the "seed" and "clip." The clip is associated with hemorrhage. The placement of these foreign devices is achieved via needling procedures, which have the potential to cause traumatic havoc to lesional tissue.

lymph node (SLN) has resulted from biologically dictated lymphovascular channel invasion or because of mechanically enabled phenomenon of epithelial displacement. Some studies have shown that the nuclei of breast carcinoma cells metastatic to lymph nodes are larger or similar in size to the nuclei of the primary breast carcinoma cells (45). Based on this hypothesis, a study by van Deurzen (46) that found the nuclear size of isolated tumor cells in SLNs of 16 patients with breast carcinoma to be significantly smaller than the nuclear size of the corresponding primary carcinoma concluded that "some of these deposits could represent benign epithelium or degenerated malignant cells lacking outgrowth potential."

It is possible that emerging novel techniques may be helpful to unequivocally differentiate the presence of displaced benign cells in lymph nodes from true nodal metastases. One array-based system for the identification of benign and malignant cells utilizes sensing strategies for the physicochemical nature of different cell surfaces with a "chemical nose-tongue approach" and may be potentially useful in this regard (47). Molecular techniques, using comparative genomic hybridization, may also be potentially helpful in establishing benign, in situ, or invasive nature of epithelial clusters in stroma or lymph nodes (48).

The *clinical significance of displaced carcinoma cells in regional lymph nodes,* sentinel or otherwise, remains uncertain. The indeterminate nature of these findings was highlighted by Carter and Page (49), who stated that they "look forward to the future development of laboratory assays that will correctly differentiate small lymph node deposits that are truly metastatic. . . from those minimal deposits that are unlikely to have any significant impact on the patient and those deposits that have been benignly transported to the lymph node as a cleanup-mechanism by the lymphatic system." Each case requires careful scrutiny that takes into consideration the histologic and immunohistochemical appearances of the primary tumor and epithelial "microdeposits" in the lymph node and the presence or absence of epithelial displacement at the primary site.

It is obvious from the foregoing that the issue of whether or not epithelial displacement following NCB procedure leads to true metastatic involvement of regional lymph node, and whether this finding has prognostic importance, has remained unsettled (50–53). The MIRROR (Micrometastases and Isolated Tumor Cells: Relevant and Robust or Rubbish?) trial showed that adjuvant therapy significantly improved disease-free survival in patients with isolated tumor cells as well as micrometastases in early breast carcinoma versus those who were not treated (54); thus, it is imperative, at a minimum, that the biologic implication of finding minute deposits of carcinoma cells in lymph node in this setting be unequivocally established.

MAJOR CLINICAL COMPLICATIONS OF NEEDLE CORE BIOPSIES

The incidence of major clinical complications after the performance of a NCB is low. Fainting, pneumothorax, significant hematoma formation, infection, and development of milk fistula have been reported, but these complications are relatively uncommon—given the ubiquity of the technique (55).

Pneumothorax is the most life-threatening complication of NCB of the breast, and the risk is greatest when the target lesion lies close to the chest wall. Inadvertent entry into the pleural space can be averted by real-time radiologic monitoring of the procedure and by angling the needle parallel to, rather than toward, the chest wall.

Compression upon completion of the procedure usually suffices to prevent *hematoma* formation. Use of anticoagulants and antithrombotics, including aspirin, may increase the likelihood of postprocedural hematoma. In this setting, the procedure should be performed with caution, and any manipulation of therapy should be carefully monitored (56,57).

Rare cases of *infection* have been reported to follow NCBs. These infections have been of the acute necrotizing (58), necrotizing fasciitis (59), and recurrent (60) types.

Direct injury to intramammary blood vessels in the course of the NCB can induce pseudoaneurysm formation (61), development of arteriovenous fistulas (62,63), and significant arterial bleeding to a degree that required emergent embolization (64).

NCB procedures of the breast are preceded by cutaneous infiltration by local anesthesia. All usual, typically minor, complications that can attend such local injections can occur in this setting; however, a remarkably rare case of *Nicolau syndrome* (embolia cutis medicamentosa) has been reported in this setting (65). This rare syndrome, presumably due to vasospasm caused by sympathetic overstimulation, occurs at an injection site and is manifested by macular rash that progresses rapidly to hemorrhagic necrosis of skin and underlying tissues.

DO NEEDLE CORE BIOPSIES INCREASE RATE OF DISTANT METASTASES?

Experimental evidence raises the possibility that NCBs might increase the rate of distant metastases, at least in the mouse model, by creating an immunosuppressive tumor microenvironment by upregulating key epithelial–mesenchymal transition genes that enable the release of circulating tumor cells (66). Additional studies to understand the biologic trails leading to metastases associated with NCB procedures need to be conducted.

REFERENCES

1. Meeuwis C, Veltman J, van Hall HN, et al. MR-guided breast biopsy at 3T: diagnostic yield of large core needle biopsy compared with vacuum-assisted biopsy. *Eur Radiol.* 2012;22:341–349.
2. Lee KC, Chan JKC, Ho LC. Histologic changes in the breast after fine-needle aspiration. *Am J Surg Pathol.* 1994;18:1039–1047.
3. Michalopoulos NV, Zagouri F, Sergentanis TN, et al. Needle tract seeding after vacuum-assisted breast biopsy. *Acta Radiol.* 2008;49:267–270.
4. McLaughlin CS, Petrey C, Grant S, et al. Displaced epithelium after liposuction for gynecomastia. *Int J Surg Pathol.* 2011;19:510–513.
5. Liberman L. Clinical management issues in percutaneous core breast biopsy. *Radiol Clin North Am.* 2000;38:791–807.
6. Kaye MD, Vicinanza-Adami CA, Sullivan ML. Mammographic findings after stereotaxic biopsy of the breast performed with large-core needles. *Radiology.* 1994;192:149–151.
7. Lamm RL, Jackman RJ. Mammographic abnormalities caused by percutaneous stereotactic biopsy of histologically benign lesions evident on follow-up mammograms. *AJR Am J Roentgenol.* 2000;174:753–756.
8. Youngson BJ, Cranor M, Rosen PP. Epithelial displacement in surgical breast specimens following needling procedures. *Am J Surg Pathol.* 1994;18:896–903.
9. Youngson BJ, Liberman L, Rosen PP. Displacement of carcinomatous epithelium in surgical breast specimens following stereotaxic core biopsy. *Am J Clin Pathol.* 1995;103:598–602.
10. Davies JD, Nonni A, Costa HFD. Mammary epidermoid inclusion cysts after wide-core needle biopsies. *Histopathology.* 1997;31:549–551.
11. Phelan S, O'Doherty A, Hill A, et al. Epithelial displacement during breast needle core biopsy causes diagnostic difficulties in subsequent surgical excision specimens. *J Clin Pathol.* 2007;60:373–376.
12. Liebens F, Carly B, Cusumano P, et al. Breast cancer seeding associated with core needle biopsies: a systematic review. *Maturitas.* 2009;62:113–123.
13. Gobbi H, Tse G, Page DL, et al. Reactive spindle cell nodules of the breast after core biopsy or fine-needle aspiration. *Am J Clin Pathol.* 2000;113:288–294.
14. Sciallis AP, Chen B, Folpe AL. Cellular spindled histiocytic pseudotumor complicating mammary fat necrosis: a potential diagnostic pitfall. *Am J Surg Pathol.* 2012;36:1571–1578.
15. Garijo MF, Val-Bernal JF, Vega A, et al. Postoperative spindle cell nodule of the breast: pseudosarcomatous myofibroblastic proliferation following endo-surgery. *Pathol Int.* 2008;58:787–791.
16. Uematsu T, Kasami M, Takahashi K, et al. Clip placement after an 11-gauge vacuum-assisted stereotactic breast biopsy: correlation between breast thickness and clip movement. *Breast Cancer.* 2012;19:30–36.
17. Samimi M, Bonneau C, Lebas P, et al. Mastectomies after vacuum core biopsy procedure for microcalcification clusters: value of clip. *Eur J Radiol.* 2009;69:296–299.
18. Thomassin-Naggara I, Lalonde L, David J, et al. A plea for the biopsy marker: how, why and why not clipping after breast biopsy? *Breast Cancer Res Treat.* 2012;132:881–893.
19. Corsi F, Sorrentino L, Sartani A, et al. Localization of nonpalpable breast lesions with sonographically visible clip: optimizing tailored resection and clear margins. *Am J Surg.* 2015;209(6):950–958. pii:S0002-9610(14)00506-6. doi:10.1016/j.amjsurg.2014.07.010.
20. Calhoun K, Giuliano A, Brenner RJ. Intraoperative loss of core biopsy clips: clinical implications. *AJR Am J Roentgenol.* 2008;190:W196–W200.
21. Bourke AG, Peter P, Jose CL. The disappearing clip: an unusual complication in MRI biopsy. *BMJ Case Rep.* 2014;2014. pii:bcr2014204092.
22. Guarda LA, Tran TA. The pathology of breast biopsy site marking devices. *Am J Surg Pathol.* 2005;29:814–819.
23. Gombos EC, Esserman LE, Odzer-Umlas SL, et al. Collagen plug metallic marker clip: mammographic and histopathologic appearance. *Breast J.* 2005;11:292–293.
24. Usami S, Moriya T, Kasajima A, et al. Pathological aspects of core needle biopsy for non-palpable breast lesions. *Breast Cancer.* 2005;12:272–278.
25. Nagi C, Bleiweiss I, Jaffer S. Epithelial displacement in breast lesions: a papillary phenomenon. *Arch Pathol Lab Med.* 2005;129:1465–1469.
26. Hoorntje LE, Schipper MEI, Kaya A, et al. Tumour cell displacement after 14G breast biopsy. *Eur J Surg Oncol.* 2004;30:520–525.
27. Gujam FJ, Going JJ, Mohammed ZM, et al. Immunohistochemical detection improves the prognostic value of lymphatic and blood vessel invasion in primary ductal breast cancer. *BMC Cancer.* 2014;14:676. doi:10.1186/1471-2407-14-676.
28. Kim S, Park HK, Jung HY, et al. ERG immunohistochemistry as an endothelial marker for assessing lymphovascular invasion. *Korean J Pathol.* 2013;47:355–364.
29. Liberman L. Impact of image-guided core biopsy on the clinical management of breast disease. In: Rosen PP, Hoda SA, eds. *Breast Pathology: Diagnosis by Needle Core Biopsy.* 2nd ed. New York, NY: Lippincott Williams & Wilkins; 2006:314–324.
30. Douglas-Jones AG, Verghese A. Diagnostic difficulty arising from displaced epithelium after core biopsy in intracystic papillary lesions of the breast. *J Clin Pathol.* 2002;55:780–783.
31. Layfield LJ, Frazier S, Schanzmeyer E. Histomorphologic features of biopsy sites following excisional and core needle biopsies of the breast. *Breast J.* 2015;21(4):370–376. doi:10.1111/tbj.12414.
32. Diaz LK, Wiley EL, Venta LA. Are malignant cells displaced by large-gauge needle core biopsy of the breast? *AJR Am J Roentgenol.* 1999;173:1303–1313.
33. Stolier A, Skinner J, Levine EA. A prospective study of seeding of the skin after core biopsy of the breast. *Am J Surg.* 2000;180:104–107.
34. Chao C, Torosian MH, Boraas MC, et al. Local recurrence of breast cancer in the stereotactic core needle biopsy site: case reports and review of the literature. *Breast J.* 2001;7:124–127.
35. Thurfjell MG, Jansson T, Nordgren H, et al. Local breast cancer recurrence cause by mammographically guided punctures. *Acta Radiologica.* 2000;41:435–440.
36. Chen AM, Haffty BG, Lee CH. Local recurrence of breast cancer after breast conservation therapy in patients examined by means of stereotactic core-needle biopsy. *Radiology.* 2000;225:707–712.
37. Uriburu JL, Vuoto HD, Cogorno L, et al. Local recurrence of breast cancer after skin-sparing mastectomy following core needle biopsy: case reports and review of the literature. *Breast J.* 2006;12:194–198.

38. Kwo S, Grotting JC. Does stereotactic core needle biopsy increase the risk of local recurrence of invasive breast cancer? *Breast J.* 2006;12:191–193.

39. Rosen PP. Tumor emboli in intramammary lymphatics in breast carcinoma: pathologic criteria for diagnosis and clinical significance. *Pathol Annu.* 1983;18(pt 2):215–232.

40. Acs G, Paragh G, Chuang ST, et al. The presence of micropapillary features and retraction artifact in core needle biopsy material predicts lymph node metastasis in breast carcinoma. *Am J Surg Pathol.* 2009;33:202–210.

41. Irie J, Manucha V, Ioffe OB, et al. Artefact as the pathologist's friend: peritumoral retraction in in situ and infiltrating duct carcinoma of the breast. *Int J Surg Pathol.* 2007;15:53–59.

42. Koo JS, Jung WH, Kim H. Epithelial displacement into the lymphovascular space can be seen in breast core needle biopsy specimens. *Am J Clin Pathol.* 2010;133:781–787.

43. Carter BA, Jensen RA, Simpson JF, et al. Benign transport of breast epithelium into axillary lymph nodes after biopsy. *Am J Clin Pathol.* 2000;113:259–265.

44. Sharek D, Zuley ML, Zhang JY, et al. Radioactive seed localization versus wire localization for lumpectomies: a comparison of outcomes. *AJR Am J Roentgenol.* 2015;204:872–877.

45. Van der Linden HC, Baak JP, Smeulders AW, et al. Morphometry of breast cancer. I: Comparison of the primary tumours and the axillary lymph node metastases. *Pathol Res Pract.* 1986;181:236–242.

46. van Deurzen CH, Bult P, de Boer M, et al. Morphometry of isolated tumor cells in breast cancer sentinel lymph nodes: metastases or displacement? *Am J Surg Pathol.* 2009;33:106–110.

47. Bajaj A, Miranda OR, Kim IB, et al. Detection and differentiation of normal, cancerous, and metastatic cells using nanoparticle-polymer sensor arrays. *Proc Natl Acad Sci U S A.* 2009;106:10912–10916.

48. Khoury T, Hu Q, Liu S, et al. Intracystic papillary carcinoma of breast: interrelationship with in situ and invasive carcinoma and a proposal of pathogenesis: array comparative genomic hybridization study of 14 cases. *Mod Pathol.* 2014;27:194–203.

49. Carter BA, Page DL. Sentinel lymph node histopathology in breast cancer: minimal disease versus artefact. *JCO.* 2006;24:1978–1979.

50. Rosser RJ. A point of view: trauma is the cause of occult micrometastatic breast cancer in sentinel axillary lymph nodes. *Breast J.* 2000;6:209–212.

51. Newman EL, Kahn A, Diehl KM, et al. Does the method of biopsy affect the incidence of sentinel lymph node metastases? *Breast J.* 2006;12:53–57.

52. Meijnen P, Oldenburg HS, Loo CE, et al. Risk of invasion and axillary lymph node metastasis in ductal carcinoma in situ diagnosed by core-needle biopsy. *Br J Surg.* 2007;94:952–956.

53. Tille JC, Loubeyre P, Bodmer A, et al. Isolated tumor cells in sentinel lymph nodes of invasive breast cancer: cell displacement or metastasis? *Breast J.* 2014;20:502–507.

54. Maaskant-Braat AJ, van de Poll-Franse LV, Voogd AC, et al. Sentinel node micrometastases in breast cancer do not affect prognosis: a population-based study. *Breast Cancer Res Treat.* 2011;127:195–203.

55. Mahoney MC, Ingram AD. Breast emergencies: types, imaging features, and management. *AJR Am J Roentgenol.* 2014;202:W390–W399.

56. Chetlen AL, Kasales C, Mack J, et al. Hematoma formation during breast core needle biopsy in women taking antithrombotic therapy. *AJR Am J Roentgenol.* 2013;201:215–222.

57. Somerville P, Seifert PJ, Destounis SV, et al. Anticoagulation and bleeding risk after core needle biopsy. *AJR Am J Roentgenol.* 2008;191:1194–1197.

58. Roque DR, MacLaughlan S, Tejada-Berges T. Necrotizing infection of the breast after core needle biopsy. *Breast J.* 2013;19:201–202.

59. Flandrin A, Rouleau C, Azar CC, et al. First report of a necrotising fasciitis of the breast following a core needle biopsy. *Breast J.* 2009;15:199–201.

60. Kasprowicz N, Bauerschmitz GJ, Schönherr A, et al. Recurrent mastitis after core needle biopsy: case report of an unusual complication after core needle biopsy of a phyllodes tumor. *Breast Care (Basel).* 2012;7:240–244.

61. Sasada S, Namoto-Matsubayashi R, Yokoyama G, et al. Case report of pseudoaneurysm caused by core needle biopsy of the breast. *Breast Cancer.* 2010;17:75–78.

62. Gregg A, Leddy R, Lewis M, et al. Acquired arteriovenous fistula of the breast following ultrasound guided biopsy of invasive ductal carcinoma. *J Clin Imaging Sci.* 2013;3:38.

63. Haider MH, Satpathy A, Abou-Samra W. Iatrogenic arteriovenous fistula of the breast as a complication of core needle biopsy. *Ann R Coll Surg Engl.* 2014;96:e20–e22.

64. Fischman AM, Epelboym Y, Siegelbaum RH, et al. Emergent embolization of arterial bleeding after vacuum-assisted breast biopsy. *Cardiovasc Intervent Radiol.* 2012;35:194–197.

65. García-Vilanova-Comas A, Fuster-Diana C, Cubells-Parrilla M, et al. Nicolau syndrome after lidocaine injection and cold application: a rare complication of breast core needle biopsy. *Int J Dermatol.* 2011;50:78–80.

66. Mathenge EG, Dean CA, Clements D, et al. Core needle biopsy of breast cancer tumors increases distant metastases in a mouse model. *Neoplasia.* 2014;16:950–960.

Processing, Pathological Examination, and Reporting of Needle Core Biopsy Specimens

SYED A. HODA

The performance of needle core biopsy (NCB) procedures for *palpable* breast lesions is currently considered the appropriate initial step in evaluating these abnormalities. NCB of *nonpalpable* radiographically detected breast lesions, under the guidance of various imaging techniques (i.e., ultrasound, stereotactic guidance, or magnetic resonance imaging [MRI]) is becoming increasingly common (1).

CORE BIOPSY TECHNIQUES AND SIZE OF NEEDLES

Two main types of NCBs are in use: cutting core type and vacuum-assisted type. It is notable that the diameter (bore) of the needle is inversely proportional to the number of needle gauge (e.g., 7-gauge is larger than 14-gauge needle). In current practice, fine needle aspiration (FNA) cytology procedures of breast typically utilize 25-gauge needles.

The *cutting (non-vacuum-assisted, spring-loaded gun)* NCB is typically used for sampling breast masses using 14-gauge needles. Needles of wider bore are used less often. The cutting NCB system is a simple, but noisy, guillotine-type device. Drawbacks of the system include the need for multiple insertions if a larger volume of tissue is to be obtained and procurement of relatively small artifact-prone specimens. The procedure is relatively inexpensive and typically takes approximately 15 minutes.

Vacuum-assisted NCB is the method of choice to sample suspicious microcalcifications without an accompanying palpable mass, and for investigating lesions considered suspicious on breast ultrasound or MRI. This technique utilizes larger (7–12 gauge) needles than those used in cutting-type biopsy instruments. An inner rotating cutting cannula is advanced into the target where it cuts a core of tissue. Vacuum delivers the sampled tissue through the needle into the collection chamber. Multiple biopsies are taken by rotating the needle without the need for multiple insertions. Vacuum-assisted biopsies yield specimens with minimum artifact. The procedure typically takes 30 to 60 minutes to perform—depending upon which guidance (stereotactic, ultrasound, or MRI) system is utilized, and is comparatively more expensive (2,3).

Stereotactic guidance is typically used for NCB performed to investigate suspicious calcifications detected on mammograms. *Ultrasound-guided core biopsies* are usually performed for solid masses or complex cystic lesions. Ultrasound guidance is particularly helpful for patients with mammary implants. *MRI-guided biopsies* are useful for lesions that are not detectable on clinical examination or on mammographic and ultrasonic evaluation. MR biopsies have a high sensitivity but poor specificity, and require sophisticated and specialized equipment and the use of contrast media (4,5).

The number of cores removed for optimal sampling should depend on the nature of the targeted lesion (i.e., calcifications, mass, etc.), particular radiographic technique employed for guidance (ultrasound, stereotactic, MRI), and size of the needle used (**Figs. 26.1 and 26.2**). An interdisciplinary group recommended at least 20 cores with 11-gauge needles for vacuum-assisted stereotactic breast biopsy (6), and at least 24 cores with 11-gauge needles for MRI-guided NCB (7). For ultrasound-guided vacuum-assisted NCB, another consensus paper recommended the removal of at least 10 cores with an 11-gauge needle and at least 6 cores with 8-gauge needles (8). Preibsch et al. (9) have devised a matrix that facilitates the implementation of German recommendations *vis a vis* required number of vacuum-assisted NCBs to be taken for different needle sizes. In summary, the authors calculated that the required minimum number of cores obtained to conform to the latest German guidelines is 20, 14, 9, and 5 for 11-, 9-, 8-, and 7-gauge needle sizes, respectively. The current German guidelines recommend a sample number of at least 12 cores with 10-gauge needle for stereotactic vacuum-assisted biopsies (9). Of note, 14-gauge needles (the least invasive needle that can be used for core biopsy purposes) are usually used in handheld ultrasound-guided vacuum-assisted NCB.

TISSUE FIXATION

Immediately after procurement, the NCB specimen should be placed in 10% *neutral buffered formalin* (10). Prompt formalin fixation preserves cytologic and architectural detail,

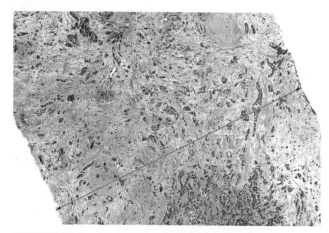

FIGURE 26.1. Histological Appearance of a Core Biopsy Obtained with a 12-Gauge Needle. Needles are available in a wide variety of outer diameters indicated by various gauge. Smaller gauge numbers of needles indicate larger outer diameters. Inner diameter of a needle depends on both gauge and wall thickness. A 12-gauge needle, typically used in a vacuum-assisted stereotactic procedure, obtains a specimen that is 1.8 mm wide (double-headed arrow equals the inner diameter of the needle). Needle wire gauge (G) scale is derived from the Birmingham Wire Gauge system.

and ensures optimal immunohistochemical (IHC) staining. *Bouin fixative* is known to degrade DNA and reduces immunoreactivity for estrogen receptor (ER) and progesterone receptor (PR). *Alcohol fixative* can interfere with hormone receptor and HER2 testing.

Ischemic time is the period of time between the time of acquisition (i.e., loss of blood supply) to the time when the biopsied sample is placed into fixative. The ischemic time

could be measured in seconds for some NCBs; however, it does not typically exceed 15 minutes in cases even when specimen radiography is performed. Prolonged ischemic time (>60 minutes) should be documented, because an extended ischemic period can affect the results of tests that utilize protein, mRNA, and DNA. Delayed tissue fixation impairs HER2 protein expression (11).

Fixation time is defined as the time from the sample being placed into fixative to commencement of tissue processing. Cross-linking occurs during the fixation period, and this process inhibits deterioration. The fixation time should be at least 6 hours and not more than 72 hours before tissue processing starts. Under-fixation (<6 hours) and over-fixation (>72 hours) can lead to suboptimal histology, false-negative results on immunohistochemistry, and problems in performing other ancillary tests. Short fixation time results in poor preservation of antigens for IHC. Prolonged fixation time results in alterations of proteins in the tissue. Extended periods of fixation may also result in the radiographic disappearance of calcifications (12).

The American Society of Clinical Oncology-College of American Pathologists (ASCO-CAP) practice guidelines recommend a minimum of 6 hours of formalin fixation for breast tissue specimens including NCB specimens (13), although some reports have suggested that shorter fixation time for NCB have no negative impact on the reliability of IHC—at least for ER and Ki67 testing, if not for all others (14,15).

Decalcification of NCB specimens may be necessary for some highly calcified specimens; however, every attempt must be made to separately process any noncalcified portions of the specimen, and minimize time in decalcifying solution. Immunostains performed on decalcified tissue ought to be interpreted with caution.

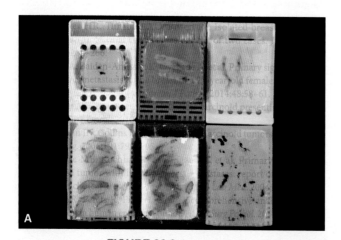
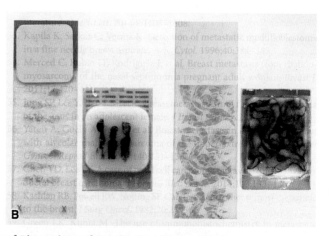

FIGURE 26.2 Demonstration of the Wide Array of Dimensions of Needle Core Biopsy (NCB) Specimens in a Random Set of Tissue Blocks. A: Note the minuscule dimension of the NCB specimen in the tissue block on the top left, and the numerous tightly packed NCB specimens in the green tissue block on the bottom right. The bottom row demonstrates haphazard placement of needle core biopsy samples in three tissue blocks rather than the orderly arrays of NCB in the top row. **B:** Two sets of tissue blocks and slides are depicted. The set on the left shows an array of needle core biopsies embedded in an orderly manner in the paraffin block. The linear arrangement of the core biopsies in the corresponding glass slide facilitates efficient microscopic review. The set on the right shows tissue block overly packed in a disorderly manner with numerous needle core biopsy samples. Microscopic examination of the corresponding glass slide can be unnecessarily time-consuming. A minute lesion could be missed in such a slide.

TABLE 26.1

Information that Should Accompany Needle Core Biopsy Specimens Targeted for a Palpable Mass or an Imaging Abnormality

Palpable Mass

Location
Size
Shape
Margins
Density
Associated calcifications
Associated features

Imaging Abnormality

Mammographic calcification
Location
Morphology
Distribution
Associated features
Mammographic architectural distortion
Location
Associated calcifications
Associated features
Mammographic asymmetry
Location
Associated calcifications
Associated features
MRI and ultrasound abnormality
Essential findings

REQUISITION FORM

The requisition form submitted with the NCB specimen should include the following information: patient name, age and gender, laterality of the specimen, indication for the procedure, clinical diagnosis, and sampled site(s). The name of the submitting physician and the date of the procedure must also be provided. The specimen container must be labeled with patient and specimen identification information that must match identifying information on the accompanying requisition form.

Specific information that should ideally accompany NCB specimens targeted for mass or imaging abnormality is listed in **Table 26.1**. The sampled site is generally indicated by a clock-face designation and distance from the nipple (e.g., right breast, 2 o'clock, N4) indicating that the specimen was taken from the upper-inner quadrant of right breast at the 2 o'clock position from a site 4 cm from the center of the nipple. Multiple palpable as well as impalpable lesions may be simultaneously sampled via NCB, safely and efficiently, and this practice favorably influences patient management (16,17).

The pathologic findings in any previously performed breast biopsy procedure must be conveyed in the requisition form. Relevant history of prior treatment (e.g., surgery, radiation, hormone modulation therapy, or chemotherapy) that could affect the histology of the breast should be provided (**Fig. 26.3**). Information regarding any known systemic disease that may also affect the breast (e.g., neoplasm at another site, diabetes mellitus, sarcoidosis, vasculitis, etc.) should be noted. Family history of breast or ovarian carcinoma, or of *BRCA1* or *BRCA2* mutations, should be included. Ideally, the instrument (cutting or vacuum-assisted) type utilized to procure NCB specimens

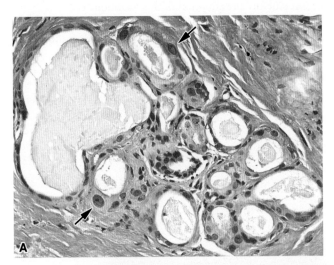
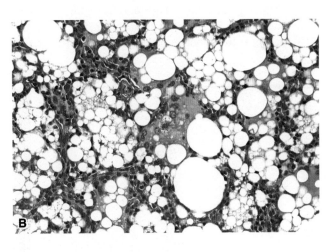

FIGURE 26.3 Significance of Clinical Information in Diagnosis of Needle Core Biopsy Specimens. A: This focus of apocrine metaplasia in a needle core biopsy shows scattered, isolated enlarged nuclei with prominent nucleoli (*arrows*) indicative of radiation effect. Clinical history of radiation was not provided, and a diagnosis of atypical hyperplasia had been rendered. **B:** The presence of foreign material represented by clear vacuoles of varying size with associated histiocytic infiltrate is diagnostic of leaked mammary implant contents. A clinical history of implant placement was not provided, and a diagnosis of organizing fat necrosis had been made.

should be stated. The image modality used for guidance to the target (e.g., stereotactic, ultrasound, or MRI) ought to be included.

As per ASCO-CAP guidelines, the ischemic time, that is, time between specimen procurement and its placement in fixative, must be recorded in the requisition form (18).

GROSS EXAMINATION AND DESCRIPTION

A gross description should be recorded for each specimen with documentation of the number of samples, the range (and *aggregate* extent) of their lengths, as well as any other notable feature (e.g., color). The entire specimen, including any accompanying blood clot, must be processed for histologic evaluation. The bottom surface of the lid of the specimen container should be routinely examined for tissue that may be stuck to it. If the material in a sample is too abundant to be placed in one tissue cassette (i.e., >10.0 cm in aggregate length), the cores should be separated into groups of approximately equal number and size **(Fig. 26.2B)**. Formalin fixation causes minimal shrinking of NCB samples (the shrinkage effect has been estimated to be 7% for 16-gauge tru-cut biopsy samples from the liver) (19). No more than four intact NCB should be placed in one cassette. The number of cassettes corresponding to each sample should be recorded, and each cassette should be labeled with a unique identifier.

Dipping of NCB specimens in dyes that are routinely available in a surgical pathology laboratory, such as methylene blue or eosin, increases the visibility of the embedded tissue in the paraffin block **(Fig. 26.4)**. Inking of breast NCB specimens at the time of gross examination has been proposed as a relatively simple, inexpensive, and effective way to reduce the possibility of specimen mix-up during the processing of the tissue in the pathology laboratory **(Fig. 26.5)**. All NCB specimens from a patient are inked with a single color. The next set of NCB specimens from another patient is inked with a different color, and so on. The color of the ink used for a case should be noted in the gross description. Three discrepancies were discovered in a study of 1,000 core biopsies that were inked sequentially with six different colors. In one instance, the error was related to switching of a tissue block. In another case, the error was related to incorrect labeling, and in a third, the error was typographic (20). Of course, no laboratory procedure can guard against the misidentification of specimens in the radiology office where NCB samples are usually obtained.

Some pathology and radiology departments weigh the NCB specimens as an objective measure of the volume sampled. In this regard, it must be kept in mind that tissue weight is proportional to tissue volume only if tissue density (i.e., weight divided by volume) is constant. Mammary tissue density, of course, is variable and depends upon the ratio of adipose, glandular, and fibrous tissue in any sampling. In spite of the foregoing, Park and Kim (2) have reported that while the 14-gauge needle collects 40 mg of tissue in each sample, the 11-gauge needle obtains 100 mg, and 8-gauge needle acquires at least 250 mg.

In general, NCB material taken for diagnostic purposes should not be taken for research studies until slides are prepared from that material. Harvesting of tissue for research should use formalin-fixed, paraffin-embedded NCB tissue rather than "fresh" tissue.

SPECIMEN PROCESSING

Routine methods of paraffin embedding, sectioning, and staining with hematoxylin and eosin (H&E) can be used for NCB specimens from the breast. A "fast-track" method for rapid processing of NCB specimens has been described (21). However, compliance with regulatory processing standards and achievement of optimal histologic and IHC staining should be ensured before the adoption of this technique (22).

The NCB samples must be embedded in a manner that positions them at approximately the same plane in the paraffin block.

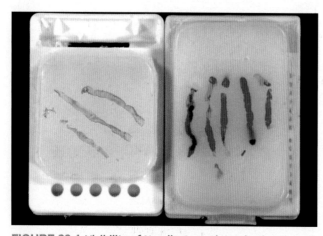

FIGURE 26.4 Visibility of Needle Core Biopsy in Tissue Blocks. Dipping the needle core biopsies in methylene blue (*left*) or eosin (*right*) renders the samples more readily visible in the tissue block. This is helpful to the histotechnologist when cutting histological sections.

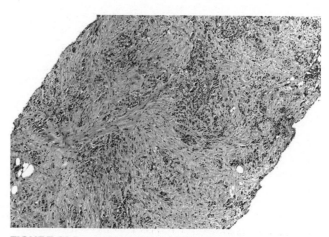

FIGURE 26.5 Inked Needle Core Biopsy Specimens. This sample was stained with blue ink at the time of gross examination. The ink is visible in the resultant histological sections shown here (H&E).

Histologic sections should be 4 to 5 μm thick. The evaluation of multiple levels (at least three "interval" levels, 50 μm apart) for NCB is standard practice in most pathology laboratories. Sectioning at lesser intervals is appropriate for samples obtained with smaller needles. Evaluation of three-step sections reportedly maximizes the chances of visualizing microcalcifications in NCB samples (23). Examination of a minimum of five levels has been recommended to ensure maximum sensitivity for detecting "atypical foci" (24) and of six levels to ensure "accurate" diagnosis (25).

The value of obtaining multiple levels for NCB performed to investigate mammographically detected calcifications has been well established **(Fig. 26.6)**; however, the routine examination of levels for NCB taken for lesions other than calcifications are of limited value. Lee et al. (26) demonstrated that the diagnosis after examining three levels was different from that in the initial level in 4 of 272 (1.5%) NCBs taken for reasons other than calcification, and in 13 of 103 (13%) NCBs taken to investigate calcifications.

It is important not to exhaust the NCB tissue in the preparation of initial histologic sections to preserve material for IHC studies that may be necessary to establish or refine a diagnosis. If laboratory resources allow, intervening sections cut between the various stained levels can be mounted unstained on labeled slides and saved for possible IHC or other ancillary studies. Such a protocol saves tissue, time, and effort that may be subsequently spent in the retrieval and processing of tissue blocks. If recuts are made at a second sitting for immunostains, one new recut slide should always be submitted for H&E staining (27).

IMAGING MODALITIES

Findings on various imaging modalities in a particular case are often communicated in the requisition. NCBs are being increasingly performed under some form of image guidance; thus, pathologists

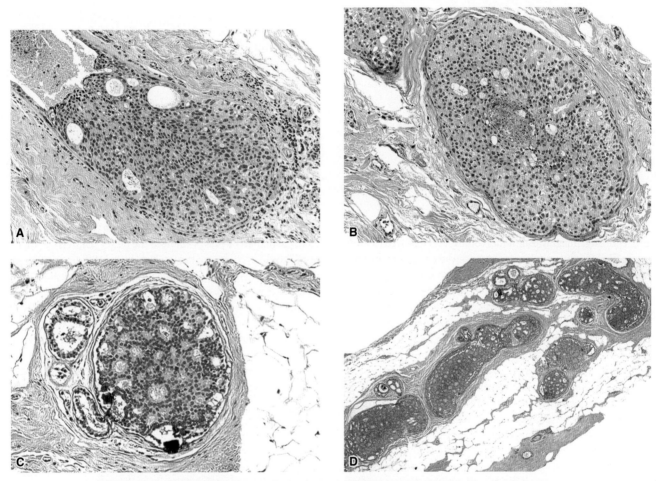

FIGURE 26.6 Facilitating a Pathological Diagnosis via Examination of "Deeper" Levels.
A, B: The initial section shows a focus of epithelial proliferation initially interpreted as atypical ductal hyperplasia **(A)**, and the deeper level shows overt ductal carcinoma in situ (DCIS) **(B)**.
C, D: The initial section shows focal atypical ductal hyperplasia with calcifications in a single duct **(C)**, and the deeper level shows unequivocal DCIS in multiple ducts **(D)**. **E, F:** The initial section shows dense calcification amid densely sclerotic tissue associated with marked lymphocytic infiltration **(E)**, and the deeper level shows rare degenerating, highly atypical ductal epithelial cells that are highly suspicious for high-grade DCIS **(F)**. **G, H:** In this case, the initial section was diagnosed as focal atypical lobular hyperplasia in a terminal duct lobular unit **(G)**, and the deeper level shows unequivocal lobular carcinoma in situ.

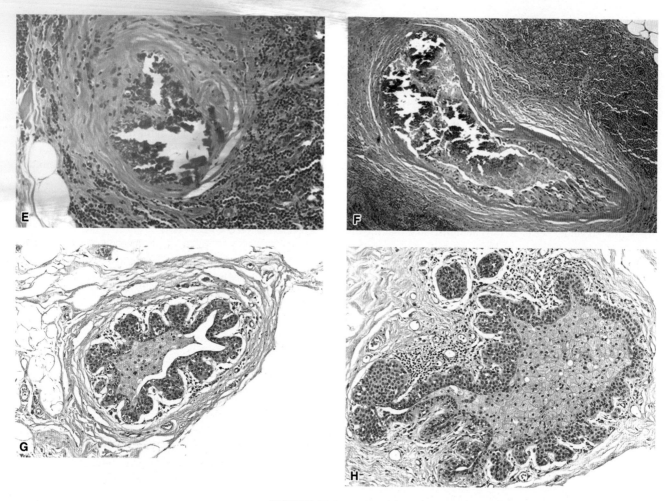

FIGURE 26.6 (continued)

ought to be acquainted with the fundamentals of breast imaging and reporting. Imaging techniques commonly employed to study the breast include mammography (including digital mammography), ultrasound, MRI, and positron emission tomography (PET). The *ACR BI-RADS* (*American College of Radiology's Breast Imaging-Reporting and Data System*) is used in reporting findings on mammography and has also been applied to the reporting of findings on other imaging modalities (**Table 26.2**).

NCB can be performed under stereotactic image (i.e., mammographic) guidance. *Stereotactic NCB* is generally used for calcifications, masses, and architectural distortion. Mammography using low-dose ionizing radiation can detect masses, architectural distortion, or calcifications. For a mammographically detected *mass* (or lesion causing architectural distortion), the radiology report usually states its density, shape, and borders. On mammography, a mass suspicious for malignancy may be dense and irregular with spiculated edges. For mammographically detected abnormal *calcifications*, the radiology report usually describes their morphology and distribution. Calcifications suspicious for malignancy may be linear ("casting-type"), branching, and/or pleomorphic. *Digital breast tomosynthesis* is an evolving, enhanced three-dimensional mammographic technique that increases lesional visibility by detecting subtle changes in the texture of parenchyma.

The *specimen radiograph* corresponding to the NCB specimen, particularly in cases wherein the target lesion is calcification, should accompany the specimen. A brief description of the abnormality seen in the specimen radiograph should be a part of the gross description.

Ultrasound imaging utilizes high-frequency sound waves to detect lesions through varying echo patterns. It is useful for determining the size and shape of masses and identifying cysts. The echogenicity of a lesion *vis a vis* that of subcutaneous adipose tissue and the orientation of the lesion in relation to the skin of the breast are usually reported in ultrasound reports. A lesion may be "isoechoic" (having the same echogenicity as adipose tissue, e.g., a lipoma), "anechoic" (e.g., a cyst), "hyperechoic" (normal fibrofatty breast tissue), or "hypoechoic" (most clinically significant lesions). On ultrasound, a lesion suspicious for carcinoma may be hypoechoic with a "taller than wide" orientation. Ultrasound is often employed to further study lesions identified on mammography and MRI. An ultrasound-guided biopsy procedure is relatively simple and quick to perform.

MRI screening is based on the premise that neoplasms incite neovascularity, which results in locally increased blood flow and permeability. MRI-guided biopsies are performed for lesions that cannot be identified by other methods. Injection

TABLE 26.2

Breast Imaging Reporting and Data System (BI-RADS) Assessment Categories and Management Recommendations[a]

Category	Assessment	Management	Likelihood of Malignancy
0	Incomplete Need additional imaging	Recall	Not applicable
1	Negative	Routine screening	Essentially 0%
2	Benign	Routine screening	Essentially 0%
3	Probably benign	Short (6 mo) interval	>0% but ≤2%
	Continued surveillance	Follow-up	
4	Suspicious	Tissue diagnosis	>2% but <95%
4A	Low suspicion for malignancy		>2%–≤10%
4B	Moderate suspicion for malignancy		>10%–≤50%
4C	High suspicion for malignancy		>50%–≤95%
5	Highly suggestive of malignancy		≥95%
6	Known biopsy-proven malignancy		Not applicable

[a]American College of Radiology's Breast Imaging Reporting and Data System. *www.acr.org/birads*. Accessed on July 1, 2016.

of contrast (intravenous gadolinium) leads to enhanced and accelerated deposition of contrast in the region of the tumor ("wash-in") and accelerated loss of contrast ("washout"). MRI can evaluate lesional morphology (shape and border) and the kinetics of contrast enhancement (initial and delayed). On MRI, a lesion suspicious for carcinoma may be irregular in outline with rim enhancement and can exhibit characteristic kinetics. MRI of the breast has diagnostic and screening applications (e.g., evaluation of occult tumor, extent of tumor, multifocality, multicentricity, response to neoadjuvant chemotherapy, recurrence, and in the screening of high-risk women). In a study of 445 MRI-guided biopsies, all performed on high-risk patients, 79% were benign (28). The technique requires sophisticated equipment, including open coil MRI and MRI compatible needles.

PET screening of the breast assesses the level of glycolysis in tissues after injecting a patient with a radiotracer with an unstable nucleus. PET scans of the breast have been used in a limited fashion with mixed results for screening in high-risk patients, for evaluating recurrences, and for evaluating response to chemotherapy or hormonal therapy.

The concordance of the clinical impression, imaging results, and pathologic findings is often referred to as the *"triple-test."* It is important to ensure that the clinical and radiographic findings are consistent with the pathologic findings on NCB. Re-biopsy with NCB or an excisional biopsy is usually recommended for discordant cases (i.e., cases that fail the "triple-test").

The histopathologic diagnosis ought to be based entirely on the microscopic appearance of the sampled tissue in the NCB specimen. The results of a pathologic interpretation that is not consistent with the clinical impression should be discussed with the submitting radiologist or responsible clinician to ensure that the sample is representative of the lesion. A written note of this discussion should be kept with the pathology records of the case. The repeated procurement of minuscule or otherwise inadequate samples (e.g., blood only) should be discussed with the appropriate clinician.

CALCIFICATIONS

NCB specimens derived from a target with calcifications, as demonstrated by mammography, should undergo specimen radiography immediately after the procedure, and the presence of calcification in the sampling should be confirmed. This process makes it possible to identify and segregate the NCB samples containing calcifications from those without visible calcifications before submission to the pathology laboratory. The cores with and without calcifications from each biopsy site can then be placed in fixative in separately labeled containers. Alternatively, the two sets of cores can be placed into separate tissue cassettes, differentiated by color and/or label, and submitted in a single container. The method chosen to separate specimens before submission to the pathology laboratory should be standardized within a given institution. The practice of separating the specimens with and without calcifications is useful for correlation with the specimen radiograph. The diagnostic yield has been reported to be higher in the segregated cores containing calcifications, although equally careful attention must be paid to samples with and without calcifications. A commercially available "tray" has been devised to facilitate radiology–pathology correlation mainly by allowing the usually fragile tissue samples to maintain their orientation and integrity **(Fig. 26.7)**. Calcifications can be visualized in X-ray images of paraffin blocks, and they remain detectable in this condition for an indefinite period.

Calcifications that are less than 100 µm (0.1 mm) in maximum dimension are unlikely to be radiographically visible (29).

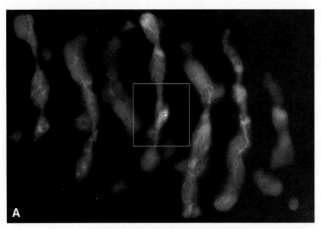

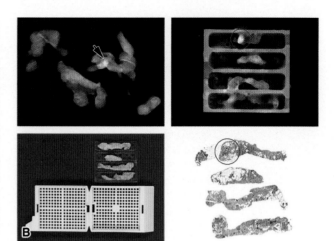

FIGURE 26.7 Radiograph of a Breast Needle Core Biopsy (NCB) Specimen. A: This NCB specimen radiograph shows a solitary focus of calcification in one (*center*) of several samples. Optimally, the radiologist should select the samples with calcifications and submit them separately from those without calcifications. **B:** Radiologic–pathologic correlation in a NCB specimen. A commercially available "tray" can facilitate radiology–pathology correlation mainly by allowing the usually fragile biopsy tissue to maintain its orientation and integrity. A set of NCB samples in a specimen radiograph. The arrow indicates the suspicious lesion (*upper left*). The individual core biopsies samples have been placed into one of the four separate slots in the "tray." This radiograph of the tray indicates the location of the lesional tissue (*upper right, circle*). The tray fits into a standard tissue cassette for histologic processing. The biopsies are embedded into the tissue block with the same orientation as in the "tray" (*lower left*). The corresponding histologic slides have the tissue samples with similar orientation, allowing ready radiologic–pathologic comparison of the circled calcifications and density (*lower right*). (Courtesy of Dr. O. Tawfik; Gallagher R, Schafer G, Redick M, et al. Microcalcifications of the breast: a mammographic-histologic correlation study using a newly designed Path/Rad Tissue Tray. *Ann Diagn Pathol*. 2012;16:196–201.)

Consequently, histologically detected calcifications of minuscule proportions cannot be assumed to represent the calcifications seen in a clinical mammogram. Whenever a biopsy procedure is performed for calcifications, the pathology report should specify whether calcific deposits are microscopically evident and the type of breast tissue in which they are located (**Fig. 26.8**).

One possible explanation for the occasional lack of histologic visualization of calcification in NCB material obtained for mammographically detected microcalcification is their loss during histologic sectioning. This may occur either due to discarding of shavings containing calcifications in the microtome or "fracturing" of the calcifications when they are hit by the microtome blade, resulting in ejection ("chipping") of shattered calcific debris, in the course of preparation of levels (**Fig. 26.9**). Radiography of histologic shavings has provided evidence for both eventualities (30,31). "Chipping" occurs more often with larger deposits of calcification (such as those in sclerotic fibroadenomas) rather than with microcalcifications. Other explanations for "missing" calcification are inadequate sampling, mislabeling of samples, and failure to recognize calcium deposits in histologic sections. This is

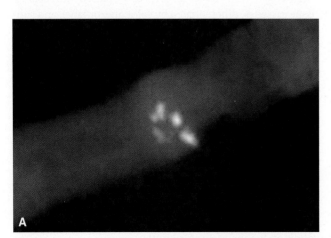

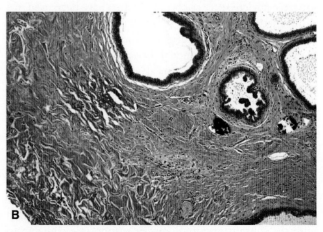

FIGURE 26.8 Radiology–Pathology Correlation of Needle Core Biopsy Samples with Calcium Phosphate Deposition. A, B: Stromal calcifications. **C, D:** Sclerosing adenosis. **E, F:** Intraductal carcinoma. **G, H:** Invasive duct carcinoma with a sclerotic and calcified duct.

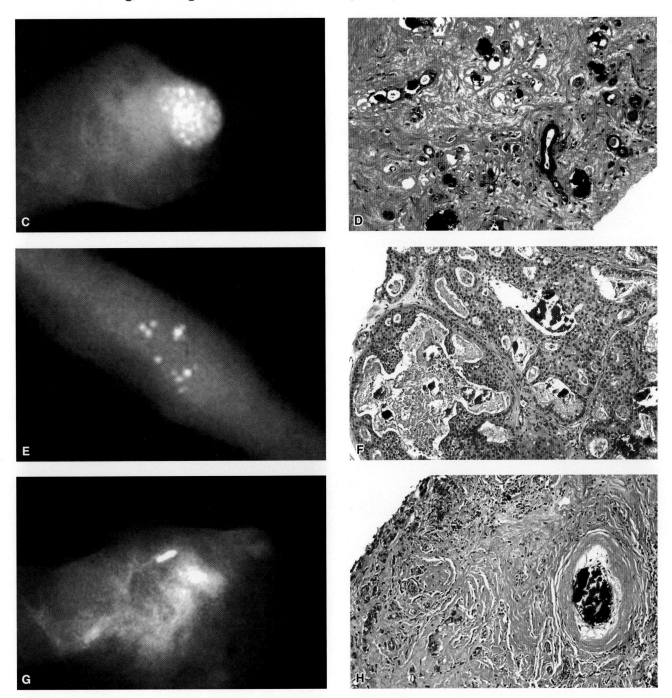

FIGURE 26.8 (*continued*)

more likely to occur with calcium oxalate than with calcium phosphate calcifications.

If calcifications are described in the radiograph of the NCB specimens and none are initially evident histologically, the slides should be examined for calcium oxalate ("weddelite") crystals. These crystals do not stain with the H&E stain but are birefringent with polarized light (32). Calcium oxalate crystals are usually located in cysts lined by apocrine epithelium and may rarely elicit a foreign body–type giant cell reaction in the cyst or in periductal stroma. Less-common types of calcifications are shown in **Figure 26.10**.

Correlation with imaging findings is crucial to the reporting of NCB specimens, as exemplified even by the seemingly innocuous finding of histologically unremarkable adipose tissue—an instance that may represent either fatty breast parenchyma, a lipoma, or a missed target. It must also be kept in mind that several noncalcium elements in breast tissue can radiologically simulate microcalcifications. In this context, suture material from prior surgical procedure is commonly encountered. Tattoo pigment used for cutaneous adornments can simulate calcifications, especially when the pigment is carried into intramammary lymphatic channels. Hemosiderin (from

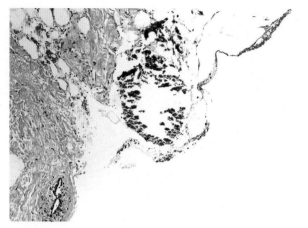

FIGURE 26.9 Displacement of Calcifications. An entire focus of calcification has become dislodged. A definitive diagnosis is not possible in such a situation.

hemorrhage at an earlier date) has been known to simulate calcifications. Injection of material into breast tissue, such as gold (injected into breast tissue for therapeutic use) and various substances (used to "lace" or "cut" recreational drugs) can also mimic calcifications radiographically.

Occasionally, calcifications are not identified in the routine slides prepared from NCB that had targeted calcifications. In such cases, the source of the specimen should be verified. This step should be followed by review of the specimen radiograph (which should ideally accompany the specimen). In most cases, radiography of the tissue block(s) can identify calcifications that have not yet been sectioned. Additional deeper levels (at least three "shallow" recuts) should be obtained from those tissue blocks that show calcifications on radiography. In exceptionally rare cases, calcifications within cysts ("milk of calcium") can be lost. This can happen by mechanical drainage of the contents

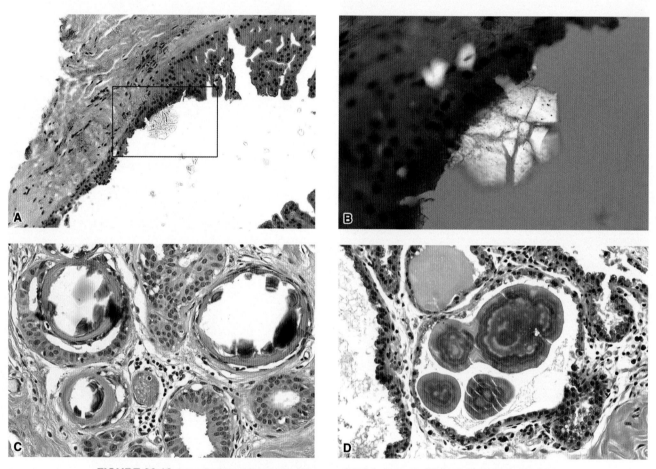

FIGURE 26.10 Less Common Types and Forms of Calcium Deposition. A: Calcium oxalate crystals are barely visible in a focus of cystic papillary apocrine hyperplasia on routine light microscopy (H&E). **B:** The birefringent calcium oxalate crystals are readily demonstrated by polarizing microscopy (H&E). **C:** "Ossifying" type of calcification in ducts with columnar cell change. **D:** "Liesegang" rings with calcifications amid pregnancy-like change. **E:** A cystically dilated duct with luminal fine "powdery" calcifications. The corresponding mammogram showed calcifications of the so-called "milk of calcium" type. **F:** A cluster of cholesterol crystals that formed a mass lesion (so-called "cholesteroloma"). **G:** Unusual pattern of calcium deposition in stroma in otherwise unremarkable breast tissue. This patient with chronic renal failure had hypercalcemia (with so-called "metastatic" depositions of calcium). Multiple amyloid stains were negative. **H:** Calcium deposition on dense fibrous tissue—possibly a senescent fibroadenoma. **I:** An unusual pattern of calcium deposition on minute stromal fibrous nodules (most likely representing obliterated lobules) in an elderly woman. There was no history of radiation treatment or chemotherapy. Various amyloid stains were negative.

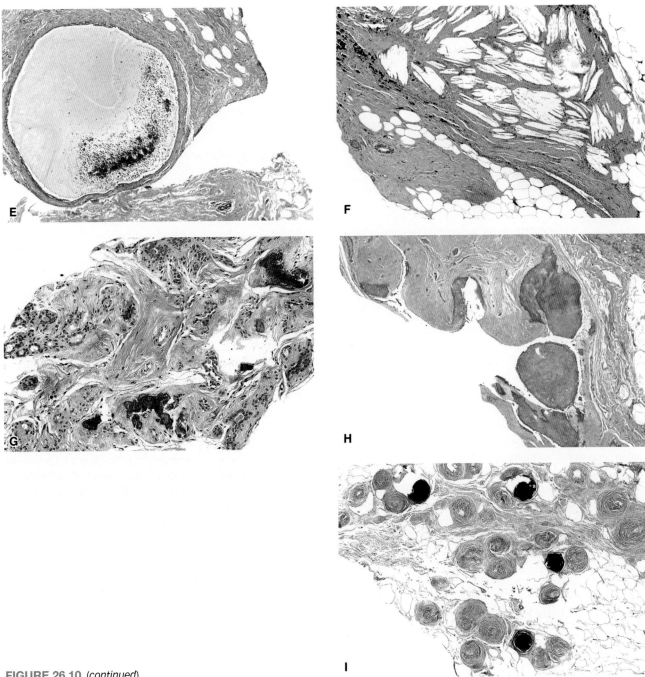

FIGURE 26.10 (continued)

when the cyst is sectioned either at the time of biopsy or at the microtome. Occasionally, the "missing" calcifications are found in the stroma (amid fibroelastic tissue) or within arterial vessels (in the pattern of Monckeberg sclerosis). Calcifications can rarely appear as minuscule "vesicles" within the stroma of some sclerotic fibroadenomas.

Well-prepared and optimally stained H&E-stained sections are crucial to rendering the correct interpretation. A definitive diagnosis should not be made on slides that are not "full face" or present extremely fragmented samples (**Fig. 26.11**). Additional "deeper" levels should be obtained in these cases, which are sometimes helpful.

FROZEN SECTION EXAMINATION

In general, frozen section examination (FSE) should not be performed on NCB samples regardless of whether they were obtained from radiographically detected nonpalpable breast lesions or from palpable tumors. This recommendation is based on the following observations: (a) interpretation of diagnostically difficult lesions is compromised by frozen section artifact, increasing the risk of misdiagnosis, and (b) significant portions of the diagnostic tissue may be exhausted in the process of preparing the frozen section slide. In spite of the foregoing, a recent study of FSE of 59 cases of ultrasound-guided NCB of

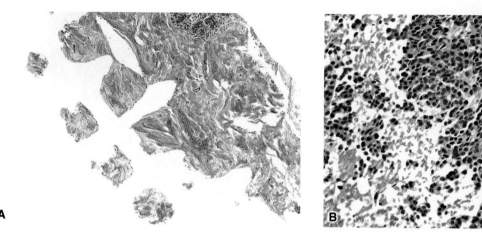

FIGURE 26.11 Artifactual Defects in Tissue. **A:** Tight packing of the tissue cassette with needle core biopsy specimens may result in the "grid" of the cassette causing artifactual geometric defects in the samples. When such a case is encountered, a "full face" deeper level should be obtained to visualize all of the tissue in the block. Furthermore, the practice of over-stuffing cassettes should be discontinued. Overly tight foam pads ("sponges") used in cassettes, to hold needle core biopsies in place and prevent them from being lost during processing, may result in a similar appearance of the tissue section. **B:** Needle core biopsy showing extreme fragmentation of the sampled tissue with proliferative epithelial cells. Additional "deeper" levels are occasionally, but not always, helpful in such cases.

breast found no false-positive and two false-negative results, with the sensitivity, specificity, positive predictive value (PPV), and negative predictive value (NPV) of this technique being 95%, 100%, 100%, and 90%, respectively, in this series (33).

In practice, FSE of an NCB specimen from a nonpalpable breast tumor is clinically warranted only in exceptionally rare and emergency situations. Optimally, a request for a FSE on an NCB specimen should be discussed with the responsible pathologist preoperatively. FSE is a particularly inappropriate method for rendering a diagnosis if nonsurgical ablation of a tumor or neoadjuvant chemotherapy is being considered. It is imperative to reach a diagnosis with "permanent", H&E-stained paraffin sections before these forms of treatment, which could radically alter the histology of the target lesion, are initiated.

TOUCH IMPRINT CYTOLOGY

Touch imprint cytology (TIC) of an NCB specimen is a technique that provides a cytologic diagnosis without the risks of tissue loss attendant on preparing a frozen section (34,35). However, this procedure substitutes the limitations of cytological preparation for those of frozen sections. Imprints are subject to drying artifacts and other distortions that may present substantial pitfalls for inexperienced, and even some experienced, pathologists.

The TIC is prepared by either "touching" (i.e., gently compressing) or "rolling" the NCB specimen on glass slides. Air-dried slides are suitable for the Diff–Quik stain. Alcohol-fixed slides may be used for either H&E or Papanicolaou stains. TIC has the potential of improving patient management in "one-stop" breast clinics by providing a prompt diagnosis. Kulkarni et al. (36) reported a 95% adequacy rate and 55% malignant rate in 819 cases in a recent series from such a setting. This method of evaluating NCB may also be of value in

the immediate assessment of specimen adequacy, thus reducing the number of insufficient specimens. The interpretation of low-grade carcinoma and fibroadenoma in a TIC preparation may be particularly challenging. Consequently, it is recommended that TIC of breast NCB specimens be undertaken only by pathologists or cytologists who examine this type of material with sufficient frequency to maintain a high level of proficiency and work in close collaboration with radiologists and surgeons who routinely perform the NCB procedure. TIC can provide same-day diagnosis (37).

"Core wash cytology" examination utilizes cells taken from the fixative fluid in which the NCB is placed. The "core wash" is subjected to liquid-based preparation and then stained by the routine Papanicolaou method. This technique has been successfully employed for the immediate diagnosis of NCB of the breast, and in a series of 30 cases was found to have better morphology and fewer insufficient diagnoses than TIC (6.6% vs 13.3%) (38). Core wash cytology entails diagnostic risks that are similar to those of TIC.

THE PATHOLOGY REPORT

The pathology report of a NCB specimen should render the diagnosis in a concise and clinically meaningful manner. A detailed microscopic description of the histologic findings is not necessary if the specific diagnosis is clearly stated. For example, it is sufficient to report "fibroadenoma" without listing the microscopic characteristics. On occasions, microscopic details may be added to the diagnosis to convey additional clinically significant information, as for example, in the diagnosis: "fibroadenoma with cellular stroma; recommend excision to rule-out phyllodes tumor." When a carcinoma is diagnosed, the presence or absence of invasion must be stated if this can be ascertained.

In Situ Carcinoma

For in situ carcinoma, the diagnosis should state the type (ductal or lobular), nuclear grade, and presence of luminal necrosis and calcification. In cases of ductal carcinoma in situ (DCIS), the architectural pattern, such as solid cribriform and micropapillary, should be mentioned. A high degree of concordance in the classification of intraductal carcinoma has been found between NCB and excisional biopsy specimens in the same patient. Jackman et al. (39) found "comedo type" of intraductal carcinoma in 91% of excisions after a diagnosis of histologically similar intraductal carcinoma in an NCB specimen and in 15% of excisions following the diagnosis of "noncomedo" intraductal carcinoma in NCB samples.

Invasive Carcinoma

The most important histologic factors that determine the prognosis of invasive breast carcinoma are lymph node involvement, tumor size, and histologic grade. Only one of these three factors, histologic grade, can be reliably assessed in NCB material.

The determination of *tumor size* on NCB material is unreliable because the samples are taken randomly and may not represent the maximum tumor extent. In one study, NCB specimens underestimated tumor size in 79% of the cases (40), and in another report tumor size determined from an NCB specimen was "upstaged" in 72% of the cases upon assessment of size in the excised tissue (41). However, it may be useful to routinely include the largest single histologically contiguous size of invasive carcinoma in a single needle core sample in an NCB specimen. This information is particularly significant in the event that little or no residual invasive carcinoma is detected in the subsequent excisional biopsy specimen. Stereotactic vacuum-assisted NCB procedures remove a "substantial quantity of tissue," and complete extirpation of the tumor may occur in 20% of nonpalpable invasive carcinomas (42). If the size of invasive carcinoma is not routinely provided prospectively, then it is important to document it retrospectively in the event that no residual invasive carcinoma is identified upon excision (i.e., include the invasive size in an addendum to the NCB specimen report and also include the size information from the NCB material in the excisional biopsy report).

It is useful to record the span of the longest histologically contiguous extent of invasive carcinoma on a core in each sampling. This measurement may determine the stage of carcinoma in cases wherein no residual invasive carcinoma (or smaller extent of invasive carcinoma) is identified in the subsequently performed excisional biopsy. In this regard, the extent of invasive carcinoma should *not* be added to the extent of invasive carcinoma on excision (43,44).

The *diagnosis of invasive carcinoma* should describe the subtype of tumor (ductal, lobular, or special type, e.g., tubular or mucinous), coexisting in situ carcinoma, presence of lymphovascular invasion, and any significant benign proliferative lesions. Information may be limited for microinvasive carcinoma. The nuclear grade of invasive tumor cells should be reported in each case (45). The presence of in situ carcinoma supports the primary mammary origin of invasive carcinoma, and this information may be clinically relevant. However, the determination of extensive intraductal component (>25% of tumor mass composed of DCIS and extension of DCIS beyond the invasive component) is not possible in an NCB specimen.

E-cadherin immunostaining should be employed in those circumstances when there is difficulty in distinguishing ductal from lobular carcinoma. This applies to in situ as well as invasive lesions (46). The cytoplasmic membranes of tumor cells are immunoreactive for E-cadherin in virtually all ductal lesions, and display fragmented, weak, or absent reactivity in lobular carcinomas. p120 catenin immunostaining may also be helpful in distinguishing ductal and lobular carcinomas (including its pleomorphic variant) (47,48). The p120 catenin immunostain is localized on the cytoplasmic membrane in ductal type of neoplastic cells and appears within the cytoplasm in lobular carcinoma cells.

The *nuclear and histologic grade* (both on a three-tier scale) can be reported for an NCB specimen of invasive carcinoma of the breast. Underestimation of grading occurs in about 20% to 33% of NCB cases (49,50); however, the agreement rate of up to 84% has been reported for poorly differentiated breast carcinomas (grade 3), the type of carcinoma most likely to benefit from neoadjuvant chemotherapy (51).

Evaluation of the *mitotic count* in NCB samples has been considered unreliable in some studies (52). Underscoring of mitotic activity, especially if fewer than four samples are available for examination, is likely (53); however, it has been shown that grading in the Nottingham system is rendered more reliable by reducing the threshold for mitotic scoring by one-half (54).

The assessment of *lymphovascular involvement* (LVI) by tumor cells in NCB specimens is not reliable owing to the limited samples obtained and the potential for retraction artifact. A sensitivity of only 8% and PPV of 87% for LVI was reported in one study (51). Adherence to established histologic criteria for LVI (i.e., location of LVI away from tumor, presence of endothelial cells around tumor, difference between the shape of tumor embolus, and space within which it lies) and confirmatory immunostains for endothelial cells such as CD31, D2-40, or WT1 may be helpful in confirming the presence of lymphovascular channel invasion (55,56).

Non-neoplastic Tissue

Some pathologists routinely resist the reporting of benign inactive breast tissue as "normal" even if it is the only histopathologic finding and yield to the temptation of using the all-encompassing rubric of "fibrocystic changes." The use of the latter term as a diagnosis without specifying the specific elements of those changes is clinically unhelpful. The report should state the *specific* fibrocystic changes that are present such as sclerosing adenosis, usual ductal hyperplasia, etc. In the absence of fibrocystic changes, a diagnosis of breast tissue with physiologic changes can be offered (e.g., atrophy) depending on the findings that are present. Prominent stromal findings, such as pseudoangiomatous stromal hyperplasia, should be reported.

STANDARDIZED REPORTING TEMPLATES

Standardized forms listing the majority of potential diagnoses are a useful method for reporting breast pathology findings in routine cases. Such a checklist is an efficient way to record the diagnosis in a comprehensive manner, and for the development of a database. The major drawback of formatted diagnoses is the rigidity of the report, which tends to give equal weightage to all components and presents the histologic findings in an inflexible sequence. In a particular case, certain diagnoses may require emphasis by being given priority in the report as well as by additional commentary. If the preformatted report does not offer sufficient latitude to rearrange the diagnostic components when necessary, the pathologist should have the option to issue a nonstructured diagnosis. This is especially important if critical information cannot be conveyed by amplifying the formatted text with comments.

In the United Kingdom, a scoring system (category classification) has been adopted for reporting NCB specimens (57). All NCB samples of the breast are classified as B1 to B5, with the assigned designation appearing prominently in each report. B1 is normal or inadequate (e.g., fibrosis), B2 is benign (e.g., sclerosing adenosis), B3 is benign with uncertain malignant potential (e.g., atypical hyperplasia), B4 is suspicious (e.g., minimal diagnostic tissue or crushed/distorted tissue), and B5 is positive (e.g., in situ or invasive carcinoma). In general, an excisional biopsy procedure might not be performed unless clinically indicated for categories B1 and B2, but local excision would follow for categories B3 to B5 (58). Although the system may appear "restrictive", it helps "concentrate the mind of the pathologist when writing a report" (42). A microscopic description or comments may be added at the pathologists' discretion. In a recent study, the B4 category was shown to have a high PPV: 74.2% (range: 62.5%–90.6%); the PPV of B5 category was more than 99%, and the PPV of the B3 category was reported to be 19.1% (59).

ROLE OF THE NEEDLE CORE BIOPSY PATHOLOGY REPORT IN PATIENT CARE

The role of pathologist in the interpretation of NCB is "limited to diagnosis," but it has a "critical role in accurately applying histological criteria and diagnostic terminology to guide risk stratification and appropriate patient management" (60).

The NCB procedure is highly accurate for the diagnosis of most breast lesions with a PPV for the diagnosis of invasive carcinoma of 98% to 99.8% (61). The pathologic diagnosis made on NCB samples can be, and often is, a key determinant in planning optimal management. Nonetheless, it cannot be relied upon to provide comprehensive data equal to that which can be obtained from an excisional biopsy specimen. In a series of 1,168 NCB specimens, there was complete histologic

agreement with the diagnosis rendered on the subsequently excised specimens in 83% of the cases (62). Consideration must be given to the potential limitations of NCB specimen diagnosis in the formulation of treatment plans. In a series of 952 consecutive cases, the overall false-negative rate of NCB specimens was 9.1%, based on the results of a standard radiology follow-up protocol for all patients (63). The pathologic report for an NCB specimen from the breast must be integrated with the clinical history, physical examination, and radiographic findings to plan the management of an individual patient.

The diagnosis rendered for an NCB specimen obviously applies only to information available from that sample. Final characterization of the lesion must be based on pathologic data from the NCB and excised specimens. It is therefore essential that the pathologist entrusted with the responsibility of diagnosing the subsequent surgical specimen have slides available from the NCB sample. It is substandard practice for a patient to undergo an excision for a lesion diagnosed in another institution on an NCB specimen without prior review of the relevant slides at the hospital where the surgical procedure is to be performed (64). It is the responsibility of the surgeon in these cases to ensure that such a review occurs.

Some diagnoses of NCB specimens could qualify for the designation of "critical." An example of this would be the unexpected diagnosis of carcinoma in an NCB specimen from a mass in a young woman that was clinically presumed to be a fibroadenoma. It has been proposed that a list of such "critical" diagnoses for various organ systems and types of biopsies should be customized for each institution (65).

SIGNIFICANCE OF ANCILLARY (ESPECIALLY ER AND HER2) TESTS ON NEEDLE CORE BIOPSY SPECIMEN

Gene expression profiling has provided a new platform for classifying breast carcinomas. This classification is based on the relative patterns of expression of genes present. Of the several gene classifiers that have been reported, the so-called "intrinsic system" has garnered the most interest and following. The St. Gallen International Breast Oncology group has not only adopted the terminology of the intrinsic system, but also supported the use of the corresponding immunohistochemical surrogates of the various molecular intrinsic subtypes (66).

The *surrogate immunohistochemical profile* mainly utilizes testing for ER, PR, HER2, and the proliferation marker Ki67. This profile divides breast carcinoma into four main groups. The largest group (constituting approximately 60% of invasive breast carcinomas) is the *luminal A-like*, which comprises tumors that are low-grade, ER-positive, PR-positive, and HER2-negative with a low proliferation rate. Each of the other three groups constitute approximately 15% of all invasive carcinomas. The *luminal B-like* group is typically ER-positive, PR-low positive, and HER2-positive or -negative with a high proliferation rate. The *HER2-enriched* group is ER-negative, PR-negative, and (as the name implies) HER2-positive. The *triple-negative* group, as the name implies, is negative for ER, PR, and HER2. The latter group is also referred to as *basal-like*, because its immunoprofile duplicates that of the myoepithelial (i.e., *basal*) cell layer in normal breast ducts and lobules.

ER-positive invasive carcinomas (approximately 70% of all breast carcinomas) can be treated by selective estrogen receptor modulators (SERMs) or aromatase inhibitors (AIs). The identification of HER2-positive carcinomas is important, because HER2-positive carcinomas can potentially be managed by HER2-targeted therapies (i.e., trastuzamab, pertuzumab, and lapatinib). ER and HER2 are not only predictive factors (i.e., predict response to treatment) but are also considered to be prognostic factors. The aforementioned discussion emphasizes the significance of testing for ER and HER2, and to a lesser extent that for PR and the proliferation rate. These tests are being increasingly, if not exclusively, performed on NCB samplings.

Current CAP regulatory guidelines dictate that when ancillary IHC testing is performed, the pathology report should specify the antibody clone, the general form of detection used, and the scoring system used. Deviations from standard processing or antigen retrieval techniques should be included. Appropriate negative and positive controls should be used and documented. The concordance rate between ancillary test results performed on NCB and excisional biopsy samples has now been established to be acceptable *(vide infra)* (67). In general, when hormone receptors are positive on NCB, they are seldom negative on excisional biopsy specimen (68). Testing for various markers on the initial NCB, prior to definitive surgery, assists in planning management—and is critical for the increasing number of cases in which neoadjuvant chemotherapy is being considered (**Fig. 26.12**). Testing for diagnostic confirmation can be performed in certain special cases on NCB samplings—such

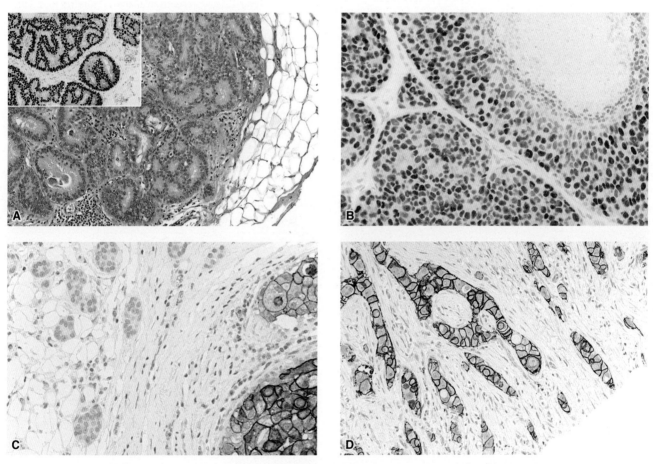

FIGURE 26.12 Ancillary Studies on Needle Core Biopsies. A: Ductal carcinoma in situ (DCIS) of the cribriform type with intermediate grade nuclei with diffuse (almost 100%) and strong immunoreactivity for estrogen receptor (ER, *inset*). **B:** ER immunostaining of DCIS of the cribriform type with intermediate grade nuclei and central necrosis. Shows diffuse (approximately 95%) and strong immunoreactivity. Note lack of ER immunoreactivity in the necrotic cells (**upper right**). **C:** Immunoreactivity of HER2 (3+, on a scale of 0 to 3+) is shown in high-grade *intraductal* carcinoma (**right**). The associated well-differentiated invasive ductal carcinoma (**left**) is negative for HER2: 0 reactivity, on a scale of 0 to 3+ (Herceptest). Only the results of HER2 staining in the invasive carcinoma cells should be reported. **D:** Positive (3+) HER2 immunoreactivity that is complete intense circumferential membrane staining in >10% (almost 100%) of cells in this invasive ductal carcinoma. **E:** ETV6 fluorescence in situ hybridization (FISH) preparation in a mammary secretory carcinoma confirming the presence of the t(12;15). The presence of the ETV6-NTRK3 fusion is demonstrated by the close proximity of a red signal (ETV6 from chromosome 12) with a green signal (NTRK3 from chromosome 15) in each cell.

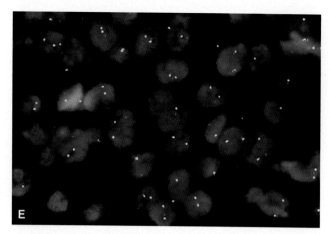

FIGURE 26.12 (*continued*)

as FISH for ETV6-NTRK3 FISH in cases wherein secretory carcinoma is in the differential diagnosis.

TESTING FOR ER (AND PR)

At present, clinical testing for ER and PR is performed using IHC. The optimal procedures for tissue handling, testing conditions, quality assurance, etc., have been outlined elsewhere (13,18). Antibodies used should have well-established specificity and sensitivity. For ER, these antibodies include 1D5, 6F11, and SP1. For PR, these include 1294, 1A6, and

312. The ASCO-CAP recommendation is that the percentage (*proportion*) of carcinoma cells showing nuclear staining as well as the average *intensity* of staining (strong, intermediate, or weak) should be reported. An interpretation (i.e., "positive" or "negative") should also be offered. The carcinoma is considered to be ER- or PR-positive if >1% of tumor cell nuclei stain regardless of intensity. This threshold for positivity applies to invasive as well as in situ carcinomas. The result can be reported using one of the two semiquantitive scoring systems: H (histochemical) score and Allred score. The H-score is derived from *multiplying* the percentage of immunostained tumor cells by the staining intensity factor (**Table 26.3**). The "Allred Score" yields the *sum* of the estimated proportion and intensity of positive tumor cells (**Table 26.4**).

Using currently available IHC techniques and antibodies, the great majority (95% or so) of all breast carcinomas are either reported as being unequivocally hormone receptor-positive or -negative. Nevertheless, presently available antibodies for ER and PR are highly sensitive, and there is concern that carcinomas being reported as being low-positive for ER and PR should be classified as triple-negative because these patients could benefit

---

TABLE 26.3

The H (Histochemical)-Score System for Quantifying Immunostaining

Obtaining the H-Score

1. Record percentage of cells staining.	0–100
2. Record staining intensity factor 0: negative, 1: weak, 2: moderate, 3: strong.	0–4
3. *Multiply* percentage of cells staining by the staining intensity factor to obtain the H (histochemical)-score.	Range: 0–300

Interpreting the H-Score

0–50	Negative
51–100	Weak-positive (1+)
101–200	Moderate-positive (2+)
201–300	Strong-positive (3+)

Based on Snead DR, Bell JA, Dixon AR, et al. Methodology of immunohistological detection of oestrogen receptor in human breast carcinoma in formalin-fixed, paraffin-embedded tissue: a comparison with frozen section methodology. *Histopathology*. 1993;23:233–238.

TABLE 26.4

The Allred Scoring System for Quantifying Immunostaining of ER and PR

This method yields the *sum* of the estimated proportion and intensity of positive tumor cells.

Obtaining the Allred Score

1. Score proportion of "positive" cell nuclei from 0 to 5.
   0: total negativity in tumor cell nuclei
   1: <1% positive cell nuclei
   2: 1%–10% positive cell nuclei
   3: 33% positive cell nuclei
   4: 66% positive cell nuclei
   5: 100% positive cell nuclei
2. Score intensity of staining from 0 to 3.
   0: no staining in tumor cells
   1: weak staining
   2: intermediate staining
   3: strong staining
3. Add proportion score and intensity score to obtain the Allred score.
   Total score could range from 0 to 8.

Interpreting the Allred Score

A score of >2 (i.e., ≥3) has been adjudged the minimum score for defining ER-positive breast carcinoma.

Based on Ellredge RM, Allred DC. Clinical aspects of estrogen and progesterone receptors. In: Harris JR, Lippman ME, Morrow M, et al, eds. *Diseases of the Breast*. Philadelphia, PA: Lippincott Williams & Wilkins; 2004:603–617; Allred DC, Harvey JM, Berardo M, et al. Prognostic and predictive factors in breast cancer by immunohistochemical analysis. *Mod Pathol*. 1998;11:155–168.
ER, estrogen receptor; PR, progesterone receptor

from treatments tailored toward the latter group. Indeed, there is growing evidence that low ER-positive carcinomas have the morphology, gene-expression profiling, and therapeutic response to chemotherapy closer to triple-negative (basal-like) carcinomas than to luminal A-like carcinomas (69–71).

Four practical caveats deserve iteration with regards to hormone receptor testing by IHC. First, positive and negative internal "controls" must not be overlooked. Ideally, hormone receptor immunoreactivity in normal breast glandular tissue, if available, should be confirmed. Second, the status of receptors cannot be reliably calculated if only a minute amount of carcinoma is present in an NCB specimen. Third, the complete absence of immunoreactivity in tissue for ER and PR (in all neoplastic and non-neoplastic breast tissue, and in control tissue) is most likely due to technical failure, such as the absence of the primary antibody or an error in technique. This finding may also be the result of loss of immunogenicity of tissue being tested due to improper fixation. In such situations, the use of vimentin or another ubiquitous antibody is helpful to assess the "immunocompetence" of the tissue. Lastly, optimal testing for prognostic markers depends on an NCB sample that is representative of a particular tumor. In tumors that show heterogeneity of grade, multifocality, or multicentricity, retesting on appropriately selected tumor tissue from excised specimens may be indicated.

Testing for ER and PR is routinely performed on all DCIS (and also LCIS of the pleomorphic and florid) types, and reported in a manner similar to that for invasive carcinoma—although the cost-effectiveness of *routine* performance of ER and PR testing on DCIS in NCB specimens has been questioned (72).

TESTING FOR HER2

The use of targeted HER2 treatment in patients with breast carcinoma relies on the reliable determination of HER2 status on tumor tissue. Approximately 15% of invasive breast carcinomas are HER2-positive. A variety of technologies exist to assess HER2 status (73), either through the detection of protein expression or through gene amplification. The former is detectable by IHC and the latter by various in situ hybridization (ISH) techniques.

Most laboratories in the United States follow the ASCO-CAP guidelines for HER2 testing, that is, use IHC for initial HER2 testing and perform FISH testing for cases with equivocal result (an IHC score of 2+). Some laboratories use FISH as the only technique for HER2 testing, and some use both testing methodologies concurrently (to prevent false-negative results, 4% in one series) (74). HER2 assessment on NCB specimens is generally considered reliable—with the important caveat that false-negative results should be prevented (75).

There are three reporting categories for HER2 testing by IHC: negative, equivocal, and positive (**Table 26.5**). In most instances, HER2 protein overexpression and gene amplification are strongly correlated. ISH assays for HER2 can use either two (dual) probes or a single probe. One of the two probes using the former, and the only probe with the latter, is for the HER2 locus on the long arm of chromosome 17. The second probe in the dual probe test is for chromosome enumerator probe 17 (CEP17) controls for the possibility that, in a minority of cases, an increase in HER2 copy number could be due to polysomy 17 rather than due to gene amplification. The criteria for reporting of single-probe and dual-probe ISH testing appears in **Tables 26.6 and 26.7**, respectively. HER2 testing can be performed by reverse transcriptase-polymerase chain reaction

TABLE 26.6
ASCO-CAP Single Probe HER2 In Situ Hybridization (ISH) Guidelines

Average HER2 Copy Number (Signals per Cell)	Result
<4.0	Negative
≥4.0 and <6.0	Equivocal[a]
≥6.0	Positive

[a]Request repeat testing on same specimen with immunohistochemistry or dual-probe ISH, or on another specimen with immunohistochemistry or dual-probe ISH.
Based on Wolff AC, Hammond MEH, Hicks DG, et al. Recommendations for HER2 testing in breast cancer: ASCO-CAP clinical practice guideline update. *J Clin Oncol*. 2013;31:3997–4013.

TABLE 26.5
ASCO-CAP Scoring System for Quantifying Immunostaining of HER2

Score, Interpretation	Criteria
0, negative	No staining observed, or incomplete faint/barely perceptible membrane staining in <10% of carcinoma cells.
1+, negative	Incomplete faint/barely perceptible membrane staining in >10% of carcinoma cells.
2+, equivocal	Weak to moderate complete membrane staining in >10% of carcinoma cells.
3+, positive	Complete intense circumferential membrane staining in >10% of carcinoma cells.

Based on Wolff AC, Hammond MEH, Hicks DG, et al. Recommendations for HER2 testing in breast cancer: ASCO-CAP clinical practice guideline update. *J Clin Oncol*. 2013;31:3997–4013; Hammond MEH, Hicks DG. ASCO-CAP HER2 testing clinical practice guideline upcoming modifications: proof that clinical practice guidelines are living documents. *Arch Pathol Lab Med*. 2015;139:970–971.

TABLE 26.7

ASCO-CAP Dual Probe HER2 In Situ Hybridization (ISH) Guidelines

HER2/CEP17 Ratio	Average HER2 Copy Number (Signals per Cell)	Category
<2.0	<4.0	Negative
<2.0	≥4.0 and <6.0	Equivocal[a]
<2.0	≥6.0	Positive
≥2.0	<4.0	Positive
≥2.0	≥4.0	Positive

[a]Request reflex testing (using same specimen using IHC, or alternative ISH chromosome 17 probe, or request new testing (new specimen if available with ISH or IHC).
Based on Wolff AC, Hammond MEH, Hicks DG, et al. Recommendations for HER2 testing in breast cancer: ASCO-CAP clinical practice guideline update. *J Clin Oncol.* 2013;31:3997–4013.

(RT-PCR) and gene-expression microarray testing; however, ASCO-CAP has "found insufficient evidence to recommend use" of these techniques for HER2 testing (76). Of note, results for ER, PR, and HER2 by RT-PCR testing has been offered as part of the OncotypeDX test results profile (Genomic Health Inc., Redwood City, CA) since 2008.

HER2 protein expression levels observed by IHC are directly, if not always consistently, related to *HER2/neu* gene amplification detected by FISH or related techniques. Variations in accuracy, reproducibility, and precision of IHC testing techniques, interobserver variation in IHC interpretation, and most importantly inconsistent IHC expression of HER2 protein in variably fixed tumor tissues have cast doubt on the reliability and efficiency of IHC even for primary "screening." For these reasons, it is more accurate (albeit more expensive) to determine HER2 status *via* techniques that detect gene amplification. These techniques include FISH, currently considered the "gold standard" for determining HER2 status, chromogenic ISH (CISH), and silver ISH (SISH). The latter two techniques are comparable to FISH and offer the advantage of being permanent, and thus available for retrospective review (77–79). FISH, CISH, and SISH techniques can all be performed on NCB material.

The 2013 ASCO-CAP guidelines for HER2 testing provide detailed recommendations for methodologies, algorithms, interpretations, and the need for retesting (76). These guidelines have undergone modifications already—proving that clinical practice guidelines need to evolve and are "living documents" (80). Two significant changes have recently been made. The first is in the important criterion for 2+ (equivocal) HER2, which has been changed to "weak to moderate complete membrane staining observed in >10% of tumor cells." The second deals with the critical issue of retesting of specimens. It is recommended that "if the initial HER2 test result in a core needle biopsy is negative, a new HER2 test **may** (*emphasis added*) be ordered on the excision specimen."

The 2015 UK guidelines for HER2 testing are, for the most part, similar to those offered by ASCO-CAP (81). It is notable that with regards to HER2 testing on NCB specimens, the UK guidelines state that "there is insufficient data to define the amount of invasive tumour tissue in core biopsy sufficient for analysis; however, this can be left to the reporting pathologist's discretion." It seems reasonable to report HER2 results even when a microinvasive (<1 mm) carcinoma is either unequivocally negative or unequivocally positive. Reporting 1+ (negative) or 2+ (equivocal) results in this setting can be misleading. Of course, carcinomas should not be definitely staged as microinvasive on NCB material, because it is possible that a larger extent of invasive carcinoma could be present in the subsequent excision. Of course, it is also possible that no additional invasive carcinoma is identified.

Lack of concordance between HER2 status assessed on NCB and surgical specimens of invasive carcinoma of the breast is usually attributable to focal amplification or levels of gene amplification around the cutoff for defining positivity (82). Certain circumstances in that ER, PR, and HER2 testing on excisional biopsy specimens should be repeated following a negative result on a NCB specimen are listed in **Table 26.8**.

TABLE 26.8

Repeat ER, PR, and HER2 Testing on Excision Following Negative Result on Needle Core Biopsy

1. Suboptimal processing of needle core biopsy (*i.e., extended ischemic time: >1 hr, suboptimal fixation: <6 hr or >72 hr, inappropriate fixative*).
2. Minimal diagnostic tissue (e.g., <0.1 cm) on needle core biopsy.
3. Lower-grade carcinoma on needle core biopsy.
4. Unexpected results on needle core biopsy. (*e.g., ER-negativity in invasive lobular carcinoma, HER2 3+ on tubular carcinoma*).
5. Equivocal (2+) HER2 results on needle core biopsy.
6. Postneoadjuvant chemotherapy.
7. "If the initial HER2 test result in a core needle biopsy of a primary breast cancer is negative, a new HER2 test *may* (emphasis added) be ordered on the excision specimen."[a]

[a]Hammond ME, Hicks DG. ASCO-CAP HER2 testing clinical practice guideline upcoming modifications: proof that clinical practice guidelines are living documents. *Arch Pathol Lab Med.* 2015;139:970–971.
ER, estrogen receptor; PR, progesterone receptor

DETERMINATION OF PROLIFERATION RATE

The proliferation rate of a carcinoma can be assessed by Ki67 (MIB1) immunoreactivity. Ki67 is expressed in the G1, S, G2, and M phases of the cell cycle and is being increasingly included in pathology reports of invasive carcinoma. There is growing evidence for the clinical utility of reporting "low" and "high" proliferation rates in invasive breast carcinomas. Carcinomas with higher proliferation rate are generally more responsive to chemotherapy, and *vice versa*. Clinical decisions should not be made on the basis of a "borderline" rate (60). The optimal cutpoints for low and high rates have not yet been established, although the St. Gallen 2013 panel has suggested a cutoff of 20% for the separation of luminal A and B tumors, with the option to also use locally established cutpoints (66). There are considerable difficulties in reliably estimating the proliferation rate in a breast carcinoma—and these difficulties are compounded in NCB specimens. In this regard, intratumoral heterogeneity, interobserver variability, and intratumoral lymphocytic infiltration are the major confounding factors (83).

OTHER ANCILLARY TESTS

Gene expression analysis on NCB specimens directed toward predicting response to chemotherapy has reported (84). Preliminary work has shown that it is possible to obtain sufficient ribonucleic acid (RNA) for transcriptional profiling by complementary deoxyribonucleic acid (cDNA) microarray from samples of breast carcinoma derived from appropriately processed NCB samples of breast carcinoma (85).

The 21-gene *Oncotype DX* test predicts the likelihood of chemotherapy benefit and the likelihood of recurrence of carcinoma primarily in women with newly diagnosed ER-positive invasive breast carcinoma. The RNA expression of 16 cancer genes (including ER, PR, and HER2) and five reference genes is analyzed. The test can be performed using formalin-fixed paraffin-embedded NCB tissue. The assay requires submission of one representative tissue block and one H&E-stained slide obtained from the same block. In general, the sample of choice for Oncotype DX testing is the tissue block corresponding to the slide prepared from *excisional biopsy* with the greatest amount (cross sectional area) of the highest grade of invasive carcinoma in a particular case. In rare cases, the diagnostic NCB material may have relatively more invasive carcinoma tissue than in the excisional biopsy specimen. The assay uses 35 to 65 microns of tissue. The Oncotype DX report includes results for ER, PR, and HER2 testing using RT-PCR methodology by measuring RNA expression of these genes ("quantitative single gene scores"). Akashi-Tanaka et al. (86) found that half of the cases of NCBs submitted for such testing yielded insufficient RNA for testing. However, the remaining specimens were "highly predictive" of response to neoadjuvant endocrine therapy.

Numerous other cancer "biomarkers" are available for testing on NCB material, including the ASCO-recommended cancer biomarker: *urokinase-type plasminogen activator* (uPA)

and its inhibitor: *plasminogen activator inhibitor (PAI-1)* (87). Extraordinary ancillary tests on NCB material may be performed for clinically valid indications at the request of the treating physician, but these will generally be part of a research protocol.

Washings from NCB specimens have been demonstrated to yield sufficient numbers of epithelial cells to allow sorting by *flow cytometry*. This methodology facilitates a variety of molecular and genetic analyses (88).

REFERENCES

1. Iwase T, Takahashi K, Gomi N, et al. Present state of and problems with needle core biopsy for non-palpable breast lesions. *Breast Cancer*. 2006;13:32–37.
2. Park HL, Kim LS. The current role of vacuum assisted breast biopsy system in breast disease. *J Breast Cancer*. 2011;14:1–7.
3. Park HL, Hong J. Vacuum-assisted breast biopsy for breast cancer. *Gland Surg*. 2014;3:120–127.
4. Plantade R. Interventional radiology: the corner-stone of breast management. *Diagn Interv Imaging*. 2013;94:575–591.
5. Ginter PS, Winant AJ, Hoda SA. Cystic apocrine hyperplasia is the most common finding in MRI detected breast lesions. *J Clin Pathol*. 2014;67:182–186.
6. Heywang-Köbrunner SH, Schreer I, Decker T, et al. Interdisciplinary consensus on the use and technique of vacuum-assisted stereotactic breast biopsy. *Eur J Radiol*. 2003;47:232–236.
7. Heywang-Köbrunner SH, Sinnatamby R, Lebeau A, et al. Interdisciplinary consensus on the uses and technique of MR-guided vacuum-assisted breast biopsy (VAB): results of a European consensus meeting. *Eur J Radiol*. 2009;72:289–294.
8. Hahn M, Krainick-Strobel U, Toellner T, et al. Interdisciplinary consensus recommendations for the use of vacuum-assisted breast biopsy under sonographic guidance: first update 2012. *Ultraschall Med*. 2012;33:366–371.
9. Preibsch H, Baur A, Wietek BM, et al. Vacuum-assisted breast biopsy with 7-gauge, 8-gauge, 9-gauge, 10-gauge, and 11-gauge needles: how many specimens are necessary? *Acta Radiol*. 2015;56:1078–1084.
10. Thavarajah R, Mudimbaimannar VK, Elizabeth J, et al. Chemical and physical basics of routine formaldehyde fixation. *J Oral Maxillofac Pathol*. 2012;16:400–405.
11. Lee AH, Key HP, Bell JA, et al. The effect of delay in fixation on HER2 expression in invasive carcinoma of the breast assessed with immunohistochemistry and in situ hybridization. *J Clin Pathol*. 2014;67:573–575.
12. Moritz JD, Luftner-Nagel S, Westerhof JP, et al. Microcalcifications in breast core biopsy specimens: disappearance at radiography after storage in formaldehyde. *Radiology*. 1996;200:361–363.
13. Hammond ME, Hayes DF, Dowsett M, et al. ASCO-CAP guideline recommendations for immunohistochemical testing of estrogen and progesterone receptors in breast cancer. *J Clin Oncol*. 2010;28:2784–2795.
14. Sujoy V, Nadji M, Morales AR. Brief formalin fixation and rapid tissue processing do not affect the sensitivity of ER immunohistochemistry of breast core biopsies. *Am J Clin Pathol*. 2014;141:522–526.
15. Kalkman S, Bulte JP, Halilovic A, et al. Brief fixation does not hamper the reliability of Ki67 analysis in breast cancer core-needle biopsies: a double-centre study. *Histopathology*. 2015;66:380–387.
16. Liberman L, Dershaw DD, Rosen PP, et al. Core needle biopsy of synchronous ipsilateral breast lesions: impact on treatment. *AJR Am J Roentgenol*. 1996;166:1429–1432.
17. Senn Bahls E, Dupont Lampert V, Oelschlegel C, et al. Multitarget stereotactic core-needle breast biopsy (MSBB)—an effective and safe diagnostic intervention for non-palpable breast lesions: a large prospective single institution study. *Breast*. 2006;15:339–346.
18. Wolff AC, Hammond ME, Schwartz JN, et al. ASCO-CAP guideline recommendations for human epidermal growth factor receptor 2 testing in breast cancer. *J Clin Oncol*. 2007;25:118–145.
19. Riley TR III, Ruggiero FM. The effect of processing on liver biopsy core size. *Dig Dis Sci*. 2008;53:2775–2777.

20. Renshaw AA, Kish R, Gould EW. The value of inking breast cores to reduce specimen mix up. *Am J Clin Pathol.* 2007;127:271–272.

21. Ragazzini T, Magrini E, Cucci MC, et al. The fast-track biopsy: description of a rapid histology and immunohistochemistry method for evaluation of pre-operative breast core biopsies. *Int J Surg Pathol.* 2005;13:247–252.

22. Yaziji H, Taylor CR. Begin at the beginning, with the tissue! The key message underlying the ASCO/CAP Task-force Guideline Recommendations for HER2 testing. *Appl Immunohistochem Mol Morphol.* 2007;15:239–241.

23. Grimes MM, Karageorge LS, Hogge JP. Does exhaustive search for microcalcifications improve diagnostic yield in stereotactic core needle breast biopsies? *Mod Pathol.* 2001;14:350–353.

24. Renshaw A. Adequate histologic sampling of breast core needle biopsies. *Arch Pathol Lab Med.* 2001;125:1055–1057.

25. Kumaraswamy V, Carder PJ. Examination of breast needle core biopsy specimens performed for screen-detected microcalcification. *J Clin Pathol.* 2007;60:681–684.

26. Lee AH, Villena Salinas NM, Hodi Z, et al. The value of examination of multiple levels of mammary needle core biopsy specimens taken for investigation of lesions other than calcification. *J Clin Pathol.* 2012;65:1097–1099.

27. Hoda SA, Rosen PP. Contemporaneous H&E sections should be standard practice in diagnostic immunopathology. *Am J Surg Pathol.* 2007;31:1627.

28. Manion E, Brock JE, Raza S, et al. MRI-guided breast needle core biopsies: pathologic features of newly diagnosed malignancies. *Breast J.* 2014;20:453–460.

29. Dahlstrom JE, Sutton S, Jain S. Histologic-radiologic correlation of mammographically detected microcalcification in stereotactic core biopsies. *Am J Surg Pathol.* 1998;22:256–259.

30. Winston JS, Geradts J, Liu DF, et al. Microtome shaving radiography: demonstration of loss of mammographic microcalcifications during histologic sectioning. *Breast J.* 2004;10:200–203.

31. Friedman PD, Sanders LM, Menendez C, et al. Retrieval of lost microcalcifications during stereotactic vacuum-assisted core biopsy. *AJR Am J Roentgenol.* 2003;180:275–280.

32. Tornos C, Silva E, el-Naggar A, et al. Calcium oxalate crystals in breast biopsies: the missing microcalcifications. *Am J Surg Pathol.* 1990;14:961–968.

33. Brunner AH, Sagmeister T, Kremer J, et al. The accuracy of frozen section analysis in ultrasound-guided core needle biopsy of breast lesion. *BMC Cancer.* 2009;9:341.

34. Carmichael AR, Berresford A, Sami A, et al. Imprint cytology of needle core-biopsy specimens of breast lesion: is it best of both worlds? *Breast.* 2004;13:232–234.

35. Kass R, Henry-Tillman RS, Nurko J, et al. Touch preparation of breast core needle specimens is a new method for same-day diagnosis. *Am J Surg.* 2003;186:737–742.

36. Kulkarni D, Irvine T, Reves RJ. The use of core biopsy imprint cytology in the 'one-stop' breast clinic. *Eur J Surg Oncol.* 2009;35:1037–1040.

37. Schulz-Wendtland R, Fasching PA, Bani MR, et al. Touch imprint cytology and stereotactically-guided core needle biopsy of suspicious breast lesions: 15-year follow-up. *Geburtshilfe Frauenheilkd.* 2016;76:59–64.

38. Wauters CA, Sanders-Eras CT, Kooistra BW, et al. Modified core wash cytology procedure for the immediate diagnosis of core needle biopsies of breast lesions. *Cancer Cytopathol.* 2009;117:333–337.

39. Jackman RJ, Nowels KW, Shepard MJ, et al. Stereotaxic large-core needle biopsy of 450 nonpalpable breast lesions with surgical correlation in lesions with cancer or atypical hyperplasia. *Radiology.* 1994;193:91–95.

40. Sharifi S, Peterson M, Baum J. Assessment of pathologic prognostic factors in breast core needle biopsies. *Mod Pathol.* 1999;12:941–945.

41. Lara JF, Abellar RG, Singh NV. Benefits and pitfalls of tumor size and/or volume determination on core needle biopsy in invasive breast cancer: a year of experience from a community hospital. *Mod Pathol.* 2005;18(Suppl 1):39A.

42. Shousha S. Issues in the interpretation of breast core biopsies. *Int J Surg Pathol.* 2003;11:167–176.

43. Ozerdem U, Hoda SA. Correlation of maximum breast carcinoma dimension on needle core biopsy and subsequent excisional biopsy: a retrospective study of 50 non-palpable imaging-detected cases. *Pathol Res Pract.* 2014;210:603–605.

44. Varma S, Ozerdem U, Hoda SA. Complexities and challenges in the pathologic assessment of size (T) of invasive breast carcinoma. *Adv Anat Pathol.* 2014;21:420–432.

45. Hoda SA, Harigopal M, Harris GC, et al. Expert opinion: what should be included in reports of needle core biopsies of breast? *Histopathology.* 2003;43:87–90.

46. Goldstein NS, Bassi D, Watts JC, et al. E-cadherin reactivity of 95 noninvasive ductal and lobular lesions of the breast: implications for the interpretation of problematic lesions. *Am J Clin Pathol.* 2001;115:534–542.

47. Dabbs DJ, Bhargava R, Chivkula M. Lobular versus ductal breast neoplasms: the diagnostic utility of p120 catenin. *Am J Surg Pathol.* 2007;31:427–437.

48. Chivkula M, Haynik DM, Brufsky A, et al. Pleomorphic lobular carcinoma in situ (PLCIS) on breast core needle biopsies: clinical significance and immunoprofile. *Am J Surg Pathol.* 2008;32:1721–1726.

49. Knuttel FM, Menezes GL, van Diest PJ, et al. Meta-analysis of the concordance of histological grade of breast cancer between core needle biopsy and surgical excision specimen [published online ahead of print on March 15, 2016]. *Br J Surg.* doi: 10.1002/bjs.10128.

50. Petrau C, Clatot F, Cornic M, et al. Reliability of prognostic and predictive factors evaluated by needle core biopsies of large breast invasive tumors. *Am J Clin Pathol.* 2015;144:555–562.

51. Harris GC, Denley HE, Pinder SE, et al. Correlation of histologic prognostic factors in core biopsies and therapeutic excisions of invasive breast carcinoma. *Am J Surg Pathol.* 2003;27:11–15.

52. Dhaliwal CA, Graham C, Loane J. Grading of breast cancer on needle core biopsy: does a reduction in mitotic count threshold improve agreement with grade on excised specimens? *J Clin Pathol.* 2014;67:1106–1108.

53. McIlhenny C, Doughty JC, George WD, et al. Optimum number of core biopsies for accurate assessment of histologic grade in breast cancer. *Br J Surg.* 2002;89:84–85.

54. Lee AH, Rakha EA, Hodi Z, et al. Re-audit of revised method for assessing the mitotic component of histological grade in needle core biopsies of invasive carcinoma of the breast. *Histopathology.* 2012;60:1166–1167.

55. Rosen PP. Tumor emboli in intramammary lymphatics in breast carcinoma: pathologic criteria for diagnosis and clinical significance. *Pathol Annu.* 1983;18(pt 2):215–232.

56. Hoda SA, Hoda RS, Merlin S, et al. Issues relating to lymphovascular invasion in breast carcinoma. *Adv Anat Pathol.* 2006;13:308–315.

57. Ellis IO, Humphrey S, Mitchell M, et al. Best practice no. 179: guidelines for breast needle core biopsy handling and reporting in breast screening assessment. *J Clin Pathol.* 2004;57:897–902.

58. Reefy S, Osman H, Chao C, et al. Surgical excision for B3 breast lesions diagnosed by vacuum-assisted core biopsy. *Anticancer Res.* 2010;30:2287–2290.

59. El-Sayed ME, Rakha EA, Reed J, et al. Predictive value of needle core biopsy diagnoses of lesions of uncertain malignant potential (B3) in abnormalities detected by mammographic screening. *Histopathology.* 2008;53:650–657.

60. Calhoun BC, Collins LC. Recommendations for excision following core needle biopsy of the breast: a contemporary evaluation of the literature. *Histopathology.* 2016;68:138–151.

61. Liberman L, Dershaw D, Rosen PP. Stereotaxic core biopsy of breast carcinoma: accuracy at predicting invasion. *Radiology.* 1995;194:379–381.

62. Crowe JP, Rim A, Patrick RJ, et al. Does core needle breast biopsy accurately reflect breast pathology? *Surgery.* 2003;134:523–528.

63. Shah VL, Raju U, Chitale D, et al. False-negative core needle biopsies of the breast: an analysis of clinical, radiologic, and pathologic findings in 27 consecutive cases of missed breast cancer. *Cancer.* 2003;97:1824–1831.

64. Rosen PP. Review of 'outside' pathology before treatment should be mandatory. *Am J Surg Pathol.* 2002;26:1235–1236.

65. Huang EC, Kuo FC, Fletcher CD, et al. Critical diagnoses in surgical pathology: a retrospective single-institution study to monitor guidelines for communication of urgent results. *Am J Surg Pathol.* 2009;33:1098–1102.

66. Goldhirsch A, Winer EP, Coates AS, et al; Panel Members. Personalizing the treatment of women with early breast cancer: highlights of the St. Gallen International Expert Consensus on the Primary Therapy of Early Breast Cancer 2013. *Ann Oncol.* 2013;24:2206–2223.

67. Chen X, Yuan Y, Gu Z, et al. Accuracy of estrogen receptor, progesterone receptor, and HER2 status between core needle and open excision biopsy in breast cancer: a meta-analysis. *Breast Cancer Res Treat.* 2012;134:957–967.

68. Loubeyre P, Bodmer A, Tille JC, et al. Concordance between core needle biopsy and surgical excision specimens for tumour hormone receptor profiling according to the 2011 St. Gallen classification, in clinical practice. *Breast J.* 2013;19:605–610.

69. Iwamoto T, Booser D, Valero V, et al. Estrogen receptor (ER) mRNA and ER-related gene expression in breast cancers that are 1% to 10% ER-positive by immunohistochemistry. *J Clin Oncol.* 2012;30:729–734.

70. Gloyeske NC, Dabbs DJ, Bhargava R. Low ER+ breast cancer: Is this a distinct group? *Am J Clin Pathol.* 2014;141:697–701.

71. Prabhu JS, Korlimarla A, Desai K, et al. A majority of low (1%–10%) ER-positive breast cancers behave like hormone receptor-negative tumors. *J Cancer.* 2014;5:156–165.

72. VandenBussche CJ, Cimino-Mathews A, Park BH, et al. Reflex estrogen receptor and progesterone receptor analysis of ductal carcinoma in situ in breast needle core biopsy specimens: an unnecessary exercise that costs the United States $35 million/year. *Am J Surg Pathol.* 2016;40(8):1090–1099.

73. Penault-Llorca F, Bilous M, Dowsett M, et al. Emerging technologies for assessing HER2 amplification. *Am J Clin Pathol.* 2009;132:539–548.

74. Kaufman PA, Bloom KJ, Burris H, et al. Assessing the discordance rate between local and central HER2 testing in women with locally determined HER2-negative breast cancer. *Cancer.* 2014;120:2657–2664.

75. Hicks DG, Fitzgibbons P, Hammond E. Core vs. breast resection specimen: does it make a difference for HER2 results? *Am J Clin Pathol.* 2015;144:533–535.

76. Wolff AC, Hammond ME, Hicks DG, et al. ASCO-CAP recommendations for HER2 testing in breast cancer: ASCO-CAP clinical practice guideline update. *Arch Pathol Lab Med.* 2014;138:241–256.

77. Van de Vijver M, Bilous M, Hanna W, et al. Chromogenic in situ hybridization (CISH) for the assessment of HER2 status in breast cancer: an international validation ring study. *Breast Cancer Res.* 2007;9:R68.

78. Shousha S, Peston D, Amo-Takyi B, et al. Evaluation of automated silver-enhanced in situ hybridization (SISH) for detection of HER2 gene amplification in breast carcinoma excision and core biopsy specimens. *Histopathology.* 2009;54:248–253.

79. Sauter G, Lee J, Bartlett JM, et al. Guidelines for human epidermal growth factor receptor 2 testing: biologic and methodologic considerations. *J Clin Oncol.* 2009;27:1323–1333.

80. Hammond ME, Hicks DG. ASCO-CAP HER2 testing clinical practice guideline upcoming modifications: proof that clinical practice guidelines are living documents. *Arch Pathol Lab Med.* 2015;139:970–971.

81. Rakha EA, Pinder SE, Bartlett JM, et al. Updated UK recommendations for HER2 assessment in breast cancer. *J Clin Pathol.* 2015;68:93–99.

82. Lee AH, Key HP, Bell JA, et al. Concordance of HER2 status assessed on needle core biopsy and surgical specimens of invasive carcinoma of the breast. *Histopathology.* 2012;60:880–884.

83. Denkert C, Budczies J, von Minckwitz G, et al. Strategies for developing Ki67 as a useful biomarker in breast cancer. *Breast.* 2015;24(Suppl 2):S67–S72.

84. Mina L, Soule SE, Badve S, et al. Predicting response to primary chemotherapy: gene expression profiling of paraffin-embedded core biopsy tissue. *Breast Cancer Res Treat.* 2007;103:197–208.

85. Symmans WF, Ayers M, Clark EA, et al. Total RNA yield and microarray gene expression profiles from fine needle aspiration biopsy and core-needle biopsy samples of breast carcinoma. *Cancer.* 2003;97:2960–2971.

86. Akashi-Tanaka S, Shimizu C, Ando M, et al. 21-gene expression profile assay on core needle biopsies predicts responses to neoadjuvant endocrine therapy in breast cancer patients. *Breast.* 2009;18:171–174.

87. Thomssen C, Harbeck N, Dittmer J, et al. Feasibility of measuring the prognostic factors uPA and PAI-1 in core needle biopsy breast cancer specimens. *JNCI.* 2009;101:1028–1029.

88. Stoler DL, Stewart CC, Stomper PC. Breast epithelium procurement from stereotactic core biopsy washings: flow cytometry-sorted cell count analysis. *Clin Cancer Res.* 2002;8:428–432.

List of Abbreviations

AdCC	adenoid cystic carcinoma	JP	juvenile papillomatosis
ADH	atypical ductal hyperplasia	LCIS	lobular carcinoma in situ
AFB	acid-fast bacilli	LGASC	low-grade adenosquamous carcinoma
AJCC	American Joint Committee on Cancer	LOH	loss of heterozygosity
ALH	atypical lobular hyperplasia	LVI	lymphovascular involvement
ALN	axillary lymph node	MALT	mucosal-associated lymphoid tissue
AME	adenomyoepithelioma	MGA	microglandular adenosis
AR	androgen receptor	MLL	mucocele-like lesion
ASCO	American Society of Clinical Oncology	MPT	malignant phyllodes tumor
BDA	blunt duct adenosis	MRI	magnetic resonance imaging
BI-RADS	Breast Imaging–Reporting and Data System	MSA	muscle-specific actin
		NHL	non-Hodgkin lymphoma
BPT	benign phyllodes tumor	OS	overall survival
BRCA	breast cancer (gene)	PAS	periodic acid-Schiff
CAP	College of American Pathology	PASH	pseudoangiomatous stromal hyperplasia
CCH	columnar cell hyperplasia	PCR	polymerase chain reaction
CEA	carcinoembryonic antigen	PET-CT	positron emission tomogram–computerized tomogram
CHH	cystic hypersecretory hyperplasia		
CIS	carcinoma in situ	PLH	pregnancy-like hyperplasia
CK	cytokeratin	PR	progesterone receptor
CSL	complex sclerosing lesion	RFS	relapse-free survival
DCIS	ductal carcinoma in situ	RR	relative risk
DFS	disease-free survival	RSL	radial sclerosing lesion (radial scar)
EGFR	epidermal growth factor receptor	SA	sclerosing adenosis
EMA	epithelial membrane antigen	SCC	small cell carcinoma
ER	estrogen receptor	SLN	sentinel lymph node
FA	fibroadenoma	SMA	smooth muscle actin
FCC	fibrocystic changes	SMM-HC	smooth muscle myosin–heavy chain
FEA	flat epithelial atypia	s/p	status-post
FISH	fluorescence in situ hybridization	SQC	squamous cell carcinoma
FNA	fine-needle aspiration	SSDH	subareolar sclerosing ductal hyperplasia
FS	frozen section	TDLU	terminal duct lobular unit
GCDFP	gross cystic disease fluid protein	TMA	tissue microarray
GMS	Gomori-Grocott methanamine silver	TNM	tumor (size), regional node (involvement), (distant) metastases
HER2	human epidermal growth factor		
HPF	high-power field	TTF1	thyroid transcription factor-1
IFDC	infiltrating ductal carcinoma	VNPI	Van Nuys prognostic index
IHC	immunohistochemistry	WHO	World Health Organization
ITC	isolated tumor cells	WT1	Wilms's tumor-1

Index

Note: Page numbers followed by *f* indicate figures; those followed by *t* indicate tables

AA. *See* Apocrine adenosis (AA)
AAA. *See* Atypical apocrine adenosis (AAA)
Aberrant E-cadherin staining, 360
Ablation therapy, pathologic effects of, 449
Abscess, bacteria-caused, 33
ACC. *See* Adenoid cystic carcinoma (ACC)
ACCH. *See* Atypical columnar cell hyperplasia (ACCH)
Acid-fast bacteria, 33
Acinic cell carcinoma, 102, 319
ACR BI-RADS. *See* American College of Radiology's Breast Imaging-
    Reporting and Data System (ACR BI-RADS)
Actinomycotic infection, 32
Adenocarcinoma, 431*f*
Adenoid cystic carcinoma (ACC), 270
  clinical presentation, 288
  differential diagnosis in needle core biopsy material
    adenomyoepithelioma, 295
    collagenous spherulosis, 295–296, 295*t*
    cribriform ductal carcinoma in situ, 294
    cylindroma and syringomatous adenoma, 295
    invasive cribriform carcinoma, 294
    microglandular adenosis, high-grade carcinoma arising in, 294
    small cell carcinoma, 294
    solid usual duct hyperplasia, 295
  immonohistochemistry, 291, 293*f*
    CD117/KIT, 292
    ER, PR, AR, and HER2, 292
    glandular component, 292
    Ki67, 292
    MYB, 293, 294*f*
    myoepithelial/basaloid cells, 292
    neuroendocrine markers, 293
  microscopic pathology
    adenoid cystic carcinoma in situ, 291
    cribriform, 289, 289*f*
    metaplastic alterations, 291
    other associated carcinomas, 291
    perineural and lymphovascular invasion, 291, 291*f*
    reticular, 289*f*, 290
    scirrhous, 290
    solid and basaloid, 290–291, 291*f*
  with neuroendocrine features, 294
  prognosis and treatment, 296
  and well-differentiated ductal carcinoma, 292*f*
Adenoid cystic carcinoma in situ, 291
Adenoid cystic hyperplasia, 50
Adenolipoma, 381*f*
Adenomatous polyposis, familial, 364
Adenomyoepithelioma (AME), 71–80, 295
  in adenosis, 73*f*
  age and gender, 72
  atypical adenomyoepithelioma, 75
  with calcifications, 77
  carcinoma (epithelial and/or myoepithelial), 75–78
  clinical presentation of, 73
  with collagenous spherulosis, 77*f*
  genetic predisposition of, 72
  imaging, 73
  with infarction, 74*f*
  microscopic pathology, 73–75
  mistaken for carcinoma, 81*f*

  myoepithelial carcinoma in, 79*f*
  with myoepithelial cell hyperplasia, 76*f*
  with myoid differentiation, 76*f*
  with sebaceous and squamous differentiation, 75*f*
  size and macroscopic feature, 73
Adenosis, 83–97
  adenomyoepithelioma in, 73*f*
  apocrine, 89–91, 90*f*
  atypical apocrine, 89–91, 90*f*
  with atypical lobular hyperplasia, 92*f*
  blunt duct, 89, 89*f*
  carcinoma and atypia in, 91
  clinical presentation, 8, 83
  differential diagnosis of, 94–95
  with dispersed pattern, 86*f*
  in fibroepithelial lesions, 93
  florid, 83, 87*f*, 88*f*
  florid papillomatosis with, 66
  LCIS and ALH in, 91–92
  lobular carcinoma in situ in, 338–339*f*
  microglandular, 97–102
  microscopic pathology, 83–93
  with myoepithelial layer, 101–102
  papilloma with, 41–42*f*
  pattern, 66
  with perineural invasion, 89*f*
  sclerosing, 83, 85*f*, 86–87*f*, 91–96*f*
  treatment and prognosis of, 95–97
  tubular, 88–89, 88*f*
  tumor, 83, 84–85*f*
Adenosquamous carcinoma. *See* Low-grade adenosquamous
    carcinoma
ADH. *See* Atypical ductal hyperplasia (ADH)
Adjacent epithelial proliferations, 219
Adjuvant chemotherapy, 296
  for adenoid cystic carcinoma, 296
  for tubular carcinoma, 212, 213
Adolescents: breast tumors
  carcinoma in, 463
  fibroepithelial lesions fibroepithelial lesions in, 460–462, 462*f*
    fibroadenoma, 460–461
    phyllodes tumor, 461–462
  gynecomastia in. *See* Gynecomastia
  imaging studies, 458
  juvenile atypical ductal hyperplasia, 460, 460*f*, 461*f*
  juvenile papillomatosis, 458–459
    age and gender, 458
    differential diagnosis in needle core biopsy material, 459
    imaging studies, 459
    microscopic pathology, 459
    predisposing factors, 459
    presenting symptoms, 459
    treatment and prognosis, 459
  nonepithelial malignant neoplasms, 463
  papilloma, 459–460
    age, gender, and symptoms, 459–460
    imaging studies, 460
    microscopic pathology, 460
    treatment and prognosis, 460
  pseudoangiomatous stromal hyperplasia, 462–463
  subsequent carcinoma, risk of, 458

Adult-type fibroadenoma, 105, 106–107*f*
Age distribution
    fibroadenoma, 104
    and incidence, in adenosis, 83
    in microglandular adenosis, 97
    PASH, 369
    phyllodes tumor, 114
    sclerosing lobular hyperplasia, 104
AJCC. *See* American Joint Committee on Cancer Staging Manual (AJCC)
Alcohol fixative, 478
ALH. *See* Atypical lobular hyperplasia (ALH)
Alveolar invasive lobular carcinoma, 355*f*, 356
AME. *See* Adenomyoepithelioma (AME)
American College of Radiology's Breast Imaging-Reporting and Data
        System (ACR BI-RADS), 482, 483*t*
American Joint Committee on Cancer Staging Manual (AJCC), 183
American Society of Clinical Oncology-College of American Pathologists
        (ASCO-CAP) practice guidelines, 478, 493–494, 493–494*t*
Amyloid tumor (AT), 27–28
Amyloidoma, 27–28
Amyloidosis, 27, 27*f*
ANA. *See* Antinuclear antibody (ANA)
Anaplastic large cell lymphoma, 419*f*
Anaplastic lymphoma kinase (ALK) immunoreactivity, 27
Androgen receptor (AR), 11, 121
    adenoid cystic carcinoma, 292
    apocrine carcinoma, 282
Angiogenesis, 188
    invasive ductal carcinoma with, 188*f*
Angiolipomas, 383, 384*f*, 390–391
    nonparenchymal, 391*f*, 392*f*
Angiomatosis, 390*f*
Angiosarcoma, 249
    growth patterns, 393
    intermediate and high-grade, 395–397*f*
    low-grade, 394–395*f*
    peripheral vascular component, 396
    radiation-related, 398
    tumor grade, 396
Antinuclear antibody (ANA), 28
Apical snouts, 10
Apocrine adenosis (AA), 89, 90*f*
Apocrine carcinoma
    atypical cystic and papillary, 280*f*
    clear cell type, 282*f*
    clinical presentation
        age and gender, 275
        genetic predisposition, 275
        incidence, 275
        presenting symptoms and imaging studies, 275
    differential diagnosis at needle core biopsy
        apocrine DCIS in sclerosing lesion mimics invasive carcinoma, 284
        granular cell tumor, 284, 286
        lymph node metastasis of breast carcinoma, 283–284
        metastasis from extramammary site, 283
        oncocytic neoplasms, 284
        radiation changes, 284
    foam cells admixed with, 280*f*
    immunohistochemistry
        ER, PR, AR, and HER2, 282
        GCDFP-15, GATA3, cytokeratins, and antigens, 282–283
        Ki67, 282
    microscopic pathology
        apocrine ductal carcinoma in situ, 276–280
        apocrine metaplasia, 275
        atypical apocrine proliferations, 275–276
        invasive apocrine carcinoma, 280–282
    with pagetoid spread mimics pleomorphic lobular carcinoma in situ,
        284
Apocrine cells, 219
Apocrine duct hyperplasia, 442, 443*f*
Apocrine ductal carcinoma in situ, 152, 153*f*, 276, 280
    intermediate-grade
        and high-grade, 278–279*f*
        in radial scar, 277–278*f*
        in sclerosing lesion, 278

    in sclerosing lesion mimics invasive carcinoma, 284, 284*f*
    treatment and prognosis, 286
Apocrine epithelium, 62
Apocrine metaplasia, 10–11, 41, 89, 118, 459*f*
    with atypia, 277*f*
    cystic and papillary, 60–64
    microscopic pathology, 275, 276*f*
    papilloma with, 43*f*
    RSL with, 53
    in sclerosing adenosis, 90*f*
Arteritis, giant cell, 28, 28*f*
ASCO-CAP. *See* American Society of Clinical Oncology-College of
        American Pathologists (ASCO-CAP) practice guidelines
Asteroid bodies, 23, 24
AT. *See* Amyloid tumor (AT)
Atrophy
    lobular, radiation-induced, 441, 441*f*
    menopausal epithelial, 6, 8*f*
    sclerosing adenosis with, 86*f*
Atypical adenomyoepithelioma, 75
Atypical apocrine adenosis (AAA), 89–91, 90*f*, 97
    treatment and prognosis, 286
Atypical apocrine proliferations. *See* Atypical apocrine adenosis (AAA)
Atypical columnar cell hyperplasia (ACCH), 141, 141–143*f*
    ductal carcinoma in situ with, 142, 143–144*f*
Atypical ductal hyperplasia (ADH), 83, 112, 132, 134–140, 135–136*f*, 453
    borderline, 138, 139*f*, 140*f*
    and breast carcinoma risk, 147
    chemoprevention of, 148
    clinical features, 125
    columnar cell, 138*f*
    cribriform, 137–138*f*
    diagnosis by needle core biopsy, 146–148
    ductal carcinoma in situ and, 143–144*f*
    gynecomastia with, 454*f*
    imaging, 125
    juvenile, 460*f*, 461*f*
    lobular extension, 137
    micropapillary, 136–137*f*, 138*f*
    papilloma with, 47*f*
    with severe cytologic atypia, 139*f*
Atypical fibroblasts, 442, 442*f*
Atypical hemangioma, 389, 389*f*
Atypical hyperplasia
    pregnancy-like, 9, 10*f*
    in sclerosing adenosis, 92*f*
Atypical lobular hyperplasia (ALH), 328*f*, 340–343, 341–342*f*, 445*f*
    in adenosis, 91–92, 95
    ductal involvement, 343*f*
    excisional biopsy and needle core biopsy diagnosis of, 345
    terminal ducts, 443, 445*f*
    terminology, 320
Atypical perilobular hemangiomas, 384
Atypical vascular lesions (AVLs), 399, 400*f*
Automated proliferation index, 167
AVLs. *See* Atypical vascular lesions (AVLs)
Axillary lymph node metastases, 434–435
Axillary nodal metastases, 448

Bartonella infection, 32
Basal cytokeratins, 194
Basal-like tumors, 193, 194*t*
Basaloid cells, 292
BDA. *See* Blunt duct adenosis (BDA)
Benign mesenchymal tumors
    angiomatosis, 390–391, 390*f*
    benign neural neoplasms, 379–380, 380*f*
    chondrolipomas, 383, 383*f*
    fibromatosis, 364–367, 365*f*, 366*f*, 377
    fibrous tumor, 367–368, 369*f*
    granular cell tumors, 378–379, 379*f*
    hamartoma, 380–381, 381*f*
    hemangiomas, 383–390
    hibernoma, 382, 382*f*
    leiomyoma, 381–382, 382*f*
    lipoma, 382–383, 383*f*

Benign mesenchymal tumors (*continued*)
  myofibroblastoma, 373–378, 373–377*f*
  nodular fasciitis, 367, 368*f*
  nonparenchymal vascular lesions, 391–392, 392*f*
  osteolipomas, 383, 383*f*
  PASH, 369–373
  tumors of nerve and nerve sheath origin, 379
Benign neural neoplasms, 379–380, 380*f*
Benign papillary tumors
  collagenous spherulosis, 50–52
  cystic and papillary apocrine metaplasia, 60–64
  florid papillomatosis of nipple, 64–66
  intraductal papilloma, 39–50
  radial sclerosing lesions, 52–59
  subareolar sclerosing duct hyperplasia, 59–60, 60*f*
  syringomatous adenoma of nipple, 66–68
Benign phyllodes tumor, 114, 116, 117, 117*f*, 121
Benign spindle cell lesions, with myxoid stroma, 271
Bicalutamide, 454
Bioresorbable embedding material, 468
Blood vessel invasion, 188
Bloody nipple discharge, 16
Blunt duct adenosis (BDA), 89, 89*f*
Borderline phyllodes tumor, 117, 118*f*
Bouin fixative, 478
*BRCA*1, 186, 235
Breast carcinoma
  atypical ductal hyperplasia, 147
  intrinsic subtypes of, 193
  lymph node metastasis of, 283–284
  in males. *See* Male breast lesions, carcinoma
  for medullary carcinoma, 236
  mortality, xx–xxi
  radiotherapy for Hodgkin disease and, 440
  standard incidence ratio for, 440
Breast-conservation therapy, 440–446
Breast-conserving surgery, 296
  DCIS treated by, xviii
Breast density, 1–2, 22
Breast development, 1
Breast glandular tissue, 1
Breast imaging, beginning of, ix
Breast irradiation, xx–xxi
Breast-specific gamma imaging (BSGI), 350
BSGI. *See* Breast-specific gamma imaging (BSGI)
Burkitt lymphoma, 416–417, 418*f*

C-kit, 121
Calcifications, 24, 83, 104, 108, 114, 483–487, 484*f*
  associated with intraductal carcinoma, 11*f*
  cystic and papillary apocrine metaplasia with, 62*f*
  displacement of, 486*f*
  in papillary carcinomas, 220, 220*f*
  pregnancy-like changes with, 9*f*
Calcium oxalate crystals, 19*f*, 485, 486–487*f*
Capillary hemangioma, 386, 387*f*
Carcinoembryonic antigen (CEA), 283, 378
Carcinoma (epithelial and/or myoepithelial), 75–78
Carcinoma cells, displaced, 474
Carcinoma in situ, 112, 113*f*
Cartilaginous metaplasia, 60
Cat-scratch disease, mammary lesions from, 32
Cavernous hemangioma, 385, 385*f*, 386*f*
CCC. *See* Columnar cell change (CCC)
CCH. *See* Columnar cell hyperplasia (CCH)
CD10, 121
CD117, 121, 292
CD34, 119
CD68 (KP1) immunoreactivity, 20
Cellular spindled histiocytic pseudotumor, 13
Central papillomas, 39
Chemoprevention, of atypical ductal hyperplasia, 148
Chemotherapy
  neoadjuvant. *See* Neoadjuvant chemotherapy
  pathologic effect, 446–449, 446*f*
    in breast, 447*f*

involving ductal carcinoma in situ, 448*f*
involving lymphatic tumor emboli, 447*f*
involving normal terminal–duct lobular unit, 448*f*
in lymph node with metastatic carcinoma, 448*f*
CHH. *See* Cystic hypersecretory hyperplasia (CHH)
Children: breast tumors
  carcinoma in, 463
  fibroepithelial lesions fibroepithelial lesions in, 462*f*
    fibroadenoma, 460–461
    phyllodes tumor, 461–462
  gynecomastia in. *See* Gynecomastia
  imaging studies, 458
  juvenile atypical ductal hyperplasia, 460, 460*f*, 461*f*
  juvenile papillomatosis
    age and gender, 458
    differential diagnosis in needle core biopsy material, 459
    imaging studies, 459
    microscopic pathology, 459
    predisposing factors, 459
    presenting symptoms, 459
    treatment and prognosis, 459
  nonepithelial malignant neoplasms, 463
  papilloma
    age, gender, and symptoms, 459–460
    imaging studies, 460
    microscopic pathology, 460
    treatment and prognosis, 460
  pseudoangiomatous stromal hyperplasia, 462–463
  subsequent carcinoma, risk of, 458
Chondrolipomas, 383, 383*f*
Chondromyolipomas, 383
Chronic inflammation, 44
CKs. *See* Cytokeratins (CKs)
Classic invasive cribriform carcinoma, 300
Classic invasive lobular carcinoma, 350–351, 350–353*f*, 355*f*
Classic lobular carcinoma in situ, 320. *See also* Lobular carcinoma in situ (LCIS)
Claudin-low tumors, 194
Clear cell ductal carcinoma in situ, 151, 152*f*
Clear cell metaplasia, 11, 11*f*
Clinging carcinoma. *See* Flat micropapillary carcinoma
Clip placement, needle core biopsy and, 468
Collagenized myofibroblastoma, 374, 374*f*
Collagenous spherulosis (CS), 50–52, 157–158, 295–296
  clinical presentation, 50
  with degenerative changes, 52*f*
  differential staining in adenoid cystic carcinoma and, 295*t*
  gross pathology, 50
  imaging studies, 50
  immunohistochemistry, 52
  with in situ carcinoma, 52*f*
  lobular carcinoma in situ in, 333, 333–334*f*
  microscopic pathology, 50–52
  in papilloma, 51*f*
  prognosis and treatment of, 52
Columnar cell change (CCC), 140, 140–141*f*
  lobular carcinoma in situ and, 144*f*
  in needle core biopsy samples, 206*f*
  tubular carcinoma and, 204, 205*f*
Columnar cell hyperplasia (CCH), 141, 141*f*
Columnar cell lesions, 132, 140–146
  atypical columnar cell hyperplasia, 141, 141–143*f*
  columnar cell change, 140, 140–141*f*
  columnar cell hyperplasia, 141, 141*f*
  flat epithelial atypia, 144
  ossifying type of calcifications in, 144, 145*f*
Comedo ductal carcinoma in situ, 158, 158–159*f*, 161, 162*f*
  grading, 166
Complex fibroadenomas, 93, 93*f*, 104, 108, 110–111*f*
Complex glandular pattern, in papillary carcinomas, 219
Complex hemangioma, 387, 388*f*
Concordant biopsy, 344
Concurrent ductal carcinoma in situ, 165
Congo red–stain, 27*f*, 28
Contralateral carcinoma, 201
Cordylobia anthropophaga infection, 36
Core wash cytology examination, 488

Coumadin anticoagulant treatment, 13
Cribriform carcinoma, 289, 289f, 301f
  clinical presentation, 300–301
  differential diagnosis, 301
  immunohistochemistry, 301
  microscopic pathology, 301
  prognosis and treatment, 302
Cribriform ductal carcinoma in situ, 157, 157f, 294
Cryoablation, 113, 449
CS. See Collagenous spherulosis (CS)
Cutaneous myiasis, 35–36
Cutting needle core biopsy, 477
Cyclosporin A, 104
Cylindroma, and syringomatous adenoma, 295
Cystic and solid papillary carcinoma. See Encapsulated papillary
        carcinomas (EPCs)
Cystic apocrine metaplasia, 60–64, 61–62f
  differential diagnosis of, 66
  prognosis and treatment of, 66
Cystic hypersecretory carcinoma
  with atypia, 308f
  clinical presentation, 305
  differential diagnosis, 308
  ductal carcinoma in situ, 306–307f
  immunohistochemistry, 308
  in lobules, 307f
  microscopic pathology, 305–308
  prognosis and treatment, 308–309
Cystic hypersecretory carcinoma in situ, 166
Cystic hypersecretory change, 307
Cystic hypersecretory hyperplasia (CHH), 9, 306f, 307
  atypia, 307, 308f
  in lobules, 307f
Cystic hypersecretory lesions, 270
Cystic neutrophilic granulomatous mastitis, 24
Cystic papilloma, 39
  with florid adenosis, 42f
Cysticercosis, 35, 35f
Cytokeratins (CKs), 13, 16, 18f, 21, 251, 282–283
  immunostaining, 448
  papillary carcinomas, 220–221
Cytologic atypia, 44, 62–63, 443

DCIS. See Ductal carcinoma in situ (DCIS)
De novo necrosis, invasive ductal carcinoma with, 194f
Degeneration, in collagenous spherulosis, 52f
Dermatobia hominis infection, 35–36
Dermatomyositis, 28
DFS. See Disease free survival
DH. See Ductal hyperplasia (DH)
Diabetic mastopathy (DM), 21–23, 22–23f
  breast density associated with, 22
  mammogram in, 22
Diffuse glandular gynecomastia, 452
Diffuse large B-cell lymphoma, 413–415, 415f
Digital breast tomosynthesis, 482
Dimorphic papillary carcinoma, 227, 227f
Dimorphic small cell carcinomas, 311
Discordant biopsy, 344
Disease free survival (DFS), 122
Distant metastases, needle core biopsies and, 475
DM. See Diabetic mastopathy (DM)
Duct carcinoma, invasive, 8f
Duct ectasia, 18–21, 18–21f
  without inflammation, 21f
  late phases of, 20f
  and mastitis, 19f
Ductal adenomas, 39
Ductal carcinoma in situ (DCIS), 83, 112, 151f, 298–299, 335t, 472, 473f
  in adenosis, 92
  ancillary studies, 167
  and atypical columnar cell hyperplasia, 143–144f, 146
  chemotherapy pathologic effect involving, 448f
  coexistent, 165, 166f
  cribriform, 294
  cystic hypersecretory carcinoma, 306–307f

diagnosis of, 89, 91
  ductal proliferative lesions and, 171–172
  Eastern Cooperative Oncology Trial, xix–xx
  extent of, 167
  frequency of, 148
  grading, 160t, 160f, 166–167
  as heterogeneous disease, xxiii
  imaging, 148–149
  inherent potential to metastasize, xxi, xxii
  intracytoplasmic mucin, 152f
  intraoperative consultation (frozen section) diagnosis, 149–150,
        149–150f
  lobular carcinoma in situ in, 337f
  lobular extension, 150f
  lumpectomy and breast irradiation for, xx–xxi
  marker/precursor, xvi–xvii
  metastases from, xxi–xxii
  microinvasive ductal carcinoma, 168–171, 169–171f
  microscopic pathology, 263
  with mucin
        differential diagnosis, 268
        neovascularization, 264f
  and myoepithelial cells, 151f
  necrosis in, 161t
  in needle core biopsy, 171, 191
  nonrandomized prospective studies of, xviii
  NSABP B-17 trial, xix
  NSABP B-24 Trial, xx
  NSABP Protocol 6, xix
  overdiagnosis and overtreatment of, xxiii
  pathology, 150–166
  principles of management of, 172–173
  with prominent lymphocytic infiltration, 193f
  recurrence after radiation, 443, 444f
  risk for progression from molecular constitution of, xxiii
  in single duct, 336f
  treatment of, xxii–xxiii
  untreated, anecdotal reports and systematic study of, xvi
  untreated, follow-up of, xvii–xviii
  with varying degrees of necrosis and calcification, 161–162f
Ductal epithelial hyperplasia, 1
Ductal hyperplasia (DH)
  atypical, papilloma with, 47f
  clinical features, 125
  collagenous spherulosis, 132, 133–134f
  florid, 128–131f, 130
  imaging, 125
  micropapillary, 128f
  with myoepithelial cells, 132f
  papilloma with, 41f
  pathology, 125–126
  in radial sclerosing lesions, 56–58
  subareolar sclerosing, 59–60
  usual, 126, 130–132
Ductal intraepithelial neoplasia, xxiii
Ductal proliferative lesions, 171–172
Ductography, 39

E-cadherin, 165, 330, 359
  stain, 37
  usage of, 489
Eastern Cooperative Oncology Trial, xix–xx
EBV. See Epstein–Barr virus (EBV)
Echinococcus granulosus, 35
EGFR. See Epidermal growth factor receptor (EGFR)
EIC. See Extensive intraductal component (EIC)
EMA. See Epithelial membrane antigen (EMA)
Embryology, 1
Embryonal rhabdomyosarcoma, metastatic, 433, 433f
EMH. See Extramedullary hematopoeisis (EMH)
EMT. See Epithelial to mesenchymal transition (EMT)
Encapsulated papillary carcinomas (EPCs), 227
  microscopic pathology, 457
Endometrial carcinoma, metastatic, 430–431, 432f, 433
EPCs. See Encapsulated papillary carcinomas (EPCs)
Epidermal growth factor receptor (EGFR), 101, 251

Epithelial atypia, 112, 113*f*
Epithelial cells, 3
    displacement, 469, 472
        carcinomatous, 472
        frequency of, 472
        long-term viability of, 472
    in papillary carcinomas, 215
Epithelial changes, in gynecomastia, 453, 454*f*
Epithelial hyperplasia, 41
    in fibroadenoma, 105, 112
    in phyllodes tumor, 116–117, 118
Epithelial hypertrophy, 5
Epithelial membrane antigen (EMA), 11, 100, 101, 299, 378
Epithelial mitoses, 89
Epithelial to mesenchymal transition (EMT), 238
Epithelioid myoepithelial hyperplasia, 335
Epithelioid myofibroblastoma, 374, 374–375*f*
Epstein–Barr virus (EBV), in medullary carcinoma, 235
ER. *See* Estrogen receptor (ER)
Erdheim–Chester disease, 13, 26, 423
Estrogen receptor (ER), 11, 121, 251, 268
    adenoid cystic carcinoma, 292
    ancillary tests for, 490–492
    apocrine carcinoma, 282
    clinical testing for, 492–493, 492*t*, 494*t*
    immunostain, invasive ductal carcinoma, 192*f*
    tubular carcinoma, 209
Ethnicity, 114
Excisional biopsy, 1, 466
    atypical lobular hyperplasia, 345
    lobular carcinoma in situ, 343–345
Extensive intraductal component (EIC), 191
Extracellular mucin, papillary carcinoma with, 220*f*
Extralobular ducts, 2
Extramedullary hematopoeisis (EMH), 385, 422

FA. *See* Fibroadenoma (FA)
Familial adenomatous polyposis (FAP), 364
FAP. *See* Familial adenomatous polyposis (FAP)
Fat necrosis, 13, 14–16*f*
FCCs. *See* Fibrocystic changes (FCCs)
FDG-PET/CT. *See* Fluorodeoxyglucose-positron emission tomography–computed tomography (FDG-PET/CT)
FEA. *See* Flat epithelial atypia (FEA)
FELs. *See* Fibroepithelial lesions (FELs)
Fibroadenoma (FA), 104–114, 460–461
    adult-type, 105, 106–107*f*
    age, 460
    with carcinoma in situ, 112, 113*f*
    clinical presentation, 104
    complex, 104, 108, 110–111*f*
    differential diagnosis in needle core biopsy material, 461
    with epithelial atypia, 112, 113*f*
    epithelial hyperplasia in, 105, 112
    growth patterns, 105, 106*f*
    imaging studies, 461
    infarcted, 109*f*
    juvenile, 112, 112*f*
    microscopic pathology, 105–112, 461
    myxoid, 108
    with myxoid stroma, 109–110*f*
    risk factors of, 104
    with sclerosing adenosis, 111*f*
    with sclerosis and calcification, 105, 106*f*
    size of, 105, 461
    stroma in, 105, 112
    symptoms, 460–461
    with telescoping of epithelium, 113*f*
    treatment and prognosis of, 112–114
    usual type, 105, 106*f*
        with sclerosis and calcification, 106*f*
        with secretory changes, 107*f*
Fibroadenomatoid mastopathy, 104, 105*f*
    clinical presentation, 104
    microscopic pathology, 104
    treatment and prognosis of, 104

Fibrocystic changes (FCCs), 108
Fibroepithelial lesions (FELs), 93, 107–108*f*, 455
    in children and adolescents, 460–462, 462*f*
        fibroadenoma, 460–461
        phyllodes tumor, 461
Fibroepithelial neoplasms
    fibroadenoma, 104–114
    fibroadenomatoid mastopathy, 104, 105*f*
    phyllodes tumor, 114–122
    sclerosing lobular hyperplasia, 104
Fibrolipomas, 383
Fibromatosis, 245, 364–367, 365*f*, 366*f*, 377
Fibrosarcoma, 405
Fibrosis, 189*f*
    periductal, in duct ectasia, 20, 20*f*
Fibrous (inactive) gynecomastia, 452
Fibrous sclerosis, 43
Fibrous tumor, 367–368, 369*f*
Fibrovascular stroma, 43, 62
Filaria dance sign, 34
Filariasis, 34, 34*f*
Fixation time, 478
Flat epithelial atypia (FEA), 144
Flat micropapillary carcinoma, 156*f*, 157–158
Florid adenosis, 83, 87*f*
    cystic papilloma with, 42*f*
    in pregnancy, 88*f*
Florid ductal hyperplasia, 128–131*f*, 130
Florid gynecomastia, 452, 453*f*, 454*f*
Florid lobular carcinoma in situ, 320, 325–326*f*. *See also* Lobular carcinoma in situ (LCIS)
Florid papillomatosis
    clinical presentation, 64
    gross pathology, 65–66
    imaging studies, 64–65
    immunohistochemistry, 66
    microscopic pathology, 65–66
    of nipple, 64–66, 65–66*f*
Florid sclerosing adenosis, 16
Fluorodeoxyglucose-positron emission tomography–computed tomography (FDG-PET/CT), 428
Foam cells, 18
Follicular lymphoma, 415–416, 417*f*
Follicular phase, 5
Foreign material, 271–272, 271*f*
Frozen section examination (FSE), 487–488
FSE. *See* Frozen section examination (FSE)
Fungal infections, 34

Galactocele, 17, 18*f*
Gastrointestinal neoplasms, 430
GATA3, 251, 282–283, 436
GCDFP-15. *See* Gross cystic disease fluid protein-15 (GCDFP-15)
GCT. *See* Granular cell tumor (GCT)
Gene expression analysis, 495
Gene expression profiling, 490
    of breast carcinomas, 194
Gene mutations, 437
Giant cells, 105
    arteritis, 28, 28*f*
    in medullary carcinoma, 235
    osteoclast-like, mammary carcinoma with, 309–311, 309*f*, 310*f*
    in phyllodes tumor, 116*f*
Glandular cells, 292
Glandular epithelium, irradiated, 284, 285*f*
Glandular structure, of breast, 3*f*
Glycogen-rich carcinoma, 314*f*
    clinical presentation, 313
    differential diagnosis, 314
    immunohistochemistry, 314
    microscopic pathology, 314
    prognosis and treatment, 315
Grading of invasive ductal carcinoma, 183–186
Granular cell tumor (GCT), 284, 285*f*, 286, 378–379, 379*f*
Granulation tissue, epithelial displacement in, 466, 467*f*
Granulomatous lobular mastitis, 23

Granulomatous lobulitis, 23, 24f
Granulomatous mastitis, 23–24
Gross cystic disease fluid protein-15 (GCDFP-15), 11, 20, 63, 100, 282–283, 436
Growth patterns
    angiosarcoma, 393
    fibroadenoma, 105, 106f
    fibromatosis, 364
    invasive lobular carcinoma, 350
    medullary carcinoma, 233, 234, 235
Gynecological organs, neoplasms of, 430–433
Gynecomastia, 1, 452–454, 454f
    age, 452
    in children and adolescents, 460
    florid, 453f, 454f
    imaging studies, 452
    immunohistochemistry, 453–454
    inactive, 453f
    intermediate, 453f
    microscopic pathology, 452–453
    predisposing factors, 452
    symptoms, 452
    treatment and prognosis, 454
Gynecomastia-like hyperplasia, 453

Hamartoma, 380–381, 381f
Hellenzellen, 11
Hemangioma, 383–390
    atypical, 389, 389f
    capillary, 386, 387f
    cavernous, 385, 385f, 386f
    complex, 387, 388f
    perilobular, 383, 384f
    venous, 386, 388f
Hemangiopericytoma, 405–407, 406f
Hematolymphoid neoplasms, 414t
Hematoma, 474
Hemorrhage
    in breast infarct, 13
    after needle core biopsy, 466, 467f
Hemosiderin, 44, 466
HER2, 121, 194, 194t, 251, 268, 282
    adenoid cystic carcinoma, 292
    ancillary tests for, 490–492
    clinical testing for, 493–494, 493–494t
    tubular carcinoma, 209
HER2/neu gene, 494
Heterologous elements, 246–249
Hibernoma, 382, 382f
High-grade malignant phyllodes, 242
Histiocytes, 4, 5f
    in duct ectasia, 18, 18–20f, 20
    in fat necrosis, 13
    lensional, 13
Histiocytic proliferations of breast, 422–424
Histiocytoid breast carcinoma, 21
Histiocytoma, malignant fibrous, 404–405, 404f
Histiocytosis X. See Langerhans cell histiocytosis
Hodgkin lymphoma, 418, 418f, 440
Holland classification system, of ductal carcinoma in situ, 167
Hormonal therapy, for adenoid cystic carcinoma, 296
Hyperelastosis, 20, 21
Hyperplasia
    apocrine duct, 442, 443f
    atypical
        ductal. See Atypical ductal hyperplasia
        pregnency-like, 9, 10f
        in sclerosing adenosis, 92f
    epithelial
        in fibroadenoma, 105, 112
        in phyllodes tumor, 116–117, 118
    lactational, 5–6f
    mild, 126, 126f
    moderate, 126, 127f
    myoepithelial cell, 73f, 76f
    pregnancy-like, 9f
    terminal ducts with atypical lobular, 443, 445f

Hyperplastic duct, squamous metaplasia in, 240f
Hyperplastic epithelial cells, 9, 21

IgG4-related disease, 27
ILC. See Invasive lobular carcinoma (ILC)
Imaging modalities, NCB specimens, 481–483
Immature breast, 1, 2f
Immunocompromised state, 32
Immunohistochemical markers, 360
Immunoperoxidase, 121
Immunostains
    in diagnosis of metastases in breast, 435–436
    Ki67, 396, 398
    p40, 131
    p63, 48, 131, 470, 471f
Implant-associated mastitis, 25f
Implantation metastases, 435, 435–436f
IMT. See Inflammatory myofibroblastic tumor (IMT)
In situ carcinoma
    history of concept, xv–xvi
    pathology report, 489
Inactive gynecomastia, 453f
Infarct
    with atypical cells, 17f
    breast, 13, 16–17
Infarction
    adenomyoepithelioma with, 74f
    in hemangiomas, 389
    in papillary tumors, 222, 223f
    papillomas with, 44, 46f
Infections
    bacterial, 32–34
    fungal, 34
    mycobacterial, 32–33
    needle core biopsies, 474
    nontuberculous bacterial, 33
    parasitic, 34–36
Infiltrating carcinoma, recurrence after radiotherapy, 445f
Infiltrating myofibroblastoma, 375, 376f
Inflammatory and reactive tumors, 29
    amyloid tumor, 27–28
    amyloidoma, 27–28
    breast infarct, 13, 16–17
    diabetic mastopathy, 21–23, 22–23f
    duct ectasia, 18–21, 18–21f
    fat necrosis, 13
    galactocele, 17, 18f
    granulomatous mastitis, 23–24
    inflammatory pseudotumor, 26–27, 26f
    mastitis related to augmentation procedures, 24–26, 25f
    plasma cell mastitis, 21, 21f
    sarcoidosis, 24, 25f
    vasculitis, 28
Inflammatory myofibroblastic tumor (IMT), 27
Inflammatory pseudotumor (IPT), 26–27, 26f, 245–246
Intermediate gynecomastia, 452
Interval carcinomas, 349
Intracystic papillary carcinoma, 225, 227, 227f
Intracystic papilloma, 39, 40f
Intracytoplasmic mucin, papillary carcinoma with, 219–220, 220f
Intraductal carcinoma
    age and symptoms, 454
    calcifications, 11f
    clinical presentation, 39
    disruption in postbiopsy excision, 469, 470f
    gross pathology, 39
    imaging studies, 39, 455
    immunohistochemistry, 48, 455
    with lobular extension in medullary carcinoma, 234–235
    with lymphatic tumor emboli, 473f
    microscopic features, 455
    microscopic pathology, 39–48, 457
    with obliterative sclerosis, 163–164f
    prognosis of, 49, 455
    treatment of, 50, 455
    tubular carcinoma with, 204, 204f

Intraductal squamous carcinoma, 240f
Intraepithelial histiocytes, 335
Intralobular carcinoma, 234–235
Intramammary blood vessels, direct injury, 475
Intramammary lymph nodes, 424
   with extramedullary hematopoiesis, 422f
   with nevus cell aggregate, 425f
Invasive apocrine carcinoma, 280f
   low nuclear grade, 279f
   with micropapillary architecture, 281f
   microscopic pathology, 280–282
   with solid papillary architecture, 281f
   treatment and prognosis, 286
   with tumor-infiltrating lymphocytes, 281f
Invasive carcinoma, 78, 94–95
   diagnosis of, 470
   displaced epithelium mistaken in needle core biopsy sample, 163f
   marker of, 345–346
   pathology report, 489
   with squamoid morphology, 239f
Invasive cribriform carcinoma, 294, 299f, 300, 301f
Invasive ductal carcinoma, 181f
   alveolar, 355f
   angiogenesis, 188, 188f
   architectural (histologic) grade, 184f
   bilaterality, 350
   classic, 350–351, 350–353f, 355f
   clinical presentation, 349
   cytologic (nuclear) grade, 185f
   differential diagnosis, 200t
   ductal carcinoma in situ, 191
   ER, PR, and HER2 testing on needle core biopsies, 192
   estrogen receptor immunostain, 192f, 360f
   frozen section, 181f
      and immediate cytologic evaluation, 179
   genetic alterations and immunohistochemistry, 359–360, 359f, 360t
   imaging, 349–350
   in male, 456f
   in situ and, 356f
Invasive lobular carcinoma (ILC)
   with de novo necrosis, 194f
   lobular carcinoma, 180f
   with lobular carcinoma in situ, 339f
   lymphovascular involvement, 186–188, 186f, 187f
   metastatic lobular carcinoma, 360–361, 361f
   microinvasive lobular carcinoma, 356f
   microscopic pathology, 350–359, 456
   mitoses, 185f
   molecular pathology aspects, 193–194
   myoepithelium, absence of, 189–191
      on immunostaining, 190–191f
      on routine staining, 190f
   nomenclature, 179
   Nottingham grading system for, 183t
   with perineural infiltration, 188–189f
   perineural invasion, 188
   plasmacytoid, 353f
   pleomorphic, 356, 357–359f
   presentation, 179–181
   prognosis, 361
   with prominent lymphocytic reaction, 353f
   pseudoangiomatous stroma, 187f
   role of needle core biopsy
      specimen in neoadjuvant chemotherapy and novel treatment modalities, 191–192
      status-post neoadjuvant chemotherapy, 193
   with signet ring cells, 357f
   size, 181–182
      grading, 183–186
      and magnetic resonance imaging, 183
      and multifocal carcinoma, 183
      and needle core biopsy samples, 182–183
   solid variant, 351, 354f
   special types of, 298–316
      cribriform carcinoma, 300–302
      cystic hypersecretory carcinoma, 305–309

glycogen-rich carcinoma, 313–315
      invasive micropapillary carcinoma, 298–300
      lipid-rich carcinoma, 315–316
      mammary carcinoma with osteoclast-like giant cells, 309–311
      secretory carcinoma, 302–305
      small cell carcinoma, 311–313
   stromal elastosis, 189, 189f
   trabecular variant, 351, 354f
   treatment, 361
   triple immunostaining, 191f
   triple negative and basal-like immunopheno-type, 195f
   tumor-infiltrating lymphocytes, 192–193
   variants of, 355t
   well differentiated, 95, 101
Invasive micropapillary carcinoma, 299f
   clinical presentation, 298
   differential diagnosis, 299–300
   microscopic pathology, 298–299
   prognosis and treatment, 300
   ultrastructure and immunohistochemistry, 299
Invasive micropapillary mucinous carcinoma, 300
Invasive papillary carcinoma, 221–222
Invasive squamous carcinoma, 240f
IPT. See Inflammatory pseudotumor (IPT)

JP. See Juvenile papillomatosis (JP)
Juvenile atypical ductal hyperplasia, 460f
Juvenile fibroadenoma, 112, 112f
Juvenile papillomatosis (JP), 458–459, 460f
   age and gender, 458
   differential diagnosis in needle core biopsy material, 459
   imaging studies, 459
   microscopic pathology, 459
   predisposing factors, 459
   presenting symptoms, 459
   treatment and prognosis, 459

Keloidal, fibromatosis, 365, 365f
Keratins, 119–120
Ki67, 121, 145, 268, 396, 398
   adenoid cystic carcinoma, 292
   apocrine carcinoma, 282
KIT, 292

Lactating adenoma, 107f
Lactating breast, uncommon findings in, 7f
Lactating glands, 7f
Lactational hyperplasia, 5–6f
Lactiferous ducts, 2
Lactiferous sinus, 2, 3f
Langerhans cell histiocytosis, 423
Laser tumor ablation, 449
LCIS. See Lobular carcinoma in situ (LCIS)
Leiomyoma, 381–382, 382f
Leiomyomatous hamartoma, 381
Leiomyosarcoma, 401, 401f
   metastatic, 433, 433f
Lesional epithelial cells, displacement of, 469
LGASC. See Low-grade adenosquamous carcinoma (LGASC)
Lipid-rich carcinoma, 315f
   clinical presentation, 315
   differential diagnosis, 315–316
   immunohistochemistry, 315
   microscopic pathology, 315
   treatment and prognosis, 316
Lipid-secreting carcinoma. See Lipid-rich carcinoma
Lipoblasts, 13
Lipofuscin pigment, 4
Lipomas, 382–383, 383f
   spindle cell, 373, 377, 383
Lipomatous myofibroblastoma, 377, 377f
Liposarcoma, 402, 402f
LN. See Lobular neoplasia (LN)
Loa loa infection, 34
Lobular cancerization, 150, 150f

Lobular carcinoma in situ (LCIS), 284, 321–323*f*, 328*f*, 330*f*
　in adenosis, 91–92, 95, 338–339*f*
　classic and florid patterns, 324–325*f*
　clinical presentation, 326
　coexistent, 165, 166*f*
　with collagenous spherulosis, 333, 333–334*f*
　and columnar cell change, 144*f*
　differential diagnosis, 335–336
　ductal involvement, 332*f*
　example of, xvi
　excisional biopsy and needle core biopsy diagnosis of, 343–345
　florid, 325–326*f*
　histopathology of, 328–333
　immunohistochemistry, 334–335, 334*t*
　incidence, 326, 328
　invasive lobular carcinoma associated with, 339*f*
　involving various lesions, 337–338*f*
　microinvasive lobular carcinoma, 339, 339*f*
　mosaic pattern, 332*f*
　in needle core biopsy samples, 206*f*
　pagetoid ductal and partial lobular involvement, 329*f*
　postmenopausal, 331*f*
　precursor lesion or marker of invasive carcinoma, 345–346
　prognosis of, 339–340
　sclerosing adenosis and, 91*f*
　in single duct, 336*f*
　terminology of "lobular" lesions, 320
　tubular adenosis with, 91*f*
　tubular carcinoma and, 204, 206*f*
　types A and B, 324*f*
　untreated, systematic study of, xvi
　in vicinity of ductal carcinoma in situ, 337*f*
Lobular gland epithelium, 11
Lobular neoplasia (LN), 320, 327*f*
Lobules, 4–5
　altered by pregnancy-like change, 6, 9
　in amid mammary adipose tissue, 2*f*
　atrophy, radiation-induced, 441, 441*f*
　cystic hypersecretory hyperplasia, 307*f*
　in fibrocollagenous stroma, 2*f*
　fully formed, 2
　mammary, 1, 2*f*
　in mammary adipose tissue, 2*f*
　myoepithelial cell layer and basement membrane in, 3*f*
　normal, 1, 2*f*
　progressive recruitment of, 5
Lobulitis
　granulomatous, 23, 24*f*
　lymphocytic, 23*f*
Low-grade adenosquamous carcinoma (LGASC)
　clinical presentation, 253
　differential diagnosis at needle core biopsy, 253–255
　imaging studies, 253
　immunoreactivity, 255
　microscopic pathology, 253
　prognosis and treatment, 256
Luminal A tumors, 193, 194*t*
Luminal B tumors, 193, 194*t*
Luminal cells, 41, 51
Lumpectomy, xx–xxi
Lung, carcinoma of, 429–430
Lupus erythematosus, 28
Lupus mastitis, 28
Luteal phase, 5
LVI. *See* Lymphovascular involvement (LVI)
Lymph node metastasis, 473*f*
　of breast carcinoma, 283–284
Lymphatic tumor emboli
　chemotherapy pathologic effect involving, 447*f*
　intraductal carcinoma, 473*f*
Lymphatics, definition of, 186
Lymphocytes, tumor-infiltrating, 192–193
Lymphocytic lobulitis, 23*f*
Lymphocytic mastitis, 23
Lymphoid and hematopoietic tumors
　histiocytic proliferations of breast, 422–424

　　Erdheim–Chester disease, 423
　　Langerhans cell histiocytosis, 423
　　Rosai–Dorfman disease, 422–423, 423*f*
　intramammary lymph nodes, 424
　　with extramedullary hematopoiesis, 422*f*
　　with nevus cell aggregate, 425*f*
　lymphomas of breast, 413–420
　　in association with implants, 418–420
　　Burkitt lymphoma, 416–417, 418*f*
　　clinical features, 413
　　differential diagnosis, 420
　　diffuse large B-cell lymphoma, 413–415, 415*f*
　　follicular lymphoma, 415–416, 417*f*
　　hematolymphoid neoplasms, 414*t*
　　Hodgkin lymphoma, 418, 418*f*
　　MALT lymphoma, 415, 416*f*
　　pathologic features and clinicopathologic correlates, 413
　　T-cell lymphomas, 417
　myeloid sarcoma, 421–422, 421–422*f*
　plasma cell neoplasms, 420
　tissue processing and ancillary studies, 424–425
Lymphoma
　of breast, 413–420
　　in association with implants, 418–420
　　Burkitt lymphoma, 416–417, 418*f*
　　clinical features, 413
　　differential diagnosis, 420
　　diffuse large B-cell lymphoma, 413–415, 415*f*
　　follicular lymphoma, 415–416, 417*f*
　　hematolymphoid neoplasms, 414*t*
　　Hodgkin lymphoma, 418, 418*f*
　　MALT lymphoma, 415, 416*f*
　　pathologic features and clinicopathologic correlates, 413
　　T-cell lymphomas, 417
Lymphoplasmacytic reaction, of medullary carcinoma, 233*f*, 235
Lymphovascular channel, 471, 471*f*, 473
Lymphovascular involvement (LVI), 186–188
　assessment of, 489
　invasive ductal carcinoma with, 186*f*
　invasive micropapillary carcinoma resembling, 187*f*
Lymphovascular spaces, displaced carcinomatous epithelium in, 473, 473*f*

Magnetic resonance imaging (MRI), 1, 13, 24, 27, 440, 482–483
　for ductal carcinoma in situ, 149
　guided biopsies, 477
　invasive ductal carcinoma, 183
　for invasive lobular carcinoma, 349–350
　for metastases in breast, 428
Male breast lesions
　carcinoma, 455–458
　　age, 455
　　differential diagnosis in needle core biopsy material, 457–458
　　imaging studies, 456
　　immunohistochemistry, 457
　　incidence and ethnicity, 455
　　invasive ductal, 456*f*
　　metastatic prostatic, 458*f*
　　microscopic pathology, 456–457
　　papillary, 457*f*
　　predisposing factors, 455–456
　　presenting symptoms, 456
　　treatment and prognosis, 458
　fibroepithelial lesions, 455
　gynecomastia, 452–454, 454*f*
　　age, 452
　　florid, 453*f*, 454*f*
　　imaging studies, 452
　　immunohistochemistry, 453–454
　　inactive, 453*f*
　　intermediate, 453*f*
　　microscopic pathology, 452–453
　　predisposing factors, 452
　　symptoms, 452
　　treatment and prognosis, 454
　intraductal papilloma, 454–455
　　age and symptoms, 454

Male breast lesions (*continued*)
    imaging studies, 455
    immunohistochemistry, 455
    microscopic features, 455
    treatment and prognosis, 455
  proliferative fibrocystic changes, 455
Malignant ductal cells, 215
Malignant fibrous histiocytoma, 404–405, 404*f*
Malignant melanoma, metastatic, 430, 430–431*f*
Malignant neoplasms, nonmammary. *See* Nonmammary malignant
    neoplasms (NMMN)
Malignant phyllodes tumor, 117, 119*f*
MALT. *See* Mucosa-associated lymphoid tissue (MALT)
Mammaglobin, 436
Mammary amyloidosis, 27, 28
Mammary carcinoma, 433
  with osteoclast-like giant cells, 309*f*, 310*f*
    clinical presentation, 309
    differential diagnosis, 310–311
    immunohistochemistry, 310
    microscopic pathology, 309–310
    prognosis and treatment, 311
Mammary ductal system, 2
Mammary epithelial cells, 46
Mammary fat necrosis, 13
Mammary glandular system, 3, 4
Mammary lobe, 2, 3*f*
Mammary lobules, 1
Mammography, 446, 473
  DCIS treated by, xviii
  for ductal carcinoma in situ, 148–149
  of fat necrosis, 13
  for invasive lobular carcinoma, 349
  low-grade adenosquamous carcinoma, 253
  male breast lesions, 452
  metaplastic carcinoma, 238, 428
  pathologic effects of, 440
Mass-forming gynecomastia, 452
Massively parallel sequencing, 437
Mastectomy, for medullary carcinoma, 236
Mastitis
  AIDS-related, 32
  augmentation procedures, related to, 24–26, 25*f*
  granulomatous, 23–24
  implant-associated, 25*f*
  lupus, 28
  plasma cell, 21
  tuberculous, 32–33, 33*f*
Mastitis obliterans, 20, 20*f*
Mastopathy, diabetic, 21–23, 22–23*f*
Matrix components, 251
MC. *See* Mucinous carcinoma (MC)
Medullary carcinoma
  clinical presentation, 232
  EBV in, 235
  giant cells in, 234*f*, 235
  gross pathology, 232
  histopathologic features of, 233
  imaging studies, 232
  immunoreactivity, 235
  intraductal carcinoma with lobular extension, 234–235
  lymphoplasmacytic reaction of, 233, 235
  metastatic, 433
  microscopic pathology, 232–235
  noninvasive microscopic circumscription, 233–234
  prognosis of, 235–236
  staging, prognosis, and treatment, 235–236
  syncytial growth pattern of, 233*f*, 234
Melanoma, 242
Memorial Sloan-Kettering Cancer Center's Nomogram, 173
Menopause, hormonal alterations during and after, 6
Menstrual phase, 5
Mesenchymal neoplasms
  benign mesenchymal tumors, 364–392
  sarcomas, 392–407
Mesothelioma, 429–430

Metaplasia, 10–11
  pseudolactational, 6
Metaplastic alterations, of adenoid cystic carcinoma, 291
Metaplastic breast carcinoma, with myxoid matrix, 271
Metaplastic carcinoma, 78
  acantholytic (pseudoangiosarcomatous) type, 249–250*f*
  clinical presentation, 238
    age, gender, and genetic predisposition, 238
    imaging studies, 238
    incidence, 238
    presenting symptoms, 238
  with high-grade morphology, 241–242*f*
  immunohistochemistry, 251
    cytokeratins, 251
    epidermal growth factor receptor, 251
    ER, PR, and HER2, 251
    GATA3, 251
    matrix components, 251
    myoepithelial antigens, 251
    snail and other EMT-related proteins, 251
    SOX10, 251
  low-grade adenosquamous type, 253–256*f*
  matrix-producing type, 247*f*, 248*f*
  microscopic pathology, 238–251
    choriocarcinomatous morphology, 249–250
    heterologous elements, 246–249
    metaplastic spindle cell carcinoma, 241–246
    metastatic to extramammary sites, 250–251
    squamous cell carcinoma, 239–241
  osteocartilaginous metaplasia, 246*f*
  with osteoid matrix production, 247–248*f*
  treatment and prognosis, 251–252
    chondroid and/or osteoid matrix, 252
    metaplastic spindle cell carcinoma, 252
    metaplastic spindle cell carcinomas with intermediate- to high-grade
      morphology, 252
Metaplastic matrix-producing carcinoma, 248*f*
Metaplastic spindle cell carcinoma (MSpCC)
  with intermediate- and high-grade morphology, 241
  microscopic pathology, 241–246
Metaplastic spindle cell carcinoma
  with chondroid and/or osteoid matrix, 252
  with intermediate- to high-grade morphology, 252
  low-grade fibromatosis-like, 243–244*f*, 252
  microscopic pathology, 241–246
Metastases
  distant, 121–122
  from extramammary neoplasm, 271
Metastases in breast
  from nonmammary malignant neoplasms
    axillary lymph node, 434–435
    clinical features, 428
    common sources, 429–433
    future directions, 436–437
    histopathologic evaluation, 428–429
    immunohistochemical approach, 437*t*
    immunostains use, 435–436
    implantation metastases, 435, 435–436*f*
    late presentation, 434
    management of, 436
    metastatic prostatic carcinoma, 434
    occult primary neoplasms, 434
    radiologic features, 428
    uncommon sources, 433
Metastatic carcinoma
  from extramammary site, 283
  in intramammary lymph node, 424
  in lymph node with metastatic carcinoma, 448, 448*f*
  mimics triple-negative apocrine breast carcinoma, 283*f*
Metastatic chondrosarcoma, 249
Metastatic disease, 457
Metastatic lobular carcinoma, 360–361, 361*f*
Metastatic prostatic carcinoma, 458*f*
MGA. *See* Microglandular adenosis
Microcalcification, 456
Microglandular adenosis (MGA), 97–102, 98–99*f*

atypical, 97, 98, 99f, 102
  carcinoma arising in, 97, 98–100
  carcinoma in situ in, 100, 100–101f, 102
  clinical presentation, 97
  differential diagnosis of, 101–102, 200t
  high-grade carcinoma arising in, 294
  invasive carcinoma arising in, 100
  microscopic pathology, 97–100
  prognosis and treatment of, 102
  tubular carcinoma and, 210–211, 211f
Microinvasive ductal carcinoma, 168–171, 169–171f, 182f, 193f
  radiotherapy, 172
  treatment for, 173
Microinvasive lobular carcinoma, 339, 339f
Micropapillary ductal carcinoma in situ, 155, 156f
Micropapillary ductal hyperplasia, 128f
Mild hyperplasia, 126, 126f
Mixed invasive cribriform carcinoma, 300
Mixed invasive micropapillary carcinoma, 298
Mixed proliferative pattern, 66
MLL. See Mucocele-like lesion (MLL)
Moderate hyperplasia, 126, 127f
Molecular alterations, 333–334
Molecular apocrine, 194
Molecular profiling, of tumors, 436
Molecular test kits, 437
Monomorphic ductal carcinoma in situ, 154
Morphology of recurrent, 118
MSpCC. See Metaplastic spindle cell carcinoma (MSpCC)
MUC-1, 299
MUC2, 268
Mucin, 268
Mucinous carcinoma (MC), 78, 249, 440
  and adenoid cystic carcinoma, 270f
  age, 259
  associated with solid and papillary carcinoma, 263
  calcifications, 260
  clinical findings, 259
  different growth patterns, 261–262f
  differential diagnosis of, 268
  ductal carcinoma in situ. See Ductal carcinoma in situ
  ethnicity, 259
  family history, 259
  gender, 259
  grade, 260
  hypocellular, 261f
  incidence, 259
  micropapillary variant of, 262–263, 263f
  mixed, 261f
  mucocele-like lesions. See Mucocele-like lesion (MLL)
  neuroendocrine differentiation, 268
  polyacrylamide gel mimics, 271f
  radiology, 259–260
  with signet ring cells, 263, 264f
  size, 260
  treatment and prognosis, 272
  type A, type B, and type AB, 260, 262, 262f
Mucocele-like lesion (MLL)
  atypia, absence of, 265–266f
  with atypical duct hyperplasia, 266f, 267f
  benign, 269–270, 269t
  differential diagnosis of, 268–269
  with intraductal carcinoma, 267f
  microscopic pathology, 263–267
Mucoepidermoid carcinoma, 270–271, 316
Mucosa-associated lymphoid tissue (MALT), 27
  lymphoma, 415, 416f
Mullerian carcinomas, 430
Multifocal invasive ductal carcinoma, 183
Multiple papillomas, 39
MYB, 293
Mycobacterial infections, 32–33
Mycobacterium abscesses, 33
Mycobacterium fortuitum, 33
Mycobacterium tuberculosis infection, 32–33
Myeloid metaplasia, 422

Myeloid sarcoma, 421–422, 421–422f
Myeloma, 21
Myiasis, cutaneous, 35–36
Myoepithelial antigens, 251
Myoepithelial carcinoma, 78
  in adenomyoepithelioma, 79–80f, 79f
  adenosis, 79f
  papilloma, 79f
Myoepithelial cells, 4–5, 11, 89, 218–219, 292
  anatomy and histology, 2–3
  ductal carcinoma in situ and, 151f
  ductal hyperplasia with, 132f
  hyperplasia, 73f
    adenomyoepithelioma with, 76f
    immunophenotype of, 71t
    invasive ductal carcinoma without, 190f
    p63 immunostain for, 470, 471f
    papillomas with, 44f
    variations in, 4f
Myoepithelial lesion, myoepithelioma, 78
Myoepithelial markers, 16, 206–209
Myoepithelial neoplasms, 71–80
Myoepithelioma, 71, 78
Myoepithelium, absence of, 189–190
Myofibroblastoma, 246, 373–378, 373–377f
  cellular variant of, 375
  epithelioid variant of, 374–375, 374–375f
  infiltrative variant of, 375–376, 376f
Myofibroblasts, in PASH, 369
Myoid differentiation, adenomyoepithelioma with, 76f
Myoid hamartoma, 381
Myoid metaplasia
  around atrophic duct, 7f
  of myoepithelial cells, 7f
  sclerosing adenosis with, 86f
Myolipomas, 383
Myxoid fibroadenomas, 108
Myxoid myofibroblastoma, 376–377, 376f
Myxoid stroma, fibroadenomas with, 109–110f

National Comprehensive Cancer Network (NCCN), 344
NCB. See Needle core biopsy (NCB)
NCB specimens. See Needle core biopsy (NCB) specimens
NCCN. See National Comprehensive Cancer Network (NCCN)
Necrosis. See also Fat necrosis
  de novo, 194f
  in ductal carcinoma in situ, 161t
Necrotic cellular debris, 130, 130f
Needle core biopsy (NCB), 1, 5–10f, 91, 96
  atypia, with and without, 269t
  atypical lobular hyperplasia, 345
  clinical complications of, 474–475
  differential diagnosis
    adenoid cystic carcinoma, 294–296
    apocrine lesions at, 283–286
    atypical ductal hyperplasia, 146–148
    fibroadenoma, 461
    juvenile papillomatosis, 459
    of low-grade adenosquamous carcinoma, 253, 255
    "low-grade" "fibromatosis-like" metaplastic spindle cell carcinoma, 245–246
    male breast lesions, 457–458
    metaplastic carcinoma with heterologous elements, 249
    of squamous cell carcinoma, 240–241
  distant metastases, 475
  ductal carcinoma in situ on, 171
  epithelial displacement, 469, 469f
  and excision specimens, 48–49
  histopathologic changes caused by, 466–474, 468–469f
  invasive carcinoma, 78
  invasive ductal carcinoma, 193
    ER, PR, and HER2 testing on, 192
    size and samples, 182–183
    specimen, role in neoadjuvant chemotherapy and novel treatment modalities, 191–192
  lesion localization, xii

Needle core biopsy (NCB) (*continued*)
  lobular carcinoma in situ, 343–345
  metaplastic carcinoma, 78
  modern techniques, xi
  mucinous carcinoma, 78
  objective of, 466
  origins of, x–xi
  phyllodes tumor, 80
  site of procedure, 467*f*
  syringomatous adenoma of nipple, 80
  upgrade rate of benign mucocele-like lesion at, 269–270
Needle core biopsy (NCB) specimens, 477–495
  ancillary tests on, 490–492, 491–492*f*, 495
  calcifications, 483–487, 484*f*, 486–487*f*
  clinical information in diagnosis of, 479*f*
  determination of proliferation rate, 495
  frozen section examination, 487–488
  gross examination and description, 480
  imaging modalities, 481–483
  inked, 480*f*
  pathologic examination of, xi–xii
  pathology report, 488–490
    invasive carcinoma, 489
    non-neoplastic tissue, 489–490
    in situ carcinoma, 489
  radiology–pathology correlation of, 484–485*f*
  requisition form, 479–480, 480*t*
  role of pathologist in interpretation, 490
  specimen processing, 480–481, 481–482*f*
  standardized reporting templates, 490
  techniques and size of needles, 477, 477*f*
  tissue fixation, 477–478
  touch imprint cytology, 488
  visibility in tissue, 480*f*
Neoadjuvant chemotherapy, 446
  invasive ductal carcinoma, 193
  needle core biopsy specimen role in, 191–192
Nerves and nerve sheath, tumors originating in, 379
Neural entrapment, 164–165
Neuroendocrine ("carcinoid") tumors, 430
Neuroendocrine markers, 152, 293
Neutral buffered formalin, 477
Neutrophils, 33
NGS. *See* Nottingham Grading System (NGS)
Nicolau syndrome, 475
Nipple, 2
  florid papillomatosis of, 64–66
  syringomatous adenoma of, 66–68
NMMN. *See* Nonmammary malignant neoplasms (NMMN)
Nodular fasciitis, 245, 367, 368*f*
Nodular mucinosis, 270
Non-Langerhans cell histiocytosis, 13
Non-neoplastic breast parenchyma, 448
Non-neoplastic tissue, pathology report, 489–490
Non-small cell carcinoma, of lung, 429
Nonepithelial malignant neoplasms, 463
Noninvasive adenoid cystic carcinoma, 166
Noninvasive microscopic circumscription, of medullary carcinoma, 233
Nonmammary malignant neoplasms (NMMN)
  metastases in breast from
    axillary lymph node, 434–435
    clinical features, 428
    common sources, 429–433
    future directions, 436–437
    histopathologic evaluation, 428–429
    immunohistochemical approach, 437*t*
    immunostains use, 435–436
    implantation metastases, 435, 435–436*f*
    late presentation, 434
    management, 436
    metastatic prostatic carcinoma, 434
    occult primary neoplasms, 434
    radiologic features, 428
    uncommon sources, 433
Nonmucinous carcinoma
  adenoid cystic carcinoma, 270

benign spindle cell lesions with myxoid stroma, 271
  cystic hypersecretory lesions, 270
  foreign material, 271–272, 271*f*
  metaplastic breast carcinoma with myxoid matrix, 271
  metastases from extramammary neoplasm, 271
  mucoepidermoid carcinoma, 270–271
  pleomorphic adenoma, 271
  secretory carcinoma, 270
  squamous cell carcinoma with prominent myxoid stroma, 271
Nonparenchymal angiolipoma, 391*f*, 392*f*
Nonparenchymal mammary hemangioma, 391
Nonparenchymal vascular lesions, 391–392, 392*f*
Nontuberculous bacterial infections, 33
Nottingham Grading System (NGS), 183, 183*t*
NSABP B-17 trial, xix
NSABP B-24 Trial, xx
NSABP Protocol 6, xix
Nuclear β-catenin, 121
Nuclear pleomorphism, 184
NY-BR-1, 436

Oat cell carcinoma. *See* Small cell carcinoma
Occult primary neoplasms, 434
Ochrocytes, 4, 5*f*, 18, 18*f*
Oncocytic carcinoma, 316
Oncocytic neoplasms, 284
Oncotype DX test, 495
Osteoclast-like giant cells, mammary carcinoma with, 309–311, 309*f*, 310*f*
Osteogenic sarcoma, 403–404, 403*f*
Osteolipomas, 383, 383*f*
Osteosarcoma, 249
Ovarian carcinoma, metastatic, 432*f*, 433

p120, 165
p40, 131
p53, 121
p63, 48, 119–120, 131, 470, 471*f*
Paget disease, 67
  of nipple, 66
Papillary apocrine metaplasia, 60–64, 61–62*f*, 63*f*
Papillary carcinoma, 216–217*f*
  carcinoma involving papilloma, 221, 222*f*
  clinical presentation, 215
  dimorphic, 227, 227*f*
  encapsulated, 227
    microscopic pathology, 457
  endocrine differentiation in, 227–230
  with extracellular mucin, 220*f*
  gross pathology, 215
  imaging studies, 215
  immunohistochemistry, 220–221
  infarction in, 222, 223*f*
  intracystic, 225, 227, 227*f*
  invasive, 221–222
  low grade, 217–218*f*
  in male, 457*f*
  microscopic pathology, 215–220
    adjacent epithelial proliferations, 219
    apocrine cells, 219
    calcifications, 220, 220*f*
    cytologic attributes, 219
    glandular pattern, 219
    intraepithelial mucin, 219–220, 220*f*
    sclerosing adenosis, 219
    stroma, 219
    types of cells, 215–219
  prognosis and treatment, 230
  with sclerotic stroma, 219*f*
  solid variant of, 223–225, 223–224*f*, 225*f*
  tall cell variant of, 230
Papillary cystadenomas, 39
Papillary ductal carcinoma in situ, 164
Papilloma, 39, 40*f*
  collagenous spherulosis in, 51*f*

with ductal hyperplasia, 41*f*
infarcted, 16, 17*f*
intraductal, 39–50
papillary carcinoma arising in, 221, 222*f*
Papillomatosis, 39
florid, of nipple, 64–66
Papillomatosis pattern, 65
Parasitic infections, 34–36
Parenchyma, 472
PAS stain. *See* Periodic acid-Schiff (PAS) stain
PASH. *See* Pseudoangiomatous stromal hyperplasia (PASH)
Pathology–radiology correlation, beginning of, ix–x
PCM. *See* Plasma cell mastitis (PCM)
Periductal fibrosis, 21
in duct ectasia, 20, 20*f*
Periductal stroma
growth of, 1
histology, 4, 5*f*, 8*f*
Perilobular hemangioma, 383, 384*f*
Perineural and lymphovascular invasion, 291, 291*f*
Perineural infiltration, invasive ductal carcinoma
with, 188–189*f*
Perineural invasion, 188–189
adenosis with, 89*f*
Periodic acid-Schiff (PAS) stain, 9
Phyllodes tumor (PT), 80, 114–122, 461–462
benign, 114, 116, 117*f*, 121
borderline, 117, 118*f*
clinical presentation, 114
diagnosis, 114
distant metastases, 121–122
epithelial hyperplasia in, 116–117, 118
epithelium in, 118–119
immunoreactivity, 121
local recurrence, 121
malignant, 117, 119*f*
with focal cytokeratin staining, 120*f*
metastatic, 119
microscopic pathology, 115–119, 461
morphologic Features of, 115*f*
with pseudoangiomatous stromal hyperplasia, 116*f*
size of, 114–115
stroma in, 115, 116–117, 121
with stromal giant cells, 116*f*
survival, 122
symptoms, 461
treatment and prognosis, 121–122, 462
Physiologic morphology, of breast, 4–10
Plasma cell mastitis (PCM), 21, 21*f*
Plasma cell neoplasms, 420
Plasmacytoma, 21, 420*f*
Plasminogen activator inhibitor (PAI-1), 495
Pleomorphic adenoma, 75, 78*f*, 249, 249*f*, 271
Pleomorphic invasive lobular carcinoma, 356, 357–359*f*
Pleomorphic variant of lobular carcinoma in situ, 320. *See also* Lobular
carcinoma in situ (LCIS)
Pneumothorax, 474
Polyarteritis, 28
Polymorphous adenocarcinoma, 316
Polyposis, familial adenomatous, 364
Positive predictive value (PPV), 39
Positron emission tomography (PET), 24, 483
Postbiopsy scar, 469*f*, 470*f*
Postirradiation atypical vascular lesions, 399–400
PPV. *See* Positive predictive value (PPV)
PR. *See* Progesterone (PR)
Precocious puberty, 1
Precursor lesion, 345
Pregnancy
florid adenosis in, 88*f*
secretory changes associated with, 5
Pregnancy-like change. *See* Pseudolactational hyperplasia
Premature thelarche, 1
Prepubertal gynecomastia, 452
Primary amyloid tumors, 27
Primary lymphoma of breast, 413, 417

Primary mammary fibromatosis, 246*f*
Primary sarcomas, 242
Procedural trauma–induced changes, in NCB site, 466
Progesterone (PR), 5, 11, 121, 251, 268
adenoid cystic carcinoma, 292
apocrine carcinoma, 282
clinical testing for, 492–493, 492*t*, 494*t*
tubular carcinoma, 209
Proliferative fibrocystic changes (FCCs), 455
Proliferative phase, 4
Prostatic carcinoma, metastatic, 434
Pseudoangiomatous stroma, 187*f*
Pseudoangiomatous stromal hyperplasia (PASH), 115, 249, 369–373, 370*f*,
452, 462–463
age distribution of, 369
fascicular, 371*f*, 372*f*
myofibroblasts in, 369
phyllodes tumor with, 116*f*
Pseudolactational hyperplasia
atypical, 9, 10*f*
with calcification, 6, 8–9*f*, 9
physiologic morphology of, 6, 9
Pseudomonas aeruginosa infection, 32
Pseudotumor, inflammatory, 26–27, 26*f*
PT. *See* Phyllodes tumor (PT)
Puberty, 1, 2*f*
Pulmonary adenocarcinoma, metastatic, 429
Pure invasive micropapillary carcinoma, 298

Radial scar, 53, 59, 211–212, 212*f*
Radial sclerosing lesions (RSLs), 52–59, 54–56*f*
with atypical duct hyperplasia, 57*f*
with carcinoma, 58*f*
clinical presentation, 53
differential diagnosis, 58
ductal carcinoma in situ in, 165, 165*f*
gross pathology, 53
imaging studies, 53
immunohistochemistry, 58
microscopic pathology, 53–56
prognosis of, 59
treatment of, 59
tubular carcinoma and, 211–212, 212*f*
Radiation, pathologic effect
apocrine duct hyperplasia, 442, 443*f*
atrophy of lobules, 441, 441*f*
atypical fibroblasts, 442, 442*f*
and breast-conservation therapy, 440–446
histologic changes, 319
and Hodgkin lymphoma, 440
recurrent carcinoma after, 443, 444*f*
recurrent ductal carcinoma in situ after, 443, 444*f*
recurrent infiltrating carcinoma, 443, 445*f*
small duct, 441, 442*f*
terminal ducts with atypical lobular hyperplasia, 443, 445*f*
vascular changes, 441–442*f*
Radiation-related angiosarcomas, 398
Radioactive seed localization, 473, 474*f*
Radiofrequency ablation, 449
Radiography, breast specimen, xi
Radiology
adenosis, 83
ductal carcinoma in situ, 172
fibroadenoma, 104–105
microglandular adenosis, 97
phyllodes tumor, 114–115
sclerosing lobular hyperplasia, 104
Recurrence
infiltrating carcinoma, 443, 445*f*
medullary carcinoma, 236
after radiotherapy, 443, 444*f*
Recurrence free survival (RFS), 121, 122
Regional lymph nodes, displaced carcinoma cells in, 474
Renal carcinoma, metastatic, 434*f*
Requisition form, NCB specimens, 479–480, 480*t*
Reticular carcinoma, 289*f*, 290

Reticulin stain, 16
Retraction artifact, 472
RFS. *See* Recurrence free survival (RFS)
Rheumatoid nodules, 23
Rosai–Dorfman disease, 422–423, 423*f*
Rosen triad, 204, 206*f*, 326, 328*f*
RSLs. *See* Radial sclerosing lesions (RSLs)

S-100, 9, 71*t*, 242
SA. *See* Sclerosing adenosis (SA)
Salmonella infection, 32
Sarcoidosis, 24, 25*f*
Sarcoma
    angiosarcoma, 393–399
    fibrosarcoma, 405
    hemangiopericytoma, 405–407, 406*f*
    leiomyosarcoma, 401, 401*f*
    liposarcoma, 402, 402*f*
    malignant fibrous histiocytoma, 404–405, 404*f*
    osteogenic and chondrosarcomas, 403–404, 403*f*
    postirradiation atypical vascular lesions, 399–400, 400*f*
Scar, 466
    epithelial displacement along healing track, 471*f*
    postbiopsy, displaced epithelium in, 471*f*
    radial. *See* Radial scar
SCC. *See* Squamous cell carcinoma (SCC)
Schaumann bodies, 23
Schistosomiasis, 35, 36*f*
Schwannoma, 380, 380*f*
Scirrhous carcinoma, 290
Scleroderma, 28
Sclerosing adenosis (SA), 83, 85*f*
    with apocrine intraductal carcinoma, 93*f*
    with atrophy, 86*f*
    atypical hyperplasia in, 92*f*
    with calcifications, 87*f*
    complex fibroadenoma with, 111*f*
    ductal carcinoma in situ in, 164, 164–165*f*
    in fibroadenoma, 93*f*
    with intraductal carcinoma, 93*f*
    with invasive pattern, 94–95*f*
    with lobular carcinoma in situ, 91–92*f*
    with microinvasive lobular carcinoma, 95*f*
    mistaken for carcinoma, 96*f*
    with myoid metaplasia, 86*f*
    with papillary carcinomas, 219
    tubular carcinoma and, 211
Sclerosing lesion, 255, 284
Sclerosing lobular hyperplasia (SLH), 104
Sclerosing lymphocytic mastitis, 23
Sclerosing papilloma, 460
Sclerosing papillomatosis, 65
Sclerosis, papilloma with, 45*f*
Sclerotic stroma, papillary carcinoma with, 219*f*
Sebaceous carcinoma, 316
Secondary lumina, 158
Secretory carcinoma, 270, 303*f*
    with apocrine cytology, 303*f*
    clinical presentation, 302
    differential diagnosis, 304–305
    immunohistochemistry and molecular studies, 305
    microscopic pathology, 302–304
    with papillary and thyroid-like architecture, 304*f*
    prognosis and treatment, 305
Secretory hyperplasia in fibroadenoma, 107*f*
Secretory phase, 5
SEER. *See* Surveillance, Epidemiology, and End Results (SEER)
Sentinel lymph node (SLN), 474
    mapping, 236
Shrinkage artefact, 291
Signet ring cells, 151, 152*f*
    invasive lobular carcinoma with, 356, 357*f*
    in lobular carcinoma in situ, 89, 91, 91*f*
Skin puncture site, excising, 472
SLH. *See* Sclerosing lobular hyperplasia (SLH)
Small cell carcinoma, 294, 312*f*

clinical presentation, 311
differential diagnosis, 313
immunohistochemistry, 312–313
of lung, 429
microscopic pathology, 311
prognosis and treatment, 313
Small cell ductal carcinoma in situ, 154, 154–155*f*
Solid adenoid cystic carcinoma, 295*f*
Solid and basaloid carcinoma, 290–291, 291*f*
Solid ductal carcinoma in situ, 158, 158*f*
Solid papillary carcinomas, 215, 223–225, 223–224*f*
    with endocrine differentiation, 227–230, 228*f*, 229*f*
    with invasion, 225–226*f*
    with mucinous and endocrine differentiation and invasion, 229*f*
Solid papilloma, 39, 42*f*
Solid usual duct hyperplasia, 295
Solid variant invasive lobular carcinoma, 354*f*, 356
Solitary papilloma, 39, 49
Sonography, metaplastic carcinoma, 238
SOX10, 251
Specimen radiograph, 482
Spindle cell
    ductal carcinoma in situ, 152, 154*f*
    lipomas, 377, 383
    neoplasms, 80
Spirometra, 35
Sporadic angiosarcoma, 393
Squamocolumnar junction, 2
Squamous cell carcinoma (SCC)
    microscopic pathology, 239–241
    with prominent myxoid stroma, 271
Squamous metaplasia, 11, 13, 16, 18, 23, 118
    in hyperplastic duct, 240*f*
    papilloma with, 44, 46, 46*f*
Standardized reporting templates, 490
Staphylococcal abscess, 33*f*
Stereotactic guidance, 477
Stereotactic needle core biopsy (stereotaxic instrument), xi, 482
Stroma, 219, 219*f*
    epithelial displacement, 469
    in fibroadenoma, 105, 112
    fibrofatty, 5
    intralobular, 2*f*
    in phyllodes tumor, 115, 116–117, 121
Stromal desmoplasia, 203*f*
Stromal elastosis, 189, 189*f*, 201, 203, 203*f*
Stromal invasion, 284
Stromal overgrowth, 115–117
Stromal reaction, 470
Subareolar sclerosing duct hyperplasia, 60*f*
    clinical presentation, 59
    gross pathology, 60
    microscopic pathology, 60
    treatment and prognosis of, 60
Surgical excision, 95–96
    of fibroadenoma, 112–114
    of phyllodes tumor, 121
Surrogate immunohistochemical profile, 490
Surveillance, Epidemiology, and End Results (SEER), 122
Syncytial growth pattern, of medullary carcinoma, 233*f*, 234
Syringoma, 255
Syringomatous adenoma of nipple, 80
    clinical presentation, 66–67
    cylindroma and, 295
    differential diagnosis of, 67–68
    gross pathology, 67
    imaging studies, 67
    immunohistochemistry, 67
    microscopic pathology, 67
    prognosis and treatment of, 68

T-cell lymphomas, 417
TA. *See* Tubular adenosis (TA)
Taenia solium infection, 35
Tall cell variant of papillary carcinoma, 230
Tamoxifen, xx, 167, 454, 458

TC. *See* Tubular carcinoma (TC)
TDLU. *See* Terminal duct lobular unit (TDLU)
Terminal duct lobular unit (TDLU), 6
Terminal ducts, with atypical lobular hyperplasia, 443, 445*f*
Terminal–duct lobular unit, 448*f*
Therapy: pathologic effect
    ablation methods, 449
    chemotherapy, 446–449
    irradiation, 440–446
        apocrine duct hyperplasia, 442, 443*f*
        atrophy of lobules, 441, 441*f*
        atypical fibroblasts, 442, 442*f*
        and breast-conservation therapy, 440–446
        and Hodgkin lymphoma, 440
        recurrent carcinoma after, 443, 444*f*
        recurrent ductal carcinoma in situ after, 443, 444*f*
        recurrent infiltrating carcinoma, 443, 445*f*
        small duct, 441, 442*f*
        terminal ducts with atypical lobular hyperplasia, 443, 445*f*
        vascular changes, 441–442*f*
TIC. *See* Touch imprint cytology (TIC)
TIL. *See* Tumor-infiltrating lymphocytes (TIL)
Tissue processing and ancillary studies, 424–425
Touch imprint cytology (TIC), 488
Touton-type giant cells, 13
Trabecular variant invasive lobular carcinoma, 354*f*, 356
Trastuzumab, 447
Trichinella infection, 35
Triple-test, 483
Tuberculosis, 32–33, 33*f*
Tuberculous mastitis, 32–33, 33*f*
Tubular adenoma, 105
Tubular adenomyoepithelioma, 71
Tubular adenosis (TA), 88–89, 88*f*
    with lobular carcinoma, 91*f*
    tubular carcinoma and, 211
Tubular carcinoma (TC), 68, 101, 201*f*
    additional morphologic features of stromal invasion, 207*f*
    atypia, columnar cell change with, 205*f*
    benign lesions
        microglandular adenosis, 210–211, 211*f*
        radial sclerosing lesion, radial scar, 211–212, 212*f*
        sclerosing and/or tubular adenosis, 211
    and calcifications, 203, 204*f*
    clinical presentation, 199–201
        age, ethnicity, and gender, 199
        contralateral carcinoma, 201
        family history, 199

        imaging studies, 199
        multifocality, 199, 201
        size, 199
        symptoms, 199
    and columnar cell change, 204, 205*f*
    differential diagnosis, 200*t*, 209–213
    and estrogen receptor, 209
    immunohistochemistry, 206, 207–209*f*, 208–209
        ER, PR, and HER2, 209
        myoepithelial markers, 206, 209
    with intracytoplasmic mucin, 201, 202–203*f*
    with intraductal carcinoma, 204, 204*f*
    and lobular carcinoma in situ, classical type, 204, 206*f*
    malignant lesions
        tubulolobular carcinoma, 210, 210*f*
        well-differentiated invasive ductal carcinoma, 209–210, 209–210*f*
    microscopic pathology, 201–206
    in needle core biopsy samples, 206*f*
    precursor lesions associated with, 204–206
    and RSL: differential diagnosis, 58
    and stromal desmoplasia, 203*f*
    and stromal elastosis, 201, 203, 203*f*
    treatment and prognosis, 212–213
Tubulolobular carcinoma, tubular carcinoma and, 210, 210*f*
Tumor-infiltrating lymphocytes (TIL), 192–193

Ultrasonography, 13, 428, 482
    for invasive lobular carcinoma, 349
    for metastases in breast, 428
Ultrasound ablation, 449
Ultrasound-guided core biopsies, 477
Ultrasound-guided vacuum-assisted percutaneous excision, 112–113
Unilateral gynecomastia, 452
University of Southern California/Van Nuys Prognostic Index (USC/VNPI), 173
Urokinase-type plasminogen activator (uPA), 495
Usual ductal hyperplasia, 126, 130–132

Vacuum-assisted needle core biopsy, 477
Van Nuys scale, of ductal carcinoma in situ, 167
Vasculitis, 28
Venous hemangioma, 386, 388*f*
Viable cells, 17

Wegener granulomatosis, 28
Well-differentiated invasive ductal carcinoma, 209–210, 209–210*f*
WT1, 268
Wuchereria bancrofti infection, 34